Visit our website

to find out about other books from W. B. Saunders
and our sister companies in Harcourt Health Sciences

Register free at
www.harcourt-international.com

and you will get

- the latest information on new books, journals and electronic products in your chosen subject areas

- the choice of e-mail or post alerts or both, when there are any new books in your chosen areas

- news of special offers and promotions

- information about products from all Harcourt Health Sciences' companies including W. B. Saunders, Churchill Livingstone, and Mosby

You will also find an easily searchable catalogue, online ordering, information on our extensive list of journals...and much more!

Visit the Harcourt Health Sciences' website today!

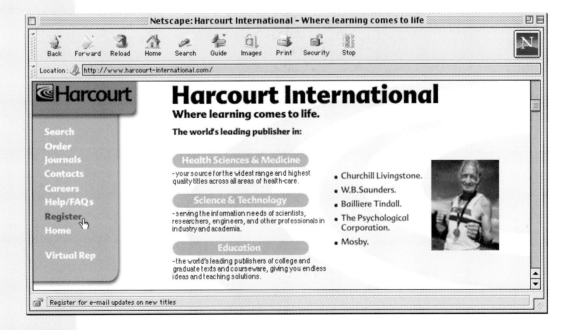

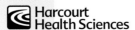

Intractable Focal Epilepsy

Commissioning Editor   Miranda Bromage
Project Development Manager   Tim Kimber
Project Manager   Rolla Couchman
Production Controller   Helen Sofio
Design and Cover Design   Deborah Gyan

Intractable Focal Epilepsy

Edited by

John M Oxbury PhD FRCP
Consultant Neurologist
Oxford University
Honorary Senior Lecturer in Clinical Neurology
Radcliffe Infirmary
Oxford, United Kingdom

Charles E Polkey MD FRCS
Professor of Functional Neurosurgery
Department of Clinical Neurosciences
King's College School of Medicine and Dentistry
London, United Kingdom

Michael Duchowny MD
Director, Neuroscience Program
Miami Children's Hospital
Clinical Professor in Neurology and Pediatrics
University of Miami School of Medicine
Miami, Florida, USA

W. B. SAUNDERS

London • Edinburgh • New York • Philadelphia • St Louis • Sydney • Toronto 2000

WB SAUNDERS
An imprint of Harcourt Publishers Limited

© Harcourt Publishers Limited 2000

First published 2000

ISBN 0 7020 2428 7

British Library Cataloguing in Publication Data
A catalogue record for this book is available from the British Library

Library of Congress Cataloguing in Publication Data
A catalogue record for this book is available from the Library of Congress

Note
Medical knowledge is constantly changing. As new information becomes available, changes in treatment, procedures, equipment and the use of drugs become necessary. The editors/authors/contributors and the publishers have taken care to ensure that the information given in this text is accurate and up to date. However, readers are strongly advised to confirm that the information, especially with regard to drug usage, complies with the latest legislation and standards of practice.

The
Publisher's
policy is to use
**paper manufactured
from sustainable forests**

Typeset by J&L Composition, Filey, North Yorkshire, UK
Printed in the United Kingdom by Bath Press Ltd, Bath

Preface

The last 15 years have seen a great expansion of interest in the management of patients with severe focal epilepsy. It has become generally accepted that surgery should be considered when the epilepsy is disabling, resistant to medication, and unlikely to remit. So, particularly when surgery is a possibility, management has become heavily dependent upon the combined skills of a multidisciplinary team including adult and pediatric neurologists, neurosurgeons, neurophysiologists, neuropsychologists, neuroradiologists, neuropathologists, nurses and social workers. An increasing number of centers are developing such multidisciplinary teams at least partly as a prelude to starting a comprehensive treatment program that includes surgery.

Our aim has been to provide an overview of the field in a single volume. We hope that it will be of particular value to epileptologists who seek information about disciplines and specialties other than their own and to those planning to set up a comprehensive treatment program. We are very fortunate to have been helped by more than 80 experts who have contributed to chapters. Their mandate was to present state-of-the-art information in an organized, concise and readable form. The book would have been impossible without their labors so generously given.

Focal epilepsy, far from being a single entity, arises from many different pathophysiologic entities whose causes are exceedingly diverse. The four introductory chapters of the book cover the general matters of diagnosis and seizure classification, epidemiology, and the risk of death that epilepsy presents. Then, the first section is concerned with seizure semeiology as a function of the locus of seizure onset and with the main clinicopathologic conditions responsible for focal epilepsy. Inevitably this is a long section. We felt it particularly important that conditions responsible for the seizures should be described in detail, because it is very probable that an ultimately rational treatment of the epilepsy will depend upon a proper understanding of the underlying pathology. Eight of the 19 chapters in this section deal with conditions that primarily affect children. That should be no surprise since severe focal epilepsy often commences in childhood and, if it can be cured, the cure should be effected as early as possible to allow normal development to occur.

The second section of 12 chapters covers the structural and metabolic imaging, neurophysiologic and neuropsychologic characteristics of the conditions that underlie the epilepsy, along with the poor quality of life imposed by the epilepsy and the psychiatric conditions that may arise in association with it. Additionally, the structural imaging of mesial temporal sclerosis and of malformations of cortical development are considered in chapters 44 and 10 respectively. Metabolic imaging is further considered in chapter 48. The third section of seven chapters deals with medical management in the broad sense. The number of available antiepileptic drugs has increased considerably during the last 10 years such that, for instance, five have been licensed for use in the UK during this period. All show some benefit, but none has been conspicuously successful for reducing seizure frequency in people whose focal epilepsy is not controlled adequately by drugs available since 1975. Furthermore, rational ideas leading to drug combinations that are reliably successful are as yet only rudimentary. So, we decided against giving a detailed account of all licensed medications and of those that may be about to be licensed. Descriptions of them can be found in at least two comprehensive textbooks published during the last five years. We have, however, attempted to cover the unwanted effects of the commonly used drugs. They all too often afflict people with severe epilepsy.

Section 4 is devoted to the selection of people for surgical treatment, to the surgery itself, and to its outcome. We make no apology that it is the longest section with 22 chapters. Surgical treatment is at its most successful when it is directed to discrete abnormalities. It has also contributed enormously to our knowledge of the pathogenesis of focal epilepsy. From the first attempts at epilepsy surgery in the late 1800s its nature has been determined by interplay between the available methods of investigation and surgical techniques on the one hand and current neuroscience knowledge on the other. The descriptions of the localization of cerebral function by Broca, Fritz, Hitzig, and Ferrier inspired Macewen and Horsley, and Krause and Foerster in Europe, to operate on discrete lesions. Penfield, after working with Foerster on the maturation of cerebral scars, began to operate upon gross cerebral lesions, exposing the brain under local anesthesia and stimulating the abnormal area to provoke seizures. In 1936 the Montreal Neurological Institute (MNI) developed the techniques of electrophysiologic investigation and electrocorticography. Over the next two or three decades the MNI made a major contribution to neurosciences from clinical observation of interictal and ictal events, neurophysiologic recording and stimulation, and follow-up of operated patients. In the 1950s and 1960s resective surgery produced data about cerebral dominance, and cognitive function including memory.

The intracranial stereotactic technique in humans was described by Spiegel and Wycis in 1947. It could be used to place electrodes accurately to try to delineate the epileptic zone. A few groups saw this as the principal tool in presurgical assessment. The most productive and longest surviving of them was started by Bancaud and Talairach in Paris. They produced a detailed map of the brain based upon the AC–PC line. This methodology allowed very detailed exploration using intracranial electrodes (stereotactic electroencephalography), combined with a multidisciplinary approach concentrating especially on seizure semeiology.

The concept of the pathology underlying focal epilepsy emerged in the 1950's and 1960's. The careful and detailed work by Murray Falconer, and his colleagues in neuropathology, revealed the pathologic substrates underlying temporal lobe epilepsy and showed that these substrates were an excellent predictor of outcome.

Direct brain imaging, by computed tomography developed in the 1970s and subsequently by magnetic resonance imaging (MRI), permits the visualization of brain pathology. Early scans only demonstrated gross brain pathology and so a concept of lesional epilepsy and lesional surgery appeared. Margerison and Corsellis in 1966 indicated that mesial temporal sclerosis is predominantly, but not exclusively, unilateral. Advances in MRI have allowed the better delineation of both mesial temporal seizures and also cortical neuronal migration disorders. At present resective surgery directed at focal epilepsies is based upon a multidisciplinary approach with a heavy emphasis on underlying pathology and direct brain imaging. Both frame-based and 'frameless' stereotactic methodology have gained a place in lesion-directed surgery.

Functional operations modify the pathophysiology of epilepsy. They are less effective than resective operations, but offer some relief to a group of patients who would otherwise be untreated. Stereotactic lesioning for epilepsy has been largely unproductive. Vagus nerve stimulation, first described by Uthman in 1990 is now a recognized technique. Callosotomy has proved useful, as has multiple subpial transection introduced by Morrell and his colleagues. The use of stereotactically directed radiosurgery as a noninvasive method for treating focal epilepsy, especially mesial temporal sclerosis, as recently described by Regis and colleagues, is another exciting development.

The appreciation that surgical success lies in the removal or destruction of pathology and the recent development of imaging techniques that will detect such pathology has provided fertile ground for both scientific and clinical advances. The clinical advances have already been of benefit to people with previously intractable epilepsy and are likely to be increasingly so in the years ahead. There is also an increasing place for surgical options that aim to modify the pathophysiology of epilepsy. For those who are thinking of starting a comprehensive treatment program including surgery, we have tried to outline the situations where the greatest success may be achieved. We hope it will be appreciated that this can be without too high an expenditure. The always, but increasingly, important matter of economics is covered in the two final chapters that constitute section 5.

Around a third of the contributors to this book have at one time or another been associated with the Guy's–Maudsley (now Kings College Hospital) Neurosurgical Unit in London or with the Neurosciences Departments at the Radcliffe Infirmary in Oxford. This is not surprising since the modern era of epilepsy surgery in the UK began with Murray Falconer's appointment in 1950 to set up the new Guy's–Maudsley Neurosurgical Unit, and there have been close neuroscience links with Oxford. Murray Falconer had been the first Nuffield Dominion Clinical Assistant to Hugh Cairns, the first University of Oxford Nuffield Professor of Surgery. One of us (Charles Polkey) was trained by Murray Falconer. The epilepsy surgery programme at the Radcliffe Infirmary was started in 1973 by Christopher Adams, who had also been trained by Murray Falconer.

Murray Falconer fully realized the advantages of surgical cure for epilepsy in childhood. The major developments in pediatric epilepsy surgery, however, began in North America. Murray Falconer had clearly shown that surgery for epilepsy in childhood results in significant improvement in seizure control and psychosocial status, but his patient pool suffered predominantly from temporal lobe epilepsy and often did not undergo surgery until the beginning of their second decade. Such patients constituted a minority of potential pediatric surgical candidates.

The comprehensive surgical management of childhood epilepsy began in the early 1990s in response to the unmet surgical needs of many children with intractable and often catastrophic epilepsy. From its inception, those involved in this initiative were keenly aware of the challenges associated with young patients and the lack of effective surgical options. The Miami Children's Hospital group emphasized the importance of detailed neurophysiologic investigations in the preoperative evaluation of neocortically-based epilepsy, particularly the deployment of chronically implanted subdural electrodes in the selection process. With the demonstration that safe and effective implantation and excisional techniques could be employed in children, a growing number of pediatric epilepsy surgical centers now seek to identify very young children with catastrophic seizures and at-risk epilepsy syndromes as early as possible.

It is doubtful whether the Miami program could have succeeded without the valuable assistance of Drs Cosimo Ajmone-Marsan and John Van Buren. Before relocating to Miami, they had been the principal epileptology–neurosurgery team at the National Institute of Health, and were thus uniquely qualified to oversee the launch of invasive electroencephalography monitoring and stimulation techniques in young patients.

Interest in pediatric epilepsy surgery was further fueled by an international pediatric epilepsy surgery symposium held in Miami in 1989. This conference marked the first time that investigators and clinicians with expertise in pediatric epilepsy and related disciplines gathered to exchange information about an emerging specialty of epilepsy treatment that had hitherto been largely unexplored. Dedicated to Murray Falconer, this symposium did much to underscore the devastating potential of unremitting childhood epilepsy and the importance of early surgical intervention. A second pediatric epilepsy surgery symposium in Bielefeld, Germany, in 1995 was widely attended and confirmed the importance of surgical treatment for intractable focal epilepsy in childhood.

We wish to express our gratitude to all our contributors. They already carry heavy loads without the additional burden of writing chapters for editors who may sometimes have been demanding. We thank them for responding to our requests. We also wish to express our gratitude to members of Harcourt Publishers, particularly Miranda Bromage, Tim Kimber, and Rolla Couchman. Without their patience and assistance we would not have managed.

John Oxbury
Charles Polkey
Michael Duchowny
2000

The editors record, with regret, the death in October 1999 of one of the contributors to this book, Professor Claudio Munari from Milan. Claudio Munari was a functional neurosurgeon with a passion for seizure semeiology. He was a careful investigator and operator with an unrivalled surgical reputation. He also had an inquiring mind that bore fruit in the number and quality of his research publications. He was much in demand around the world as a speaker and presenter. His presence and influence will be sorely missed both in his native Italy and in international epileptology.

Contents

SECTION 1: SEMEIOLOGY OF FOCAL SEIZURES AND UNDERLYING CAUSES

COLOUR PLATES

List of Color Plates

The color plates lie between pages 268 and 269.

Contributors

Jane Elizabeth Adcock BMed FRACP
Epilepsy Research Foundation
   Desmond Pond Fellow
Department of Neurology
Radcliffe Infirmary
Oxford, United Kingdom

Adriano Aguzzi MD MRCPath
Director, Institute for Neuropathology
University Hospital
Zurich, Switzerland

Jean Aicardi MD
Honorary Professor of Child
   Neurology
Institute of Child Health
Great Ormond Street Hospital for
   Children
London, United Kingdom

Rustam Al-Shahi MA MRCP
Medical Research Council Clinical
   Training Fellow
Department of Clinical Neurosciences
Western General Hospital
Edinburgh, United Kingdom

Frederick Andermann MD FRCP(C)
Professor of Neurology and Pediatrics
McGill University Faculty
Montreal Neurological Institute and
   Hospital
Montreal, Quebec, Canada

Philip Anslow FRCR
Consultant Neuroradiologist
The Radcliffe Infirmary
Oxford, United Kingdom

Gus Anthony Baker BA PhD
   MClinPsychol CClinPsychol FBPS
Senior Lecturer in Clinical
   Neuropsychology
The Walton Centre for Neurology
   and Neurosurgery
Liverpool, United Kingdom

Fabrice Bartolomei MD PhD
Neurophysiologist
Laboratoire de Neurophysiologie
Hôpital de la Timone
Marseille, France

Sallie Ann Baxendale BSc MSc PhD
   CPsychol
Principal Neuropsychologist
Epilepsy Research Group
Institute of Neurology
London, United Kingdom

Emilia Berta MD
Aluto-Neurochirurgia
Centro Regionale per la Chirurgia
   dell'Epilessia
Ospedale Niguarda-Padiglione
   Rossini
Milan, Italy

Colin D Binnie MD FRCP
Professor of Neurophysiology
Department of Clinical
   Neurophysiology
King's College Hospital
London, United Kingdom

Victoria Burch MA MEd
Senior Psychologist
Department of Psychology
St Piers School
Lingfield, United Kingdom

Hilary Cass BSc FRCPCH MRCP(Paediat)
Consultant in Paediatric Disability
Director, Postgraduate Medical
   Education
Great Ormond Street Hospital for
   Children
London, United Kingdom

Fernando Cendes MD PhD
Assistant Professor
Department of Neurology
FCM Unicamp
Cidade Universitaria
Campinas, São Paulo, Brazil

Christopher Chandler FRCS(SN)
Consultant Neurosurgeon
Department of Neurological Surgery
King's College Hospital
London, United Kingdom

Patrick Chauvel MD
Neurophysiologist
Laboratoire de Neurophysiologie
Hôpital de la Timone
Marseille, France

Diane C Chugani PhD
Associate Professor of Pediatrics and
   Radiology
PET Center
Children's Hospital of Michigan
Wayne State University
Detroit, Michigan, USA

Harry T Chugani MD
Professor of Neurology, Pediatrics and
   Radiology
PET Center
Children's Hospital of Michigan
Wayne State University
Detroit, Michigan, USA

Carolyn M Cowey BSc PhD ClinPsyD
Clinical Psychologist
Department of Psychology
Warneford Hospital
Oxford Mental Healthcare NHS Trust
   and Oxford Learning Disabilities Trust
Oxford, United Kingdom

Pamela M Crawford MD FRCP
Consultant Neurologist and Director
   of the Special Centre for Epilepsy
York District Hospital
York, United Kingdom and
Visiting Professor in Neurological
   Studies
Leeds Metropolitan University
Leeds, United Kingdom

J Helen Cross MB ChB PhD MRCP(UK)
   FRCPCH
Consultant and Honorary Senior
   Lecturer in Paediatric Neurology
The Institute of Child Health
Great Ormond Street Hospital for
   Children
London, United Kingdom

Anthony S David MD MSc MPhil FRCP
   FRCPsych
Professor of Cognitive
   Neuropsychiatry
Institute of Psychiatry
Guy's, King's and Thomas' School of
   Medicine
London, United Kingdom

Darryl C De Vivo MD
Sidney Carter Professor of Child
   Neurology
The Neurological Institute of New
   York
College of Physicians and Surgeons
Columbia University
New York, New York, USA

Patricia Dean ARNP MSN
Clinical Nurse Specialist
Program Manager
Comprehensive Epilepsy Center
Miami Children's Hospital
Miami, Florida, USA

Michael Duchowny MD
Director, Neuroscience Program
Miami Children's Hospital
Clinical Professor in Neurology and
   Pediatrics
University of Miami School of
   Medicine
Miami, Florida, USA

Roderick Duncan MD PhD FRCP
Consultant Neurologist
Institute of Neurological Sciences
Southern General Hospital
Glasgow, United Kingdom

Christian E Elger FRCP
Direktor der Klinik für Epileptologie
Universtät Bonn
Bonn, Germany

Robert DC Elwes MD FRCP
Consultant Clincial Neurophysiologist
Department of Clinical Neurosciences
Guy's, King's and Thomas' School of
   Medicine
London, United Kingdom

Peter BC Fenwick DPM (London)
   FRCPsych
Senior Lecturer, Institute of
   Psychiatry
London, United Kingdom and
Consultant Neuropsychiatrist
Radcliffe Infirmary
Oxford, United Kingdom

Jamie T Gilman PharmD
Director, Neuropharmacology
Department of Neuroscience
Miami Children's Hospital
Miami, Florida, USA

Laura Hilary Goldstein BSc PhD MPhil
Reader in Neuropsychology
Department of Psychiatry
Institute of Psychiatry
London, United Kingdom

Achim Gooss MD
Senior Clinician
Institute for Neuropathology
University Hospital
Zurich, Switzerland

Renzo Guerrini MD
Professor of Epileptology
Guy's, King's and Thomas' School of
   Medicine
London, United Kingdom

Marketa Hajek MD
Senior Clinician
Neurology Clinic
Department of Epileptology and
   Electroencephalography
University Hospital
Zurich, Switzerland

William Harkness FRCS
Consultant Neurosurgeon
Department of Neurosurgery
Great Ormond Street Hospital for
   Children
London, United Kingdom

Yvonne Hart MD FRCP
Consultant Neurologist
Department of Neurology
Atkinson Morley's Hospital
London, United Kingdom

A Simon Harvey MD FRACP
Director, Children's Epilepsy Program
Department of Neurology
Royal Children's Hospital
Melbourne, Victoria, Australia

Susie Henley MSc
Research Assistant
Department of Clinical
  Neuropsychology
Radcliffe Infirmary
Oxford, United Kingdom

Penelope B Hewitt MB BS LRCP DA
  FRCA
Consultant Anaesthetist and
Honorary Senior Lecturer
Neuroscience Unit
Guy's, King's and Thomas' School of
  Medicine
London, United Kingdom

Gregory L Holmes MD
Consultant Pediatric Neurologist
Childhood Epilepsy Program
Division of Epilepsy and Clinical
  Neurophysiology
Department of Neurology
Children's Hospital
Harvard Medical School
Boston, Massachusetts, USA

Mrinalini Honavar MBRS MD FRCPath
Director of Anatomic Pathology
Hospital Pedro Hispano
Matosinhos, Portugal and
Consultant Neuropathologist
Institute of Psychiatry
London, United Kingdom

Elizabeth B Isaacs PhD
Senior Research Fellow
Wolfson Centre
Developmental Cognitive
  Neuroscience Unit
Institute of Child Health
Great Ormond Street Hospital for
  Children
London, United Kingdom

Ann Jacoby BA(Hons) PhD
Professor of Medical Sociology
Department of Primary Care
University of Liverpool
Liverpool, United Kingdom

Prasanna Jayakar MD PhD
Director, Neuroscience Center
Miami Children's Hospital
Miami, Florida, USA

Robin Peter Kennett BSc MD FRCP
Consultant Neurophysiologist
Department of Clinical
  Neurophysiology
Radcliffe Infirmary
Oxford, United Kingdom

Fenella J Kirkham MB ChB PhD
  MRCP(UK) FRCPCH
Senior Lecturer and Honorary
  Consultant in Paediatric Neurology
The Institute of Child Health
Great Ormond Street Hospital for
  Children
London, United Kingdom

Eve S Knight BSc ClinPsyD
Clinical Psychologist in Child
  Neuropsychology
Radcliffe Infirmary
Oxford, United Kingdom

Michelle Vanessa Lambert MBChB
  MRCPsych MSc
Clinical Lecturer in Neuropsychiatry
Institute of Psychiatry
Guy's, King's and Thomas' School of
  Medicine
London, United Kingdom

Susan L Lannon RN BS MA
Clinician Instructor
Epilepsy Clinician
Department of Neurology
University of North Carolina
Chapel Hill, North Carolina, USA

Janet Lees MPhil
Speech and Language Therapist
The Institute of Child Health
Great Ormond Street Hospital for
  Children
London, United Kingdom

Lori E Lovitz BA
Research Associate
Jefferson Comprehensive Epilepsy
  Center
Thomas Jefferson University Hospital
Philadelphia, Pennsylvania, USA

Christopher John McEvedy BA
  MBBS MRCPsych
Consultant Psychiatrist
Paterson Centre
St Mary's Hospital
London, United Kingdom

Eliane Correa Miotto PhD
Department of Neuropsychology
National Hospital
London, United Kingdom

Mortimer Miskin PhD
Chief, Section on Cognitive
  Neuroscience
Laboratory of Neuropsychology
National Institute of Mental Health
Bethesda, Maryland, USA

Robin Guy Morris MA MSc PhD
Reader in Neuropsychology
Neuropsychology Unit
Institute of Psychiatry
London, United Kingdom

Claudio Munari MD
Late Professor of Neurosurgery
Centro Regionale per la Chirurgia
 dell'Epilessia
Ospedale Niguarda-Padiglione Rossini
Milan, Italy

Lina Nashef MBChB MRCP MD
Consultant Neurologist
Kent and Canterbury Hospital NHS
 Trust
Honorary Senior Lecturer
Guy's, King's and Thomas' School of
 Medicine
London, United Kingdom

Brian GR Neville MB BS FRCP
Professor of Paediatric Neurology
Institute of Child Health
University College London
Great Ormond Street Hospital for
 Children
London, United Kingdom

Anna Christina Nobre PhD
Lecturer in Experimental Psychology
Department of Experimental
 Psychology
University of Oxford
Oxford, United Kingdom

Douglas R Nordli Jr MD
Director, Children's Epilepsy Center
Children's Memorial Hospital
Chicago, Illinois, USA

John M Oxbury PhD FRCP
Consultant Neurologist
Oxford University Honorary Senior
 Lecturer in Clinical Neurology
Radcliffe Infirmary
Oxford, United Kingdom

Susan M Oxbury MA
Consultant Clinical Psychologist
Oxford University Honorary Senior
 Lecturer in Clinical Neurology
Radcliffe Infirmary
Oxford, United Kingdom

Lucio Parmeggiani MD
Consulant Neurologist
Institute of Child Neurology and
 Psychiatry
University of Pisa and Institute for
 Medical Research
Stella Maris Foundation
Pisa, Italy

Charles E Polkey MD FRCS
Professor of Functional Neurosurgery
Department of Clinical Neurosciences
Guy's, King's and Thomas' School of
 Medicine
London, United Kingdom

Anling Rao BM PhD
Research Assistant
Department of Experimental
 Psychology
University of Oxford
Oxford, United Kingdom

James J Riviello Jr MD
Director, Childhood Epilepsy
 Program
Division of Epilepsy and Clinical
 Neurophysiology
Department of Neurology
Children's Hospital
Harvard Medical School
Boston, Massachusetts, USA

Richard C Roberts MA DPhil BM BCL
 FRCP
Senior Lecturer in Neurology
University of Dundee
Department of Neurology
Ninewells Hospital and Medical
 School
Dundee, United Kingdom

Peter Rothwell MD MRCP
Oxford University Clinical Lecturer
 in Neurology
Honorary Consultant Neurologist
Radcliffe Infirmary
Oxford, United Kingdom

Jagdish R Shah MD
Assistant Professor of Neurology
University Health Center
Detroit, Michigan, USA

Herbert Silfvenius MD PhD
Professor of Neurosurgery
Section of Epilepsy
Department of Neurosurgery
University Hospital
Umea, Sweden

Sanjay M Sisodiya PhD MRCP
Senior Lecturer in Neurology and
 Honorary Consultant Neurologist
National Hospital for Neurology and
 Neurosurgery
London, United Kingdom

O Carter Snead III MD FRCP(C)
Chair in Pediatric Neuroscience
Bloorview Children's Hospital
 Foundation
Hospital for Sick Children;
Professor of Pediatrics, Medicine
 (Neurology) and Pharmacology
University of Toronto;
Senior Scientist and Director
Brain and Behaviour Program
 Research Institute;
Head, Division of Neurology
Hospital for Sick Children
Toronto, Ontario, Canada

Michael R Sperling MD
Baldwin Keyes Professor of Neurology
Department of Neurology
Jefferson Comprehensive Epilepsy
 Center
Thomas Jefferson University Hospital
Philadelphia, Pennsylvania, USA

Marian V Squier MRCP FRCPath
Consultant Neuropathologist
The Radcliffe Infirmary
Oxford, United Kingdom

Hermann Stefan MD PhD
Professor of Neurology
Zentrum Epilepsie Erlangen
Department of Neurology
Der Universität Nuremberg
Nuremberg, Germany

Gerald F Tuite MD
Neurosurgeon
All Children's Hospital
St Petersburg, Florida, USA

Faraneh Vargha-Khadem BA MPsychol
  PhD
Professor of Cognitive Neuroscience
The Wolfson Centre
Cognitive Neuroscience Unit
Institute of Child Health
Great Ormond Street Hospital for
  Children
London, United Kingdom

Kate Watkins PhD
Post Doctoral Research Fellow
Cognitive Neuroscience Unit
Montreal Neurological Institute
Montreal, Quebec, Canada

Heinz-Gregor Wieser MD
Professor of Neurology
Neurology Clinic
Department of Epileptology and
  Electroencephalography
University Hospital
Zurich, Switzerland

Shelly Karen Weiss MD FRCPC
Assistant Professor
Department of Pediatrics and
  Medicine (Neurology)
University of Toronto
Division of Neurology
The Hospital for Sick Children
Toronto, Ontario, Canada

Peter D Williamson MD
Director, Dartmouth Epilepsy
  Program
Professor of Medicine, Dartmouth
  Medical School
Dartmouth-Hitchcock Medical Center
Lebanon, New Hampshire, USA

Geoffrey DS Wright FRCP
Honorary Consultant Neurologist
Radcliffe Infirmary
Oxford, United Kingdom

Zenobia Zaiwalla MBBS MRCP FRCP
  FRCPCH
Consultant in Paediatric Clinical
  Neurophysiology
The Park Hospital for Children
Oxford, United Kingdom

Introduction

JM OXBURY, CE POLKEY, AND M DUCHOWNY

The physician who first sees an epileptic patient should set himself two questions: Where is the focus? What is the cause? The first and most important clue to the anatomical localisation of a seizure is the pattern of the attack.

Wilder Penfield and Herbert Jasper, 1954

For Penfield and Jasper (1954), *focal epilepsy* was a condition in which the seizures begin with 'a neuronal discharge in the vicinity of a demonstrably abnormal focus' within the brain. These seizures contrasted with a second variety, 'centrencephalic seizures,' that were regarded as originating in the central integrating system of the upper brain stem. *Focal seizures* were subdivided into a number of categories (motor, sensory, autonomic, psychical, etc.) according to the nature of the initial symptom that was itself taken to indicate the anatomic site of the initial electrical discharge. The focal epilepsies, that is the syndromes of which the seizures were a feature, were divided into two main categories, *symptomatic* and *cryptogenic*, according to whether or not a pathologic cause could be found. Thus, a seizure could be specified according to its symptoms, the locus of its origin and, for symptomatic seizures, the nature of the pathologic substrate. The causes and consequences, and the diagnosis and treatment, of *intractable seizures* of this type, in conjunction with their pathologic substrates, are the subject of this book. The matter of intractability is discussed in Chapters 2 and 35. In brief, we have defined it operationally for adults as the situation in which seizure control has yet to be achieved more than 2 years after the initiation of treatment with optimal

doses of at least three of phenobarbitone, phenytoin, carbamazepine, sodium valproate, and lamotrigine, either individually or in combination. The two-year rule is not always applicable for children who are clinically deteriorating.

The currently popular term *partial seizures* was introduced by the Commission on Terminology of the International League Against Epilepsy (ILAE) (Gastaut *et al* 1964). The definition evolved over subsequent proposals (Gastaut 1970; Commission on Classification and Terminology of the ILAE 1981) and can now be taken as applying to seizures in which the first clinical and EEG changes 'indicate initial activation of a system of neurones limited to part of one cerebral hemisphere.' The Commission proposed the term *generalized seizures* for those in which first clinical changes indicate involvement of both hemispheres at seizure onset and the initial ictal EEG pattern is bilateral. Current views on the classification of partial seizures and epilepsies are described in Chapter 2. The Commission's definition of partial seizures is clearly very close to the definition of focal seizures given by Penfield and Jasper (1954). We have adopted the term *focal* for the title of this book because we feel that it is more descriptive of the pathophysiology that probably underlies these epilepsies.

Indeed, for more than a century, studies of the pathophysiology of focal seizures have made major contributions to the understanding of cerebral organization. Throughout the text, however, the two terms focal and partial are used interchangeably.

Intractable focal epilepsy afflicts 14 000–15 000 people in the UK and 50 000–55 000 in the USA, let alone millions elsewhere. Thus, it poses both an intellectual fascination and a major therapeutic challenge. Many facets of the condition must be understood if the challenge is to be met. Our aim has been to gather together a group of authors capable of presenting reliable information concerning these many facets to a wide multidisciplinary readership drawn from neurology, neurosurgery, neurophysiology, neuropsychology, neuroradiology, neuropathology, and other professions in contact with people with epilepsy. The content has been restricted almost entirely to clinical matters. The basic neuroscience deserves a textbook to itself rather than an obligatory chapter in an essentially clinical text that could but touch on the topic superficially. Nevertheless, we hope that neuroscientists working in the field of epilepsy will find here a clear description of clinical problems that need basic neuroscience solutions. Our aim has also been to emphasize broad principles and to give general guidance as well as appropriate detail. We are particularly keen to attract as readers those who are proposing to enter the field of treating this therapeutically challenging and intellectually taxing branch of epileptology.

The early chapters give an overview of the diagnosis, classification, and epidemiology of focal seizures and the intractable focal epilepsy syndromes. The chapter 'Death from intractable focal epilepsy' appears in this introductory section to emphasize the serious nature of the condition and to underline that it can have very severe consequences. There then follows a section devoted to seizure symptoms according to their cortical site of origin and to the clinicopathologic conditions that underlie the epilepsy. Many of these chapters are concerned with conditions that effect, primarily, children or whose manifestations often commence during childhood. We have tried throughout to span the artificial divide between children and adults. In much of epilepsy, as for Wordsworth in *My Heart Leaps Up*, 'the child is father of the man.' Thus, disability in adult life often arises against the background of failure to gain control of an epileptic seizure disorder that has become intractable during childhood. Focal epilepsy is not a unitary condition and it is essential that accurate diagnosis should precede the creation of treatment plans. Decisions about treatment must be based on prognosis, and a realistic prognosis is only possible given correct diagnosis. In this respect surgery in childhood for a condition that has a very low probability of

remitting spontaneously but is known to have a high probability of 'cure' with surgery can restore normality that is then carried through into an adult life not blighted by disability. In this situation the surgery justifies risks that it may carry. On the other hand, surgery for a condition likely to remit spontaneously is to be strictly avoided. This is why fourteen chapters have been devoted to the clinicopathologic conditions associated with intractable focal epilepsy.

Section 2 is concerned with investigation of the epilepsy and its pathologic substrate in the broadest sense, including evaluation of the consequences of the disorder. There are chapters not only on neurophysiology and neuroimaging but also on quality of life and psychosocial evaluation, on the neuropsychologic features that may accompany the epilepsy, and on the neuropsychiatric conditions that may arise. Since the mid 1980s enormous developments in structural, metabolic, and functional imaging of the brain have revolutionized approaches to the diagnosis of the focal epilepsy disorders and especially their surgical treatment. At the time of the 1986 Palm Desert Conference on the Surgical Treatment of Epilepsy, MRI was included as one of the new techniques 'that could considerably expand the methods of presurgical evaluation' (Sperling *et al* 1987). Twelve years on, MRI and, to a lesser extent, metabolic imaging with positron emission tomography (PET) and single-photon emission computed tomography (SPECT) pervade discussion of the focal epilepsy disorders. Section 2 contains chapters on diagnostic neuroradiology, PET, and SPECT. Much discussion, especially of MRI, also appears elsewhere, especially in the Section 4 chapters on the 'Radiological Evaluation of Hippocampal Sclerosis' and on 'Functional Imaging: PET and MRI' and in the Section 2 chapters on various clinicopathologic conditions.

Since the early 1970s it has been clear that the secret to successful epilepsy surgery lies in the removal of pathology, greater success coming with some forms of pathology than with others (Falconer 1971; Bruton 1988). Developments in imaging have allowed this principle to be more easily put into operation with a parallel reduction in the need for complex neurophysiology. It is no surprise, therefore, that the number of chapters devoted to imaging equals the number devoted to neurophysiology. Also since the mid 1980s there has been an enormous expansion of research into both the neuropsychologic accompaniments to the symptomatic localization-related epilepsy syndromes (and specific pathology-related syndromes) prior to any surgical intervention and into the quality-of-life issues. At the time of the first Palm Desert Conference, Rausch (1987) justly summarized the position with the statement that 'neuropsychological research directed towards the preoperative work-up of the epileptic patient is sparse,' despite much research having taken place with such patients postoperatively. The change since then is reflected here in four chapters devoted to neuropsychologic and quality-of-life issues not directly related to surgical treatment. Change in neuropsychologic function as a result of surgery and in quality of life has rightly become one of the important parameters in the equation for deciding whether surgery should be undertaken. It can only be used meaningfully if there is clear understanding of how to measure preoperative baseline levels.

Sections 3 and 4 are concerned with treatment – the former with medical, psychologic and dietary aspects and the latter with surgical. Unfortunately, newly developed medications rarely provide freedom from seizures for people whose focal epilepsy has been intractable. There is no temptation, therefore, to devote many chapters to drugs and it is only to be hoped that this might become necessary in the near future. On the other hand, appropriately directed surgery can give complete freedom from seizures and a return to normal life. Consequently, nearly twenty chapters are devoted to the selection of patients for surgery, the surgery itself and the surgical outcome. The specifics of preoperative evaluation methods, surgical techniques and postoperative seizure, neuropsychologic and quality-of-life outcome, and unwanted effects are covered in seventeen chapters. A further three chapters are devoted to 'Syndromes Amenable to Surgery,' 'Surgical Options,' and 'Rational Preoperative Investigation Programmes and Patient Selection.' We very much hope that these will be helpful to those wishing to refer their patients for possible surgical treatment or planning to set up a surgical treatment facility in an already established medical unit. We hope we can show that the latter requires assiduous attention to detail and a multidisciplinary team including the *sine qua non* of a neurosurgeon with specific training, but that it can be achieved with equipment available in most clinical neurosciences centers.

Inevitably, in the current era it is also necessary to have an understanding of the economic implications of both the continuing epilepsy and the treatments. This topic is covered in Section 5.

EPIDEMIOLOGY

The *raison d'être* for this book lies in the epidemiologic data, which are presented in detail in Chapter 3. Essentially, intractable focal epilepsy is a major cause of disability among all age groups. The age-adjusted incidence of epilepsy in Western industrialized communities is in the region of 45/100 000 persons per year (Joensen 1986; Forsgren 1990; Hauser *et al* 1993; Olafsson *et al* 1996). Around 50% of them have developed focal seizures or a focal epilepsy syndrome (Loiseau *et al* 1990). This applies across all age groups, the incidence of focal seizures being remarkably constant from infancy through to 65 years. Thereafter, the incidence of focal seizures that involve altered consciousness (complex partial seizures) rises sharply among people aged >65 years (Hauser *et al* 1993), although there is little change in the incidence of focal seizures without altered consciousness. Approximately 15% of people who develop focal seizures are unlikely to achieve a period of 3 years remission within 9 years of the onset of their epilepsy and around 30% are unlikely to achieve a 5-year remission (Cockerell *et al* 1995). It is estimated that around 10% of the incident cases of focal epilepsy become truly intractable with frequent seizures despite 'optimal' drug therapy (Hauser and Hesdorffer 1996).

A population of one million will each year generate around 35 new cases of chronic epilepsy manifest by a focal epilepsy syndrome, and 15–20 of these will have severe intractable epilepsy resistant to modern drug therapy. Furthermore, the prevalence of cases with focal seizures causing altered consciousness or convulsions that will not remit even in the long term has been estimated at around 265 persons/million population. It is not surprising, therefore, that epilepsy is second only to migraine or headache in precipitating referral to a neurologist in the UK (Hopkins *et al* 1989b) and third only to prolapsed lumbar disk and cerebrovascular disease among neurologic conditions leading to referral to hospital (Hopkins 1989a). Many of those who have first consultations will, of course, need continuing care long term in the clinic.

CHILDREN

The incidence and diversity of seizures in children is greater than at any other age. For this reason, many chapters are devoted exclusively, or nearly so, to issues of pediatric diagnosis and treatment. Maturational factors are potent modifiers of early epileptic phenomena, influencing the expression of both partial and generalized disorders. A full appreciation of partial seizures in pediatric patients therefore requires a clear understanding of the basic mechanisms of epileptogenesis in the immature brain.

The spectrum of focal epilepsy is particularly diverse in the first decade of life. The seizure presentation ranges from relatively mild and medically responsive conditions such as benign partial seizures in infancy (Watanabe *et al* 1990, 1993) and partial epilepsy with centrotemporal spikes (Loiseau and Beaussart 1973), to catastrophic disturbances associated with frank developmental regression. Infants with recurrent partial seizures have a particularly high risk for long-term seizure persistence and neurologic handicap (Chevrie and Aicardi 1978, 1979). In fact, the guarded prognosis of early-onset partial seizures rivals that of infants with status epilepticus and is poorer than for infants with infantile spasms. Given such extremes in partial seizure presentation, considerable care should be exercised before counseling parents, choosing medical therapy, or referring for surgical therapy.

The tendency to misdiagnose or misinterpret the clinical signs of partial seizures is an important clinical pitfall in dealing with the young child. Whereas adults usually characterize their own auras and are able to report both simple and complex sensory phenomena, preverbal or nonverbal children cannot describe internal experiences, and even the most fluent child may be unable to elaborate subtle sensory phenomena. Parental anxiety surrounding the seizures further interferes with full descriptions of symptoms, and brief disturbances of behavior are readily overlooked. Partial seizures in younger children tend to last significantly longer than in older children and to display a spikier morphology in their EEG seizure patterns (Yamamoto *et al* 1987). Partial seizures in early life also show an increased tendency to secondarily generalize, presumably owing to immaturity of inhibitory safeguards against access to motor pathways. Motor convulsive patterns are more likely to occur early in the ictal sequence, often coinciding with or immediately following clinical onset of seizures. Video-EEG analysis may be the only way to confidently differentiate secondary from primary generalized patterns. Rapid secondary generalization may present as tonic, atonic, or myoclonic movements that terminate the ictal event. In conjunction with the difficulties associated with sensory reporting, rapid spread to motor pathways obscures other symptoms making the accurate diagnosis of partial seizures extremely difficult in very young children (Oller-Daurella and Oller 1989).

Blume (1989) studied the clinical profile of partial seizures beginning in the first four years of life in children without perinatal cerebral insult. Of 46 patients 33 (72%) had complex partial seizures, while 11 patients (24%) had simple partial attacks; 37 (80%) had ictal motor phenomena, which were unilateral in only 14 patients. There was good correlation between the lobe of interictal spiking and surgically proven origin of the seizures. Not surprisingly, malformations of cortical development were the most common known cause of seizures, a finding confirmed in two surgical series involving infants (Wyllie 1996;

Duchowny *et al* 1998). Malformations of cortical development account for a high proportion of cryptogenic and symptomatic partial seizures in children, and underlie many medically refractory cases. Advances in EEG and neuroimaging techniques have been especially helpful for evaluating these disorders and high-resolution anatomic and functional imaging has been particularly useful for detecting subtle abnormalities. In surgical cases, invasive EEG recording with subdural electrodes has dramatically increased the ability to localize seizure origin and to map the cortical surface functionally.

The changing semeiology of partial seizures over the first decade is another distinctive clinical feature. While partial seizures in the school-age child might include auras and automatisms similar to those of adolescents and adults, infants and toddlers are more likely to exhibit highly stereotyped gross motor automatisms (gestural and oroalimentary) in conjunction with motor symptomatology (Jayakar and Duchowny 1990). Motionless staring, while characteristic of many partial seizures in childhood, is easily overlooked in very young patients and may be discerned only during video-EEG monitoring. The increasing complexity of seizure semeiology probably reflects the development of enhanced cortical and subcortical connections rather than strict anatomic variability or 'migration' of the seizure focus.

The inherent complexity of partial seizure manifestations in infants and young children has led to proposals that standard ILAE criteria for seizure classification be modified for these age groups (Nordli *et al* 1997). For example, the occurrence of bilateral tonic stiffening in infants with partial seizures and the association of infantile spasms and generalized EEG abnormalities with small regions of cortical dysgenesis suggest that partial seizures in infancy may not fit the standard nomenclature. Evidence for subcortical involvement in seizure expression reinforces the concept that complex mechanisms of seizure expression are caused by different patterns of excitation and inhibition in immature cortex (Chugani *et al* 1994). This issue is presently under review by the ILAE.

Partial seizures in childhood are also more likely to occur in the context of specific epilepsy syndromes. Many of these are included in this volume. Most are recognized as developmentally and genetically based disorders such as the tuberous sclerosis complex, Sturge–Weber syndrome and hemimegalencephaly. They may produce deterioration and have a known long-term prognosis. When regression occurs rapidly, there may be an urgent need to refer for prompt surgical intervention. Thus, the caveat often applied to adults that seizures should be given an 'adequate' trial of many antiepileptic drugs over two years before referring for surgical consideration requires revision in the infant with catastrophic partial epilepsy.

Other syndromes are clearly age-related, their onset at certain ages coinciding with critical periods of brain maturation. In some patients, the disappearance of one syndrome is followed by the appearance of another. For example, the age-dependent early epileptic encephalopathies, Ohtahara, West, and Lennox–Gastaut syndromes, may present at different ages in the same patient (Donat 1992). Evidence of focality can be demonstrated in a high proportion of affected individuals even though partial seizures are not necessarily a cardinal feature.

Despite the challenges posed by partial seizures in preadolescent patients, innovative strategies for diagnosis and intervention, many of which are reviewed in this volume, provide hope for the future. Newer medical, surgical, and dietary treatments are increasingly available, and careful epidemiologic, clinical, anatomic, functional, genetic and neuropsychologic studies provide a greater understanding of brain functioning in the epileptic child than ever before. As the sophistication of different investigative methods increases, a fuller understanding of basic mechanisms and of clinical expression of partial epilepsy in the child seems to be just over the horizon.

CONDITIONS

Fourteen chapters are devoted to a description of the clinical features of pathologic conditions that commonly include intractable focal epilepsy among their manifestations. A precise diagnosis of the epilepsy syndrome responsible for the focal seizures, and of the pathologic substrate that will be found in around 85% of cases, is an essential prerequisite to prognosis and to any decision concerning the probability that surgical treatment will be successful. Such diagnosis is based on the clinical presentation and investigation results. It can occasionally also guide rational drug therapy, although unfortunately as yet only too rarely.

Detailed chapters are devoted to hippocampal sclerosis (HS)/mesial temporal lobe sclerosis (MTS) and to malformations of cortical development (MCD). These are core conditions. They accounted for the MRI-detected pathology in around 35% and 15%, respectively, of the cases examined by Cook and Stevens (1995). MCD might well account for a higher proportion of a series restricted to children. Both may occur in isolation or they may exist together, and either may occur in combination with a third pathology, particularly a dysembryoplastic neuroepithelial tumor.

Some discussion of terminology is necessary. In current parlance the terms hippocampal sclerosis and mesial temporal sclerosis are often used synonymously. That is not strictly correct. The term *mesial temporal sclerosis* (MTS) was introduced by Murray Falconer and his colleagues in the epilepsy surgery group at the Maudsley Hospital during the 1960s (Falconer *et al* 1964) to describe the appearances commonly seen in specimens excised by anterior temporal lobectomy to treat chronic temporal lobe epilepsy. They pointed out that the severity of the histologic abnormality that they labeled MTS varied. At its mildest there was simply a loss of neurons in the CA1 sector of the hippocampus with some gliosis in the amygdala. At the other end of the continuum, severe MTS, there was marked neuronal loss and gliosis throughout the hippocampus, except for relative sparing in CA2, along with neuronal loss in the amygdala, hippocampal and fusiform gyri, and elsewhere. At much the same time, Margerison and Corsellis (1966), on the basis of an autopsy study, defined classical *Ammon's horn sclerosis* (AHS) as neuronal loss and gliosis in CA1 and in variable portions of CA3–5 and in the dentate gyrus. AHS was considered distinct from end folium sclerosis where the neuronal loss and gliosis were confined to CA3–5.

Margerison and Corsellis (1966) used the term *hippocampal sclerosis* to embrace both AHS and end folium sclerosis. There was a statistically powerful association between the pathologic features of hippocampal sclerosis and the clinical and electroencephalographic features of temporal lobe epilepsy. They noted that the mean age at the onset of the epilepsy was in childhood for AHS compared to adolescence with end folium sclerosis. They also commented that the AHS seen in the post-mortem specimens was identical to the state of the hippocampus in many of the excision specimens obtained by Murray Falconer. This latter observation has been confirmed by data subsequently presented by Bruton (1988). Margerison and Corsellis also noted that in their study population around 20% of those with AHS on one side had it on the opposite side also, and a further 35% had a lesser degree of sclerosis on the opposite side. This is of considerable importance to decisions about surgical treatment for patients with AHS, particularly with respect to the chances of achieving complete seizure relief and to the possibility that a severe amnesic syndrome might ensue. It should also be borne in mind when interpreting neuropsychologic test data, particularly the results of memory tests.

Also at much the same time, Ounsted *et al* (1966) advanced the hypothesis that the severe neuronal loss and gliosis of AHS is due to a bout of status epilepticus occurring in a child, especially one genetically predisposed to febrile convulsions. They posited that the temporal lobe damage so induced is the cause of the subsequent intractable temporal lobe epilepsy. Thirty years on there is still uncertainty about the precise cause of AHS, as defined by Margerison and Corsellis, but the strong association with an episode of childhood status epilepticus or some other brain insult has been amply confirmed (Sagar and Oxbury 1987; Mathern *et al* 1995). Lesser degrees of hippocampal neuron loss, however, may be simply the consequence of long-term chronic epilepsy (Mouritzen Dam 1980, 1982) rather than its cause.

Falconer (1971) was fully aware that the chances of what has now come to be known as the syndrome of *mesial temporal lobe epilepsy* (Wieser *et al* 1993) being relieved by surgery were good if the pathologic substrate was hippocampal sclerosis, or MTS as he called it, associated with a history of a prolonged convulsion in early childhood. Attempts were made to define the EEG characteristics of the condition so that it might be more easily diagnosed (Engel *et al* 1975). However, reliable investigational evidence to support a clinical diagnosis of hippocampal sclerosis did not become available until the advent of MRI (see Chapter 44 on 'Radiologic Evaluation of Hippocampal Sclerosis') and the definition of the neuropsychologic profile associated with the condition (see review by Oxbury and Oxbury, 1998). It is some 50 years since Falconer (1953) described the en bloc temporal lobectomy that, by providing good specimens for histopathologic analysis, was the initial step towards recognizing the mesial temporal lobe epilepsy syndrome (MTLE) associated with severe hippocampal sclerosis and the effectiveness of its surgical treatment. Nevertheless, this common condition still often goes undiagnosed, so that many who could be offered surgery without complex preoperative neurophysiologic investigation are denied the opportunity of treatment. We hope that the material contained in some of the chapters of this book will lead to more of the unfortunate individuals afflicted by disabling epilepsy from this pathology receiving effective treatment.

In contrast to MTLE, understanding of the epilepsy associated with malformations of cortical development (MCD), which may in reality be as common a cause of intractable focal epilepsy as hippocampal sclerosis, is only in its infancy. This pathology poses one of the next major challenges to the therapeutically inclined epileptologist. The classification of these malformations is complex (see Chapter 10 dealing with malformations of cortical development), their diagnosis can be difficult, although it is being eased by developments in MR technology, and their surgical treatment has not been conspicuously successful. The epilepsy seems to arise from the disordered and disorganized neurons that constitute the pathology, and these are often situated diffusely. It is likely, therefore, that therapeutic advances will have to await an understanding of the mechanisms underlying the epileptogenicity of dysplastic tissue sufficient to permit the development of specific counteracting drugs.

TREATMENTS

As has been mentioned above, it is unfortunate that recently introduced antiepileptic drugs have done little to increase the proportion of people with intractable focal epilepsy who can be rendered seizure free by modification of their drug regimen (Marson *et al* 1996). Adjustments of medication may bring about some reduction in the frequency of the seizures, and may give a more acceptable side-effect profile, but they rarely bring about a cure.

It is inevitable, therefore, that hope most often lies in surgery regardless of the reality that only a small proportion of people with intractable focal epilepsy fall into a category amenable to successful surgical treatment. Even so, surgery is underutilized partly because of failure to recognize that the epilepsy is due to a surgically treatable cause and partly because of a fear that surgery, and particularly presurgical evaluation, is unduly complicated and expensive. Needless to say, any unit that sets out to treat patients surgically requires a multidisciplinary team. There should be, for both children and adults, at least a neurologist, a neurosurgeon, a neurophysiologist, a neuroradiologist, a neuropsychologist, a neuropsychiatrist, and a neuropathologist, along with specialist nursing and technical support staff and appropriate investigational facilities (Wallace *et al* 1997). We very much hope that the descriptions in this book of the conditions amenable to surgery, and of the approach to presurgical evaluation, will stimulate more units to form such groups. By so doing they will relieve a considerable burden of disability. The level of expertise required varies according to the complexity of the case and for a number of reasons special expertise is necessary to treat children.

The place of surgery in the treatment of focal epilepsy was firmly established by the 1986 and 1992 Palm Desert International Conferences on the Surgical Treatment of the Epilepsies organized by Professor Jerome Engel (Engel 1987, 1993). The first conference celebrated the centennial anniversary of Victor Horsley's classic paper 'Brain surgery' published in the *British Medical Journal* of 1886. The second was dedicated to Wilder Penfield and to the Montreal Neurological Institute. The Institute had recently celebrated the fiftieth anniversary of the establishment of its EEG laboratory by Herbert Jasper. Contributions to the 1986 conference made it clear that at least some forms of surgery were very effective and that considerable numbers of patients were being operated on at various centers across the world. By the time of the 1992 conference there had been a great increase in the number of centers worldwide providing epilepsy surgery, and in the number of patients operated on, and also in improved efficacy (Engel *et al* 1993).

The evolution of surgical treatment from the early work of Foerster and Penfield, which was based on gross pathology, direct brain stimulation, and later brain recording, is elegantly summarized in *Epilepsy and The Functional Anatomy of the Human Brain* (Penfield and Jasper 1954). This was followed by the realization that the nature of the pathology was also important, as pioneered by Falconer and his collaborators (Falconer *et al* 1964; Falconer 1971; Bruton 1988) and subsequently emphasized by the methods of direct brain imaging that became available in the mid 1970s and 1980s. Resective surgery, especially in the temporal lobe, is now a well-recognized and safe technique for the treatment of drug-resistant partial epilepsy. The same applies in the extratemporal cortex, although there the chances of success are less and the possibility of morbidity is greater. However, even along this well-trodden path, apart from variations in surgical technique, there remain a number of unsolved problems.

First, there is the question of whether and when it is necessary to resect functionally abnormal tissue that may appear to be structurally normal. The concept of the epileptogenic zone and its concomitant areas described by Luders (Luders and Awad 1992) has to be reckoned with. The second question relates to the identification of pathology. It is becoming clear from imaging studies that there may be multiple pathology in two senses. The first is when there is pathology of one type but it is multifocal. The second is when there are coexisting pathologies, best exemplified by the dual pathology, such as a dysembryoplastic neuroepithelioma and mesial temporal sclerosis, described in the temporal lobe (Cascino *et al* 1993). Patients who are clearly unsuitable for resective surgery may benefit from some form of functional intervention. These interventions include lesioning, the division of fiber tracts, and direct or indirect brain stimulation. It is more difficult to set down the indications for these procedures, and they are less effective than the majority of resective operations. Nevertheless, they will give some patients better control of their seizures and a better quality of life.

The first part of the section on surgery begins with chapters describing the surgical options and the epilepsy syndromes particularly amenable to surgery before going on to describe the methods of presurgical evaluation. This part ends with a chapter dealing with rational preoperative assessment intended as a guide to how to investigate and select patients for the options available. The second part includes three chapters, dealing with the common cortical areas of resection in some detail, written in a manner that should not be rapidly outdated. These chapters cover the indications for surgery, surgical technique, and outcome. The 'nonsurgical' methods of tissue ablation such as stereotactic radiosurgery and thermocoagulation are discussed in relation to temporal lobe surgery. Two chapters are concerned with functional surgery. The rationale for this kind of surgery is often of a hybrid nature derived partly from empirical observation of patients who have undergone the surgery and partly from notions arising out of animal experiments. The potential of lesioning and the division of fiber tracts may not have been fully realized. This is because our understanding of the pathophysiology of epilepsy is still very crude. It will be intriguing to see whether new methods for investigating brain function such as PET, SPECT, functional MRI and MR spectroscopy will improve our understanding of the pathophysiology sufficiently to enable the application of these techniques to be extended. For instance, multiple subpial transection applied to multiple foci might open up a completely new field of treatment for patients suffering from cognitive defects associated with epilepsy. A chapter is devoted to brain stimulation as first proposed by Cooper (1973). Controlled trials could not establish his method as valuable. Thalamic stimulation, as proposed by Velasco, seems to have more substance (Velasco *et al* 1993, 1995). The most recent proposal – stimulation of the brain through the vagus nerve – also gives significant results and has the potential to be more valuable.

The surgical section ends with chapters considering the outcome of surgery in a broad sense. The effects on seizure control are covered, as are the physical, neuropsychologic and psychiatric morbidity together with the effects on quality of life.

The book ends with two chapters, written by two very well-established experts, on the economic considerations that are essential in this age in all countries of the world.

REFERENCES

Blume WT (1989) Clinical profile of partial seizures beginning at less than four years of age. *Epilepsia* **30**:813–819.

Bruton CL (1988) *The Neuropathology of Temporal Lobe Epilepsy*, Institute of Psychiatry Maudsley Monographs 31. Oxford: Oxford University Press.

Cascino GD, Jack CR Jr, Parisi JE *et al* (1993) Operative strategy in patients with MRI-identified dual pathology and temporal lobe epilepsy. *Epilepsy Research* **14**:175–182.

Chevrie JJ, Aicardi J (1978) Convulsive disorders in the first year of life: neurological and mental outcome and mortality. *Epilepsia* **19**:67–74.

Chevrie JJ, Aicardi J (1979) Convulsive disorders in the first year of life: persistence of epileptic seizures. *Epilepsia* **20**:643–649.

Chugani HT, Rintahaka PJ, Shewmon DA (1994) Ictal patterns of cerebral glucose utilization in children with epilepsy. *Epilepsia* **35**:813–822.

Cockerell OC, Johnson AL, Sander JWAS, Hart YM, Shorvon SD (1995) Remission of epilepsy: results from the National General Practice Study of Epilepsy. *Lancet* **346**:140–144.

Commission on Classification and Terminology of the International League Against Epilepsy (1981) Proposal for revised clinical and electroencephalographic classification of epileptic seizures. *Epilepsia* **22**:489–501.

Cook M, Stevens JM (1995) Imaging in epilepsy. In: Hopkins A, Shorvon S, Cascino G (eds) *Epilepsy*, 2nd edition, pp 143–169. London: Chapman and Hall.

Cooper I (1973) Chronic stimulation of the paleo-cerebellum in humans. *Lancet* **i**:206.

Donat J (1992) The age-dependent epileptic encephalopathies. *Journal of Child Neurology* **7**:7–21.

Duchowny M, Jayakar P, Resnick T *et al* (1998) Epilepsy surgery in the first three years of life. *Epilepsia* **39**:737–743.

Engel J (ed.) (1987) *Surgical Treatment of the Epilepsies*. New York: Raven Press.

Engel J (ed.) (1993) *Surgical Treatment of the Epilepsies*, 2nd edn. New York: Raven Press.

Engel J, Driver MV, Falconer MA (1975) Electrophysiological correlates of pathology and surgical results in temporal lobe epilepsy. *Brain* **98**:129–156.

Engel J, Van Ness PC, Rasmussen T, Ojemann LM (1993) Outcome with respect to epileptic seizures. In: Engel J (ed.) *Surgical Treatment of the Epilepsies*, 2nd edn, pp 609–622. New York: Raven Press.

Falconer MA (1953) Discussion on the surgery of temporal lobe epilepsy: surgical and pathological aspects. *Proceedings of the Royal Society of Medicine* **46**:971–975.

Falconer MA (1971) Genetic and related aetiological factors in temporal lobe epilepsy: a review. *Epilepsia* **12**:13–31.

Falconer MA, Serafetinides EA, Corsellis JA (1964) Etiology and pathogenesis of temporal lobe epilepsy. *Archives of Neurology* **10**:233–248.

Forsgren L (1990) Prospective incidence study and clinical characterization of seizures in newly referred adults. *Epilepsia* **31**:292–301.

Gastaut H (1970) Clinical and electroencephalographic classification of epileptic seizures. *Epilepsia* **11**:102–113.

Gastaut H, Caveness WF, Landolt H *et al* (1964) A proposed international classification of epileptic seizures. *Epilepsia* **5**:297–306.

Hauser WA, Hesdorffer DC (1996) The natural history of seizures. In: Wyllie E (ed.) *The Treatment of Epilepsy: Principles and Practice*, 2nd edn, pp173–178. Baltimore: Williams and Wilkins.

Hauser WA, Annegers JF, Kurland LT (1993) Incidence of epilepsy and unprovoked seizures in Rochester, Minnesota: 1935–1984. *Epilepsia* **34**:453–468.

Hopkins A (1989a) Lessons for neurologists from the United Kingdom Third National Morbidity Survey. *Journal of Neurology, Neurosurgery and Psychiatry* **52**:430–433.

Hopkins A, Menken M, De Friese G (1989b) A record of patient encounters in neurological practice in the United Kingdom. *Journal of Neurology, Neurosurgery and Psychiatry*, **52**:436–438.

Jayakar P, Duchowny MS (1990) Complex partial seizures of temporal lobe origin in early childhood. In: Duchowny MS, Resnick TJ, Alvarez LA (eds) *Pediatric Epilepsy Surgery*, pp 41–46. New York: Demos.

Joensen P (1986) Prevalence, incidence, and classification of epilepsy in the Faroes. *Acta Neurologica Scandinavica* **74**:150–155.

Loiseau P, Beaussart M (1973) The seizures of benign childhood epilepsy with Rolandic paroxysmal discharges. *Epilepsia* **14**:381–389.

Loiseau J, Loiseau P, Guyot M, Duche B, Dartigues J-F, Aublet B (1990) Survey of seizure disorders in the French Southwest. I. Incidence of epileptic syndromes. *Epilepsia* **31**:391–396.

Luders H, Awad IA (1992) Conceptual considerations. In: Luders H (ed.) *Epilepsy Surgery*, pp 51–62. New York: Raven Press.

Margerison JH, Corsellis JAN (1966) Epilepsy and the temporal lobes. A clinical, electroencephalographic and neuropathological study of the brain in epilepsy with particular reference to the temporal lobes. *Brain* **89**:499–530.

Marson AG, Kadir ZA, Chadwick DW (1996) New antiepileptic drugs: a systematic review of their efficacy and tolerability. *British Medical Journal* **313**:1169–1174.

Mathern GW, Babb TL, Vickrey BG, Melendez M, Pretorius JK (1995) The clinical-pathogenic mechanisms of hippocampal neuron loss and surgical outcomes in temporal lobe epilepsy. *Brain* **118**:105–118.

Mouritzen Dam A (1980) Epilepsy and neuron loss in the hippocampus. *Epilepsia* **21**:617–629.

Mouritzen Dam A (1982) Hippocampal neuron loss in epilepsy and after experimental seizures. *Acta Neurologica Scandinavica* **66**:601–642.

Nordli DRJ, Bazil CW, Scheuer ML, Pedley TA (1997) Recognition and classification of seizures in infants. *Epilepsia* **38**:553–560.

Olafsson E, Hauser WA, Ludvigsson P, Gudmundsson G (1996) Incidence of epilepsy in rural Iceland: a population-based study. *Epilepsia* **37**:951–955.

Oller-Daurella L, Oller LF (1989) Partial epilepsy with seizures appearing in the first three years of life. *Epilepsia* **30**:820–826.

Ounsted C, Lindsay J, Norman R (1966) *Biological Factors in Temporal Lobe Epilepsy*, Clinics in Developmental Medicine 22. London: The Spastics Society Medical Education and Information Unit and William Heinemann Medical Books.

Oxbury JM, Oxbury SM (1998) Memory and the human temporal lobes. In: Milner AD (ed.) *Comparative Neuropsychology*, pp 95–108. Oxford: Oxford University Press.

Penfield W, Jasper H (1954) *Epilepsy and the Functional Anatomy of the Human Brain*. Boston: Little, Brown.

Rausch R (1987) Psychological evaluation. In: Engel J Jr (ed.) *Surgical Treatment of the Epilepsies*, pp 181–211. New York: Raven Press.

Sagar HJ, Oxbury JM (1987) Hippocampal neuron loss in temporal lobe epilepsy: correlation with early childhood convulsions. *Annals of Neurology* **22**:334–340.

Sperling MR, Sutherling WW, Nuwer MR (1987) New techniques for evaluating patients for epilepsy surgery. In: Engel J Jr (ed.) *Surgical Treatment of the Epilepsies*, pp 235–257. New York: Raven Press.

Velasco M, Velasco F, Velasco AL, Velasco G, Jimenez F (1993) Effect of chronic electrical stimulation of the centromedian thalamic nuclei on various intractable seizure patterns: II. Psychological performance and background EEG activity. *Epilepsia* **6**:1065–1074.

Velasco F, Velasco M, Velasco AL, Jimenez F, Marquez I, Rise M (1995) Electrical stimulation of the centromedian thalamic nucleus in control of seizures: long-term studies. *Epilepsia* **36**:63–71.

Wallace H, Shorvon SD, Hopkins A, O'Donoghue M (1997) *Adults with Poorly Controlled Epilepsy.* London: The Royal College of Physicians of London.

Watanabe K, Yamamoto N, Negoro T, Takahashi I, Aso K, Maehara M (1990) Benign infantile epilepsy with complex partial seizures. *Journal of Clinical Neurophysiology* 7:409–416.

Watanabe K, Negoro T, Aso K (1993) Benign partial epilepsy with secondarily generalized seizures in infancy. *Epilepsia* **34**:635–638.

Wieser H-G, Engel J Jr, Williamson PD, Babb TL, Gloor P (1993) Surgically remediable temporal lobe syndromes. In: Engel J Jr (ed.) *Surgical Treatment of the Epilepsies*, 2nd edn, pp 49–63. New York: Raven Press.

Wyllie E (1996) Surgery for catastrophic localization-related epilepsy in infants. *Epilepsia* **37**:S22–25.

Yamamoto N, Watanabe K, Negoro T *et al* (1987) Complex partial seizures in children: ictal manifestations and their relation to clinical course. *Neurology* **37**:1379–1382.

Diagnosis and classification

JM OXBURY AND M DUCHOWNY

The term *epilepsy* embraces a constellation of seizures and syndromes, each manifest by recurrent epileptic seizures. An epileptic seizure is defined as a transient episode of neurological dysfunction brought about by abnormal, synchronous and excessive discharges of cerebral neurons (Hopkins 1987; Chadwick 1994; Engel and Pedley 1998). An *epileptic syndrome* has been defined as 'an epileptic disorder characterized by a cluster of signs and symptoms customarily occurring together' (Commission on Classification and Terminology of the International League Against Epilepsy (ILAE) 1985, 1989). Features that could be in the cluster include the seizure type and the anatomic locus of onset. The etiology and the prognosis could also be included but they need not necessarily be so.

A clinician asked to advise on the diagnosis and treatment of a person with presumed epilepsy should first obtain a precise description of the episodic symptoms that are experienced, that is of the presumed epileptic seizures. The patient should describe all the features of the attacks that he or she can remember from personal experience. Great care should be taken to distinguish between what are truly remembered symptoms and what are features known to the patient as a consequence of the description of observers. A description of what is observed should also be obtained from a reliable witness, usually a family member, who has seen a number of the attacks. The first witnessed manifestation or internal experience is highly important as it often localizes seizure origin.

Epileptic seizures essentially have a stereotyped pattern of symptoms within an individual. The individual may have seizures of more than one type but the number of types is nevertheless small, rarely amounting to more than three. An apparently greater number of types should raise the suspicion that the seizures are propagating to distant regions or that at least some may not be epileptic.

The information derived from the descriptions of the patient and of an observer, taken along with data from routine interictal scalp EEG recordings, should make it possible to classify the patient's seizures, in terms of the seizure classification given below. Occasionally additional information derived from ictal video-telemetry may be necessary.

Sometimes seizures cannot be classified even after a detailed evaluation. The pattern of the attacks, or in modern parlance the type of the focal (partial) seizures experienced by the patient, gives a clue to the anatomic source of the epilepsy. Further information must be obtained from EEG and brain imaging before a more definite diagnosis of the source can be established. Also, other aspects of the history including the family history and the findings on physical examination must be considered before the nature of the epileptic syndrome can be suggested. It is worth emphasizing, however, that the diagnosis is ultimately a clinical judgment.

In the final analysis, it should be possible to specify the type and frequency of the patient's seizures and the nature of the underlying epilepsy syndrome. It should also be possible to specify the anatomic site or sites of origin of the seizures and, especially in the case of the symptomatic localization-related epilepsies, the nature of the underlying pathology. Only then can a proper treatment plan be defined.

SEIZURE CLASSIFICATION

The classification of seizures is along two major axes.

The first axis is anatomically organized into partial seizures, primary generalized seizures, including unclassified seizures, and prolonged or repetitive seizures (status epilepticus) – see Table 2.1 based on the classification proposed by the ILAE (Commission on Classification and Terminology of the ILAE 1981). *Partial seizures* are defined as those where, in general, the first clinical and EEG changes indicate initial activation of a system of neurons restricted to a part of one cerebral hemisphere; that is to say they are focal. Partial seizures are divided into three categories (simple partial, complex partial, and partial evolving to secondary generalization) and each is further subdivided. *Primary generalized seizures* are those whose first clinical change indicates initial involvement of both cerebral hemispheres simultaneously, and whose initial EEG pattern is bilateral and presumed to reflect neuronal discharges widespread throughout both

Table 2.1 Seizure classification. Derived from the Commission on Classification and Terminology of the International League Against Epilepsy (1981).

I. Partial (focal, local) seizures
    (A) Simple partial seizures
        • motor
        • sensory
        • autonomic
        • psychic
    (B) Complex partial seizures
        • with simple partial onset
        • without simple partial onset, altered awareness/memory from onset
    (C) Partial seizures (simple or complex) evolving to secondary generalization
II. Primary generalized (convulsive or nonconvulsive)
    (A) Absence seizures
    (B) Myoclonic seizures
    (C) Clonic, tonic, and tonic–clonic seizures
    (D) Atonic seizures
III. Unclassified seizures
IV. Prolonged or repetitive seizures (status epilepticus)

hemispheres. It must be stressed that this is a classification of seizures only and not a classification of epilepsy syndromes. A patient may have more than one seizure type. Thus, for instance, a person prone to primary generalized seizures may, during a seizure, suffer a head injury causing frontal lobe damage, due to a hematoma, that becomes the source of partial seizures evolving to secondary generalization. This person will then be prone to two types of seizure.

The second axis is defined by etiology. Seizures are *idiopathic* when the etiology is presumed to be genetic, even if linkage studies have not yet been performed. *Cryptogenic* seizures are believed to have a structural cause that is not really defined by available diagnostic techniques. For all practical purposes, cryptogenic seizures result from intrauterine-acquired disorders of cortical development. *Symptomatic* seizures are attributable to a known postnatally acquired antecedent such as trauma, infection, etc. Looked upon as a temporal continuum, idiopathic, cryptogenic and symptomatic epilepsies define seizures due to familial, prenatal and postnatal factors, respectively.

The concern of this chapter is only with partial ('focal' or 'localization-related') seizures.

PARTIAL SEIZURES

SIMPLE PARTIAL SEIZURES

These are seizures in which awareness is preserved and memory for the seizure symptoms is well retained after the seizure has terminated. So, the patient can describe the content of such seizures from the memory of his/her personal experience. These seizures are subdivided into those with: motor signs; sensory symptoms; autonomic symptoms or signs; and psychic symptoms.

An *aura* is the initial part of a partial seizure, at onset, that is remembered after the seizure has terminated. The symptoms are usually sensory, autonomic or psychic as defined below. It is not uncommon for a patient to experience these symptoms sometimes in isolation as an *isolated aura*, which is in reality a simple partial seizure, and sometimes as the onset to a complex partial seizure or to a partial seizure with secondary generalization.

Seizures with motor signs

These have their onset in, or involve propagation to, the central rolandic cortex or the supplementary motor area of one cerebral hemisphere (see Chapter 5). They have been divided into:

1. Focal motor without a march. These are the commonest variety. They usually consist of clonic jerking movements involving a part or the whole of one side of the body. There may be a brief initial tonic phase. The body parts most often involved, in decreasing order of frequency, are the hand, especially the thumb and index finger, the face and tongue, and the foot.
2. Focal motor with a march (Jacksonian seizure). The first manifestation is usually clonic jerking of one side of the face or of a thumb or index finger associated with seizure discharges in the contralateral sensorimotor (rolandic) cortex. Spread of the seizure discharges to contiguous parts of the cerebral cortex results in a sequential involvement of body parts in the clonic movements, the order within the sequence being determined by the geographic relationships within the precentral gyrus.

    Focal motor seizures, irrespective of whether a march is involved, may be followed by a weakness of the involved muscle groups that lasts for up to several hours (*Todd's paralysis*).
3. Versive. These consist of tonic-sustained, or clonic-jerking, and turning of the head and eyes, and sometimes of the whole body, to one side. The turning may be the first feature of a partial seizure that evolves to secondary generalization. The direction of movement is usually, but not always, away from the side of the seizure focus that may be in the frontal cortex or in the parietooccipital region. Versive turning is organized in motor cortex anterior to the precentral gyrus (areas 4 and 6). Versive head and eye deviation is characteristic of seizures originating in the supplementary motor area (interhemispheric area 6). The seizures consist of bilateral tonic postures with contraversive head and eye movement. As consciousness is fully preserved, these seizures consist of bilateral motor phenomena with preserved consciousness. Bilateral motor manifestations may be confused with true generalized epilepsy and are easily mistaken for psychogenic attacks by the unwary.
4. Postural. These are the manifestation of tonic-sustained muscle contraction leading to a posture being maintained. The whole body may be involved, such as when a statuesque position is adopted, or there may simply be an altered position of one limb. The supplementary motor area is believed to play an important part in these seizures.
5. Phonatory. These may involve vocalization or speech arrest. They may arise from seizure discharges in either hemisphere.

Seizures with somatosensory or special-sensory symptoms (simple hallucinations)

1. Somatosensory. Such seizures are relatively rare. They often arise from the contralateral (but sometimes ipsilateral) central rolandic region and they may show a Jacksonian march as with focal motor seizures. The symptoms may be bilateral when there is involvement of the second sensory area. They are usually manifest by numbness/tingling, and sometimes by pain, particularly in one hand (see Chapter 7). These symptoms may be the prelude to a Jacksonian motor seizure.
2. Visual. Simple ictal visual symptoms include positive phenomena, such as flickering or zig-zag lights that may be colored, and negative phenomena such as field defects or patches of darkness. These sensations may occur in central vision or in the half-field contralateral to the seizure discharges.
3. Auditory. Simple ictal auditory symptoms are sounds such as roaring, humming, or ringing noises, or tones. They are particularly associated with seizure discharges in the region of Heschl's gyrus and may be heard in the contralateral ear or bilaterally.
4. Olfactory. The smell experienced as an ictal olfactory sensation is more often unpleasant than pleasant and is often described as being of a 'chemical' nature or a 'burning sensation'.
5. Gustatory. As with olfactory sensations, simple ictal gustatory sensations are more often unpleasant than pleasant and are often described as 'metallic'.
6. Vertiginous. These sensations include true vertigo, body tilt sensations, unsteadiness and vague dizziness. The symptoms are often regarded initially as of vestibular or brainstem origin.

Seizures with autonomic symptoms or signs

These include abdominal sensations which may have a rising quality, cephalic and thoracic sensations including pain, breathlessness and altered breathing rhythm, altered heart rhythm, pallor or flushing, sweating, pilo-erection, pupillary dilatation, vomiting, salivation, thirst, urinary incontinence and genital sensations or orgasm.

An abdominal or cephalic sensation is an especially common component of a simple partial seizure or aura (Currie *et al* 1971; Taylor and Locherty 1987) and the former is particularly common in medial temporal lobe epilepsy (MTLE, see below) due to mesial temporal sclerosis (Duncan and Sagar 1987; Fried *et al* 1998). This epilepsy syndrome occasionally presents as episodic abdominal pain

(Peppercorn *et al* 1978), particularly in young children, leading to extensive gastrointestinal investigation before the diagnosis of epilepsy is established. For many patients the abdominal sensation is either unpleasant or accompanied by fear. Seizures may also be associated with frank vomiting ('ictus emeticus'). This symptom is particularly common in children with occipital seizures and presumably reflects spread anteriorly to the temporal lobe.

Seizures with psychic symptoms

These have been divided into six categories but there is often considerable overlap, particularly between altered affect, dysmnesic symptoms, dreamy states, and structured hallucinations.

1. Dysphasic alteration of language function. Dysphasic language during the course of a seizure, or in the immediate postictal period, is strongly associated with seizure origin from the language-dominant side (see Chapters 5 and 6). Postictal dysphasia may be of a nonfluent variety accompanied by dysarthria or it may be fluent with paraphasias and impaired comprehension (Ardila and Lopez 1988). It must be distinguished from postictal confusion. Prolonged ictal aphasia can occur as a form of complex partial status epilepticus (Rosenbaum *et al* 1986).

    Both ictal vocalization and nondysphasic speech during the course of a seizure appear to be without any lateralizing or localizing significance.
2. Dysmnesic alterations of memory. *Déjà vu* ('already seen') is the commonest of these. It is the sensation that some new scene has been witnessed on a previous occasion. It is often accompanied by a strong sense of familiarity and sometimes by a feeling that it is possible to know what will happen next. It is relatively common as an aura to temporal lobe onset seizures when it may coincide with other ictal symptoms or be part of an experiential hallucination and/or a dreamy state. Isolated *déjà vu* is also relatively common as an occasional experience of people who have no other manifestations of epilepsy, particularly adolescents and young adults, and it is a feature of various psychiatric conditions (Rooth 1987).

    Déjà entendu is the auditory equivalent of *déjà vu*. *Jamais vu* (*jamais entendu*) is the converse feeling that a familiar experience is novel or that an experience has not actually occurred.

    Pure amnesic seizures have been defined as seizures

during which the only clinical manifestation is inability to retain in memory what occurs during the seizure (Palmini *et al* 1992). Cognition and ability to interact normally with the environment is retained. These seizures usually last for <5 min but may last longer (Zeman *et al* 1998). They are rarely if ever the patient's only seizure type.

3. Dreamy states and distortions of time sense. The term *dreamy state* was introduced by Hughlings Jackson to refer to an elaborate ictal state of mind shortly after seizure onset, and sometimes constituting the whole of the seizure, that the patient is usually unable to subsequently recall fully. The patient may say that there have been feelings of strangeness or of unreality or particularly of heightened reality. The condition has elements of dysmnesia, especially *déjà vu*, and of illusions or experiential hallucinations and sometimes of altered affect. There may be what is described as depersonalization or a feeling of being 'out of body' (autoscopy). Thoughts may feel forced and subjected to unavoidable intrusions. Despite having no more than fragmentary recall of the ictal experience, some patients feel that it is always the same, whereas others feel that it varies from seizure to seizure. The electrophysiological studies of Gloor (1990) and of Bancaud *et al* (1994) suggest that both the medial temporal lobe structures and lateral temporal neocortex are activated during both dreamy states and structured experiential hallucinations which cannot be considered as separate and distinct.
4. Altered affect. A feeling of fear is the most common. Its intensity can vary from mild anxiety to sheer terror and it may be accompanied by autonomic symptoms/signs. These manifestations are commonly observed in seizures both of anterior frontal lobe origin and of medial temporal lobe origin. Ictal depression is less common but may be prolonged and has been described as lasting for up to one hour (Williams 1956). Other feelings include anxiety, anger, sadness, and less often pleasurable feelings such as elation, exhilaration, and satisfaction.
5. Illusions. Apparent alterations of object size (macropsia/micropsia), shape or distance probably indicate involvement of visual association cortex. Color may be altered and objects may be seen as multiple. Similarly, sounds may be perceived as louder or softer or as more or less distant. Phantom sensations and body part agnosia have been described as ictal symptoms (Sveinbjornsdottir and Duncan 1993) as have false impressions of movement and feelings that a limb is shrinking or swelling.
6. Structured hallucinations. These are more often visual

scenes than auditory. Visual hallucinations may be extremely complex and usually consist of places and people, and complex auditory hallucinations consist of voices or music. They are often experiential in that they are recollections of past happenings and they have what Gloor (1990) described as 'a compelling immediacy similar to or sometimes even more vivid than those occurring in real life'. As with dreamy states, the hallucinations are often accompanied by altered affect and by dysmnesia, especially *déjà vu*.

Wilder Penfield's review of 520 cases of temporal lobe epilepsy (Penfield and Perot 1963) revealed 21 with purely visual and 12 with purely auditory ictal experiential hallucinations. No such hallucinations were reported in 612 further cases of extratemporal epilepsy. Penfield and Perot felt that experiential hallucinations arose from seizure discharges in lateral temporal neocortex. The electrophysiological findings of Gloor (1990) and his colleagues and of Bancaud *et al* (1994), however, suggest that activation of the medial temporal lobe structures is of at least equal importance. The dual nature of activation suggests that these symptoms are organized in a radial fashion.

There is much overlap between the separately described elements of these seizures with psychic symptoms. The 'dreamy states' particularly seem to involve at least some alteration of awareness, with subsequent inability to fully remember the content, thereby making it difficult to know whether they should be classified as complex partial rather than simple partial. Patients often regard their symptoms negatively and desire relief through medication or surgery.

COMPLEX PARTIAL SEIZURES

These are seizures in which *consciousness* is impaired but there is no progression to a generalized tonic–clonic convulsion. Impairment of consciousness is the factor that constitutes the fundamental distinction from a simple partial seizure. The term consciousness refers to the degree of *awareness* (the patient's contact with events and the ability to recall them subsequently) and/or *responsiveness* (the ability to carry out simple commands or willed movements). Impaired consciousness is defined as 'the inability to respond normally to exogenous stimuli by virtue of altered awareness and/or responsiveness' (the Commission on Classification and Terminology of the ILAE 1981). Observers sometimes believe that a person in a complex partial seizure may obey a simple command and people who experience complex partial seizures may sometimes feel that they have an awareness of some simple event during the

course of the seizure. In general, however, people who experience complex partial seizures are not able to recall the content of their seizures.

Complex partial seizures are subdivided according to whether or not they commence with the features of a simple partial seizure and according to whether or not they incorporate an automatism. Thus:

1. (a) Simple partial features followed by impaired consciousness without automatism.
   (b) Simple partial features followed by an automatism.
2. (a) Impaired consciousness only without preceding simple partial features.
   (b) Automatism without preceding simple partial features.

For these purposes, an *automatism* is taken as a 'more or less coordinated adapted involuntary motor activity occurring during the state of clouding of consciousness … and usually followed by amnesia for the event' (Commission on Classification and Terminology of the ILAE 1981). An automatism usually lasts for 2–5 min but is then mostly followed by a period of postictal confusion and/or amnesia. Automatisms were subdivided into:

1. Oropharyngeal. These consist of lip-smacking, chewing, repetitive swallowing and drooling of saliva and there may be other autonomic components such as borborygmi.
2. Expression of emotion. Most often the appearance is of fear but there may be laughter, anger or rage and sexual behavior has been described. Unprovoked violence is extremely rare and poorly documented (Fenwick 1985).
3. Gestural. Tonic, clonic or tonic–clonic movements of one side of the face are common but should not be regarded as gestural. Otherwise hand and/or arm movements are common. They may be simple, such as tapping or rubbing another body part, or elaborate such as making flag-waving movements. There may be whole body movements.
4. Ambulatory. These include activities such as walking/running and jumping out of moving cars that may put the person at considerable risk.
5. Verbal. These consist of recognizable nonaphasic speech, often a single word or a brief phrase that is usually out of context. This type of verbal behavior, unlike dysphasic ictal speech, does not have any lateralizing significance.

The behavior during some automatisms is complex, for instance undressing which is relatively common, and cannot easily be placed in any of the above categories. It has been suggested that ictal automatisms should be distinguished from the postictal automatisms following severe tonic–clonic convulsions but this may be difficult because automatisms may occur at any point in the ictal sequence including the terminal part.

PARTIAL SEIZURES EVOLVING TO SECONDARY GENERALIZATION

These are seizures that commence with the features of a simple partial or a complex partial seizure but evolve to a generalized tonic–clonic convulsion. They are subdivided according to the features before the onset of the convulsion. Thus:

1. Simple partial evolving to secondary generalization.
2. Complex partial evolving to secondary generalization.
3. Simple partial evolving to complex partial evolving to secondary generalization.

PROLONGED OR REPETITIVE SEIZURES (STATUS EPILEPTICUS)

Status epilepticus is the term applied to seizures that are prolonged, usually beyond 30 min, or that recur at a frequency too rapid to permit proper recovery of consciousness between the individual seizures. A number of varieties are recognized in both children and adults including convulsive, petit mal absence, complex partial, and simple partial of which epilepsia partialis continua is a form. Only complex partial status and epilepsia partialis continua are considered here. Varieties confined to children include febrile and electrical status epilepticus during slow wave sleep as part of the Landau–Kleffner syndrome (see Chapters 9 and 22).

Complex partial status has been defined as an epileptic episode that is prolonged beyond 30 min during which focal fluctuating or frequently recurring electrographic epileptic discharges arising out of the temporal or extratemporal regions result in a confusional state with variable clinical symptoms (Cockerell *et al* 1994). It is often recurrent and it may be prolonged over days or weeks. The diagnosis is often suspected clinically in patients with prolonged confusional episodes. The scalp EEG may be nonspecific. It must be differentiated from primary generalized absence status, postictal confusion, and from other neurologic and psychiatric causes of confusion.

Epilepsia partialis continua (see also below) is manifest by simple partial motor seizures, with repetitive regular or irregular clonic jerks of cortical origin, on a part of one side

of the body without loss of consciousness. It may progress to secondarily generalized convulsive status.

CLASSIFICATION OF EPILEPTIC SYNDROMES

As has been mentioned above, an epileptic syndrome (or an 'epilepsy') has been defined as 'an epileptic disorder characterized by a cluster of signs and symptoms customarily occurring together'. An abbreviated and modified version of

Table 2.2 Classification of epileptic syndromes. Derived from the Commission on Classification and Terminology of the International League Against Epilepsy (1989) but with modifications/additions.

1. Localization-related (focal, local, partial) epilepsies and syndromes
   1.1. Idiopathic
      - Benign localization-related epilepsies of childhood
        – childhood epilepsy with centrotemporal spike
        – childhood epilepsy with occipital paroxysms
      - Autosomal dominant nocturnal frontal lobe epilepsy
      - Familial temporal lobe epilepsy
      - Primary reading epilepsy
   1.2. Symptomatic
      - Chronic progressive epilepsia partialis continua of childhood (Kojewnikow's syndrome)
      - Syndromes characterized by seizures with specific modes of precipitation
      - Temporal lobe epilepsies
      - Frontal lobe epilepsies
      - Parietal lobe epilepsies
      - Occipital lobe epilepsies
   1.3. Cryptogenic
      - Hot water epilepsy
      - Musicogenic epilepsy
      - Eating epilepsy
2. Generalized epilepsies and syndromes
   2.1. Idiopathic
      - Benign neonatal familial convulsions
      - Benign neonatal convulsions
      - Benign myoclonic epilepsy of childhood
      - Childhood absence epilepsy
      - Juvenile absence epilepsy
      - Juvenile myoclonic epilepsy
      - Epilepsy with grand mal seizures on awakening
      - Other generalized idiopathic epilepsies
      - Epilepsies with seizures precipitated by specific modes of activation
   2.2. Cryptogenic or symptomatic
      - West syndrome
      - Lennox–Gastaut syndrome
      - Epilepsy with myoclonic–astatic seizures
      - Epilepsy with myoclonic absences
   2.3 Symptomatic
3. Epilepsies and syndromes undetermined whether focal or generalized
4. Special syndromes

the classification of epileptic syndromes as proposed by the Commission on Classification and Terminology of the ILAE (1989) is shown in Table 2.2.

The concern here is with the *localization-related (focal, local, partial) epilepsies and syndromes*. These are the epilepsies manifest by partial or focal seizures as opposed to the generalized epilepsies that are manifest by primary generalized seizures. Both major groups (localization-related and generalized) are subdivided on an etiological basis into idiopathic, symptomatic and cryptogenic. The term *idiopathic* is applied to epilepsies that are presumed to have a genetic etiology. The term *symptomatic* is applied to epilepsies that are considered to be due to known brain pathology. The term *cryptogenic* is applied to epilepsies that are presumed to be due to brain pathology that is occult or hidden and not yet established.

IDIOPATHIC LOCALIZATION-RELATED EPILEPSIES

These are conditions characterized by focal seizures without detectable underlying cerebral pathology but with a strong family history suggesting that there is a major genetic factor in their etiology. The benign localization-related epilepsies of childhood are described in detail in Chapter 20. Autosomal dominant nocturnal frontal lobe epilepsy, familial temporal lobe epilepsy and primary reading epilepsy are described in Chapter 21. The conditions will be mentioned only in brief outline here.

BENIGN LOCALIZATION-RELATED EPILEPSIES OF CHILDHOOD

This group includes benign childhood epilepsy with centrotemporal spike and childhood epilepsy with occipital paroxysms. Photosensitive occipital lobe epilepsy and benign frontal lobe epilepsy might also be included if the latter is indeed a unitary syndrome (Gobbi and Guerrini 1998). They carry a good prognosis and are not a form of intractable drug-resistant disorder.

AUTOSOMAL DOMINANT NOCTURNAL FRONTAL LOBE EPILEPSY

Autosomal dominant nocturnal frontal lobe epilepsy (Scheffer *et al* 1995; Oldani *et al* 1998) typically begins in childhood and persists throughout adulthood. The brief motor seizures, with features characteristic of frontal lobe onset, occur in clusters arising during dozing or shortly before waking. Neurologic, neuropsychologic, and neuroimaging examinations are normal. Several families with many affected members have been described. The pattern of inheritance appears to be autosomal dominant with gene locus heterogeneity between the families.

FAMILIAL TEMPORAL LOBE EPILEPSY

People with this condition typically experience simple partial seizures or isolated auras, especially with psychic and/or autonomic features, occasional complex partial seizures and occasional seizures with secondary generalization. The condition appears to be inherited as an autosomal dominant with a penetrance of around 60% (Berkovic and Scheffer 1997).

PRIMARY READING EPILEPSY

Primary reading epilepsy is a disorder where seizures are triggered by reading and in some cases also by other language-related higher cognitive functions (Koutroumanidis *et al* 1998). The seizures typically consist of jaw or orofacial myoclonus sometimes spreading to the arms. A less common variety consists of reading-induced dyslexia that may evolve to a secondarily generalized convulsion.

SYMPTOMATIC LOCALIZATION-RELATED EPILEPSIES

The semeiology of the symptomatic localization-related epilepsies is described in detail in Chapters 5, 6, 7 and 8. The medial temporal lobe epilepsy associated with hippocampal and/or amygdala sclerosis is detailed in Chapter 11. Consequently only brief descriptions are given here. Seizure onset is considerably more often frontal, frontoparietal (central/rolandic), or temporal than from more posterior parts of 'a' cerebral hemisphere (Manford *et al* 1992).

EPILEPSIA PARTIALIS CONTINUA (EPC)

EPC is relatively rare (see also Chapter 5). A study based on data collected in the UK by the British Neurological Surveillance Unit suggests an annual incidence in the region of one case per million people (Cockerell *et al* 1996). The condition consists of clonic jerking of cortical origin of a muscle or muscle group that continues unabated for periods of hours, days or weeks and sometimes longer. Rasmussen encephalitis and virus encephalitis in general are the commonest causes in children in industrialized countries. Cerebral vascular pathology is the commonest cause in adults (Schomer 1993). A number of other causes are listed in Table 2.3. Around half of those who develop EPC also experience seizures of other types. EPC sometimes resolves spontaneously but in general it responds poorly to antiepileptic drugs and surgical resection of underlying focal pathology in the rolandic region may be necessary (Biraben and Chauvel 1998).

TEMPORAL LOBE EPILEPSY

Temporal lobe epilepsy is currently subdivided into *lateral (neocortical) temporal lobe epilepsy* and *medial temporal lobe epilepsy*. It is said that fewer than 10% of patients prone to temporal lobe seizures without any circumscribed nonatrophic temporal lobe pathology have the seizures arising from temporal lobe neocortex (Williamson *et al* 1998). The seizure semeiology of lateral temporal lobe epilepsy is not clearly different to that of medial temporal lobe epilepsy (see Chapter 6). A vertiginous aura and *déjà vu* may, however, be more common with the former and an abdominal aura may be more common with the latter (Duncan and Sagar 1987; Gil-Nagel and Risinger 1997; Fried *et al* 1998).

The term medial temporal lobe epilepsy is used sometimes to refer to seizures arising from the medial temporal lobe structures irrespective of the underlying pathology, but more often to refer to the syndrome of epilepsy arising as a consequence of mesial temporal sclerosis. This syndrome has been recognized for several decades (for instance, Ounsted *et al* 1966) but it is only since the introduction of magnetic resonance imaging (MRI), allowing clear detection of unilateral hippocampal atrophy, that it has been widely

accepted. The primary features of the mesial temporal lobe epilepsy syndrome (see Chapter 11) are:

1. A history of a prolonged convulsion in early childhood, or some other cerebral insult, prior to the onset of the habitual epilepsy is common as is a family history of febrile convulsions (Maher and McLachlan 1995).
2. The seizures usually commence in childhood or adolescence and the prognosis for achieving adequate control with medication is <60%.
3. The typical pattern consists of partial seizures, particularly an epigastric-rising sensation associated with psychic phenomena such as fear, and complex partial seizures, especially oroalimentary and gestural automatisms, sometimes with secondary generalization.
4. Characteristic investigation findings are:
   (a) hippocampal smallness and increased T2 signal on MRI (see Chapter 44);
   (b) interictal blunt sharp waves predominating at the basal anterior electrodes on scalp EEG, and a generalized attenuation of background rhythms and disappearance of interictal spikes at seizure onset, and fairly regular θ-rhythms of about $5\,\text{s}^{-1}$ ictally with a crescendo-like increase of amplitude and slowing of discharge rhythms;
   (c) ipsilateral temporal lobe hyperperfusion on ictal single-photon emission computed tomography (SPECT);
   (d) ipsilateral temporal lobe hypometabolism on interictal positron emission tomography (PET);
   (e) variable degrees of memory and learning deficit.
5. Unilateral resection of the atrophic medial temporal lobe structures from those with predominantly unilateral hippocampal sclerosis renders 80% seizure-free, or virtually so, without producing additional clinically relevant deficits.

Table 2.3 Causes of epilepsia partialis continua.

Cause	Reference
Rasmussen's syndrome	Hart and Andermann (Chapter 18)
Tick-borne encephalitis (Russian spring-summer encephalitis)	Asher and Gajdusek (1991)
Focal rolandic pathology	
• infarction, hemorrhage	
• cortical vein thrombosis	
• arteriovenous malformation	
• trauma	
• tumor (rarely)	
Malformations of cortical development (rarely)	
Mitochondrial encephalopathy (MERRF)	Berkovic *et al* (1989)
Multiple sclerosis	Matthews (1991)
Nonketotic hyperglycemia	Singh and Strobos (1980)
Sjögren's syndrome	Bansal *et al* (1987)
Tuberculoma	Juul-Jensen and Denny-Brown (1966)

FRONTAL LOBE EPILEPSY

The frontal lobes are second only to the temporal lobes as the site of seizure onset in adults. In general, the seizures arise explosively, are brief, and end suddenly with little postictal confusion. They show a predilection for nocturnal onset. Also, they can be very frequent with >100 month^{-1} being not uncommon, whereas it is very unusual for temporal lobe seizures to be so frequent. Nevertheless, a recent comparison of frontal and temporal lobe onset seizures found no significant differences in frequency or duration or postictal duration (Manford *et al* 1996). Seizures that were very frequent (>50 day^{-1}) or very brief (<10s) were, however, more likely to be frontal than temporal.

Focal clonic movements and asymmetric tonic posturing are common features of frontal lobe seizures as is speech arrest. Somatosensory symptoms, autonomic symptoms/ signs and psychic symptoms are all relatively common with spread to other regions. There may be bizarre behavior and complex gestural motor activity with vocalizations in frontal lobe seizures arising in premotor cortex. Manford *et al* (1996) have reiterated that a reliable differentiation between frontal and temporal lobe seizures can be difficult on the basis of semeiology alone. In their analysis, early focal tonic posturing or head turning and general motor agitation were particularly associated with frontal onset seizures whereas auras, particularly fear and experiential, often followed by an oropharyngeal automatism, were particularly associated with a temporal lobe onset. The semeiology of frontal lobe epilepsy is described in detail in Chapter 5.

PARIETAL LOBE EPILEPSY

Parietal lobe seizures are relatively uncommon and there are few pathognomonic features. Numbness/tingling is the most frequently reported ictal sensation. Pain, usually a burning dysesthesia, may be felt. There may be a Jacksonian march as with focal motor seizures. Often symptoms do not commence until the seizure has propagated beyond the parietal lobe when the features are those of the area to which it has spread. The semeiology of parietal lobe epilepsy is described in detail in Chapter 7.

OCCIPITAL LOBE EPILEPSY

The semeiology of occipital lobe onset seizures and their underlying pathology/syndromes are described in Chapter 8. Simple visual phenomena, either positive or negative, are the most common initial symptom. The seizures may propagate to the frontal lobe where they produce turning of the head and/or eyes.

THE UNDERLYING PATHOLOGY

A detailed history of the epilepsy and of any related symptoms along with high-quality MRI are the keystones to establishing the nature of the underlying pathology in patients with intractable focal epilepsy. All such patients merit examination using the radiological techniques outlined in Chapter 24.

Table 2.4 Causes of chronic intractable focal epilepsy.

Mesial temporal sclerosis
Cerebral developmental disorders, including:
- Cortical dysplasia and neuronal migration defects
- Sturge–Weber syndrome
- Tuberous sclerosis
Brain tumor
- Oligodendroglioma and low-grade astrocytoma
- Dysembryoplastic neuroepithelioma
- Ganglioglioma
- Hamartoma
Cerebral vascular disease
- Cerebral infarction/hemorrhage, including intrauterine/perinatal stroke and hemiconvulsions-hemiplegia-epilepsy syndrome (HHE) syndrome
- Arteriovenous malformations
- Cavernous angioma
- Aneurysmal subarachnoid hemorrhage
CNS infection
- Subdural empyema and cerebral abscess
- Viral encephalitis, especially arborviruses, cytomegalovirus, herpes simplex, human immunodeficiency virus, Japanese B, measles
- Bacterial meningitis, including tuberculous and tuberculoma
- Other infections, especially cysticercosis
Brain trauma
Chronic alcoholism
Alzheimer's disease
Multiple sclerosis

This should enable pathology to be detected in at least 85% of cases. The usual causes of the condition are listed in Table 2.4. Descriptions of the neuroradiologic features of many of them will be found in Chapter 24. Hippocampal atrophy (34%) was the most common pathology detected in the MRI study of Cook and Stevens (1995), followed by a malformation of cortical development (16%), tumor (16%), and vascular malformation (10%). Pathology was detected more often in those with temporal lobe epilepsy (>90%) than in those with an extratemporal epilepsy (65%). The proportion of patients in whom no pathology can be defined may well fall even lower with improving MRI technology and the application of increasingly sophisticated techniques such as quantitative block analysis to detect areas of cerebral maldevelopment (Sisodiya *et al* 1995). Accurate diagnosis is an essential prelude to a proper treatment plan.

The underlying causes in children are often developmental in origin and consist of disordered cortical development. Disorders of neuronal migration, cortical dysplasia, phakomatous disorders, glial-neuronal hamartomas, and developmental tumors (gangliogliomas, dysembryoplastic neuroepitheliomas, gangliocytomas) account for a high proportion of partial seizures beginning in the first decade of life.

MESIAL TEMPORAL SCLEROSIS

The essential features of the medial temporal lobe epilepsy syndrome due to mesial temporal sclerosis have been outlined above. The condition is described in detail in Chapter 11 and the neuroradiologic features are described in Chapter 44. The pathology *is responsible for* the epilepsy in the medial temporal lobe epilepsy syndrome. In other situations, hippocampal sclerosis may be *consequent upon* the epilepsy (Mouritzen Dam 1980, 1982; Barr *et al* 1997).

CEREBRAL DEVELOPMENTAL DISORDERS

The classification, clinical features and radiologic appearances of cortical dysplasia and the neuronal migration defects are described in Chapter 10. Cortical dysplasia is not infrequently combined with other pathology, particularly hippocampal sclerosis, as part of 'dual pathology'. It may be more prevalent in people with epilepsy than has as yet been recognized. Indeed, there is a recent description of radiologic appearances suggestive of dysplasia in association with typical idiopathic primary generalized epilepsy syndromes (Woermann *et al* 1998) which could call into question the definition of these syndromes.

Sturge–Weber syndrome and tuberous sclerosis are described in Chapter 17.

BRAIN TUMOR

Brain tumors are described in detail in Chapter 15. Slowly progressive glioma such as oligodendroglioma may cause intractable epilepsy that continues over many years even in the absence of other neurologic deficit. Dysembryoplastic neuroepithelioma, ganglioglioma and hamartoma are the most frequent tumors in centers treating intractable epilepsy by surgery, especially those operating on children and adolescents.

CEREBRAL VASCULAR DISEASES

These conditions are described in Chapter 12 for adults and for children in Chapter 13. Cerebral vascular disease was the commonest cause of focal epilepsy in a general population study (Manford *et al* 1992). It has been estimated that around 3% of people who suffer a cerebral infarction develop intractable epilepsy. The risk of intractable epilepsy is higher after lobar hemorrhage (see Chapter 12). As is mentioned above, vascular disease is a prominent cause of epilepsia partialis continua. Intrauterine and perinatal cerebral infarction is the most frequent cause of the infantile hemiplegia with epilepsy syndrome.

The risk of developing intractable epilepsy in association with a cerebral arteriovenous malformation is greatest if the malformation has bled and/or if it is large (Crawford *et al* 1986; Piepgrass *et al* 1993). Cavernous angioma is a relatively common cause among patients requiring surgical treatment for epilepsy, although only relatively few patients with a cavernous angioma develop intractable epilepsy (Kondziolka *et al* 1995). As many as 25% of survivors of aneurysmal subarachnoid hemorrhage may develop epilepsy (Hauser 1999).

CNS INFECTION

The relationship between infection and intractable epilepsy is discussed in Chapter 16. Around 30–60% of survivors of subdural empyema or cerebral abscess develop epilepsy that may become intractable. This applies to around 10–15% of survivors of viral encephalitis and around 5–10% of survivors of bacterial meningitis. Cysticercosis and tuberculosis are particularly common causes of intractable focal epilepsy in some geographic areas.

BRAIN TRAUMA

The epilepsy risks arising from brain trauma are described in Chapter 14. The risk of subsequent epilepsy that may become intractable is increased by a number of factors including penetrating injury, depressed skull fracture and intracranial hemorrhage.

OTHER CONDITIONS

Other common conditions associated with an increased risk of focal epilepsy that may become intractable include chronic alcoholism (Leone *et al* 1997), Alzheimer's disease (Hesdorffer *et al* 1996) and multiple sclerosis (Engelsen and Gronning 1997; Hauser 1999).

NONEPILEPTIC DISORDERS

For most patients the key to establishing whether or not the continuing 'attacks' are likely to be epileptic lies in an accurate description of precisely what happens in the attacks both from the patient, for the aura, and from an observer who has seen many of them. Video-telemetry should be undertaken if doubt remains.

Many conditions may produce symptoms that mimic epileptic seizures. Some that may need to be considered in the differential diagnosis of epilepsy are listed in Table 2.5.

Table 2.5 Nonepileptic conditions that may mimic some aspects of epilepsy.

Nonepileptic attack disorder
Syncope
- Cardiogenic syncope (Stokes–Adams attacks and other cardiac arrhythmias, AS, MV prolapse, hypertrophic cardiac myopathy) +/– secondary anoxic seizures
- Cough syncope
- Micturition syncope
Cataplexy
Parasomnias – night terrors, sleepwalking
Dyscontrol syndrome
Vertebrobasalar ischemia
Idiopathic drop attacks
Paroxysmal dystonia, hemifacial spasm, dyskinesias
Multiple sclerosis tonic spasms
Metabolic – hypocalcemia, hypomagnesemia
Hyperekplexia
Tics
Breath-holding
Shuddering attacks

Relatively few of them, however, are relevant to the differential diagnosis of drug-resistant epilepsy defined as epileptic seizures that have continued uncontrolled over at least 2 years despite treatment with 'optimum' doses of at least three main line antiepileptic drugs. The condition that most often creates difficulty is the *nonepileptic attack disorder* especially since some patients do have both epileptic and nonepileptic seizures. The condition is discussed in Chapter 34. Very occasionally periods of neurologic dysfunction due to *cardiac arrhythmia* take the form of a complex partial seizure, in which case the correct diagnosis may be established only from the ECG trace during video-telemetry, but this is very rare. *Parasomnias*, particularly *sleepwalking* and *night terrors*, are occasionally mistaken for complex partial seizures. Both occur most often in children and arise out of stage 3–4 non-REM sleep usually during the first part of the night. 'Sleepwalking' usually consists of the child sitting up and making repetitive nonpurposeful movements but walking may happen. With a night terror there is often a scream followed by hyperkinetic automatic behavior with tachycardia, sweating and other features of autonomic over activity.

KEY POINTS

1. The term epilepsy embraces a constellation of seizures and syndromes each manifest by recurrent epileptic seizures. An epileptic seizure is defined as a transient episode of neurologic dysfunction brought about by abnormal, synchronous and excessive discharges of cerebral neurons. The diagnosis is essentially clinical but may be helped by EEG.

2. The classification of seizures is along two major axes. The first is anatomically organized into partial seizures, primary generalized seizures, including unclassified seizures, and prolonged or repetitive seizures. The second axis is defined by etiology, with idiopathic, cryptogenic and symptomatic seizures due, respectively, to familial, prenatal and postnatal factors.

3. Partial seizures (focal seizures) are defined as those in which, in general, the first clinical and EEG changes indicate initial activation of a system of neurons restricted to a part of one cerebral hemisphere. The first witnessed manifestation of an epileptic seizure, or the first internal experience, is highly important as it often localizes seizure origin. Partial seizures are divided into three categories – simple, complex and evolving to secondary generalization.

4. Simple partial seizures (isolated auras) are those in which awareness is preserved and memory for the seizure symptoms is well retained after the seizure has terminated. Complex partial seizures are those in which awareness is impaired but there is no progression to a generalized tonic–clonic convulsion. Partial seizures evolving to secondary generalization are those that commence with the features of a simple partial or a complex partial seizure but evolve to a generalized tonic–clonic convulsion.

5. Simple partial seizures have been subdivided into those with motor signs; sensory symptoms; autonomic symptoms or signs; and psychic symptoms. Those with psychic symptoms may manifest one or more of the elements of dysphasia, dysmnesia, altered affect, illusion, structured hallucination or a dreamy state.

6. Complex partial seizures often incorporate an automatism defined as a 'more or less coordinated adapted involuntary motor activity occurring during the state of clouding of consciousness … and usually followed by amnesia for the event'. An automatism usually lasts for 2–5 min but is then mostly followed by a period of postictal confusion and/or amnesia. Automatisms have been subdivided into oropharyngeal, expressions of emotion, gestural, ambulatory and verbal categories.

7. An epileptic syndrome is defined as an epileptic disorder characterized by a cluster of signs and symptoms customarily occurring together. Localization-related (focal, local, partial) epilepsy syndromes are manifest by partial seizures and are

KEY POINTS

subdivided on an etiologic basis into idiopathic, symptomatic and cryptogenic.

8. The ideopathic localization-related syndromes are conditions without detectable underlying cerebral pathology, but with a strong family history, including the benign localization-related epilepsies of childhood, autosomal dominant nocturnal frontal lobe epilepsy, familial temporal lobe epilepsy and primary reading epilepsy. The symptomatic localization-related syndromes are divided into epilepsia partialis continua, and then on an anatomic basis into temporal lobe epilepsy (medial and lateral varieties), frontal lobe epilepsy, parietal lobe epilepsy and occipital lobe epilepsy.

9. The common forms of pathology underlying the symptomatic localization-related conditions are cerebral developmental disorders, mesial temporal sclerosis, brain tumor, cerebral vascular diseases, CNS infections and brain trauma. Establishing the diagnosis, which is an essential prelude to a proper treatment plan, is dependent upon a detailed history and high-quality neuroimaging and should be possible in 85% of cases. Disorders of neuronal migration, cortical dysplasia, phakomatous disorders, glial-neuronal hamartomas and developmental tumors (gangliogliomas, dysembryoplastic neuroepitheliomas, gangliocytomas) account for a high proportion of partial seizures beginning early in the first decade of life.

10. Many conditions may produce symptoms that mimic epileptic seizures. Relatively few are relevant to the differential diagnosis of drug-resistant epilepsy defined as epileptic seizures that have continued uncontrolled over at least 2 years despite treatment with 'optimum' doses of at least three main line antiepileptic drugs. The condition that most often creates difficulty is the nonepileptic attack disorder especially since some patients do have both epileptic and nonepileptic seizures.

REFERENCES

Ardila A, Lopez MV (1988) Paroxysmal aphasias. *Epilepsia* 29: 630–634.

Asher DA, Gajdusek DC (1991) Virological studies in chronic encephalitis. In: Andermann F (ed.) *Chronic Encephalitis and Epilepsy. Rasmussen's Syndrome*, pp 147–158. Boston: Butterworth-Heinemann.

Bancaud J, Brunet-Bourgin F, Chauvel P, Halgren E (1994) Anatomical origin of *déjà vu* and vivid 'memories' in human temporal lobe epilepsy. *Brain* 117:71–90.

Bansal SK, Sawhney IMS, Chopra JS (1987) Epilepsia partialis continua in Sjogren's syndrome. *Epilepsia* 28:362–363.

Barr WB, Ashtari M, Schaul N (1997) Bilateral reduction in the hippocampal volume in adult with epilepsy and a history of febrile convulsions. *Journal of Neurology, Neurosurgery, and Psychiatry* 63:461–467.

Berkovic SF, Scheffer IE (1997) Genetics of human partial epilepsy. *Current Opinion in Neurology* 10:110–114.

Berkovic SF, Carpenter S, Evans A *et al* (1989) Myoclonus epilepsy and ragged-red fibres (MERRF). 1. A clinical, pathological, biochemical, magnetic resonance spectrographic and positron emission tomographic study. *Brain* 112:1231–1260.

Biraben A, Chauvel P (1998) Epilepsia partialis continua. In: Engel J Jr, Pedley TA (eds) *Epilepsy: A Comprehensive Textbook*, Vol 3, pp 2447–2453. Philadelphia: Lippincott-Raven Publishers.

Chadwick D (1994) Epilepsy. *Journal of Neurology, Neurosurgery and Psychiatry* 57:264–277.

Cockerell OC, Walker MC, Sander JWAS, Shorvon SD (1994) Complex partial status epilepticus: a recurrent problem. *Journal of Neurology, Neurosurgery, and Psychiatry* 57:835–837.

Cockerell OC, Rothwell J, Thompson PD, Marsden CD, Shorvon SD

(1996) Clinical and physiological features of epilepsia partialis continua. Cases ascertained in the UK. *Brain* 119: 393–407.

Commission on Classification and Terminology of the International League Against Epilepsy (1981) Proposal for revised clinical and electroencephalographic classification of epileptic seizures. *Epilepsia* 22:489–501.

Commission on Classification and Terminology of the International League Against Epilepsy (1985) Proposal and classification of epilepsies and epileptic syndromes. *Epilepsia* 26:268–278.

Commission on Classification and Terminology of the International League Against Epilepsy (1989) Proposal for revised classification of epilepsies and epileptic syndromes. *Epilepsia* 30:389–399.

Cook M, Stevens JM (1995) Imaging in epilepsy. In: Hopkins A, Shorvon S, Cascino G (eds) *Epilepsy*, pp 143–169. London: Chapman and Hall.

Crawford PM, West CR, Shaw MD, Chadwick DW (1986) Cerebral arteriovenous malformations and epilepsy: factors in the development of epilepsy. *Epilepsia* 27:270–275.

Currie S, Heathfield KWG, Henson RA, Scott DF (1971) Clinical course and prognosis of temporal lobe epilepsy. A survey of 666 patients. *Brain* 94:173–190.

Duncan JS, Sagar HJ (1987) Seizure characteristics, pathology, and outcome after temporal lobectomy. *Neurology* 37:405–409.

Engel J Jr, Pedley TA (1998) Introduction: what is epilepsy? In: Engel J Jr, Pedley TA (eds) *Epilepsy: A Comprehensive Textbook*, Vol 1, pp 1–7. Philadelphia: Lippincott-Raven Publishers.

Engelsen BA, Gronning M (1997) Epileptic seizures in patients with multiple sclerosis. Is the prognosis of epilepsy underestimated? *Seizure* 6:377–382.

Fenwick P (1985) Introduction – Regina v Sullivan: the trial and the judgment. In: Fenwick P, Fenwick E (eds) *Epilepsy and the Law – a Medical Symposium on the Current Law*, pp 3–8. London: Royal Society of Medicine.

Fried I, Spencer D, Spencer S (1998) The anatomy of epileptic auras: focal pathology and surgical outcome. *Journal of Neurosurgery* **83**:60–66.

Gil-Nagel A, Risinger MW (1997) Ictal semiology in hippocampal versus extrahippocampal temporal lobe epilepsy. *Brain* **120**:183–192.

Gloor P (1990) Experiential phenomena of temporal lobe epilepsy. Facts and hypotheses. *Brain* **113**:1673–1694.

Gobbi G, Guerrini R (1998) Childhood epilepsy with occipital spikes and other benign localisation-related epilepsies. In: Engel J Jr, Pedley TA (eds) *Epilepsy: A Comprehensive Textbook*, Vol 3, pp 2315–2326. Philadelphia: Lippincott-Raven Publishers.

Hauser WA (1999) Risk factors for epilepsy. In: Kotagal P, Luders HO (eds) *The Epilepsies: Etiologies and Prevention*, pp 1–11. San Diego: Academic Press.

Hesdorffer DC, Hauser WA, Annegers JF, Kokmen E, Rocca WA (1996) Dementia and adult-onset unprovoked seizures. *Neurology* **46**:727–730.

Hopkins A (1987) Definitions and epidemiology of epilepsy. In: Hopkins A (ed.) *Epilepsy*, pp 1–17. London: Chapman and Hall.

Juul-Jensen P, Denny-Brown D (1966) Epilepsia partialis continua. *Archives of Neurology* **15**:563–578.

Kondziolka D, Lunsford LD, Kestle JR (1995) The natural history of cerebral cavernous malformations. *Journal of Neurosurgery* **83**:820–824.

Koutroumanidis M, Koepp MJ, Richardson MP *et al* (1998) The variants of reading epilepsy. A clinical and video-EEG study of 17 patients with reading-induced seizures. *Brain* **121**:1409–1427.

Leone M, Bottacchi E, Beghi E *et al* (1997) Alcohol use is a risk factor for a first generalized tonic–clonic seizure. The AL.C.E. (Alcohol and Epilepsy) Study Group. *Neurology* **48**:614–620.

Maher J, McLachlan RS (1995) Febrile convulsions. Is seizure duration the most important predictor of temporal lobe epilepsy? *Brain* **118**:1521–1528.

Manford M, Hart YM, Sander JWAS, Shorvon SD (1992) National General Practice Study of Epilepsy (NGPSE): partial seizure patterns in a general population. *Neurology* **42**:1911–1917.

Manford M, Fish DR, Shorvon SD (1996) An analysis of clinical seizure patterns and their localizing value in frontal and temporal lobe epilepsies. *Brain* **119**:17–40.

Matthews WB (1991) Clinical aspects. Symptoms and signs. In: Matthews WB, Compston A, Allen IV, Martyn CN (eds) *McAlpine's Multiple Sclerosis*, 2nd edn, pp 43–77. Edinburgh: Churchill Livingstone.

Mouritzen Dam A (1980) Epilepsy and neuron loss in the hippocampus. *Epilepsia* **21**:617–629.

Mouritzen Dam A (1982) Hippocampal neuron loss in epilepsy and after experimental seizures. *Acta Neurologica Scandinavica* **66**:601–642.

Oldani A, Zucconi M, Asselta R *et al* (1998) Autosomal dominant nocturnal frontal lobe epilepsy. A video-polysomnographic and genetic appraisal of 40 patients and delineation of the epileptic syndrome. *Brain* **121**:205–223.

Ounsted C, Lindsay J, Norman R (1966) Biological factors in temporal lobe epilepsy. *Clinics in Developmental Medicine No. 22*. London: Spastics Society Medical Education and Information Unit in association with Heinemann Medical.

Palmini AL, Gloor P, Jones-Gotman M (1992) Pure amnestic seizures in temporal lobe epilepsy. Definition, clinical symptomatology and functional anatomical considerations. *Brain* **115**:749–769.

Penfield W, Perot P (1963) The brain's record of auditory and visual experience. A final summary and discussion. *Brain* **86**:595–696.

Peppercorn MA, Herzog AG, Dichter MA, Mayman CI (1978) Abdominal epilepsy. A cause of abdominal pain in adults. *Journal of the American Medical Association* **240**:2450–2451.

Piepgrass DG, Sundt T Jr, Ragoowansi AT, Stevens L (1993) Seizure outcome in patients with surgically treated cerebral arteriovenous malformations. *Journal of Neurosurgery* **78**:5–11.

Rooth FG (1987) *Déjà vu*. In: Gregory RL, Zangwill OL (eds) *The Oxford Companion to The Mind*, pp 182–184. Oxford: Oxford University Press.

Rosenbaum DH, Siegel M, Barr WB, Rowan AJ (1986) Epileptic aphasia. *Neurology* **36**:822–825.

Scheffer IE, Bhatia KP, Lopes-Cendes I *et al* (1995) Autosomal dominant nocturnal frontal lobe epilepsy. A distinctive clinical disorder. *Brain* **118**:61–73.

Schomer D (1993) Focal status epilepticus and epilepsia partialis continua in adults and children. *Epilepsia* **34** (Suppl 1):S29–S36.

Singh BM, Strobos RJ (1980) Epilepsia partialis continua associated with nonketotic hyperglycaemia: clinical and biochemical profile of 21 patients. *Archives of Neurology* **8**:155–160.

Sisodiya SM, Free SL, Stevens JM, Fish DR, Shorvon SD (1995) Widespread cerebral structural changes in patients with cortical dysgenesis and epilepsy. *Brain* **118**:1039–1050.

Sveinbjornsdottir S, Duncan JS (1993) Parietal and occipital lobe epilepsy: a review. *Epilepsia* **34**:493–521.

Taylor DC, Locherty M (1987) Temporal lobe epilepsy: origin and significance of simple and complex auras. *Journal of Neurology, Neurosurgery, and Psychiatry* **50**:673–681.

Williams D (1956) The structure of emotions reflected in epileptic experience. *Brain* **79**:29–67.

Williamson PD, Engel J Jr, Munari C (1998) Anatomic classification of localisation-related epilepsies. In: Engel J Jr, Pedley TA (eds) *Epilepsy: A Comprehensive Textbook*, Vol 3, pp 2405–2416. Philadelphia: Lippincott-Raven Publishers.

Woermann FG, Sisodiya SM, Free SL, Duncan JS (1998) Quantitative MRI in patients with idiopathic generalized epilepsy. Evidence of widespread cerebral structural changes. *Brain* **121**:1661–1667.

Zeman AZJ, Boniface SJ, Hodges JR (1998) Transient epileptic amnesia: a description of the clinical and neuropsychological features in 10 cases and a review of the literature. *Journal of Neurology, Neurosurgery, and Psychiatry* **64**:435–443.

Epidemiology of intractable focal epilepsy

3

PM CRAWFORD

There have been many epidemiological studies looking at epilepsy but there is a comparative paucity of information relating to the epidemiology of focal epilepsies. This is partly because of the difficulties associated with classification of seizure disorders in population-based studies. In this chapter an attempt is made to summarize the available literature to give a clearer picture of the epidemiology of the focal epilepsies. However, it is rarely possible to look specifically at the epidemiology of *intractable* focal epilepsies.

There are many problems inherent in undertaking studies to examine the epidemiology of seizure disorders. Thus, in 1993, the Commission on Epidemiology and Prognosis of the International League Against Epilepsy (ILAE) published guidelines that established the basic principles for epidemiologic studies of epilepsy (Table 3.1) and also proposed the definitions which are used in this chapter. The current ILAE classification of seizures and epileptic syndromes relies on the use of clinical and EEG criteria (Commission on Classification and Terminology of the International League Against Epilepsy 1981, 1989), but in many field surveys of epilepsy the EEG is unavailable or not practical. It has been suggested that an attempt should be made to classify seizure types into generalized, partial, and unclassifiable according to the ILAE classification (Commission on Epidemiology and Prognosis of the International League Against Epilepsy 1993). However it is clear from review of the epidemiologic literature that many secondarily generalized tonic–clonic seizures have probably been labeled incorrectly as 'generalized' rather than 'partial onset.'

Table 3.1 ILAE guidelines for epidemiological studies of epilepsy.

In field studies, the screening instrument should be adapted to the population at risk

The specificity and sensitivity of the questionnaire must be tested and validated and the methods used clearly described

The diagnosis of epilepsy should be clinical, based on a history of epileptic seizures

This diagnosis should be confirmed by a health professional with an expertise in epilepsy, using the medical history, seizure description, and neurologic examination to do so

Standardized methods should be used to obtain the information and, if available, use made of EEG records and other diagnostic tools

EPIDEMIOLOGIC STUDIES

Each epidemiologic study has slightly different methods of case ascertainment and classification of seizure disorders. The four major studies that have looked at the epidemiology of focal epilepsies are summarized below.

Rochester, Minnesota

The population from Olmsted County, Rochester, Minnesota, which is predominantly white and middle class, has been studied in great detail over the last 50 years. All medical contacts for seizures were identified over the period 1934–1984 (Hauser *et al* 1993). Cases were classified by etiology into two groups: (a) remote symptomatic, defined as individuals with unprovoked seizure(s) and a history of a CNS insult before (and temporally remote from) the first unprovoked seizure; and (b) idiopathic, defined as individuals with unprovoked seizures occurring in the absence of an historical insult demonstrated to increase greatly the risk of unprovoked seizures, but not necessarily without lesions of uncertain etiology identified on neuroimaging. The majority of patients with remote symptomatic seizures will have had a focal onset to their seizures as these included posttraumatic epilepsy and epilepsy secondary to a variety of CNS insults, such as cerebrovascular disease, CNS infections and neoplasms, neurologic deficits present at birth, and degenerative and metabolic neurologic disorders. However some patients with focal seizures will have had an idiopathic etiology in that they had no known antecedent insult predisposing towards epilepsy. In the Rochester study, seizures were classified as partial when there was clinical evidence of a partial onset, according to the ILAE classification (Commission on classification and Terminology of the International League Against Epilepsy 1981). However in some patients it was difficult to be certain whether the seizures were simple or complex partial. These were classified as 'partial seizures of uncertain type.' The interictal EEG was not used to modify the seizure classification, as it was not routinely used until the late 1940s. This may explain why so many tonic–clonic seizures in the elderly have been classified as part of a 'generalized' seizure disorder (Hauser *et al* 1993).

Department of Gironde, Bordeaux, France

This epidemiologic study by Loiseau *et al* (1990a,b) was of people resident in the department of Gironde who had their first epileptic seizure in the period between 1 March 1984 and 28 February 1985 and came to medical attention. In the 1982 census there were 1 128 164 residents. The seizures were classified into epileptic syndromes according to the ILAE classification (Commission on Classification and Terminology of the International League Against Epilepsy 1989).

National General Practice Study of Epilepsy, UK

The National General Practice Study of Epilepsy (NGPSE) was a prospective population-based cohort study of 1195 patients with suspected epileptic seizures; 594 cases proved to have newly diagnosed epilepsy. The 275 UK general practitioners who took part in the study notified the study panel whenever a new case of epilepsy was suspected in any patient on their lists during the period June 1984 to October 1987 (Sander *et al* 1990). The seizures were classified initially using a classification similar to that used by the Rochester study, but the study also used the ILAE's classification of epileptic seizures and syndromes.

Aarhus, Denmark

Since 1863, a register has been kept of all people with seizures in Greater Aarhus, Denmark, which has a population of 244 800. Retrospective data have been collected from medical records dating back to 1940. The register comprises all patients who have been admitted to hospital with an epileptic or febrile convulsion up to 1 April 1977 (Juul-Jensen and Foldsprang 1983). The World Health Organization classification of seizures was used with modifications to classify the seizure disorders (Alving 1978).

INCIDENCE OF EPILEPSY

Most studies agree that the peak incidences of epilepsy are at the extremes of life. In the first year of life, there is a high incidence particularly of generalized epilepsies and this incidence decreases during childhood. The second rise is in old age, mainly as a consequence of cerebrovascular disease (Hopkins and Shorvon 1995).

In the 50-year period of the Rochester study, 880 individuals received a new diagnosis of epilepsy. The incidence of epilepsy (both partial and generalized) for this period was 44/100 000 person-years adjusted to the population of the USA in 1970. The age-adjusted incidence of epilepsy for males (49/100 000 person-years) was significantly higher than that for women (41/100 000 person-years) and the same gender difference obtained for partial epilepsies (28 and 24/100 000 person-years, respectively) (Hauser *et al* 1993). For patients with partial epilepsies (Table 3.2), the majority had complex seizures (64%) or simple partial seizures (24%). Epilepsy with uncertain partial seizures accounted for 12% of cases. The age-adjusted incidence for complex partial epilepsy was 16/100 000 person-years, for simple partial

Table 3.2 Incidence of epilepsy per 100 000 person-years in Rochester, Minnesota, 1935–1984, age adjusted to the population of the USA in 1970. (Data from Hauser *et al* 1993)

	Male	*Female*	*Total*
Population	900 475	1 002 882	1 903 357
All epilepsy	49	41	44
All partial seizures	28	24	25
Simple	7	5	6
Complex	18	15	16
Unknown	3	3	3
Secondarily generalized	17	13	15
All generalized seizures	20	15	17

A population-based study of childhood epilepsy in northern Sweden again found a higher incidence of generalized seizures, particularly in the first year of life. The incidence of partial seizures increased with age up to the age of 10 (Table 3.3); 14% of the children with partial seizures had benign childhood epilepsy with centrotemporal spikes (incidence 19.7/100 000) (Sidenvall *et al* 1993). A Finnish study that examined the prevalence of childhood epilepsy produced similar findings. Generalized seizures and epilepsies were commoner amongst children aged 0–6 years, whilst localization-related epilepsies were commoner in those aged 6–15 years (Eriksson and Koivikko 1997). In Rochester the incidence of focal epilepsy was relatively stable throughout childhood and adult years but increased considerably in the elderly, particularly in men (Figs 3.2 and 3.3). Secondarily generalized seizures occurred in about 60% of people with partial epilepsies. The proportion of cases with secondarily generalized seizures was slightly lower among those with simple partial seizures (54%) compared with those with complex partial and uncertain partial epilepsy (61%) (Hauser *et al* 1993).

In Bordeaux 153 patients at diagnosis had symptomatic localization-related epilepsies, defined as disorders in which seizure semeiology or findings at investigation disclosed a localized origin of the seizures, giving an annual incidence rate of 13.6/100 000 (Table 3.4) (Loiseau *et al* 1990a,b). However at 1 year, this rate had risen slightly to 17.11/100 000 because some patients originally classified as having an isolated unprovoked seizure then went on to have further seizures. There were 19 patients with idiopathic partial epilepsy, giving an annual incidence rate of 1.7/100 000; 16 of these had benign childhood epilepsy with centrotemporal spikes. A total of 804 patients were considered to have had a first nonfebrile

epilepsy 6/100 000 person-years, and for unclassified partial epilepsy 5/100 000 person-years (Hauser *et al* 1993). In Rochester the age-specific incidence showed different patterns for generalized and partial epilepsies. The generalized epilepsies demonstrated the highest incidence in the first year of life. For partial epilepsies there was a relatively constant rate of about 20/100 000 throughout childhood and adult years up to the age of 65. In people above the age of 65, there was a dramatic increase in the incidence of partial epilepsy. In those over the age of 75, the incidence of partial epilepsy was 98/100 000, a five-fold increase over that observed in earlier years (Hauser *et al* 1993). When the age-specific incidences of generalized and partial epilepsies in Rochester are compared (Fig. 3.1), the incidence of generalized epilepsies was higher than that of partial epilepsies in the first 5 years of life, then similar from the age of 6 to 24. After this age the incidence of partial epilepsy was at least twice that of generalized epilepsy (Hauser *et al* 1993).

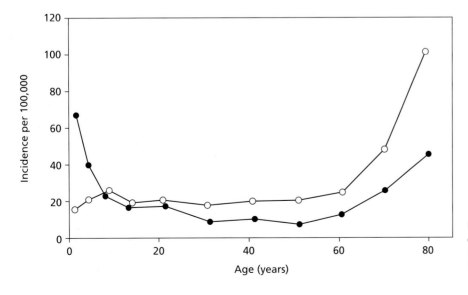

Fig. 3.1 Age-specific incidence of generalized onset (●) and partial onset (○) epilepsies in Rochester, Minnesota, 1935–1984. (Redrawn from Hauser *et al* 1993.)

Table 3.3 Annual incidence of childhood seizures per 100 000 children at risk in northern Sweden. (Data from Sidenvall *et al* 1993.)

| Type of seizure | Total | Age at initial seizure | | | |
| | | 1–12 months | 1–5 years | 6–10 years | 11–15 years |
	(n = 66)	(n = 8)	(n = 20)	(n = 22)	(n = 16)
Partial	32.0	20.8	35.0	46.4	18.0
Without secondary generalization	14.2	20.8	15.6	19.3	7.2
With secondary generalization	17.8	–	19.5	27.1	10.8
Generalized	44.0	145.6	38.9	34.8	39.7
Unclassifiable	2.4		3.9	3.9	
Total	78.5	166.4	77.8	85.1	57.7

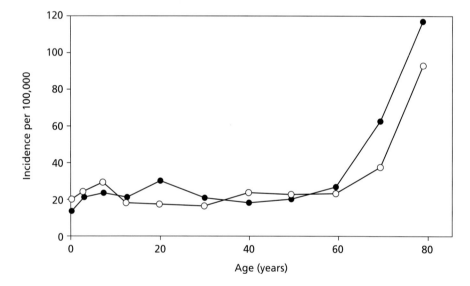

Fig. 3.2 Age- and gender-specific incidence of partial epilepsy in Rochester, Minnesota, 1935–1984. ●, Male; ○, female. (Redrawn from Hauser *et al* 1993.)

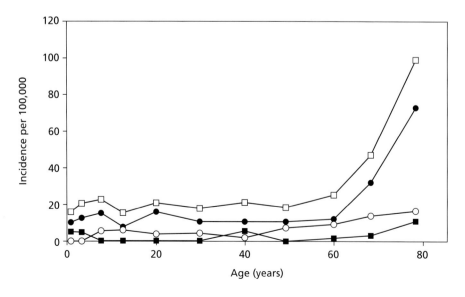

Fig. 3.3 Age-specific incidence of partial epilepsy by subcategory in Rochester, Minnesota, 1935–1984. ●, Complex partial; ○, simple partial; ■, partial unclassified; □, total. (Redrawn from Hauser *et al* 1993.)

Table 3.4 Bordeaux study: patients classified according to the ILAE classification of epileptic syndromes. (Data from Loiseau et al 1990a.)

Classification	Incidence rates at 1 year
Localization-related epilepsies	
Idiopathic (with age-related onset)	1.7/100 000
Symptomatic	17.1/100 000
Cryptogenic	0
Generalized epilepsies and syndromes	7.8/100 000
Epilepsies undetermined whether focal or generalized	2.9/100 000
Acute symptomatic (situation-related) epilepsy	25.4/100 000

seizure during the recording period and of these 284 (35%) were aged 60 or older. The annual incidence rate for partial seizures was 33.2/100 000 in those aged 60 years or above (Table 3.5). Incidence rates increased with age and were higher in men (56.5/100 000 vs. 17.3/100 000).

A retrospective study in Frederiksberg, Denmark examined the incidence of epileptic seizures in people above the age of 60 who were admitted to hospital over a 5-year period (Luhdorf et al 1986). The mean annual incidence rate at 60 years or older was 104/100 000. However if only definite cases of epilepsy were considered, the annual incidence rate was 77/100 000 at age 60 or over. A similar annual overall incidence of seizures (117/100 000) was found in people over the age of 60 in a primary care study in the UK. The incidence of epilepsy increased from 76/100 000 in those aged 60–69 to 159/100 000 in those aged 80 and above (Tallis et al 1991).

Studies from the developing world have shown a high incidence of epilepsy. A random cluster sample survey from Tanzania reported an annual incidence of 73.3/100 000, 32% of whom had partial seizures (Rwiza et al 1992). A door-to-door survey in rural central Ethiopia found a lower annual incidence of 64/100 000, 20% of whom had partial seizures (Tekle-Haimanot et al 1997). A survey from Chile found a very high annual incidence of 113/100 000, 54% of whom had partial seizures (Levados et al 1992).

Table 3.5 Age-specific annual incidence rate of epileptic syndromes in elderly patients per 100 000 population in Bordeaux. (Data from Loiseau et al 1990b.)

Age	Symptomatic localization-related epilepsies	Undertermined epilepsies	Isolated seizures
60–69	35.5	1.0	14.6
70–79	37.3	0	18.0
80+	20.3	2.2	15.8

CUMULATIVE INCIDENCE

Using the annual rates of new seizure cases per 1000 of the population it is possible to make an estimate of the number of people who are likely to have a seizure of some sort during their lifetime (Crombie et al 1960).

In a longitudinal study of a national population sample in the UK of all children born in one week in 1958, the cumulative incidence of epilepsy of all types was 0.41% by age of 11 (64 cases in 15 496 children), 0.6% by the age of 16, and 0.84% by the age of 23 (Ross et al 1980; Kurtz et al 1998). Of these patients 69% were classified as having a localization-related epilepsy (Kurtz et al 1998). A similar cumulative incidence of 0.43% by the age of 10 was found by the 1970 cohort of the UK Child Health and Education Study, 30% of whom had partial seizures (Verity et al 1992).

In the Rochester study, the slope of the cumulative incidence curve increases sharply with age (Fig. 3.4), and at the older ages the risk of a seizure is greater for men than women. The cumulative incidence of epilepsy for men was 3.4% and 2.8% for women by the age of 74. The cumulative incidence by the age of 75 was 1.8% for partial epilepsies compared with 1.3% for generalized epilepsies (Hauser et al 1993).

A general practice-based study in the UK of 6000 patients supported these high cumulative incidence figures, with epilepsy affecting 1.67% of the population at one time. As many of the population were children or young adults, the lifetime incidence will be even higher than this. Of these patients 35% had partial epilepsies (Hopkins and Shorvon 1995; Goodridge and Shorvon 1983a,b).

In the Danish Aarhus study, the cumulative incidence was 2.44% for a person having some form of epileptic seizure some time during their lives. If febrile seizures are excluded the cumulative incidence falls to 2.033%, and to 1.274% if only epilepsy is considered. The cumulative incidence for the different types of focal seizures was 88/100 000 for simple partial seizures (Fig. 3.5), 239/100 000 for complex partial seizures (Fig. 3.6) and 457/100 000 for secondarily generalized seizures (Fig. 3.7) (Juul-Jensen and Foldsprang 1983).

PREVALENCE OF PARTIAL SEIZURES

The prevalence of epilepsy at different ages is the balance between age of onset and duration of epilepsy before remission or death. Studies looking at the prevalence of different seizure types use many different methods of case ascertainment and definitions of seizure

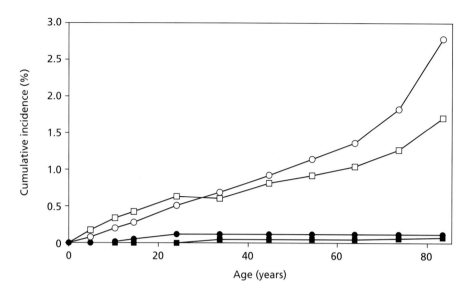

Fig. 3.4 Cumulative incidence by seizure type (%) in Rochester, Minnesota, 1935–1984. ○, Partial epilepsy; □, all generalized onset epilepsy; ●, absence; ■, myoclonic. (Redrawn from Hauser *et al* 1993.)

activity, making comparisons difficult. The ILAE classifications of seizure disorders and epileptic syndromes, which are designed to take advantage of modern methods of investigation, are difficult to use in epidemiological studies particularly in the developing world.

For the accurate classification of both seizure type and epileptic syndrome, EEG and imaging studies are required as well as a detailed clinical appraisal. Few epidemiologic studies have attempted all this. The population characteristics will determine the prevalence of the different seizure types and epilepsy syndromes. In the developing world there is a higher incidence of bacterial and parasitic intracranial infections as well as poorer obstetric care, leading to a higher prevalence of symptomatic partial seizure disorders (Table 3.6).

A Finnish epidemiologic study reported a prevalence rate of epilepsy of 7.01/1000 in people over the age of 15. The seizure type was classifiable in 82.5%. Of the 56% who had partial seizures, 25.5% had secondarily generalized tonic–clonic seizures, 23% complex partial seizures, and 7.5% simple partial seizures. A simple partial onset was seen in 56% of those with complex partial seizures and 92% of those with secondarily generalized tonic–clonic seizures (Table 3.7) (Keranen *et al* 1988). The prevalence rate for intractable focal epilepsy (defined as seizures at least once a month) was 0.78/1000 (Keranen and Riekkinen

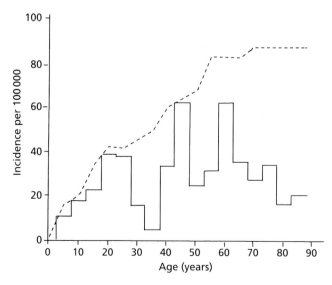

Fig. 3.5 Cumulative incidence (broken line) and prevalence (solid line) of simple partial epilepsy in Aarhus, Denmark. (From Juul-Jensen and Foldsprang 1983.)

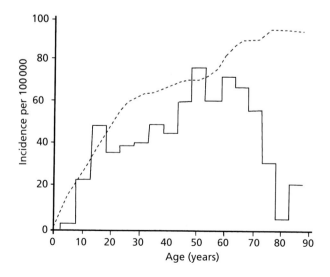

Fig. 3.6 Cumulative incidence (broken line) and prevalence (solid line) of complex partial epilepsy in Aarhus, Denmark. (From Juul-Jensen and Foldsprang 1983.)

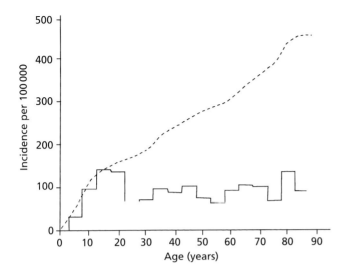

Fig. 3.7 Cumulative incidence (broken line) and prevalence (solid line) of partial epilepsy with secondary generalization in Aarhus, Denmark. (From Juul-Jensen and Foldsprang 1983.)

amongst patients with chronic epilepsy or, less likely, that epilepsy in some patients may become less severe with advancing age. Keranen and Riekkinen (1988) also confirmed earlier reports that patients with intractable focal epilepsies are more commonly male and have a high frequency of associated neurologic deficits and learning difficulties (Rodin 1968).

Another Finnish prevalence study that examined childhood seizure disorders found a total point prevalence rate of 3.94/1000 in children aged 0–15 years with a prevalence rate of 1.68/1000 for partial seizure disorders (Table 3.8); 41% had localization-related epilepsies (Table 3.9) (Eriksson and Koivikko 1997). A population-based survey of childhood epilepsy in children under the age of 10 in Okayama Prefecture, Japan was able to classify the seizure disorders in 79% of children with epilepsy, 56% having localization-related epilepsies (Oka *et al* 1995).

In the prospective population-based study of 594 cases of newly diagnosed epilepsy (NGPSE), it was only possible to place 33.6% into diagnostic ILAE epilepsy categories (Table 3.10). Overall, 31% of patients had localization-related epilepsies but in only 24% of all patients could the onset of seizure activity be localized to a single ILAE proposed site of origin (Table 3.11), and of these best clinically

1988). The age-adjusted rate for men (0.93/1000) was significantly higher than that for women (0.64/1000). The age-related prevalence rates for intractable focal epilepsy peaked during the fourth decade of life and declined in older age groups (Figs 3.8 and 3.9) (Keranen and Riekkinen 1988). This may be due to an increased mortality

Table 3.6 Prevalence of epilepsy in different countries.

Reference	Method	Country	Population studied	Prevalence	Active epilepsy	Partial seizures (%)
Mendizabal and Salguero (1996)	Cross-section	Rural Guatemala	2111	8.5/1000	5.8/1000	CPS, 37.5 SPS, 6.2
Muir *et al* (1996)	General practice patients on treatment	UK	145 609	7.2/1000		39
Levados *et al* (1992)		Chile	17 694	17.7/1000		54.1
Cornaggia *et al* (1990)	Males on military service	Italy	54 520	4.7/1000		29
Bharucha *et al* (1988)	House to house	India	14 010	4.7/1000	3.6/1000	54.5
Aziz *et al* (1994)	House to house	Pakistan	24 130	Age-specific: 9.99/1000 Urban: 7.4/1000 Rural: 14.8/1000		SPS, 5 CPS, 6 SGS, 18
Rwiza *et al* (1992)	Random cluster sample survey	Tanzania	18 000 from 11 villages	Varied between 5.1/1000 and 37.1/1000 in a village		31.9

CPS, complex partial seizures; SGS, secondarily generalized seizures; SPS, simple partial seizures.

Table 3.7 Percentage distribution of seizure types in community studies.

	Classification in children (age 0–15 years)[a]	Dominant prevalent seizure type (age > 15 years)[b]	Classification at 6 months (NGPSE) (all ages)[c]
Classifiable	89	82.5	91
Generalized seizures	44	26.5	39
Partial seizures	45	56.0	52
Simple	10	7.5	3
Complex	23	23.0	11
Partial evolving to secondarily generalized	9	25.5	27
Mixed partial	–	–	12

[a] Data from Eriksson and Koivikko (1997).
[b] Data from Keranen et al (1988).
[c] Data from Hopkins and Shorvon (1995).

Table 3.8 Percentage distribution of childhood seizures in different age groups in a prevalence study in Finland. (Data from Eriksson and Koivikko 1997.)

Seizure classification	Prevalence rate	Age (years)			Total
		0–5	6–10	11–15	
All partial seizures	1.68/1000	21	45	50	45
Simple partial		4	17	7	10
Complex partial		12	17	33	23
Secondarily generalized		4	11	10	9
Generalized seizures	1.73/1000	55	43	39	44
Mixed	0.37/1000	18	7	7	9
Unclassified	0.17/1000	6	5	3	4

localized cases 14% had discordant imaging or EEG (Manford *et al* 1992a,b). In the NGPSE (see Table 3.7) 184 patients exhibited clinical evidence of partial seizures, 56 of whom had secondarily generalized tonic–clonic seizures; 38

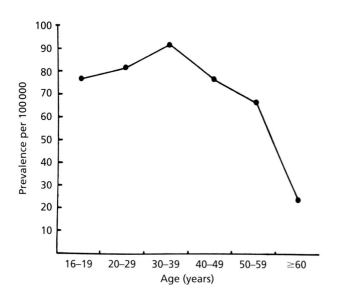

Fig. 3.8 Age-specific prevalence rates of adult patients with severe complex partial seizures, Finland. (From Keranen and Riekkinen 1988.)

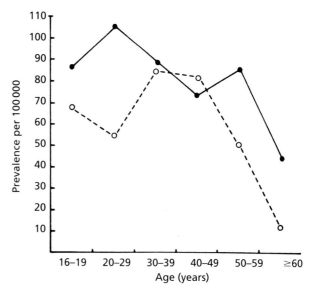

Fig. 3.9 Age-specific prevalence rates of severe complex partial seizures for adult men (●) and women (○), Finland. (From Keranen and Riekkinen 1988.)

Table 3.9 Percentage distribution of childhood epilepsies and epileptic syndromes in a prevalence study in Finland. (Data from Eriksson and Koivikko 1997.)

Type of epilepsy	Age (years)			Total
	0–5	*6–10*	*11–15*	
Localization-related epilepsies/syndromes	21	45	47	41
Idiopathic	–	10	11	8
Symptomatic	8	10	13	11
Cryptogenic	13	25	24	22
Generalized epilepsies/syndromes	66	45	43	48

Table 3.10 NGPSE study: patients classified according to the ILAE classification of epileptic syndromes. (Data from Manford et al 1992a.)

Classification	No. of cases (%)
Localization-related epilepsies	252 (31)
Idiopathic (with age-related onset)	7 (0.9)
Symptomatic	96 (11.8)
Cryptogenic	146 (17.9)
Generalized epilepsies and syndromes	66 (8.1)
Epilepsies undetermined whether focal or generalized	190 (23.3)
Special syndromes	306 (37.6)

Table 3.11 NGPSE study: proposed sites of partial seizure onset of localization-related epilepsies. (Data from Manford et al 1992a.)

Site of onset	No.
Localized to a single site	50
Motor cortex	31
Supplementary motor area	6
Lateral temporal	3
Parietal	10
Overlapping neighboring regions	110
Frontal	30
Central	21
Frontotemporal	9
Temporal	40
Posterior cortex	10
Lateralized only	3
Unlocalized	92

Table 3.12 Classification of partial seizures in 1505 patients with epilepsy from Aarhus, Denmark. (Data from Juul-Jensen and Foldsprang 1983.)

	Male	*Female*	*Total*
Partial seizures	279	281	560 (37.2%)
Simple partial	42	28	70 (4.7%)
Complex partial	123	146	269 (17.9%)
With secondary generalization	114	103	217 (14.4%)
Benign rolandic	0	4	4 (0.2%)

had simple partial seizures, of whom five also had complex partial seizures and 16 secondarily generalized seizures; 146 patients had complex partial seizures, of whom 38 also had secondarily generalized seizures (Manford *et al* 1992b). In the study from Aarhus, 37% of patients had partial seizures and 14% of these seizures became secondarily generalized (Table 3.12) (Juul-Jensen and Foldsprang 1983).

The prevalence and incidence of epilepsy and partial seizure disorders does appear to vary from country to country (see Table 3.6). In part this is due to different methods of case ascertainment, although rates do appear to be substantially higher in the developing world. This is partly due to an increased incidence of birth and head trauma, and parasitic and other intracranial infections, leading to an increased prevalence of partial seizures in particular (Hopkins and Shorvon 1995). In the USA, one study that examined the risk of epilepsy in childhood found an increased risk of epilepsy in black children compared with white children and an excess incidence in low socioeconomic areas (Shamansky and Glaser 1979). However another study in Colombia failed to show a difference in the prevalence of epilepsy in different social classes (Gomez *et al* 1978).

Most studies have shown a slight excess of males with epilepsy. Studies of seizures in early childhood have shown a differential effect of seizures on the brains of infant boys and girls at different maturational ages (Hopkins and Shorvon 1995). However this excess of males may in part be accounted for by their different occupational exposures to epileptogenic insults, such as head trauma and alcohol. Surprisingly a study from Colombia showed a greater prevalence in females (Gomez *et al* 1978).

ETIOLOGY

The introduction of new investigative techniques such as magnetic resonance imaging (MRI) has led to a much greater understanding of the etiology of partial seizure disorders. However MRI is a relatively recent technique and postdates the majority of epidemiologic studies; even in countries such as the UK it is not always available for all patients developing partial seizure disorders.

In the Rochester study, 64% of all partial cases were classified as idiopathic. Idiopathic cases accounted for a higher proportion of cases in childhood than at older ages. The etiology of the seizure disorder tends to influence the prognosis (Hauser *et al* 1993). Among the children with a presumed etiology, most cases of epilepsy were associated with neurologic deficits present at birth (learning difficulties and/or cerebral palsy). In those with an identified etiology in the 15–34 age group, CNS tumors, CNS infections, neurologic deficits from birth, and cerebral trauma were identified as antecedents with equal frequency. In those aged 35–64 with a presumed cause, cerebrovascular lesions preceded the onset of epilepsy in 15% of patients diagnosed, and were the presumed cause in 35% with an identified etiology. About 10% of patients had epilepsy as a result of a brain tumor; in another 10% epilepsy was secondary to a head injury (Hauser *et al* 1993). In the oldest age group (above 65 years of age), the majority of cases were associated with a remote symptomatic etiology. The most frequently identified antecedent was cerebrovascular disease, which accounted for 28% of all cases in this age group and two-thirds of those with presumed etiology. About 20% of cases with presumed etiology were associated with degenerative CNS diseases (Hauser *et al* 1993).

In the Bordeaux study 153 patients had symptomatic localization-related epilepsies. An etiologic factor could be identified in 125 patients: cerebrovascular disease (51), perinatal anoxia (12), head trauma (8), CNS infection (4), after intracranial surgery (3), brain tumor (39), arteriovenous malformation (4) and arachnoid cyst (4). The other 28 patients had experienced partial seizures but there were no apparent etiologic factors (Loiseau *et al* 1990a). A cause could be identified in 68 of the 284 Bordeaux patients with a first seizure at age 60 or above (Table 3.13). Cerebrovascular disease was again the most frequently recognized etiologic factor and was found in 36.6% of patients with spontaneous seizures and in 53.9% of patients with established epilepsy. The sex-specific incidence was higher in men. Of the 93 patients who had seizures within the acute phase of a stroke 62 (66.7%) died, 13 within the first week, 17 within the first month, and 22 within the first year after stroke. A total of 41 patients had late vascular epilepsy, 30 of whom had ischemic lesions, three had had a previous intracerebral hematoma, while the nature of the lesion was not documented in the remaining eight patients. A brain tumor was found in 22.3% of these elderly patients with spontaneous seizures, 10 patients having a glioblastoma and 11 having metastases. The incidence of brain tumors was four times higher in men (Loiseau *et al* 1990b).

In the NGPSE study, of the 252 patients with localization-related epilepsy, a cause was identified in 32% (Table 3.14). In 16 patients the epilepsy was secondary to cerebrovascular disease, 11 had a primary brain tumor, and five had metastases. Birth trauma and congenital disease accounted for another six cases and five patients developed posttraumatic epilepsy (Manford *et al* 1992a,b).

However none of these studies take account of the recent advances in imaging for epilepsy. Developmental anomalies were once thought to be an unusual cause of epilepsy but are now recognized as an important determinant of seizures, especially seizure disorders that are refractory to antiepileptic therapy (Schachter 1995). Their incidence amongst people with focal epilepsies is not known. The older literature is based on pathologic studies from either patients who had died or who had surgery for epilepsy. Various surgical studies have reported neurodevelopmental lesions in lobectomy specimens in 7–21% of patients (Green 1991) and in 42% of temporal neocortex specimens in patients with intractable epilepsy (Hardiman *et al* 1988). In a more recent study, 25% of children undergoing surgery for partial epilepsy had MRI and pathologic findings indicative of cortical dysplasia or agyria/pachygyria (Kuzniecky *et al* 1993).

Developmental cerebral anomalies may be diffuse or localized and there is a wide spectrum of cognitive involvement, MRI abnormalities, and seizure disorders. The MRI findings for a group of 146 patients with intractable focal epilepsy are summarized in Table 3.15 (Cook and Stevens

Table 3.13 Causes of symptomatic localization-related epilepsies in 284 patients with a first seizure at age 60 or above in Bordeaux. (Data from Loiseau *et al* 1990b.)

Etiology	No. of cases (%)	Incidence rate		
		Men	Women	Total
Vascular	41 (55.4)	29.9	10.5	18.4
Tumor	25 (33.8)	19.9	5.3	11.2
Traumatic	2 (2.7)	1.1	0.8	0.9
Unknown	6 (8.1)	5.5	0.8	2.7

Table 3.14 Etiologic factors in 51 patients with localization-related epilepsies (NGPSE). (Data from Manford *et al* 1992a.)

	Definitely significant	Probably significant
Congenital disease	5	0
Birth trauma	1	0
Meningitis	0	1
Cerebral infarction	15	1
Glioma	10	0
Meningioma	1	0
Metastasis	4	1
Space-occupying lesion, uncertain type	3	0
Acute trauma	2	0
Remote trauma	0	3
Encephalitis	1	1
Other	1	1

Table 3.15 Imaging abnormalities in 146 patients with focal epilepsy (four patients had two lesions). (Data from Cook and Stevens 1995.)

Pathology	
Hippocampal atrophy	34%
Dysembryoplastic neuroepithelioma	8%
Glioma	8%
Focal cortical dysplasia	14%
Heterotopia	2%
Traumatic	3%
Vascular malformation	10%
Cystic lesion	3%
White matter lesion with overlying focal cortical atrophy	3%
Focal lesion, uncertain nature	1%
Epidermoid	1%
Tuberous sclerosis	1%
No lesion demonstrated	15%

1995). These abnormalities were detected using volumetric imaging with hippocampal volume studies and reformatting. Over 90% had a previous normal CT scan, and nearly 25% a previous MRI scan that had been regarded as normal (Cook and Stevens 1995).

PROGNOSIS

Epidemiologic data clearly show that for most patients who develop epileptic seizures the prognosis is excellent for eventual seizure control in that the prevalence rate for active epilepsy is fairly consistent at about 0.6% while the lifetime prevalence is between 2 and 5% (Sander 1993). Therefore about 70–80% of the people developing epilepsy

will eventually achieve remission, whilst 20–30% will continue to have recurrent seizures despite antiepileptic therapy. The most important factor in the prognosis is the underlying etiology. In newly diagnosed patients, a less favorable outcome is seen in patients with simple or complex partial seizures or multiple seizure types, associated neurologic deficits, and behavioral or psychiatric disturbances. The prognosis for people developing partial seizure disorders, especially those with only simple or complex partial seizure disorders, is poorer than for generalized epilepsy. Only a small percentage of these patients with intractable focal epilepsy can be rendered seizure-free by surgery or the use of new antiepileptic drugs (Sander 1993).

Remission of a seizure disorder is defined as a period of freedom from seizures, usually for at least 2 years. Retrospective population-based studies have shown that between 65 and 75% of patients achieve at least a 2-year remission (Annegers *et al* 1979; Goodridge and Shorvon 1983b). A Finnish prevalence study of childhood seizure disorders looked at the prognosis of localization-related epilepsies (Table 3.16). The prognosis was defined as good if the child was seizure-free for 1–2 years; partial control was defined as 1–11 seizures per year and poor control as one or more seizures per month (Eriksson and Koivikko 1997). Fewer than half achieved the 'good' category.

In the prospective NGPSE, of 292 patients with partial seizures 39% achieved a 3-year remission by 3 years and 80% and 63% achieved a 3-year and 5-year remission respectively by 9 years after onset. Within the group with remote symptomatic seizures, the remission rate differed substantially between patients with epilepsy secondary to tumors (43% remission rate at 9 years) compared to those with cerebrovascular disease (78% remission rate at 9 years) (Cockerell *et al* 1995). Only 11% of 76 patients with simple or complex partial seizures and 40% of 151 patients with secondarily generalized tonic–clonic seizures were seizure-free at 1 year after the onset of treatment; by 3 years control had deteriorated, with 6% and 28% respectively seizure-free. The pattern and frequency of seizures did not show any difference between the different sites of onset of seizure activity. Frequent seizures were seen in only 7% of patients with partial seizures and 28% only had rare seizures. Of those with frequent seizures, the seizure disorder was secondary to a CNS tumor in four, cerebrovascular disease in two and of unknown etiology in the remaining five patients (Cockerell *et al* 1995).

A general practice population-based study in the UK examined the number and pattern of seizures from the onset of epilepsy to the time of the survey (Table 3.17). Overall, by 15 years after the onset of epilepsy 50% had entered a remission of 4 years or more. Of the 21

Table 3.16 Seizure control in localization-related epilepsies in a Finnish study of the prevalence of childhood epilepsies. (Data from Eriksson and Koivikko 1997).

Type of epilepsy	Percentage of patients	Percentage control of seizure disorder		
		Poor	Partial	Good
All localization-related epilepsies	40	3	9	27
Benign epilepsy	7	–	–	7
Localization-related, symptomatic	10	1	3	6
Localization-related, cryptogenic	23	2	6	14

patients who had partial seizures, three had had a single seizure and 11 repeated seizures followed by remission to the date of the study (burst pattern); another five patients had continuous and repeated seizures, whilst the remaining two patients had repeated seizures with at least one period of remission (intermittent pattern) (Goodridge and Shorvon 1983b). Another UK study, which prospectively randomized adults and children with newly diagnosed epilepsy to treatment with either carbamazepine, phenytoin, or sodium valproate, found that about 40% of patients remained seizure-free over the first 12 months of therapy and at 3 years 75% had achieved a 1-year remission. The prognosis was better for tonic–clonic seizures than partial seizures. There were no differences in efficacy between the drugs (DeSilva *et al* 1989; Heller *et al* 1995).

The Italian Collaborative Group for the Study of Epilepsy examined newly referred patients with partial seizures (78) and found that 44% of patients with partial seizures relapsed by 1 year. However relapse only occurred in 40% of those whose initial treatment after diagnosis was the study drug.

Table 3.17 Type, number, and pattern of seizures from onset of epilepsy to time of survey in 122 patients. (Data from Goodridge and Shorvon 1983b.)

	Partial epilepsies	Generalized epilepsies
No. of seizures		
1	3	15
2–10	10	43
11–49	4	7
50–99	1	0
> 100	5	6
Pattern		
Single	3	13
Burst	11	38
Continuous	5	9
Intermittent	2	10

The prognosis was worse for patients who developed epilepsy before the age of 10, had a high number of seizures, had a long duration of epilepsy before treatment was started, and had etiologic factors and/or EEG abnormalities (Beghi and Tognoni 1988).

In the Aarhus study, 269 (17.9%) patients had complex partial seizures; however only 28% were seizure-free for 2 years or more whilst 27% had severe epilepsy (Juul-Jensen and Foldsprang 1983). Secondarily generalized tonic–clonic seizures occurred in 217 (14.4%) patients and here the prognosis was better in that 49% were seizure-free and only 12% had severe epilepsy (Table 3.18) (Juul-Jensen and Foldsprang 1983).

In the USA, two prospective studies of 1102 adults with newly diagnosed localization-related epilepsy investigated the prognosis for total seizure control (Mattson *et al* 1996). At 1 year, 70% and 61% of patients with secondarily generalized tonic–clonic seizures had no further tonic–clonic seizures on treatment and 55% and 48% entered a 1-year remission. Of those with complex partial seizures 23% and 26% had no further seizures. Those patients with both complex partial and secondarily generalized tonic–clonic seizures had an intermediary prognosis, with 32% and 25% being seizure-free at 1 year. The authors concluded that the best prognosis for total control at 1 year was for those with secondarily generalized tonic–clonic seizures and the poorest prognosis was for those with only complex partial seizures ($P < 0.0001$) (Figs 3.10–3.12). Most seizure recurrences occurred in the first year after starting treatment, with 50% occurring within 3 months. Of those who developed a recurrence of their complex partial seizures, virtually all did this within the first year. In 5% of patients with complex partial seizures and 10% of those with secondarily generalized tonic–clonic seizures a new seizure type developed within the first year of follow-up. However the prognosis for short-term control at any point in time was considerably better. Many patients with partial seizures entered a period

Table 3.18 Prognosis in patients with partial epilepsies in Aarhus, Denmark. (Data from Juul-Jensen and Foldsprang 1983.)

	Simple partial (%)	Complex partial (%)	Tonic–clonic (%)
Seizure-free	43	28	49
Mild/moderate	33	38	24
Severe	11	27	12
Unassessable	13	7	15

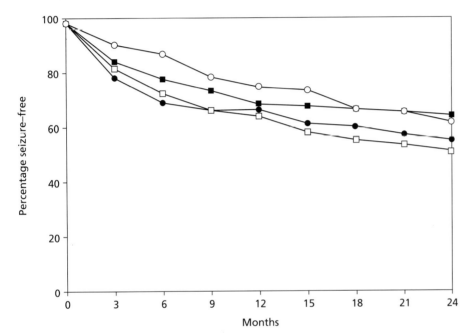

Fig. 3.10 Cumulative percentage remaining free of secondarily generalized tonic–clonic seizures in two studies (VA-118, VA-264). ○, Secondarily generalized tonic–clonic seizures, study VA-118; ●, multiple types of partial seizures, study VA-118; □, secondarily generalized tonic–clonic seizures, study VA-264; ■, multiple types of partial seizures, multiple types of partial seizures, study VA-264. (Redrawn from Mattson *et al* 1996.)

of remission despite having one or more seizures during their first year of therapy. One year after initiating therapy, 60–65% of patients were not having seizures (Mattson *et al* 1988, 1990, 1996).

All studies therefore suggest that a considerable proportion of those with partial seizures do not achieve complete seizure control with currently available antiepileptic drugs. Patients with simple or complex partial seizures have a greater risk of developing intractable focal seizures than those with other seizure disorders. The etiology, failure to respond to the initial antiepileptic drug, and a history of seizures for more than 1 year before beginning therapy increase the likelihood of intractable seizures.

CONCLUSIONS

The incidence and prevalence of focal seizure disorders varies from country to country and increases with increasing age. The incidence of focal seizure disorders is relatively stable throughout childhood and in early adult life but increases fivefold with increasing age. The cumulative incidence of partial seizures increases sharply in old age and reaches at least 1.8% by the age of 75. The prevalence of partial seizures is greater in the developing world. About half the patients reported in prevalence studies have focal seizure disorders. The prevalence of intractable focal seizures is reported in a Finnish study as being 0.78/1000. The age-related prevalence rates for intractable focal epilepsy appear to peak in the fourth decade of life and decline in older age groups. This may in part be due to an increased mortality from sudden unexpected death in epilepsy (SUDEP) amongst patients with intractable secondarily generalized seizures (Keranen and Riekkinen 1988).

Etiology, failure to respond to an initial antiepileptic drug, and a history of seizures for more than 1 year before beginning therapy increase the likelihood of developing intractable focal epilepsy. Seizures secondary to cerebrovascular disease have a better outlook for remission compared with those secondary to cerebral tumors or neurologic deficits present at birth. The best prognosis is for those

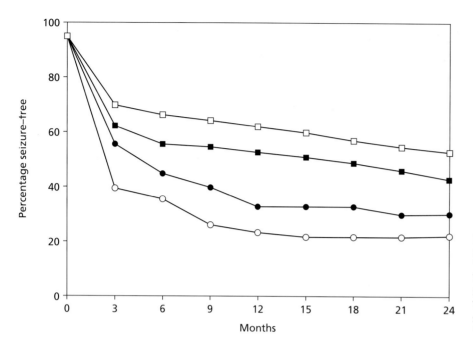

Fig. 3.11 Cumulative percentage remaining free of complex partial seizures in two studies (VA-118, VA-264). ○, Complex partial seizures, study VA-118; □, multiple types of partial seizures, study VA-118; ●, complex partial seizures, study VA-264; ■, multiple types of partial seizures, study VA-264. (Redrawn from Mattson et al 1996.)

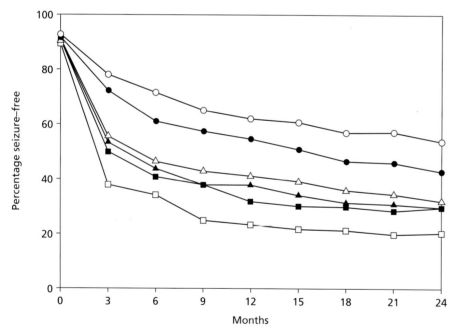

Fig. 3.12 Cumulative percentage remaining free of secondarily generalized tonic–clonic seizures and complex partial seizures in two studies (VA-118, VA-264). ○, Secondarily generalized tonic–clonic seizures, study VA-118; □, complex partial seizures, study VA-118; △, multiple types of partial seizures, study VA-118; ●, secondarily generalized tonic–clonic seizures, study VA-264; ■, complex partial seizures, study VA-264; ▲, multiple types of partial seizures, study VA-264. (Redrawn from Mattson et al 1996.)

developing secondarily generalized tonic–clonic seizures and the poorest for those with complex partial seizures. Most seizure recurrences occur within the first year after starting treatment. There is also an increased mortality amongst patients with intractable focal seizures, related both to the underlying etiology of the seizure disorder and SUDEP. People with intractable secondarily generalized seizures are at greatly increased risk from SUDEP.

KEY POINTS

1. The incidence of focal seizure disorders is around 20/100 000 per year, made up of 64% complex partial seizures and 24% simple partial seizures. The incidence remains approximately the same from childhood to age 65 years but then rises with increasing age.

2. The prevalence of focal seizure disorders is around 3.92/1000, with complex partial seizures in 41% and secondarily generalized tonic–clonic seizures in 46%.

3. The prevalence of intractable focal seizure disorders with at least one seizure per month is around 0.78/1000. The rate is higher for men than for women and it peaks at ages 30–40 and then declines, perhaps because of increased mortality amongst people with chronic intractable epilepsy.

4. The site of onset of focal seizures is most often the temporal lobe; the next most common sites are the frontal lobe and the rolandic area.

5. The pathology underlying focal epilepsy varies according to patient age: 'benign' CNS tumor, CNS infection, trauma (birth and after birth), and CNS developmental abnormalities are common causes amongst those aged < 35 years; tumor, cerebrovascular disease, and degenerative CNS disease are common causes amongst the elderly.

6 At least 20% of people who develop a partial seizure disorder will not achieve a 3-year remission within 9 years of onset.

REFERENCES

Alving J (1978) Classification of the epilepsies. *Acta Neurologica Scandinavica* **58**:205–212.

Annegers JF, Hauser WA, Elveback LR (1979) Remission of seizures and relapse in patients with epilepsy. *Epilepsia* **20**:729–737.

Aziz H, Ali SM, Frances P *et al* (1994) Epilepsy in Pakistan: a population based epidemiologic study. *Epilepsia* **35**:950–958.

Beghi E, Tognoni G (1988) Prognosis of epilepsy in newly referred patients: a multicentre prospective study. *Epilepsia* **29**:236–243.

Bharucha NE, Bharucha EP, Bharucha AE *et al* (1988) Prevalence of epilepsy in the Parsi community of Bombay. *Epilepsia* **29**:111–115.

Cockerell OC, Johnson A, Sander JWAS *et al* (1995) Remission of epilepsy: results from the National General Practice Study of Epilepsy. *Lancet* **346**:140–144.

Commission on Classification and Terminology of the International League Against Epilepsy (1981) Proposal for the revised clinical and electroencephalographic classification of epileptic syndromes. *Epilepsia* **22**:489–501.

Commission on Classification and Terminology of the International League Against Epilepsy (1989) Proposal for the revised classification of epilepsies and epileptic syndromes. *Epilepsia* **30**:389–399.

Commission on Epidemiology and Prognosis of the International League Against Epilepsy (1993) Guidelines for epidemiologic studies on epilepsy. *Epilepsia* **34**:592–596.

Cook M, Stevens JM (1995) Imaging in epilepsy. In: Hopkins A, Shorvon S, Cascino G (eds) *Epilepsy*, 2nd edn, pp 143–170. London: Chapman & Hall Medical.

Cornaggia CM, Canevini MP, Christe W *et al* (1990) Epidemiologic survey of epilepsy among army draftees in Lombardy, Italy. *Epilepsia* **31**:27–32.

Crombie DL, Cross KW, Fry J *et al* (1960) A survey of the epilepsies in general practice: a report by the research committee of the College of General Practitioners. *British Medical Journal* **2**:416–422.

DeSilva M, McGowan M, Neville BR *et al* (1989) A prospective randomised comparative monotherapy clinical trial in childhood epilepsy. In: Chadwick D (ed) *Proceedings of the Fourth International Symposium on Sodium Valproate and Epilepsy*, pp 81–86. London: Royal Society of Medicine Services.

Eriksson KJ, Koivikko MJ (1997) Prevalence, classification and severity of epilepsy and epileptic syndromes in children. *Epilepsia* **38**:1275–1282.

Gomez JG, Arciniegas E, Torres J (1978) Prevalence of epilepsy in Bogota, Columbia. *Neurology* **28**:90–94.

Goodridge DMG, Shorvon SD (1983a) Epileptic seizures in a population of 6000. I. Demography, diagnosis and classification, and role of the hospital services. *British Medical Journal* **287**:641–644.

Goodridge DMG, Shorvon SD (1983b) Epileptic seizures in a population of 6000. II. Treatment and prognosis. *British Medical Journal* **287**:645–647.

Green RC (1991) Neuropathology and behavior in epilepsy. In: Devinsky O, Theodore WH (eds) *Epilepsy and Behavior*, p 345. New York: Alan R Liss.

Hardiman O, Burke T, Phillips J *et al* (1988) Microdysgenesis in resected temporal neocortex: incidence and clinical significance in focal epilepsy. *Neurology* **38**:1041.

Hauser WA, Annegers JF, Kurland LT (1993) Incidence of epilepsy and unprovoked seizures in Rochester, Minnesota: 1935–1984. *Epilepsia* **34**:453–468.

Heller AJ, Chesterman P, Elwes RDC *et al* (1995) Phenobarbitone, phenytoin, carbamazepine or valproate for newly diagnosed adult epilepsy: a randomised comparative trial. *Journal of Neurology, Neurosurgery and Psychiatry* **58**:40–50.

Hopkins A, Shorvon S (1995) Definitions and epidemiology of epilepsy. In: Hopkins A, Shorvon S, Cascino G (eds) *Epilepsy*, 2nd edn, pp 1–24. London: Chapman & Hall Medical.

Juul-Jensen P, Foldsprang A (1983) Natural history of epileptic seizures. *Epilepsia* **24**:297–312.

Keranen T, Riekkinen P (1988) Severe epilepsy: diagnostic and epidemiological aspects. *Acta Neurologica Scandinavica* **78** (Suppl):7–14.

Keranen P, Sillanpaa M, Riekinnen PJ (1988) Distribution of seizure types in an epileptic population. *Epilepsia* **29**:1–7.

Kurtz Z, Tookey P, Ross E (1998) Epilepsy in young people: 23 year follow up of the British National Child Development Study. *British Medical Journal* **316**:339–342.

Kuzniecky R, Murro A, King D *et al* (1993) Magnetic resonance imaging in childhood intractable partial epilepsies: pathologic correlations. *Neurology* **43**:681.

Levados J, Germain L, Morales A *et al* (1992) A descriptive study of epilepsy in the district of El Salvador Chile, 1984 to 1988. *Acta Neurologica Scandinavica* **89**:249–256.

Loiseau J, Loiseau P, Guyot M *et al* (1990a) A survey of epileptic disorders in Southwest France: I. Incidence of epileptic syndromes. *Epilepsia* **31**:391–396.

Loiseau J, Loiseau P, Duché BI *et al* (1990b) A survey of epileptic disorders in Southwest France: seizures in elderly patients. *Annals of Neurology* **27**:232–237.

Luhdorf K, Jensen LK, Plesner AM (1986) Epilepsy in the elderly: incidence, social function and disability. *Epilepsia* **27**:135–141.

Manford M, Hart YM, Sander JWAS *et al* (1992a) National General Practice Study of Epilepsy (NGPSE): partial seizure patterns in a general population. *Neurology* **42**:1911–1917.

Manford M, Hart YM, Sander JWAS, Shorvon SD (1992b) National General Practice Study of Epilepsy: the syndromic classification of the International League Against Epilepsy applied to epilepsy in a general population. *Archives of Neurology* **49**:801–808.

Mattson RH, Cramer JA, Collins JF (1988) Time of next seizure after starting an antiepileptic drug. *Epilepsia* **29**:704.

Mattson RH, Cramer JA, and the VA Epilepsy Cooperative Study Group (1990) Seizure remission after active epilepsy. *Epilepsia* **31**:648.

Mattson RH, Cramer JA, Collins JF (1996) Prognosis for total control of complex partial and secondarily generalised tonic clonic seizures. *Neurology* **47**:68–76.

Mendizabal JE, Salguero LF (1996) Prevalence of epilepsy in a rural community in Guatemala. *Epilepsia* **37**:373–376.

Muir TM, Bradley A, Wood SF *et al* (1996) An audit of treated epilepsy in Glasgow. *Seizure* **5**:1059–1061.

Oka E, Ishida S, Ohtsuka Y, Ohtahara S (1995) Neuroepidemiological study of childhood epilepsy by application of international classification of epilepsies and epileptic syndromes (ILAE 1989). *Epilepsia* **36**:658–661.

Rodin E (1968) *The Prognosis of Patients with Epilepsy*. Springfield, IL: Charles C Thomas.

Ross EM, Peckham CS, West PB *et al* (1980) Epilepsy in childhood: findings from the National Child Development Study. *British Medical Journal* **280**:207–210.

Rwiza HT, Kilonzo GP, Haule J *et al* (1992) Prevalence and incidence of epilepsy in Ulanga, a rural Tanzanian district: a community based study. *Epilepsia* **33**:1051–1056.

Sander JWAS (1993) Some aspects of prognosis in the epilepsies: a review. *Epilepsia* **34**:1007–1016.

Sander JWAS, Hart YM, Johnson AL, Shorvon SD (1990) National General Practice Study of Epilepsy: newly diagnosed epileptic seizures in a general population. *Lancet* **336**:1267–1271.

Schachter SC (1995) The neurobiology of epilepsy: developmental biology and clinical aspects. In: Hopkins A, Shorvon S, Cascino G (eds) *Epilepsy*, 2nd edn, pp 25–34. London: Chapman & Hall Medical.

Shamansky SL, Glaser GH (1979) Socioeconomic characteristics of seizure disorders. *Epilepsia* **20**:457–474.

Sidenvall R, Forsgren L, Blomquist HK, Heijbel J (1993) A community based prospective incidence study of epileptic seizures in children. *Acta Paediatrica Scandinavica* **82**:60–65.

Tallis R, Hall G, Craig I, Dean A (1991) How common are epileptic seizures in old age? *Age and Ageing* **20**:442–448.

Tekle-Haimanot R, Forsgren L, Ekstedt J (1997) Incidence of epilepsy in rural central Ethiopia. *Epilepsia* **38**:541–546.

Verity CM, Ross EM, Golding J (1992) Epilepsy in the first 10 years of life: findings of the Child Health and Education Study. *British Medical Journal* **305**:857–861.

Death from intractable focal epilepsy

4

L NASHEF

Mortality is increased in epilepsy compared with the general population, with overall standardized mortality ratios (SMRs) in population-based cohorts of 2–3 (Hauser and Hesdorffer 1990; Nashef *et al* 1995a). (Standardized mortality ratio is the ratio of deaths observed in a group to the number of deaths that would be expected to have occurred during a follow-up period if the group in question had experienced the same age- and sex-specific death rates as in the control population.)

Interest in death during and from epilepsy has waxed and waned over the years and has recently undergone a revival. The aim of documenting the extent of the problem is to arrive at effective, widely applicable strategies for prevention of avoidable mortality. This chapter reviews causes of death in epilepsy and focuses, where appropriate, on mortality in focal epilepsy.

MORTALITY PRIOR TO MODERN ANTIEPILEPTIC DRUG THERAPY

Epileptologists at the turn of the century were well aware of the dangers from seizures and recognized that seizure deaths could be accidental or due to intrinsic mechanisms during a single seizure or serial seizures and status (Nashef 1995). Their experience was based on direct observation at epilepsy colonies prior to the era of modern antiepileptic drug therapy. While residents at such colonies are not considered representative of the general population with epilepsy, at the time a larger proportion of those affected resided in institutions.

Early authors who addressed mortality included Delasiauve (1854), Geysen (1895), Bacon (1868), Gowers (1885), Munson (1910), and Spratling (1904). Like now, there was no agreed classification of causes of death in epilepsy (Bacon 1868). Terminology differed from that used today. The term 'sudden death,' for example, often encompassed traumatic fatalities. Different writers described similar causes of death and all except Gowers considered epilepsy a grave danger to life.

Delasiauve (1854) in his *Treatise on Epilepsy* addressed outcome, including mortality. He classified 52 deaths based on his personal experience and that of other authors, describing four categories: (a) fortuitous seizure-related deaths totalling nine (two from trauma, five from suffocation, one from obstruction of food, and one from cardiac rupture); (b) deaths from serial seizures or status (total 13); (c) deaths from apoplexy or meningism (total 15); and (d) unrelated deaths (15) including, among others, pulmonary causes. He thus distinguished between deaths occurring as a consequence of a single seizure of diverse mechanisms, those due to serial seizures and status epilepticus, those most likely to be due to underlying disease, and deaths from other causes. That he reported more deaths from serial seizures and status than from all causes in a single seizure was consistent with the experience of other authors at the time and, indeed, from a more recent report of an under-treated population (Snow *et al* 1994). Interpretation of this interesting observation is difficult without accurate knowledge of underlying etiology.

Bacon (1868) classified deaths in epilepsy as occurring from 'the long continued effect of the disease on the body,' 'after a rapid succession of fits,' 'sudden deaths in a fit,' and 'accidents due to fits.' He stated that deaths in a fit were more rare than after a series of fits and ascribed cause of death to 'asphyxia' (violence of the spasm with venous congestion), 'loss of nervous power' (heart or its nerves), and 'suffocation' (face buried in something soft, impaction of food, aspiration, etc.). He stated that suffocation in bed, which at the time was widely considered the cause of death in nocturnal epileptic deaths, was 'far from uncommon in asylums.' Suffocation was revisited by Wilson in 1973.

Gowers (1885), in the section on prognosis in his textbook on epilepsy, stated that 'the danger to life in epilepsy is not great. Alarming as is the aspect of a severe epileptic fit … it is extremely rare for a patient to die during a fit.' Despite this reassurance, he added that 'the chief danger of death in an attack is the liability to accidental asphyxia, in consequence of the occurrence of an attack during a meal, when food may get into the air passages, or of vomiting during the attack with the same result, or in consequence of the patient, in bed, after an attack turning on to the face and being suffocated in the post-epileptic insensibility.' He also considered that there was some risk of death by other forms of accident to which the attacks expose the patient, such as burns and drowning, and considered the latter the commonest mode of accidental death in epilepsy.

The discrepancy between Gower's viewpoint that the danger to life from epilepsy was not great and that of others was noted by Spratling in 1904 in his textbook on epilepsy. Spratling's interpretation of this discrepancy reflects a difference in outlook between expectations then and now. He stated that 'a disease which destroys life suddenly and without warning through a single, brief attack, unaided by an accident to the patient at the moment, such as suffocation or fracture of the skull from falling, and does so in from 3 to 4 per cent. of all who suffer from it … [may not be considered] of excessively high mortality.' However, if deaths in epilepsy from additional causes were considered it becomes a 'serious affection.'

Spratling and later Munson (1910), based on their experience at the Craig Colony, were in no doubt that epilepsy constituted a risk to life. In Munson's series, some 40 deaths out of every 100 were epilepsy related and status

deaths were relatively common. Nocturnal deaths were considered accidental and amenable to intervention. Munson also described deaths that would be classified currently as sudden unexpected death in epilepsy (SUDEP) (see below). He noted that there was 'a definite and fairly large group where neither accident of any kind nor suffocation can be assigned as the cause of death which seemed to be intrinsic rather than extrinsic.' He highlighted the frequent presence of pulmonary edema, which he considered 'a frequent dangerous condition following all forms of the epileptic attack, even single grand mal seizures.' He concluded 'that death is imminent at the time of seizures, unless help is at hand. The cause may be traumatic, suffocation may take place, or deaths may occur without any apparent cause … the moral … [being that] the epileptic should be by himself as little as possible.'

Many years and numerous publications later our knowledge, although perhaps more sophisticated, is not all that different from that cited above.

CAUSES OF DEATH IN EPILEPSY

Deaths in epilepsy are classified as apparently unrelated to the epilepsy, related to underlying or associated disease, and related to epilepsy and its treatment (Table 4.1). Classification in an individual case is not always easy. For example, an unwitnessed accident may be secondary to a seizure or entirely unrelated. In the older population, death from associated ischemic heart disease may be precipitated by a severe generalized seizure. The relative contribution of the epilepsy in a given case of suicide may be uncertain. Nevertheless, mortality data show that certain causes of death are overrepresented in epilepsy cohorts (Hauser and Hesdorffer 1990; Nilsson *et al* 1997).

Table 4.1 Causes of death in epilepsy.

Death from underlying/associated disease
Epilepsy related
  Seizure related
    Status epilepticus
    Trauma, burns, or drowning consequent to a seizure
    The majority of sudden unexpected deaths in epilepsy
    Deaths in a seizure with severe aspiration or airway obstruction by food, etc.
    Deaths provoked by habitual seizures due to coexisting cardiorespiratory disease
  Deaths as a consequence of medical or surgical treatment of epilepsy
  Suicides

DEATH FROM UNDERLYING DISEASE VS. EPILEPSY

In their review of the subject in 1990, Hauser and Hesdorffer stated that 'Studies suggest that the underlying conditions rather than the epilepsy itself may explain most of the increased relative risk in younger patients.' In support of this statement are observations in population-based studies: (a) excess mortality is highest during the first few years after diagnosis (Table 4.2); (b) the breakdown of causes of death seen in these studies (Hauser *et al* 1980; Cockerell *et al* 1994); and (c) the higher SMRs observed in symptomatic epilepsies. Epilepsy-related deaths, which can occur early or late in the course of the disease, also contribute to the excess mortality as shown by the observed smaller increase in SMR in cryptogenic or idiopathic cohorts (Table 4.3; Henriksen *et al* 1970; Hauser *et al* 1980; Cockerell *et al* 1994), although not all studies have shown such an increase (Olafsson *et al* 1998). Remission rates are high in population-based studies of incident cases and the above observations should not be extrapolated to cohorts with chronic intractable epilepsy, where the impact of epilepsy-related deaths is most marked. In one cohort of young people with generally severe epilepsy and learning disability, epilepsy-related deaths constituted 74% of the total (overall SMR 15.9 [10.6–23.0]); in another adult cohort from a tertiary center, at least 58% of deaths were considered epilepsy-related (overall SMR 5.1 [3.3–7.6]) (Nashef *et al* 1995b,c). The risk will depend on the severity and frequency of the seizures and social factors.

SUICIDE

Although an excess of suicides was not observed in the population-based Rochester study, with only three suicides reported in 8233 person-years (Hauser *et al* 1980), it is generally agreed that both self-poisoning and suicides are increased among patients with epilepsy, particularly in certain subgroups such as those with temporal lobe epilepsy. The subject has been reviewed by Barraclough (1987) and Mathews and Barabas (1981). Overall, suicide rates are increased four to five times in cohorts with epilepsy compared with the general population. In proportional mortality series they constituted 2–10% of total deaths (Nashef *et al* 1995a). In the Warsaw study a higher incidence was observed among those in the community compared with institutionalized patients (Zielinski 1974). A younger age at suicide than in the general population and an association with more severe epilepsy has also been reported (Force *et al* 1989). Suicides are reported after temporal lobectomy, particularly in the first few years (Taylor and Marsh 1977). Mendez and Doss (1992) suggest a greater association with psychotic behavior and psychic symptoms than with major depression or the psychosocial burden of having epilepsy. This is in keeping with a much higher risk in those with a diagnosis of temporal lobe epilepsy, estimated to be 25 times that of the general population (Barraclough 1987). Of interest are differences observed between right and left temporal lobe epilepsy. Depression is reportedly more common in left temporal lobe epilepsy, while it has been suggested that postoperative depression is more common following right temporal lobe resections (see Chapter 52).

Suicides are potentially preventable. Vigilance, early treatment of depression, input from psychiatric services, and awareness of the effect of different antiepileptic drugs on mood are all important in this context (Robertson 1998). Careful follow-up is also required following surgery for epilepsy.

Table 4.2 Population-based study of epilepsy in Rochester, USA: standardized mortality ratios (SMRs) for all patients with epilepsy (1935–1974) in relation to years of follow-up. (Adapted from Hauser *et al* 1980.)

Years of follow-up	SMR	95% confidence interval
0–1	3.8	2.8–5.0
2–4	2.4	1.7–3.3
5–9	2.0	1.4–2.7
10–14	1.4	0.8–2.2
15–19	1.4	0.7–2.5
20–24	1.8	0.7–3.0
25–29	3.9	1.8–7.6

Table 4.3 Population-based studies of epilepsy: overall standardized mortality ratios with 95% confidence intervals in parentheses.

	Rochester, USA (Hauser et al 1980)	NGPSE, UK (Cockerell et al 1994)
Overall	2.3 (1.9–2.6)	2.5 (2.1–2.9)
Idiopathic/cryptogenic	1.8 (1.4–2.3)	1.6 (1.0–2.4)

NGPSE, National General Practice Study of Epilepsy.

ACCIDENTAL DEATH: DROWNING, TRAUMA, AND BURNS

Two main risk factors for injury are seizure frequency and seizure type, i.e. generalized tonic–clonic seizures (Buck *et al* 1997). This highlights the importance of controlling seizures. Patients also need to be informed of potentially hazardous situations, with the extent of precautionary measures taken dependent on the control of their epilepsy. Other relevant factors include drug-related ataxia and osteoporosis. A recent study reported that treatment with antiepileptic drugs was one of the risk factors for hip fracture in white women (Cummings *et al* 1995).

Deaths from nonintentional drowning constitute 1.8–10% of deaths in epilepsy (Nashef *et al* 1995a). The increased risk of drowning in epilepsy is dependent on exposure, is greater in the absence of supervision, and is amenable to prevention (Orlowski *et al* 1982; Smith *et al* 1991; Diekema *et al* 1993; Kemp and Sibert 1993; Ryan and Dowling 1993). All patients with epilepsy should be given appropriate advice. Baths should be avoided; sit-down showers with thermostat-controlled water temperatures are considered the safest option. Swimming should be supervised by an informed person capable of giving assistance. Unprotected waterfronts need to be avoided in the same way as heights; flotation devices need to be worn during water-sports and the patient accompanied.

Other accidental deaths are known to be increased in cohorts with epilepsy. The Rochester and Warsaw population-based studies reported that 5–6% of deaths in people with epilepsy were caused by accidents (Zielinski 1974; Hauser *et al* 1980). In proportional mortality studies, nondrowning accidental deaths constitute up to 18% of total deaths (Nashef *et al* 1995a). Driving restrictions aim to limit driver-related vehicle accidents due to epilepsy. Regulations vary considerably between countries; in some countries no regulations have been in force (Bener *et al* 1996). In the UK, in police-reported road traffic accidents due to driver collapse, 39% of drivers had suffered tonic–clonic seizures confirmed by witnesses, although it is unknown how many of these would have satisfied the regulations in force at the time (Taylor 1993). Seizures themselves may result in potentially fatal head injuries, cervical trauma, or limb fractures. In one study, the incidence of

Table 4.4 Measures to prevent accidental injury and death in epilepsy.

Avoid all situations that are potentially dangerous in the event of a
  seizure, including
    unprotected heights
    unprotected waterfronts
    proximity to fires
    proximity to dangerous machinery
Have sit-down showers with thermostat-controlled water
    temperature rather than baths
Follow driving regulations
Take care as a pedestrian and cyclist, avoiding traffic
Take care with cooking, hot water, and home appliances
In severe epilepsy, with frequent drop attacks, consider helmet or
    wheelchair use

seizures that resulted in injury requiring treatment at an emergency department was 29.5/100 000 of the population (Kirby and Sadler 1995). Another study of a cohort of patients with more severe epilepsy showed that the risk of serious head injury per seizure was relatively low (Russell-Jones and Shorvon 1989). However this study was of residents in a sheltered environment and is likely to have underestimated the risk, particularly since nondrowning accidents in a mortality study at the same center constituted only 0.8% of total deaths (Klenerman *et al* 1992). These observations underline the preventable nature of these accidental deaths (Table 4.4).

STATUS EPILEPTICUS

That status epilepticus constitutes a risk to life has long been known. In the eleventh century Avicenna (b. 980, d. 1037) wrote that epileptic attacks are fatal if linked ('Wa itha ittassalat nawa' ib a(l)-sara' qatalat').

Status epilepticus is more common in children but mortality is higher in adults. In 12 series reviewed by Shorvon (1994) mortality was 18% of all cases, 7% of children and 28% of adults. Reports from tertiary centers indicate that deaths in status in that setting are primarily due to the neurologic insult precipitating status, with only some 2% of deaths considered due to the status itself. Such reports should not undermine the view that convulsive status epilepticus remains a life-threatening medical emergency where prompt treatment is essential. In various series of treated cohorts with epilepsy, status epilepticus is listed as the cause in 10% or less of epilepsy deaths. The accuracy of these figures is uncertain as in the past, in the UK at least, unwitnessed deaths that would be currently classified as SUDEP were often certified as status epilepticus. Although Hauser has observed that overall mortality from status in a population-based study has not altered in recent years, the inclusion of proportionately more cases with acute neurologic insults in older age groups is one likely explanation for this apparent discrepancy. Interestingly, however, Hauser also observed that those with epilepsy who present with, or who are susceptible to, status, even in the idiopathic/cryptogenic category, have a greater medium- and long-term overall mortality and are a group at special risk (WA Hauser, personal communication).

SUDDEN UNEXPECTED DEATH

Problems with definitions

Otherwise well patients with epilepsy sometimes die unexpectedly, with post-mortem examination showing pulmonary or other organ congestion but not the cause of death (Jay and Leestma 1981; Schwender and Troncoso 1986; Leestma *et al* 1989; Lathers and Schraeder 1990; Leestma 1990; Wannamaker 1990; Brown 1992; Lip and Brodie 1992; Nashef and Sander 1996). The definition of SUDEP, the acronym frequently used to denote this category, has been subject to debate and the following working definition has been proposed: sudden, unexpected, witnessed or unwitnessed, nontraumatic and nondrowning death in epilepsy, with or without evidence for a seizure and excluding documented status epilepticus, where post-mortem examination does not reveal a cause for death. These deaths are difficult to investigate as they are often unwitnessed.

Controversies regarding definitions center on (a) the inclusion or otherwise of nontraumatic and nondrowning seizure-related deaths and (b) the difficulties in classifying deaths in epilepsy, particularly the level of certainty required, given the often limited information on the circumstances of death and occasional absence of autopsy data. These issues are discussed in detail in Nashef and Brown (1997). Researchers in the USA, perhaps partly because of lower autopsy rates, have defined levels of probability that are very useful in defining the limits of risk in epidemiologic studies (Table 4.5).

Epidemiology

SUDEP rates need to be compared with sudden deaths rates in the general population. Based on the Rochester, Minnesota study (Elveback *et al* 1981), Annegers (1997) concludes that sudden unexpected death in the general population is extremely rare in young adults (< 45 years), with an incidence of 5–10/100 000 person-years (Fig. 4.1). He also quotes a study from Allegheny County, Pennsylvania (Neuspiel and Kuller 1985) where there were 108 sudden deaths in the age range 14–21, 25 in people with epilepsy, from 1972 to 1980, or an overall rate of 5.6/100 000 person-years. Using a prevalence figure for

Table 4.5 Definition of SUDEP, with categories denoting level of certainty. (Adapted from Annegers 1997.)
Sudden unexpected death of someone suffering from epilepsy (defined as recurrent, unprovoked, epileptic seizures) occurring while the victim is in a reasonable state of health, during normal activities, and in benign circumstances, with no other obvious medical cause of death found
Definite SUDEP: meets above criteria, with sufficient description of death circumstances and post-mortem
Probable SUDEP: as above but no post-mortem
Possible SUDEP: either case is suggestive of SUDEP but information incomplete, or there is a competing plausible explanation for the death, e.g. bath death
Not SUDEP: either other cause of death clearly established or circumstances make SUDEP highly improbable

epilepsy of 0.7/1000, the incidence of sudden death for individuals with epilepsy was estimated at 188.6/100 000 compared with only 4.6/100 000 for the general population, a relative risk that was 40-fold higher for younger individuals with epilepsy compared with the general population. There is thus no doubt of the significantly elevated risk of sudden death in epilepsy among younger age groups (adolescents and young adults). With the increasing incidence of sudden death from all causes the relative contribution of epileptic sudden deaths becomes smaller in older age.

There have been a number of recent studies of sudden death in epilepsy and these have been reviewed (Nashef and Sander 1996; Annegers 1997; O'Donaghue and Sander 1997). Incidence rates depend on the cohort under study. Data from the Medical Research Council Antiepileptic Drug Withdrawal Study Group (1991) suggest that patients in remission, whether as a result of treatment or inherently less severe disease, have an extremely low risk of sudden death. Those in the general population are estimated to carry a risk of approximately 1/500 to 1/1000 per year. Those with more severe epilepsy seen at specialized units have a risk of about 1/250 per year, while those being

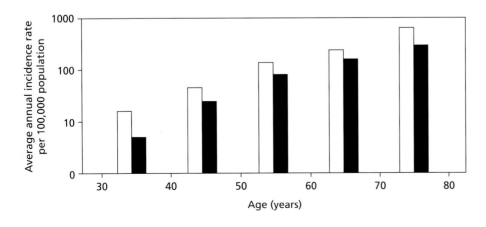

Fig. 4.1 Sudden unexpected death in Rochester, Minnesota, 1955–1959 (open box) and 1970–1975 (black box). (Originally adapted from Elverback *et al* 1981.)

considered for epilepsy surgery have a risk of 1/100 per year or more. Those rejected for epilepsy surgery and those with failed surgery are at particularly high risk. These data also support the view that those with focal epilepsies are more at risk than those with idiopathic epilepsy as they tend to constitute the majority of such cohorts.

Increased rates of sudden death in intractable cohorts should not be understood to mean that such deaths do not occur in those with less severe epilepsy, albeit at a lower rate. There are many anecdotal reports of people dying who had been considered to have only 'mild' epilepsy; indeed the records of the self-help group Epilepsy Bereaved? (Wantage, UK) suggest that such cases, including those with a recent diagnosis of epilepsy, are not infrequent (Hanna 1997). In the detailed interview study of bereaved relatives, 8/26 SUDEP cases had experienced less than 10 generalized tonic–clonic seizures in a lifetime (Nashef *et al* 1998). Hauser argues that 'Most SUDEP events will occur in those not yet identified as being at risk, with only 30% occurring in intractable cases' (Hauser 1997). More data is required on incidence in children and the elderly (Luhdorf *et al* 1987; Keeling and Knowles 1989; Harvey *et al* 1991).

Risk factors

Descriptive studies have highlighted a number of risk factors, which have not yet been confirmed by case–control studies; such studies are ongoing (Hauser 1997; Tomson and Kenneback 1997; Y Langan, personal communication). These factors include youth (second, third, and fourth decade), uncontrolled epilepsy, a history of generalized tonic–clonic seizures, unwitnessed seizures, nocturnal seizures, remote symptomatic epilepsy, male sex, a history of psychotropic drug prescriptions, and noncompliance or abrupt drug withdrawal. The finding of low post-mortem antiepileptic drug levels has also been listed as a risk factor in the past; however, apart from excluding overdose, the significance of this result is uncertain (Bowerman *et al* 1978; Lund and Gormsen 1985). Levels of certain drugs are dependent on timing of the sample collection after death and many patients achieve control on so-called 'sub-therapeutic' levels. Since this chapter was first written, a case control study of SUDEP has been published showing an increased relative risk of seizures, polytherapy, and frequent medication changes. (Nilsson *et al* 1999).

Mechanisms

Many investigators believe, myself amongst them, that the majority of these deaths occur during or soon after convulsive epileptic seizures when potentially life-threatening cardiorespiratory changes are known to occur, although this view is not unanimous. A recent report of detailed interviews of relatives of SUDEP patients gives indirect evidence in favor of the majority of SUDEP cases being seizure related (Nashef *et al* 1998). Similarly, in an ongoing case–control study of 150 SUDEP cases, of the 15 (10%) witnessed cases 12 were in the context of a convulsive seizure (Y Langan, personal communication). The different mechanisms responsible for SUDEP are not mutually exclusive and indeed may be contributory in a given case. There is strong evidence in favor of hypoventilation being a common occurrence in epileptic seizures and this is likely to be a significant mechanism in SUDEP. The frequent presence of pulmonary edema (almost a *sine qua non*) argues against an instantaneous primary cardiac arrhythmia in the majority. Systematic studies of ambulatory ECG, both ictally (Blumhardt *et al* 1986) and interictally, have generally shown malignant arrhythmias to be rare, although, as reviewed by Jallon (1997a,b), there are a number of case reports of severe bradyarrhythmias with secondary syncope in complex partial seizures of temporal lobe origin. Of 18 cases, 10 were right-sided, five were left-sided, and three undetermined. Such cases probably constitute a special subgroup at risk but are not likely to account for the majority of SUDEP cases, although they are clearly more relevant to patients with focal epilepsy.

Animal and stimulation studies support an important role for apnea/hypoventilation, known for many years to occur commonly during seizures (Simon 1997). In Simon's sheep model of ictal sudden death, animals that died were those with a greater rise in pulmonary vascular pressure and hypoventilation, thought to be central rather than obstructive. In a further study of tracheostomized sheep, where an obstructive element was excluded, central apnea and hypoventilation were observed in all eight animals. This caused or contributed to death in two; a third animal also developed heart failure with significant pathologic cardiac ischemic changes (Johnston *et al* 1997).

Systematic ictal recordings in humans with techniques used in polysomnography (Nashef *et al* 1996; Walker and Fish 1997) show that central apnea is observed commonly during seizures, including complex partial seizures, and is infrequently accompanied by transient bradycardia. Obstructive apnea is also observed but less commonly. Studies in telemetry units are likely to underestimate intrinsic/positional and extrinsic obstructive apnea because of intervention from attending staff. In the interview study referred to above, while only 5/26 were found face down on a pillow, in 11/26 (including these five) the position of the head was such that obstructive apnea is likely to have contributed to death (Nashef *et al* 1998). In an EEG/video-recorded case of death in a seizure (Bird *et al* 1997), respiratory parameters were not recorded, although the persistence of pulse artifact seen on one of the intracranial depth EEG electrode channels for 120 s after complete EEG flattening indicated adequate perfusion until the late stages of the terminal event. This was therefore consistent with apneic death after the ictal discharge due to, or occurring concurrently with, cessation of all brain activity.

Thus obstructive and central apnea, which may be amenable to intervention by an observer, occurs not only as part of an ictal discharge but also postictally. Emphasizing the role of apnea in SUDEP does not exclude an important role for cardiac autonomic changes. These may occur in association with apnea due to the same ictal discharge, as a secondary event as part of cardiorespiratory reflexes, or indeed independently of apnea as in the cases of severe bradycardia/sinus arrest in temporal lobe epilepsy cited above. Mameli's animal data, where cardiac autonomic changes with activation of brainstem arrhythmogenic trigger zones were recorded, showed that cardiac changes were transient and not life-threatening unless accompanied by alteration in metabolic parameters (Mameli *et al* 1993; Mameli 1997).

Ongoing studies of heart rate variability (HRV) may shed light on the risk factors identified in the descriptive studies outlined below. Changes in HRV have been shown to be strong predictors of mortality in other patient groups. At a simplified level, the various components of HRV are thought to reflect the sympathetic (low frequency) and parasympathetic (high frequency) autonomic systems and the relationship between them (low frequency/high frequency ratio). It is certainly possible, and probably likely, that there are specific changes in HRV where there is involvement of the limbic system and that such changes are influenced by laterality. Of interest in future studies are differences between nocturnal and daytime recordings, the influence of the epilepsy syndrome, left and right temporal discharges, and antiepileptic drugs (Massetani *et al* 1997; Tomson and Kenneback 1997).

On a different level, however, and as pointed out by Hauser (1997), a strict definition of SUDEP has limitations. He points out that current definitions preclude assessment of risk in the older population by excluding those where post-mortem findings show significant pathology in other systems. Cardiac mechanisms for example are likely to be particularly important in older age groups with ischemic heart disease who may be at risk of sudden death from their cardiac disease during habitual seizures.

Cardiac mechanisms are also important in cases of misdiagnosis of cardiac syncope as epilepsy (Hordt *et al* 1995). While undoubtedly such deaths can be, and are, misdiagnosed as sudden epileptic deaths, they cannot account for the majority of deaths as seen in well-documented series. On the other hand, the finding that channelopathies underline certain idiopathic epilepsy syndromes raises the possibility that an individual may be predisposed to both epilepsy and sudden cardiac death, or indeed of being more likely to die during a severe seizure. There are reasons for believing that the latter explanation would apply to a subgroup only. The risk of SUDEP appears to be more common in the severe symptomatic and focal epilepsies, a lower incidence of SUDEP is observed in controlled cohorts irrespective of drug treatment, and a lower mortality is observed following successful surgery for epilepsy (Sperling *et al* 1996).

General and neuropathologic changes

Pulmonary edema and congestion of other organs are frequently seen in SUDEP cases at post-mortem. The presence of pulmonary edema is a pathologic hallmark, almost a *sine qua non* of SUDEP (Terrence *et al* 1981). This finding is also observed in Simon's sheep model of sudden death (Johnston *et al* 1997; Simon 1997). Findings of cardiac perivascular and interstitial fibrosis (Natelson *et al* 1998) and of increased heart weight relative to height have been observed, the increase being significant in males (Leestma 1990). There have been no large systematic studies of specialized cardiac pathology in SUDEP cases compared with an epilepsy control group dying of other causes. It is uncertain if such a study would yield useful information but this needs to be performed. Neuropathologic studies indicate a higher incidence of macroscopic abnormalities in SUDEP cases (Freytag and Lindenberg 1964; Leestma 1990; Thom 1997). This suggests a greater risk for focal epilepsies and is in keeping with the higher risk reported in remote symptomatic epilepsy. Whether localization of abnormalities is important or whether this observation mainly reflects that such epilepsies tend to be more severe is uncertain.

Ischemic changes are generally not seen in SUDEP cases on neuropathologic examination, and would not be expected with a brief terminal event. However, such changes are occasionally observed in unwitnessed cases that would otherwise fulfill the definition stated above, again suggesting that some of these deaths occurred over a longer time course than a few minutes (Fig. 4.2).

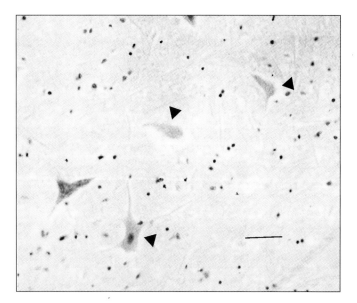

Fig. 4.2 Neuropathologic findings in a 29-year-old male SUDEP victim. Macroscopically the brain was unremarkable but histologically there were occasional nerve cells in both cerebral hemispheres and brainstem showing acute neuronal necrosis. The photomicrograph illustrates scattered motor cells in the XIIth nucleus of the brainstem, showing acute neuronal changes (arrowheads) indistinguishable from ischemic damage. Luxol Fast Blue/Nissl preparation. Bar = 40 μm. (Courtesy of Dr Maria Thom, Department of Neuropathology, Institute of Neurology, Queen Square, London, UK.)

DEATH SECONDARY TO MEDICAL AND SURGICAL TREATMENT

Antiepileptic drugs: potentially fatal idiosyncratic reactions

Idiosyncratic reactions to antiepileptic drugs, generally viewed as rare, may be life-threatening and include skin eruptions, blood dyscrasias, hepatic failure, and sinus arrest. The exact magnitude of risk with established antiepileptic drugs is uncertain but is considered very low compared with the risk inherent in uncontrolled epilepsy. However, the risk is unknown in any newly introduced drug as, at the time of licensing, the total number of individuals exposed to a new treatment is usually small. Thus the risk of a potentially life-threatening idiosyncratic reaction, even one occurring relatively commonly, would not have been excluded. Many of the relatively new antiepileptic drugs have already passed 100 000 person-years of prescribing and we now have a reasonable measure of their safety profile, an altogether different issue from tolerability. Postmarketing surveillance and caution on the part of the prescribing clinician is essential with any new drug. The relatively common occurrence of liver failure and aplastic anemia with the use of Felbamate is salutary (Kaufman *et al* 1997). The clinician needs to take into account the severity

of the epilepsy, including the risk of injury and death before recommending a relatively untried antiepileptic drug. Vigilance is also required when any antiepileptic drug, new or old, is first prescribed, particularly in the first few weeks or months.

An association between antiepileptic drugs and an increased long-term risk of secondary neoplasia has been suggested. In a study of over 2000 residents with epilepsy, White *et al* (1979) defined the limits of an overall increase in risk for cancer (excluding the CNS) at 1.1–1.8 times the average. Clemmesen *et al* (1974) and Shirts *et al* (1986) found no such overall increase. A study of 7864 patients with epilepsy from Denmark showed no overall increased risk when brain cancers were excluded (Olsen *et al* 1989). The available evidence suggests that once CNS neoplasms are excluded, any excess reported is small or borderline, although doubt remains regarding neoplasms of the lung and nonHodgkin's, lymphomas (Anthony 1970; Friedman 1981).

Temporal lobectomy

In surgical candidates, the relatively low mortality from presurgical assessment and from surgery itself needs to be balanced against the risks associated with intractable epilepsy. It may be expected that late mortality would decline after surgery for epilepsy.

Two older series report elevated long-term mortality after surgery for epilepsy, with some half to two-thirds of deaths related to seizures or suicides (Jensen 1975; Taylor and Marsh 1977). In a recent cohort of 248 people who underwent diagnostic evaluation for epilepsy surgery (Vickery 1997), those not operated on had a significantly higher mortality than the surgical group. Furthermore, a significantly higher proportion of those who died were noted to have ongoing seizures at the last recorded follow-up compared with survivors. Sperling *et al* (1996) observed that a seizure-free state following temporal lobectomy was associated with reduced mortality and increased employment. So far there have been no published studies of long-term follow-up reporting on deaths in relation to person-years under observation.

In Polkey's personal series of 299 traced temporal resections for refractory epilepsy (including 165 with mesial temporal sclerosis) performed at the Maudsley Hospital, London, there were 20 deaths (17 late) with a follow-up period of 2729 person-years (MJ Hennessy, in press). Long-term mortality was raised, with an SMR of 3.7 (2.5–5.3). Although elevated, this is less than would be expected in a severe intractable cohort. Of the 17 late deaths, four were not considered epilepsy related and included one death from alcohol-related drowning, one from suicide, one from cancer, and one from ischemic heart disease. The 13 epilepsy-related deaths included two from aspiration of vomitus, one road traffic accident, two probable drownings, two deaths from status epilepticus, and six sudden unexpected deaths (four among the group with right mesial temporal sclerosis, one in the group with left mesial temporal sclerosis, and one nonspecific). SUDEP constituted the largest single category, with three of the six cases still experiencing generalized convulsive seizures prior to death, although some had experienced an improvement in the overall control of their epilepsy. One of the two 'seizure-free' SUDEP cases was thought to be undergoing withdrawal of medication. Of particular note is that, despite a decrease in overall seizure frequency, a change in seizure type to more severe generalized or more prolonged attacks might have increased the risk in a few individuals. A higher mortality from all causes was observed in the group with right mesial temporal sclerosis. The reason for this is uncertain.

Vagal nerve stimulation

As would be expected in any cohort with severe intractable epilepsy, excess mortality has been observed in those having vagal nerve stimulation. The raised SMR observed in patients treated were comparable with studies of young adults with intractable epilepsy, as was the rate of definite/probable SUDEP of 4.5/1000 person-years (6/1000 if possible cases were included) reported by Annegers *et al* (1998). Details of fatalities were not provided. However, as with any newly introduced treatment, continuous monitoring is essential.

Epilepsy treatment: the potential to make epilepsy worse

An important concept relevant to treatment interventions that is not often emphasized is the potential for treatment to make epilepsy worse (Genton and McMenamin 1998; Perucca *et al* 1998), in particular the potential for a medication or surgery to alter seizure severity, including the postictal phase, thus altering the risk to life associated with an individual seizure. So far, scales of seizure severity have not addressed the cardiorespiratory distress that occurs during seizures (e.g. cyanosis or severe change in respiratory pattern), although the potential for injury has been included (Baker *et al* 1991; O'Donoghue *et al* 1996). Also relevant to treatment are risks related to noncompliance and abrupt drug changes.

THE POTENTIAL FOR PREVENTION OF EPILEPSY-RELATED DEATHS

In addition to avoiding seizure-related injury, the potential for prevention of excess mortality related to epilepsy lies in the response to an individual seizure and in the prevention of seizures, particularly generalized convulsions (Table 4.6). This emphasizes the need to treat epilepsy aggressively and the importance of compliance with medical treatment, avoiding precipitated seizures such as those associated with sleep deprivation, alcohol, or photosensitivity. It also highlights the need to improve seizure control for those with epilepsy. The issue of assistance at the time of seizures could be addressed further. Advice is usually given about cushioning the fall, protection from sharp objects, and placing the individual in the recovery position following the event. There is little discussion on the need for supervision to ensure assistance is available should a seizure occur or on more specific resuscitative measures. The former, with its potential to curtail independence, should be based on informed individual choice. In my view, timely assistance at the time of a seizure is likely to reduce the risk of death or injury. There is some evidence in support of this statement. Supervision has been shown to be helpful in preventing fatal drowning, and the same would logically apply to other accidental deaths. With regard to sudden unexpected deaths, it is worth emphasizing that the majority of these are unwitnessed. In the largest series so far, about 10% of over 150 cases were witnessed (Y Langan, personal communication). A likely explanation for this is that unwitnessed seizures carry a higher risk of death. A significant proportion of SUDEP cases are nocturnal (also unwitnessed), and there may be physiologic reasons why a nocturnal seizure may lead to death, such as higher likelihood of respiratory compromise or increased vagal tone. The observations in a cohort of pupils with epilepsy and learning difficulty at a special residential school are of interest (Nashef *et al* 1995b). During the period under study no SUDEP cases occurred while the pupils were under the supervision of the school (866 person-years); however, 14 SUDEP cases occurred either after the pupils had left the school or during holidays or weekend leave (3269

Table 4.6 Prevention of epilepsy-related deaths.

Prevention of injury and drowning
Prevention of seizures
Reduction in seizure severity
Detection and treatment of psychiatric comorbidity
Choice of treatment appropriate for severity of epilepsy

person-years). While the difference did not reach statistical significance there was certainly a strong trend, supporting the premise that supervision at the school was providing some protection despite the pupils having very severe epilepsy and very frequent seizures. The pupils were supervised constantly, including at night where four night staff,

an on-call resident nurse, and a sound-monitoring system insured a prompt response to seizures. Compliance in that environment was also assured. Similar experience has been noted at Lingfield School in the UK (F Besag, personal communication).

KEY POINTS

1. Mortality is increased in people with epilepsy compared with the general population.
2. The SMR is higher in symptomatic than in idiopathic cases.
3. The main categories of increased and potentially preventable mortality, other than any underlying pathology, are suicides, drowning, accidents, status epilepticus, and SUDEP.
4. SUDEP is mostly seizure related and is more common in severe symptomatic/focal and intractable epilepsies, youth, generalized convulsions, noncompliance, and rapid drug withdrawal. Obstructive and central apnea may be important factors. Pulmonary edema is a frequent post-mortem finding.
5. Treatments that control the epilepsy (e.g. surgery) may reduce mortality but may themselves carry a small finite mortality.

REFERENCES

Annegers JF (1997) United States perspective on definitions and classifications. *Epilepsia* **38**(Suppl 11):S9–S12.

Annegers JF, Coan SP, Hauser WA, Leestma J, Duffell, Taverner B (1998) Epilepsy, vagal nerve stimulation by the NCP system, mortality and sudden unexpected unexplained death. *Epilepsia* **39**:206–212.

Anthony JJ (1970) Malignant lymphoma associated with hydantoin drugs. *Archives of Neurology* **22**:450–454.

Avicenna (1993) *The Canon of Medicine*, Arabic edition, Vol 2, Book 3, p 907. Beirut: Izziddin Printing and Publishing Company.

Bacon GM (1868) On the modes of death in epilepsy. *Lancet* i:555–556.

Baker GA, Nashef L, Van Hout BA (1991) The impact of frequent seizures on cost of illness, quality of life and mortality. Current issues in the management of epilepsy. *Epilepsia* **38** (Suppl 1):S1–S8.

Barraclough BM (1987) The suicide rate of epilepsy. *Acta Psychiatrica Scandinavica* **76**:339–345.

Bener A, Murdoch JC, Achan NV, Karama AH, Sztriha L (1996) The effect of epilepsy on road traffic accidents and casualties. *Seizure* **5**:215–219.

Bird JM, Dembny KAT, Sandeman D, Butler S (1997) Sudden unexplained death in epilepsy: an intracranially monitored case. *Epilepsia* **38** (Suppl 11):S52–S56.

Blumhardt LD, Smith PEM, Owen L (1986) Electrographic accompaniments of temporal lobe epileptic seizures. *Lancet* i:1051–1055.

Bowerman DL, Levinsky JA, Urich RW, Wittenberg PH (1978) Premature deaths in persons with seizure disorders: subtherapeutic levels of anticonvulsant drugs in postmortem blood specimens. *Journal of Forensic Science* **23**:522–526.

Brown SW (1992) Sudden death and epilepsy: clinical review. *Seizure* **1**:71–73.

Buck D, Baker G, Jacoby A *et al* (1997) Patients' experience of injury as a result of epilepsy. *Epilepsia* **38**:439–444.

Clemmesen J, Fuglsang-Frederiksen V, Plum C (1974) Are anticonvulsants oncogenic? *Lancet* i:705–707.

Cockerell OC, Johnson AL, Sander JWAS, Hart YM, Goodridge DMG, Shorvon SD (1994) Mortality from epilepsy: results from a prospective population-based study. *Lancet* **344**:918–921.

Cummings SR, Nevitt MC, Browner WS *et al* (1995) Risk factors for hip fracture in white women. *New England Journal of Medicine* **332**:767–773.

Delasiauve (1854) Terminaisons. In: *Traite de L'Epilepsie*, pp 165–173. Paris: Victor Masson.

Diekema DS, Quan L, Holt VL (1993) Epilepsy as a risk factor for submersion injury in children. *Pediatrics* **91**:612–616.

Elveback LR, Connolly DC, Kurland LT (1981) Coronary heart disease in residents of Rochester Minnesota. Mortality, incidence and survivorship, 1950–1975. *Mayo Clinic Proceedings* **56**:665–672.

Force L, Jallon P, Hoffman JJ (1989) Suicide and epilepsy. *Advances in Epileptology* **17**:356–358.

Freytag E, Lindenberg R (1964) Medicolegal autopsies on epileptics. *Archives of Pathology* **78**:274–286.

Friedman GD (1981) Barbiturates and lung cancer in humans. *Journal of the National Cancer Institute* **67**:291–295.

Genton P, McMenamin J (1998) Can antiepileptic drugs aggravate epilepsy? Proceedings of a symposium held at the 22nd International Epilepsy Congress, 29 June 1997, Dublin, Ireland. *Epilepsia* **39** (Suppl 3).

Geysen MH (1895) *De la mort inopinee ou rapide chez les epileptiques*. Thesis, Faculte de Medicine et de Pharmacie de Lyon.

Gowers WR (1885) Prognosis. In: *Epilepsy and Other Chronic Convulsive Diseases: Their Causes, Symptoms and Treatment*, pp 199–200. New York: Dover Publications.

Hanna J (1997) Epilepsy and sudden death: a personal view. *Epilepsia* **38** (Suppl 11):S3–S5.

Harvey AS, Hopkins IJ, Nolan TM, Carlin JB (1991) Mortality in children with epilepsy: an epidemiological study. *Epilepsia* **32** (Suppl 3):54.

Hauser WA (1997) Sudden unexpected death in patients with epilepsy: issues for further study. *Epilepsia* **38** (Suppl 11):S26–S29.

Hauser WA, Hesdorffer DC (1990) Mortality. In: Hauser WA, Hesdorffer DC (eds) *Epilepsy: Frequency, Causes and Consequences*, pp 297–326. Maryland: Epilepsy Foundation of USA.

Hauser WA, Annegers JF, Elveback LR (1980) Mortality in patients with epilepsy. *Epilepsia* **21**:399–412.

Hennessy MJ, Langan Y, Elwes RDC, Binnie CD, Polkey CE, Nashef L (in press) A study of mortality following temporal lobe epilepsy surgery. *Neurology*.

Henriksen B, Juul-Jensen P, Lund M (1970) The mortality of epileptics. In: Brackenridge RDC (ed) *Proceedings of the 10th International Congress of Life Assurance Medicine*, pp 139–148. London: Pitman.

Hordt M, Haverkamp W, Oberwittler C *et al* (1995) The idiopathic QT syndrome as a cause of epileptic and nonepileptic seizures. *Nervenarzt* **66**:282–287.

Jallon P (1997a) Epilepsy and the heart. *Revue Neurologique* **153**:173–184.

Jallon P (1997b) Arrhythmogenic seizures. *Epilepsia* **38** (Suppl 11):S43–S47.

Jay GW, Leetsma JE (1981) Sudden death in epilepsy. A comprehensive review of the literature and proposed mechanisms. *Acta Neurologica Scandinavica* **63** (Suppl 82):5–66.

Jensen I (1975) Temporal lobe epilepsy. Late mortality in patients treated with unilateral temporal lobe resections. *Acta Neurologica Scandinavica* **52**:374–380.

Johnston SC, Siedenberg R, Min JK, Jermone EH, Laxer KD (1997) Central apnea and acute cardiac ischemia in a sheep model of epileptic sudden death. *Annals of Neurology* **42**:588–504.

Kaufman DW, Kelly JP, Anderson T, Harmon DC, Shapiro S (1997) Evaluation of case reports of aplastic anaemia among patients treated with Felbamate. *Epilepsia* **38**:1265–1269.

Keeling JW, Knowles SAS (1989) Sudden death in childhood and adolescence. *Journal of Pathology* **159**:221–224.

Kemp AM, Sibert JR (1993) Epilepsy in children and the risk of drowning. *Archives of Disease in Childhood* **68**:684–685.

Kirby S, Sadler RM (1995) Injury and death as a result of seizures. *Epilepsia* **36**:25–28.

Klenerman P, Sander JWAS, Shorvon SD (1992) Mortality in patients with epilepsy: a study of patients in long term residential care. *Journal of Neurology, Neurosurgery and Psychiatry* **56**:149–152.

Lathers CM, Schraeder PL (eds) (1990) *Epilepsy and Sudden Death*. New York: Marcel Dekker.

Leetsma JE (1990) A pathological review. In: Lathers CM, Schraeder PL (eds) *Epilepsy and Sudden Death*, pp 61–88. New York: Marcel Dekker.

Leestma JE, Walczak T, Hughes JR, Kalelkar MB, Teas SS (1989) A prospective study on sudden unexpected death in epilepsy. *Annals of Neurology* **26**:195–203.

Lip GYH, Brodie MJ (1992) Sudden death in epilepsy: an avoidable outcome? *Journal of the Royal Society of Medicine* **85**:609–611.

Luhdorf K, Jensen LK, Plesner AM (1987) Epilepsy in the elderly: life expectancy and causes of death. *Acta Neurologica Scandinavica* **76**:183–190.

Lund A, Gormsen H (1985) The role of antiepileptics in sudden death in epilepsy. *Acta Neurologica Scandinavica* **72**:444–446.

Mameli O (1997) Discussion. *Epilepsia* **38** (Suppl 11):S58.

Mameli O, Melis F, Giraudi D *et al* (1993) The brainstem cardioarrhythmogenic triggers and their possible role in sudden epileptic death. *Epilepsy Research* **15**:171–178.

Massetani R, Strata G, Galli R *et al* (1997) Alterations of cardiac function in patients with temporal lobe epilepsy: different roles of EEG–ECG monitoring and spectral analysis of RR variability. *Epilepsia* **38**:363–369.

Mathews WS, Barabas G (1981) Suicide and epilepsy: a review of the literature. *Psychosomatics* **22**:515–524.

Medical Research Council Antiepileptic Drug Withdrawal Study Group (1991) Randomized study of antiepileptic drug withdrawal in patients in remission. *Lancet* **337**:1175–1180.

Mendez MF, Doss RC (1992) Ictal and suicidal aspects of suicide in epileptic patients. *International Journal of Psychiatry in Medicine* **22**:231–237.

Munson JF (1910) Death in epilepsy. *Medical Record* 8 January: **77**:58–62.

Nashef L (1995) *Sudden unexpected death in epilepsy: incidence, circumstances and mechanisms.* MD thesis, University of Bristol.

Nashef L, Brown S (eds) (1997) Epilepsy and sudden death. Proceedings of the International Workshop on Sudden Death in Epilepsy, London, 28 October 1996. *Epilepsia* **38** (Suppl 11).

Nashef L, Sander JWAS (1996) Sudden death in epilepsy. Where are we now? *Seizure* **5**:235–238.

Nashef L, Sander JWAS, Shorvon SD (1995a) Mortality in epilepsy. In: Pedley TA, Meldrum BS (eds) *Recent Advances in Epilepsy*, Vol 6, pp 271–287. Edinburgh: Churchill Livingstone.

Nashef L, Fish DR, Garner S, Sander JWAS, Shorvon SD (1995b) Sudden death in epilepsy: a study of incidence in a young cohort with epilepsy and learning difficulty. *Epilepsia* **36**:1187–1194.

Nashef L, Fish DR, Sander JWAS, Shorvon SD (1995c) Incidence of sudden unexpected death in an adult out-patient population cohort with epilepsy at a tertiary referral centre. *Journal of Neurology, Neurosurgery and Psychiatry* **58**:462–464.

Nashef L, Walker F, Allen P, Sander JWAS, Shorvon SD, Fish DR (1996) Apnoea and bradycardia during epileptic seizures: relation to sudden death in epilepsy. *Journal of Neurology, Neurosurgery and Psychiatry* **60**:297–300.

Nashef L, Garner S, Sander JWAS, Fish DR, Shorvon SD (1998) Circumstances of death in sudden death in epilepsy: interviews of bereaved relatives. *Journal of Neurology, Neurosurgery and Psychiatry* **64**:349–352.

Natelson BH, Suarez RV, Terrence CF, Turizo R (1998) Patients with epilepsy who die suddenly have cardiac disease. *Archives of Neurology* **55**:857–860.

Neuspiel DR, Kuller LH (1985) Sudden and unexpected natural death in childhood and adolescence. *Journal of the American Medical Association* **254**:1321–1325.

Nilsson L, Tomson T, Farahmand BY, Diwan V, Persson PG (1997) Cause specific mortality in epilepsy: a cohort study of more than 9,000 patients once hospitalised for epilepsy. *Epilepsia* **38**:1062–1068.

Nilsson L, Farahmand BY, Persson PG *et al* (1999) Risk factors for sudden unexpected death in epilepsy: a case control study. *Lancet* **353**:888–893.

O'Donaghue MF, Sander JWAS (1997) The mortality associated with epilepsy, with particular reference to sudden unexpected death: a review. *Epilepsia* **38** (Suppl 11):S15–S19.

O'Donaghue MF, Duncan JS, Sander JW (1996) The national hospital seizure severity scale: a further development of the seizure severity scale. *Epilepsia* **37**:563–571.

Olafsson E, Hauser WA, Gudmundsson G (1998) Long-term survival in people with unprovoked seizures: a population based study. *Epilepsia* **39**:89–92.

Olsen JH, Boice JD, Jensen JPA, Fraumeni JF (1989) Cancer among epileptic patients exposed to antiepileptic drugs. *Journal of the National Cancer Institute* **81**:803–809.

Orlowski JP, Rothner DA, Lueders H (1982) Submersion accidents in children with epilepsy. *American Journal of Diseases of Children* **136**:777–780.

Perucca E, Grant L, Avanzini G, Dulac O (1998) Antiepileptic drugs as a cause of worsening seizures. *Epilepsia* **39**:5–17.

Robertson M (1998) Mood disorders associated with epilepsy. In:

McConnel HW, Snyder PJ (eds) *Psychiatric Co-morbidity in Epilepsy*, pp 133–167. Washington: American Psychiatric Press.

Russell-Jones DL, Shorvon SD (1989) The frequency and consequences of head injury in epileptic seizures. *Journal of Neurology, Neurosurgery and Psychiatry* **52**:659–662.

Ryan CA, Dowling G (1993) Drowning deaths in people with epilepsy. *Canadian Medical Association Journal* **148**:781–784.

Schwender LA, Troncoso JC (1986) Evaluation of sudden death in epilepsy. *American Journal of Forensic Medicine and Pathology* **7**:283–287.

Shirts SB, Naaegers JF, Hauser AW, Kurland LT (1986) Cancer incidence in a cohort of patients with seizure disorders. *Journal of the National Cancer Institute* **77**:83–87.

Shorvon SD (1994) Prognosis and outcome of status epilepticus. In: *Status Epilepticus*, pp 293–301. Cambridge: Cambridge University Press.

Simon RP (1997) Epileptic sudden death: animal models. *Epilepsia* **38**(Suppl 11):S35–S36.

Smith NM, Byard RW, Bourne AJ (1991) Death during immersion in water in childhood. *American Journal of Forensic Medicine and Pathology* **12**:219–221.

Snow RW, Williams REM, Rogers JE, Mung'ala VO, Peshu N (1994) The prevalence of epilepsy among a rural Kenyan population: its association with premature mortality. *Tropical and Geographical Medicine* **46**:175–179.

Sperling M, O'Conner M, Saykin A, Plummer C (1996) Temporal lobectomy for refractory epilepsy. *Journal of the American Medical Association* **276**:470–475.

Spratling WP (1904) Prognosis. In: *Epilepsy and its Treatment*, p 304. Philadelphia: WB Saunders.

Taylor DC, Marsh SM (1977) Implications of long-term follow-up studies in epilepsy: with a note on the cause of death. In: Penry JK (ed.) *Epilepsy: the Eighth International Symposium*, pp 27–34. New York: Raven Press.

Taylor J (1993) Epilepsy and driving. In: Duncan JS, Gill JQ (eds) *Lecture Notes: 4th Epilepsy Teaching Weekend*. International League Against Epilepsy (British Branch): pp 275–278.

Terrence CF, Rao GR, Perper JA (1981) Neurogenic pulmonary edema in unexpected unexplained death of epileptic patients. *Annals of Neurology* **9**:458–464.

Thom M (1997) Neuropathologic findings in postmortem studies of sudden death in epilepsy. *Epilepsia* **38** (Suppl 11):S32–S34.

Tomson T, Kenneback G (1997) Arrhythmia, heart rate variability and antiepileptic drugs. *Epilepsia* **38** (Suppl 11):S48–S51.

Vickery BG (1997) Mortality in a consecutive cohort of 248 adolescents and adults who underwent diagnostic evaluation for epilepsy surgery. *Epilepsia* **38**(Suppl 11):S67.

Walker F, Fish DR (1997) Recording respiratory parameters in patients with epilepsy. *Epilepsia* **38** (Suppl 11):S41–S42.

Wannamaker BB (1990) A perspective on death of persons with epilepsy. In: Lathers CM, Schraeder PL (eds) *Epilepsy and Sudden Death*, pp 27–37. New York: Marcel Dekker.

White SJ, McLean AEM, Howland C (1979) Anticonvulsant drugs and cancer. A cohort study in patients with severe epilepsy. *Lancet* **ii**:458–460.

Wilson JB (1973) Suffocation in epilepsy (letter). *British Medical Journal* **4**:173–174.

Zielinski JJ (1974) Epilepsy and mortality rate and cause of death. *Epilepsia* **15**:191–201.

Semeiology of focal seizures and underlying causes

Seizure symptoms and cerebral localization: frontal lobe and rolandic seizures

F BARTOLOMEI AND P CHAUVEL

In the past 10 years, significant progress has been achieved in the identification and classification of the semeiology of frontal lobe seizures (FLS), as reflected in the publications from two symposia dedicated to this topic (Chauvel *et al* 1992a; Jasper *et al* 1995). However, the clinical manifestations of FLS remain far less known than those of temporal lobe seizures (TLS). The best defined subtypes are seizures arising from the posterior part of the frontal lobe, i.e. from the premotor or supplementary motor areas and the precentral area. In contrast, seizures involving other regions of the frontal lobe are less easy to systematize.

The difficulty in delineating the features of FLS is due to several factors. First, patients with FLS are less common than those with TLS, even though FLS represent the second most commonly reported subtype of seizures in surgical series (Rasmussen 1975; Williamson *et al* 1985; Talairach *et al* 1992; Laskowitz *et al* 1995). Second, the frontal lobe covers a large territory of cerebral cortex (40% of the mass of the hemispheres), it is grossly divided into three main regions each with distinct cortico-subcortical organizations (Goldman-Rakic, 1995) and numerous cortico-cortical connections with the temporal and parietal cortices. In these circumstances, it requires particularly fine analysis to make correlations between ictal signs and symptoms and the anatomofunctional organization of the frontal lobe. Third, the high speed of seizure propagation to other

frontal or extrafrontal areas often limits the possibility of establishing these correlations.

Previous studies have underlined some general characteristics of FLS, in particular the so-called 'partial complex seizures of frontal lobe origin' (Williamson *et al* 1985; Delgado-Escueta *et al* 1987). The best spatiotemporal and dynamic descriptions of the seizures are based on intracranial recordings using video-telemetry. In particular stereo-EEG appears to be the best suited method (Chauvel *et al* 1992a,b; 1995). The main limitation of stereo-EEG is in the cerebral volume sampled, especially in the frontal lobe. Therefore, the results of stereo-EEG investigation must be validated by the results of surgery in the same patients.

GENERAL CHARACTERISTICS OF FRONTAL LOBE SEIZURES

Several clinical seizure characteristics suggest frontal lobe origin (Williamson *et al* 1985; Williamson and Engel 1997): rapid secondary generalization, focal clonic motor activity, prominent asymmetric tonic posturing, explosive onset and sudden ending, minimal postictal confusion, and frequent and brief seizures, often occurring in clusters. The semeiology of seizures originating in the anterior part of the frontal lobe is often puzzling and it can be difficult to establish the differential diagnosis between epilepsy and psychiatric or movement disorders.

In addition, in frontal lobe epilepsy the seizures occur most often during sleep especially when compared with patients with temporal lobe epilepsy (Crespel *et al* 1998; So 1998). This aspect has frequently raised questions on differential diagnosis with sleep disorders. For example, the classical nocturnal paroxysmal dystonia, long considered as sleep disorder, is now recognized as a type of FLS (Tinuper *et al* 1990).

ANALYTICAL SEMEIOLOGY OF FRONTAL LOBE SEIZURES

Chauvel has recently reported the semeiological analysis of frontal lobe seizures, which is now summarized here (Chauvel *et al* 1995).

SUBJECTIVE MANIFESTATIONS

As reported by the patient, these are:

Sensory manifestations

Somatosensory sensations are present in half of the cases. Cephalic sensations are frequently described as 'oppression', sensation of 'frontal striction', cephalalgia, or 'electrical sensation in the head'. When located in the limbs, they are often bilateral and vague: 'discharge in the whole body', 'sensation of body heat', or 'vertebral column shivering'. They are indeed more frequent in patients with seizures from the central region.

Visual symptoms are rare, nonlateralized and nonspecific. Generally, they consist in a global change in ambient brightness, or in contrast ('blurred vision', 'as in the fog', 'darkening', 'illumination'). True hallucinations or illusions ('persistence of images') are exceptional. Other patients may report 'psychical' illusions with visual character ('inability to recognize objects', sensation of 'unreality'), gustatory sensation ('bad taste') or miscellaneous sensation (diffuse sensations, polysensory, described as 'dizziness').

Autonomic symptoms

They are particularly frequent (noted in more than 50% of the patients). Various viscerosensory signs can be found: digestive (sensation of striction, in abdomen or in the throat); respiratory (thoracic oppression, choking sensation); cardiovascular (palpitations, praecordial sensations, cephalic migraine-like sensations); urogenital (urination, sexual sensations).

Emotional manifestations

These are frequent (in approximately 20%) and are described as sensations of fear, distress, dread, terror, etc. Discriminating whether an observed behavior disturbance (evoking intense fear) actually corresponds to a real experienced emotion can be difficult.

Excitation, contentment, and euphoria may be also observed. Similarly, to determine if smile and laughter are expressions of an experienced happiness is questionable.

Forced thinking and ideational manifestations

This is the more characteristic, but less frequent (less than 20%) 'psychical' symptom in FLS. Such an obsessive thought which imposes itself is often oriented towards an act to achieve or gaze attraction: the patient can report that he or she was 'forced to fix something with the eyes', or that 'the brain commanded something that he should not do', or a 'sensation of being forced to open the eyes'.

OBJECTIVE MANIFESTATIONS

Autonomic symptoms

Several visceromotor signs may be observed: digestive (salivation, swallowing); respiratory (tachypnea, bradypnea, apnea); cardiovascular (tachycardia, pallor, face flush); ocular intrinsic muscles (mydriasis); urogenital (urination, erection, complex sexual behavior).

Somatomotor and postural

These are the most frequent manifestations. They are observed in more than 90% of the patients. They may occur in isolation or in association with other manifestations.

All the varieties of paroxysmal motor signs can be noted. They can be schematically divided into three categories.

1. Seizures with predominant involvement of limb musculature: various focal signs can be observed (clonic, tonic, or tonic–clonic movements) on one side, or in one limb, or in both superior or inferior limbs or at the four extremities.
2. Seizures with predominant postural manifestations including adversion (ipsi- or contralateral turning of the eyes and the head, sometimes of the trunk). Adversion

can be isolated but more often is associated with loss of consciousness and other motor signs or automatisms.

3. Seizures with initial head and trunk flexion: forward propulsion of the head and the trunk is a frequent manifestation followed or not by other motor or gestural manifestations.

Oral, verbal, and nonverbal manifestations

Speech arrest is frequently seen in two-thirds of patients. In this case, the patient is able to obey simple commands and to recall them after the seizure; sometimes, he or she may report that it was impossible to express himself or herself orally. It is often difficult to distinguish speech arrest from a disturbance of consciousness. This sign has no lateralizing value.

Vocalization is less frequent. It can be simple (roaring, moaning, howl, scream) or complex (incomprehensible sounds or words, rhythmical sounds or syllables, palilalia).

Complex motor manifestations, 'automatisms', and gestural manifestations

Bizarre behavior and complex motor activities (gestural manifestations) have been increasingly described in FLS. In contrast to automatisms seen in temporal lobe epilepsy, in FLS these manifestations occur early in the seizure - and they are brief and repetitive (Riggio and Harner 1995). Impairment of consciousness is not constant and the association with tonic and postural manifestations is frequent. There are often changes in facial expression associated with gestural symptomatology: an expressionless face, a stupefied mask, fixed gaze or 'staring', with speech arrest and inhibition of gestures, or with automatisms; smiling, laughter, with simple gestural stereotypes or complex gestural sequences; a facial expression of fear or dread, sometimes accompanied by a peculiar vocalization, often integrated in a complex and global gesticulation. Some gestural stereotypes are simple; for example, rhythmical and discrete finger movements, seemingly adapted to the context (kneading of an object or a cloth, crumbling, snapping of the fingers, rubbing one's hands, buttoning and unbuttoning one's coat), periodic movements of waddling, flexion and extension, crossing and uncrossing of the legs. Verbal stereotypes (echolalias) can be associated. Gestural manifestations can be more complex; they can be violent, less rhythmical, asymmetrical or unilateral: gripping something or somebody, slapping one's thigh, tapping on one's foot, kicking, rubbing the leg with the hand, or rubbing the genitals.

Geier *et al* (1977) first used the term 'eupraxic' forced actions to describe the behavioral disturbance characteristic of these seizures. Gaze and gestures of the upper limbs appear to be attracted by some object in the immediate environment, which orients a pseudointentional sequence of catching, touching, putting in order, or playing with the hands.

These forced actions may seem to be goal-directed: aggressive facial expression, with a complex vocalization (menaces, insults, obscenities), preceding a sequential gestural pattern. For instance, standing up, then running around the table, spitting, tapping on the table, seeming to speak to somebody; or jumping or pedalling movements with rhythmic joyful vocalization. Their onset is often marked by alternating head deviations as if oriented towards an external stimulus. In other cases, they consist of much more complex and bizarre gesticulations, seemingly aimless, or apparently running away from some frightening situation, possibly as a reaction to 'unconscious' hallucinations. Often occurring during sleep, they are characterized by a facial expression of fear or terror, a powerful vocalization (screaming), agitation of the upper limbs as if struggling or tearing out something, manipulation of the genitals accompanying pelvic movements, pedalling movements, or kicking.

Finally, forced actions could be placed in two main categories: the first is characterized by obsessive manual activity centered on the personal space, or object-oriented in an 'utilization behavior', associated with postural adjustments or automatisms; the second category is of complex sequences of disorganized and nonsense gesticulations involving the whole body and often directed towards extrapersonal space, or seemingly reacting to hallucinations or emotions such as fear.

Disturbance of consciousness

Although, classically, impairment of consciousness is usual during FLS, it is not a constant feature. All degrees of impairment of consciousness are seen with FLS: from the complete loss of consciousness which accompanies the generalized phase which often ends seizures originating in the lateral premotor cortex, through the relatively preserved consciousness, but with loss of contact, seen in seizures originating in the central and medial premotor areas, to the altered consciousness with preserved contact seen in seizures from the ventromedial prefrontal areas. However, as already stated, anterior frontal lobe seizures are often brief and recovery of consciousness is generally rapid in the postictal period.

ANATOMIC CLASSIFICATION OF FRONTAL LOBE SEIZURES

Evidence from anatomic and functional studies and from the observed effects of lesions in patients allows the frontal lobe to be subdivided into precentral, premotor, and prefrontal cortex, also including limbic and paralimbic areas. This functional organization of frontal lobe regions is based on distinct thalamocortical systems and distinct patterns of cortico-cortical connectivity (Pandya and Yeterian 1985). In addition, strong medial-lateral interactions determine fast propagation, for instance from the anterior supplementary motor area (SMA) to lateral area 6 and from the anterior cingulate area to the dorsolateral and ventrolateral prefrontal areas. The symptoms of FLS depend on the involvement of these several distinct regions during a seizure and this explains why individual signs or groups of signs are of little localizing value. Except in the case of primary areas, a given sign is not necessarily produced by a discharge from a single area.

There is no definitive anatomic categorization of FLS (Chauvel and Bancaud 1994; Jasper *et al* 1995; Williamson *et al* 1997). The proposed schemes are preliminary because of the lack of sufficient data to define the different subtypes. We can distinguish three principal categories of FLS schematically: precentral seizures, premotor seizures, and prefrontal seizures.

PRECENTRAL SEIZURES

Symptoms of precentral seizures

The epileptogenic zone is confined to the primary motor cortex and the semeiology is mainly represented by partial clonic or tonic–clonic seizures. The classical model is the Jacksonian seizure, corresponding to a seizure starting with focal clonic movements of a limited part of the body musculature that progressively extends to adjacent segments. Precentral seizures are characterized by a high incidence of contralateral clonic movements, always unilateral, often purely clonic (46% of the cases in the St Anne's series (Chauvel *et al* 1992b)) and they can present with several patterns:

1. Partial myoclonus, predominantly distal.
2. Simple partial motor seizures, tonic–clonic with or without Jacksonian march.
3. Tonic postural motor seizures, associated with clonic movements: unilateral, or bilateral and asymmetric.
4. Partial unilateral clonic seizures.

The preferential locations are in decreasing order: distal upper limb, lower limb, and face. Clonic jerks can be associated with tonic postural signs and can be bilateral but asymmetric. Isolated focal tonic manifestation is rarely observed (Chauvel *et al* 1992b).

Epilepsia partialis continua

One particular type of seizure arising from the motor cortex is epilepsia partialis continua (EPC) (Biraben and Chauvel 1997). The characteristic clinical feature of EPC is focal myoclonus usually involving the distal part of one extremity that may last for hours, days, and even years. Any muscle group may be affected by this shock-like contraction, but distal musculature is more commonly involved. In some patients, the clonic movement may be confined to one group of muscles, in others the spatial distribution of the jerks may be larger, involving several limb segments which are synchronously engaged in the myoclonus. In the myoclonic jerks of EPC, agonists and antagonists are coactivated, unilaterally, and they are, by definition, spontaneous; but movement or sensory stimuli may exacerbate the motor symptomatology. Association of myoclonus with partial simple motor seizures is common. Long controversial, the origin of myoclonus in EPC from the precentral cortex was first demonstrated by stereo-EEG studies (Bancaud 1992) and also by a noninvasive approach using 'back-averaging' techniques. This method may reveal a reproducible EEG potential arising from the contralateral motor region and preceding the electromyogram burst by a short interval appropriate to conduction through the corticonuclear pathway (Cockerell *et al* 1996). A variety of etiologic factors have been implicated in EPC (Biraben and Chauvel 1997). Immunologic factors could be particularly implicated in the genesis of EPC both in Rasmussen encephalitis or in other more recently described conditions (Guillon *et al* 1997; Bartolomei *et al* 1999).

Reflex-triggered motor seizures

Several types of reflex seizures arising from the perirolandic cortex are known (Vignal *et al* 1998): seizures triggered by cutaneous stimulation, seizures provoked by movement, cortical reflex myoclonus, and startle epilepsy.

Seizures triggered by cutaneous stimulation

Several reports have focused on sensorimotor seizures provoked by the repeated stimulation of a cutaneous trigger zone. Tooth-brushing triggered seizures are a good example of this condition. Seizures generally start with somatosensory symptoms (dysesthesic sensations) located in the trigger zone. Motor signs are delayed, generally tonic, rarely clonic. Stereo-EEG study has proved the origin of the discharge in the postcentral somatosensory cortex and the rapid spread to the precentral motor cortex, illustrating the direct links between these two regions.

Seizures triggered by movement

In this situation, seizures are triggered by movements of a large joint or many small joints, always in the same location for a given patient. The nature of the movement is highly variable (starting to walk, catching the foot on a obstacle, putting on a shirt) and can be complex (manipulation of an object). There is no absolute requirement that the movement be sudden, but sudden movements are often the most effective. The common mechanism is probably the activation of the joint position receptors of one or more joints.

Seizures induced by movement are often characterized by early sensory symptoms (with possible Jacksonian march and close to the joints involved) but they may be purely motor. The motor manifestations are tonic, localized to one limb or bilateral with the adoption of a tonic posture, and may be associated with more delayed clonic jerks signs of frontal opercular involvement (vocalization, facial jerks). They are typically brief (20–30 s) and spontaneous seizures with similar semeiology may occur. Some patients have seizures triggered by cutaneous stimulation and by movement.

From the few published cases (reviewed in Vignal *et al* 1998) and the monkey model (Lamarche and Chauvel 1978), one can assume that seizures provoked by movements are related to a hyperexcitability of the sensorimotor rolandic cortex through a paroxysmal evoked response to afferent impulses, arising from proprioceptive sensory stimulations of the involved muscles and joints.

Cortical reflex myoclonus

Reflex myoclonus refers to myoclonic jerks (or cessation of muscle contraction in the case of negative myoclonus) provoked by touch or stretching a body part or by visual or auditory stimulation. Cortical reflex myoclonus is related to a sensorimotor cortex discharge and may be associated with other types of central seizures, particularly EPC (Obeso *et al* 1985).

Startle epilepsy

Startle seizures occur in a particular clinical context since they are observed in patients with infantile hemiplegia (Alajouanine and Gastaut 1955; Chauvel *et al* 1992b). The typical neuroradiologic lesion is a porencephalic cyst affecting the sensorimotor cortex. The effective trigger may be proprioceptive, somatosensory, auditory, visual or, more rarely, emotional.

The same subject may be reactive to several sensory modalities. The key point is that the stimulus must be sudden and unexpected. These conditions are similar to those provoking a physiologic startle. Indeed, polygraphic recordings have shown that such seizures begin with a startle response (generally asymmetrical) and are followed by a motor tonic seizure. This motor tonic seizure begins with a contraction of the paralyzed arm (flexion and abduction), an extension of the ipsilateral leg and a flexion of the trunk and head. Speech arrest is constant and the seizure generally continues in a tonic–clonic or clonic fashion. The level of consciousness is often altered. The seizures are brief (30–60 s) and may also occur spontaneously.

Startle seizures arise from both precentral and premotor areas including SMA (Chauvel *et al* 1992b) and subsequently spread to the mesial frontal area and the parietal cortex. The electrographic pattern is a fast discharge preceded by a high-amplitude evoked response localized to the motor or premotor (SMA) cortex. Alternative pathophysiologic hypotheses involve either a direct pathologic response of motor or premotor cortex to sensory afferents or an indirect response mediated by proprioceptive afferents initiated by the startle reflex.

PREMOTOR SEIZURES

Seizures from the premotor areas are mainly characterized by tonic and postural phenomena, predominant in the upper limbs, with adversion which can be contralateral or ipsilateral and symmetrical or asymmetrical. When there is a propagation to the primary motor cortex, clonic jerks may be associated with the seizure.

SMA seizures have often been confounded with the results of electrical stimulation of the SMA (Penfield and Welch 1951). Pure classical SMA seizures (emerging from the mesial premotor region) are rare (Morris *et al* 1988; Chauvel *et al* 1992a). They are mainly postural, with bilateral, generally asymmetric involvement of limb girdles (i.e. shoulder and pelvis) adversion (possibly alternating) of the head and eyes, speech arrest, or vocalization. Complex incoordinated movements of the four limbs can coincide with, or follow, these main signs. The tonic signs of these seizures (especially adversion) are due to discharge spread to the dorsolateral cortex of areas 6 and 8 (Chauvel *et al* 1996). Some patients experience subjective symptoms including bilateral, ipsilateral, or contralateral sensations of numbness or tingling (Williamson *et al* 1997). When the propagation remains purely mesial, the consciousness is preserved. Seizures are brief, generally lasting less than 1 min, and are often nocturnal.

A separate group is represented by seizures arising from both precentral and premotor areas. These seizures generally occur in patients with large lesions in these regions; such lesions are usually atrophic due to perinatal hypoxia or after trauma (Chauvel *et al* 1992a) (see startle epilepsy above). Their propagation involves the medial and lateral parts of these areas simultaneously. The motor semeiology is tonic postural, unilateral or bilateral, adversion is constant, and generalization is frequent. All the motor patterns, except pure unilateral clonic movements, can be observed. They are clinically very difficult to localize. The existence of lesions seems to coincide with a faster propagation.

In addition, some seizures can initially involve the posterior part of the inferior frontal gyrus (frontal operculum). The semeiology is characterized by speech arrest (or dysarthria and/or vocalization in the dominant hemisphere), facial clonic jerks (contra- or ipsilateral), tonic–clonic movements of arms and face, salivation, deglutition, and some other autonomic symptoms.

PREFRONTAL SEIZURES

The symptoms of prefrontal seizures are various and the two best individualized patterns of these seizures are as follows (Chauvel and Bancaud 1994).

Dorsal FLS

Some symptoms are suggestive of seizure onset in this region: 'forced thinking', 'eye directed' automatism and pseudocompulsive behavior, or tonic deviation of the eyes preceding head deviation (frontal eye field involvement). As has already been described above, complex visual hallucinations can be observed. Some complex sequences of disorganized and nonsense gesticulations involving the whole body and often directed towards extrapersonal space, also described above, are produced by seizures originating in ventrolateral prefrontal areas, spreading to dorsolateral areas. When the discharge secondarily involves premotor and motor areas, secondary generalization is frequent.

Ventral FLS

These seizures correspond well to the pattern described as 'complex partial seizures of frontal origin' (Williamson *et al*

1985). They are characterized by sudden onset with loss of contact and more or less elaborate automatism (Geier *et al* 1977): complex gestural sequences with bizarre gesticulations and eupraxic pseudointentional behavior and other features as described above. Some seizures start by vocalization, intense fear (or appearance of fear) and violent movements mimicking a frightening behavior or hallucination. This emotional (or pseudoemotional) behavior is associated with autonomic signs (facial flush, mydriasis, respiratory changes). Peri-ictal urination is typical in these seizures. Some patients may report an olfactory hallucination at the onset of seizures. However, olfactory hallucinations are not specific for these seizures since they are also observed in seizures primarily involving limbic temporal structures implicated in olfactory function (Acharya *et al* 1998).

CONCLUSION

Although a classification of FLS is certainly premature, nevertheless, general trends appear along the anteroposterior and mediolateral axes of anatomic organization. The majority of autonomic and emotional symptoms and signs arise from ventromedial anterior (prefrontal) regions, certain parts of which are in close relation with limbic and paralimbic systems. The motor semeiology associated with those symptoms seems pseudointentional and oriented towards personal space.

Progressing more posteriorly brings to the clinical tableau more postural and tonic components. Whereas the features of some seizures generated in the dorsolateral area appear to react with the external environment, some of the seizures generated in the dorsomedial area are completely independent of the external environment. It can be debated as to whether the posterior medial and ventromedial areas (SMA and cingulate gyrus) are responsible for elementary postural or more complex and elaborate motor semeiology.

Finally, there is a general agreement to consider the precentral region as responsible for pure and elementary motor signs, even though their variable grouping and the discharge frequency may be misleading and generate tonic complex patterns which could have been taken for premotor or parietal semeiology. Furthermore, the precentral epilepsies are rarely pure, and most of them must be considered as 'central', with somatosensory symptoms intermingled with motor signs.

KEY POINTS

1. Frontal lobe (FL) and central seizures are the second most commonly reported subtypes of seizures in surgical series.
2. The FL can be subdivided into the primary motor cortex, the premotor cortex, and the prefrontal cortex (that also includes limbic and paralimbic areas) covering a large territory of cerebral cortex (40% of the mass of the hemispheres).
3. The extent of the frontal lobe and the high speed of seizure propagation often limits the possibility to definitely establish the correlations between symptoms and the anatomo-functional organization of the paroxysmal discharge.
4. FL seizures can be schematically subdivided into precentral seizures, premotor/SMA seizures, and prefrontal seizures.
5. The best-defined subtypes are seizures arising from the posterior part of the frontal lobe (premotor/supplementary motor area, precentral cortex).
6. Precentral seizures are characterized by a high incidence of contralateral clonic movements, always unilateral, often purely clonic. Several types of reflex seizures arising from perirolandic cortex are known.
7. Supplementary motor area (SMA) seizures must not be confounded with the results of electrical stimulation of SMA.
8. Pure classical SMA seizures emerge from the mesial premotor region and are mainly postural, with bilateral generally asymmetric involvement of limb girdles, adversion of the head and eyes, speech arrest, or vocalization.
9. The symptoms of prefrontal seizures (pre-FLS) are various, and can be divided into dorsal pre-FLS and ventral pre-FLS.
10. Some symptoms are suggestive of dorsal pre-FLS: 'forced thinking', 'eye directed', automatism, and tonic deviation of the eyes preceding head deviation (frontal eye field involvement).
11. Orbito FLS correspond well to the pattern described as 'complex partial seizures of frontal origin', characterized by loss of contact and more or less elaborate automatism (Geier et al 1977): complex gestural sequences with bizarre gesticulations, eupraxic, and pseudointentional behavior.

REFERENCES

Acharya V, Acharya J, Luders H (1998) Olfactory epileptic auras. *Neurology* **51**:56–61.

Alajouanine T, Gastaut H (1955) La syncinesie-sursaut et l'épilepsie sursaut à déclanchement sensoriel ou sensitif inopiné. *Review of Neurology* **93**:29–41.

Bancaud J (1992) Kojewnikow's syndrome (epilepsia partialis continua) in children. In: Roger J, Bureau M, Dravet C, Dreiffus F, Perret A, Wolf P (eds) *Epileptic Syndromes in Infancy, Childhood and Adolescence*, pp 363–380. London: John Libbey.

Bartolomei F, Gavaret M, Dhiver C *et al* (1999) Isolated, chronic, epilepsia partialis continua in an HIV-infected patient. *Archives of Neurology* **56**:111–114.

Biraben A, Chauvel P (1997) Epilepsia partialis continua. In: Engel J, Pedley T (eds) *Epilepsy: a Comprehensive Textbook*, pp 2447–2453. New York: Lippincott-Raven.

Chauvel P, Bancaud J (1994) The spectrum of frontal lobe seizures: with a note on frontal lobe syndromatology. In: Wolf P (ed.) *Epileptic Seizures and Syndromes*. London: John Libbey.

Chauvel P, Delgado-Escueta A, Halgren E, Bancaud J (1992a) Frontal lobe seizures and epilepsies. *Advances in Neurology*, Vol 57. New York: Raven Press.

Chauvel P, Trottier S, Vignal J, Bancaud J (1992b) Somatomotor seizures of frontal lobe seizures. *Advances in Neurology*, **57**:185–232.

Chauvel P, Kliemann F, Vignal J, Chodkiewicz J, Talairach J, Bancaud J (1995) The clinical signs and symptoms of frontal lobe seizures. Phenomenology and classification. In: Jasper H, Riggio S, Goldman-Rakic P (eds) *Epilepsy and the Functional Anatomy of the Frontal Lobe*, pp 115–125. New York: Raven Press.

Chauvel P, Rey M, Buser P, Bancaud J (1996) What stimulation of the supplementary motor area in humans tells about its functional organization. *Advances in Neurology* **70**:199–209.

Cockerell C, Rothwell J, Thompson P, Marsden C, Shorvon S (1996) Clinical and physiological features of epilepsia partialis continua. *Brain* **119**:393–407.

Crespel A, Baldy-Moulinier M, Coubes P (1998) The relationship between sleep and epilepsy in frontal and temporal lobe epilepsies: practical and physiopathologic considerations. *Epilepsia* **39**:150–157.

Delgado-Escueta A, Swartz B, Maldonado H, Walsh G, Rand R, Halgren E (1987) Complex partial seizures of frontal origin. In: Wieser H, Elger C (eds) *Presurgical Evaluation of Epileptics*, pp 268–299. New York: Springer-Verlag.

Geier S, Bancaud J, Talairach J, Bonis A, Szikla G, Enjelvin M (1977) The seizures of frontal lobe epilepsy. A study of clinical manifestations. *Neurology* **27**:951–958.

Goldman-Rakic P (1995) Anatomical and functional circuits in prefrontal cortex of nonhuman primates. Relevance to epilepsy. *Advances in Neurology* **66**:51–65.

Guillon B, Ferron E, Feve J *et al* (1997) Simple partial status epilepticus and antiglycolipid IgM antibodies: possible epilepsy of autoimmune origin. *Archives of Neurology* **54**:1194–1196.

Jasper H, Riggio S, Goldman-Rakic P (1995) *Epilepsy and the Functional Anatomy of the Frontal Lobe*. New York: Raven Press.

Lamarche M, Chauvel P (1978) Movement epilepsy in the monkey with an experimental motor focus. In: Cobb WA, van Duijn H. (eds) *Contemporary Clinical Neurophysiology*, pp 323–328. Amsterdam: Elsevier.

Laskowitz D, Sperling M, French J, O'Connor M (1995) The syndrome of frontal lobe epilepsy: characteristics and surgical management. *Neurology* **45**:780–787.

Morris H, Dinner D, Lüders H, Wyllie E, Krainer R (1988) Supplementary motor area seizures: clinical and electroencephalographic findings. *Neurology* **38**:1075–1082.

Obeso J, Rothwell J, Marseden C (1985) The spectrum of cortical myoclonus: from focal reflex jerks to spontaneous motor epilepsy. *Brain* **108**:193–224.

Pandya DN, Yeterian EH (1985) Architecture and connections of cortical association areas. In: Peters A, Jones EG (eds) *Cerebral Cortex*, Vol 4, pp 3–6. New York: Plenum Press.

Penfield W, Welch K (1951) The supplementary motor area of the cerebral cortex: a clinical and experimental study. *Archives of Neurology and Psychiatry* **66**:289–317.

Rasmussen T (1975) Surgery of frontal lobe epilepsy. In: Purpura D, Penry J, Walter R (eds) *Neurosurgical Management of the Epilepsies*, pp 197–205. New York: Raven Press.

Riggio S, Harner R (1995) Repetitive motor activity in frontal lobe epilepsy. *Advances in Neurology* **66**:153–164.

So N (1998) Mesial frontal epilepsy. *Epilepsia* **39** (Suppl 4):S49–S61.

Talairach J, Bancaud J, Geier S *et al* (1992) Surgical therapy of frontal epilepsies. *Advances in Neurology* **57**:707–732.

Tinuper P, Cerullo A, Cirignotta F, Cortelli P, Lugaresi E, Montagna P (1990) Nocturnal paroxysmal dystonia with short-lasting attacks: three cases with evidence for an epileptic frontal origin. *Epilepsia* **31**:549–556.

Vignal J, Biraben A, Chauvel P, Reutens D (1998) Reflex partial seizures of sensorimotor cortex (including cortical reflex myoclonus and startle epilepsy). In: Zifkin B, Andermann F, Beaumanoir A, Rowan A (eds) *Reflex Epilepsies and Reflex Seizures*, pp 207–226. New York: Lippincott-Raven.

Williamson P, Engel J (1997) Complex partial seizures. In: Engel J (ed.) *Epilepsy: a Comprehensive Textbook*. New York: Lippincott-Raven.

Williamson P, Spencer D, Spencer S, Novelly R, Mattson R (1985) Complex partial seizures of extra temporal origin. *Annals of Neurology* **18**:497–504.

Williamson P, Engel J, Munari C (1997) Anatomic classification of localization-related epilepsies. In: Engel J, Pedley T (eds) *Epilepsy: a Comprehensive Textbook*. New York: Lippincott-Raven

Semeiology of temporal lobe seizures

CE ELGER

The term 'psychomotor seizures' of older classifications was regarded as indicating seizures arising within a temporal lobe. These seizures were so designated because temporal lobe epilepsy (TLE) dominated epilepsy surgery, and seizures arising within a temporal lobe had to be differentiated from motor seizures without mental symptoms. Later, terminology changed and the term 'psychomotor seizures' was replaced by 'complex partial seizures' indicating that this type of seizure is accompanied by a loss of consciousness. The latter is not a clearly assessable sign, however, because consciousness is not 'all or none' but varies in time, as pointed out later.

The increasing use of epilepsy surgery, with its extensive presurgical assessment, has generated data showing that seizures with 'psychomotor' semeiology may well arise from regions outside the temporal lobes, e.g. the frontal pole, the fronto-orbital cortex, or the cingulate gyrus. Phenomena during an epileptic event are due to cellular discharges within certain brain structures. The first part of this chapter deals with this principle. The second part describes the different symptoms of temporal lobe seizures with respect to whether they arise from the mesial or the extramesial parts of the temporal lobe, their time course, and whether they constitute lateralizing signs. Finally, specific phenomena of childhood TLE are described.

PRINCIPLES UNDERLYING SEIZURE PHENOMENA

Since the early investigations of intracellular activity during experimental seizures, there has been agreement that *paroxysmal depolarization shift* (PDS) can be considered the equivalent of epileptic activity at the level of single neurons. The PDS consists of high-frequency discharges of action potentials followed by depolarization. During a seizure the PDS occurs continuously in a tonic–clonic pattern. If the seizure arises in the primary motor cortex, where neurons are monosynaptically or oligosynaptically connected with motoneurons, the discharge pattern is transmitted in a one-to-one manner leading to the typical sequence of motor seizures with clonic and tonic phenomena. Motor phenomena that arise from areas rostral to the primary motor cortex can be explained similarly. The oligosynaptic connection to the motor strip results in a 'smoothing' of clonic activity. Thus, the whole event is dominated by tonic or clonic movements with very high frequencies, leading to body posturing. Both states are more or less 'unphysiologic.'

In contrast, psychomotor seizures exhibit 'physiologic' signs like chewing, lip smacking, explorative movements, and even complex sensations such as *déjà vu*. These phenomena cannot be generated by a PDS because simple burst discharges do not lead to complex physiologic movements or such sensations. Analysis of the intracerebral EEG during a seizure shows that changes in the EEG pattern do not run simultaneously with the seizure signs. Several investigations have shown that EEG discharges precede subjective and objective clinical signs by several seconds (Delgado Escueta 1979; Delgado Escueta *et al* 1979). It can be assumed, therefore, that the neuroelectrical seizure activity responsible for generating temporal lobe seizures has a different locus to that underlying symptoms of the seizure. This is in contrast to simple motor seizures (Fig. 6.1), as had been suspected by Penfield and Jasper (1954).

In this context, it is noteworthy that electrical stimulation of the insular cortex results in an epigastric sensation equivalent to that occurring as an early symptom of mesiotemporal attacks. Consequently, the discharges of neurons involved in seizure activity can lead to phenomena generated at a distance and even to the release of stored motor programs. Furthermore, similar symptoms may result from seizures arising in different parts of the temporal lobe.

In what follows, therefore, a differentiation is made only between mesial and extramesial temporal lobe areas. This is the most relevant differentiation with respect to temporal lobe surgery. The Bonn group adopts complete seizure control following resection of the mesial or extramesial temporal lobe structures as the gold standard for localizing seizure onset. Reports from elsewhere do not always use this strict criterion. For example, some authors report correlations between seizure phenomena and extracerebral, or sometimes intracerebral, recordings. Caution is necessary with this approach. Intracerebral recordings are extremely focused, precluding the assessment of electrical activity in neighboring areas. On the other hand, extracerebral EEG is very coarse, so that a precise differentiation between mesial and extramesial seizure activity is usually impossible. Extracerebral EEG is, however, very helpful for seizure lateralization.

SEIZURES OF MESIAL TEMPORAL LOBE ONSET IN ADULTS

The mesial structures of the temporal lobe consist of the amygdala, the hippocampus, and the entorhinal cortex. They are highly sensitive to external and/or internal noxious stimuli causing sclerosis of the hippocampus and/or the amygdala, which is the commonest pathology underlying TLE of mesial origin. Mesial TLE (MTLE) responds well to temporal lobe surgery, regardless of whether a two-thirds resection or a selective amygdalohippocampectomy (SAH) is performed. However, cognitive outcome is better after SAH and so it is the operation of choice when pathology is confined to these mesial structures. Consequently, it is rational to differentiate between mesial and extramesial seizure semeiology and to use this differentiation, along with magnetic resonance imaging and EEG data, in deciding which surgical procedure should be performed (two-thirds anterior temporal lobe resection vs. SAH).

Table 6.1 Percentage incidence of semeiologic signs in temporal lobe epilepsy from an analysis of 126 seizures (89 of mesial origin and 37 of extramesial origin) from 107 patients: 64 with sclerosis of Ammon's horn, 10 with mesially situated tumors, and 33 with extramesial pathology.

	Mesial		Extramesial	
	Left	*Right*	*Left*	*Right*
Aura	87.3	65.7	50.0	50.0
Staring	32.7	40.0	40.0	37.5
Arrest reaction	27.3	5.7	15.0	6.3
Oroalimentary automatisms	25.5	51.4	45.0	43.8
Restlessness	38.2	45.7	40.0	56.3
Head deviation, right	10.9	25.7	10.0	56.3
Head deviation, left	27.3	8.6	20.0	12.5
Finger automatism	0.0	0.0	10.0	0.0
Dystonic arm, right	38.2	2.9	25.0	6.3
Dystonic arm, left	3.6	37.1	0.0	18.8
Escape reaction	12.7	2.9	10.0	12.5
Ictal laughter	3.6	2.9	0.0	12.5
Stereotyped movement right	9.1	17.1	5.0	12.5
Stereotyped movement, left	12.7	2.9	10.0	0.0
Hand automatism	0.0	8.6	5.0	12.5
Leg automatism	5.5	8.6	0.0	25.0
Unformed vocalization	32.7	40.0	30.0	50.0
Grimacing	16.4	17.1	5.0	6.3
Lip smacking	3.6	0.0	5.0	0.0

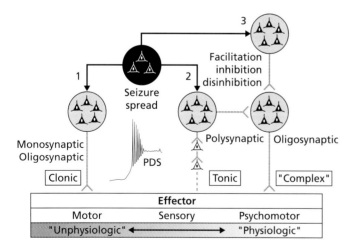

Fig. 6.1 Generation of semeiologic phenomena in seizures. The neuronal discharge (PDS) results in different phenomena according to the type of connection: I, monosynaptic/oligosynaptic; II, polysynaptic; III, connection via neuronal networks.

Table 6.2 Semeiologic signs in temporal lobe epilepsy (listed in descending order of incidence).

	Mesial		Extramesial	
	Left	Right	Left	Right

Initial signs	Aura
	Staring
	Arrest reaction
		Aura
		Restlessness
		Oroalimentary
		  automatisms
		Staring
		Head deviation
		  to the right
			Aura
			Oroalimentary
			  automatisms
			Finger automatisms
			Dystonic right arm
			Escape reaction
			Staring
				Aura
				Ictal laughter
				Staring
				Stereotypic movements
				Restlessness

Late signs	Arrest reaction
	Restlessness
	Oroalimentary
	  automatisms
	Head deviation
	  to the left
	Staring
		Restlessness
		Oroalimentary
		  automatisms
		Staring
		Dystonic left arm
		Head deviation
		  to the right
		Arrest reaction
			Restlessness
			Oroalimentary
			  automatisms
			Staring
			Manual automatisms
			Leg automatisms
			Dystonic right arm
			Eye deviation
			  to the left
				Restlessness
				Oroalimentary
				  automatisms
				Vocalization
				Head deviation
				  to the right
				Stereotypic movements
				  of the right hand

Review of the literature

It seems generally accepted that seizures from the mesial temporal lobe usually start with a restricted and subjective seizure symptom described as an aura. Most often an epigastric sensation is experienced (Fried *et al* 1995). Gustatory or olfactory auras and auras with experiential contents, such as *déjà vu* or *jamais vu*, are less frequent (Gil-Nagel and Risinger 1997). The commonest objective phenomenon of MTLE is an oroalimentary automatism, which occurs in 70% of patients (Gil-Nagel and Risinger 1997). Other symptoms include arrest reactions, vocalizations, and other motor involvements; these have not, however, been related to ictal discharges on intracranial EEG or to postoperative seizure outcome. According to Gil-Nagel and Risinger (1997), they do not reliably differentiate between a mesial and a nonmesial temporal lobe seizure origin.

Our investigations

We analyzed 89 seizures in 74 patients with MTLE who became seizure-free after SAH: 29 with right-sided sclerosis of Ammon's horn (30 seizures), 35 with left-sided sclerosis of Ammon's horn (46 seizures), four with right mesial tumors (five seizures), and six with left mesial tumors (eight seizures). Seizures were analyzed by split-screen recordings with intracranial EEG and thorough visual inspection of the seizure semeiology; the patient was tested by a qualified person during both the seizure and the postictal state.

The results are summarized in Tables 6.1 and 6.2. An aura occurred in 78% of the patients. Epigastric auras were

most frequent; fearful auras and unspecified sensations were less frequent. Other forms of aura occurred only in single cases. The initial objective seizure phenomena were staring, motor restlessness, oroalimentary automatisms (early and late sign), and a nonforced head deviation. These early signs were followed by either an arrest reaction or motor restlessness, head deviation or staring, if these had not already occurred during the very early phase. Dystonic posturing might start at this phase but usually dominated later stages of the seizure. Hypersalivation was a rare characteristic of mesial-onset seizures. The postictal state was characterized by phenomena such as reorientation or dysphasia, and occasionally by coughing. Figure 6.2 shows ictal phenomena in three different phases of a temporal lobe seizure.

Consciousness is difficult to test. Two-thirds of the patients reacted to testing during their seizures but their reactions were not always specific. Nevertheless, it indicates that their consciousness was not severely affected. The level of consciousness showed considerable variability (see below).

Lateralizing signs

It is generally accepted that ictal dystonic posturing indicates, with considerable reliability, that the seizure originated in the contralateral temporal lobe (Bleasel *et al* 1997). However, the sign occurred in only 30% of cases, and there was no differentiation between mesial and nonmesial TLE. Gil-Nagel and Risinger (1997) reported the sign in only 20% of patients with MTLE, always contralateral to the seizure onset.

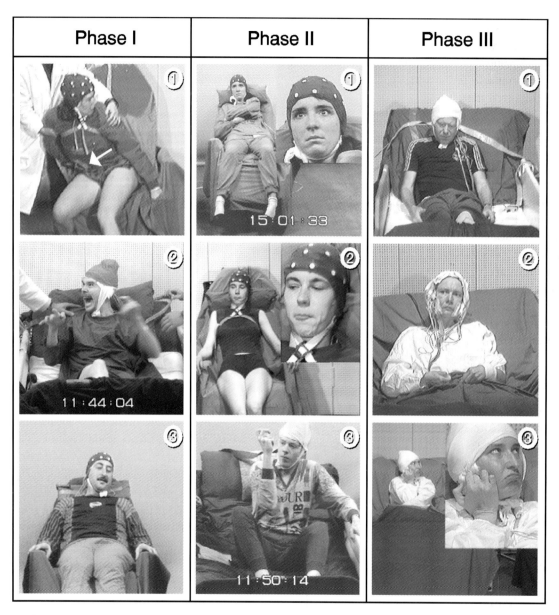

Fig. 6.2 The main phenomena during three phases of temporal lobe seizures. Phase I: 1, epigastric aura; 2, fear; 3, aura with positive sensations. Phase II: 1, staring; 2, oroalimentary automatisms; 3, dystonic arm. Phase III: 1, hand automatisms; 2, bilateral tonic arm posture; 3, head and eye deviation.

Analysis of our own cases has shown relevant differences between seizures of right and left mesial origin. Impaired consciousness, if clearly present, pointed to the left side (left/right, 44%/20%). Arrest reactions were typical of left MTLE (left/right, 20%/4%). Escape reactions were rare, but when they occurred they related to left MTLE (left/right, 10%/2%). Auras were more frequent in patients with left than right MTLE (left/right, 65%/45%). Fearful auras occur more often in patients with left MTLE than in those with right MTLE (Markand *et al* 1994; Bleasel *et al* 1997). Hyperventilation during the seizure occurred only with left mesial onset but was rare. In contrast, vocalizations, motor restlessness, and staring did not lateralize.

Furthermore, stereotypic movements of one extremity did not point to the contralateral temporal lobe. In contrast to findings reported in the literature, postictal aphasia was found in both right and left MTLE, possibly due to the spread of seizure discharges from right to left.

SEIZURES OF EXTRAMESIAL TEMPORAL LOBE ONSET IN ADULTS

Differentiation between mesial and extramesial temporal lobe seizures is difficult, because mesial seizures spread to the lateral and/or basal parts of the temporal lobe. Mesial and extramesial seizure origins cannot be differentiated by surface EEG recordings. Clear descriptions in cases with only lateral resections and intracranial EEG are rare. Only early signs are reported here.

Review of the literature

The careful study of Gil-Nagel and Risinger (1997) showed that auras with experiential contents (*déjà vu*, *jamais vu*) occur only in nonmesial seizures. Other authors describe auras consisting of acoustic, gustatory, and vestibular phenomena, hallucinations, receptive aphasia, and sensory–motor phenomena (Wieser 1983; Williamson and Wieser 1987). Initial signs are motor phenomena without oroalimentary automatisms (Fried *et al* 1995). An early involvement of the contralateral upper extremity was often seen by others (Gil-Nagel and Risinger 1997). Further carefully performed studies are not available.

Our investigations

We investigated 37 seizures of extramesial temporal lobe origin in 33 patients. Auras were rare (15%). The phenomena varied from patient to patient. This might be because seizures originating from any extramesial part of the temporal lobe were included. Clonic movements of facial muscles, grimacing, finger and hand automatisms, dystonic posturing of an upper extremity, oroalimentary automatisms, leg automatisms, restlessness, and unformed vocalizations were seen. More frequent, and clearly differentiating between extramesial and mesial seizures, was a rotation of the whole body. Eye blinking, aggressive behavior, dystonic posturing, swallowing, lip smacking, late oroalimentary automatisms, and hypersalivation, although typical of MTLE, did not occur with nonmesial onset. Impairment of consciousness was different to that seen in MTLE and was generally less pronounced.

Lateralizing signs

Contralateral dystonic posturing in right-sided seizures is described in the literature as a helpful sign for lateralizing the seizure onset (Kotagal *et al* 1989; Kotagal 1991; Bleasel *et al* 1997). Postictal dysphasia is thought to be a clear pointer to a dominant hemisphere seizure onset.

In our evaluation, only a limited loss of consciousness during the seizure was a useful indicator of a nondominant hemisphere origin. Leg automatisms were only seen during right-sided seizures. The rare phenomenon of ictal laughter occurred in only those patients with right extramesial

seizures, although in the literature it has been described as often having its origin in the dominant temporal lobe and less frequently in a frontal lobe (Sethi and Rao 1976; Sackeim *et al* 1982; Luciano *et al* 1993). Retching is rare, but if it occurs it is predominantly during right MTLE. Vomiting seems to have its origin during seizure activity of the lateral temporal lobe (Kramer *et al* 1988).

TEMPORAL LOBE SEIZURES IN CHILDREN

In children, especially young children, the nervous system is not fully developed. This is especially true of the motor system, which is responsible for many seizure phenomena. Even in children with a congenital lesion of one hemisphere, such as a porencephalic cyst, reduced motor function develops gradually and is only seen after the first year. Furthermore, the course of seizure spread is different in the immature nervous system. Auras cannot be reported by the young and as yet no study has differentiated between mesial and nonmesial seizures.

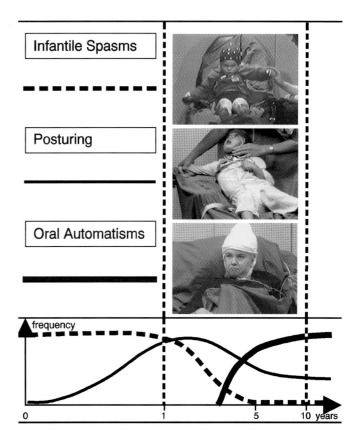

Fig. 6.3 Age-related time course of development and frequency of phenomena of temporal lobe seizures in children. The lines in the diagram correspond to the phenomena in the upper part of the figure.

It seems that typical phenomena of temporal lobe seizures occur only in children older than 5 or 6 years. Young children show more simple automatisms and a reduced responsiveness. Older children show phenomena similar to those seen in adults (Wyllie *et al* 1993). Nordli *et al* (1997) investigated young children up to the age of 26 months. They found with decreasing incidence, bilateral clonic movements, unilateral clonic movements, oral automatisms, bilateral tonic phenomena, and infantile spasms, thus demonstrating a clear difference to the seizure signs in adults. In our own study the change from nonspecific motor signs to typical seizures of temporal lobe origin was also shown to be a function of age (Brockhaus and Elger 1995). Typical temporal lobe seizures occurred only beyond the age of 6 years. The development of these phenomena is shown in Fig. 6.3.

KEY POINTS

1. Temporal lobe seizures show signs that often display physiologic phenomena.
2. Loss of consciousness, which is the core symptom for the classification of complex vs. simple seizures, is not seen in all seizures from the right temporal lobe (or perhaps the nondominant temporal lobe).
3. Further lateralizing signs are contralateral dystonic posturing and, a less valid sign, postictal aphasia.
4. A clear differentiation between mesial and nonmesial seizures is often not easy because of seizure spread.
5. Aura phenomena are very helpful.
6. In young children temporal lobe seizures may look very nonspecific since simple motor signs dominate.

REFERENCES

Bleasel A, Kotagal P, Kankirawatana P, Rybicki L (1997) Lateralizing value and semiology of ictal limb posturing and version in temporal lobe and extratemporal epilepsy. *Epilepsia* **38**:168–174.

Brockhaus A, Elger CE (1995) Complex partial seizures of temporal lobe origin in children of different age groups. *Epilepsia* **36**:1173–1181.

Delgado Escueta AV (1979) Epileptogenic paroxysms: modern approaches and clinical correlations. *Neurology* **29**:1014–1022.

Delgado Escueta AV, Nashold B, Freedman M *et al* (1979) Videotaping epileptic attacks during stereoelectroencephalography. *Neurology* **29**:473–489.

Fried I, Spencer D, Spencer S (1995) The anatomy of epileptic auras: focal pathology and surgical outcome. *Journal of Neurosurgery* **83**:60–66.

Gil-Nagel A, Risinger MW (1997) Ictal semiology in hippocampal versus extrahippocampal temporal lobe epilepsy. *Brain* **120**:183–192.

Kotagal P (1991) Seizure symptomatology of temporal lobe epilepsy. In: Lüders H (ed) *Epilepsy Surgery*, pp 143–156. New York: Raven Press.

Kotagal P, Lüders H, Morris HH (1989) Dystonic posturing in complex partial seizures of temporal lobe onset. *Neurology* **39**:1270–1271.

Kramer R, Lüders H, Goldstick L (1988) Ictus emeticus. An electroclinical analysis. *Neurology* **38**:1048–1052.

Luciano D, Devinsky O, Perrine K (1993) Crying seizures. *Neurology* **43**:2113–2117.

Markand ON, Salanova V, Worth RM, Park HM, Wellman HH (1994) Ictal brain imaging in presurgical evaluation of patients with medically intractable complex partial seizures. *Acta Neurologica Scandinavica* Suppl **152**:137–144.

Nordli DR, Bazil CW, Scheuer ML, Pedley TA (1997) Recognition and classification of seizures in infants. *Epilepsia* **38**:553–560.

Penfield W, Jasper H (1954) *Epilepsy and the Functional Anatomy of the Brain*. Boston: Little, Brown.

Sackeim H, Greenberg M, Weiman A (1982) Hemispheric asymmetry in the expression of positive or negative emotions. *Archives of Neurology* **39**:210–218.

Sethi P, Rao T (1976) Gelastic, quiritarian and cursive epilepsy. *Journal of Neurology, Neurosurgery and Psychiatry* **39**:823–828.

Wieser HG (1983) *Electroclinical features of the psychomotor seizure*. New York: G Fischer.

Williamson P, Wieser HG (1987) Clinical characteristics of partial seizures. In: Engel J (ed) *Surgical Treatment of the Epilepsies*, pp 101–120. New York: Raven Press.

Wyllie E, Chee M, Granstrom ML *et al* (1993) Temporal lobe epilepsy in early childhood. *Epilepsia* **34**:859–868.

Parietal lobe epilepsy

PD WILLIAMSON

INTRODUCTION

The enormous growth in centers specializing in the management of epilepsy that include surgical intervention have served to emphasize the importance of differentiating the varieties of localization-related epilepsy (Lüders 1992; Engel 1993). Perhaps in agreement with the early writings of John Hughlings Jackson (Jackson 1874), traditional attempts to subclassify these epilepsies have related to the lobe of origin. While it could legitimately be argued that such a method of classification is largely artificial, since seizures do not respect anatomic boundaries that themselves are partially artificial, this anatomic classification does serve a purpose: it allows investigators in the field to develop a system of communication and comparison. For example, it has long been recognized that most complex partial (psychomotor, temporal lobe) seizures begin in the temporal lobes (Penfield and Jasper 1954; Ajmone-Marsan and Ralston 1957; Bancaud *et al* 1965; Rasmussen 1975a). The syndrome of mesial temporal lobe epilepsy (MTLE) has been identified and well defined as the single, most common type of localization-related epilepsy encountered in adult populations (French *et al* 1993; Williamson *et al* 1993, 1998; Engel *et al* 1997). Similarly, various seizures originating in the frontal lobes have clinical characteristics that differentiate them from the more common temporal lobe seizures (Williamson *et al* 1985, 1997; Waterman *et al* 1987; Bancaud and Talairach 1992; Wieser *et al* 1992; Williamson 1995; Williamson and Engel 1997). Previous reports have described early signs and symptoms that help identify seizures originating in the occipital lobes, recognizing that multiple different potential spread patterns will define subsequent clinical events (Blume 1991; Salanova *et al* 1992; Williamson *et al* 1992a). The topic of this chapter, parietal lobe epilepsy, has proven more difficult to define accurately (Williamson *et al* 1992b; Cascino *et al* 1993).

PARIETAL LOBE EPILEPSY

Parietal lobe seizures are rare, constituting no more than 5% of all partial seizures reported from comprehensive surgical series (Rasmussen 1975b). While the epileptic significance of localized paresthesias has been recognized since antiquity (Temkin 1945), localizing and lateralizing significance have only been documented more recently (Penfield and Jasper 1954). Several reports and reviews have examined the clinical seizure characteristics, electroencephalographic findings, and results of neuroimaging studies in patients with carefully documented parietal lobe origin of seizure (Williamson *et al* 1992b; Cascino *et al* 1993; Ho *et al* 1994). In two of these studies (Williamson 1992b; Cascino *et al*

1993), all patients had circumscribed epileptogenic lesions, but in the third report, parietal lobe seizure origin was based upon ictal SPECT (single-photon emission computed tomography) results (Ho *et al* 1994). Ictal SPECT can, however, produce misleading data (Thadani *et al* 1995).

Most partial seizures consist of subjective and objective components. In parietal lobe seizures, the most common subjective sensations or auras are paresthesias, usually numbness and tingling but also a 'pins and needles' sensation, and rarely crawling or itching. Ictal paresthesias, however, occurred in less than half of patients reported in recent parietal lobe epilepsy series (Williamson *et al* 1992b; Cascino *et al* 1993). Furthermore, these somatosensory symptoms were not always lateralized. Even when lateralized, they were not always contralateral to the side of seizure origin, presumably reflecting activity in secondary sensory systems (Williamson *et al* 1992b).

Pain as a subjective ictal phenomenon has been recognized for over 100 years (Reynolds 1861; Gowers 1901). Young and Blume (1983) examined ictal pain in patients with this symptom as part of their seizures and identified three types of pain. The most common variety of pain was a burning dysesthesia. This involved part or all of the hemibody contralateral to the parietal lobe of seizure origin. Abdominal pain was the second most common type and was associated with temporal lobe seizure origin. Abdominal pain has also been associated with parietal lobe seizure origin (Cascino *et al* 1993; Sveinbjornsdottir and Duncan 1993). Ictal head pain was the least common variety and had no localizing value. A recent report examined epileptic pain and reported contralateral peripheral dysesthesias and abdominal pain, and unilateral head pain in seizures with parietal seizure origin (Siegel *et al* 1999).

Sveinbjornsdottir and Duncan (1993) extensively reviewed parietal lobe seizures. They described paresthetic, dysesthetic, and painful symptoms. They also described additional parietal lobe symptoms, including sexual sensations, apraxias, and disturbances of body image. Gustatory hallucinations have been associated with seizure activity in the parietal operculum, but also with seizures or stimulation in the insula and the amygdala (Hauser-Hauw and Bancaud 1987). Conversely, much of the parietal lobe may be clinically silent in terms of seizure manifestations or only demonstrable during extraordinary circumstances. For example, while undergoing electrocorticography under local anesthesia, a patient from the Montreal program had an electrically induced seizure that remained restricted to the parietal lobe (Penfield and Jasper 1954, p 724). During the seizure, two-point discrimination was impaired in the contralateral hand but returned to normal when the seizure was over. The patient was unaware of any specific symptoms.

Episodes with diagnostic criteria for panic attacks have been described in patients with parietal lobe seizure origin (Alemayehu *et al* 1995). Rarely, parietal lobe seizures can be precipitated by complex somatosensory afferent input (Williamson *et al* 1992b) (see patient 1 reported below).

There are few conceivable objective manifestations of seizures confined to the parietal lobes. Seizures confined to the dominant parietal lobe could produce disturbances in language function, demonstrable by specific testing. One of our patients with a neurocytoma in the parietal lobe had inhibitory motor seizures or ictal hemiplegia (patient 2). Most objective manifestations of parietal lobe seizures, however, would reflect seizure spread outside of the parietal lobe – (1) anteriorly into the frontal lobe; (2) inferiorly into the temporal lobe; or (3) posteriorly into the occipital lobe — with seizure characteristics corresponding to the direction of spread. As such, tonic motor activity, automatisms, or both can occur in patients with parietal lobe seizure origin. Asymmetrical tonic posturing was shown to be due to spread from parietal lobe to supplementary motor area (SMA) during a depth electrode study (Williamson *et al* 1992b), but this was specifically not observed in another study of parietal lobe seizures using invasive monitoring (Geier *et al* 1977).

Seizures originating in the parietal lobes that spread to medial temporal structures have been well documented using intracranial recording (Geier *et al* 1977; Williamson *et al* 1992b). When this happens, the clinical seizure characteristics will resemble temporal lobe seizures. Two patients with unsuspected parietal lobe seizure origin underwent unsuccessful temporal lobe surgeries in the Yale series (Williamson *et al* 1992b), as did two patients from the series reported by Ho (Ho *et al* 1994). In the two patients from the Yale series, parietal lobe seizure origin was considered likely after parietal lobe lesions were detected using previously unavailable MRI, and was verified following successful surgery that removed the lesion and limited surrounding brain. Ictal SPECT was used to determine parietal lobe seizure origin in the study of Ho and colleagues. This included the two patients with prior unsuccessful temporal lobectomies.

The region of seizure origin within the parietal lobe may correspond with certain clinical characteristics. Seizures beginning in the anterior part are more often associated with contralateral sensorimotor phenomena, while posterior parietal origin is associated with automatisms, unresponsiveness, and other complex clinical manifestations (Cascino *et al* 1993; Ho *et al* 1994). These posteriorly originating seizures were also described as 'psychoparetic,' which implied a psychic aura such as *déja vu* or fear followed by impairment of consciousness and motor arrest

(Ho *et al* 1994). Some patients with parietal lobe seizure origin had elementary visual hallucinations or ictal amaurosis as initial seizure symptoms, indicating spread to the occipital lobe from 'silent' posterior parietal foci (Williamson *et al* 1992b; Cascino *et al* 1993).

Scalp electroencephalograms were evaluated in a series of patients with well-documented parietal lobe epilepsy (Williamson *et al* 1992b). In most patients, the interictal EEGs were either normal, nonspecific, or misleading. EEGs were clearly localized or lateralized to the side of seizure origin in only one patient.

All patients from two studies of parietal lobe epilepsy had probable epileptogenic lesions detected with MRI (Williamson *et al* 1992b; Cascino *et al* 1993). Signs and symptoms of parietal lobe seizures were analyzed retrospectively. Although some findings suggested parietal lobe seizures, most patients had no clinical seizure manifestations until after seizures had spread beyond the parietal lobe. This observation leads to two conclusions. First, most of the parietal lobe is clinically silent in terms of seizures, and second (following from the first conclusion) most patients with parietal lobe seizure origin consequently will not have a clinically localizable form of localization-related epilepsy. These observations, coupled with misleading scalp EEG findings, almost certainly explain some of the surgical failures in patients with normal neuroimaging studies, including those studied with invasive EEG, but without coverage of the parietal lobe.

ILLUSTRATIVE CASE REPORTS

PATIENT 1

This 41-year-old woman began having seizures when 13 years old. The first episode consisted of left-side numbness and left hemianopsia that lasted several minutes and was followed by a headache. She was diagnosed with migraine. Typical episodes ultimately evolved into generalized tonic–clonic seizures, and the diagnosis of epilepsy was established. After initiation of treatment with antiepileptic drugs, the seizures changed. She no longer had somatosensory symptoms. She experienced complete visual loss before some, but not all, seizures. She then had generalized tonic, but not clonic motor activity. In most seizures consciousness was lost, but in some it was not. When aware during seizures, she could hear but reported that she could not see or speak. Seizures were brief, lasting about 15 seconds, but were frequent, occurring many times a day. Several times a month, seizures would occur almost continuously for

several hours. If standing, she would fall and sustain injuries, some near fatal. Multiple antiepileptic drugs, alone and in combination, failed to control her seizures and she was evaluated for surgery. Interictal scalp EEG revealed an active right parietal spike focus (Fig. 7.1). This was the only patient from the Yale series (Williamson *et al* 1992b) who had a relatively well-localized and lateralized EEG. There were less active independent sharp wave foci in the right temporal and left frontal regions. Ictal scalp recordings were obscured by muscle artifact. Videotaped seizures revealed tonic contraction of facial muscles producing a grimace or pucker, and tonic contraction of the hands and arms with clenched fists and with both arms held in flexion across her chest. Both legs were held in tonic extension. There was consistent right head deviation. During monitoring, seizures frequently occurred when she was trying to open a container or package. Only then was it learned that the patient was well aware that this type of kinesthetic input frequently precipitated seizures. Cranial CT was normal. Retrospectively, MRI from an early research 0.3 T machine revealed a possible right parietal convexity lesion. Subdural and depth electrodes were placed to sample the left and right medial frontal regions, right medial and lateral occipital regions, right medial and lateral parietal regions, and right medial and anterior temporal lobe regions. Numerous

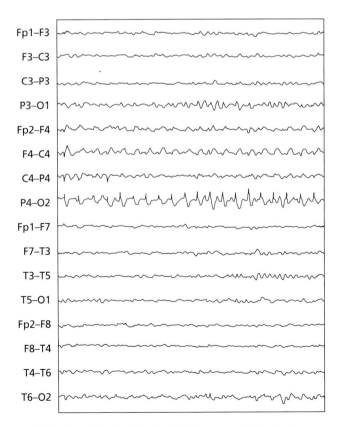

Fig. 7.1 Patient 1. Active interictal right parietal (P4) spike focus.

subclinical and typical clinical seizures were recorded. Subclinical seizures were well localized to the right parietal convexity, but clinical seizures were associated with rapid spread to both supplementary motor areas. Early occipital lobe seizure spread occurred in some seizures, but ictal amaurosis was not described during intracranial recording. At surgery, an intra-axial lesion was found in the middle of the right parietal convexity. Pathologic diagnosis was hamartoma. She had a few brief seizures during the first postoperative year, but then became seizure-free and has remained so for 14 years.

Comment

This patient, whose initial presentation was strongly suggestive of migraine, was ultimately found to have parietal lobe epilepsy. She had the unusual finding of kinesthetic precipitation of seizures. She also clearly described ictal amaurosis at the onset of some of her seizures, a symptom most often associated with occipital lobe seizure origin (Williamson *et al* 1992a). Presumably, this was due to posterior seizure spread, but we were unable to document this during invasive monitoring. Finally, the consistent asymmetrical tonic seizures, while more typical of frontal lobe seizure origin, have been described in well-documented parietal lobe epilepsy both with and without evidence of spread to the supplementary motor area (Geier *et al* 1977; Williamson *et al* 1992b).

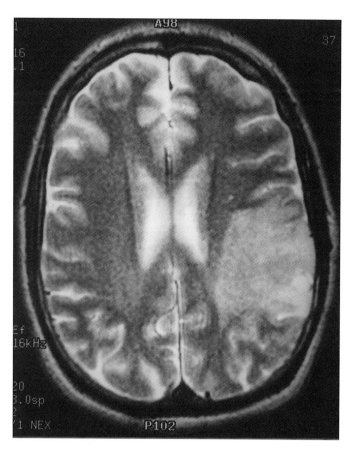

Fig. 7.2 Patient 2. T2-weighted MRI with lesion and surrounding edema in left parietal lobe (left on right).

PATIENT 2

This 37-year-old, right-handed man had a 3-month history of recurrent spells consisting of an unpleasant burning sensation in his right hand that would spread up his arm and into his face. His trunk and right leg were not involved. As soon as he experienced the painful dysesthesia, he developed right-sided weakness and could not speak. Occasionally, he would also develop clonic twitching in his right face, but no other tonic or clonic activity. The ictal aphasia and right hemiplegia would persist for as long as 10 minutes during the postictal period.

MRI showed a lesion in the left parietal lobe that extended into the left posterior frontal lobe (Fig. 7.2). He was evaluated for surgery. Recorded seizures were as described with ictal hemiplegia and aphasia associated with burning dysesthesias on the right, followed by prolonged right postictal hemiplegia and aphasia. There was no tonic or clonic motor activity. Interictal and ictal scalp EEGs provided no useful information. An 8 × 8 subdural grid was placed over the lesion for functional mapping and recording of seizures. Resection of the entire lesion could not be done because of the risks to language and motor function. The region of brain and underlying lesion in the parietal lobe from which the intracranially recorded seizures appeared to originate consistently was resected. Pathologic diagnosis was a neurocytoma. Although post operative seizures initially occurred very infrequently, he was re-admitted 1 year after surgery, having seizures without pain, but otherwise typical, occurring every 30 minutes. He was ultimately much better controlled with medications. Four years after surgery, he continues to have one mild seizure per month.

Comment

This patient provides an example of lateralized ictal pain in seizures originating in the parietal lobe. The elimination of pain, but not the seizures, following a limited parietal cortical resection would suggest that this symptom of pain was of parietal lobe origin. The ictal and postictal aphasia are not surprising findings, but ictal hemiplegia is an uncommon phenomenon.

PATIENT 3

Sixteen years before examination, this 57-year-old man began having seizures consisting of 1-minute periods of confusion and disorientation. He was found to have a large right-sided meningioma overlying the parietal lobe adjacent to the midline. The meningioma was resected. Four months later he had two generalized convulsive seizures. These were controlled with medication, but he then developed very unusual seizures consisting of nausea, an 'alien hand' on the left that he did not recognize as his own, loss of motor control on the left, and mild confusion. Four years before his most recent surgery, the character of the seizures changed dramatically. They began as described, but he would then develop severe cramping, left-sided abdominal pain, and intense 'pins and needles' sensations in his left hand, arm, trunk, and leg, sparing the face. The seizures occurred weekly and would last for hours or until given benzodiazepines intravenously. Seizures were otherwise not controlled with a variety of antiepileptic drugs, alone or in combination. He was evaluated for surgery. MRI revealed encephalomalacia in the right high parietal convexity extending to the midline (Fig. 7.3a,b). Scalp EEG revealed continuous interictal sharp and slow activity over the right parietal lobe (Fig. 7.4). Ictal SPECT was strongly positive in the right parietal region (Fig. 7.5). During the evaluation, the alien hand sensation was described during the seizures, and the agonizing left abdominal pain was dramatically documented. He underwent resection of the gliotic parietal tissue after intracranial subdural grid recording documented limited parietal lobe seizure origin. Immediately post surgery, he developed touch-sensitive left-sided choreoathetosis that resolved spontaneously in 1 week. Six weeks after surgery, he developed a progressive left hemiparesis over several days, culminating in an isolated left focal motor clonic seizure that was followed by hemiparesis with a strong apractic component. MRI showed postoperative changes and right centroparietal edema. This complication, which was thought to be due to a cerebral venous occlusion, resolved completely over 3 weeks. There have been no habitual seizures during the year since surgery.

Comment

This patient provides a dramatic example of parietal lobe seizures with severe abdominal pain. This very stoic former tractor-trailer driver was in such excruciating pain during seizures that reviewing his videotaped events was an unpleasant experience. The ictal symptom of an alien hand is extremely uncommon. The unusual postoperative complications were not expected, but fortunately they resolved completely over time.

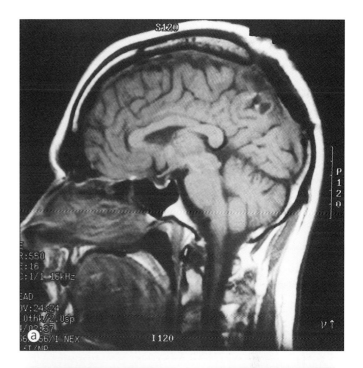

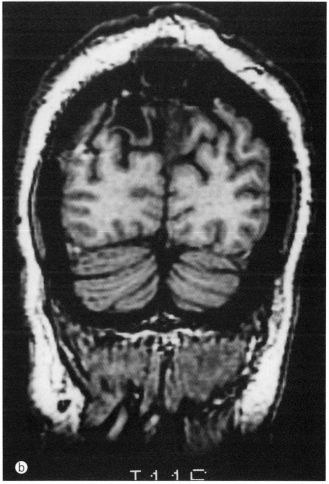

Fig. 7.3 Patient 3. (a) MRI showing lesion in right medial parietal lobe. (b) MRI showing cross-section of lesion through the right parietal lobe (right on left).

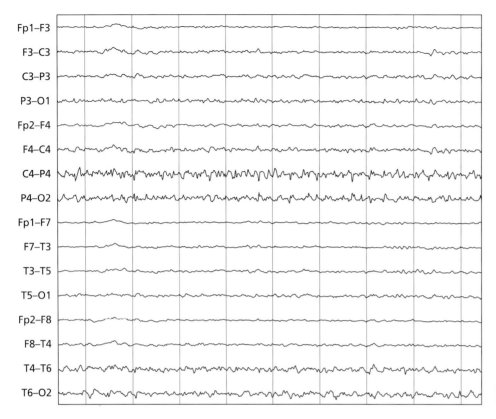

Fig. 7.4 Patient 3. Active right parietal (P4) sharp and slow focus.

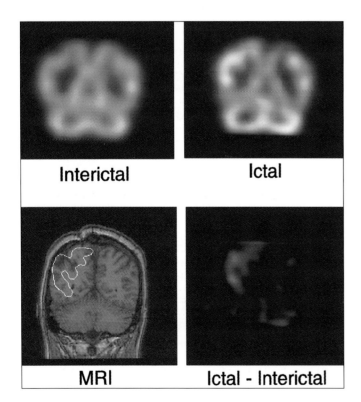

Fig. 7.5 Patient 3. SPECT study. Upper left and right: interictal and ictal SPECT scans Lower right: SPECT subtraction study. Lower left: SPECT subtraction study coregistered with MRI.

SUMMARY AND CONCLUSIONS

When symptoms such as lateralized paresthesias or pain occur prominently and early in partial seizures, parietal lobe seizure origin should be suspected. However, most patients with parietal lobe seizures have no symptoms or signs suggesting the parietal lobe. In the absence of detectable epileptogenic lesions, these patients without clinical seizure characteristics that suggest parietal lobe origin can present with very misleading findings, resulting in erroneous localization that can, in turn, lead to ineffective surgical intervention (Williamson *et al* 1992b; Ho *et al* 1994). Although ictal SPECT might provide vital evidence of parietal lobe seizure origin (Ho *et al* 1994), as noted previously, this technology can also produce misleading data in some patients (Thadani *et al* 1995).

Even when parietal lobe seizure origin is suspected, documenting this with invasive monitoring can be difficult in the absence of a structural lesion. The parietal lobes, like the frontal lobes, are large, diffuse structures, and the potential for sampling error is high (Williamson 1992). Spread patterns are unpredictable and can result in false localization (Williamson *et al* 1992b). Even with extensive and repetitive invasive studies, localization can prove elusive

(Siegel, to be published in *Epilepsia*). In the modern literature there are no well-documented series of patients with nonlesional parietal lobe epilepsy who have been cured by surgery, owing to a combination of the rarity of the condition and the lack of correct recognition, as well as the difficulty of localization.

Patients with medically intractable parietal lobe seizures can experience excellent surgical results (Williamson *et al* 1992b; Cascino *et al* 1993). Postoperative parietal lobe findings, even when extreme, are usually not enduring (patient 3). However, one of our patients did develop a chronic pain syndrome (Siegel, 1999).

KEY POINTS

1. Parietal lobe seizures are rare.
2. Many patients with parietal lobe seizure origin have no signs or symptoms to indicate parietal lobe origin.
3. In the absence of detectable parietal lobe lesions, parietal lobe seizure origin is often not suspected.
4. Lateralized ictal pain is a symptom of parietal lobe seizure origin.

REFERENCES

Ajmone-Marsan C, Ralston BL (1957) *The Epileptic Seizure. Its Functional Morphology and Diagnostic Significance*, pp 211–215. Springfield, IL: Charles C. Thomas.

Alemayehu S, Bergey GK, Barry E *et al* (1995) Panic attacks as ictal manifestations of parietal lobe seizures. *Epilepsia* **38**:824–830.

Bancaud J, Talairach J (1992) Clinical semiology of frontal lobe seizures. In: Chauvel P, Delgado-Escueta AV, Halgren E, Bancaud J (eds) *Frontal Lobe Seizures and Epilepsies*, pp 3–58. New York: Raven Press.

Bancaud J, Talairach J, Bonis A *et al* (1965) *La Stereo Electroencephalographie dans l'Epilepsie*. Paris: Masson.

Blume WT (1991) Occipital lobe epilepsies. In: Lüders H (ed) *Epilepsy Surgery*, pp 167–171. New York: Raven Press.

Cascino GD, Hulihan JF, Sharbrough FW, Kelly PK (1993) Parietal lobe lesional epilepsy: electroclinical correlation and operative outcome. *Epilepsia* **34**:522–527.

Engel J Jr (1993) *Surgical Treatment of the Epilepsies*, 2nd edn. New York: Raven Press.

Engel J Jr, Williamson PD, Wieser HG (1997) Mesial temporal lobe epilepsy. In: Engel J Jr, Pedley TA (eds) *Epilepsy: A Comprehensive Textbook*, pp 2417–2426. Philadelphia: Lippincott-Raven.

French JA, Williamson PD, Thadani VM *et al* (1993) Characteristics of medial temporal lobe epilepsy I. Results of history and physical examination. *Annals of Neurology* **34**:774–780.

Geier S, Bancaud J, Talairach J, Bonis A, Hossard-Bouchard H, Enjelvin M (1977) Ictal tonic postural changes and automatisms of the upper limb during epileptic parietal lobe discharges. *Epilepsia* **18**:517–524.

Gowers W (1901) *Epilepsy and Other Chronic Convulsive Disorders: Their Causes, Symptoms and Treatment* pp. 29–58. London: Churchill.

Hauser-Hauw C, Bancaud J (1987) Gustatory hallucinations in epileptic seizures: electrophysiological, clinical and anatomical correlates. *Brain* **110**:339–359.

Ho SS, Berkovic SF, Newton MR, Austin MC, McKay WJ, Bladin PF (1994) Parietal lobe epilepsy: clinical features and seizure localization by ictal SPECT. *Neurology* **44**:2277–2284.

Jackson JH (1874) *Selected Writings of John Hughlings Jackson*. London: Staples Press.

Lüders HO (1992) *Epilepsy Surgery*. New York: Raven Press.

Penfield W, Jasper H (1954) *Epilepsy and the Functional Anatomy of the Human Brain*. Boston: Little, Brown.

Rasmussen T (1975a) Surgical treatment of patients with complex partial seizures In: Penry JK, Daly DD (eds) *Complex Partial Seizures and Their Treatment*, pp 415–449. New York: Raven Press.

Rasmussen T (1975b) Surgery for epilepsy arising in regions other than the temporal and frontal lobes. In: Purpura DP, Penry JK, Walter RD (eds) *Neurosurgical Management of the Epilepsies*, pp. 207–226. New York: Raven Press.

Reynolds JR (1861) *Epilepsy: Its Symptoms, Treatment and Relation to Other Chronic Convulsive Diseases*. London: J & A Churchill.

Salanova V, Andermann F, Olivier A, Rasmussen T, Quesney LF (1992) Occipital lobe epilepsy: electroclinical manifestations, electrocorticography, cortical stimulation and outcome in 42 patients treated between 1930 and 1991. *Brain* **115**:1655–1680.

Siegel AM, Williamson PD, Roberts DW, Thadani VM, Darcey TM (1999) Localized pain associated with seizures originating in the parietal lobe. *Epilepsia* **40**(7):845–855.

Sveinbjornsdottir S, Duncan JS (1993) Parietal and occipital lobe epilepsy: a review. *Epilepsia* **34**:493–521.

Temkin O (1945) *The Falling Sickness*. Baltimore: Johns Hopkins Press.

Thadani VM, Darcey TM, Williamson PD, Lewis PJ, Siegel A (1995) Consistent and inconsistent findings with ictal SPECT. *Epilepsia* **36**:14.

Waterman K, Purves SJ, Kosaka B, Strauss E, Wada JA (1987) An epileptic syndrome caused by mesial frontal lobe foci. *Neurology* **37**:577–582.

Wieser HG, Swartz BE, Delgado-Escueta AV *et al* (1992) Differentiating frontal lobe seizures from temporal lobe seizures. In: Chauvel P, Delgado-Escueta AV (eds) *Frontal Lobe Seizures and Epilepsies*, Vol 57, Advances in Neurology, pp 267–285. New York: Raven Press.

Williamson PD (1992) Frontal lobe seizures: problems of diagnosis and classification. In: Chauvel P, Delgado-Escueta AV, Halgren E, Bancaud J (eds) *Frontal Lobe Seizures and Epilepsies*, Vol 57, Advances in Neurology, pp. 289–309. New York: Raven Press.

Williamson PD (1995) Frontal lobe epilepsy: some clinical characteristics. In: Jasper HH, Riggio S, Goldman-Rakic PS (eds) *Epilepsy and the Functional Anatomy of the Frontal Lobe*, pp 127–152. New York: Raven Press.

Williamson PD, Engel J Jr (1997) Complex partial seizures. In: Engel J Jr, Pedley TA (eds) *Epilepsy: A Comprehensive Textbook*, pp 557–566. Philadelphia: Lippincott-Raven.

Williamson PD, Spencer DD, Spencer SS, Novelly RA, Mattson RH

(1985) Complex partial seizures of frontal lobe origin. *Annals of Neurology* **18**:497–504.

Williamson PD, Thadani VM, Darcey TM, Spencer DD, Spencer SS, Mattson RH (1992a) Occipital lobe epilepsy: clinical characteristics, seizures spread patterns and results of surgery. *Annals of Neurology* **31**:3–13.

Williamson PD, Boon PA, Thadani VM *et al* (1992b) Parietal lobe epilepsy: diagnostic considerations and results of surgery. *Annals of Neurology* **31**:193–201.

Williamson PD, French JA, Thadani VM *et al* (1993) Characteristics of medial temporal lobe epilepsy II. Interictal and ictal scalp electroencephalography, neuropsychological testing, neuroimaging, surgical results and pathology. *Annals of Neurology* **34**:781–787.

Williamson PD, Engle J Jr, Munari C (1997) Anatomic classification of localization-related epilepsies. In: Engel J Jr, Pedley TA (eds) *Epilepsy: A Comprehensive Textbook*, pp 2405–2416. Philadelphia: Lippincott-Raven.

Williamson PD, Thadani VM, French JA *et al* (1998) Medial temporal lobe epilepsy: videotape analysis of objective clinical seizure characteristics. *Epilepsia* **39**(1):1182–1188.

Young GB, Blume WT (1983) Painful epileptic seizures. *Brain* **106**:537–554.

Occipital seizures

R GUERRINI, L PARMEGGIANI, E BERTA, AND C MUNARI[1]

8

Patients with occipital seizures diagnosed by means of clinical and electrographic criteria, including idiopathic occipital epilepsies, constitute about 8% of those referred to epilepsy centers (Gibbs and Gibbs 1953). Those submitted to surgical treatment represent no more than 5% of large epilepsy surgery series (Talairach *et al* 1974; Rasmussen 1975; Williamson *et al* 1992). There was no patient with pure occipital lobe epilepsies in the 59 consecutive patients operated on by Kahane and colleagues (1993) but four patients had multilobar epileptogenic zones including the occipital lobe. In a recently reported series of 35 patients operated on for occipital lobe epilepsy (Aykut-Bingol *et al* 1998), neuropathologic examination demonstrated that developmental and neoplastic lesions form the overwhelming majority of the underlying types of pathology, accounting for 40% and 37% of structural lesions, respectively. Birth injury was reported in one-fourth of 42 patients with occipital lobe epilepsy operated at the Montreal Neurological Institute (Salanova *et al* 1992). Although such figures are influenced by a selection bias linked to surgical recruitment, these three etiological groupings account for the most significant proportion of symptomatic occipital epilepsies.

Despite representing only 10% of cerebral matter, for various and often poorly understood reasons the occipital lobes are the elective site of a number of epileptogenic structural abnormalities that can lead to well-defined anatomic clinical syndromes. Therefore, when a patient's clinical seizure semeiology is clearly indicative of occipital origin, investigations should first aim to determine whether the epilepsy can be described in terms of a recognizable syndrome. Clinical seizure semeiology, per se, does not necessarily show distinctive patterns that can be of assistance in differentiating an idiopathic epilepsy from a symptomatic form (Van den Hout *et al* 1997). Investigations designed to study the etiology in greater depth are almost always appropriate.

---

[1] Late Professor Claudio Munari.

ETIOLOGY

ISCHEMIC BRAIN LESIONS

Perinatal occlusion of the posterior cerebral artery produces atrophy of the occipitoposterior temporal region that may result in occipital and temporal seizures, with onset from infancy to adulthood (Remillard *et al* 1974; Roger *et al* 1977; Deonna and Prodhom 1980). Unsuspected small cerebral infarctions involving the posterior brain regions are not uncommon both in children and adults. Multifocal ischemic lesions resulting from systemic perfusion failure predominate in the posterior watershed brain areas, and are frequently accompanied by occipital seizures (Fig. 8.1a).

Ulegyria, a peculiar configuration of the gyri in which the depth of the gyrus is more shrunken than the superficial portion, creating a mushroom appearance, is most commonly seen in the boundary zone between the anterior and middle, or middle and posterior cerebral arteries (Friede 1989; Barkovich 1995). It results from hypoxic–ischemic injuries occurring in the full-term newborn and should be carefully looked for in the MRI of patients with parietooccipital seizures of apparent cryptogenic origin.

ECLAMPSIA

Occipital lobe epilepsy can represent a rare complication of eclampsia (Plazzi *et al* 1994a). In this condition, transient clinical and structural occipital lobe involvement presenting

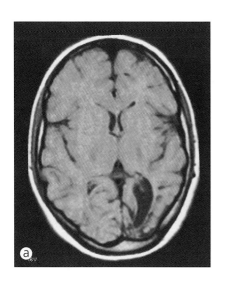
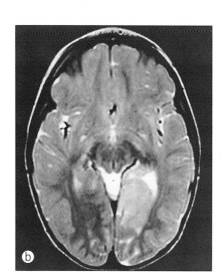
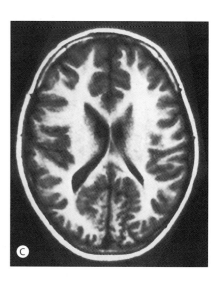
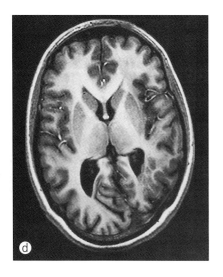
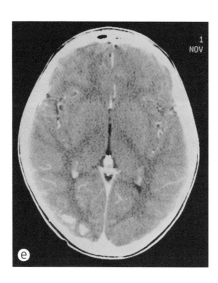

Fig. 8.1 (a) Axial T1-W MRI of a girl with a history of perinatal suffering producing an ischemic lesion in the region of the left posterior cerebral artery. Note the atrophic lesion involving the left occipital and posterior temporal cortex. (b) Axial T2-W MRI of an infant with a large area of cortical dysplasia involving the left occipital and inferior temporal cortex. (c) Axial IR-W MRI. Bilateral parasagittal parietooccipital polymicrogyria. (d) Axial FSPGR-W MRI. Gray-matter heterotopia involving the left occipital and posterior temporal lobes, which are reduced in size. Areas of heterotopia are scattered from the wall of the occipital horn of the left lateral ventricle to the overlying subcortex. (e) CT scan of a boy with celiac disease and occipital calcifications. This CT scan was performed after the onset of visual seizures that brought the child to medical attention. Later investigations (antigliadin antibodies and jejunal biopsy) confirmed the clinical suspicion of celiac disease).

the characters of hypertensive encephalopathy is frequently observed (Raroque *et al* 1990). Only rarely is this followed by occipital epilepsy, which is possibly correlated with an increased risk of border zone cerebral damage accompanying excessively vigorous treatment of hypertension (Plazzi *et al* 1994a).

MALFORMATIONS OF CORTICAL DEVELOPMENT

Most malformations involving the occipital lobe(s) are diffuse and may lead to multiple seizure types. However, some malformations, such as focal cortical dysplasia (Taylor *et al* 1971) (Fig. 8.1b), polymicrogyria (Guerrini *et al* 1997a) (Fig. 8.1c) or gray-matter heterotopia (Tampieri *et al* 1996) (Fig. 8.1d), may be limited to or predominant in the occipital lobe(s) (Guerrini *et al* 1997a; Aykut Bingol *et al* 1998; Kuzniecky 1998). Although characteristics of clinical seizures are generally similar to those of patients with other structural lesions involving the occipital lobe, most patients with bilateral occipital malformations present with seizures characterized by sudden loss of contact without warning and late or no automatisms (Guerrini *et al* 1997a). It has been suggested that occipital lobe developmental lesions may less frequently lead to visual field defects than do other types of lesions (Kuzniecky 1998). However, there was no difference in the rate of visual field defects between patients with developmental lesions and those with tumors in the series reported by Aykut-Bingol and colleagues (1998). The most likely explanation is that destructive (vascular) occipital lesions are consistently accompanied by a visual field defect while nondestructive lesions may not be.

TUMORS

Low-grade astrocytomas and oligodendrogliomas are the types of tumors most frequently found in surgical series of patients affected by occipital seizures (Rasmussen 1975; Aykut-Bingol *et al* 1998). This is consistent with the overall distribution of epileptogenic tumors (Kim 1995; Kuzniecky and Jackson 1995). However, occipital lobe localization appears to be correlated with lower epileptogenicity with respect to other localizations (Paillas *et al* 1959). As it is generally observed in epilepsy symptomatic of brain tumors, occipital neoplasias have been associated with seizure onset more strictly localized within the lobe and with a much better postoperative seizure outcome than in the other etiologic groups (Cascino *et al* 1992; Britton *et al* 1994; Aykut-Bingol *et al* 1998).

STURGE–WEBER SYNDROME

Sturge–Weber syndrome is a rare, sporadic, mesodermic phakomatosis including venous malformation of leptomeninges (100% of cases) accompanied by nevus flammeus of the skin supplied by the trigeminal nerve (port-wine stain; 90% of cases) and, less often, by choroidal angioma and glaucoma. Although angiomatosis can be localized anywhere in the brain, it occurs more frequently in the occipital region. There may be progressive accumulation of calcium in the outer cortical zone and in the subependymal spaces of capillaries and small vessels, producing extensive cortical gliosis (Alexander 1972; Rasmussen *et al* 1972). This disorder has a potentially progressive course. Bilateral involvement is correlated with earlier seizure onset and worse developmental prognosis.

About 90% of patients have their first seizure within the first 3 years of life (Dulac and Roger 1980; Erba and Cavazzuti 1990; Rochkind *et al* 1990). Almost all the early seizures qualify as status epilepticus, and subsequent seizures are similar to the initial ones. Most patients have partial motor seizures, but occipital seizures are also reported (Rochkind *et al* 1990). Outcome after the first seizure is variable, but long-term follow-up has shown that seizures are often well controlled (Erba and Cavazzuti 1990). Neurologic deterioration and progressive parenchymal atrophy can occur even if epilepsy is not severe (Arzimanoglou and Aicardi 1992).

Isolated reports suggest that prophylactic treatment with barbiturates, starting from infancy, may be useful (Dulac *et al* 1982), but prospective studies are not available.

Interictal EEG in Sturge–Weber syndrome shows focal or unilateral depression of background activity over the area of leptomeningeal angiomatosis (Brenner and Sharbrough 1976; Sassower *et al* 1994). Polymorphic delta slowing is the next most frequent EEG abnormality and correctly lateralizes the angiomatosis when it is unilateral (Arzimanoglou and Aicardi 1992). Focal epileptiform abnormalities are infrequent (Sassower *et al* 1994).

Gadolinium-enhanced MRI is the best method for imaging pial angiomatosis, provided it is performed at least 3 weeks after status epilepticus (Aicardi 1994). MRI is also very sensitive for detecting parenchymal atrophy. Enhanced CT scanning permits imaging of the angioma and a hypertrophic choroid plexus (Welch *et al* 1980).

Surgery should be considered early when medical treatment fails. The earlier the surgery with respect to seizure onset, the less the chance of increased neurologic deterioration (Ogunmekan *et al* 1989). Approximately 40% of affected patients are surgical candidates. Only a minority of patients have been treated with occipital lobectomy for intractable seizures (Rosen *et al* 1984; Rochkind *et al*

1990), while most surgically treated patients undergo hemispherectomy for treatment of rapidly progressing unilateral disease (Hoffmann *et al* 1979). Seizure control is better achieved with larger resections (Rochkind *et al* 1990). The results of surgery are encouraging, with surgically treated patients having significantly better seizure control, no statistically different motor function, and much higher incidence of normal or borderline intelligence compared to conservatively treated children (Rochkind *et al* 1990).

EPILEPSY WITH OCCIPITAL CALCIFICATIONS

The association of unilateral (Fig. 8.1e) or bilateral occipital calcification and epilepsy has been reported by numerous authors (Sammaritano *et al* 1985 Gobbi *et al* 1988, 1992; Ambrosetto *et al* 1992; Magaudda *et al* 1993; Pascotto *et al* 1994). About 77% of patients with this picture have celiac disease (Gobbi *et al* 1997). Moreover, some patients with celiac disease may have occipital epilepsy without brain calcification (Ambrosetto *et al* 1992; Gobbi *et al* 1997). Whether patients with occipital calcification and without apparent celiac disease are carriers of a latent form of the disease is still a matter of debate (Lambertini *et al* 1997). Preferential involvement of the occipital lobe in patients with celiac disease and epilepsy, with or without calcification, remains unexplained. Since the occipital calcification bear resemblance to those observed in Sturge–Weber syndrome, a common origin has been suggested (Tiacci *et al* 1993). Pathologic findings obtained in two patients having occipital calcification who were operated on for intractable occipital lobe seizures (Bye *et al* 1993; Plazzi *et al* 1994b; Tinuper 1997) revealed confluent cortical microcalcification predominating in the deep cortical layers, small calcification in contact with the endothelium of intracortical capillaries, and a few foci of pial angiomatosis, with cortical blurring and neuronal loss (Tinuper 1997). These findings were distinct from those referring to Sturge–Weber syndrome, in which cortical architecture is better preserved. Children treated with X-rays and antifolate for leukemia may develop similar cerebral calcification (Young *et al* 1977), often accompanied by occipital epilepsy (Guerrini *et al* 1990).

Patients with posterior calcifications and epilepsy have varying clinical characteristics and outcome. An exhaustive review of published cases (Gobbi *et al* 1997) showed that age at onset of epilepsy, which was always partial, ranged between 1 and 28 years in the syndrome of celiac disease epilepsy and cerebral calcifications. Most patients had occipital seizures, which often became severe after an insidious onset. An additional feature of progression was rapid growth of calcification in patients not following a gluten-free diet. Early gluten-free diet seems to lead to seizure control, with arrest of growth of calcification. In other patients, good seizure outcome resembling benign occipital epilepsy could be achieved even without a gluten-free diet. Other types of partial seizures have been reported, often related to development of frontal lobe calcification (Gobbi *et al* 1992). The clinical picture is similar when epilepsy and occipital or parietooccipital calcification is observed in patients without celiac disease. However, it is unclear whether a gluten-free diet can influence outcome in the latter group.

In patients operated on for intractable occipital lobe seizures, calcification was unilateral in one (Plazzi *et al* 1994b), in whom surgery was unsuccessful (Tinuper 1997), but bilateral in the other (Bye *et al* 1989, 1993), in whom remission of seizures was achieved.

OCCIPITAL LOBE SEIZURES ASSOCIATED WITH MITOCHONDRIAL DISEASES

Patients with MELAS (mitochondrial encephalopathy, lactic acidosis, and strokelike episodes) and MERRF (myoclonus epilepsy with ragged red fibers) have heterogeneous ages at onset of symptoms, clinical presentation, and progression of the disease. Some of them may present with occipital lobe seizures (Montagna *et al* 1988; So *et al* 1989) having ictal visual phenomena as the presenting symptom. In MELAS, initial occipital seizures are often easily controllable and are accompanied by migrainous attacks. With disease progression, multiple types of neurologic deficits occur, seizures become intractable and may be accompanied by development of epilepsia partialis continua. Bilateral occipital ischemic lesions may determine cortical blindness. Both MELAS and MERRF patients are often photosensitive (So *et al* 1989).

LAFORA BODY DISEASE

Lafora body disease is transmitted in an autosomal recessive fashion; the gene has been localized to chromosome 6 (Serratosa *et al* 1995) but the exact mechanism involved in the disease has not yet been elucidated. Onset of symptoms occurs between age 6 and 19 years, with variable speed of disease progression (Roger *et al* 1992). Visual seizures with elementary hallucinations or scotomas are considered to occur in about half of patients as an early manifestation (Roger *et al* 1983; Tinuper *et al* 1983). There follows a severe myoclonic syndrome, rapidly accompanied by mental deterioration.

HYPERGLYCEMIA

Seizures are common in hyperglycemia and may be the presenting symptom, especially in nonketotic hyperglycemia. Although most patients present with partial motor seizures (Grant and Warlow 1985), occipital seizures with visual or versive symptoms have also been described (Duncan *et al* 1991; Harden *et al* 1991). Seizures disappear following correction of abnormal glucose levels, without need for antiepileptic drug treatment. Neuroimaging shows no abnormalities in these patients.

EARLY ICTAL MANIFESTATIONS AND SYMPTOMS RELATED TO EXTRAOCCIPITAL SEIZURE SPREAD

The clustering of symptoms and signs typical of occipital lobe seizure onset is usually recognizable by clinical characteristics (Williamson *et al* 1997). The ictal discharge originating in the occipital cortex may spread to anterior areas, above and below the sylvian fissure, both ipsilateral and contralateral to the occipital lobe of seizure origin (Ajmone-Marsan and Ralston 1957; Talairach *et al* 1974; Williamson *et al* 1992). Thus a potential for multiple patterns of spread may be observed even in the same patient (Bancaud *et al* 1961; Williamson *et al* 1992). This characteristic appears to be more pronounced in seizures of occipital origin than in those originating from other lobes (Williamson and Spencer 1986). Ictal recordings show that spreading may be either rapid or remarkably slow and can occur after many minutes of discharge limited to the occipital lobe (Jasper 1954; Naquet *et al* 1960, 1987; Aso *et al* 1988). When spread is rapid, early clinical features related to occipital lobe origin tend to be overshadowed by the most prominent manifestations resulting from involvement of extraoccipital structures.

Almost all patients experiencing subjective symptoms describe visual phenomena as the initial ictal manifestation. These are usually described as bright, colorful or multicolored, or occasionally dark rings or spots or simple geometric forms that are continuous or flashing, usually but not necessarily in the periphery of the contralateral visual field, rotating or moving slowly to the opposite side across the visual field (Penfield and Jasper, 1954; Rusell and Whitty, 1955; Davidson and Watson, 1956; Bancaud 1969; Ricci and Vigevano, 1993; Guerrini *et al* 1994, 1995; Williamson *et al* 1992). Initial symptoms are usually in the field contralateral to the side of seizure origin, sometimes in a quadrant or without a clear lateralization. Ictal amaurosis,

blindness, or severe blurring of vision, limited to one hemifield or quadrant or involving the entire visual field, may follow the visual hallucinations but may occasionally be the first symptom (Huott *et al* 1974; Aso *et al* 1988; Maeda *et al* 1990; Bauer *et al* 1991; Salanova *et al* 1992; Williamson *et al* 1992). Hemianopia and quadrantanopia have highly localizing value. However, sometimes it may be impossible to distinguish between ictal and postictal blindness. It is of paramount importance to test visual avoidance when witnessing a patient experiencing ictal or postictal visual symptoms.

More complex visual hallucinations include complex scenes often related to past experiences. They may be accompanied by macropsia, micropsia, or perception of scenes of peoples or animals described as static or moving horizontally, approaching or moving away (Blume 1991; Williamson *et al* 1992; Sveinbjornsdottir and Duncan 1993). Hallucinations may also include letters or numerals (Gastaut and Zifkin 1984; Sowa and Pituck, 1989). Patients are usually aware of the hallucinatory nature of the perception. Ictal activity producing complex hallucinations involves the occipital association cortex and the posterolateral temporal cortex.

Visual illusions of different kinds involving part or the whole of the visual field may be experienced during occipital lobe seizures (Sveinbjornsdottir and Duncan 1993). The simpler forms may feature alterations in the size, shape or motion of objects, or change in color quality with monochrome vision or lack of color (achromatopsia). More complex illusions may result in altered perception of objects in space, accentuating distance or proximity (Critchley 1949). Ictal palinopsia, i.e. the persistence or recurrence of visual images once the real object of perception is no longer present, is reported fairly frequently (Robinson and Watt 1947; Critchley 1951; Lefebre and Koelmel 1989). As this phenomenon often occurs with hallucinations, there may be difficulty in distinguishing the two components. (Aspects of differential diagnosis between occipital and parietal ictal manifestations have been reviewed by Bancaud *et al* 1991.)

Visual phenomena are often accompanied or followed by 'conscious' tonic or, rarely, clonic eye or eye and head deviation, usually but not always toward the side of the initial visual symptoms (in other words, contralateral to the side of seizure origin) (Bancaud 1969; Beun *et al* 1984; Munari *et al* 1984; Kanazawa *et al* 1989; Furman *et al* 1990; Salanova *et al* 1992; Williamson *et al* 1992; Guerrini *et al* 1995; Harris 1997). Clinically, it may be impossible to determine whether eye and head turning is part of the seizure or is related to attempts by the patient to follow the images and hallucinatory figures. However, ictal eye deviation has an initial tonic phase, corresponding to the sustained high-frequency ictal discharge, followed by a clonic phase, with eye jerks corresponding to the bursts of fast ictal activity interrupted by periods of electrical silence. Oculoclonic movements were defined by Gastaut as 'epileptic nystagmus' (Gastaut and Roger 1954; Gastaut 1960).

Eyelid flutter or forced blinking and a sensation of eye pulling represent further seizure manifestations that have been correlated with occipital localization of seizure discharges (Bancaud 1969; Holtzman and Goldensohn 1977; Munari *et al* 1984; Williamson *et al* 1992).

If a patient is able to recall visual symptoms this indicates the initial localization of the ictal discharge near the calcarine fissure, followed by slow propagation to adjacent areas. When the discharge is occipitotemporal at the onset, visual phenomena cannot usually be recalled (Munari *et al* 1993).

Spread of seizure activity to the contralateral occipital cortex is responsible for visual phenomena, both positive and negative, involving the entire visual field.

Infrasylvian propagation to mesiotemporal limbic structures, possibly through the inferior longitudinal fasciculus, is frequent (Jones and Powell 1970; Olivier *et al* 1982) and accompanied by automatisms typical of temporal lobe epilepsy (Bancaud *et al* 1961; Takeda *et al* 1969; Salanova *et al* 1992; Williamson *et al* 1992). The most frequent ictal pattern is a sequence of epigastric discomfort, unresponsiveness, and automatisms. Some patients experience vomiting, which seems to be particularly frequent in the course of prolonged seizures triggered by photic stimulation (Guerrini *et al* 1994, 1995).

Propagation to lateral occipital cortex and temporal neocortex is responsible for complex visual and auditory hallucinations (Penfield and Perot, 1963; Geier *et al* 1973; Munari *et al* 1993)

Suprasylvian propagation to the lateral motor cortex is accompanied by focal motor or hemiclonic activity and propagation to the supplementary sensorimotor cortex by asymmetric tonic posturing. (Jasper 1954; Naquet *et al* 1960; Davidoff and Johnson 1963; Fischer-Williams *et al* 1964; Takeda *et al* 1969; Babb *et al* 1981; Williamson and Spencer 1986; Aso *et al* 1988; Ricci and Vigevano 1993). Secondary generalization is very frequent when suprasylvian spread occurs.

Analysis of seizure semeiology and corticocortical spread indicates that about one-third of patients with occipital lobe seizure onset show frontal lobe-type seizure manifestations suggesting suprasylvian spread and one-third show temporal lobe-type manifestations suggesting infrasylvian spread (Williamson *et al* 1992). In addition, one-third of all patients have more than one seizure type, indicating multiple spread patterns (Salanova *et al* 1992; Williamson *et al* 1992; Aykut-Bingol *et al* 1998). Manifestations of seizure spread are often the most prominent clinical feature and tend to overshadow findings indicating occipital origin (Williamson *et al* 1997). According to Ajmone-Marsan and Ralston (1957), infrasylvian seizure spread occurs more frequently when seizure origin is below the calcarine fissure, while suprasylvian spread is most often related to supracalcarine seizure origin. However, analysis of the relationships between seizure spread patterns and site of seizure origin within the occipital lobe revealed no correlation in the study by Aykut-Bingol *et al* (1998) who, however, could demonstrate occipital seizure onset using

Fig. 8.2 (a) Stereo-EEG investigation, adapted to the anatomo-electro-clinical characteristics of this individual patient (Munari *et al* 1994b), by means of stereotactically implanted electrodes (lateral view). This procedure should allow verification of the origin of the ictal discharges in the lesion and its immediate periphery: electrode O investigates the lesion, the subcalcarine mesial occipital cortex, the white matter and the lateral occipital cortex; electrode Q investigates the supracalcarine cortex and the superior lateral occipital cortex; electrodes F, Z, P, and S investigate the parietal involvement up to the suprasylvian opercular cortex (electrode R); electrodes E, D, and T give information about the temporal involvement. (b) For investigated anatomic structures, see (a). Interictal recording. Background activity is normal in the mesial and lateral parietal cortex (S1, S3, and Z1), posterior part of the superior temporal gyrus (T1) and suprasylvian opercular region (R1). Subcontinuous theta–delta activity is recorded in the inferior lateral parietal cortex (P4, F3), posterior part of the second temporal gyrus (D3), and occipital lateral cortex (Q3). Continuous fast spiking is recorded in the supracalcarine (Q1) and subcalcarine (lesional) occipital cortex (O1). Activity recorded from the inferior lateral parietal cortex (P4) and the posterior part of the superior temporal gyrus (T1) is remarkably different, despite the proximity of the electrodes. Abnormalities in the lateral occipital cortex are discrete. EYES = electroculogram; SCMR = right sternocleidomastoideus muscle (c) For investigated anatomic structures, see (a). Immediately after the acceleration of the spikes in the occipital intralesional cortex, the patient reports a subjective symptom accompanying his habitual seizures. The acceleration of the discharge (2) concerns only mesial occipital cortex (O1, Q1) and the temporooccipital junction (E1), slightly affecting the lateral parietal cortex (F3, P4, T1) and lateral inferior occipital cortex (O3). Q3 and E3 are spared. Also note how the internal occipital discharge is appreciable on the right occipital region (see scalp EEG). Upper parietal areas remain indifferent as well as the opercular region. EYES = electroculogram; SCMR = right sternocleidomastoideus muscle. (d) For investigated anatomic structures, see (a). The evolution of the discharge is very similar in O1 and E1, whereas in the supracalcarine cortex (Q1) the rapidity decreases earlier. At the end of the discharge, note the major depression of the electrical activity in O1, E1, and Q1 but not in the cortical areas, which are only secondarily affected. EYES = electroculogram; SCMR = right sternocleidomastoideus muscle.

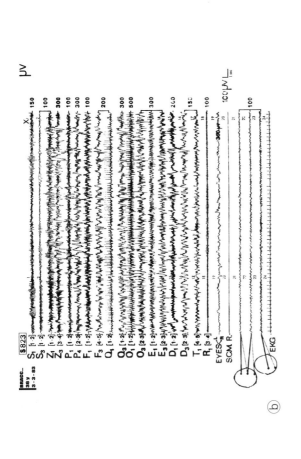

(b)

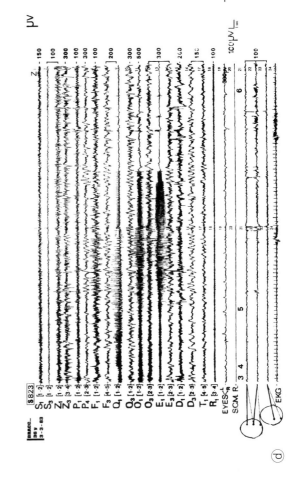

(d)

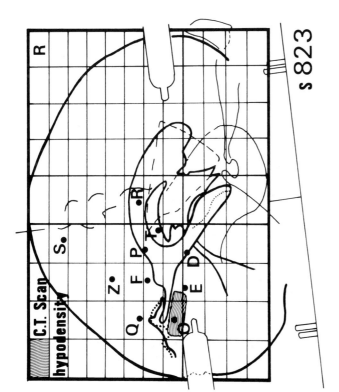

(a)

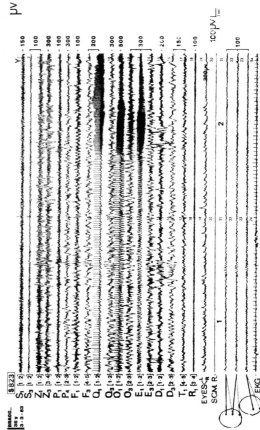

(c)

invasive monitoring in a limited number of patients. Furthermore, these authors observed no significant differences in seizure types between patients with developmental lesions and those with tumors or other structural abnormalities. Such findings were at variance with studies suggesting that developmental lesions are associated with multiple types of seizures (Palmini *et al* 1991).

There is very little information about the participation of the occipital lobe in patients with multi-lobar epilepsy. If the patients undergoing various types of hemispherectomy (Krynauw 1950, Rasmussen 1983, Olivier 1991) are included then such procedures account for 2.5–11% of the operations in the largest published epilepsy surgery series. In such series the commonest etiologies in patients undergoing these hemispherectomy variations are malformative-hamartomous lesions, encephalomalacia as a sequel to a severe hypoxic-ischemic episode (Farrel 1992) and Rasmussen's encephalitis. In a recent series of 23 consecutive patients with multi-lobar epilepsies in 1/11 cryptogenic patients and in 4/12 symptomatic patients the occipital lobe was included in the epileptogenic zone (Luders *et al* 1993, Munari *et al* 1994). This relatively high rate of occipital involvement (5/23: 22%) is similar to that observed by Salanova *et al* (1992) who reported that 14/42 multilobar resections included the occipital lobe.

PRECIPITATION OF OCCIPITAL SEIZURES BY VISUAL STIMULATION

Photosensitivity has predominantly been correlated with generalized epileptogenesis and identified, with few exceptions, within idiopathic generalized epilepsies. However, in about 20% of patients sensitive to photic stimulation, visually induced seizures are focal, originating from reflex activation in the occipital neocortex (Guerrini *et al* 1997b). Widespread exposure to television screens, computer monitors, and videogames has increased the time spent before such triggers and the number of observations. Photic triggering of partial seizures is also possible in the presence of epileptogenic lesions of the occipital cortex, producing both spontaneous and reflex seizures (Naquet *et al* 1960; Guerrini *et al* 1994). Isolated seizures provoked by intermittent photic stimulation (IPS) during EEG performed for reasons other than epilepsy have been reported in healthy subjects, as well as in alcoholic patients and in patients with migraine, cerebral palsy, and brain malformations (Bickford 1949; Davidoff and Johnson 1963; Courjon *et al* 1968; Beaumanoir and Jekiel 1987; Ricci and Vigevano 1993).

An idiopathic epileptic syndrome characterized by reflex occipital seizures has been identified (Guerrini *et al* 1995). This represents a form of pure focal reflex epilepsy with a specific mode of seizure precipitation, typical of adolescence. Correlation with other idiopathic partial epilepsies is suggested by the rolandic seizures or rolandic spikes seen in some patients (Guerrini *et al* 1997c), and by the giant visual evoked potentials (Guerrini *et al* 1997b). Photically induced occipital seizures are often characterized by the succession of visual and vegetative symptoms, sometimes with headache (Guerrini *et al* 1994, 1995). These seizures can be mistaken for migraine, especially if ictal activity does not spread above the sylvian fissure and no motor manifestations are recognizable.

In exceptional cases, visual stimuli have been demonstrated to induce mesiotemporal seizures without evidence of preceding ictal activity in the occipital lobe on either surface (Guerrini *et al* 1997b) or depth electrode (Isnard *et al* 1998) recordings.

INVESTIGATION OF PATIENTS WITH OCCIPITAL LOBE SEIZURES

When a patient's clinical seizure semeiology is clearly indicative of occipital origin, investigations should first aim to determine whether the epilepsy can be defined in terms of a recognizable syndrome. Clinical seizure semeiology, per se, may not show distinctive patterns that can be of assistance in differentiating an idiopathic epilepsy from a symptomatic (Van den Hout *et al* 1997).

VISUAL FIELD

Visual field assessment should be performed in every patient with occipital seizures. Visual field defects have been reported in over 50% of patients in several recent surgical series (Salanova *et al* 1992; Williamson *et al* 1992). A possible ascertainment bias should be taken into account, since patients referred for surgical treatment are more likely to have structural lesions.

INTERICTAL EEG

Routine EEG recordings in patients with clinically suspected occipital lobe seizure origin should always be performed using a median occipital electrode (Oz) as well as conventional 10–20 system electrodes (Guerrini *et al* 1995). In addition to improving the detection rate of abnormalities originating from the mesial surface, such a technique facilitates evaluation of background activity and of the many physiological activities whose maximum expression occurs in the occipital lobes (α rhythm, λ, posterior slowing in children). Although interictal paroxysmal EEG activity is commonly seen when occipital lobe seizures are present, only in a minority of these patients is such activity localized in the occipital lobes on scalp EEG recordings (Paillas *et al* 1959; Salanova *et al* 1992; Williamson *et al* 1992; Munari *et al* 1993; Aykut-Bingol *et al* 1998). In most patients spike or sharp waves are recorded over the temporal lobes and are bilateral independent in about one-fourth and bilaterally synchronous in more than one-third (Salanova *et al* 1993). Increase in posterior discharges upon eye closure is frequent in occipital epilepsies, both lesional and idiopathic. Intermittent photic stimulation may produce asymmetric photic driving, usually, but not necessarily, depressed on the side of the structural abnormality. A photoparoxysmal EEG response may be observed in about one-third of patients (Ludwig and Ajmone-Marsan 1975; Guerrini *et al* 1997b).

ICTAL EEG

Ictal recordings with surface electrodes may be electrically silent (Bancaud 1969) but frequently show regional discharges involving the occipital lobes as well as the posterior temporal lobes (Bancaud 1969; Williamson *et al* 1992; Munari *et al* 1993; Salanova *et al* 1993). Since clear-cut focal occipital involvement is seen in a minority of patients, scalp EEG findings are considered to be of little avail and often misleading for occipital lobe localization. Many authors believe that invasive EEG studies are necessary to clarify seizure origin and spread (Munari *et al* 1994b) (Fig. 8.2 a–d). Depth electrode studies confirm that, even when the clinical semeiology is strongly indicative of occipital origin, ictal discharges can involve the mesial temporal structures or the parietal cortex immediately or may originate either in occipital or extraoccipital structures (Williamson *et al* 1992; Munari *et al* 1993). The origin of the occipital discharge is more frequently pericalcarine, but there may also be simultaneous involvement of the lateral occipital cortex (Munari *et al* 1993).

KEY POINTS

1. Patients with occipital seizures constitute around 8% of those referred to epilepsy centers.
2. Developmental abnormalities, including Sturge–Weber syndrome, tumors, and birth trauma underlie most of the symptomatic epilepsies. Other causes include: ischemic lesions; occipital calcification, mostly in association with celiac disease; celiac disease without occipital calcification; mitochondrial disorders; hyperglycemia; and Lafora body disease.
3. Photic stimulation can precipitate seizures by activation of occipital cortex. An idiopathic epilepsy syndrome of reflex occipital seizures, representing a form of pure focal reflex epilepsy, has been identified. It is characterized by visual and vegetative symptoms, sometimes with headache, and it can be mistaken for migraine.
4. Ictal discharges originating in the occipital cortex have a potential for multiple spread patterns even in the same patient. Spread may be to cortex dorsal or ventral to the sylvian fissure, both ipsilateral and contralateral.
5. Visual phenomena are usually the first ictal feature in patients who experience subjective symptoms. When the spread is rapid, such symptoms may be overshadowed by manifestations arising from extraoccipital structures. Thus around 30% patients show frontal lobe-type seizure manifestations, aound 30% show temporal lobe-type manifestations, and around 30% have more than one seizure type.
6. Visual field assessment should be performed in every patient with occipital seizures.
7. Routine EEG recording should always use a median occipital electrode, in addition to the conventional 10–20 system, when occipital seizures are suspected. Interictal spike/sharp waves are recorded over the temporal lobes more often than occipitally and are frequently bilateral. Increase in posterior discharges on eye closure is common with occipital epilepsies.
8. Scalp EEG findings are often misleading for occipital lobe localization.

REFERENCES

Aicardi J (1994) *Epilepsy in Children*. New York: Raven Press.

Ajmone-Marsan C, Ralston B (1957) *The Epileptic Seizure: Its Functional Morphology and Diagnostic Significance*, pp 211–215. Springfield: Thomas.

Alexander GL (1972) Sturge–Weber syndrome. In: Vinken PJ, Bruyn GW (eds) *Handbook of Clinical Neurology*, vol 14, pp 223–240. Amsterdam: Elsevier.

Ambrosetto G, Antonini L, Tassinari CA (1992) Occipital lobe seizures related to clinically asymptomatic celiac disease in adulthood. *Epilepsia* 33:476–481.

Arzimanoglou A, Aicardi J (1992) The epilepsy of Sturge–Weber syndrome: clinical features and treatment in 23 patients. *Acta Neurologica Scandinavica* 86 (suppl. 140):18–22.

Aso K, Watanabe K, Negoro T *et al* (1988) Photosensitive partial seizure: the origin of abnormal discharges. *Journal of Epilepsy* 1:87–93.

Aykut-Bingol CA, Bronen RA, Kim JH *et al* (1998) Surgical outcome in occipital lobe epilepsy: implications for pathophysiology. *Annals of Neurology* 44:60–69.

Babb TL, Halgren E, Wilson C *et al* (1981) Neuronal firing patterns during the spread of an occipital lobe seizure to the temporal lobes in man. *Electroencephalography and Clinical Neurophysiology* 51:104–107.

Bancaud J (1969) Les crises épileptiques d'origine occipitale (étude stéréo électroencéphalographique). *Révue d'oto-neuroophthalmologie* 41:299–311.

Bancaud J, Bonis A, Morel P *et al* (1961) Epilepsie occipitale à expression 'rhinencéphalique' prévalente (corrélations électrocliniques à la lumière des investigations fonctionnelles stéréotaxiques). *Révue Neurologique* 105:219–220.

Bancaud J, Talairach J, Munari C, Giallonardo T, Brunet P (1991) Introduction à l'étude cliniques des crises épileptiques rétro-rolandiques. *Canadian Journal of Neurological Sciences* 18 (suppl. 4):566–569.

Barkovich AJ (1995) *Pediatric Neuroimaging*, 2nd edn. New York: Raven Press.

Bauer J, Schuler P, Feistel H, Hilz MJ, Stefan H (1991) Blindness as an ictal phenomenon: investigations with EEG and SPECT in two patients suffering from epilepsy. *Journal of Neurology* 238:44–46.

Beaumanoir A, Jekiel M (1987) Electrographic observations during attacks of classical migraine. In: Andermann F, Lugaresi E (eds) *Migraine and Epilepsy*, pp. 163–180. Boston-London: Butterworths.

Beun AM, Beintema DJ, Binnie CD, Debets RMC, Overweg J, Van Heycop ten Ham MW (1984) Epileptic nystagmus. *Epilepsia* 25:609–614.

Bickford RG (1949) Electroencephalographic and clinical responses to light stimulation in normal subjects. *Electroencephalography and Clinical Neurophysiology* 1:126 (abstract).

Blume WT (1991) Occipital lobe epilepsies. In: Lüders H (ed) *Epilepsy Surgery*, pp 167–171. New York: Raven Press.

Brenner RP, Sharbrough FW (1976) Electroencephalographic evaluation in Sturge–Weber syndrome. *Neurology* 26:629–632.

Britton JW, Cascino GD, Sharbrough FW, Kelly PJ (1994) Low-grade glial neoplasms and intractable partial epilepsy: efficacy of surgical treatment. *Epilepsia* 35:1130–1135.

Bye AME, Matheson JM, Mackenzie RA (1989) Epilepsy surgery in Sturge–Weber syndrome. *Australian Paediatric Journal* 25:103–105.

Bye AM, Andermann F, Robitaille Y, Oliver M, Bohane T, Andermann E (1993) Cortical vascular abnormalities in the syndrome of celiac disease, epilepsy, bilateral occipital calcifications, and folate deficiency. *Annals of Neurology* 34:399–403.

Cascino GD, Kelly PJ, Sharbrough FW *et al* (1992) Long-term follow up of stereotactic lesionectomy in partial epilepsy: predictive factors and EEG results. *Epilepsia* 33:639–644.

Courjon J, Moene Y, Revol M, Gerin P (1968) A propos des crises occipitales déclenchées par la SLI. *Révue Neurologique* 118:523–525.

Critchley M (1951) Types of visual preservation: 'palinopsia' and 'illusory visual spread'. *Brain* 74:267–299.

Critchley M (1949) Metamorphosia of central origin. *Transactions of the Ophthalmological Society of the UK* 69:111–121.

Davidoff RA, Johnson LC (1963) Photic activation and photoconvulsive responses in a nonepileptic subject. *Neurology* 13:617–621.

Davidson S, Watson CW (1956) Hereditary light sensitive epilepsy. *Neurology* 6:235–261.

Deonna T, Prodhom LS (1980) Temporal lobe epilepsy and hemianopsia in childhood of perinatal origin. An overlooked and potentially treatable disease? Report of two cases, one with a demonstrable etiology. *Neuropediatrie* 11:85–90.

Dulac O, Roger J (1980) Sémiologie de la maladie de Sturge–Weber pendant les deux premières années de la vie. In: Gastaut H, Pinsard N (eds) *Pathologie cérébrale du nourrisson, XXIVème Colloque de Marseille*, pp 203–209. Marseille: Lamy.

Dulac O, Larregue M, Roger J *et al* (1982) Maladie de Sturge–Weber. Intérêt de l'analyse topographique de l' angiome cutanée pour le diagnostic d'angiome pial associé. *Archives Françaises de Pédiatrie* 39:155–158.

Duncan MB, Jabbari B, Rosenberg ML (1991) Gaze-evoked visual seizures in nonketotic hyperglycemia. *Epilepsia* 32:221–224.

Erba G, Cavazzuti V (1990) Sturge–Weber syndrome: natural history and indications for surgery. *Journal of Epilepsy* 3(suppl):287–291.

Farrel MA, DeRosa MJ, Curran JG *et al* (1992). Neuropathologic findings in cortical resections (including hemispherectomies) performed for the treatment of intractable childhood epilepsy. *Acta Neuropathologica* 83:246–259.

Fischer-Williams M, Bickford RG, Whisnant JP (1964) Occipito-parieto-temporal seizure discharge with visual hallucinations and aphasia. *Epilepsia* 5:279–292.

Friede RL (1989) *Developmental Neuropathology*. Berlin: Springer–Verlag.

Furman JMR, Crumrine PK, Reinmuth OM (1990) Epileptic nystagmus. *Annals of Neurology* 27:686–688.

Gastaut H (1960) Un aspect méconnu des décharges neuroniques occipitales: la crise oculoclonique ou 'nystagmus épileptique'. In: T. Alajouanine (ed) *Les grandes activités du lobe occipital*, pp 169–85. Paris: Masson.

Gastaut H, Roger A (1954) Formes inhabituelles de l'épilepsie: nystagmus épileptique. *Révue d'Electroéncéphalographie et de Neurophysiologie Clinique* 90:130–132.

Gastaut H, Zifkin BG (1984) Ictal visual hallucinations of numerals. *Neurology* 34:950–953.

Geier S, Bancaud J, Talairach J, Bonis A, Szikla G, Enjelvin M (1973) Signification des correlations electro-cliniques au cours de crises visuelles enregistrées en tele-S.E.E.G. *Révue d'Electroéncéphalographie Neurophysiologie Clinique* 3:355–359.

Gibbs FA, Gibbs EL (1953) *Atlas of Electroencephalography*, vol 2: *Epilepsy*, pp 201–225. Cambridge MA: Addison-Wesley.

Gobbi G, Sorrenti G, Santucci M *et al* (1988) Epilepsy with bilateral occipital calcification: a benign onset with progressive severity. *Neurology* 38:913–920.

Gobbi G, Ambrosetto P, Zaniboni MA, Lambertini A, Ambrosioni G, Tassinari CA (1992) Celiac disease, posterior cerebral calcifications and epilepsy. *Brain Development* 14:23–29.

Gobbi G, Bertani G, and the Italian Working Group on Coeliac Disease and Epilepsy (1997) Coeliac disease and epilepsy. In: Gobbi G, Andermann F, Naccarato S, Bianchini G (eds) *Epilepsy and Other Neurological Disorders in Coeliac Disease*, pp. 65–79. London: John Libbey.

Grant C, Warlow C. (1985) Focal epilepsy in diabetic nonketotic hyperglycemia. *British Medical Journal* 290:1204–1205.

Guerrini R, Vigliano P, Battaglia A *et al* (1990) Epilessia e calcificazioni cerebrali dopo trattamento della leucemia linfoblastica acuta. *Bollettino lega Italiana contro l'Epilessia* 70/71:243–246.

Guerrini R, Ferrari AR, Battaglia A *et al* (1994) Occipitotemporal seizures with ictus emeticus induced by intermittent photic stimulation. *Neurology* 44:253–259.

Guerrini R, Dravet C, Genton P *et al* (1995) Idiopathic photosensitive occipital lobe epilepsy. *Epilepsia* 36:883–891.

Guerrini R, Dubeau F, Dulac O *et al* (1997a) Bilateral parasagittal parieto-occipital polymicrogyria and epilepsy. *Annals of Neurology* 41:65–73.

Guerrini R, Bonanni P, Parmeggiani L *et al* (1997b) Induction of partial seizures by visual stimulation. *Advances in Neurology* 75:159–178.

Guerrini R, Bonanni P, Parmeggiani L *et al* (1997c) Adolescent onset of idiopathic photosensitive occipital epilepsy after remission of benign rolandic epilepsy. *Epilepsia* 38:777–781.

Harden CL, Rosenbaum DH, Daras M (1991) Hyperglycemia presenting with occipital seizures. *Epilepsia* 32:215–220.

Harris W (1997) Hemianopia, with especial reference to its transient varieties. *Brain* 20:308–364.

Hoffman HJ, Hendrick EB, Dennis M, Armstrong D (1979) Hemispherectomy for Sturge–Weber syndrome. *Child's Brain* 5:233–248.

Holtzman RNN, Goldensohn ES (1977) Sensations of ocular movement in seizures originating in occipital lobe. *Neurology* 27:554–556.

Huott AD, Madison DS, Niedermeyer E (1974) Occipital lobe epilepsy: a clinical and electroencephalographic study. *European Neurology* 11:325–339.

Isnard J, Guénot M, Fischer C, Mertens P, Sindou M, Mauguière F (1998) A stereoelectroencephalographic (SEEG) study of light-induced mesiotemporal epileptic seizures. *Epilepsia* 39:1098–1103.

Jasper H (1954) Electroencephalography. In: Penfield W, Jasper H (eds) *Epilepsy and the Functional Anatomy of the Human Brain*, pp 569–666. Boston: Little Brown.

Jones EG, Powell TPS (1970) An anatomical study of converging sensory pathways within the cerebral cortex of the monkey. *Brain* 93:793–820.

Kahane P, Francione S, Tassi L *et al* (1993) Traitement chirurgical des épilepsies partielles graves pharmaco-résistantes: approches diagnostiques et thérapeutiques. *Epilepsies* 5:179–204.

Kanazawa O, Sengoku A, Kawai I (1989) Oculoclonic status epilepticus. *Epilepsia* 30:121–123.

Kim JH (1995) Pathology of seizure disorders. *Neuroimaging Clinics of North America* 5:527–545.

Krynauw RA (1950) Infantile hemiplegia treated by removing one cerebral hemisphere. *Journal of Neurology, Neurosurgery and Psychiatry* 13:243–267.

Kuzniecky R (1998) Symptomatic occipital lobe epilepsy. *Epilepsia* 39 (suppl. 4):S24–S31.

Kuzniecky RI, Jackson GD (1995) Occipitoparietal epilepsy. In: Kuzniecky RI, Jackson GD (eds) *Magnetic Resonance in Epilepsy*, pp. 203–212. New York: Raven Press.

Lambertini A, Zaniboni MG, Mayer M, Città A, Ventura A (1997) Epilepsy and cerebral calcifications with normal jejunal mucosa: latent coeliac disease? In: Gobbi G *et al* (eds) *Epilepsy and Other Neurological Disorders in Coeliac Disease*, pp. 83–87. London: John Libbey.

Lefebre C, Koelmel HW (1989) Palinopsia as an epileptic phenomenon. *European Neurology* 29:323–327.

Lüders HO, Engel J Jr, Munari C (1993) General principles. In: Engel J Jr (ed) *Surgical Treatment of the Epilepsies*, 2nd edn, pp. 137–153. New York: Raven Press.

Ludwig BI, Ajmone-Marsan C (1975) Clinical ictal patterns in epileptic patients with occipital electroencephalographic foci. *Neurology* 25:463–471.

Maeda Y, Kurokawa T, Sakamoto K, Kitamoto I, Ueda K, Tashima S (1990) Electroclinical study of video-game epilepsy. *Developmental Medicine and Child Neurology* 32:493–500.

Magaudda A, Dalla Bernardina B, De Marco P *et al* (1993) Bilateral occipital calcification, epilepsy and coeliac disease: clinical and neuroimaging features of a new syndrome. *Journal of Neurology, Neurosurgery and Psychiatry* 56:885–889.

Montagna P, Gallassi R, Medori R *et al* (1988) MELAS syndrome. Characteristic migrainous and epileptic features and maternal transmission. *Neurology* 38:751–754.

Munari C, Bonis A, Koehen S *et al* (1984) Eye movements and occipital seizures in man. *Acta Neurochirurgica* 33 (suppl.):47–52.

Munari C, Tassi L, Francione S *et al* (1993) Occipital seizures with childhood onset in severe partial epilepsy: a surgical perspective. In: Andermann F, Beaumanoir A, Mira L, Roger J, Tassinari CA (eds) *Occipital Seizures and Epilepsies in Children*, pp. 203–211. London, Paris: John Libbey Eurotext.

Munari C, Francione S, Kahane P *et al* (1994a) Multilobar resections for control of epilepsy. In Schmidek HH, Sweet WJ (eds) *Operative Neurosurgical Techniques*, 3rd edn, pp. 1323–1339. London: WB Saunders.

Munari C, Hoffmann D, Francione S *et al* (1994b) Stereo-electroencephalography methodology: advantages and limits. *Acta Neurologica Scandinavica* 89 (suppl. 152):56–67.

Naquet R, Fegersten L, Bert J (1960) Seizure discharges localized to the posterior cerebral regions in man, provoked by intermittent photic stimulation. *Electroencephalography and Clinical Neurophysiology* 12:305–316.

Naquet R, Menini Ch, Riche D, Silva-Barrat C, Valin A (1987) Photic epilepsy problems raised in man and animals. *Italian Journal of Neurological Science* 8:437–447.

Ogunmekan AO, Hwang PA, Hoffman HJ (1989) Sturge–Weber–Dimitri: role of hemispherectomy in prognosis. *Canadian Journal of Neurological Sciences* 16:78–80.

Olivier A (1991) Extratemporal cortical resections: principles and methods. In: Lüders HO (ed) *Epilepsy Surgery*, pp 559–568. New York: Raven Press.

Olivier A, Awad IA (1993) Extratemporal resections. In: Engel J Jr (ed) *Surgical Treatment of the Epilepsies*, 2nd edn, pp 489–500. New York: Raven Press.

Olivier A, Gloor P, Andermann F, Ives J (1982) Occipitotemporal epilepsy studied with stereotaxically implanted depth electrodes and successfully treated by temporal resection. *Annals of Neurology* 11:428–432.

Paillas JE, Vigouroux G, Darcourt G, Naquet R (1959) Considérations sur l'épilepsie occipitale (A propos de 12 observations de lésions occipitales opérées). *Neuro-Chirurgie* 5:3–16.

Palmini A, Andermann F, Olivier A, Tampieri D, Robitaille Y (1991) Focal neuronal migration disorders and intractable partial epilepsy: a study of 30 patients. *Annals of Neurology* 30:741–749.

Pascotto A, Coppola G, Ecuba P, Liguori G, Guandalini S (1994) Epilepsy and occipital calcifications with or without celiac disease: report of four cases. *Journal of Epilepsy* 7:130–136.

Penfield W, Jasper H (1954) *Epilepsy and the Functional Anatomy of the Human Brain*. Boston: Little Brown

Penfield W, Perot P (1963) The brain's record of auditory and visual experience: a final summary and discussion. *Brain* 86:595–616.

Plazzi G, Tinuper P, Cerullo A, Provini F, Lugaresi E (1994a) Occipital lobe epilepsy: a chronic condition related to transient occipital lobe involvement in eclampsia. *Epilepsia* 35:644–647.

Plazzi G, Tinuper P, Provini F *et al* (1994b) Epilepsy, occipital calcifications and coeliac disease: anatomopathologic findings and response to a gluten-free diet. *Epilepsia* 35:81–82.

Raroque HGJ, Orrison WW, Rosenberg GA (1990) Neurologic involvement in toxemia of pregnancy: reversible MRI lesions. *Neurology* 40:167–169.

Rasmussen T (1975) Surgery for epilepsy arising in regions other than the temporal and frontal lobes. *Advances in Neurology* **8**:207–225.

Rasmussen T (1983) Hemispherectomy for seizures revisited. *Canadian Journal of Neurological Sciences* **10**:71–78.

Rasmussen T, Mathieson G, Le Blanc F (1972) Surgical treatment of typical and forme fruste variety of the Sturge–Weber syndrome. *Archives Suisse de Neurologie, Neurochirurgie, Psychiatrie* **3**:393–409.

Remillard GM, Ethier R, Andermann F (1974) Temporal lobe epilepsy and perinatal occlusion of the posterior cerebral artery. A syndrome analogous to infantile hemiplegia and a demonstrable etiology in some patients with temporal lobe epilepsy. *Neurology* **24**:1001–1009.

Ricci S, Vigevano F (1993) Occipital seizures provoked by intermittent light stimulation: ictal and interictal findings. *Journal of Clinical Neurophysiology* **10**:197–209.

Robinson PK, Watt AC (1947) Hallucinations of remembered scenes as an epileptic aura. *Brain* **70**:440–448.

Rochkind S, Hoffman HJ, Hendrick EB (1990) Sturge–Weber syndrome: natural history and prognosis. *Journal of Epilepsy* **3** (suppl.):293–304.

Roger J, Gastaut JL, Dravet C, Tassinari CA, Gastaut H (1977) Epilepsie partielle à sémiologie complexe et lésions atrophiques occipito-pariétales. Intérêt de l'examen tacoencéphalographique. *Revue Neurologique* **133**:41–53.

Roger J, Pellissier JF, Bureau M, Dravet C, Revol M, Tinuper P (1983) Le diagnostic précoce de la maladie de Lafora. Importance de manifestations paroxystiques visuelles et intérêt de la biopsie cutané. *Revue Neurologique* **139**:115–124.

Roger J, Genton P, Bureau M, Dravet C (1992) Progressive myoclonus epilepsies in childhood and adolescence. In Roger J, Bureau M, Dravet Ch, Dreifuss FE, Perret A, Wolf P (eds) *Epileptic Syndromes in Infancy, Childhood and Adolescence*, 2nd edn, pp 381–400. London: John Libbey.

Rosen I, Salford L, Stark L (1984) Sturge–Weber disease. Neurophysiological evaluation of a case with secondary epileptogenesis successfully treated with lobectomy. *Neuropediatrics* **15**:95–98.

Russell WR, Whitty CWM (1955) Studies in traumatic epilepsy: 3, visual fits. *Journal of Neurology, Neurosurgery and Psychiatry* **18**:79–96.

Salanova V, Andermann F, Olivier A, Rasmussen T, Quesney LF (1992) Occipital lobe epilepsy: electroclinical manifestations, electrocor-ticography, cortical stimulation and outcome in 42 patients treated between 1930 and 1991. *Brain* **115**:1655–1680.

Salanova V, Andermann F, Rasmussen TB. (1993) Occipital lobe epilepsy. In: Wyllie E (ed) *The Treatment of Epilepsy: Principles and Practice*, pp. 533–40. Philadelphia: Lea and Febiger.

Sammaritano M, Andermann F, Melanson D *et al* (1985) The syndrome of epilepsy and bilateral occipital cortical calcifications. *Epilepsia* **26**:532 (abstract).

Sassower K, Duchowny M. Jayakar P *et al* (1994) EEG evaluation in children with Sturge–Weber syndrome and epilepsy. *Journal of Epilepsy* **7**:285–289.

Serratosa JM, Delgado-Escueta AV, Posada I *et al* (1995) The gene for progressive myoclonus epilepsy of the Lafora type maps to chromosome 6q. *Human Molecular Genetics* **4**:1657–1664.

So N, Berkovic S, Andermann F, Kuzniecky R, Gendron D, Quesney LF (1989) Myoclonus epilepsy and ragged-red fibres (MERRF). *Brain* **112**:1261–1276.

Sowa MV and Pituck S (1989) Prolonged spontaneous complex visual hallucinations and illusions as ictal phenomena. *Epilepsia* **30**:524–526.

Sveinbjornsdottir S, Duncan S (1993) Parietal and occipital lobe epilepsy: a review. *Epilepsia* **34**:493–521.

Takeda A, Bancaud J, Talairach J, Bonis A, Bordas-Ferrer M (1969) A propos des accès épileptiques d'origine occipitale. *Revue Neurologique* **121**:306–315.

Talairach J, Bancaud J, Szikla G, Bonis A, Geier S (1974) Approche nouvelle de la neurochirurgie de l'épilepsie. Méthodologie stéréotaxique et résultats thérapeutiques. *Neurochirurgie* **20** (suppl. 1):1–240.

Tampieri D, Dubeau F, Leblanc R, Melançon D, Andermann F (1996) Imaging of heterotopic gray matter. In: Guerrini *et al* (eds) *Dysplasias of Cerebral Cortex and Epilepsy*, pp. 163–168. Philadelphia: Lippincott-Raven.

Taylor DC, Falconer MA, Bruton CJ, Corsellis JAN (1971) Focal dysplasia of the cerebral cortex in epilepsy. *Journal of Neurology, Neurosurgery and Psychiatry* **34**:369–387.

Tiacci C, D'Alessandro P, Catisani TA *et al* (1993) Epilepsy with bilateral occipital calcifications: Sturge–Weber variant or a different encephalopathy? *Epilepsia* **34**:528–539.

Tinuper P (1997) Pathological findings of coeliac disease, epilepsy and cerebral calcifications. In: Gobbi G *et al* (eds) *Epilepsy and Other Neurological Disorders in Coeliac Disease*, pp. 181–184. London: John Libbey.

Tinuper P, Aguglia P, Pellissier JF, Gastaut H (1983) Visual ictal phenomena in a case of Lafora disease proven by skin biopsy. *Epilepsia* **24**:214–218.

Van den Hout B, Van der Meij V, Wieneke G, Van Huffelen A, Van Nieuwenhuizen O (1997) Seizure semiology of occipital lobe epilepsy in children. *Epilepsia* **38**:1118–1191.

Welch K, Naheedy MH, Abroms LF, Strand RD (1980) Computed tomography of Sturge–Weber syndrome in infants. *Journal of Computer Assisted Tomography* **4**:33–36.

Williamson PD, Spencer S (1986) Clinical and EEG features of complex partial seizures of extratemporal origin. *Epilepsia* **27** (suppl. 2):S46–S63.

Williamson PD, Thadani VM, Darcey TM, Spencer DD, Spencer SS, Mattson H (1992) Occipital lobe epilepsy: clinical characteristics, seizure spread patterns, and results of surgery. *Annals of Neurology* **31**:3–13.

Williamson PD, Engel J, Munari C (1997) Anatomic classification of localization-related epilepsies. In: Engel J Jr, Pedley TA (eds) *Epilepsy: A Comprehensive Textbook*, pp. 2405–2416. Philadelphia: Lippincott-Raven

Young LW, Jequier S, O'Gorman AM (1977) Intracerebral calcifications in treated leukemia in a child. *American Journal of Disease in Childhood* **131**:1283–1285.

Seizures associated with multilobar pathology

Z ZAIWALLA

The Commission on Classification and Terminology of the International League Against Epilepsy in 1989 proposed a revised classification of epilepsies and epileptic syndromes. There was tentative description of anatomic localization-related epilepsy syndromes, based predominantly on seizure semeiology as judged from data obtained during studies including intracranial recordings. Since then, some authors have supported this approach to seizure classification while others have pointed out its limitations, particularly as the same symptoms and signs can occur with seizures starting from many different parts of the brain (Manford *et al* 1996; Spencer 1998). In clinical practice, especially in children, many of the localization-related epilepsies occur with multilobar pathology that may be either unilateral or bilateral. The semeiology of seizures in this group of patients can be very variable.

Seizure semeiology in patients with multilobar pathology depends to some extent on the nature of the pathology. For example, cortical dysplasia is intrinsically epileptogenic (Palmini *et al* 1995) and the seizures that it causes may assume features characteristic of the cortical function of areas from which they arise (Spencer 1998). On the other hand, acquired pathology, such as infarction, trauma, or hypoxic ischemia is not intrinsically epileptogenic; rather, intact neurons are needed for seizures to occur and the epileptogenic region is likely to be the adjacent, intact, but dysfunctional cortex.

The substance of this chapter draws on data, including preoperative video-EEG recordings, obtained from a consecutive series of 50 hemispherectomy procedures carried out in Oxford as treatment for intractable epilepsy, mainly on children with unilateral multilobar pathology (Table 9.1). These patients, who are extensively investigated, provide a unique opportunity to study the semeiology of seizures arising from both developmental and acquired fixed multilobar cortical pathology, and from progressive unilateral multilobar pathology as occurs in Rasmussen syndrome. Data have also been derived from an analysis of video-EEG recordings from children with other intractable epilepsy syndromes due to multilobar pathology referred to our epilepsy center.

MATURATIONAL ASPECTS OF SEIZURE SEMEIOLOGY

As in unifocal pathology, seizure semeiology in multilobar pathology depends on age. The systems required for the full clinical presentation of easily recognizable automatisms of

Table 9.1 Underlying pathology and seizure types in 50 consecutive cases of intractable epilepsy due to multilobar pathology treated by anatomic hemispherectomy (Adams modified)

Pathology

33	Prenatal or early-life cerebral infarction
8	Cerebral developmental malformation
6	Rasmussen syndrome
2	Sturge–Weber syndrome
1	Perinatal cerebral hemorrhage

Seizure types

33		Predominantly motor seizures
	21	focal involving contralateral limbs
	6	epilepsia partialis continua
	2	'fencing' type, suggesting supplementary motor area onset
	2	complex, suggesting cingulate onset
	2	startle attacks
6		Predominantly complex partial
10		Motor and complex partial mixed
14		Atypical absence (1 as sole seizure type)
7		Nonconvulsive status epilepticus
1		Continuous spike–wave in slow-wave sleep

complex partial seizures are not yet developed in the immature brain (Luders *et al* 1989). Also, as a number of authors have pointed out, determining an alteration of consciousness, which is essential for the classification of an attack as a complex partial seizure, is difficult in infants (Duchowny 1987; Dravet *et al* 1989; Nordli *et al* 1997). Luna *et al* (1989) attempted to assess consciousness by comparing unsuccessful efforts to attract the child's attention during discharges with the reappearance of visual contact and purposeful behavior after the seizures, but this cannot be regarded as a reliable method. Hence, the semeiology of focal seizures in neonates and infants is often simple.

Developmental malformations, hypoxic–ischemic insults, CNS infections, infarcts, and intracranial hemorrhage are all associated with multilobar pathology and are included in the etiology of neonatal seizures. Evans and Levene (1998) pointed out that seizures in a neonate may be the first manifestation of neurologic dysfunction. They classified the seizure semeiology in neonates as

Subtle	including eye deviation, mouthing, apnea, and unstable blood pressure,
Clonic	with rhythmic jerking either focal or multifocal
Myoclonic	with bilateral or focal limb jerks
Tonic	with extension of the lower limbs accompanied by pronation of the arms and clenching of the fists

None of these seizure types has localizing reliability and all will occur in both unifocal and multilfocal lesions. The only

exception is focal clonic movements of the limbs, or one side of the face, which usually suggests a contralateral focal lesion involving the central area.

Neonatal seizures may be transient, with or without recurrence later in life, in association with acquired perinatal insults. Of the 33 children in our hemispherectomy series who had suffered a middle cerebral artery territory infarct, 4 had neonatal seizures that were transient, the habitual seizures appearing after an interval ranging from 5 months to 11 years. These children, all had nonlocalizing seizures as neonates with arching, episodes of cyanosis and apnea, sucking, and throat sounds or brief tonic seizures. In contrast, 4 of the 7 children with a unilateral developmental malformation had seizures starting in the neonatal period that persisted, without a seizure-free interval. In three, the seizures were localizing with clonic movements of the limbs contralateral to the side of the pathology.

Seizures that start during the first year of life continue to have simple seizure semeiology. Wyllie *et al* (1996), in their paper on epilepsy surgery in infants, described the seizure semeiology in 12 children with unilateral multilobar pathology. A third had arrest or marked reduction of behavioral motor activity, with an unclear level of consciousness, which they termed 'hypomotor seizures.' Some of these seizures involved subtle limb movements and oroalimentary (sucking, chewing) activity. Head turning was observed both toward and away from the hemisphere of seizure onset. This hypomotor phase was followed by generalized atonia with head drops or slumping in some of the children. As in the neonatal seizures, children who had focal clonic seizures had perirolandic electrographic seizure localization. A quarter of the children had predominantly bilateral tonic seizures, sometimes progressing to clonic jerking, with or without head and eye version, with a variable localization - of the cortical pathology, as seen on MRI, to frontal, parietal or temporo-parieto-occipital areas. Similar seizure semeiology was observed by other authors evaluating children with partial seizures in infancy (Blume 1989; Dravet *et al* 1989; Duchowny *et al* 1990; Nordli *et al* 1997).

West syndrome is an age-dependent epileptic encephalopathy of infancy with a characteristic seizure semeiology consisting of a clinical triad of infantile spasms, mental retardation, and hypsarrhythmic EEG (Donat 1992). The peak age of onset is from 3 to 7 months, and usually before 1 year of age. The syndrome may occur in children with focal pathology involving adjacent lobes (Chugani *et al* 1990), although the usual causes are neonatal asphyxia, cerebral malformations, and tuberous sclerosis indicative of diffuse multifocal disease. Infantile spasms consist of a very brief sudden myoclonic or tonic flexor contraction of the limbs, often tending to occur in clusters over several seconds or a few minutes. Gaily *et al* (1995) studied video-EEG recordings of 60 children with infantile spasms. They found that 25% were asymmetric and 7% asynchronous (spasm involved one side of the body before the other). Mostly asymmetrical or asynchronous spasms were significantly associated with unilateral central pathology, and never with focal pathology exclusively involving the temporal lobe or posterior to the central area. Yamamoto *et al* (1988) reported partial seizures in the neonatal period associated with cessation of activity, eye deviation, autonomic disturbance and laughter evolving to infantile spasms, with the partial seizure semeiology often preceding the spasm.

Infantile spasms may be the first manifestation of a symptomatic epileptic encephalopathy, as in children with tuberous sclerosis, or may evolve from neonatal encephalopathies as in *Ohtahara syndrome*[1], or they may follow transient neonatal seizures due to perinatal conditions such as birth asphyxia or cerebral infarction. Two of the four children with perinatal unilateral cerebral infarction who had transient neonatal seizures in our hemispherectomy series developed infantile spasms at around 6–7 months of age.

Lennox–Gastaut syndrome can occur with unilateral multilobar pathology although it is generally associated with diffuse or multifocal cerebral disease. The clinical triad of the syndrome consists of intractable seizures, mental retardation, and generalized slow spike and wave discharges on EEG. The peak incidence of the appearance of this syndrome is between 1 and 7 years of age, but most commonly it is at around 2 years of age (Donat 1992). The seizures include the following.

- *Tonic* seizures involving sudden flexion of the neck and body, with raising of the arms in a semiflexed or an extended position, extension of the legs, contraction of the face muscles, apnea and facial flushing, which may lead to a fall with or without a brief alteration in consciousness. Tonic seizures are particularly frequent from slow-wave sleep.
- *Atypical absence seizures*, which are often difficult to detect because they begin and end progressively and alteration of consciousness is incomplete. These atypical absences may be accompanied by a decrease in muscle tone that may cause the head to drop forward with the mouth open and drooling or with collapse of the whole body.
- *Massive myoclonias, myoclonia, atonia, or atonic seizures* associated with a sudden head drop or whole body fall (Beaumanoir and Dravet 1992).

Not all patients with multilobar pathology present in the early years with severe encephalopathies such as West syndrome or the Lennox–Gastaut syndrome. The seizures may remain focal motor with or without secondary generalization, or with age the more subtle behaviors with prominent motor semeiology in the very young evolve to the behaviors associated with complex partial seizures in adults. Dravet *et al* (1989), in their study of seizure semeiology in 40 children under 3 years of age, classified 11 children as having complex partial seizures and mention one child who was diagnosed as having generalized epilepsy until 18 months of age when complex partial seizures appeared. Brockhaus and Elger (1995), studying seizure semeiology in temporal lobe epilepsy, observed that children aged over 6 years had features similar to those of adults. In the preschool age group (1.5–6 years), the typical semeiology included symmetric motor phenomena of limb posturing similar to frontal lobe seizures in adults, and also head nodding as in infantile spasms. In our experience, children with multilobar pathology show an evolution of their seizure semeiology similar to that described by Brockhaus and Elger (1995) except that the bilateral semeiology including bilateral spasms may persist into the first decade if the disturbance of cortical function is severe. In children without severe learning difficulty, the characteristic features of complex partial seizures can be recognized by 3–4 years of age. Thus, the child who experiences fear seeks out the parent, or is able to describe an aura, before altered consciousness occurs.

Clinical experience suggests that seizure semeiology remains fairly stable from 6 years into adult life except that with age the patient is better able to verbalize the aura and the preseizure experiences. However, Tinuper *et al* (1996) studied seizure semeiology in 58 patients aged over 60 years who had been epileptic for 23–85 years. Twenty-three percent had lesional epilepsy due to head injury, previous infection, or Sturge–Weber syndrome. They found that, in 84%, the secondarily generalized convulsions that had been present at the onset of the epilepsy had disappeared. Furthermore, in 38% (including three patients with lesional epilepsy) there was a progressive change in seizure semeiology between 48 and 70 years of age. In these patients, the initial ictal phenomena remained the same, but older patients had fewer automatisms, in particular gestural and semipurposeful behavior. Instead, they had only brief loss of contact with slight confusion. Hence it appears that in some

---

[1] *Ohtahara syndrome* is the severest type of neonatal encephalopathy with a uniformly poor diagnosis. It is usually due to either bilateral brain malformations or metabolic disorder. The baby presents in the first 10 days after birth with repetitive tonic spasms of less than 10 seconds duration, with the characteristic burst suppression pattern in the EEG (Donat 1992).

patients, even with multilobar pathology, the seizure semeiology may became simpler in old age, with less tendency to secondary generalization.

MOTOR SEIZURES AND COMPLEX PARTIAL SEIZURES

When the pathology is extensive, the rapid spread of seizure activity to involve adjacent lobes leads to difficulties in classifying the seizure type by semeiology. Within these limitations, we attempted to classify the seizure semeiology in our hemispherectomy series by dividing the cases into three groups:

- Those with predominantly motor seizures (suggesting involvement of the rolandic area, and frontal lobe)
- Those with predominantly complex partial seizures, usually with an aura or alteration in consciousness and complex automatisms (suggesting temporal/parietal/occipital involvement)
- Those with both seizure types occurring equally frequently.

MOTOR SEIZURES

Of our 50 hemispherectomy cases, 33 had predominantly motor seizures. Of these, 21 had destructive pathology due to middle cerebral artery territory infarction; 2 had the Sturge–Weber syndrome; 4 had a unilateral cortical dysplasia; and 6 had Rasmussen syndrome. Twenty-one of the 33 had focal seizures involving the contralateral limbs, characterized by limb stiffening and focal jerking, often with facial distortion and twitching. Four of them also had attacks with sudden falls when either the legs gave way or the falls were associated with bilateral limb stiffening. In another four some of the seizures were associated with bilateral rhythmic jerks of both upper limbs.

Two of the 33 had frequent brief seizures with 'fencing' posturing, suggestive of supplementary motor area involvement. Two had more complex motor automatisms, including vocalization with writhing and thrashing movements of the limbs, suggesting cingulate involvement. A further two had seizures mainly precipitated by startle, and perirolandic electrographic onset, resembling attacks described by Oguni *et al* (1998).

The remaining six had *epilepsia partialis continua*, which is usually a symptom of an acute or progressive focal lesion (Mitchell 1996), and consists of localized epileptic jerks with more or less continuous Jacksonian seizures (Bancaud 1992). All six patients had Rasmussen encephalitis. None of those with either vascular pathology or focal cortical dysplasias had epilepsia partialis continua, unlike the series of Palmini *et al* (1991) in which this seizure type was seen in two patients with focal neuronal migrational disorder. Fusco and Vigevano (1991) have also reported a reversible operculum syndrome with progressive epilepsia partialis continua in a child with a left hemimegalencephaly, due to discharge spreading to the contralateral central area.

COMPLEX PARTIAL SEIZURES

In contrast to the number of patients who had predominantly motor seizures, only six had predominantly complex partial seizures. Of these, three had seizures starting with an abdominal sensation, suggesting a temporal lobe onset. The seizure semeiology in the others suggested a parietooccipital onset. One patient was frightened by 'seeing things look funny,' before becoming unresponsive and talking gibberish. One child habitually called out 'I am going to be sick,' and appeared to have visual hallucinations of seeing spiders during the attack. One child had stereotyped seizures in which he looked frightened, held on to the parent as he turned his head and eyes to the side of the hemiplegia, and briefly became unresponsive. In four of these six patients the habitual seizures often progressed to involve the motor cortex, with facial distortion and stiffening of the hemiplegic limb.

Frequent secondarily generalized tonic–clonic convulsions occurred in 12 of the 50 patients, irrespective of whether their predominant seizure type was focal motor, complex, or mixed partial. When the seizures occurred from the awake state there was usually clinical evidence of focal onset, either the habitual aura, or focal limb jerking, or the patient momentarily holding the hemiplegic arm, as if having a sensory experience, before the generalized tonic–clonic convulsion. However, one patient with a vascular pathology following neonatal meningitis, had infrequent but fairly long (15–45 minutes) tonic–clonic convulsions only. The EEG showed bilateral spike discharges, but more often lateralized to the anterior quadrant, contralateral to the hemiplegic side.

Hence, in our series with multilobar unilateral pathology, 66% had predominantly motor seizures. Detailed seizure semeiology in other comparable series of unilateral multilobar pathology is not available. Palmini *et al* (1991), however, found that 71% of patients with neuronal migrational disorders had partial motor seizures with the occurrence of drop attacks when the pathology involved the central regions. Thirty percent of their patients had generalized or partial motor epileptic status. They point out that this incidence is higher than in either nonselected populations or patients with brain tumors, leading them to suggest that partial or generalized motor status is most frequently associated with extensive structural abnormality involving two or more lobes. In contrast, only 8% in our series had episodes of convulsive status (two had focal motor status and two had generalized convulsive status). None of our eight children with a cortical malformation had episodes of convulsive status, though this may simply reflect the small number with this pathology.

UNILOBAR SEIZURES

It is easy to assume that patients with multilobar pathology will have multiple seizure types. In practice they not uncommonly present with seizures that are stereotyped, clinically and electrographically, appearing to arise from a limited cortical area.

Three of our patients with a unilateral destructive pathology in the middle cerebral artery territory had clinically and electrographically frontal lobe seizures on video-EEG studies. Another three had stereotyped complex partial seizures, clinically localizing to the parietooccipital cortex, but as there was rapid involvement of the adjacent posterior temporal cortex, the lobar localization was less reliable.

When the cortical damage is very extensive, it is understandable that seizures can be sustained from only a limited area of the residual cortex, either frontal or parietooccipital or inferior temporal. However, the cortical damage does not have to be near-total for seizures to arise from a localized epileptogenic area, despite multilobar pathology. Patients with developmental malformations, both unilateral and bilateral, may present with a single seizure type. Two of our patients with widespread unilateral cortical dysplasia, who subsequently became seizure-free following hemispherectomy, had focal motor seizures that were stereotyped and electrographically localized over a single lobe. The attacks of one child, who had a predominantly left frontal abnormality on MRI, usually occurred with abrupt arousal from sleep. The right arm would elevate with the head and eyes turned to the left; about 12 seconds later, repeated jerks occurred with flexion of the right arm and elevation of the left arm, as both shoulders came forward, with extension and abduction of the right leg. The limbs were held in this posture for 4 seconds before relaxing, the movements repeating every 4 seconds. Electrographically, the seizures localized over the left midfrontocentral area. Another child with focal pachygyria and widespread focal ectopia in the right hemisphere presented with focal jerking of the contralateral arm on the eighth day after birth, later progressing to bilateral arm jerks. The ictal recording showed a localized seizure onset, over the right parietal area. The MRI scan was not localizing, showing diffuse loss of normal grey–white differentiation on the right, but with a normal gyral pattern.

Two patients with band heterotopia both presented with single seizure types. One had attacks of violent thrashing movements from sleep, resembling frontal lobe seizures, but with no visible scalp EEG change (the interictal spike discharge was over the left parietooccipital, posterior temporal areas). The other had attacks with posturing of the limbs, resembling attacks from the mesial frontal lobe, with the arms abducted and elevated, as the head and eyes turned to the left, recovering with a grimace in <60 seconds. Again the ictal EEG recordings were not localizing.

Patients with tuberous sclerosis usually have multiple bilateral tubers and intractable epilepsy, assumed to be multifocal. Infantile spasms are the commonest type of seizure in this syndrome. However, Curatolo (1991) noted that when the seizures start at an age greater than 2 years, the children usually have complex partial seizures or secondarily generalized seizures. Perot et al as long ago as 1966 reported on patients with tuberous sclerosis who became seizure-free after focal cortical resection. Bebin et al (1993) operated on nine patients with tuberous sclerosis. Five had complex partial seizures, one had a combination of left partial motor seizures and complex partial seizures, one had generalized tonic–clonic seizures, one had left partial motor seizures, and one had persistent infantile spasms. Ictal EEG recordings confirmed that the seizures were occurring from a single region, corresponding to a prominent lesion on neuroimaging in eight patients, though three of these had multifocal and generalized interictal discharges. On a mean follow-up of 35 months, four patients were seizure-free on antiepileptic drugs and two were seizure-free without medication. The Cleveland Clinic surgical experience on six patients with tuberous sclerosis suggests that if the habitual seizures arise from one temporal lobe, the patient has a good chance of becoming seizure-free, while their one patient who had an occipital resection had no reduction in seizures (Kotagal and Tuxhorn 1997).

When the seizure semeiology suggests unifocal seizure onset in a patient with cortical dysplasia, there is concern that focal resection will be followed by recurrence of seizures from other dysplastic areas, some of which may be outside the MRI-visible lesion (Sisodiya et al 1995). It is not known whether the epileptogenicity of various lesions arises independently, depending on local factors including the size of the lesion and/or the state of regional cortical maturation (Chugani et al 1987), or whether there is interaction between potentially epileptogenic areas so that a dominant epileptic focus suppresses epileptic activity in other areas, which may be released once the dominant focus is excised. We have certainly seen children who have a multifocal seizure potential and in whom one lesion is more epileptogenic, both clinically and electrographically, but after a period another lesion dominates while the initial epileptogenic area appears to be relatively dormant. It is difficult to predict the interval before another lesion will become epileptogenic with or without resection of the primary epileptogenic lesion. However, the interval may be long because good results can be achieved with resection of circumcised lesions in some patients (Holthausen *et al* 1997).

MULTIPLE SEIZURE TYPES

When multiple seizure types are reported it is important to try to tease out whether the seizure semeiology reflects variable propagation of ictal activity from a single focus or multiple seizures from independent foci. After excluding the various seizure types produced by variable propagation from the perirolandic cortex, and the complex partial seizures that spread to the motor cortex, and the absences due to secondary generalization of discharge (see below), only 10 of the 50 in our series had frequent motor and complex partial seizures occurring independently. Even then there was some overlap of the two seizure types.

Although, clinically, the different seizure types appeared to start from independent cortical areas, this could not always be confirmed with video-EEG studies. Even when both seizure types were recorded, the almost continuous or multifocal discharges over the affected hemisphere, which were sometimes bilaterally synchronous, made it difficult to identify seizure onset electrographically, especially during focal motor seizures. At best, ictal EEG studies aided lateralization but were of little use for lobar localization. Eight of these 10 patients with multiple seizure types had vascular pathology, one had hemimegalencephaly, and one had a combination of developmental malformation and perinatal acquired damage.

Of the 50 in our series, 14 had clinical absences (atypical with indistinct onset and end, and alteration in consciousness) confirmed to coincide with secondarily generalized spike–wave discharges of varying duration. Absences occurred in seven patients with predominantly motor seizures, one with complex partial seizures, and five with both seizure types. One patient had absences as the sole seizure type. *Absence attacks*, with arrest of activity, staring, unresponsiveness for several seconds, and sometimes with simple automatisms, may be difficult to diagnose. These behaviors in patients with multilobar pathology and learning difficulties may not be epileptic and can simply reflect poor concentration or drowsiness. If epileptic, the arrest of activity may be the initial phase of a complex partial seizure and electrographically will be associated with a focal discharge or EEG change similar to that seen at the start of the habitual seizures. More often in patients with multilobar pathology, the absence attacks are associated with secondarily generalized paroxysms or bilateral synchronicity of the multifocal discharges, producing diffuse slow spike–wave discharge.

Tukel and Jasper in 1952 pointed out that secondary generalization, especially from a frontal focus, can produce clinical and electrographic absences, indistinguishable from idiopathic absence epilepsy. We have seen secondary generalization of discharges producing clinical absences in association with epileptic foci, involving in particular the parasagittal cortex, presumably aided by rapid callosal spread of the discharge. Tinuper *et al* (1995), studying bilateral synchrony in 41 patients, showed focal discharges localizing to the frontotemporal area in 16, temporal in 5, parietooccipital in 5 and multiple independent in 15. While the absence seizure type in this patient group may not have localizing significance, Tinuper *et al* found bilateral synchronicity of discharge to be significantly associated with drug-resistant epilepsy, drop attacks, mental deterioration, and progressive background EEG slowing, suggesting poor cognitive outcome.

Reports of seizure semeiology in focal cortical dysplasia (Palmini *et al* 1991; Guerrini 1997) describe multiple seizure types. However, closer scrutiny of some of the published work suggests that seizure semeiology variability may reflect propagation to adjacent cortex. For example, of the 10 patients described by Kuzniecky *et al* (1997) with parietooccipital lobe developmental malformations, 6 had ictal visual symptoms and initial bilateral eye blinking occurred in one, followed by contralateral eye and head deviation. Contralateral motor dystonic posturing of the upper extremity was observed in two patients. However, three had initial behavioral arrest followed by stereotyped automatisms suggesting early temporal lobe involvement. Multiple seizure types with semeiology suggestive of ictal onset from functionally different cortical areas (frontal, mesolimbic, parietal, temporooccipital) were reported by Battaglia *et al* (1997) in patients with both unilateral and bilateral periventricular nodular heterotopia. However, the interictal discharges were localized in the unilateral group and localized or bitemporal in the bilateral group, and the two patients who had ictal recording suggested seizure onset localized to one posterior temporal area.

The above discussion does not exclude the occurrence of multiple seizure types from independent foci in some patients with multilobar pathology. Preoperative and post-operative video-EEG monitoring in patients who continue to have seizures following surgery provides an opportunity to study semeiology of seizures from more than one non-adjacent area and may indicate that there is a dynamic inter-action between multifocal epileptogenic areas in some patients with bilateral multilobar pathology.

NONCONVULSIVE STATUS EPILEPTICUS

Nonconvulsive status epilepticus (NCSE) consists of a pro-longed seizure state, predominantly affecting mental func-tion. Doose (1983) classified nonconvulsive status epilepticus into NCSE occurring in the primary generalized epilepsies and partial epilepsies with or without secondary generalization. In our study (Stores *et al* 1995) of 50 children in nonconvulsive status, 12 had intractable partial epilepsy usually due to unilateral multilobar pathology. We found that the effect on mental function with this con-tinuous epileptic state was subtle in some children, with periods when the child was more forgetful or less moti-vated, to gross when the child was described as 'zombie like' or apparently 'deaf and dumb.' The effect on mental state was also associated with unsteadiness, frequent falls, and low-amplitude, often only palpable, myoclonic jerks. The cause for the deterioration in mental state could go unrecognized for months when this epileptic state occurred in children with preexisting developmental delay and learn-ing difficulties.

Seven children in our hemispherectomy series had a his-tory suggestive of periods in nonconvulsive status, or were in nonconvulsive status when first referred to our epilepsy surgery program. Four had vascular pathology, one had hemimegalencephaly and two had an unilateral neuronal migrational disorder with pachygyria, lissencephaly and laminar heterotopia. Seizure onset was from the neonatal period to $2\frac{1}{2}$ years. The precise duration in this state, before treatment, was not always ascertainable, but was at least 6 months in one child and 2 years in another. One child had two prolonged episodes of being 'almost comatose' and another showed diurnal variation, being unsteady and con-fused for the first 4 hours each morning. Below are some descriptions given by the carers when the patients were in nonconvulsive status.

Unsteady and confused for 4 hours on waking. Feels sick, not able to see well. Improves as day goes on, like a 'curtain goes up' later in the day.

Two years in a dreamy state. Lost skills, including speech. Most days cannot stand or sit unsupported and soils. On good days appears more alert and can stand and take a few steps.

Frequent periods of unresponsiveness occurring every 3 to 4 minutes, lasting 1 to 2 minutes with twitching of limbs, and eye flickering.

After chickenpox, less alert, jerking and unsteady for long periods of time. Unable to stand. Moves around only by crawling.

Periods when he appears like a zombie. Walks through doors. Alternates with periods of alertness.

Prolonged periods in detached state.

Long periods when unresponsive. 'Nearly comatosed' during two peri-ods at ages 12 and 14.

CONTINUOUS SPIKE–WAVE IN SLOW-WAVE SLEEP (CSWS)

Patry *et al* (1971) described an epileptic condition charac-terized by continuous spike–wave occurring in sleep, coin-ciding with cognitive decline. Initially the authors used the term 'subclinical electrical status' to describe the condition, but later Tassinari *et al* (1977) called it electrical status epilepticus during sleep (ESES), and later continuous spike and wave during slow sleep (CSWS). A number of reports of this condition in children with epilepsy have been pub-lished during the last 25 years (Morikawa *et al* 1985; Bureau 1995).

Many of the children who develop CSWS have idio-pathic partial epilepsy resembling benign epilepsy of child-hood, with centrotemporal spikes. In a report of 29 cases of CSWS by Tassinari *et al* (1992), however, 14 children had neuroradiologically identified brain abnormality. Six had unilateral atrophy, five had diffuse atrophy, two had diffuse atrophy and porencephaly and one had localized pachy-gyria. Epileptic seizures appeared between 8 months and 12 years of age. They were predominantly unilateral motor seizures and generalized tonic–clonic convulsions in sleep. EEG findings in wake at the onset of the epilepsy varied from generalized spike–wave bursts, focal interictal spikes or slow spikes over the frontotemporal or centrotemporal regions, to multifocal discharges without generalized spike–wave bursts. With the appearance of CSWS (continu-ous discharge in more than 85% of non-REM stage 3 and stage 4 sleep), at average age of 8 years (3 years 1 month to 15 years 1 month), there was increase in the interictal epileptiform activity while awake. The appearance of CSWS was associated with increase in the focal motor seizures with or without atypical absences. In 12 of the 14 lesional patients in the study of Tassinari *et al* (1992), the seizures increased in frequency during the period of CSWS from several a week to several a day. Neuropsychologic deterioration, including of language function, with temporospatial disturbance, mental impairment, and psychiatric disturbance was the most prominent clinical change coinciding with CSWS.

Tassinari *et al* (1992) and other authors (e.g. Morikawa *et al* 1992) emphasize that seizures ultimately disappear in all cases, including those with demonstrable multilobar cortical lesions, the total duration of the epilepsy being around 12 years (4 years 1 month to 17 years 8 months). In four of the lesional cases reported by Tassinari *et al* the seizures disappeared either before or at the time of the end of CSWS. In a few, infrequent seizures, either absences or generalized tonic–clonic convulsions persisted from 7 months to 4 years 8 months after the end of CSWS. Global neuropsychologic improvement, but to a variable degree, coincided with the end of the epileptiform discharge in wakefulness and the progressive reduction in CSWS. However, only 7 of the 15 children with sufficient follow-up data available were described as living normally.

Guerrini *et al* (1996) reported on seven patients with localized polymicrogyria who developed CSWS. Guerrini (1997) suggests that CSWS occurs only in patients with polymicrogyria and not in those with any other types of cortical dysplasia. He points out that the evolution of the epilepsy is benign in all the cases (as in the other lesional cases reported by Tassinari *et al* 1992 and Morikawa *et al* 1992). The seizures may be very frequent, including atypical absences, and are often accompanied by marked atonic component producing drop attacks, though focal motor seizures are infrequent. In our series, CSWS has been associated not only with polymicrogyria but also with unilateral vascular pathology (see also Wolff *et al* 1995).

CONCLUSIONS

Ictal scalp EEG recordings are of limited value for establishing the anatomic locus of seizure onset in patients with multilobar pathology. At best they help in lateralization. To make use of seizure semeiology in clinical practice it is essential to be aware of the pitfalls and to be prepared to analyze the semeiology critically in relation to propagation of seizure discharge.

Maturational factors are clearly important in seizure semeiology in both unifocal and multifocal pathology. Seizure semeiology in neonates and infants is simple, even in the presence of multilobar pathology, because the immature cortex lacks the substrate for the complex automatisms used to identify localization-related epilepsy syndromes in older children and adults. Furthermore, rapid bilateral spread of seizure discharges is more common in the immature cortex. Hence infants, even with localized pathology, may present with bilateral seizure semeiology suggesting a generalized onset including myoclonic jerks and even infantile spasms. There is some evidence (Tinuper *et al* 1996) that, after the age of 50 years, there is a change in seizure semeiology with less secondary generalization.

Seizure semeiology may depend on the underlying pathology. With destructive lesions, as in children with congenital hemiplegia due to cerebral infarction, the remaining cortical mantle may be too thin in some regions to sustain seizure activity, so that only a single seizure type may occur despite the widespread lesion. Multiple lesions in focal cortical dysplasia and tuberous sclerosis have a potential for multifocal independent epileptogenesis. Even in this patient group, however, one epileptogenic area may be most active at a given time and a single seizure type may predominate despite multifocal interictal discharges. It is not known how long it takes for other epileptogenic areas to become active, if at all, following resection of one lesion. However, at least short-term good seizure outcome in some patients with tuberous sclerosis and focal cortical dysplasia suggests that the interval may be long.

Focal motor, suggesting involvement of the perirolandic area, is the most common seizure type in patients with focal cortical dysplasia and in those with unilateral vascular pathology. Seizure semeiology with involvement of this region can be variable and includes contralateral jerking of face and limbs, single limb jerks, bilateral limb jerks, drop attacks, and even the operculum syndrome with signs of pseudobulbar palsy, in addition to the secondarily generalized tonic–clonic convulsions. Multiple seizure types that can be correlated with multiple independent anatomic locations of onset are relatively infrequent. More often, seizures apparently starting at the temporal or parietooccipital lobes have a semeiology suggesting spread to adjacent cortex, especially the perirolandic area, resulting in focal motor seizures. Some seizures in which the initial symptamotology is lost due to the rapid spread of seizure discharges result in predominantly motor or generalized convulsive seizures.

Convulsive epileptic status episodes are infrequent, although Palmini *et al* (1991) have suggested a particular predisposition to status in patients with focal cortical dysplasia. Patients with multilobar pathology are, however, particularly susceptible to nonconvulsive status and to CSWS, with consequent deterioration of mental functioning. These epileptic states with predominant effects on mental function may be missed unless their possibility is considered and EEG studies are carried out. Guerrini (1997) suggests that patients with polymicrogyria are particularly prone to develop CSWS.

Secondary generalization of discharges and bilateral synchrony are more common in patients with multilobar pathology with both unifocal and multifocal interictal discharges (Tinuper *et al* 1995). The clinically atypical absences produced by the bilateral synchronous discharges have no localizing value, but it is important to identify them as they are associated with poor cognitive outcome.

KEY POINTS

1. Seizure semeiology in multilobar pathology varies with age.

2. During infancy, seizure types include clonic jerks, flexor spasms, myoclonias and atonia, cessation of activity, eye deviation, autonomic disturbance, and apnea. Only clonic limb and/or face jerks are localizing (to the contralateral perirolandic region).

3. Symptoms characteristic of complex partial seizures at older ages emerge at 3–4 years and the semeiology of these remains stable from around 6 years through adulthood. After 50 years of age the semeiology may change and secondarily generalized convulsions become less frequent.

4. After infancy, focal motor seizures (>80% cases) are the most common seizure type, followed by complex partial seizures (30–35% cases). Epilepsia partialis continua is common with Rasmussen syndrome and may be seen with disorders of cortical development.

5. Around 25% patients have frequent secondarily generalized convulsions. Multiple seizure types (including focal motor and/or complex partial and/or atypical absence) occur in 20–40%, but it can be very difficult to establish that these arise from separate foci and are not simply due to variable propagation of ictal activity.

6. Nonconvulsive status epilepticus may occur and may remain unrecognized as the cause for a child's mental deterioration over many months.

7. Continuous spike–wave in slow-wave sleep with cognitive decline, accompanied by predominantly unilateral motor seizures ± atypical absences and generalized tonic–clonic convulsions in sleep, can occur as a manifestation of multilobar pathology especially polymicrogyria.

REFERENCES

Bancaud J (1992) Kojewnikow's syndrome (epilepsia partialis continua) in children. In: Roger J, Bureau M, Dravet Ch, Dreifuss FE, Perret A, Wolf P (eds) *Epileptic Syndromes in Infancy, Childhood and Adolescence*, 2nd edn, pp 363–379. London: John Libbey.

Battaglia G, Granata T, Farina L, D'Incerti L, Franceschetti S, Avanzini G (1997) Periventricular nodular heterotopia: epileptogenic findings. *Epilepsia* 38(11):1173–1182.

Beaumanoir A, Dravet C (1992) The Lennox–Gastaut syndrome. In: Roger J, Bureau M, Dravet Ch, Dreifus FE, Perret A, Wolf P (eds) *Epileptic Syndromes in Infancy, Childhood and Adolescence*, 2nd edn, pp 115–132. London: John Libbey.

Bebin EM, Kelly PJ, Gomez MR (1993) Surgical treatment for epilepsy in cerebral tuberous sclerosis. *Epilepsia* 34(4):651–657.

Blume WT (1989) Clinical profile of partial seizures beginning at less than four years of age. *Epilepsia* 30(6):813–819.

Brockhaus A, Elger CE (1995) Complex partial seizures of temporal lobe origin in children of different age groups. *Epilepsia* 36(12):1173–1181.

Bureau M (1995) 'Continuous spikes and waves during slow sleep' (CSWS): definition of the syndrome. In: Beaumanoir A, Bureau M, Deonna T, Mira L, Tassinari CA (eds) *Continuous Spikes and Waves during Slow Sleep*, pp 17–26. London: John Libbey.

Chugani HT, Phelps ME, Mazziotta JC (1987) Positron emission tomography. Study of human brain functional development. *Annals of Neurology* 22:487–497.

Chugani HT, Shields WD, Shewmon DA, *et al* (1990) Infantile spasms: I. PET identifies focal cortical dysgenesis in cryptogenic cases for surgical treatment. *Annals of Neurology* 27:406–413.

Commission on Classification and Terminology of the International League Against Epilepsy (1989) Proposal for Revised Classification of Epilepsies and Epileptic Syndromes. *Epilepsia* 30(4):389–399.

Curatolo P (1991) Epilepsy in tuberous sclerosis. In: Ohtahara S, Roger J (eds) *New Trends in Paediatric Epileptology*, pp 86–93. Okayama: Okayama University Medical School.

Donat JF (1992) The age-dependent epileptic encephalopathies. *Journal of Child Neurology*, 7:7–21.

Doose H (1983) Nonconvulsive status epilepticus in childhood: clinical aspects and classification. In: Delgado-Escueta AV, Wasterlain CG, Treiman DM, Porter RJ (eds) *Advances in Neurology*, Vol 34: *Status Epilepticus*, pp 83–92. New York: Raven Press.

Dravet C, Catani C, Bureau M, Roger J (1989) Partial epilepsies in infancy: a study of 40 cases. *Epilepsia* 30(6):807–812.

Duchowny MS (1987) Complex partial seizures of infancy. *Archives of Neurology* 44:911–914.

Duchowny M, Resnick TJ, Lewis A, Alvarez LA, Morrison G (1990)

Focal resection for malignant partial seizures in infancy. *Neurology* **40**:980–984.

Evans D, Levene M (1998) Neonatal seizures. *Archives of Disease in Childhood, Fetal and Neonatal Edition* **8**:70–75.

Fusco L, Vigevano F (1991) Reversible operculum syndrome caused by progressive epilepsia partialis continua in a child with left hemimegalencephaly. *Journal of Neurology, Neurosurgery and Psychiatry* **54**:556–558.

Gaily EK, Shewmon DA, Chugani HT, Curran JG (1995) Asymmetric and asynchronous infantile spasms. *Epilepsia* **36**(9):873–882.

Guerrini R (1997) Clinical epilepsy syndromes in focal cortical dysplasias. In Tuxhorn I, Holthausen H, Boenigk H (eds) *Paediatric Epilepsy Syndromes and Their Surgical Treatment*, pp 170–184. London: John Libbey.

Guerrini R, Parmeggiani A, Bureau M, et al (1996) Localised cortical dysplasia: good seizure outcome after sleep related electrical status epilepticus. In: Guerrini R, Andermann F, Canapicchi R, Roger J, Zifkin B, Pfanner P (eds) *Dysplasias of Cerebral Cortex and Epilepsy*, pp 329–335. Philadelphia: Lippincott–Raven.

Holthausen H, Teixeira VA, Tuxhorn I, et al (1997) Epilepsy surgery in children and adolescents with focal cortical dysplasia. In: Tuxhorn I, Holthausen H, Boenigk H (eds) *Paediatric Epilepsy Syndromes and Their Surgical Treatment*, pp 199–215. London: John Libbey.

Kotagal P, Tuxhorn I (1997) Epilepsy surgery in tuberous sclerosis and other phakomatoses. In: Tuxhorn I, Holthausen H, Boenigk H (eds) *Paediatric Epilepsy Syndromes and Their Surgical Treatment*, pp 371–376. London: John Libbey.

Kuzniecky R, Gilliam F, Morawetz R, Faught E, Palmer C, Black L (1997) Occipital lobe developmental malformations and epilepsy: clinical spectrum, treatment and outcome. *Epilepsia* **38**(2):175–181.

Luders H, Wyllie E, Rothner DA, Bourgeois B, Kotagal P (1989) Surgery of localisation related epilepsies in children. *Brain and Development* **11**:98–101.

Luna D, Dulac O, Plouin P (1989) Ictal characteristics of cryptogenic partial epilepsies in infancy. *Epilepsia* **30**(6):827–832.

Manford M, Fish DR, Shorvon SD (1996) An analysis of clinical seizure patterns and their localising value in frontal and temporal lobe epilepsies. *Brain* **119**:17–40.

Mitchell WG (1996) Status epilepticus and acute repetitive seizures in children, adolescents, and young adults: etiology, outcome, and treatment. *Epilepsia* **37**(Suppl 1):S74–S80.

Morikawa T, Seino M, Osawa T, Kazuichi Y (1985) Five children with continuous spike wave discharges during sleep. In: Roger J, Bureau M, Dravet Ch, Dreifuss FE, Perret A, Wolf P (eds) *Epileptic Syndromes in Infancy, Childhood and Adolescence*, pp 205–212. London: John Libbey.

Morikawa T, Seino M, Yagi K (1992) Long-term outcome of four children with continuous spike-waves during sleep. In: Roger J, Bureau M, Dravet Ch, Dreifuss FE, Perret A, Wolf P (eds) *Epileptic Syndromes in Infancy, Childhood and Adolescence*, 2nd edn, pp 257–265. London: John Libbey.

Nordli DR Jr, Bazil CW, Scheuer ML, Pedley TA (1997) Recognition and classification of seizures in infants. *Epilepsia* **38**(5):553–560.

Oguni H, Hayashi K, Usui N, Osawa M, Shinizu H (1998) Startle epilepsy with infantile hemiplegia: report of two cases improved by surgery. *Epilepsia* **39**(1):93–98.

Palmini A, Andermann F, Olivier A, et al (1991) Focal neuronal migration disorders and intractable partial epilepsy: a study of 30 patients. *Annals of Neurology* **30**:741–749.

Palmini A, Gambardella A, Andermann F, et al (1995) Intrinsic epileptogenicity of human dysplastic cortex as suggested by corticography and surgical results. *Annals of Neurology* **37**:476–487.

Patry G, Lyagoubi S, Tassinari CA (1971) Subclinical 'electrical status epilepticus' induced by sleep in children. *Archives of Neurology* **4**:242–252.

Perot P, Weir B, Rasmussen T (1966) Tuberous sclerosis. *Archives of Neurology* **15**:498–506.

Sisodiya AM, Free SL, Stevens JM, Fish DR, Shorvon SD (1995) Widespread cerebral structural changes in patients with cortical dysgenesis and epilepsy. *Brain* **118**:1039–1050.

Spencer SS (1998) Substrates of localisation-related epilepsies: biologic implications of localising findings in humans. *Epilepsia* **39**(2):114–123.

Stores G, Zaiwalla Z, Styles E, Hoshika A (1995) Non-convulsive status epilepticus. *Archives of Disease in Childhood* **73**:106–111.

Tassinari CA, Terzano G, Capocchi G, et al (1977) Epileptic seizures during sleep in children. In: Penry JK (ed) *Epilepsy. The 8th International Symposium*, pp 345–354. New York: Raven Press.

Tassinari CA, Bureau M, Dravet C, Dalla Bernardina B, Roger J (1992) Epilepsy with continuous spikes and waves during slow sleep – otherwise described as ESES (epilepsy with electrical status epilepticus during slow sleep). In: Roger J, Bureau M, Dravet Ch, Dreifuss FE, Perret A, Wolf P (eds) *Epileptic Syndromes in Infancy, Childhood and Adolescence*, 2nd edn, pp 245–256. London: John Libbey.

Tinuper P, Cerullo A, Riva R, et al (1995) Clinical and EEG features of partial epilepsy with secondary bilateral synchrony. *Journal of Epilepsy* **8**:210–214.

Tinuper P, Provini F, Marini C, et al (1996) Partial epilepsy of long duration: changing semeiology with age. *Epilepsia* **37**(2):162–164.

Tukel K, Jasper H (1952) The electroencephalogram in parasagittal lesions. *Electroencephalography and Clinical Neurophysiology* **4**:481–494.

Wolff M, Bureau M, Bartolomei F, Dravet Ch, Genton P (1995) Case reports: In: Beaumanoir A, Bureau M, Deonna T, Mira L, Tassinari CA (eds) *Continuous Spikes and Waves during Slow Sleep*, pp 189–193. London: John Libbey.

Wyllie E, Comair YG, Kotagal P, Raja S, Ruggieri P (1996) Epilepsy surgery in infants. *Epilepsia* **37**(7):625–637.

Yamamoto N, Watanabe K, Negoro T, et al (1988) Partial seizures evolving to infantile spasms. *Epilepsia* **29**(1):34–40.

Malformations of cortical development

SM SISODIYA, MV SQUIER, AND P ANSLOW

Malformations of cortical development (MCD) were once identified almost only in post-mortem specimens from subjects with gross developmental disorders or severe childhood epilepsy. They can now be revealed *in vivo* by imaging studies. Although their true incidence is unknown, they are an important cause of refractory epilepsy in adults (Li *et al* 1995), children, and subjects with mental retardation (Brodtkorb *et al* 1992). Some pathologic studies suggest a comparatively high prevalence of these changes in the brains of patients with epilepsy (Meencke and Veith 1999). Interest in MCD has grown because of their possible genetic causation, the understanding of epileptogenesis they may afford, the light they shed upon normal cerebral development, and the refractory nature of the epilepsy that they may cause.

Many varieties of MCD are recognized on morphologic grounds, although their discrimination and labeling are debated. We consider the following: focal cortical dysplasia; microdysgenesis; polymicrogyria; lissencephaly; schizencephaly (also known as cleft); heterotopia, both periventricular and subcortical; hemimegalencephaly; and hamartomas. There is currently no satisfactory definition or classification of cortical dysplasias, due mainly to our incomplete understanding of their etiology and to their wide phenotypic variability. In its broadest definition the term encompasses structural changes of the cortex resulting from disruption of its development. There are many causes, including genetic, metabolic, traumatic, infectious, and hypoxic–ischemic insults, and the final structural nature of the malformation is largely dependent on the precise time in development when the insult occurred. In order to understand how such lesions arise it is necessary to review the basic steps of normal human cortical development.

HUMAN CORTICAL DEVELOPMENT

Development of the cerebral cortex occurs in an orderly sequence of precisely timed stages involving cell proliferation, migration, differentiation, and programmed cell death.

Cell proliferation

The neurons of the cerebral cortex originate in the germinal matrix, a dense mass of mitotically active precursor cells found just beneath the ependymal lining of the ventricular system. Cell proliferation takes place at an enormous rate in early gestation to produce neuronal precursors. During the second half of gestation glial cells are produced and the germinal matrix involutes by about 36 weeks.

Cell migration

All neuronal precursors have to leave the germinal matrix and migrate to reach their final destination in the mature cortex. They do this with the guidance of radial glial cell processes. These specialized glial cells align themselves radially and extend long processes to span the developing brain wall, with one foot process on the ventricular lining and the other on pial membrane at the surface of the brain. The migrating neuroblasts attach themselves to these radial glial guides and migrate along them to the cortical plate (Fig. 10.1). Migration is both spatially and temporally ordered. Cells tend to remain in radial units and their position in the cortex usually overlies the sector of the germinal zone in which they originated, although some tangential migration may occur (Rakic 1988). Neuronal migration begins just before 7 weeks and is essentially complete by 20 weeks (Marin-Padilla 1995).

Cortical lamination

The first cells to arrive form the preplate, which is subsequently split into superficial and deep layers by the arrival of neurons destined to form the definitive cortical plate. The superficial (marginal) zone contains large horizontally orientated neurons (Cajal–Retzius cells). They are a transient population that cannot be identified in normal postnatal cortex. They express a protein called reelin and appear to play a crucial role in cortical lamination (Flint and Kriegstein 1997). All newly arriving neurons make contact with these cells before descending to their destined layer of the cortex. Cells arriving subsequently migrate through earlier formed laminae to reach the Cajal–Retzius cells and then form more superficial layers so that the cortex develops 'inside-out' with the earliest migrating cells forming the deep cortical layers and the latest migrating cells forming the most superficial layers. The deep layer of the original preplate becomes the subplate, another transient structure that involutes during the first months of postnatal life. The role of the subplate appears to be one of guiding axons into the developing cortex (Molnar and Blakemore 1995). Thus the position of a cell in the cortex depends on both its position in the germinal matrix and the time at which it migrated from the matrix. Disorders of cortical structure may be determined even before neuroblasts have begun their migration (Fig. 10.2).

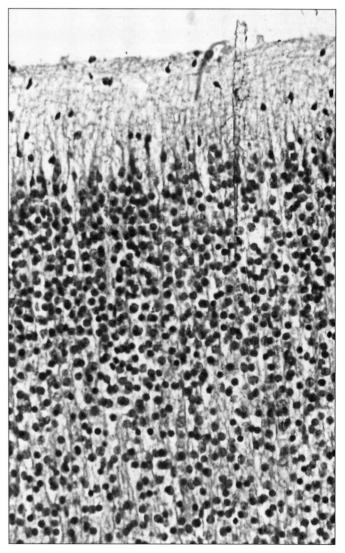

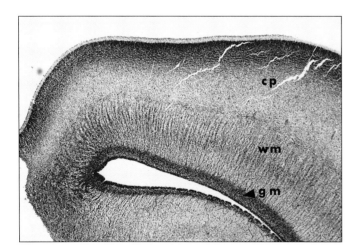

Fig. 10.1 Neuronal migration: normal cerebral mantle at 19 weeks of gestation. Neurons are seen migrating through the primitive white matter (wm) in radial columns. The cortical plate (cp) already has a distinct marginal zone. gm, germinal matrix. Hematoxylin and eosin ×20.

Fig. 10.2 Neuronal migration: high-power magnification of cortical plate at 20 weeks of gestation. A cell-poor marginal layer is seen. Primitive neurons of the cortex are aligned along radial glial fibers. Hematoxylin and eosin ×300.

Cell differentiation

The final specific phenotype of a neuron is only achieved once it has reached the cortex and established synaptic contacts with other cells. Neurons of the human cortex all have recognizable phenotypes by the time of birth (Marin-Padilla 1995).

Programmed cell death

During the formation of the brain there is a massive over-production of cells, which are subsequently pruned by programmed cell death. This is a form of cell death (termed 'apoptosis') that involves activation of a series of intracellular enzymes, some dependent on gene transcription and translation, which break down nuclear DNA. The cells have a characteristic morphology, with shrunken, densely staining, rounded nuclei. This form of cell death is responsible for involution of transient structures such as the subplate (Ferrer *et al* 1992a).

Control of cortical development

The control of brain development is extremely complex, involving half of the human genome. In the earliest stages of brain formation, soluble factors or morphogens secreted by mesoderm or notochord are responsible for induction of the early neural tube. They act by inducing families of transcription factors which subsequently influence downstream genes responsible for the cellular phenotype of the primitive neural tube cells. A series of genes, including *Hox*, *Pax*, and *sonic hedgehog*, are responsible for craniocaudal and dorsoventral patterning of the neural tube. The position of a cell in the neural tube at this very early stage determines its later position and differentiation. A protein called HES-1 is expressed in proliferative cell layers and appears to be involved in signaling the beginning of migration and maturation of neuroblasts (Scotting and Rex 1996).

Neuronal migration depends on the complex interaction between neuroblasts, radial glia, and extracellular matrix components. Several distinct molecules have been described at sites of neuroblast–glial interaction that appear to be crucial in permitting neuronal migration. They include astrotactin, which is expressed on early post-mitotic neurons (Zhang *et al* 1996), NJPA1, and D4 (Flint and Kriegstein 1997). Neural cell adhesion molecules, chondroitin sulfate proteoglycans, neurotransmitters, and calcium may all influence neuronal migration (Gressens *et al* 1996; Blackshear *et al* 1997; Flint and Kriegstein 1997) (Fig. 10.3).

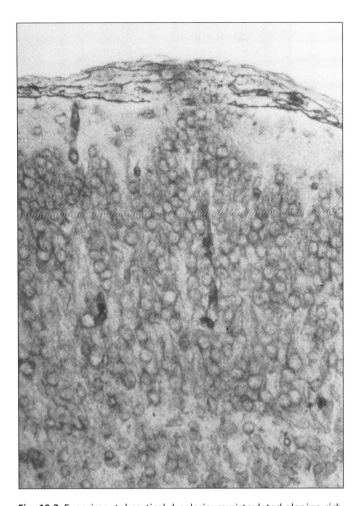

Fig. 10.3 Experimental cortical dysplasia: myristoylated alanine-rich C-kinase substrate deficient mouse. There is a focal disruption in the pial barrier and neurons are streaming up from layer II of the cortex into the leptomeninges to form a focal glioneuronal leptomeningeal heterotopia. Note the irregularity of the border between layers I and II and the large neurons (Cajal–Retzius cells) in layer I, the molecular layer. Reticulin ×450. (Courtesy of Professor Perry Blackshear.)

CLASSIFICATION OF MALFORMATIONS OF CORTICAL DEVELOPMENT

For the purposes of this chapter we have adopted a scheme based on the morphologic appearances of the dysplastic brain. Morphologic descriptions are used in radiology but even the increasingly detailed images produced by new magnetic resonance imaging (MRI) techniques cannot always define the precise nature of cortical dysplasias. Indeed, some malformations of cortical structure may be extremely hard to identify even at the histologic level. Subtle disorganization of neuronal structure or orientation may be focal and involve only a few layers of the cortex (Ying *et al* 1998) and so are readily missed. Recent studies suggest that immunocytochemistry which labels specific neuronal subtypes may be a far more sensitive marker of disorganization of the cortex than routine histologic stains (Spreafico *et al* 1998, Hannan *et al* 1999). Eventually it is hoped that clinical studies and information from genetics, molecular biology, imaging, neurophysiology, and pathology will converge to produce a rational classification.

Cortical dysplasia is essentially a disorganization of cortical structure resulting from disturbance of one or more of the processes of its development. It is not synonymous with *neuronal migration disorder*, as many other developmental processes may be involved. The process may be extensive and obvious macroscopically and on MRI scans, or it may be a subtle cytoarchitectural change visible only at a microscopic level.

A spectrum of histologic changes may be seen. Mischel *et al* (1995) have defined nine characteristic features of the dysplastic cortex that may be seen singly or together.

Cortical laminar disorganization is the most consistent histologic finding (Mischel *et al* 1995). Other features include loss of the clear margin between layer I (the molecular layer) and layer II, and irregularity or blurring of the deep cortical border with the white matter (Figs 10.4 and 10.5). These features most probably result from disruption of neuronal migration to the cortex. However, more subtle neuronal disorganization may occur later, after cortical plate formation. Marin-Padilla (1997) has shown that cytoarchitectural rearrangement in the cortex may result

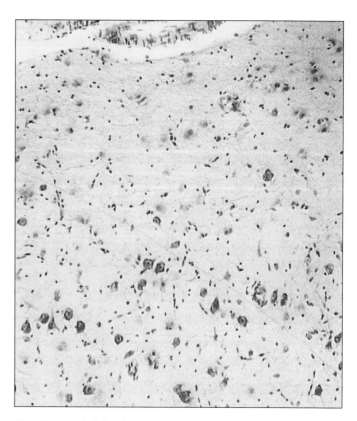

Fig. 10.5 Cortical dysplasia: the boundary between layer I (molecular layer) and layer II is ragged and large neurons are seen in the molecular layer. There is also gliosis of the molecular layer, secondary to repeated seizures. Luxol Fast Blue and cresyl violet ×170.

from partial isolation, such as occurs in surviving cortex overlying areas of white matter damage. Deafferented neurons may develop complex hypertrophic axonal sprouts that contribute to increased neuropil between neuronal cell bodies, thus altering their spatial rearrangement.

Single neurons in the white matter are frequently seen in the infant brain without other abnormality. Their significance depends on their number and site: they are much less frequent in the adult white matter and their numbers vary between the lobes of the brain. Quantitative studies have shown increased white matter neuronal counts to be significantly associated with epilepsy (Meencke 1983; Hardiman *et al* 1988). While ectopic white matter neurons may result from incomplete migration at mid gestation, it is equally possible that they represent subplate neurons that have failed to undergo programmed cell death, in which case they may represent a disruption in late gestation or the first months of postnatal life (Chun and Shatz 1989) (Fig. 10.6).

White matter neuronal heterotopias are groups of neurons in the white matter rather than isolated single cells.

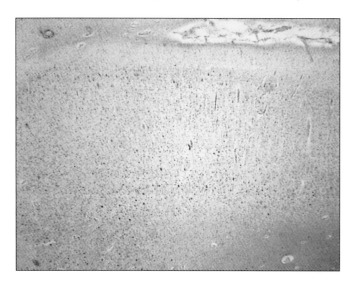

Fig. 10.4 Cortical dysplasia: edge of a dysplastic focus; the cortex on the right of the picture is normal. It becomes thickened, with blurring of its deep border with the white matter. Neuronal lamination is lost and large deeply stained neurons are scattered through all layers. There is fusion of the pial surface with an adjacent gyrus. Luxol Fast Blue and cresyl violet ×20.

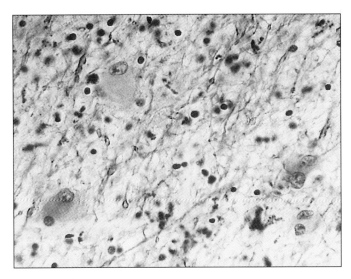

Fig. 10.6 White matter neurons: neurons and abnormal balloon cells in the white matter in hemimegalencephaly. Luxol Fast Blue and cresyl violet ×700.

Neuronal heterotopias may be focal and nodular, or diffuse. Nodular heterotopias may be seen beneath the ependyma, beneath the cortex, or elsewhere in the white matter. Band heterotopias are less clearly defined and usually form a dense layer beneath the cortex, giving the impression of a 'double cortex.' Neuronal heterotopias are probably the result of failed migration in the second trimester (Fig. 10.7).

Leptomeningeal glioneuronal heterotopia is clusters of neurons and glial cells found in the leptomeninges. It is found in brains with a variety of malformations, and is a characteristic finding in the fetal alcohol syndrome. There may be tiny nests of cells or more extensive sheets in association with underlying malformation of the cortex (Fig. 10.8). The disorder appears to result from excessive migration of cells through a damaged pial–glial barrier (Barth 1987).

Molecular layer neurons are encountered occasionally in most normal brains. However they may be more numerous than usual in the context of cortical dysplasia. The cells are often horizontally orientated and possibly represent persistent Cajal–Retzius cells that have not undergone programmed cell death. Specific markers allow their identification as neurons and distinguish them from reactive astrocytes.

Persistent subpial granule layer. The subpial granule cell layer (subpial layer of Brun) is a transient fetal structure seen in the human cerebral cortex between 12 weeks of gestation and the first months of postnatal life (Friede 1989).

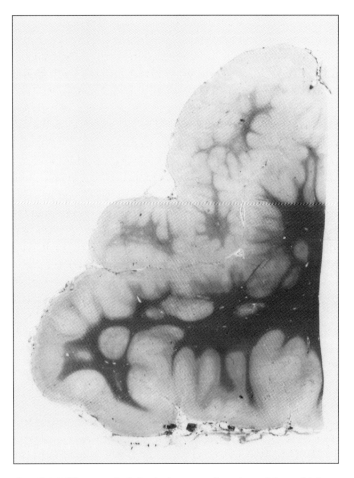

Fig. 10.7 Diffuse cortical dysplasia: coronal section of frontal lobe showing extensive dysplasia, mainly polymicrogyria. Note several large nodular heterotopias in the subcortical white matter. Luxol Fast Blue and cresyl violet ×2.5.

In the dysplastic cortex, remnants of this layer are seen as a row of small regular cells in the immediate subpial zone.

Neuronal cytomegaly is characterized by abnormally enlarged neurons that are irregularly shaped and often contain cytoplasmic neurofibrillary tangles (De Rosa *et al* 1992). Several groups have demonstrated increased DNA in these cells, suggesting polyploidy (Bignami *et al* 1968; Manz *et al* 1979). This has led to the suggestion that these cells result from disruption very early on in development when the cells are in the periventricular zone. However, cells deprived of their normal connections may also undergo enlargement and phenotypic alterations (Marin-Padilla 1997), indicating much later origin.

Balloon cells have massively enlarged, hyaline, eosinophilic cytoplasm that displaces the nucleus to one side of the cell (Fig. 10.9). Some cells are ambiguous in their staining patterns, expressing markers of both immature and mature

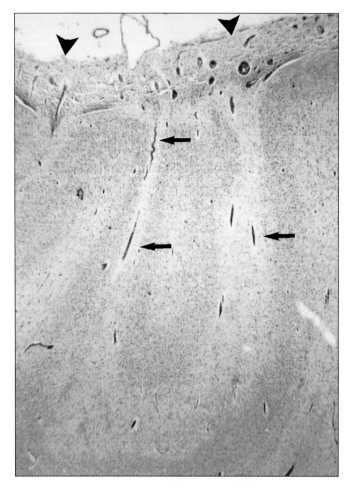

Fig. 10.8 Glioneuronal leptomeningeal heterotopia: polymicrogyria. The cortex consists of a sweeping band of neurons beneath fused molecular layers, marked by large blood vessels (arrows). Note the thickened leptomeninges (arrowheads) containing glial cells and neurons that have migrated through breaks in the pia. Phosphotungstic acid and hematoxylin ×34.

glial cells as well as neuronal markers (De Rosa *et al* 1992; Farrell *et al* 1992), indicating interference with differentiation.

Focal polymicrogyria is a frequent component of cortical dysplasia but is also seen alone in other clinical and pathologic contexts. Macroscopically, the cortex appears to have too many small gyri but the diagnosis can only be confirmed by histologic examination. The essential finding is of fusion of the surface layers of adjacent gyri with disruption of underlying neuronal layers, which may take several forms (Fig. 10.10). These are described in more detail below.

The above changes may be seen in any combination in dysplastic cortex, and may give some indication of the time at which development was disrupted.

FOCAL CORTICAL DYSPLASIA

This term was first introduced by Taylor *et al* in 1971 to describe macroscopically evident focal lesions in which they noted loss of cortical lamination, the presence of abnormal giant cells, and heterotopic white matter neurons (Fig. 10.11). The term has been used for describing extensive macroscopically evident lesions seen on MRI scans, as well as subtle cytoarchitectural changes restricted to only a few cortical layers. There is clinical and histologic evidence that further lesions may exist beyond macroscopically evident areas of focal cortical dysplasia. As Janota and Polkey (1992) have indicated, cortical dysplasia need be neither focal nor cortical.

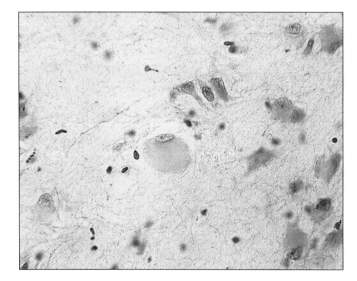

Fig. 10.9 Cortical dysplasia: a balloon cell among irregularly arranged cells of astrocytic and neuronal appearance. Luxol Fast Blue and cresyl violet ×700.

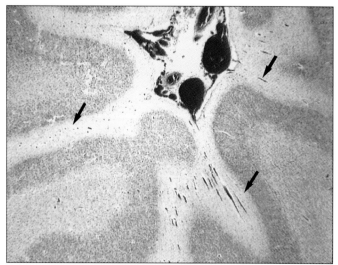

Fig. 10.10 Polymicrogyria: a band of neurons forms festoons beneath fused molecular layers. Prominent blood vessels are seen at the seam line of adjacent gyri (arrows). Hematoxylin and eosin ×34.

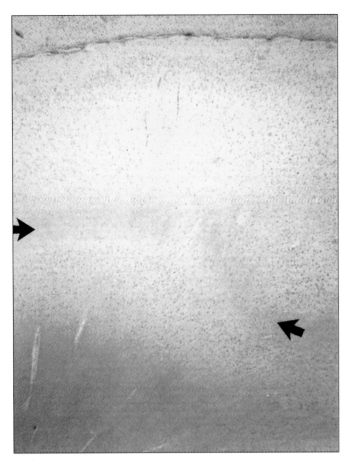

Fig. 10.11 Focal cortical dysplasia: the cortex lacks normal lamination. A transverse band of myelinated fibers (arrows) separates the irregular lower border of the cortex from a band of heterotopic neurons. Luxol Fast Blue and cresyl violet ×68.

MICRODYSGENESIS

Microdysgenesis is a term applied to minor diffuse changes, including increased neurons in the molecular layer, single white matter neurons, and abnormal clustering of cortical neurons (Meencke and Janz 1984; Hardiman *et al* 1988). Although there has been controversy about the significance of these findings in relation to epilepsy (Lyon and Gastaut 1985), careful quantitative studies indicate that they do appear to occur more frequently in patients with epilepsy (Hardiman *et al* 1988).

The use of immunocytochemistry to identify neuronal subtypes in the cortex adds much more information. This technique may show abnormal neuronal clustering not readily identified with conventional stains (Spreafico *et al* 1998; Hannan *et al* 1999), and it may also demonstrate alteration in the proportions of excitatory and inhibitory cells (Ying *et al* 1998), which has significance in relation to epileptogenesis. The technique is a very helpful adjunct to carefully controlled quantitative studies in establishing the significance of microdysgenesis in epilepsy.

POLYMICROGYRIA

This is a frequent cortical malformation associated with ischemic, traumatic, genetic, and infectious etiologies. The cortex may appear to have small irregular and closely packed gyri. The cut surface (and also the MRI appearance) may show the cortex to be thicker than normal. Diagnosis can only be confirmed by histologic examination.

The constant histologic finding is fusion of the pial surfaces of adjacent gyri, the seam often being marked by a row of large occluded meningeal vessels. Beneath this there may be a variety of patterns of neuronal disorganization. Two main forms are described. In the 'unlayered' form, the neurons typically produce a band that is thrown into folds or festoons beneath the fused molecular layers. This form is thought to arise before the cortical plate is fully formed and has been associated with injuries at 13–16 weeks of gestation. The second commonly described form is the 'four-layered' which is thought to result from selective loss of cortical layers III–V after formation of the cortical plate and has been described at 24 weeks of gestation (Barth 1987).

Polymicrogyria only arises before 28 weeks of gestation. There may be a band of myelinated fibers beneath the pial surface and widespread thickening of the leptomeninges with increased numbers of blood vessels. The polymicrogyric cortex may be found over small areas of the cortex, bordering porencephalic cysts, or may be extensive involving the majority of the brain surface. The commonest site for partial polymicrogyria is in the sylvian fissure (Fig. 10.12).

LISSENCEPHALY (SMOOTH BRAIN)

In lissencephaly all, or a major part, of the cerebral hemispheres lacks gyri. Lissencephaly encompasses agyria and pachygyria, which are macroscopic or MRI descriptions of areas of cortex that lack gyri or that are thickened, with reduced numbers of coarse gyri. There is no specific histologic correlate with these macroscopic terms. Any of the histologic patterns of cortical dysplasia may be found. In contrast, diffuse and extensive lissencephaly may be differentiated into two specific subtypes on the basis of the histologic findings, supported by genetic associations that confirm their specific identities.

Type I (classical) lissencephaly

The cortex is thick and smooth. The neuronal content is very poor, with no laminar pattern and an indistinct inferior border with the white matter. There may be a large volume of residual germinal matrix, indicating failure of

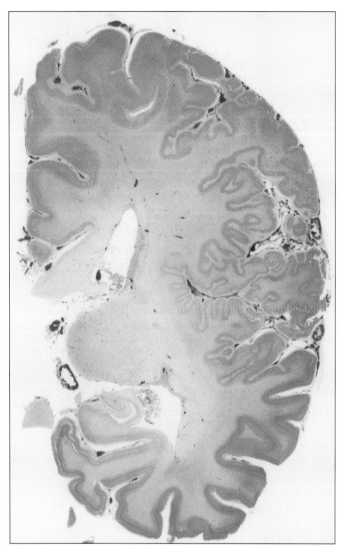

Fig. 10.12 Polymicrogyria: section of a hemisphere showing extensive polymicrogyria, most marked in the sylvian fissure. Phosphotungstic acid and hematoxylin.

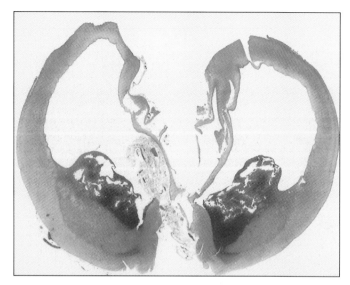

Fig. 10.13 Type I lissencephaly: coronal section of a term brain showing completely smooth cerebral surface, indistinct cortex, and widely dilated lateral ventricles. There is a large mass of residual germinal matrix. Hematoxylin and eosin ×2.4.

neurons to migrate. The lateral ventricles are enlarged, particularly the occipital horns (Fig. 10.13). Type I lissencephaly occurs alone in the isolated lissencephaly sequence or in association with other malformations as part of the *Miller–Dieker syndrome*. The gene responsible for both conditions (*LIS-1*) has been found on chromosome 17p13.3 (Reiner *et al* 1993).

Type II (cobblestone) lissencephaly

In this form of lissencephaly the cortical dysplasia appears to result from overmigration of neurons, which stream through the pial barrier into the leptomeninges (Squier 1993). The resultant proliferation of blood vessels and fibrous tissues causes the ectopic neurons to become trapped in irregular masses separated by fibrovascular bands, which obliterate the subarachnoid space and become incorporated into the outer part of the cortex (Fig. 10.14). There may be focal polymicrogyria and fusion of the medial surfaces of the frontal lobes. The malformation is usually very extensive and may even involve the cerebellum (Fig. 10.15). The surface of the brain is smooth or 'cobblestone' in appearance.

Type II lissencephaly is an important component of three syndromes involving malformation of muscle, eye, and brain. *Fukuyama congenital muscular dystrophy* is an autosomal recessive disease found mainly in Japan; muscle involvement is severe. Mutations at chromosome 9q31–33 are described (Dobyns and Truwit 1995). *Walker–Warburg syndrome* is also autosomal recessive but brain and eye manifestations are much more severe. *Muscle–eye–brain disease* has manifestations of intermediate severity. Neither Walker–Warburg syndrome nor muscle–eye–brain disease are associated with mutations at 9q31–33 and it has been suggested that these disorders are allelic (Dobyns and Truwit 1995), although there are differences in the severity of the pathology between them. All three diseases exhibit disturbances in components of the basement membrane that guide cell migration, which may explain malformations in muscle, eye, and brain (Haltia *et al* 1997) (Fig. 10.16).

HETEROTOPIA

Neuronal heterotopia is clusters of irregularly orientated neurons found in the white matter that result from failure of neuronal migration before 20 weeks of gestation.

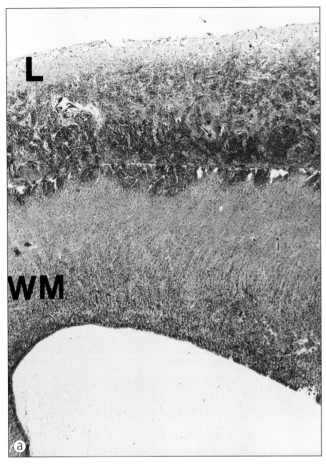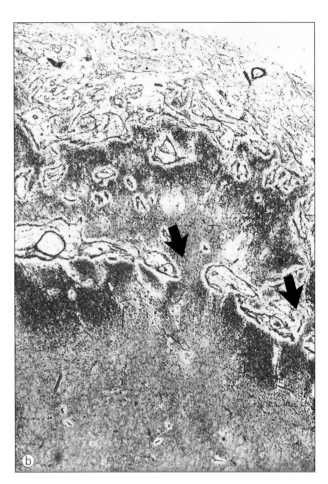

Fig. 10.14 Type II lissencephaly. (a) Disordered, excessive migration in the cerebral wall of a fetus at 18 weeks of gestation. Note massive thickening of the leptomeninges (L), which contain masses of heterotopic neurons and proliferating blood vessels and connective tissues. Reticulin ×20. WM, white matter. (b) At higher power, breaks in the pial barrier are seen (arrows) with fountains of neurons migrating through them with the leptomeninges. Reticulin ×60.

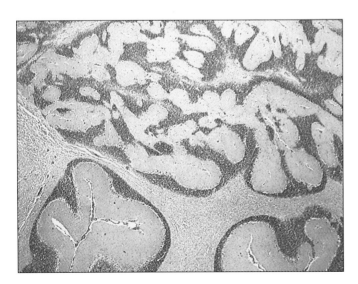

Fig. 10.15 Type II lissencephaly: a large area of cerebellar cortical dysplasia is seen in the upper part of the picture. Compare with normal cerebellar cortex below. Hematoxylin and eosin ×30.

Immunohistochemical studies have shown the nodules to comprise both γ-aminobutyric acid (GABA)-containing and excitatory pyramidal neurons with limited connectivity to each other and adjacent tissues (Hannan *et al* 1999). The morphology of the neurons within these nodules suggests that they are immature compared with the overlying cortex, with few, short, simple processes. It is suggested that these immature cells act in an excitatory fashion and may thus be capable of generating epileptic activity.

Focal nodular heterotopias may be single or multiple and found in subcortical or periventricular locations (Fig. 10.17). They are usually sporadic and may be seen in association with ischemic or traumatic damage (Fig. 10.18). Groups of heterotopic nodules frequently underlie areas of dysplastic cortex. *Bilateral periventricular nodular heterotopia* is a distinct and fascinating entity. It is characterized by nodular masses of heterotopic gray matter, often contiguous, lining the walls of the lateral ventricles and bulging into the ventricular lumen.

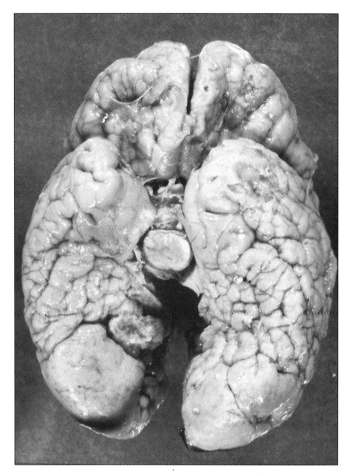

Fig. 10.16 Focal agyria: muscle–eye–brain disease. Base of the brain of a female aged 9 years, showing focal agyria of the occipital poles and coarse gyri over the temporal poles. Elsewhere the gyral pattern is irregular.

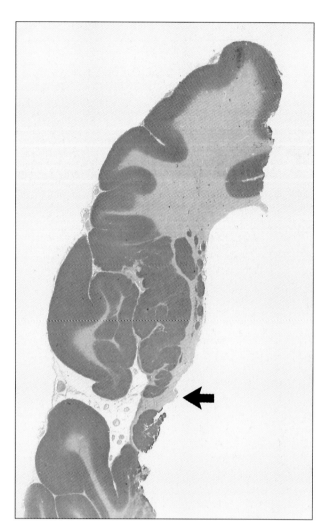

Fig. 10.18 Cortical dysplasia: nodular heterotopias. Coronal section of a hemisphere removed at hemispherectomy from a male aged 8 years. There is a large area of dysplastic cortex adjacent to a defect caused by penetration during amniocentesis at 17 weeks of gestation (arrow). There are multiple nodules of heterotopic neurons in the underlying white matter. Stained with the neuronal marker synaptophysin ×2.

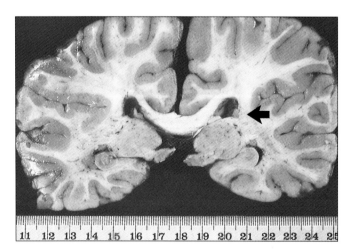

Fig. 10.17 Single nodular heterotopia: coronal slice of the brain of a female aged 5 years showing a single subependymal heterotopic nodule (arrow).

The neurons in the nodules are irregularly orientated and are separated into groups by glial cells or bands of myelinated fibers. The overlying cortex is usually normal in females with this malformation. However a small number of males have been described in which there is extensive polymicrogyria in the overlying cortex (Fig. 10.19), together with a variety of other malformations within and outside the nervous system (Dobyns *et al* 1997). *Subcortical heterotopia* may be single or multiple or may form a contiguous band separated from the overlying cortex by a thin, indistinct band of myelinated white matter. *Band heterotopia* appear on MRI scans as a 'double cortex.' The band contains irregularly arranged neurons separated from the deep margin of the cortex by a thin and

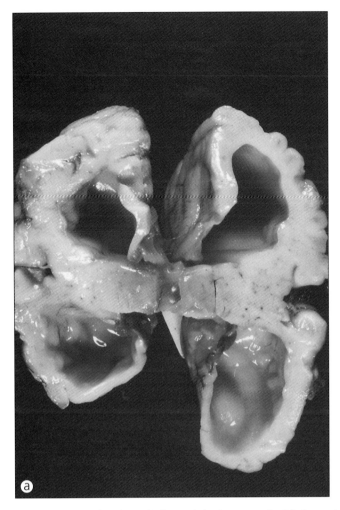
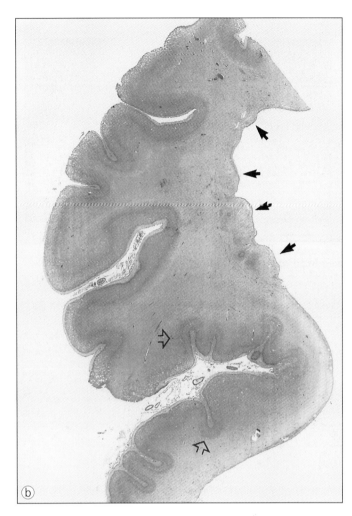

Fig. 10.19 Bilateral periventricular nodular heterotopia. (a) Coronal slice through the brain of a male neonate. Multiple masses are seen protruding into the walls of the very dilated lateral ventricles. Cortical gyration is abnormal. (b) Section of the brain in (a) showing contiguous clusters of subependymal heterotopias (arrows) and polymicrogyria in the cortex (open arrows). Luxol Fast Blue and cresyl violet ×4.

irregular strip of white matter (Fig. 10.20). The overlying cortex may be normal or dysplastic.

SCHIZENCEPHALY

Schizencephaly is a complete cleft through the brain wall that extends from the ventricle to the brain surface. The cleft is usually fully or partially lined by cortex, which is often dysplastic. This lesion is probably the result of a destructive injury in early development involving the entire thickness of the brain wall and synonymous with *porencephaly* (Friede 1989; Barkovich *et al* 1992). Indeed, MRI appearances of collapsed porencephalic cysts conform to the definition of schizencephaly. Schizencephaly was originally thought to be the result of early migration failure not associated with destructive lesions (Yakovlev and Wadworth 1946a,b). Recently, mutations of the homeobox gene *EMX2* have been described in patients with schizencephaly

(Granata *et al* 1997) and schizencephaly has been described in two children with cytomegalovirus infection (Iannetti *et al* 1998). These recent findings suggest a multifactorial etiology during early development.

HEMIMEGALENCEPHALY

This fascinating malformation has been the subject of much pathologic study. The macroscopic appearances are of enlargement of most or all of one cerebral hemisphere, with broad, coarse gyri, a thickened cortex and dilatation of the lateral ventricle, and a variety of changes in the white matter. The cortex shows the entire spectrum of dysplastic change, while the white matter may be gliotic, calcified, and cystic (Renowden and Squier 1994) (Fig. 10.21). In a few cases of hemimegalencephaly where whole brains have been studied, minor dysplastic changes have been described in the contralateral hemisphere (Robain *et al* 1988). Some

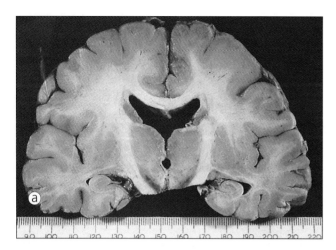

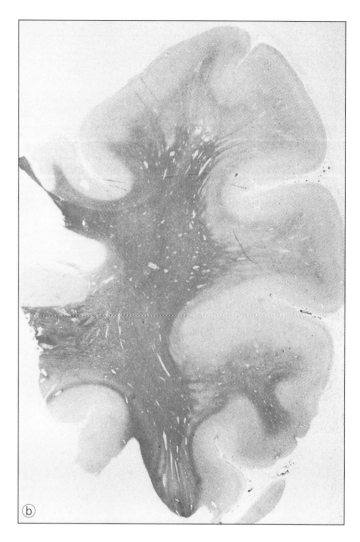

Fig. 10.20 Band heterotopia 'double cortex.' Coronal slice of the fixed brain of a female aged 45 years. Note the poorly defined junction between cortex and white matter where there is a diffuse band of heterotopic neurons. (b) Coronal section of brain in (a). Note the subcortical band of heterotopic neurones, in some areas faintly demarcated from the cortex by an irregular band of myelinated fibers. Luxol Fast Blue and cresyl violet.

children have associated skin lesions on the ipsilateral side of the body (Pavone *et al* 1991).

The etiology is quite unknown. The presence, in many cases, of bizarre giant neurons has suggested heteroploidy (Mischel *et al* 1995; see above). In some cases, gliosis, dystrophic calcification, and iron deposition in neurons indicate a destructive lesion (De Rosa *et al* 1992) and frequent coexistence of polymicrogyria and heterotopias would indicate damage in the second trimester (Barkovich 1996). Recently, hemimegalencephaly has been described in association with cytomegalovirus encephalitis (Jay *et al* 1997). The possibility that hemimegalencephaly represents a tumor or hamartoma has also been raised (Townsend *et al* 1975; Barkovich 1996). The enlargement of the damaged hemisphere has not been explained. However, individual cells may enlarge and develop masses of new sprouting processes, thus expanding the neuropil, after destructive damage in adjacent white matter (Marin-Padilla 1997). Further, it has been demonstrated that the neonatal brain is capable of growth and regeneration after a perinatal insult

(Rutherford *et al* 1997). Thus hemimegalencephaly may represent an unusual regeneration and overgrowth following a variety of insults during intrauterine life.

TUMORS/HAMARTOMAS

Tumors may undoubtedly be the cause of focal intractable epilepsy. Some of them have features in common with cortical dysplasia. Rare cases are described where tumors and cortical dysplasia coexist. Ganglioglioma, dysembryoplastic neuroepithelial tumor, and low-grade astrocytoma, as well as tuberous sclerosis, have all been described in association with cortical dysplasia (Prayson *et al* 1993; Prayson and Estes 1995). This coexistence is rare, perhaps because cortical dysplasia is unlikely to be sought, or is overlooked, in the presence of obvious tumor. Both ganglioglioma and dysembryoplastic neuroepithelial tumor are very slow growing tumors of mixed cellularity and may represent hamartomas or tumorous dysplasias (Prayson and Estes 1995). Due to the similarity of the histology of these lesions

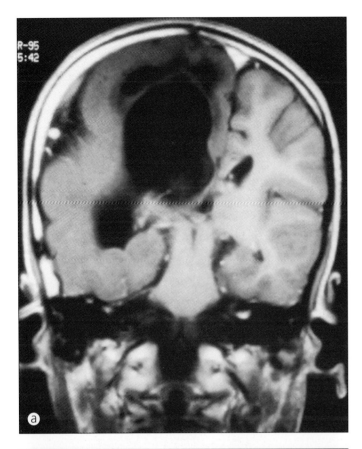

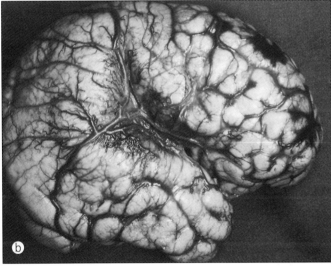

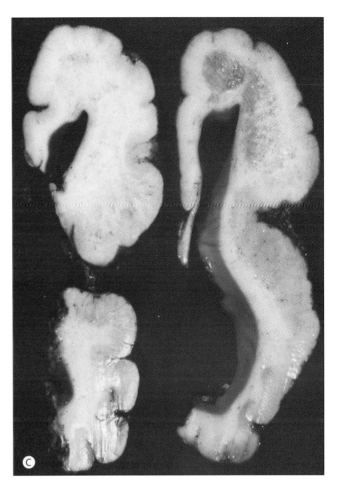

Fig. 10.21 Hemimegalencephaly. (a) Coronal CT scan showing enlargement of the right hemisphere with dilatation of the lateral ventricle, cysts in the white matter, and a thickened partly agyric cortex. (b) Hemispherectomy specimen showing abnormal gyration around the posterior sylvian fissure and parietooccipital regions. (c) Coronal slices of fixed hemispherectomy specimen showing a thickened dysplastic cortex. The white matter had extensive spongy microcystic change and contained many small nodular neuronal heterotopias. The cortex showed dysplasia with extensive polymicrogyria.

to dysplastic cortex, these unusual tumors may only be distinguished from dysplasia by their mass.

GENETIC FACTORS

Both environmental and genetic causes of MCD are recognized (Barth 1987; Sarnat 1993; Norman *et al* 1995). Many possible environmental culprits are known, although finding

definite causes in individual cases is difficult in practice (Barkovich et al 1995a). Nevertheless, a history of prenatal and perinatal events must always be sought, as positive findings may have implications for therapy, counseling, and prevention.

An increasing number of genes are known to affect cerebral development. The field is rapidly advancing, as shown by the discovery of at least four human mutations involved in MCD since the publication of a detailed review of the subject by Rorke (1994). Although the precise mechanism of action of mutations is not always understood, most seem to affect higher-order genes that control development. Four genes controlling neuronal migration have been found in mammals: *reelin, LIS1, disabled,* and *doublecortin.*

Schizencephaly, a rare malformation, is usually sporadic and rarely familial (Robinson 1991; Hosley *et al* 1992; Hilburger *et al* 1993; Haverkamp *et al* 1995; Packard *et al* 1997). In sporadic schizencephaly, germline mutations in a homeobox gene (*EMX2*) were identified by Boncinelli's group, extrapolating from studies of murine cerebral development (Brunelli *et al* 1996). A different mutation in the same gene was found in a pair of affected brothers (Faiella *et al* 1997). The phenotype was not identical in these sibs, possibly implicating an environmental contribution to the phenotype. In addition, these brothers were unusual in not manifesting epilepsy, although this might reflect their ages at the time of imaging.

The X-linked dysgenesis that manifests as lissencephaly in males and subcortical heterotopia in females (Dobyns *et al* 1996; Des Portes *et al* 1997) has recently been shown to be due to mutations in a novel gene, *doublecortin,* that is highly expressed in fetal development. The mechanism of action of this gene is under scrutiny, but it may be involved in intracellular signal transduction (Des Portes *et al* 1998a; Gleeson *et al* 1998). That homozygous males with a mutation in this gene are more severely affected than heterozygous females is ascribed to lyonization and the absence of a normal copy of the gene in the male. The *doublecortin* gene is believed to be the major gene involved in familial and sporadic subcortical laminar heterotopia (Des Portes *et al* 1998b).

Familial periventricular nodular heterotopia is a similar X-linked dysgenesis (DiMario *et al* 1993). In these kindreds, there is a relative lack of male births and an excess fetal loss, ascribed to a prenatal lethality in homozygous males. The gene responsible, and human linkage data suggest that only one is involved, has been linked to Xq28 (Eksioglu *et al* 1996); a duplication within this region was detected in a sporadic male with mental retardation and bilateral periventricular nodular heterotopia (Fink *et al* 1997). There are known to be environmental causes of periventricular nodular heterotopia in animals (Jensen and Killackey 1984).

Most patients with Miller–Dieker syndrome, who have type I lissencephaly as part of the phenotype, have abnormalities of 17p13.3. Within this region, Reiner *et al* (1993) isolated a gene called *LIS1* that is deleted in patients with Miller–Dieker syndrome. The *LIS1* gene has 99% homology with brain platelet-activating factor (PAF) acetylhydrolase (Hattori *et al* 1994). Recent work suggests that PAF acetylhydrolase inactivates PAF, activation of PAF receptors regulating neuronal cytoskeletal structure. Thus activation of PAF receptors *in vitro* leads to a dose-dependent

decrease in granule cell migration (Adachi *et al* 1997; Bix and Clark 1998). PAF acetylhydrolase may also take part in the prevention of catastrophic microtubule collapse and thus may play a direct role in neuronal migration (Sapir *et al* 1997). Although understanding of the generation of the structural abnormality in Miller–Dieker syndrome may not lead directly to treatment, it will contribute to genetic diagnosis and counseling.

Knowledge of the genetic basis of dysgenesis is progressing rapidly. Both sporadic and familial cases may have genetic mutations (germline or somatic). Only further correlative studies of patients whose clinical, electrical, neuroimaging, and genetic attributes have been established will define the full extent of genetic involvement. Future functional classifications of individual patients may need imaging and genetic components. Genetic information will be important for counseling patients with dysgenesis, and may also provide patients with some explanation of their condition. Whether it will aid the treatment of an individual patient's epilepsy remains uncertain.

EPILEPTOGENESIS AND NORMAL FUNCTION

Recent studies have confirmed the long-held association between structural abnormalities and focal epilepsy and have begun to explore its pathophysiologic basis. An understanding of the underlying epileptogenic mechanisms of MCD is essential to its rational treatment.

MRI studies have shown that MCD are relatively common in people with refractory epilepsy. Conversely, there have been very few reports of dysgenesis being found by chance during the investigation of nonepileptic disorders (Kuzniecky *et al* 1993; Dubeau *et al* 1995; Granata *et al* 1997; Miller *et al* 1998). That epilepsy in association with MCD has an age-dependent expression suggests that some of the apparently nonepileptic cases may have been imaged at an age before the development of seizures. Very few reports of completely asymptomatic MCD have been published (Raymond *et al* 1995a) despite the fact that several thousand neurologically normal individuals have been scanned across the world. This is powerful circumstantial evidence for the epileptogenicity of MCD.

An animal model of symptomatic subcortical heterotopia has been generated (Lee *et al* 1997). Rats with this structural abnormality (termed telencephalic internal structural heterotopia) had electrographic and behavioral seizures. Increased perilesional excitatory activity and reduced intralesional inhibitory activity were demonstrated in freeze-induced polymicrogyria (Jacobs *et al* 1996). *In vitro* hyperexcitability of radiation-induced dysgenesis in rats has been revealed by pharmacologic intervention (Roper *et al* 1997). An animal model of microdysgenesis has also been created (Amano *et al* 1996). These and other novel models demonstrate the epileptogenicity of MCD in animals and should speed progress in understanding the basic mechanisms of epileptogenesis in humans.

More direct evidence in humans comes from functional studies, both electrical and imaging. Functional imaging studies have shown that areas of MCD show appropriate increases in regional cerebral blood flow on activation (Hatazawa *et al* 1996), and utilize glucose (De Volder *et al* 1994), although the pattern of more complex metabolic activity may be abnormal (Kuzniecky *et al* 1997a). Proton magnetic resonance spectroscopy has revealed abnormalities within heterotopic gray matter (Marsh *et al* 1996; Li *et al* 1998); Marsh and colleagues interpreted this as reflecting either the persistence of immature neuronal tissue or increased cellular activity within the ectopic tissue. Abnormalities of binding of neuroactive ligands, such as flumazenil, have been shown in patients with MCD, within both visually abnormal and visually normal areas as identified on MRI scans (Richardson *et al* 1996).

Direct perioperative or chronic intracranial electrical recording has detected activity compatible with epileptogenesis in cases of periventricular nodular heterotopia, subcortical heterotopia, and focal cortical dysplasia (Francione *et al* 1994; Dubeau *et al* 1995; Palmini *et al* 1995). Such recordings do not, of themselves, prove that the lesions are the cause of epilepsy, but they do show that the regions are capable of generating seizures. *In vitro* study of tissue resected from people with heterotopia (Preul *et al* 1997) showed sustained repetitive burst discharges after pharmacologic activation. The authors interpreted the recorded field potentials, similar to those seen *in vitro* from temporal neocortex, as demonstrating some degree of neuronal organization within the dysgenesis. Mattia *et al* (1995) induced 'seizure-like' discharges from resected human neocortical dysplastic tissue to which 4-aminopyridine had been added; such discharges could not be elicited from temporal neocortex from patients with sclerosis of Ammon's horn. Though the authors postulated 'morphologic and functional changes in synaptic interconnectivity' as the cause of this activity, they did not subject the tissue they had studied to histology.

The cessation of seizures in some cases following focal resective surgery, and the unexpected finding of MCD in some resections guided by electrical studies, ascribe a pivotal role to MCD in epileptogenesis since it is very probable that if fits stop following resection of a given brain region, then that region must have been necessary for overt epileptogenesis. This extensive body of investigation demonstrates that MCD can be intrinsically epileptogenic.

Several authors have reported on aspects of the histopathology of MCD relevant to the causation of epilepsy (Manz *et al* 1979; Ferrer *et al* 1992b; Duong *et al* 1994; Battaglia *et al* 1996; Yamanouchi *et al* 1996; Crino *et al* 1997). There is a suggestion that an imbalance of excitatory to inhibitory influences may contribute to the epileptogenic potential of MCD. It has been shown in four cases that GABAergic neurons within subcortical and periventricular heterotopia appear to have excitatory rather than inhibitory characteristics (Hannan *et al* 1999). The nodules are connected to other regions of the brain, allowing spread of nodular epileptogenic activity. Of particular interest, two of our subjects with heterotopia had increased epileptic activity following treatment with vigabatrin, which increases GABAergic influence in the brain (Petroff *et al* 1996). As these cases exhibit immature and excitatory GABAergic neurons, enhancement of their function with the use of vigabatrin might explain its deleterious effect. This emphasizes the clinical importance of understanding the anatomy and neurochemistry of dysgenesis.

Spreafico *et al* (1998) also postulated that epileptogenicity in cortical dysplasia might be due to an imbalance of excitation over inhibition. They studied three cases of focal cortical dysplasia. All three had an increased number of giant (excitatory) pyramidal neurons, a decrease in inhibitory GABAergic neurons, and abnormal baskets of parvalbumin-positive terminals around presumed excitatory neurons in the dysgenetic regions. The authors suggested that additional, progressive tissue changes may have occurred over time, creating an epileptogenic network by positive feedback. Ying *et al* (1998) have demonstrated alterations in glutamate receptor subtype in dysplastic neurons, suggesting that they are hyperexcitable. Connectivity was not studied, nor were the inhibitory components of neuronal networks.

Mischel *et al* (1995) studied 77 cases of MCD, of a variety of types and syndromes, all of whom had undergone surgical treatment for refractory epilepsy. Based on morphologic criteria (e.g. detection of balloon cells, neuronal cytomegaly, white matter heterotopia, etc.), these authors proposed a grading of pathologic severity and were able to demonstrate correlations between the grading and seizure frequency and age at resection. A weak correlation was found between grading and developmental delay, but none with neurologic deficit. Prudently, these fascinating findings were interpreted cautiously by the authors. For example, there is inherent uncertainty in measuring seizure frequency or developmental delay; though a more clear-cut measure, surgical outcome is prey to other factors, such as completeness of resection, the distribution of primary pathology, and the presence of secondary changes.

Most cases of MCD treated by surgery fail to become seizure-free. It has been suggested that this is not because resected tissue is unimportant, but rather that epileptogenesis in MCD is distributed in additional abnormal tissue. Taylor *et al* (1971) stated that 'it may well be that other, if less ostentatious, areas of cortical dysplasia have been left behind,' sentiments since echoed (e.g. Awad *et al* 1991). Such occult areas might be undetected by both routine MRI and EEG (Palmini *et al* 1997). Positron emission tomography (PET) and quantitative MRI neuroimaging studies support this concept (Sisodiya *et al* 1995, 1997; Richardson *et al* 1996; Li *et al* 1997, 1998). Several histologic examples of the phenomenon, i.e. noncontiguous areas of dysgenesis removed from the presumed focus of epilepsy, have been published (Robain *et al* 1988; Jahan *et al* 1997). It is difficult to imagine that histologically demonstrated widespread manifest areas of dysgenesis are kindled, and it is thought that widespread areas of structural abnormality demonstrated by quantitative MRI also reflect primary pathology rather than kindled changes. To view most cases of dysgenesis as isolated lesions may be erroneous.

In addition to the perhaps widely distributed pathology of MCD, some cases may have a quite distinct, visible second pathology that is itself capable of generating seizures, i.e. 'dual pathology.' An MRI study suggests that 15% of cases of MCD may also have hippocampal sclerosis (Cendes *et al* 1995). Ho *et al* (1998) showed that of 30 patients with temporal lobe developmental malformations, nine had unilateral and 17 bilateral abnormalities of the mesial temporal structures; therefore 87% had 'dual pathology.' From their poor results of temporal lobectomy for hippocampal sclerosis associated with periventricular heterotopia, Li *et al* (1997) suggested that there are three possible interactions: (a) the nodules of periventricular heterotopia may be the epileptogenic source with secondary involvement of the temporal lobe; (b) there may be dual pathology with independent epileptogenic sources, from both the periventricular heterotopic tissue and the temporal lobe; and (c) the periventricular heterotopia may be part of a more widespread epileptogenic source. In the case of periventricular heterotopia, quantitative MRI studies suggest that in males any of these three options are feasible, while in females it seems that the nodules are themselves sufficient for epileptogenesis, with or without independent activity from associated hippocampal sclerosis

(Sisodiya *et al* 1999). Although the same considerations might be applied to other MCD with hippocampal sclerosis, Prayson *et al* (1996) reported that five cases of hippocampal sclerosis with MCD found in the operative specimen did well after surgery. Larger series are required, with better dissection of the precise contributions of MCD and hippocampal sclerosis.

It is clear that histologic study will continue to provide results of fundamental importance. Sutula (1998), in a recent editorial, states that 'preliminary observations (of immunohistochemical changes) clearly require additional quantitative analysis and confirmation by other groups … It is hoped that epilepsy surgery groups with access to human dysplastic cortex … will continue to pursue detailed anatomic and physiologic studies of the neuronal and circuit alterations.' Detailed clinical, neuropsychologic, neurophysiologic, and imaging studies will be required in addition if histologic findings are to be completely understood. Only such studies may explain why a practically invisible area of focal cortical dysplasia may cause life-threatening status epilepticus, while a patient with a large cleft and polymicrogyria may remain asymptomatic. It can be seen that the epileptogenesis of MCD is both definite and complex. Its study has direct clinical implications, especially with respect to the choice of drug treatment and surgical planning.

An important converse issue is whether normal function may be harbored within dysgenetic tissue. Total disruption of function normally ascribed to a given cortical region is often seen clinically and on investigation (Brown *et al* 1993; Calabrese *et al* 1994). However, specific function normally ascribed to an affected region may persist, albeit in a modified fashion. Thus extensive bilateral posterior dysgenesis was revealed in a patient with refractory epilepsy; three-dimensional rendering of her MRI scan revealed the extent of the abnormalities, which encompassed both occipital lobes. This patient had normal visual fields and function, as far as could be determined. Raymond *et al* (1997) recorded detectable, if distorted, somatosensory evoked potentials (P20 and N20 waveforms) in 5 of 13 patients with dysgenesis affecting the appropriate central regions. Leblanc *et al* (1995) demonstrated that electrocortical stimulation over a dysgenetic posterior temporal gyrus led to interference with speech. Duchowny *et al* (1996) demonstrated that language representation and developmental abnormalities may overlap in some cases, with no language displacement. Therefore, although MCD may cause functional derangement, some contribution to a function may be made by dysgenetic cortex. The complexities of the mixture of normal and abnormal neurons within the lesion (Preul *et al* 1997), of the neuronal connections, and of the timing of the development of dysgenesis with respect to synaptogenesis and functional development may explain why cortical function is not reallocated to other regions. The structural substrate of the function may be more dispersed than usual, confounding investigation dependent on spatial density of information or signal changes.

The role of microdysgenesis in idiopathic primary generalized epilepsies remains controversial. Meencke has reported increased numbers of dystopic neurons within the frontal lobe, particularly in patients with both juvenile myoclonic and childhood absence epilepsies (Meencke 1983). The significance of these findings has been disputed (Lyon and Gastaut 1985; Meencke and Janz 1985). There is additional quantitative MRI evidence in favor of structural changes in the brains of patients with idiopathic generalized epilepsies (Savic et al 1998; Woermann et al 1998).

CLINICAL FEATURES AND NATURAL HISTORY

The true prevalence of MCD is difficult to determine because MCD causing tractable epilepsy may remain undiscovered if the patient is not scanned. Among selected cases, periventricular nodular heterotopia seems to be the most common. In surgical cases, already preselected, focal cortical dysplasia is probably the commonest variety.

Most cases present with epilepsy that is often refractory to medical treatment. The seizures are of a wide variety of types and not usually specific to the actual MCD. Most present with partial seizure syndromes, of any localization, with or without secondary generalization. Focal cortical dysplasia is a recognized cause of focal motor status (Desbiens et al 1993), and status epilepticus may be relatively more common in MCD than in other primarily epileptogenic conditions; it occurred in 30% of patients in the Montreal series (Palmini et al 1994). Rarely, MCD, and periventricular nodular heterotopia in particular, may present with what appears to be an idiopathic generalized seizure disorder (Dubeau et al 1995; Raymond et al 1995b). MCD may also present with specific syndromes, such as West syndrome (Meencke and Veith 1999), Ohtahara's syndrome (Pedespan et al 1995; Aicardi 1996), and Lennox–Gastaut syndrome (Ricci et al 1992).

Some individuals have no seizures (Raymond et al 1995a) or have seizures responsive to medication (Ambrosetto 1993). MCD may present in a number of other ways, developmental delay or cognitive impairment, progressive neurologic decline in children, and fixed neurologic deficits in adults being among the more common.

Clinical features that should lead to a search for MCD include a positive family history of epilepsy, mental retardation, miscarriages, or an excess of female births; developmental delay; dysmorphism or any other congenital abnormalities, such as microcephaly; associated neurologic findings (e.g. pseudobulbar palsy, hemiparesis, and hemiatrophy, including isolated facial hemiatrophy); presentation with focal motor status epilepticus.

The range of clinical and seizure manifestations is diverse, and has been extensively reviewed elsewhere (Sarnat 1993; Norman et al 1995; Guerrini et al 1996). Only the salient clinical features are highlighted here. It should be appreciated that different forms of MCD may occur together in the same individual.

FOCAL CORTICAL DYSPLASIA

Focal cortical dysplasia may present with focal motor status or epilepsia partialis continua, with an apparently normal scan. This is an important, potentially fatal mode of presentation and may occur either *de novo* or with a previous history of epilepsy. In some cases, surgical resection offers the only hope of controlling seizure activity, even at the cost of hemiplegia (Desbiens et al 1993). It is the commonest MCD found in pathologic specimens, although this may reflect selection bias. However, it may be the most common MCD in general, as subtle examples are probably missed even with the most sophisticated imaging. Epilepsy is the most common manifestation, presenting at almost any age to adulthood. Mental retardation may be found in some cases.

POLYMICROGYRIA

Patients with polymicrogyria can present with neurologic signs or developmental delay, or just with epilepsy and a hemisyndrome. One specific condition is *congenital bilateral perisylvian polymicrogyria*. Specific components of the presentation include abnormal tongue movements, dysarthria, dysphagia, absent gag reflex, drooling, pyramidal signs, club feet, and arthrogryposis multiplex congenita (Kuzniecky et al 1993). Mirror movements may be seen. *Bilateral parasagittal parietooccipital polymicrogyria* has also been mooted as a separate entity (Guerrini et al 1997). However, the absence of common clinical, electrographic, or etiologic characteristics raises some doubts about the status of this finding as a separate entity. Overall, polymicrogyria is probably the second commonest MCD detected on MRI. The timing of seizure onset is variable. Familial cases are very rare.

SCHIZENCEPHALY

Schizencephaly is a rare MCD often associated with developmental delay, which may be marked and may include language delay. Hemiparesis is sometimes seen. Median age at seizure onset in one series was 13 months. Hydrocephalus may lead to presentation, usually in association with the open-lip variety; shunting may lead to reduction in the size of the cleft and apparent cortical expansion (Capra *et al* 1996; Packard *et al* 1997). The extent of the cleft varies, and the developmental delay or degree of handicap seems to correlate with this extent, varying from complete normality to the most severe delay in those with bilateral open-lip clefts. The condition may be associated with septooptic dysplasia or multiple congenital abnormalities.

LISSENCEPHALY

Patients with lissencephalies are often severely delayed in all aspects of their development. They may have mixed spasticity and hypotonia, feeding difficulties, and shortened lifespan (Pilz and Quarrell 1996). Additional dysmorphic features and the early onset of epilepsy (earlier than 6 months in more than 85% of cases), possibly with a family history, may point to the diagnosis. Type II lissencephalies may be associated with arthrogryposis multiplex congenita, as well as multiple other abnormalities. Associations include Miller–Dieker, Walker–Warburg, and Fukuyama syndromes.

HETEROTOPIA

Periventricular nodular heterotopia

This is associated with a number of specific clinical findings. Epilepsy, the commonest manifestation (80–90%), usually begins in the second decade or later; occasionally it may take the form of a primary generalized epilepsy. There may be a family history of seizures and strokes in female relatives (Huttenlocher *et al* 1994), an excess of spontaneous abortions, and a dearth of live male births, suggesting an X-linked disorder with prenatal lethality for homozygous males (Raymond *et al* 1994; Dubeau *et al* 1995). Affected females are often, though not always (Musumeci *et al* 1997), of normal intelligence and manifest neither mental retardation nor abnormal neurologic signs. Males manifesting seizures at an earlier age may have additional features, such as mental retardation, frontonasal dysplasia, syndactyly, short-gut syndrome, absence of the corpus callosum, or nephrosis (Dobyns *et al* 1997).

Subcortical heterotopia

This may also present with many seizure types, ranging in age of onset from 2 months to 14 years, with combinations of developmental delay and neurologic signs (hypotonia, poor motor control, spasticity, orofacial weakness), and a family history of lissencephaly in males and laminar (band) subcortical heterotopia in females. Those with diffuse laminar (band) heterotopia tend to be the most severely affected (Barkovich and Kjos 1992). However, patients may have above-average intellectual function and relatively late onset of seizures (Calabrese *et al* 1994).

HEMIMEGALENCEPHALY

Hemimegalencephaly is very rare. It may be associated with scalp lesions, linear nevus of Jadassohn, tuberous sclerosis, neurofibromatosis, incontinentia pigmenti, hypomelanosis of Ito, hemicrania or macrocrania, and hemisomatic hypertrophy; it is almost always associated with hemideficits of motor or sensory function and mental retardation (King *et al* 1985; Vigevano *et al* 1996). The reason for the phenotypic variation in this condition is unclear, although it may reflect the wide variation in underlying pathology. Seizure onset is usually neonatal.

CLINICAL INVESTIGATION

ELECTROENCEPHALOGRAPHY

The scalp EEG features of MCD are diverse and rarely unique. They may change with age, drug treatment, and surgery. They must reflect properties of the presumed intrinsic epileptogenicity of MCD, even if in some cases the findings are more generalized than expected.

Rarely, the EEG is normal even with extensive MCD (Raymond *et al* 1995b). In baseline recordings, findings include:

1. preservation of normal background rhythms and reactivity, possibly even over areas appearing abnormal on neuroimaging, with intrusion of other features;
2. high-amplitude (>100 μV) rhythmic activity, which when abnormally rapid and large (>400 μV) for age is considered pathognomonic of lissencephaly (Gastaut *et al* 1987);
3. asymmetric high-amplitude activity in hemimegalencephaly;
4. abnormal fast rhythms, usually nonspecific;

5. focal slow activity or continuous slow discharges, either of which may be polymorphic (Raymond and Fish 1996);
6. continuous spike-and-wave activity during sleep;
7. widespread or multifocal spiking activity, thought to represent extensive underlying pathology;
8. repetitive trains of 10–14 Hz spikes in sleep (Bureau *et al* 1996).

Abnormal findings may not appear until later in development, may be more marked during sleep, and are often visually unresponsive. Though often overlying structural abnormalities, epileptiform activity may be spatially more or less extensive than the visualized underlying changes, and may shift its focus during development (Raymond *et al* 1995b). Noncongruence of EEG abnormalities and structural changes may be due to the limitations of scalp EEG, the presence of structural changes not visible on MRI (Otsubo *et al* 1993; Palmini *et al* 1997), or the depth of MCD, activity of which is modulated before recording on the surface.

Acute or chronic intracranial recordings of MCD have rarely been made. Acutely, all MCD may show ictal and interictal features typical of an epileptogenic focus. Some workers maintain that electrocorticography may reveal specific abnormalities. Palmini *et al* (1995) recorded 'ictal/continuous epileptogenic discharges' from the surface of the cortex in patients with MCD, and in some cases from surrounding cortex that appeared normal on inspection but was subsequently proven histologically to be dysgenetic. Completeness of the resection of cortex evincing ictal or continuous epileptogenic discharges was correlated with a better outcome. Although in need of confirmation, especially with regard to specificity, these findings support the existence of pathogenic dysgenetic tissue beyond the visualized abnormalities. Electrocorticographic findings may also be widespread, as are scalp EEG changes on occasion (Palmini *et al* 1991; Hirabayashi *et al* 1993; Otsubo *et al* 1993). Chronic recordings may show independent epileptiform activity in MCD, spreading activity from other epileptogenic tissue (e.g. coexistent hippocampal sclerosis), or changes spreading from otherwise normal-appearing regions (Francione *et al* 1994; Dubeau *et al* 1995; Munari *et al* 1996). Resection of all epileptiform activity recorded peroperatively has not always been considered essential for the best outcome from surgery (McBride *et al* 1991), although these differences may reflect varying anesthetic milieu and underlying pathologies.

Of especial interest, some MCD may generate surface EEG data compatible with idiopathic generalized epilepsy. Thus cases of periventricular heterotopia (Raymond *et al* 1994) or microdysgenesis (Meencke and Veith 1999) may be mistaken for idiopathic generalized epilepsy in adulthood, opercular macrogyria for benign epilepsy of childhood with centrotemporal spikes (Ambrosetto 1993), and other focal MCD for idiopathic generalized epilepsy (Guerrini *et al* 1992; Bureau *et al* 1996). That there may be underlying pathogenic similarities is supported by the poor response to vigabatrin seen in both idiopathic generalized epilepsy and in some cases of periventricular heterotopia. The pathologic basis of this phenomenon is being explored (Hannan *et al* 1999).

EEG findings are rarely pathognomonic of MCD; conversely MCD enters into the differential diagnosis of many abnormal EEG findings. EEG should be seen as an investigational tool, but not one that defines the condition. Neuroimaging remains of paramount importance.

Magnetoencephalography has been used to locate an epileptogenic focus that proved to be focal cortical dysplasia (Paetau *et al* 1992), although there were no features on recording that seemed specific to this disorder.

STRUCTURAL IMAGING

Numerous studies have shown the superiority of MRI to CT scanning (e.g. Barkovich *et al* 1987; Raymond *et al* 1995a), and the MRI features of MCD have been well described. In appropriate studies, the presence of MCD is best established by application of the following principles.

1. Multiple sequences, including T1 weighted, T2 weighted, fast FLAIR (Wieshmann *et al* 1996), and proton density, help to confirm the nature of ectopic tissue, allow good discrimination of gray and white matter, and identification of foci of T2 prolongation (seen typically with polymicrogyria and focal cortical dysplasia).
2. Volumetric acquisition with thin (≤1.5 mm) partition size enables complete coverage and reformatting in any plane (Barkovich *et al* 1995b) for detailed visualization of data and three-dimensional reconstruction (Sisodiya *et al* 1996).
3. The use of surface coils improves discrimination by increasing the signal-to-noise ratio (Grant *et al* 1997). Magnification techniques and phased-array coils may enable detection of subtle abnormalities (Barkovich 1996).
4. The entire dataset and electroclinical localizing data are made available for careful study by experienced neuroradiologists. Attention should be paid to the pattern of gyration, sulcal depth and cortical thickness, and to the pattern and definition of the gray–white interface. The discovery of one area of MCD should prompt detailed

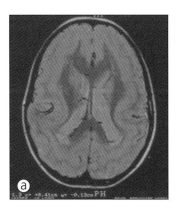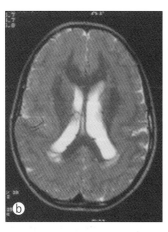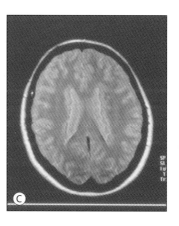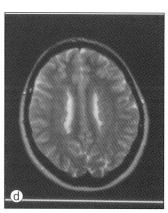

Fig. 10.22 Nodular heterotopia. (a) Axial proton density and (b) T2 weighted scans show numerous nodules of heterotopic gray matter lining the walls of the lateral ventricles. Laminar heterotopia. (c) axial proton density and (d) T2 weighted scans show a thick region of arrested grey matter paralleling the cortical surface. Note the very simple cortex as a consequence.

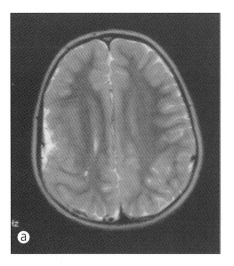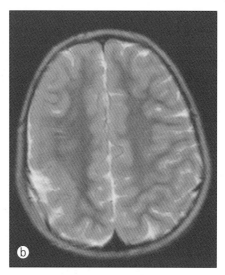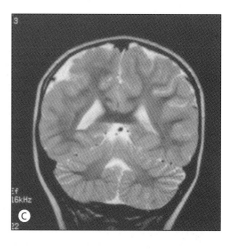

Fig. 10.23 Cortical malformation (a & b) axial T2 weighted scans reveal a small malformation in the right posterior frontal – anterior parietal cortex. Note the thickened malformed cortex with poor definition of the gray-white interface. There is an enlarged CSF space over the malformation. (c) Coronal T2 weighted scan shows the same features.

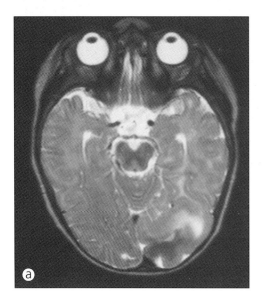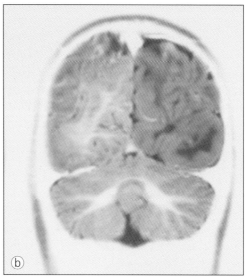

Fig. 10.24 Cortical malformation (a) axial T2 weighted scan. Shows left occipital malformation. The lesion is of low signal and was calcified on CT scans. Note also the subcortical high signal in the white matter. (b) Coronal video inverted, inversion recovery T2 weighted scan. This shows a more extensive malformation affecting the whole of the left occipital region. Note the subcortical signal change (Dark on this video inverted image)

study of the rest of the brain to exclude other macroscopically visible abnormalities. The importance of examining all the data cannot be overemphasized. Regions that appear abnormal need to retain that attribute in multiple planes and in more than one slice, e.g. apparent heterotopia may turn out to be merely a deep but normal invagination of cortex, or narrow clefts may be missed if the only plane of imaging examined is parallel to the cleft.

Figures 10.22–10.24 demonstrate the features of MCD seen on MRI: thickened cortex; alteration of the complexity of the gray–white interface; blurring of this interface; increased signal intensity of underlying white matter on T2 or proton-density images, possibly in a taper pointing to, and reaching, the ventricle; static appearance over time of suspicious areas; heterotopic gray matter; loss of white matter volume. Heterotopic gray matter is diagnosed by its identity with normal gray matter on all sequences (Barkovich *et al* 1992). Occasionally, additional CT scanning may be required: fewer than 10% of MCD are calcified. Anomalous venous drainage may also occur and needs consideration in order to avoid misdiagnosis and mistreatment. Enlarged gyri seen on MRI may be caused by a number of histopathologies (including focal cortical dysplasia, polymicrogyria, lissencephaly) and is therefore not diagnostic.

Some patients with electroclinical features suggestive of an underlying structural abnormality, perhaps MCD, do not have any visible changes on MRI (25% in the report of Li *et al* 1995). This group of patients presents a challenge. Other methods for analyzing MRI data have been devised to tackle the problem (Sisodiya *et al* 1995; Fig. 10.25).

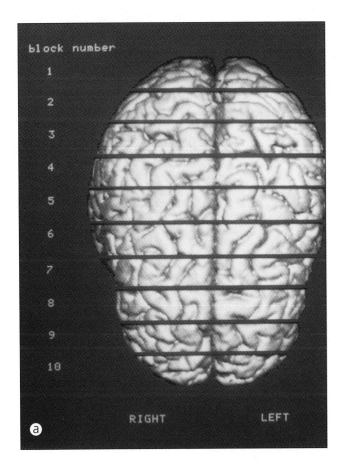

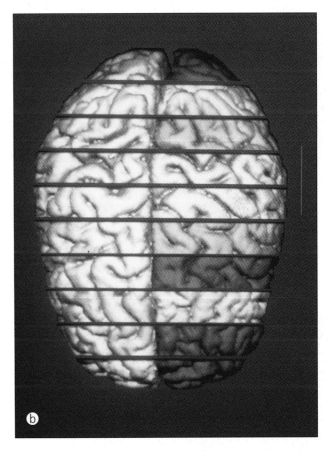

Fig. 10.25 A quantitative method of analysis of MRI data that has been devised in an attempt to detect structural changes not visible on inspection alone. Gray and white matter are semiautomatically isolated on each slice of a high-resolution MRI scan. The isolated regions are reconstructed into volumes of interest (or 'blocks'), in this case each extending for one-tenth of the anterior–posterior extent of the respective hemisphere, as shown in (a), a vertical view of a brain divided into blocks. The volume of gray and white matter in each block can be measured and corrected for brain size. Corrected volumes in patients are compared with normal ranges obtained from a control group. Abnormal volumes can be identified and their position in the brain noted, for example with respect to known pathology. Thus in (b), also viewed from the vertex, the darker blocks are of abnormal value and mark structural abnormalities in areas of brain that appeared completely normal on inspection alone; the line beside the brain marks the extent of the sclerosed hippocampus that was seen on inspection and that was thought to be the only abnormality present on the scan. The additional abnormalities detected correlate with a poor outcome after temporal lobectomy. For details see Sisodiya *et al* (1995).

FUNCTIONAL IMAGING

Some workers have encouraged the use of PET (Chugani *et al* 1993; Wyllie *et al* 1994), particularly in patients with apparently normal MRI. The place of such investigational modalities in imaging the brain in epilepsy has been comprehensively reviewed by Duncan (1997).

TREATMENT

Not all individuals with MCD have epilepsy, nor is epilepsy associated with MCD always refractory to medical treatment. Nevertheless, it is probably true to say that the treatment of epilepsy in most patients with MCD is unsatisfactory. Treatment may be with drugs or surgery.

MEDICATION

No single antiepileptic drug has any special efficacy for any particular MCD. Further neuropathologic and receptor studies are required to understand drug resistance and perhaps to allow the design of more specific agents. In some cases, the detection of underlying MCD should prompt early surgical treatment, and time, especially for cognitive development, should not be wasted on prolonged trials of antiepileptic drugs (King *et al* 1985).

SURGERY

Surgery for MCD may take the form of subpial transection, focal resection, hemispherectomy, or callosal section. Seizure outcome, for example as measured on the Engel scale (Engel *et al* 1987), is not the only important outcome. Improvement in quality of life needs particular consideration in individuals whose epilepsy may not be the only burden (e.g. those with additional learning, behavioral, and physical disabilities) and in whom a reduction in the overall burden of illness may be of value even if seizures are not completely abolished.

Resection of an apparently focal area of developmental abnormality is sometimes offered. The rationale of this treatment is based on the idea that the lesion is probably intrinsically epileptogenic. While this is partly correct, it may be an oversimplification of the underlying biologic reality. This may explain why surgery is generally not as effective as in other lesional epilepsies (Fish *et al* 1993). Nevertheless, surgery for MCD may achieve a useful degree of improvement or render otherwise intractable epilepsy tractable. Hemispherectomy is based on the idea that the dysgenetic hemisphere is already mostly nonfunctional and that continuing seizures disable the development of the contralateral hemisphere, although given the proclivity of MCD to be diffuse the possibility that the contralateral hemisphere may go on to generate seizures must be borne in mind.

Table 10.1 cites the only cases published in the English literature, of which there are remarkably few, with adequate individual documentation, an outcome of class I on Engel's scale, and a minimum of a 2-year follow-up. There are many reasons for this paucity of data, some intrinsic to the pathology and some iatrogenic. Devising a prospective randomized controlled trial of different surgical protocols for MCD is very difficult because the lesions are rarely operated upon, they may be pathologically unique (Jay *et al* 1993), and they can be positioned such that the surgical strategy must be flexible. Inevitably, different centers have different philosophies, methodologies, and reporting systems, thwarting meaningful comparisons. There are a number of difficulties with published outcome data: (a) inadequate data or only abstract presentation; (b) too short a duration of follow-up (< 24 months), though a long-term follow-up showed that 27% of surgically operated cases, with unspecified pathology, developed medically tractable epilepsy more than 10 years postoperatively (Paillas *et al* 1983); (c) data that do not allow determination of the duration of follow-up of individual patients because of grouping of results and the presentation of mean values; (d) multiple presentation of data that does not allow adequate discrimination of new from previously published cases; and (e) difficulties of definition of pathology and nomenclature changes over time.

Prolonged follow-up is the single most important parameter. Broad follow-up scales, with some reflection of eventual quality-of-life assessment, should be employed. Detailed analysis of operated cases may give the best guide to management, given that controlled trials of surgical treatment may not be feasible. The establishment of a central registry might be of value, as there is inevitably a bias against publishing negative results. It can only be hoped that future collaborations between centers operating on such patients will take place. This is an important issue. Some epilepsy centers are not performing surgery on patients with MCD in the belief that such surgery is ineffective. Only thorough reporting of postoperative follow-up will enable such centers to determine whether their policy is justified. These caveats not withstanding, some general principles can be made.

The likelihood of good outcome is increased by complete resection of the pathology (Awad *et al* 1991; Palmini *et al* 1991, 1994, 1995; Hirabayashi *et al* 1993) and more complete resection of the epileptogenic zone as determined by intracranial EEG (Jayakar *et al* 1997). Poor outcome has

Table 10.1 Patients free from seizures after surgery for MCD.

Main pathology	Reference	No. of patients seizure-free
Focal cortical dysplasia	Taylor *et al* (1971)	4
	Bruton (1988)	3
	Palmini *et al* (1991)	2
	Al Rodhan *et al* (1992)	1
	Chugani *et al* (1993)	2 + 2 (additional heterotopia)
	Bass *et al* (1995)	1
	Montes *et al* (1995)	2 (2)[a]
	Raymond *et al* (1995a)	1
	Saint Martin *et al* (1995)	1
	Guerrini *et al* (1996)	1
	Wyllie *et al* (1996)	1 (1)[a]
	Kilpatrick *et al* (1997)	1
	Kuzniecky *et al* (1997b)	2
	Barkovich *et al* (1998)	1
	Oxford series (1998)	6 (4)[a]
Polymicrogyria	Bruton (1988)	1
Schizencephaly	Silbergeld and Miller (1994)	1
Lissencephaly	Hirabayashi *et al* (1993)	2 (localized lesion)
Heterotopia	Verity *et al* (1982)	1[a], [b]
	Lindsay *et al* (1987)	1[a], [b]

[a]Number in parentheses represents those patients treated by hemispherectomy.
[b]Precise pathology unspecified.

been associated with MCD situated outside the frontal or temporal lobes (Hirabayashi *et al* 1993; Palmini *et al* 1994), with EEG factors such as widespread slowing, non-focal spikes, and generalized paroxysmal discharges (Hirabayashi *et al* 1993), and with PET evidence of abnormalities beyond the apparent epileptogenic zone (Chugani *et al* 1993). On the other hand, outcome is not necessarily influenced by the precise nature of the MCD, provided that it is fully resected (Taylor *et al* 1971), or by low IQ preoperatively (Kuzniecky *et al* 1995). An apparently good outcome initially may not be maintained with prolonged follow-up (Bruton 1988).

Other reports are less complete or describe the outcome in only isolated or small numbers of cases (Hardiman *et al* 1988; Kuzniecky *et al* 1991, 1993; Leblanc *et al* 1991; Rougier *et al* 1992; Salanova *et al* 1992, 1994; Fish *et al* 1993; Jay *et al* 1993; Otsubo *et al* 1993; Cascino *et al* 1994; Khanna *et al* 1994; Wyllie *et al* 1994; Prayson and Estes 1995; Sawhney *et al* 1995; Brännströmm *et al* 1996; Olivier *et al* 1996; Prayson *et al* 1996; Wyllie 1996; Gilliam *et al* 1997; Li *et al* 1997; Maehara *et al* 1997; Udani *et al* 1997).

The variation in seizure and quality-of-life outcome after surgery is illustrated by the results from our own series treated in Oxford. Of 13 patients with adequate follow-up (a minimum of 2 years), six were seizure-free (Table 10.2). It is clear that the empirically derived prognostic factors given above do not explain all the variation in outcome. Thus, although some patients might have been expected to do well given the nature and location of their pathology,

others with pathology generally associated with a better outcome (e.g. focal cortical dysplasia) did poorly despite extensive resection, including hemispherectomy. In some cases, poor outcome is associated with preoperative evidence of extensive dysfunction, as witnessed by developmental delay or widespread preoperative EEG changes. Poor outcome in another patient was associated with resolution of the preoperative EEG focus and the development of a novel focus, possibly representing the uncovering of a preexisting focus by removal of a dominant 'pacemaker.' Apparently complete resection of a visualized abnormality, whether by complete lobar resection or indeed hemispherectomy, was not always associated with a seizure-free outcome, although in another case with very similar pathology, hemispherectomy did give relief from seizures. Detailed study of similar cases may prove rewarding. For example, it is of interest that in one case the semeiology of persistent seizures remained unchanged despite hemispherectomy, suggesting that 'distributed matrices' of neurons may be involved in epileptogenesis (Gloor 1990), which possibly have been entrained by seizure activity and are capable of causing seizures of unchanged manifestation despite removal of part of the network.

Patients with hemimegalencephaly usually have hemiparesis of varying severity in association with refractory epilepsy. Localized resections have little useful effect (Palmini *et al* 1994). Vigevano *et al* (1989) reported results of surgical treatment in two cases: one was seizure-free with improved functioning during 11 months of follow-up,

Table 10.2 The Oxford series of patients with MCD treated with surgery.

Patient no./sex/age at surgery/duration of epilepsy	Clinical details and seizure type	EEG	Operation	Outcome on Engel scale and follow-up duration (years)	Pathology	Other outcome details
1/M/11/5	Developmental delay; left hemisyndrome; multiple seizure types and episodes of status	Right temporal spikes; diffusely slow background	Right temporal lobectomy	IV 2	Focal cortical dysplasia and subcortical heterotopia; incomplete resection	No worthwhile benefit
2/M/36/19	Complex partial seizures	Right temporal focus	Right temporal lobectomy	I 5	At least bifocal cortical dysplasia	Long seizure-free survival
3/F/9/8	FSIQ 65; frontal lobe syndrome; complex partial seizures	Low amplitude spike–wave activity right central region	Right frontal lobectomy	IC 6	Large area of focal cortical dysplasia	Psychologic improvement to preoperative level with halt in decline
4/M/14/14	Development delay; right hemiparesis; unprovoked rages; complex partial seizures; secondary generalized seizures	Left rolandic focus; independent right sharp wave focus	Left hemispherectomy	IIIA 5	Polymicrogyria, dyslamination, subependymal calcification	Infrequent seizures; parents report improvement in quality of life
5/M/3/3	Development delay; left hemisyndrome; multiple seizure types	Irregular spike–wave activity right central region; electrical status in early life, resolved	Right hemispherectomy	IA 5	Lissencephaly; subcortical heterotopia	Off antiepileptic drugs for 4 years
6/M/8/8	Mental age 2 years; left hemisyndrome; poor behavior; absences, secondary generalized seizures, drops	Right centrotemporal spiking; less frequent bilateral spikes; bilateral slow background	Right hemispherectomy	IIIA 5	Focal cortical dysplasia	Seizures continue, but no drops or secondary generalized seizures; improved quality of life judged by parents; small cognitive improvement
7/M/10/9	Developmental delay; ritualistic; complex partial seizures; secondary generalized seizures	Runs of sharp/slow waves over right hemisphere	Right temporal lobectomy	IIIA 5	Microdysgenesis and hippocampal sclerosis	Improvement in behavior, but not in cognitive function; far fewer seizures

Table 10.2 (contd)

Patient no. sex/age at surgery/duration of epilepsy	Clinical details and seizure type	EEG	Operation	Outcome on Engel scale and follow-up duration (years)	Pathology	Other outcome details
8/M/19/16	FSIQ 74; complex partial seizures; frequent secondary generalized seizures	Ictal focus at C4; occasional independent	Partial right parietal lobectomy	IVB 5	Focal cortical dysplasia	No change in seizure semeiology, frequency, or quality of life; shift in ictal focus to right centrotemporal region with extinction of previous focus
9/M/14/9	FSIQ 110; partial right homonymous hemianopia; complex partial seizures with occipital semeiology	Background rhythms over left posterior quadrant replaced by irregular components; left posterior quadrant spike/slow waves	Left occipital lobectomy	IIIA 2	Cortical dysplasia	Preoperative focus resolved; new focus more anteriorly; fewer seizures with improved behavior and independence
10/M/10/9	Developmental delay; left hemisyndrome; multiple seizure types; developmental regression	Slow background on right; normal on left; long runs of high-amplitude spike–wave discharge over right	Right hemispherectomy	IA 3	Frontotemporoparietal polymicrogyria, cleft and subcortical heterotopia	Improvement in behavior: much more manageable; off antiepileptic drugs for 3 years
11/F/12/2	VIQ 78; PIQ 102; complex partial seizures; ictal and interictal language disorder	Bitemporal changes on scalp EEG; intracranial record showed left mesial temporal onset	Left temporal lobectomy	IA 3	Focal cortical dysplasia	Improvement in speech
12/M/9/8	Developmental delay; behavioral disorder; left hemisyndrome; right hemispheric amniocentesis injury; multiple seizure types	Continuous right parietotemporal rhythmic slow/sharp waves; no independent left-sided activity	Right hemispherectomy	IA 2.5	Polymicrogyria, subcortical heterotopia, dyslamination, glioneuronal meningeal heterotopia	Educational improvement; drug reduction; postoperative EEG showed no epileptiform activity over left
13/F/11/10	Developmental delay and regression; left hemisyndrome, hemianopia; multiple seizure types; frequent generalized seizures	Widespread bursts of high-amplitude spike–wave activity; independent active left centrotemporal focus, but right hemisphere pushed across midline	Right hemispherectomy	IA 2	Polymicrogyria, heterotopia, dyslamination and giant neurons	Improved communication; persistent left hemisphere focus though no seizures on antiepileptic drugs

FSIQ, Full scale IQ; PIQ, Performance IQ; VIQ, Verbal IQ.

while the other was seizure-free during 5 months of follow-up. Hemispherectomy may be curative (Guerrini *et al* 1996). DiRocco (1996) reported that 10 of 11 patients became free of seizures after hemispherectomy but the duration of follow-up was not specified in any case. Neurologic, cognitive, and social functioning was improved in many of those who became seizure-free. The true indication for surgery is the intractability of the seizure disorder. This is often accompanied by developmental arrest or even regression. Whether earlier surgery ought to be contemplated is unclear, but given the poor response to therapy and the deleterious effect on the apparently normal contralateral hemisphere (though not always, see Jahan *et al* 1997), there must be a case for early consideration of surgery (King *et al* 1985).

Section of the corpus callosum has been employed, especially in the treatment of tonic or atonic seizures leading to falls. A few reports have been published of callosal section in patients with MCD. Stearns *et al* (1989) reported marked improvement in atonic seizure frequency during an 8-month follow-up after total callosal section in an 8-year-old girl with subcortical and subependymal heterotopia. Landy *et al* (1993) reported section of the anterior two-thirds of the callosum in a 15-year-old girl with bilateral band heterotopia, with definite improvement in the frequency of disabling atonic seizures during 16 months of follow-up. Marked improvement in atonic seizure frequency was reported in seven patients with congenital bilateral perisylvian syndrome (Kuzniecky *et al* 1993), and in atonic seizures due to hemimegalencephaly (Vigevano *et al* 1996). Marchal *et al* (1989) report a favorable outcome during a 2-year follow-up in one patient with 'generalised cortical dysplasia,' further supported by the report of Palmini *et al* (1994). However, some workers consider callosotomy to be contraindicated in patients with diffuse or bilateral MCD, especially lissencephaly, as section is associated with neurologic or neuropsychologic decline without benefit to seizures (Pinard *et al* 1996). It is difficult to draw conclusions on the basis of such a small number of patients, most of whom have additional compromise of cognitive or motor function.

The factors detracting from a favorable outcome probably all reflect the distributed nature of the underlying epileptogenic lesions of MCD, and the difficulty achieving a complete removal of such parcellated pathology. The factors favoring a good outcome might be interpreted in the same light. The better outcome after temporal resection may be because lesions in the temporal lobes are fundamentally different from those elsewhere, perhaps in their developmental origin. Similarly, it may be that focal cortical dysplasia is much more likely than other pathologies to be

Table 10.3 Factors related to outcome after surgery.

Factors associated with a poor outcome
Incomplete resection of lesion (visible or invisible)
Extratemporal or extrafrontal lesion
Widespread EEG changes or generalized cognitive dysfunction
Location in eloquent cortex, limiting resection
Pathologic grading (may reflect only extent of lesion)

Factors associated with a favorable outcome
Complete resection
Temporal location
Complete resection of area from which ictal-like electrocorticographic recording found

Irrelevant factors
Variety of dysgenesis (discounting effect this has on extent of change)
Sex of patient
Duration of epilepsy
Age at onset of surgery

truly focal and nondisseminated. However, these features do not explain the variation in outcome completely. It is still more difficult to predict outcome in patients with MCD than in patients with other 'focal' pathologies, such as isolated hippocampal sclerosis or dysembryoplastic neuroepithelial tumor. The factors affecting outcome are summarized in Table 10.3.

The explanation of a particular outcome must lie with the biology of dysgenesis and is most probably due to subtle extension of epileptogenic pathology (kindled or primary), as reflected in generalized cognitive dysfunction, widespread EEG changes, and extensive corticographic abnormalities. Until the biology of MCD is better understood the empirical findings above may remain the best available predictors of outcome. Interim strategies to improve patient selection may become available, and may depend on more detailed analysis of preoperative MRI data in an attempt to identify other structural abnormalities during preoperative assessment (Sisodiya *et al* 1997).

CONCLUSIONS

From this brief review it is clear that the conditions grouped under the heading of MCD are biologically complex. Although major advances in the detection of MCD have occurred as a result mainly of MRI, much about these conditions remains obscure. Thus a microscopic area of focal cortical dysplasia, invisible on even high-resolution MRI, may cause life-threatening status epilepticus, while much larger areas of maldevelopment may not cause any symptom.

Malpositioning of neurons alone is not enough to explain the occurrence of seizures. Systems analysis of networks of individually malfunctioning neurons may be required to understand epileptogenesis in the whole individual.

It is unlikely that abnormality of structure alone will explain epileptogenesis, as shown by the reeler mouse which, despite having total inversion of its cortical neuronal lamination, does not have seizures. Coexistent abnormalities of neurotransmission and connection are more likely to explain the generation of seizures, and the recently demonstrated links between primitive neurotransmission and neuronal migration may hint at parallel phenomena in abnormalities of structure and function.

The treatment of patients with MCD remains difficult. Most fail to respond adequately to drugs, while the outcome after surgery seems to be poor. Here, emphasis again needs to be placed on detailed reporting of individual cases, perhaps via a central registry. In this way it may be possible to determine prognosis on an empirical basis and, until the biology of MCD is better understood, such data may provide the sole guide to surgical treatment.

The opportunities offered by the study of MCD ought not to be underestimated. It is only such pursuit that is likely to reward us with rational treatment options for this most disadvantaged group of patients, whether treatment is medical, surgical, or even genetic (Freese *et al* 1997). Genetic studies in patients with MCD are in their infancy, but they should contribute to sensible genetic counseling and prevent the paternalistic denial of procreation to individuals who may carry no genetic risk.

Walsh's group have demonstrated that familial cases of periventricular heterotopia are due to mutations in the gene encoding filamin, a cytoskeletal protein (Fox et al 1998).

KEY POINTS

1. MCD are the second commonest cause of adult refractory epilepsy.
2. MCD are usually well demonstrated on detailed high-resolution MRI studies, but may require sophisticated imaging techniques to reveal their full extent.
3. MCD may be associated with dysmorphism, developmental delay, learning disability, or a family history, but do not usually have pathognomonic semeiologic features.
4. Epilepsy caused by MCD is poorly understood and usually responds poorly to drugs.
5. Surgery may have a role to play in treatment, but requires further study. Surgery is most likely to be curative for focal cortical dysplasia in a temporal location.
6. MCD may have a genetic etiology and its discovery should prompt consideration of genetic factors.
7. MCD are an area of active research and rapid developments.

REFERENCES

Adachi T, Aoki J, Manya H, Asou H, Arai H, Inoue K (1997) PAF analogues capable of inhibiting PAF acetylhydrolase activity suppress migration of isolated rat cerebellar granule cells. *Neuroscience Letters* **235**:133–136.

Aicardi J (1996) Aicardi syndrome. In: Guerrini R, Andermann F, Canapicchi R, Roger J, Zifkin BG, Pfanner P (eds) *Dysplasias of Cerebral Cortex and Epilepsy*, pp 211–216. New York: Lippincott-Raven.

Al Rodhan NR, Kelly PJ, Cascino GD, Sharbrough FW (1992) Seizure outcome in computer-assisted stereotactic resection of intraaxial cerebral lesions for epilepsy. *Stereotactic and Functional Neurosurgery* **58**:172–177.

Amano S, Ihara N, Uemara S *et al* (1996) Development of a novel rat mutant with spontaneous limbic-like seizures. *American Journal of Pathology* **149**:329–336.

Ambrosetto G (1993) Treatable partial epilepsy and unilateral opercular neuronal migration disorder. *Epilepsia* **34**:604–608.

Awad I, Rosenfeld J, Ahl J, Hahn J, Luders H (1991) Intractable epilepsy and structural lesions of the brain: mapping, resection strategies, and seizure outcome. *Epilepsia* **32**:179–186.

Barkovich AJ (1996) Magnetic resonance imaging of lissencephaly, polymicrogyria, schizencephaly, hemimegalencephaly, and band heterotopia. In: Guerrini R, Andermann F, Canapicchi R, Roger J,

Zifkin BG, Pfanner P (eds) *Dysplasias of Cerebral Cortex and Epilepsy*, pp 115–130. New York: Lippincott-Raven.

Barkovich AJ, Chuang SH (1990) Unilateral megalencephaly: correlation of MR imaging and pathologic characteristics. *American Journal of Neuroradiology* **11**:523–531.

Barkovich AJ, Kjos BO (1992) Nonlissencephalic cortical dysplasia: correlation of imaging findings with clinical deficits. *American Journal of Neuroradiology* **13**:95–103.

Barkovich AJ, Chuang SH, Norman D (1987) MR of neuronal migration anomalies. *American Journal of Neuroradiology* **8**:1009–1017.

Barkovich AJ, Gressens P, Evrard P (1992) Formation, maturation, and disorders of brain neocortex. *American Journal of Neuroradiology* **13**:423–446.

Barkovich AJ, Rowley H, Bollen A (1995a) Correlation of prenatal events with the development of polymicrogyria. *American Journal of Neuroradiology* **16**:822–827.

Barkovich AJ, Rowley HA, Andermann F (1995b) MR in partial epilepsy: value of high-resolution volumetric techniques. *American Journal of Neuroradiology* **16**:339–343.

Barkovich AJ, Kuzniecky R, Bollen AW, Grant PE (1998) Focal transmantle dysplasia: a specific malformation of cortical development. *Neurology* **49**:1148–1152.

Barth PG (1987) Disorders of neuronal migration. *Canadian Journal of Neurological Sciences* **14**:1–16.

Bass N, Wyllie E, Comair Y, Kotagal P, Ruggieri P, Holthausen N (1995) Supplementary sensorimotor area seizures in children and adolescents. *Journal of Pediatrics* **126**:537–544.

Battaglia G, Arcelli JG, Granata T *et al* (1996) Neuronal migration disorders and epilepsy: a morphological analysis of three surgically treated patients. *Epilepsy Research* **26**:49–58.

Bignami A, Palladini G, Zappella M (1968) Unilateral megalencephaly with cell hypertrophy. An anatomical and quantitative histochemic study. *Brain Research* **9**:103–114.

Bix GJ, Clark GD (1998) Platelet-activating factor receptor stimulation disrupts neuronal migration *in vitro*. *Journal of Neuroscience* **18**:307–318.

Blackshear PJ, Silver J, Nairn A *et al* (1997) Widespread neuronal ectopia associated with secondary defects in cerebrocortical chondroitin sulfate proteoglycans and basal lamina in MARCKS-deficient mice. *Experimental Neurology* **146**:46–61.

Brännströmm T, Silfvenius H, Olivecrona M (1996) The range of disorders of cortical organisation in surgically treated epilepsy patients. In: Guerrini R, Andermann F, Canapicchi R, Roger J, Zifkin BG, Pfanner P (eds) *Dysplasias of Cerebral Cortex and Epilepsy*, pp 57–64. New York: Lippincott-Raven.

Brodtkorb E, Nilsen G, Smevik O, Rinck PA (1992) Epilepsy and anomalies of neuronal migration: MRI and clinical aspects. *Acta Neurologica Scandinavica* **86**:24–32.

Brown MC, Levin BE, Ramsay RE, Landy HJ (1993) Comprehensive evaluation of left hemisphere Type I schizencephaly. *Archives of Neurology* **50**:667–669.

Brunelli S, Faiella A, Capra V *et al* (1996) Germline mutations in the homeobox gene EMX2 in patients with severe schizencephaly. *Nature Genetics* **12**:94–96.

Bruton CJ (1988) *Neuropathology of Temporal Lobe Epilepsy*. Oxford: Oxford University Press.

Bureau M, Genton P, Guerrini R, Roger J (1996) Sleep EEG in cortical dysplasias. In: Guerrini R, Andermann F, Canapicchi R, Roger J, Zifkin BG, Pfanner P (eds) *Dysplasias of Cerebral Cortex and Epilepsy*, pp 247–254. New York: Lippincott-Raven.

Calabrese P, Fink GR, Markowitsch HJ *et al* (1994) Left hemispheric neuronal heterotopia: a PET, MRI, EEG and neuropsychological investigation of a university student. *Neurology* **44**:302–305.

Capra V, De Marco P, Moroni A *et al* (1996) Schizencephaly: surgical features and new molecular genetic results. *European Journal of Pediatric Surgery* **6** (Suppl 1):27–29.

Cascino GD, Sharbrough FW, Trenerry MR *et al* (1994) Extratemporal cortical resections and lesionectomies for partial epilepsy: complications of surgical treatment. *Epilepsia* **35**:1085–1090.

Cendes F, Cook MJ, Watson C *et al* (1995) Frequency and characteristics of dual pathology in patients with lesional epilepsy. *Neurology* **45**:2058–2064.

Chugani HT, Shewmon DA, Shields WD *et al* (1993) Surgery for intractable seizures. *Epilepsia* **34**:764–771.

Chun JJM, Shatz CJ (1989) Interstitial cells of the adult neocortical white matter are the remnant of the early generated subplate neuron population. *Journal of Comparative Neurology* **282**:555–569.

Crino PB, Trojanowski JQ, Eberwine J (1997) Internexin, MAP1B, and nestin in cortical dysplasia as markers of developmental maturity. *Acta Neuropathologica* **93**:619–627.

De Rosa MJ, Secor DL, Barsom M, Fisher RS, Vinters HV (1992) Neuropathologic findings in surgically treated hemimegalencephaly: immunohistochemical, morphometric, and ultrastructural study. *Acta Neuropathologica* **84**:240–260.

Desbiens R, Berkovic SF, Dubeau F *et al* (1993) Life-threatening focal status epilepticus due to occult cortical dysplasia. *Archives of Neurology* **50**:695–700.

Des Portes V, Pinard J-M, Smadja D *et al* (1997) Dominant X-linked subcortical laminar heterotopia and lissencephaly syndrome (XSCLH/LIS): evidence for the occurrence of mutation and mapping of a potential locus in Xq22. *Journal of Medical Genetics* **34**:177–183.

Des Portes V, Pinard JM, Billuart P *et al* (1998a) A novel CNS gene required for neuronal migration and involved in X-linked subcortical laminar heterotopia and lissencephaly syndrome. *Cell* **92**:51–61.

Des Portes V, Francis F, Pinard JM *et al* (1998b) doublecortin is the major gene causing X-linked subcortical laminar heterotopia. *Human Molecular Genetics* **7**:1063–1070.

De Volder AG, Gadisseux J-FA, Michel CJ *et al* (1994) Brain glucose utilization in band heterotopia: synaptic activity of 'double cortex'. *Pediatric Neurology* **11**:290–294.

DiMario FJ, Cobb RJ, Ramsby GR, Leicher C (1993) Familial band heterotopia simulating tuberous sclerosis. *Neurology* **43**:1424–1426.

DiRocco C (1996) Surgical treatment of hemimegalencephaly. In: Guerrini R, Andermann F, Canapicchi R, Roger J, Zifkin BG, Pfanner P (eds) *Dysplasias of Cerebral Cortex and Epilepsy*, pp 295–304. New York: Lippincott-Raven.

Dobyns WB, Truwit CL (1995) Lissencephaly and other malformations of cortical development: 1995 update. *Neuropediatrics* **26**:132–147.

Dobyns WB, Andermann E, Andermann F *et al* (1996) X-linked malformations of neuronal migration. *Neurology* **47**:331–339.

Dobyns WB, Guerinni R, Czapansky-Beilman DK *et al* (1997) Bilateral periventricular nodular heterotopia with mental retardation and syndactyly in boys: a new X-linked mental retardation syndrome. *Neurology* **49**:1042–1047.

Dubeau F, Tampieri D, Lee N *et al* (1995) Periventricular and subcortical nodular heterotopia. A study of 33 patients. *Brain* **118**:1273–1287.

Duchowny M, Jayakar P, Harvey AS *et al* (1996) Language cortex representation: effects of developmental versus acquired pathology. *Annals of Neurology* **40**:31–38.

Duncan JS (1997) Imaging and epilepsy. *Brain* **120**:339–377.

Duong T, DeRosa MJ, Poukens V, Vinters HV, Fisher RS (1994) Neuronal cytoskeletal abnormalities in human cerebral cortical dysplasia. *Acta Neuropathologica* **87**:493–503.

Eksioglu YZ, Scheffer IE, Cardenas P *et al* (1996). Periventricular heterotopia: an X-linked dominant epilepsy locus causing aberrant cerebral cortical development. *Neuron* **16**:77–87.

Engel J Jr, Van Ness PC, Rasmussen TB, Ojemann LM (1987) Outcome with respect to epileptic seizures. In: Engel J Jr (ed) *Surgical Treatment of the Epilepsies*, pp 553–571. New York: Raven Press.

Faiella A, Brunelli S, Granata T (1997) A number of schizencephaly patients including 2 brothers are heterozygous for germline mutations in the homeobox gene EMX2. *European Journal of Human Genetics* **5**:186–190.

Farrell MA, DeRosa MJ, Curran JG *et al* (1992) Neuropathologic findings in cortical resections (including hemispherectomies) performed for the treatment of intractable childhood epilepsy. *Acta Neuropathologica* **83**:246–259.

Ferrer I, Soriano E, del Rio JA, Alcantara S, Avladell C (1992a) Cell death and removal in the cerebral cortex during development. *Progress in Neurobiology* **39**:1–43.

Ferrer I, Pineda M, Tallada M (1992b) *et al* Abnormal local-circuit neurons in epilepsia partialis continua associated with focal cortical dysplasia. *Acta Neuropathologica* **83**:646–652.

Fink JM, Dobyns WB, Guerrini R, Hirsch BA (1997) Identification of a duplication of Xq28 associated with bilateral periventricular nodular heterotopia. *Journal of Medical Genetics* **61**:379–383.

Fish DR, Smith SJ, Quesney LF, Andermann F, Rasmussen T (1993) Surgical treatment of children with medically intractable frontal or temporal lobe epilepsy: results and highlights of 40 years' experience. *Epilepsia* **34**:244–247.

Flint AC, Kriegstein AR (1997) Mechanisms underlying neuronal migration disorders and epilepsy. *Current Opinion in Neurology* **10**:92–97.

Fox JW (1998) Mutations on *FLM1* prevent migration of cerebal cortical neurons in human periventricular heterotopia. *Neuron* **21**:1315–1325.

Francione S, Kahane P, Tassi L *et al* (1994) Stereo-EEG of interictal and ictal electrical activity of a histologically proved heterotopic grey matter associated with partial epilepsy. *Electroencephalography and Clinical Neurophysiology* **90**:284–290.

Freese A, Kaplitt MG, O'Connor WM *et al* (1997) Direct gene transfer into human epileptogenic hippocampal tissue with an adeno-associated virus vector: implications for a gene therapy approach to epilepsy. *Epilepsia* **38**:759–766.

Friede RL (1989) Gross and microscopic development of the central nervous system. In: *Developmental Neuropathology*. Berlin: Springer.

Gastaut H, Pinsard N, Raybaud C, Aicardi J, Zifkin B (1987) Lissencephaly (agyria–pachygyria): clinical findings and serial EEG studies. *Developmental Medicine and Child Neurology* **29**:167–180.

Gilliam F, Wyllie E, Kashden J *et al* (1997) Epilepsy surgery outcome: comprehensive assessment in children. *Neurology* **48**:1368–1374.

Gleeson JG, Allen KM, Fox JW *et al* (1998) Doublecortin, a brain-specific gene mutated in human X-linked lissencephaly and double cortex syndrome, encodes a putative signaling protein. *Cell* **92**:63–72.

Gloor P (1990) Experiential phenomena of temporal lobe epilepsy. Facts and hypotheses. *Brain* **113**:1673–1694.

Granata T, Farina L, Faiella A *et al* (1997) Familial schizencephaly associated with EMX2 mutation. *Neurology* **48**:1403–1406.

Grant PE, Barkovich AJ, Wald LL *et al* (1997) High-resolution surface coil MR of cortical lesions in medically refractory epilepsy: a prospective study. *American Journal of Neuroradiology* **18**:291–301.

Gressens P, Marret S, Evrard P (1996) Developmental spectrum of the excitotoxic cascade induced by ibotenate: a model of hypoxic insults in fetuses and neonates. *Neuropathology and Applied Neurobiology* **22**:498–502.

Guerrini R, Dravet C, Raybaud C *et al* (1992) Epilepsy and focal gyral anomalies detected by MRI: electroclinical–morphological correlations and follow-up. *Developmental Medicine and Child Neurology* **34**:706–718.

Guerrini R, Dravet C, Bureau M *et al* (1996) Diffuse and localised dysplasias of the cerebral cortex: clinical presentation, outcome, and proposal for a morphologic MRI classification based on a study of 90 patients. In: Guerrini R, Andermann F, Canapicchi R, Roger J, Zifkin BG, Pfanner P (eds) *Dysplasias of Cerebral Cortex and Epilepsy*, pp 255–270. New York: Lippincott-Raven.

Guerrini R, Dubeau F, Dulac O *et al* (1997) Bilateral parasagittal parietooccipital polymicrogyria and epilepsy. *Neurology* **41**:65–73.

Haltia M, Leivo I, Somer H *et al* (1997) Muscle–eye–brain disease: a neuropathological study. *Annals of Neurology* **41**:173–180.

Hannan AJ, Servotte S, Katsnelson A *et al* (1999) Characterization of neuronal heterotopia in children. *Brain* **122**:219–238.

Hardiman O, Burke T, Phillips J *et al* (1988) Microdysgenesis in resected temporal neocortex. *Neurology* **38**:1041–1047.

Hatazawa J, Sasajima T, Shimosegawa E (1996) Regional cerebral blood flow response in gray matter heterotopia during finger tapping: an activation study with positron emission tomography. *American Journal of Neuroradiology* **17**:479–482.

Hattori M, Adachi H, Tsujimoto M, Arai H, Inoue K (1994) Miller–Dieker lissencephaly gene encodes a subunit of brain platelet-activating factor. *Nature* **370**:216–218.

Haverkamp F, Zerres K, Ostertun B, Emons D, Lentze MJ (1995) Familial schizencephaly: further delineation of a rare disorder. *Journal of Medical Genetics* **12**:242–244.

Hilburger AC, Willis JK, Bouldin E, Henderson-Tilton A (1993) Familial schizencephaly. *Brain and Development* **15**:234–236.

Hirabayashi S, Binnie CD, Janota I, Polkey CE (1993) Surgical treatment of epilepsy due to cortical dysplasia: clinical and EEG findings. *Journal of Neurology, Neurosurgery and Psychiatry* **56**:765–770.

Ho SS, Kuzniecky RI, Gilliam F, Faught E, Morawetz R (1998) Temporal lobe developmental malformations and epilepsy. Dual pathology and bilateral hippocampal abnormalities. *Neurology* **50**:748–754.

Hosley MA, Abroms IF, Ragland RL (1992) Schizencephaly: case report of familial incidence. *Pediatric Neurology* **8**:148–150.

Huttenlocher PR, Taravath S, Mojtahedi S (1994) Periventricular heterotopia and epilepsy. *Neurology* **44**:51–54.

Iannetti P, Nigro G, Spalice A, Faiella A, Boncinelli E (1998) Cytomegalovirus infection and schizencephaly: case reports. *Annals of Neurology* **43**:123–127.

Jacobs KM, Gutnick MJ, Prince DA (1996) Hyperexcitability in a model of cortical maldevelopment. *Cerebral Cortex* **6**:514–523.

Jahan R, Mischel PS, Curran JG (1997) Bilateral neuropathologic changes in a child with hemimegalencephaly. *Pediatric Neurology* **17**:344–349.

Janota I, Polkey CE (1992) Cortical dysplasia in epilepsy: a study of material from surgical resections for intractable epilepsy. In: Pedley TA, Meldrum BS (eds) *Recent Advances in Epilepsy*, pp 37–49. Edinburgh: Churchill Livingstone.

Jay V, Becker LE, Otsubo H *et al* (1993) Pathology of temporal lobectomy for refractory seizures in children. *Journal of Neurosurgery* **79**:53–61.

Jay V, Otsubo H, Hwang P, Hoffman HJ, Blaser S, Zielenska M (1997) Coexistence of hemimegalencephaly and chronic encephalitis: detection of cytomegalovirus by the polymerase chain reaction. *Child's Nervous System* **13**:35–41.

Jayakar P, Udani V, Yaylali I *et al* (1997) Surgical outcome in cortical dysplasia. *Epilepsia* **38** (Suppl 8):53.

Jensen KF, Killackey HP (1984) Subcortical projections from ectopic neocortical neurons. *Proceedings of the National Academy of Sciences of the USA* **81**:964–968.

Khanna S, Chugani HT, Messa C, Curran JG (1994) Corpus callosum agenesis and epilepsy: PET findings. *Pediatric Neurology* **10**:221–227.

Kilpatrick C, Cook M, Kaye A, Murphy M, Matkovic Z (1997) Non-invasive investigations successfully select patients for temporal lobe surgery. *Journal of Neurology, Neurosurgery and Psychiatry* **63**:327–333.

King M, Stephenson JBP, Ziervogel M, Doyle D, Galbraith S (1985) Hemimegalencephaly: a case for hemispherectomy? *Neuropediatrics* **16**:46–55.

Kuzniecky R, Garcia JH, Faught E, Morawetz RB (1991) Cortical dysplasia in temporal lobe epilepsy: magnetic resonance imaging correlations. *Annals of Neurology* **29**:293–298.

Kuzniecky R, Andermann F, Guerrini R (1993) Congenital bilateral perisylvian syndrome: study of 31 patients. *Lancet* **341**:608–612.

Kuzniecky R, Morawetz R, Faught E, Black L (1995) Frontal and central lobe focal dysplasia: clinical, EEG and imaging features. *Developmental Medicine and Child Neurology* **37**:159–166.

Kuzniecky R, Hetherington H, Pan J *et al* (1997a) Proton spectroscopy imaging at 4T in patients with malformation of cortical development and epilepsy. *Neurology* **48**:1018–1024.

Kuzniecky R, Gilliam F, Morawetz R, Faught E, Palmer C, Black L (1997b) Occipital lobe developmental malformations and epilepsy: clinical spectrum, treatment and outcome. *Epilepsia* **38**:175–181.

Landy HJ, Curless RG, Ramsay ER (1993) Corpus callosotomy for seizures associated with band heterotopia. *Epilepsia* **34**:79–83.

Leblanc R, Tampieri D, Robitaille Y, Feindel W, Andermann F (1991) Surgical treatment of intractable epilepsy associated with schizencephaly. *Neurosurgery* **29**:421–429.

Leblanc R, Robitaille Y, Andermann F, Ptito A (1995) Retained language in dysgenic cortex: case report. *Neurosurgery* **37**:992–997.

Lee KS, Schottler F, Collins JL *et al* (1997) A genetic model of human neocortical heterotopia associated with seizures. *Journal of Neuroscience* **17**:6236–6242.

Li LM, Fish DR, Sisodiya SM, Shorvon SD, Alsanjari N, Stevens JM (1995) High resolution magnetic resonance imaging in adults with partial or secondary generalised epilepsy attending a tertiary referral unit. *Journal of Neurology, Neurosurgery and Psychiatry* **59**:384–387.

Li LM, Dubeau F, Andermann F *et al* (1997) Periventricular nodular heterotopia and intractable temporal lobe epilepsy: poor outcome after temporal lobe resection. *Annals of Neurology* **41**:662–662.

Li LM, Cendes F, Cunha Bastos A *et al* (1998) Neuronal metabolic dysfunction in patients with cortical developmental malformations. *Neurology* **50**:755–759.

Lindsay J, Ounsted C, Richards P (1987) Hemispherectomy for childhood epilepsy: a 36-year study. *Developmental Medicine and Child Neurology* **29**:592–600.

Lyon G, Gastaut H (1985) Considerations of the significance attributed to unusual cerebral histological findings recently described in eight patients with primary generalised epilepsy. *Epilepsia* **26**:365–367.

McBride MC, Binnie CD, Janota I, Polkey CE (1991) Predictive value of intraoperative electrocorticograms in resective epilepsy surgery. *Annals of Neurology* **30**:526–532.

Maehara T, Shimuzu H, Nakayama H, Oda M, Arai N (1997) Surgical treatment of epilepsy from schizencephaly with fused lips. *Surgical Neurology* **48**:507–510.

Manz HJ, Phillips TM, Rowden G, McCullough DC (1979) Unilateral megalencephaly, cerebral cortical dysplasia, neuronal hypertrophy, and heterotopia: cytomorphometric, fluorometric cytochemical, and biochemical analyses. *Acta Neuropathologica* **45**:97–103.

Marchal G, Andermann F, Tampieri D (1989) Generalised cortical dysplasia manifested by diffusely thick cerebral cortex. *Archives of Neurology* **46**:430–434.

Marin-Padilla M (1995) Prenatal development of human cerebral cortex: an overview. *International Pediatrics* **10** (Suppl 1):6–15.

Marin-Padilla M (1997) Development neuropathology and impact of perinatal brain damage. II: White matter lesions of the neocortex. *Journal of Neuropathology and Experimental Neurology* **56**:219–235.

Marsh L, Lim KO, Sullivan EV, Lane B, Spielman D (1996) Proton magnetic resonance spectroscopy of a grey matter heterotopia. *Neurology* **47**:1571–1574.

Mattia D, Olivier A, Avoli M (1995) Seizure-like discharges recorded in human dysplastic cortex maintained *in vitro*. *Neurology* **45**:1391–1395.

Meencke H-J (1983) The density of dystopic neurone in the white matter of the gyrus frontalis inferior in epilepsies. *Journal of Neurology* **230**:171–181.

Meencke H-J, Janz D (1984) The significance of microdysgenesis in primary generalised epilepsy: an answer to the considerations of Lyon and Gastaut. *Epilepsia* **26**:368–371.

Meencke H-J, Veith G (1999) The relevance of slight migrational disturbances (microdysgenesis) to the etiology of the epilepsies. *Adv Neurol* **79**:123–131.

Miller SP, Shevell M, Rosenblatt B *et al* (1998) Congenital bilateral perisylvian polymicrogyria presenting as congenital hemiplegia. *Neurology* **50**:1866–1869.

Mischel PS, Nouyen LP, Vinters H (1995) Cerebral cortical dysplasia associated with pediatric epilepsy. Review of neuropathologic features and proposal for a grading system. *Journal of Neuropathology and Experimental Neurology* **54**:137–153.

Molnar Z, Blakemore C (1995) How do thalamic axons find their way to the cortex? *Trends in Neurosciences* **18**:389–397.

Montes JL, Rosenblatt B, Farmer JP *et al* (1995) Lesionectomy of MRI detected lesions in children with epilepsy. *Pediatric Neurology* **22**:167–73.

Munari C, Francione S, Kahane P *et al* (1996) Usefulness of stereo-EEG investigations in partial epilepsy associated with cortical dysplastic lesions and gray matter heterotopia. In: Guerrini R, Andermann F, Canapicchi R, Roger J, Zifkin BG, Pfanner P (eds) *Dysplasias of*

Cerebral Cortex and Epilepsy, pp 383–394. New York: Lippincott-Raven.

Musumeci SA, Ferri R, Elia M *et al* (1997) A new family with periventricular nodular heterotopia and peculiar dysmorphic features. A probable X-linked trait. *Archives of Neurology* **54**:61–64.

Norman MG, McGillivray BC, Kalousek DK, Hill A, Poskitt KJ (eds) (1995) *Congenital Malformations of the Brain*. New York: Oxford University Press.

Olivier A, Andermann F, Palmini A, Robitaille Y (1996) Surgical treatment of cortical dysplasias. In: Guerrini R, Andermann F, Canapicchi R, Roger J, Zifkin BG, Pfanner P (eds) *Dysplasias of Cerebral Cortex and Epilepsy*, pp 351–366. New York: Lippincott-Raven.

Otsubo H, Hwang Pa, Jay V *et al* (1993) Focal cortical dysplasia in children with localisation-related epilepsy: EEG, MRI and SPECT findings. *Pediatric Neurology* **9**:101–107.

Packard AM, Miller VS, Delgado MR (1997) Schizencephaly: correlations of clinical and radiologic features. *Neurology* **48**:1427–1434.

Paetau R, Kajola M, Karhu J *et al* (1992) Magnetoencephalographic localisation of epileptic cortex: impact on surgical treatment. *Annals of Neurology* **32**:106–109.

Paillas JE, Gastaut H, Sedan R *et al* (1983) Long-term results of conventional surgical treatment for epilepsy. Delayed recurrence after a period of 10 years. *Surgical Neurology* **20**:189–193.

Palmini A, Andermann F, Olivier A *et al* (1991) Focal neuronal migration disorders and intractable partial epilepsy: a study of 30 patients. *Annals of Neurology* **30**:741–749.

Palmini A, Gambardella A, Andermann F *et al* (1994) Operative strategies for patients with cortical dysplastic lesions and intractable epilepsy. *Epilepsia* **35** (Suppl 6):S57–S71.

Palmini A, Gambardella A, Andermann F *et al* (1995) Intrinsic epileptogenicity of human dysplastic cortex as suggested by corticography and surgical results. *Annals of Neurology* **37**:476–487.

Palmini A, Costa da Costa J, Andermann F (1997) 'New' seizures from unsuspected, imaging-negative, remote epileptogenic cortex, after surgical excision of apparently well-localised cortical dysplastic lesions (CDLs). *Epilepsia* **38** (Suppl 8):75.

Pavone L, Curatolo P, Rizzo R *et al* (1991) Epidermal nevus syndrome: a neurologic variant with hemimegalencephaly, gyral malformation, mental retardation, seizures, and facial hemihypertrophy. *Neurology* **41**:266–271.

Pedespan JM, Loiseau H, Vital A, Marchal C, Fontan D, Rougier A (1995) Surgical treatment of an early epileptic encephalopathy with suppression-bursts and focal cortical dysplasia. *Epilepsia* **36**:37–40.

Petroff OA, Rothman DL, Behar KL, Collins TL, Mattson RH (1996) Human brain GABA levels rise rapidly after initiation of vigabatrin therapy. *Neurology* **47**:1567–1571.

Pilz DT, Quarrell OW (1996) Syndromes with lissencephaly. *Journal of Medical Genetics* **33**:319–323.

Pinard J-M, Delalande O, Dulac O (1996) Hemispherotomy and callosotomy for cortical dysplasia in children: technique and postoperative outcome. In: Guerrini R, Andermann F, Canapicchi R, Roger J, Zifkin BG, Pfanner P (eds) *Dysplasias of Cerebral Cortex and Epilepsy*, pp 375–382. New York: Lippincott-Raven.

Prayson RA, Estes ML (1995) Cortical dysplasia: a histopathological study of 52 cases of partial lobectomy in patients with epilepsy. *Human Pathology* **26**:493–500.

Prayson RA, Estes ML, Morris HH (1993) Coexistence of neoplasia and cortical dysplasia in patients presenting with seizures. *Epilepsia* **34**:609–615.

Prayson RA, Reith JD, Najm IM (1996) Mesial temporal sclerosis. A clinicopathological study of 27 patients, including 5 with coexistent cortical dysplasia. *Archives of Pathology and Laboratory Medicine* **120**:532–536.

Preul MC, Leblanc R, Cendes F *et al* (1997) Function and

organisation in dysgenic cortex. *Journal of Neurosurgery* **87**:113–121.

Rakic P (1988) Specification of cerebral cortical areas. *Science* **241**:170–176.

Raymond AA, Fish DR (1996) EEG features of focal malformations of cortical development. *Journal of Clinical Neurophysiology* **13**:495–506.

Raymond AA, Fish DR, Stevens JM, Sisodiya SM, Alsanjari N, Shorvon SD (1994) Subependymal heterotopia: a distinct neuronal migration disorder associated with epilepsy. *Journal of Neurology, Neurosurgery and Psychiatry* **57**:1195–1202.

Raymond AA, Fish DR, Sisodiya SM, Alsanjari N, Stevens JM, Shorvon SD (1995a) Abnormalities of gyration, heterotopias, tuberous sclerosis, focal cortical dysplasia, microdysgenesis, dysembryoplastic neuroepithelial tumours and dysgenesis of the archicortex in epilepsy. Clinical, electroencephalographic and neuroimaging features in 100 adult patients. *Brain* **118**:629–660.

Raymond AA, Fish DR, Boyd SG, Smith SJM, Pitt MC, Kendall R (1995b) Cortical dysgenesis: serial EEG findings in children and adults. *Electroencephalography and Clinical Neurophysiology* **94**:389–397.

Raymond AA, Jones SJ, Fish DR, Stewart J, Stevens JM (1997) Somatosensory evoked potentials in adults with cortical dysgenesis and epilepsy. *Electroencephalography and Clinical Neurophysiology* **104**:132–142.

Reiner O, Carrozzo R, Shen Y et al (1993) Isolation of a Miller–Dieker lissencephaly gene containing G protein β-subunit-like repeats. *Nature* **364**:717–721.

Renowden S, Squier MV (1994) Unusual MRI and neuropathological findings in hemimegalencephaly: case report. *Developmental Medicine and Child Neurology* **36**:357–369.

Ricci S, Cusmai R, Fariello G, Fusco L, Vigevano F (1992) Double cortex: a neuronal migration disorder as a possible cause of Lennox–Gastaut syndrome. *Archives of Neurology* **49**:61–64.

Richardson MP, Koepp MJ, Brooks DJ, Fish DR, Duncan JS (1996) Benzodiazepine receptors in focal epilepsy with cortical dysgenesis. *Annals of Neurology* **40**:188–198.

Robain O, Floquet J, Heldt N, Rozenberg F (1988) Hemimegalencephaly: a clinicopathological study of four cases. *Neuropathology and Applied Neurobiology* **14**:125–135.

Robinson RO (1991) Familial schizencephaly. *Developmental Medicine and Child Neurology* **33**:1010–1014.

Roper SN, King MA, Abraham LA, Boillot MA (1997) Disinhibited *in vitro* neocortical slices containing experimentally induced cortical dysplasia demonstrate hyperexcitability. *Epilepsy Research* **26**:443–449.

Rorke LB (1994) A perspective: the role of disordered genetic control of neurogenesis in the pathogenesis of migration disorders. *Journal of Neuropathology and Experimental Neurology* **53**:105–117.

Rougier A, Dartigues J-F, Commenges D et al (1992) A longitudinal assessment of seizure outcome and overall benefit from 100 cortectomies for epilepsy. *Journal of Neurology, Neurosurgery and Psychiatry* **55**:762–767.

Rutherford MA, Pennock JM, Cowan FM, Dubowitz LMS, Hajnal JV, Bydder GM (1997) Does the brain regenerate after perinatal infarction? *European Journal of Pediatric Neurology* **1**:13–17.

Saint Martin C, Adamsbaum C, Robain O, Chiron C, Kalifa G (1995) An unusual presentation of focal cortical dysplasia. *American Journal of Neuroradiology* **16** (Suppl 4):840–842.

Salanova V, Andermann F, Olivier A, Rasmussen T, Quesney LF (1992) Occipital lobe epilepsy: electroclinical manifestations, electrocorticography, cortical stimulation and outcome in 42 patients treated between 1930 and 1991. *Brain* **115**:1655–1680.

Salanova V, Quesney LF, Rasmussen T, Andermann F, Olivier A (1994) Reevalauation of surgical failures and the role of reoperation in 39 patients with frontal lobe epilepsy. *Epilepsia* **35**:70–80.

Sapir T, Elbaum M, Reiner O (1997) Reduction of microtubule catastrophe events by LIS1, platelet-activating factor acetylhydrolase subunit. *EMBO Journal* **16**:6977–6984.

Sarnat HB (1993) *Cerebral Dysgenesis*. New York: Oxford University Press.

Savic I, Seitz RJ, Pauli S (1998) Brain distortions in patients with primarily generalized tonic–clonic seizures. *Epilepsia* **39**:364–370.

Sawhney IMS, Robertson IJA, Polkey CE, Binnie CD, Elwes RDC (1995) Multiple subpial transection: a review of 21 cases. *Journal of Neurology, Neurosurgery and Psychiatry* **58**:344–349.

Scotting PJ, Rex M (1996) Transcription factors in early development of the central nervous system. *Neuropathology and Applied Neurobiology* **22**:469–481.

Silbergeld DL, Miller JW (1994) Resective surgery for medically intractable epilepsy associated with schizencephaly. *Journal of Neurosurgery* **80**:820–825.

Sisodiya SM, Free SL, Stevens JM, Fish DR, Shorvon SD (1995) Widespread cerebral structural changes in patients with cortical dysgenesis and epilepsy. *Brain* **118**:1039–1050.

Sisodiya SM, Stevens JM, Free SL, Fish DR, Shorvon SD (1996) The demonstration of gyral abnormalities in patients with cryptogenic partial epilepsy using three-dimensional MRI. *Archives of Neurology* **53**:28–34.

Sisodiya SM, Moran N, Free SL et al (1997) Correlation of widespread preoperative MRI changes with unsuccessful surgery for hippocampal sclerosis. *Annals of Neurology* **43**:490–496.

Sisodiya SM, Free SL, Thom M, Everitt AE, Fish DR, Shorvon SD (1999) Evidence for nodular epileptogenicity and gender differences in periventricular nodular heterotopia. *Neurology* **52**:336–341.

Spreafico R, Battaglia G, Arcelli P et al (1998) Cortical dysplasia: an immunocytochemical study of three patients. *Neurology* **50**:27–36.

Squier MV (1993) Development of the cortical dysplasia of type two lissencephaly. *Neuropathology and Applied Neurobiology* **19**:209–214.

Stearns M, Wolf AL, Barry E, Bergey G, Gellad F (1989) Corpus callosotomy for refractory seizures in a patient with cortical heterotopia: case report. *Neurosurgery* **25**:633–636.

Sutula T (1998) A glimpse into abnormal cortical development and epileptogenesis at epilepsy surgery. *Neurology* **50**:8–10.

Taylor DC, Falconer MA, Bruton CJ, Corsellis JAN (1971) Focal dysplasia of the cerebral cortex in epilepsy. *Journal of Neurology, Neurosurgery and Psychiatry* **34**:369–387.

Townsend JJ, Nielsen SL, Malamud N (1975) Unilateral megalencephaly: hamartoma or neoplasm? *Neurology* **25**:448–453.

Udani V, Jayakar P, Duchowny M, Resnick TJ, Alvarez L (1997) Excisional surgery of perirolandic epilepsy in children. *Epilepsia* **38** (Suppl 8):74.

Verity CM, Strauss EH, Moyes PD, Wada JA, Dunn HG, Lapointe JS (1982) Long term follow-up after cerebral hemispherectomy: neurophysiologic, radiologic, and psychologic findings. *Neurology* **32**:629–639.

Vigevano F, Bertini E, Boldrini R et al (1989) Hemimegalencephaly and intractable epilepsy. *Epilepsia* **30**:833–843.

Vigevano F, Fusco L, Granata T, Fariello G, Di Rocco C, Cusmai R (1996) Hemimegalencephaly: clinical and EEG characteristics. In: Guerrini R, Andermann F, Canapicchi R, Roger J, Zifkin BG, Pfanner P (eds) *Dysplasias of Cerebral Cortex and Epilepsy*, pp 285–294. New York: Lippincott-Raven.

Wieshmann U, Free SL, Everitt AD et al (1996) Magnetic resonance imaging in epilepsy with a fast FLAIR sequence. *Journal of Neurology, Neurosurgery and Psychiatry* **61**:357–361.

Woermann F, Sisodiya SM, Free SL, Duncan JS (1998) Quantitative MRI in patients with idiopathic generalised epilepsy (IGE): evidence of widespread cerebral structural changes. *Brain* **121**:1661–1667.

Wyllie E (1996) Surgery for catastrophic localisation-related epilepsy in infants. *Epilepsia* **37**: (Suppl 1):S22–S25.

Wyllie E, Baumgartner C, Prayson R et al (1994) The clinical spectrum of focal cortical dysplasia and epilepsy. *Journal of Epilepsy* **7**:303–312.

Wyllie E, Comair Y, Ruggieri P, Raja S, Prayson R (1996) Epilepsy surgery in the setting of periventricular leukomalacia and focal cortical dysplasia. *Neurology* **46**:839–841.

Yakovlev PI, Wadworth RC (1946a) Schizencephalies: a study of the congenital clefts in the cerebral mantle I. Clefts with fused lips. *Journal of Neuropathology and Experimental Neurology* **5**:116–130.

Yakovlev PI, Wadsworth RC (1946b) Schizencephalies: a study of the congenital clefts in the cerebral mantle II. Clefts with hydrocephalus and lips separated. *Journal of Neuropathology and Experimental Neurology* **5**:169–206.

Yamanouchi H, Zhang W, Jay V, Becker LE (1996) Enhanced expression of microtubule-associated protein 2 in large neurons of cortical dysplasia. *Annals of Neurology* **39**:57–61.

Ying Z, Babb TL, Comair YG *et al* (1998) Induced expression of NMDAR2 proteins and differential expression of NMDAR1 splice variants in dysplastic neurons of human epileptic cortex. *Journal of Neuropathology and Experimental Neurology* **57**:47–63.

Zhang C, Heintz N, Hatten ME (1996) CNS gene encoding astrotactin, which supports neuronal migration along glial fibers. *Science* **272**:417–419.

Mesial temporal lobe epilepsy syndrome with hippocampal and amygdala sclerosis

HG WIESER, M HAJEK, A GOOSS, AND A AGUZZI

In 1880 John Hughlings Jackson described the symptoms of 'dreamy states,' and in 1889 other variants of 'uncinate fits,' as 'a particular variety of epilepsy.' In 1938 these were called 'psychomotor seizures' by Gibbs *et al* (1938) and then 'temporal lobe seizures' by Jasper and Kershman (1941). Anderson (1886), and Jackson and Beevor (1890), had noted the association of temporal lobe tumors with olfactory hallucinations and dreamy states, but it was the post-mortem finding of a small cystic lesion restricted to the uncinate gyrus in a patient who had suffered from seizures with dreamy states, elaborated automatisms, and amnesia (Jackson and Colman 1898) that led Jackson and Stewart (1899) to the concept of 'uncinate fits' with 'origin of the discharge ... in a region of which this gyrus (i.e. the gyrus uncinatus) is part.'

Jackson and Stewart (1899) gave a masterly description of the most characteristic symptoms of mesial temporal lobe seizures. Indeed, modern neurology and epileptology can add little of substance to their pioneering observations. Nevertheless, verification of the close relationship between certain temporal lobe structures, in particular the anterior mesial ones, and a particular variety of symptoms and signs had to await the era of epilepsy surgery and its associated electrical brain stimulation, EEG, pathologic, anatomic, and physiologic studies (Penfield and Erickson 1941; Paillas and Subirana 1950; Penfield and Kristiansen 1951; Feindel *et al* 1952; MacLean 1952; Penfield 1952, 1954, 1959; Bickford *et al* 1953; Feindel and Penfield 1954; Penfield and Jasper 1954; Penfield and Rasmussen 1957; Baldwin and Bailey 1958; Daly 1958; Talairach *et al* 1958; Adey 1959; Gloor 1960; Jasper 1960; Lennox 1960; Feindel 1961; Crandall *et al* 1963; Gloor and Feindel 1963; Green 1964; Bancaud *et al* 1965; Robb 1965; Margerison and Corsellis 1966; Ounstead *et al* 1966; Schneider *et al* 1969; Williams 1969; Mark and Irvine 1970; Wieser 1983a).

With regard to the pathology of mesial temporal lobe epilepsy, as early as 1825 Bouchet and Cazauvieilh presented very important autopsy data showing pathology in Ammon's horn in 7 of 18 patients who suffered from epilepsy and psychiatric symptoms.

TYPES OF TEMPORAL LOBE EPILEPSY

A variety of conditions associated with partial seizures of presumed temporal lobe origin have been termed temporal lobe epilepsy. The 1989 International Classification of Epilepsies and Epileptic Syndromes divided symptomatic localization-related epilepsies according to the cerebral lobe of their origin and recognized two types of temporal lobe epilepsy or seizures, namely *hippocampal* (mesiobasal limbic or primary rhinencephalic psychomotor) and *lateral* temporal, and defined them purely on an anatomic basis (Commission on Classification and Terminology of the International League Against Epilepsy 1989).

Problems arise because the term 'temporal lobe epilepsy' has also been used to refer to conditions where:

1. the primary epileptogenic region is outside the temporal lobe, but discharges preferentially propagate to the temporal lobe to produce typical complex partial seizures (CPS);
2. an old and initially epileptogenic lesion outside the temporal lobe leads to the development of an active temporal lobe 'focus', in the sense of an 'independent secondary focus,' despite the extratemporal lesion itself having lost its epileptogenic properties (sometimes called 'secondary temporalization');
3. the epileptogenic region is in the lateral temporal lobe and gives rise only to neocortical type seizures.

Pure descriptive terms, such as 'psychomotor seizures' and 'temporal pseudo-absences' for CPS consisting of impaired consciousness only, have obvious limitations. Psychomotor seizures can originate outside the temporal lobes (Wieser 1983a), as indeed can CPS; and most epileptologists associate the term 'absence' with generalized 3 per sec petit mal absences. The term 'temporal pseudo-absence' is therefore unfortunate and is better replaced by 'arrest reaction.'

Given the lack of unanimously accepted terminology, many epileptologists prefer an etiologic approach and divide temporal lobe epilepsy into three types:

1. mesial temporal epilepsy, associated with hippocampal sclerosis;
2. lesional temporal lobe epilepsy, defined by lesions, other than hippocampal sclerosis, in the temporal lobe;
3. cryptogenic temporal lobe epilepsy.

Both simple partial and complex partial seizures can be encountered, and a distinction is increasingly made between limbic partial seizures and neocortical partial seizures, although their semeiology does overlap in many respects.

THE SYNDROME OF MESIAL TEMPORAL LOBE EPILEPSY

The syndrome of mesial temporal lobe epilepsy (MTLE) is now widely recognized and accepted. It is common and often resistant to antiepileptic drugs but surgically remediable. Its clinical features are relatively homogeneous, as are the findings on investigational tests such as histology, magnetic resonance imaging (MRI), positron emission tomography (PET), and EEG. It can be characterized in terms of genetic and environmental factors, natural history, pathogenesis, and prognosis. Most important, however, is its association with the histopathologic finding of hippocampal sclerosis (Engel 1992; Wieser *et al* 1993; Engel *et al* 1997).

EPIDEMIOLOGY: INCIDENCE AND PREVALENCE

Precise epidemiologic data are not available because MTLE has only recently been clearly defined, and even then usually only in the context of the medically refractory variant referred for surgery. Nevertheless, MTLE is probably the most common human epileptic syndrome.

About 40–50% of newly diagnosed cases and almost 60% of prevalence cases have partial seizures, most often CPS. However, not all patients with CPS have MTLE. Overall, antiepileptic drugs can achieve complete seizure control in 60–70% of patients with newly diagnosed CPS, and many patients can discontinue medication successfully after a small number of years. MTLE has a less favorable prognosis. Although no good data are presently available, it is undisputed that patients with MTLE experience a high rate of failure with antiepileptic drug treatment. At the same time there is often an aggravation of seizure problems, an accentuation of personality and behavior problems, and a decline of memory. Patients with MTLE who are adequately controlled with drugs might bear some relationship to the recently described syndrome of benign familial temporal lobe epilepsy (Berkovic *et al* 1994).

GENETICS AND PATHOPHYSIOLOGY

Childhood febrile seizures, especially when prolonged, have been incriminated as one important factor in the development of temporal lobe epilepsy associated with mesial temporal sclerosis (Falconer *et al* 1964), although this issue does remain controversial (Lee *et al* 1981). The rate of febrile seizures in surgical series ranges from 9 to 50% (Paillas 1958; Green 1967; Jensen 1976; Lindsay *et al* 1984). In a neuropathologic study, Margerison and Corsellis (1966) found hippocampal sclerosis in 22 of 26 cases thought to have temporal lobe epilepsy on clinical grounds. However, such series are likely to be significantly biased by case selection. In prospective cohort studies of children with febrile seizures the risk of developing epilepsy varied from 2 to 7% (Annegers *et al* 1979), although only 2.4% of those children without prior neurologic disease developed epilepsy in later life, 90% of them within the first 3 years of life (4% before 6 months) and 6% after 6 years of age. There is evidence for an association between a history of childhood febrile seizures and hippocampal sclerosis, but the explanation is disputed. Likewise, there is a relationship between a history of childhood febrile seizures and hippocampal sclerosis that has been demonstrated by hippocampal volume loss on volumetric MRI (Cendes *et al* 1993a,b; Kuks *et al* 1993) and histopathologically (Sagar and Oxbury 1987). Davies *et al* (1996) have found a significant inverse correlation between the severity of hippocampal sclerosis and the age of onset of the epilepsy, but no definite relationship between hippocampal sclerosis and the duration of epilepsy. These results replicate earlier studies of Trenerry *et al* (1993) and imply that hippocampal sclerosis is not the consequence of longstanding seizures but rather that the hippocampus exhibits an age-specific sensitivity to whatever causes the sclerosis. Other initially precipitating events are found in about 33% patients (Abou-Khalil *et al* 1993; Mathern *et al* 1995a,b).

The prevalence of a positive family history of febrile convulsions is higher in patients with late seizure recurrence and in patients with temporal lobe epilepsy treated surgically. It is assumed that the tendency to febrile seizures is to a large extent genetically determined and inherited in a multifactorial way.

THE SEIZURES OF MTLE

The clinical course of MTLE typically starts with the onset of seizures at around 10 years of age. First attacks may present as CPS or (secondary) generalized seizures. Initially the seizures respond well to antiepileptic drugs, although they usually recur in adolescence or early adulthood and tend to become refractory to these drugs. In our amygdalohippocampectomy series, patients with MTLE and only slight gliosis histopathologically had recurrence of seizures at age 12 years, those with moderate gliosis had recurrence at age 11 years, and those with severe gliosis had recurrence at age 5 years (Siegel 1990).

SEIZURE SEMEIOLOGY

Seizures in MTLE are typically characterized by auras evolving into CPS with initial arrest (motionless stare), followed by oroalimentary and other automatisms. Vegetative–autonomic signs and symptoms are prominent. Auras frequently occur in isolation and typically consist of epigastric-rising sensations associated with olfactory, gustatory, and psychic phenomena (fear, dreamy states, *déjà vu*, *déjà vecu*, *déjà entendu*, other kinds of recollections) and alterations of self-perception (in time and space), as well as emotional and affective changes (Wieser 1983a,b, 1986a, 1987, 1991a; Wieser and Williamson 1993). Kotagal *et al* (1989) have pointed out that posturing of one extremity can occur and is then a valid lateralizing sign pointing to contralateral ictal onset. Automatisms may be ictal or postictal, *de novo* or reactive. Ictal automatisms frequently consist of oroalimentary symptoms, such as lip-smacking and swallowing, and gestures, such as picking, fumbling, and aimless movements. Consciousness, typically, is gradually lost or at least clouded. Marked reactive automatisms may be seen in the postictal phase. Varying degrees of postictal confusion with amnesia for the ictal events, and persistent postictal memory deficit, are very characteristic. Postictal aphasia is also typical with left temporal lobe seizures. Secondary generalization can occur, particularly in children, but is relatively infrequent in adults receiving standard antiepileptic drugs.

The ictal semeiology of seizures involving the limbic system is particularly rich, a phenomenon well expressed by the French term *elaboré*. Unfortunately the English term 'elaborate' does not have exactly the same meaning. Consequently, in 1964 the Commission on Classification and Terminology of the International League against Epilepsy decided to use the term 'partial seizures with complex symptomatology.' In a later report a footnote is included explaining that the term 'complex' implies an 'organised, high level cerebral activity' (Commission on Classification and Terminology of the International League Against Epilepsy 1969). If impairment of consciousness is used as a major criterion for classifying such seizures, then operationally it refers to the patient's degree of awareness and/or responsiveness to external stimuli.

The clinical overall *gestalt* of mesiobasal limbic seizures can be best described within the following groups. First there are those seizures that to an observer appear absence-like (*fausses absences*, Paillas *et al* 1949). A second group is characterized by psychomotor symptoms and automatisms. Third, there is a group of seizures with predominant psychosensory and/or pure psychic intellectual, cognitive, and emotional symptoms. It is tempting to correlate these seizure types with the localization-related subtype classification (Wieser 1983a), but as yet only some relatively vague correlations have been established. Many symptoms seem to depend on a characteristic seizure discharge constellation, i.e. they depend on the type of propagation along preferential pathways and appear as part of a characteristic 'march of symptoms'.

Absence-like seizures

Absence-like seizures express themselves with an initial motionless stare, the arrest reaction (Wieser 1983a), and are more or less identical with the 'type I CPS' of Delgado-Escueta and Walsh (1985). Clinically one observes clouded consciousness associated with a stare of 10–20 s, often with an expression of fearful astonishment, followed by abrupt and restless looking around and discrete tongue movements. Without EEG the differentiation from true 3 per sec spike–wave absences can sometimes be difficult. However, CPS with the arrest reaction usually lack the palpebral cloni and the sursum-vergens of the bulbi seen in true petit mal absence seizures. Moreover, during the latter the patient usually has a vacant and dull rather than a fearful and tense look.

Automatisms

Automatisms usually start with a short arrest reaction, which then evolves rapidly into the 'automatic' phase. Clouding of consciousness is usually more pronounced than with absence-like seizures and recovery is slower. Automatisms have been classified into eupraxic (well adapted) and dyspraxic (maladapted), although in practice this division is not very helpful.

Gastaut and Gastaut (1951) divided automatisms into (a) those that represent a continuation of the previous activity and (b) *de novo* automatisms. Within *de novo* automatisms one can distinguish:

1. reactions of the already confused patient to environmental stimuli – these stimuli are inadequately interpreted and so the patient's reactions are usually maladapted;
2. reactions to ictal experiences (reactive automatisms);
3. the release of archaic motor patterns.

Antisocial and aggressive behaviors may occur (Wieser 1983b), but are extremely rare. Eupraxic urination or defecation and spitting automatisms are described (Hecker et al 1972).

Some clinicians prefer a symptomatic classification that differentiates automatisms into oroalimentary, mimic, gestural, verbal, and ambulatory. In MTLE the oroalimentary automatisms are most frequent and consist of swallowing, lip-smacking, lip-pursing, chewing, and swallowing. Prominent autonomic symptoms usually accompany oroalimentary automatisms and both correlate fairly well with epileptic discharges in the amygdala and periamygdalar region. It is important to note that automatisms are not confined to temporal lobe seizures. They can also be seen with frontal and parietal onset seizures, although they then have different characteristics (Geier *et al* 1976, 1977; Walsh and Delgado-Escueta 1984).

Seizures with predominant psychosensory symptoms

These manifest by illusions and hallucinations that affect one (unimodal) or more than one (polymodal) sense, either simultaneously or in succession. Consciousness must be intact, in a global sense, if the patient is to recognize and subsequently recall psychosensory, and also pure psychic, symptoms. These symptoms are therefore usually reported very early in the course of a seizure as an aura or a 'primictal' (signal) symptom.

Psychosensory symptoms are classified according to their nature into elementary (simple) or structured (i.e. complex, elaborate, formed) and according to their sensorial quality: visual, auditory, somesthetic, vertiginous, olfactory, gustatory. Moreover, 'positive' and 'negative' symptoms can be differentiated. As a rule, in MTLE, elementary hallucinations do not occur and well-structured hallucinations are rare. Delusions are more common.

Visual illusions

Visual illusions may express themselves as distorted perceptions of an object's size (macropsia–micropsia) and distance (teleopsia). An object may appear with an inclination (plagiopsia), or flattened and elongated (dysplatopsia). The object's contour may be perceived as undulating or indistinct, eventually fragmented, or as being replaced by a halo. The objects may be perceived as without color (achromatopsia) or with an unnatural color, most often red (erythropsia) or yellow (xanthopsia). The three-dimensional perception of an object might be absent (astereognosia) or enhanced. An object may be perceived as doubled or even multiplied (monocular diplopia, polyopia) and can perseverate (paliopsia). Finally the movement of an object can be judged as being accelerated (quick-motion) or slowed down (slow-motion).

Auditory illusions

Auditory illusions follow a similar pattern. Sounds can be apperceived more intensely (macroakusia) or less intensely (microakusia). They can be perceived as coming closer while becoming louder (macropreakusia) or as moving away while decreasing in intensity (microtelakusia). Their rhythm, tonality, and timbre can be experienced as altered; and sounds can be experienced as perserverating (paliakusia). Rarely the illusion of an echoing of the patient's own phrases may be reported.

Somesthetic illusions

Somesthetic illusions may refer to parts of the body or to its entirety. The perception of size, form, and weight may be altered (statoesthetic illusions) or the patient may have the feeling of a displacement of a body part, which is in reality immobile (kinesthetic illusion), or may have no experience at all of a real movement.

Vertiginous illusions

Vertiginous illusions are often described as a sensation of instability of the body and true vertigo is relatively rare, but ictal vertigo has been documented with neocortical temporal posterior seizure onset (Wieser 1987).

Olfactory illusions

Olfactory illusions are typically confined to hyperosmias and parosmias. Ictal olfactory hallucinations in patients with temporal lobe epilepsy are often combined with gustatory hallucinations. They are usually unpleasant, often reported as having a metallic character. Gustatory sensations can be classified as hypergeusia or pargeusia. Olfactory auras are more often associated with tumoral than with nontumoral temporal lobe epilepsies.

As a general rule elementary illusions and hallucinations point to an ictal onset in or near the primary sensory areas, whereas complex ictal hallucinations are typical of seizure onset in association areas. As Penfield (1952) and Gloor *et al* (1982) have pointed out, most complex ictal hallucinations, produced either by electrical stimulation or occurring spontaneously with epileptic discharges, are *experiential phenomena* in the sense of being recollections of past experiences.

Seizures with predominant psychic symptoms

These can be differentiated, following Jackson's classical description, into those with either intellectual or affective–emotional phenomena. Jackson's description of the 'dreamy state' (*état de rêve*) includes:

1. recollections in the sense of *déjà vu, déjà entendu, déjà vécu*;
2. unfamiliarity or unreality (*jamais vu, jamais entendu, jamais vécu*);
3. forced thinking, including what the French called *pensée parasite*;
4. the rapid recollection of the past, the so-called 'panoramic vision.'

Emotional auras are relatively rarely reported. Gowers (1885) stated that he found them in 15 of 505 patients with auras. The most common is fear often associated with restlessness and irritability. Sadness (*aura de tristesse*; Offen *et al* 1976) and pleasure, elation, exhilaration, satisfaction, and the 'eureka feeling' are well documented. According to Lennox (1960) about 0.9% of auras have a pleasurable quality. Some aura symptoms may not have a counterpart in human experience and cannot be described. This 'strange feeling' is in fact very often reported. Moreover some patients have experienced auras in the past but no longer do so. For example, during monitoring, a patient will consistently press the alarm button at the beginning of a seizure, yet deny any warning afterwards. This could be due to seizure-related retrograde amnesia (Engel 1989; Engel *et al* 1997) and may indicate the development of a contralateral 'mirror focus.'

Ictal autonomic phenomena

These can be divided into *visceromotor* symptoms and *viscerosensitive* sensations. Measurable autonomic visceromotor changes occur during the course of most temporal lobe seizures. When these changes characterize the clinical picture, the terms 'visceral' or 'autonomic' seizures were used by Penfield and Jasper (1954) and Gastaut (1973). According to the effector systems, one can distinguish between cardiovascular, respiratory, pupillary, sudomotor and pilomotor, salivatory, gastrointestinal, and genito-urinary symptoms.

Cardiovascular symptoms

Cardiovascular symptoms are very frequent and include tachycardia and bradycardia, as well as arrhythmias, hypertension, flushing, or pallor. A vast amount of experimental work has shown the importance of the amygdala, in particular its central nuclear group, and of the functionally connected perifornical HACEAR (hypothalamic area controlling emotional responses; Ben-Ari 1981; Smith and DeVito 1984). Although the direction and type of heart rate and blood pressure changes during seizures, electrostimulation, and induced after discharges vary considerably, in our experience a slowing of the heart rate predominates in association with amygdalar discharges (Stodieck and Wieser 1986).

Respiratory symptoms

A short respiratory arrest or a deep inspiration is common in the initial seizure phase and can be reproduced by mesiobasal limbic electrical stimulation (Nelson and Ray 1968; Wieser 1983a). In the later course of CPS, hyperpnea as well as hypopnea and apnea may occur.

Pupillary symptoms

Pupillary dilatation, i.e. mydriasis, is a very common symptom associated with the arrest reaction. Mydriasis is sometimes asymmetric (Wieser 1987). Miosis and hippus pupillae are observed.

Sudomotor, pilomotor, and salivatory symptoms

A feeling of 'shivering cold' is sometimes associated with piloerection. Salivation is common, but lacrimation and nasal secretion are more rarely encountered.

Gastrointestinal symptoms

Gastrointestinal symptoms, such as vomiting, borborygmus, and eructation, are often major seizure symptoms (Jacome and Fitzgerald 1982). Ictal vomiting has been related to right temporal lobe seizure onset (Kotagal 1991).

Genitourinary and hormonal symptoms

There are occasional reports of penile erection or even ejaculation during partial seizures (Stoffels et al 1981). Hormonal changes, most consistently an increase of prolactin, are observed and can, to some extent, be helpful in the differentiation between epileptic seizures and 'pseudoseizures.' An increase in serum prolactin could be reproduced by amygdala stimulation in humans (Pritchard et al 1983).

SEIZURE DISTRIBUTION

Seizures typically occur at random with a frequency of a few seizures per month to a few per week. There is no marked circadian preponderance of seizure occurrence, but drowsiness and light sleep (non-REM sleep stage I) usually facilitate seizures. Sleep deprivation and all kinds of stress may exacerbate seizures. In females the seizures of MTLE may be exacerbated by certain phases of the menstrual cycle.

OTHER CLINICAL FEATURES OF MTLE

Neurologic examination is usually normal. Endocrine functions are also usually normal, but some women may report irregularities of the menstrual cycle or changes in the sexual sphere. In particular hyposexuality is often reported. Often, however, it is difficult to attribute these changes to the epileptic process *per se* and to differentiate them from possible side-effects of antiepileptic drugs, in particular high-dose carbamazepine.

Patients with MTLE may be at greater risk of developing certain personality and behavioral pecularities. Waxman and Geschwind (1974, 1975) described an 'interictal behavioural and personality syndrome of TLE' consisting of irritability, lower stress tolerance, 'stickiness' and sometimes hypergraphia, 'hyperreligiosity,' and changes of sexuality with altered self-perception, as a kind of 'sensory–limbic hyperconnection' syndrome (Bear and Fedio 1977; Bear 1979) due to kindling-like mechanisms. Depression and psychosis-like states in the sense of schizophrenia-like psychosis (Slater and Beard 1963; Slater et al 1965) have also been associated with MTLE, although the nature of the association remains controversial (Flor-Henry 1969, 1972; Ferguson and Rayport 1984; Trimble and Bolwig 1992).

DIFFERENTIAL DIAGNOSIS

BENIGN CHILDHOOD EPILEPSY WITH CENTROTEMPORAL SPIKES

As with this condition, MTLE can begin in childhood with generalized seizures. However, the partial seizures of benign childhood epilepsy with centrotemporal spikes usually have sensory and/or motor lateralized symptoms localized around the mouth and/or the upper extremity. Interictal EEG spikes are also different in the two conditions: the broad centrotemporal EEG spike is located more posteriorly and superiorly and has a characteristic transverse dipole, whereas in MTLE the spike or spike–wave discharges are located more anteriorly and basally with a characteristic oblique dipole direction.

EPILEPSY DUE TO OTHER LESIONS IN OR CLOSE TO THE MESIAL TEMPORAL LOBE

Differentiation of these conditions is usually easy by MRI. Clinical signs and symptoms may be similar, although in MTLE the age of seizure onset is often earlier and there is often a history of complicated febrile seizures as well as an increased incidence of family members with seizures. CPS of extratemporal origin often have an aura consisting of symptoms pointing more closely to the primary epileptogenic area involved.

SO-CALLED CRYPTOGENIC TEMPORAL LOBE EPILEPSY

Temporal lobe epilepsies without a pathologic substrate can be listed under this category. At present it is difficult to estimate their prevalence. Available figures from surgical series are heavily biased, as are the figures for the recently identified familial temporal lobe epilepsy syndrome with a benign course (Berkovic *et al* 1994). Whereas in Mathieson's (1975) surgical series no histopathologic abnormality was found in 173 of 857 resected temporal lobes, in our Zurich study only 2% of 224 available mesial temporal lobe tissue specimens were without pathology (Plate *et al* 1993). Since the surgical outcome of patients without pathology is usually less good, it is possible that the temporal lobe was not the site of seizure origin in those without histopathologic abnormalities who did not become seizure-free following temporal lobe resection. This cryptogenic category becomes progressively smaller as the sophistication of investigation increases and it may disappear in the near future, at least from surgical series.

LATERAL NEOCORTICAL TEMPORAL LOBE SEIZURES

Seizures originating in the lateral neocortical temporal lobe cortex are rare in comparison with seizures originating in the mesial temporal lobe structures. Furthermore, they are usually associated with a structural lesion involving the lateral temporal cortex alone or in combination with the insula. Nevertheless, seizures of lateral temporal origin do exist without a gross morphologic lesion and have been documented by stereo-EEG (Wieser and Müller 1987). Such seizures, as a rule, spread to the ipsilateral mesial temporal structures, which may act as a kind of 'amplifier' sustaining and prolonging the seizure discharges. Clinical signs and symptoms indicative of seizures arising from the lateral temporal neocortex commonly derive from epileptic discharges involving the cortex of more than one lobe. There

are no symptoms and signs that are absolutely specific for lateral temporal seizure onset, but the following are most frequently encountered.

1. Ictal aphasia occurs if the dominant hemisphere is involved.
2. Auditory hallucinations occur if the posterior insula (Heschl's gyrus) and the superior temporal gyrus are involved (Wieser 1980; Wieser and Williamson 1993).
3. Vestibular hallucinations have been documented with posterior temporal–parietal discharges (Wieser 1987).
4. Visual hallucinations, in particular macropsia and micropsia, as well as teleopsia, plagiopsia, dysplatopsia, achromatopsia or erythropsia and xanthopsia, loss or enhancement of three-dimensional perception, polyopia, paliopsia, and quick-motion as well as slow-motion, can occur with discharges in the temporoparietooccipital junction and inferotemporal cortex (Wieser 1987).
5. Motor symptoms, with contralateral tonic–clonic manifestations and head–eye deviation, are seen in neocortical lateral onset seizures more frequently than in mesiobasal seizures, whereas dystonic posturing occurs more frequently (in about 40% of patients) with mesial temporal lobe onset seizures.

ANATOMY AND PHYSIOLOGY OF THE MESIOTEMPORAL LIMBIC STRUCTURES

The phylogenetically oldest parts of the cortex, known as the allocortex, are different from the six-layered isocortex or neocortex. The allocortex consists of the archicortex (hippocampus and subiculum), the paleocortex (in essence, olfactory cortex), and the periarchicortex (in essence, area entorhinalis, regio retrosplenialis and cingularis). At the base of the temporal lobe the fissura rhinalis represents the border between allocortex and isocortex.

Functionally, the most important difference between allocortex and neocortex is that the allocortex does not receive direct thalamic afferents, whereas the neocortex does (Creutzfeldt 1983). The efferent pyramidal cells of the allocortex receive their input directly from the afferent fibers, i.e. the output neurons are at the same time the input neurons. Phylogenetically, in parallel with increasing neocorticalization, the percentage of allocortex in relation to the total cortex steadily decreases and is restricted to the medial–ventral border zone (lat. limbus) of the cortical mantle. In the older anatomic literature, for example

Campbell (1905), the term 'limbus corticalis' denotes the border between cortex and the corpus callosum. Broca (1878) coined the term *grand lobe limbique* for that region but without giving cytoarchitectonic references. In humans the allocortex comprises only 4% of the total cortex, whereas in primitive insectivores, such as the hedgehog and the shrew-mouse, it comprises 75% of the total. A part of the allocortex and its pathways has close anatomic and functional relations to the bulbus olfactorius and is therefore called the rhinencephalon. In the older literature the term 'rhinencephalon' was used to refer to the whole of the allocortex and its subcortical connections. In the narrow sense, however, the rhinencephalon comprises only the bulbus olfactorius to the regio praepiriformis, the amygdala, and regio septalis and periseptalis.

The term 'limbic system' is more comprehensive and, according to the original definition of Papez (1937), includes the allocortex and the connections of the hippocampus, i.e. the fornix, the corpus mamillare, and further on via the Vicq d'Azyr bundle (tractus mamillothalamicus), the anterior thalamic nucleus. From the thalamus there are projections to the anterior cingulate cortex, and from the cingulum back to the hippocampus. Thus this limbic circuit, which was proposed as a kind of reverberating circuit, includes the cingulate gyrus, which receives thalamic inputs and thus represents neocortex, or 'transitional' cortex. Within the concept of the limbic system, the hippocampal–cingulate connections are considered to be of less importance and several authors emphasize the connections of the limbic core structures to the hypothalamic regions and, via the nucleus accumbens, to the striopallidar system which controls motor functions.

Initially Papez (1937) proposed the limbic circuit as a kind of 'mediator of emotions'; later he coined the term 'visceral brain' (Papez 1958). Nauta (1958) enriched the limbic system concept with the term 'limbic midbrain area.'

NUCLEI AMYGDALAE (FIGS 11.1 AND 11.2)

The amygdalae are located directly above the temporobasal cortex and ventrorostral to the tip of the temporal horn of the lateral ventricle and are usually separated into three main nuclear groups: the phylogenetically older corticomedial group, the younger basolateral group, and a central group. In essence the corticomedial group receives afferents from various areas of the olfactory cortex, in particular the periamygdalar cortex, whereas the basolateral group receives its afferents from the inferotemporal neocortex (Broca's area 20). In the rhesus monkey nearly all cortical areas of the temporal lobe, major parts of the frontal lobe,

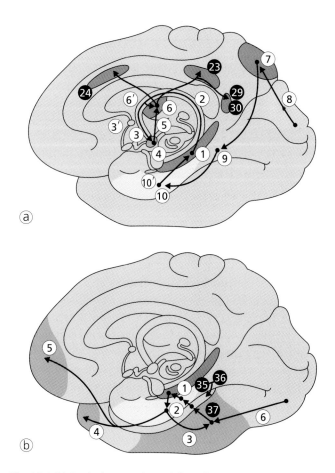

Fig. 11.1 (a) Cortical connections of the polysynaptic intrahippocampal pathway. Hippocampal output fibers to the cortex: arising from the hippocampus (1), fibers successively reach the body (2) and column (3) of the fornix (3', anterior commissure), the mamillary body (4), and, via the mamillothalamic tract (5), the anterior thalamic nucleus (6); some fibers reach this nucleus directly (6'); from the anterior thalamic nucleus, the main cortical projections are the posterior cingulate (area 23) and the retrosplenial (areas 29, 30) cortices; some fibers may project to the anterior cingulate cortex (area 24). Input fibers from the cortex to hippocampus: the posterior parietal area association cortex (7) in relation to the superior visual system (8) projects via the parahippocampal gyrus (9) to the entorhinal area (10); 10', perforant fibers. (b) Cortical connections of the direct intrahippocampal pathway. 1, Intrahippocampal circuitry. Hippocampal output fibers to the cortex: from the deep layers of the entorhinal cortex (2), fibers reach the inferior temporal association cortex (3), the temporal pole (4), and the prefrontal cortex (5). Input fibers from the cortex to the hippocampus: the main origin of these fibers is the inferior temporal association cortex (area 37) in relation to the inferior visual system (6), reaching the entorhinal cortex through the perirhinal cortex (areas 35 and 36). (From http://muskingum.edu/~biology/ hippocp/anatomy/cortconn.htm and http://muskingum.edu/~biology/hippocp/anatomy/directcn.htm; Duvernoy 1998).

and the insular cortex project to the amygdala (Ben-Ari 1981). These projections have a differential distribution within the amygdala. Some parts of some amygdaloid nuclei receive several cortical sensory projections. The lateral part of the central nucleus, the laterobasal nucleus, and the dorsomedial part of the lateral nucleus are areas where

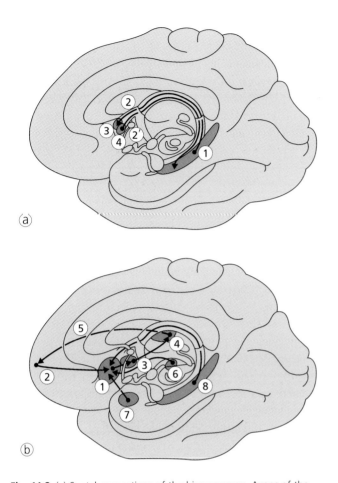

Fig. 11.2 (a) Septal connections of the hippocampus. Axons of the cornu Ammonis (1), via the precommissural fornix (2), reach the lateral septal nucleus (3). The fibers from the medial septal nucleus (4) return to the hippocampus the same way; 2′, anterior commissure. (b) Ventral (limbic) striatal loop. The ventral striatum (nucleus accumbens) (1) receives fibers from the prefrontal cortex (2) and controls the ventral pallidum (3). The ventral pallidum projects to the dorsomedial thalamic nucleus (4), whose fibers return to the prefrontal cortex (5). The ventral tegmental area (6) (the dopaminergic mesolimbic system A10), the amygdala (7) and the hippocampus (8) control the ventral striatal loop. (From http://muskingum.edu/~biology/hippocp/anatomy/septalcn.htm and http://muskingum.edu/~biology/hippocp/anatomy/vent.htm; Duvernoy 1998.)

substantial convergence of cortical input occurs. It is well documented that visual, auditory, olfactory, and, to some extent, taste information reaches the amygdala. Somatic sensory input is less clear, but there is reason to believe that all five modalities have some convergence in the dorsomedial part of the lateral nucleus. For example, the dorsomedial part of the lateral nucleus receives projections from the orbitofrontal area, which responds to olfactory stimulation, and this part is also the major amygdaloid projection zone of the cortical taste area. In addition there are posterior insular cortex projections to this area carrying visceral and probably other somatic information. Moreover, auditory input from the temporal polar cortex projects strongly to

this region. Visual projections are directed primarily to the dorsolateral part of the lateral nucleus. All types of cortex (isocortex, proisocortex, periallocortex, and allocortex) project to the amygdala, although proisocortical projections dominate over all others. Finally it is very important to remember that some corticoamygdaloid projections can be induced to sprout and to reinnervate deafferented parts of the amygdala (Rosene and Van Hoesen 1987).

The efferent fibers from the amygdala are the stria terminalis and, to a lesser extent, the ventrofugal bundle, with overlapping targeting areas in the medial and rostral hypothalamus (nuclei ventromedialis and dorsomedialis hypothalami, regio praeoptica), the regio septalis (nucleus lateralis septi, 'bed nucleus' of the stria terminalis, diagonal band), and the posterior part of the magnocellular nucleus dorsomedialis thalami. The latter connects the amygdala with the orbitofrontal cortex and constitutes a part of the second 'basolateral limbic circuit' formulated by Yakovlev (1948) and reemphasized by Livingston and Escobar (1971).

HIPPOCAMPAL FORMATION

In 1587 Arantius described the hippocampus, comparing the protrusion on the floor of the temporal horn to a seahorse (*Hippocampus*); Winslow in 1732 suggested 'ram's horn.' Garengeot (1742, cited in Duvernoy 1988) probably introduced the term 'cornu Ammonis' by analogy with the Egyptian god Ammon (Ammun Knegh). Currently the terms 'cornu Ammonis' and 'pes hippocampus' are usually used synonymously. The term 'hippocampus' applies to the entire ventricular protrusion and consists of two cortical laminae, rolled up one inside the other: the cornu Ammonis and the gyrus dentatus. The subiculum and entorhinal area represent a transitional cortex between the cornu Ammonis and the rest of the temporal lobe and are sometimes conceptually linked to the hippocampus to form a functional unit, the hippocampal formation (Chronister and White 1975). From its deepest level to the surface, i.e. from the ventricle towards the hippocampal sulcus, the cornu Ammonis is divided into six layers: alveus, stratum oriens, stratum pyramidale, stratum radiatum, stratum lacunosum, and stratum moleculare (Fig. 11.3).

A striking feature of the connectivity of the hippocampal formation is that its afferent connections are entirely through the entorhinal cortex, which is itself a link in numerous multisensory corticocortical networks.

Hippocampal connections

The intrinsic wiring of the hippocampal formation is mainly unidirectional. The predominantly superficial layers of the

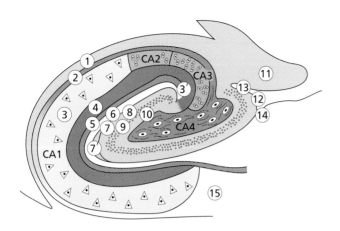

Fig. 11.3 Structure of the hippocampus, coronal section CA1–CA4, fields of the cornu Ammonis. Cornu Ammonis: 1, alveus; 2, stratum oriens; 3, stratum pyramidale; 3′, stratum lucidum; 4, stratum radiatum; 5, stratum lacunosum; 6, stratum moleculare; 7, vestigial hippocampal sulcus (note a residual cavity, 7′). Gyrus dentatus: 8, stratum moleculare; 9, stratum granulosum; 10, polymorphic layer; 11, fimbria; 12, margo denticulatis; 13, fimbriodentate sulcus; 14, superficial hippocampal sulcus; 15, subiculum. (From http://muskingum.edu/~biology/hippocp/anatomy/linanat.html; Duvernoy 1998.)

entorhinal cortex give rise to a powerful excitatory projection called the perforant path (which 'perforates' the subiculum to reach the hippocampus). The perforant path is composed of glutaminergic fibers to the dentate gyrus. The axons of the granule cells of the dentate gyrus, the mossy fibers, have a large content of zinc (McLardy 1962). Mossy fibers project to the CA3 and CA4 zones of the cornu Ammonis. Axons of CA3–CA4 enter the alveus and then the fimbria, but they first emit the Schaffer collaterals, which reach the apical dendrites of CA1 in the stratum radiatum and stratum lacunosum. The axons of CA1, by entering the alveus, produce collaterals that reach the subiculum. The subiculum emits the glutaminergic fibers of the principal efferent pathways, which are routed via the fimbria, the crus, the body of the fornix and the postcommissural fornix (behind the anterior commissure) to reach the anterior thalamic nuclei, either directly or via the mamillary bodies.

The entorhinal cortex receives inputs from the sensory association areas of the temporal lobe that convey visual, auditory, somatosensory, gustatory, nociceptive, and olfactory signals (Van Hoesen and Pandya 1975; Insausti *et al* 1987a,b). These inputs are distributed along the rostrocaudal extent of the entorhinal cortex, with the olfactory inputs occupying the most rostral part. Fibers from layers II and III that form the origin of the perforant path are further differentiated: fibers from layer II are distributed almost exclusively to the dentate gyrus and CA3, whereas fibers from layer III project exclusively to CA1 and the

subiculum. Thus, the perforant path is the main afferent pathway to the hippocampus. A second path, the alvear path, was described by Ramon y Cajal (1909–11) but its existence is currently questioned (Hjorth-Simonsen and Jeune 1972). Although the core elements of this neuronal chain, i.e. entorhinal area, gyrus dentatus, cornu Ammonis, and subiculum are of disparate anatomy, they constitute a single functional unit and are therefore rightly grouped together as the hippocampal formation (Powell and Hines 1975; Squire 1986).

FUNCTIONAL ANATOMY OF THE HIPPOCAMPAL FORMATION

Work with hippocampal slices, in both animals and humans, has been a cornerstone of the investigation of basic mechanisms of epileptogenesis, and has clarified the functional anatomy of the hippocampal formation. The trisynaptic pathway (Fig. 11.4) is tightly restricted in the rostrocaudal dimension so that separate lamellae can be identified. According to this scheme, the hippocampal formation is organized in a series of functional lamellae arranged perpendicular to the longitudinal axis of the hippocampal formation and operating independently of each other. The lamellar organization allows thin slices to be cut so that at least some important functions of the hippocampus can be maintained *in vitro*. Hippocampal slice studies have been critical to our current understanding of cellular and synaptic mechanisms of epileptiform, interictal, and ictal discharges. For example, such studies have demonstrated that CA3 pyramidal cells, but not those in CA1, become pacemakers for interictal spiking. This disparity can be accounted for by certain intrinsic membrane conductances in CA3 pyramidal cells (Johnston *et al* 1980) along with recurrent excitatory connections between CA3 pyramidal cells, both of which are lacking in CA1. On the other hand, ictal events develop in CA1 but not CA3 (Lothman 1991). The dentate gyrus thus serves as a critical control point for the regulation of epileptogenesis.

The biochemistry and morphology of the dentate granule cells are also altered as a function of epilepsy. In the kindled animal, these granule cells undergo a persistent decrease in calbindin (a calcium-binding protein) (Baimbridge *et al* 1985). Mody and Heinemann (1987) found that dentate granule cells in the kindled animal are more sensitive to agonists that activate the N-methyl-D-aspartate (NMDA) type of glutamate receptor than are dentate granule cells in nonkindled animals. Binding studies indicate that dentate granule cells have abundant receptors for NMDA (Bekenstein *et al* 1990), and that their expression and operation are altered after kindling (Yeh *et al* 1989).

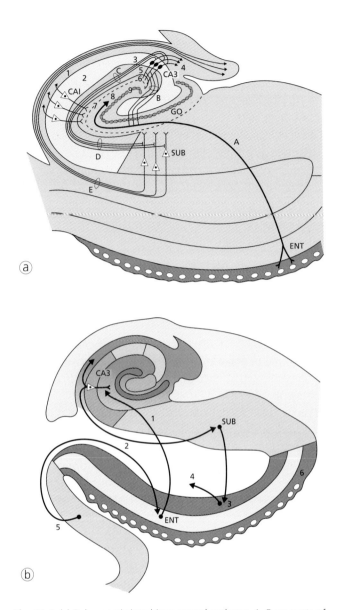

(a)

(b)

Fig. 11.4 (a) Polysynaptic intrahippocampal pathway. A–E are parts of the neural chain forming the polysynaptic intrahippocampal pathway. Layer II of the entorhinal area (ENT) is the origin of this chain; its pyramidal neurons are grouped in clusters, giving a granular aspect at the entorhinal surface. 1, alveus; 2, stratum pyramidale; 3, Schaffer collaterals (Schaffer 1892); 4, axons of pyramidal cells (mainly to septal nuclei); 5, stratum lacunosum and stratum radiatum; 6, stratum moleculare; 7, vestigial hippocampal sulcus; 8, gyrus dentatus stratum moleculare; 9, gyrus dentatus stratum granulosum; SUB, subiculum. CA1 and CA3 are fields of cornu ammonius. (b) Direct hippocampal pathway. The entorhinal area (ENT) (layer III) projects directly (1) on to CA1 pyramidal neurons, which innervate (2) the subiculum (SUB). Subicular axons project back to the deep layers of the entorhinal cortex (3). The neurons of these layers send axons to the association cortex (4). The direct pathway receives inputs through the perirhinal cortex (5). (From http://muskingum.edu/~biology/hippocp/anatomy/intrapat.htm and http://muskingum.edu/~biology/hippocp/anatomy/directhp.htm; Duvernoy 1998.)

These findings are, of course, very interesting in the light of experimental results which show that maximal dentate activation and the changes that take place during such

activation can be opposed by NMDA antagonists (Stringer and Lothman 1990). Morphologic changes of dentate granule cells as a consequence of epilepsy were first reported by Tauck and Nadler (1985) who demonstrated sprouting of axons (mossy fiber sprouting) in animals. Several laboratories have now documented that this occurs also in the human epileptic brain (Sutula *et al* 1988, 1989). It is reasonable to assume that mossy fiber sprouting contributes significantly to epileptogenesis by providing recurrent excitation of adjacent cells.

The ultimate stimulus to chronic alterations of the dentate granule cells probably acts at the genomic level. Through translation and transcription this would lead to alterations in protein expression. After seizures the expression of early–intermediate genes in dentate cells is activated (Dragunow and Robertson 1987a,b) and expression of the glial fibrillary acidic protein gene in the hippocampus is upregulated (Steward *et al* 1991). The latter finding is important since it addresses the glia, which constitute the second most important cellular compartment of the brain.

FUNCTIONAL LOOPS BETWEEN THE BASAL GANGLIA AND THE TEMPORAL LOBE

The connections of the temporal lobes with the basal ganglia are important with respect to some well-known features of temporal lobe seizures, such as *déjà vu, jamais vu*, macropsia, micropsia, delusions of familiarity, depersonalization, and the recently rediscovered contralateral tonic or dystonic posturing (Magnus *et al* 1954; Ajmone-Marsan and Ralston 1957; Kotagal *et al* 1989; Newton *et al* 1992).

The basal ganglia, i.e. the caudate, putamen, and ventral striatum, are known to receive inputs from frontal, parietal, and temporal lobes. The output from the basal ganglia via the thalamus is known to access the frontal motor and prefrontal cortex. Basal ganglia loops with the cortex have been thought to 'funnel' or collect information from diverse cortical areas in order to direct motor output and the executive functions of the frontal lobe. Recently, evidence has been provided that the output nucleus of the basal ganglia, the substantia nigra pars reticulata, projects via the thalamus to inferotemporal cortex (area TE), thereby targeting at least one visual area critically involved in the visual recognition and discrimination of objects (Middleton and Strick 1996). Dysfunction of the basal ganglia–inferotemporal cortex loop could underlie alterations in visual perception, including visual hallucinations. Mishkin and colleagues (Bachevalier and Mishkin 1994; Brown *et al* 1995; Malkova *et al* 1995) have proposed that visuomotor associations including 'habit memories' involve the 'visual striatum,' i.e. the tail of the caudate, and caudal–ventral portions of the putamen. These findings explain how damage to the basal ganglia impairs visual perception that results in deficits in the recognition and discrimination of faces and facial expressions in the early stages of Huntington's disease. They also explain visual hallucinations produced by lesions in the substantia nigra pars reticularis or by brainstem compression (peduncular hallucinosis, i.e. seeing fully formed images of or animals), and possibly also the visual hallucinations seen as a major side-effect of the use of L-dopa or other dopaminergic agents.

These findings may also account for dystonic posturing, which is an important lateralizing sign and occurs in 15–70% of patients with mesial temporal lobe seizures (Kotagal *et al* 1989; Fakhoury & Abou-Khalil 1995). Indeed ictal single-photon emission computed tomography (SPECT) studies have equated this dystonic posturing with increased blood flow in the basal ganglia ipsilateral to the seizure onset (Newton *et al* 1992).

PATHOLOGY

DEFINITIONS

Neuropathology plays an important role in the evaluation of hippocampal structural damage but many aspects remain unclear. Furthermore, the nomenclature applied to hippocampal pathology during the last century is confusing. The terms 'mesial temporal sclerosis' (Falconer *et al* 1964) and 'Ammon's horn sclerosis' have been used synonymously with 'hippocampal sclerosis' (Margerison and Corsellis 1966). Although the most common pathologic substrate of temporal lobe epilepsy is hippocampal sclerosis (Bratz 1899; Babb and Brown 1987), it is important to distinguish carefully the specific types of hippocampal pathology associated with such seizures.

Although the terms 'mesial temporal sclerosis,' 'Ammon's horn sclerosis,' and 'hippocampal sclerosis' have been used synonymously, strictly they imply different degrees of anatomic involvement (Armstrong and Bruton 1987). The term 'mesial temporal sclerosis' has advantages because it takes into account that the amygdala often shows pathology, consisting of neuronal loss and gliosis, equally severe to that in the hippocampus (Gloor 1991).

HIPPOCAMPAL SCLEROSIS

The most characteristic pathologic substrate of MTLE is hippocampal sclerosis. The term should only be used for the specific type of hippocampal cell loss consisting of marked neuronal depletion in the CA1 and hilar regions with some loss in the endfolium (CA3/CA4) but relative sparing of CA2. The subicular complex, entorhinal cortex, and other transitional cortex and the temporal gyri are relatively resistant to cell loss (Fig. 11.5). Hippocampal sclerosis is associated with other characteristic features, such as mossy fiber sprouting (Sutula *et al* 1989) and selective loss of somatostatin- and neuropeptide Y-containing neurons (De Lanerolle *et al* 1992), and is found in up to 70% of patients with medically refractory temporal lobe epilepsy undergoing surgery (Babb and Brown 1987).

In a normal hippocampus the granule cell layer in the dentate gyrus is relatively narrow and the cell bodies are closely approximated. In epilepsy specimens, however, the granule cell layer is often wider and disorganized (Houser 1990). Dispersed granule cells may extend into the surrounding molecular layer and sometimes show a bilaminar pattern (Fig. 11.6). Other cerebral diseases can also cause hippocampal damage but usually show a different pattern, with variable involvement of particular subfields but most often involving CA2.

The association between epilepsy and a sclerotic hippocampus was first described by Bouchet and Cazauvieilh (1825) following gross pathologic examination of the brains of patients with 'mental alienation seizures.' These lesions were believed to be an effect, rather than a cause, of the epilepsy. Jackson (1931–32) recognized limbic-type seizures and associated them with lesions in mesial temporal structures but not with Ammon's horn sclerosis. Sommer (1880) and Bratz (1899) suggested that Ammon's horn sclerosis might be an epileptogenic lesion, and since then evidence has accumulated that distinctive structural damage, i.e. hippocampal sclerosis, is typical of temporal lobe epilepsy. The pathology was accurately described and illustrated by Bratz, who showed destruction of the pyramidal cells in Sommer's sector (CA1) with preservation of the cells in the neighboring subiculum, cell loss in the hilus of the dentate gyrus and adjacent sector CA3, but preservation of neurons in sector CA2 and of the dentate granule cells.

The pathology of MTLE is not completely uniform. Gliosis may involve the anterior mesial temporal lobe structures in addition to the hippocampus. Moreover, hippocampal sclerosis is very often a bilateral condition, although frequently with a preponderance on one side (Margerison and Corsellis 1966). The precise cause of hippocampal sclerosis is not known, but there is no doubt that its epileptogenicity results from loss of specific hippocampal neurons and synaptic reorganization, with resulting hypersynchronization and hyperexcitability (Engel *et al* 1997).

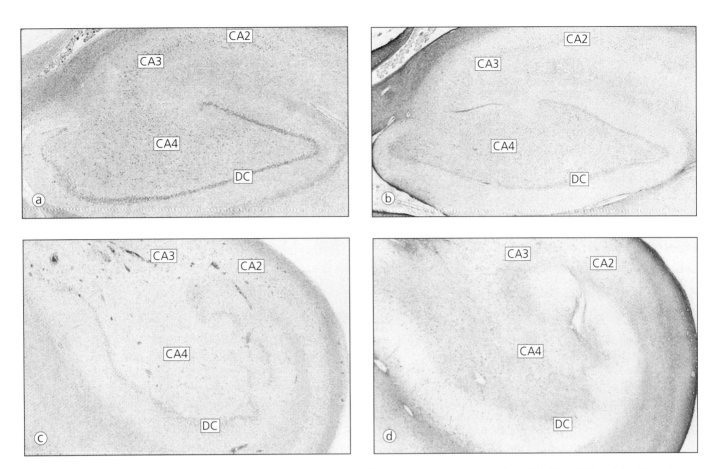

Fig. 11.5 Representative histopathologic examples of human hippocampus. (a) Normal autopsy control: regions CA2, CA3, CA4, and dendritic cell layer (DC). Hematoxylin and eosin ×15. (b) The same specimen stained for glial fibrillary acidic protein (GFAP) ×15. (c) Hippocampal sclerosis: note the dispersed granule cell layer (DC), severe damage and neuron loss in CA4 and CA3; there are some neurons left in CA2. Hematoxylin and eosin ×15. (d) The same specimen stained for GFAP: note the strong astrogliosis compared with (b). ×15.

Nevertheless, not every damaged hippocampus is epileptogenic and there are studies showing autopsy specimens of hippocampal pathology without antemortem seizures (Vogt and Vogt 1937; Corsellis 1957; Haymaker *et al* 1958; Meencke and Veith 1991; Verdi *et al* 1994). Conversely, other autopsy studies have shown that not every person with severe epilepsy has hippocampal sclerosis (Meencke and Veith 1991).

DUAL PATHOLOGY

Only a proportion of patients with temporal lobe epilepsy have 'classical' hippocampal sclerosis. Hippocampal sclerosis associated with some other temporal lobe pathology is referred to as dual pathology (Levesque *et al* 1991). Such associated pathology includes cortical microdysgenesis and cortical dysplasia, hamartomas, small tumors, and cavernomas. In these circumstances it may not be clear which pathology is responsible for the seizure disorder. Numerous studies have analyzed the neuropathologic findings in patients with temporal lobe epilepsy retrospectively (Mathieson 1975; Duncan and Sagar

1987; McMillan *et al* 1987; Bruton 1988; Estes *et al* 1988; Plate *et al* 1993; Wolf *et al* 1993). Table 11.1 provides a literature survey on the incidence of neoplasms reported in such patients and contains preliminary results from our Zurich study on 405 patients who underwent selective amygdalohippocampectomy.

THEORIES OF CAUSATION OF MESIAL TEMPORAL SCLEROSIS

Developments in contemporary chemical neuroanatomy can resolve the question as to whether hippocampal sclerosis is the cause or the consequence of seizures, and also settle part of the well-known controversy between Spielmeyer's vascular theory (Spielmeyer 1927) and the Vogt's specific cellular vulnerabilities within the pathoclisis theory (Vogt 1925; Vogt and Vogt 1937) (see Fig. 11.7). The vulnerability of CA1 can be attributed to the richness of the glutamate receptor, NMDA, while that of the hilus

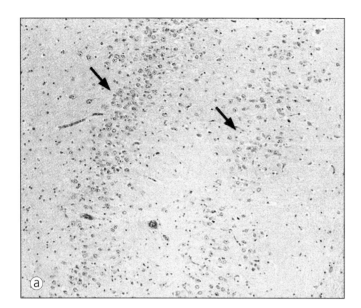
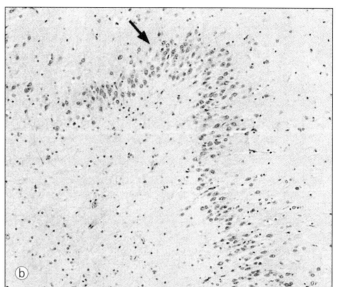

Fig. 11.6 Two examples of the dentate gyrus from a patient with epilepsy. (a) Dispersed granule cells form a bilaminar pattern (arrows) with a relatively neuron-free zone between the two layers. ×25. (b) Granule cell somata are dispersed (arrow) and extend into the molecular layer. ×25.

of the dentate gyrus and CA3 can be attributed to kainate receptors. These receptors, when powerfully activated by glutamate or aspartate, cause an excessive influx of calcium ions into the postsynaptic pyramidal neurons that may damage them irreversibly. Since the calcium-buffering protein calbindin is not present in the CA3 pyramidal cells and occurs in only small concentrations in the CA1 pyramidal cells, these areas are particularly vulnerable. On the other hand, calbindin is present in the CA2 pyramidal cells and in the dentate granule cells. Likewise, chromogranin A, another calcium-binding protein, shows a distribution that matches the profile of hippocampal sclerosis very well, being absent in the vulnerable sectors CA1 and CA3 and

present in the resistant sector CA2 and in the dentate gyrus granule cells and their axons, the mossy fibers. GABAergic neurons are also protected against calcium-induced damage by either calbindin or parvalbumin, and the sparing of the subiculum can be explained by its much lower content of NMDA receptors (Gloor 1991).

Hippocampal sclerosis is most commonly found in patients with a history of febrile seizures or status epilepticus in childhood, and has a lesser but significant correlation with birth trauma (Bruton 1988) reminiscent of the concept of incisural sclerosis proposed by Earle *et al* (1953). A common theme of the many authors who have considered these relationships is that there may be a particular time

Table 11.1 Neuropathologic findings in patients with temporal lobe epilepsy. (Modified from Plate *et al* 1993, © Springer-Verlag.)

Reference	Neoplasms (%)	Vascular malformations (%)	Hamartomas (%)	Hippocampal sclerosis/gliosis (%)	Other pathologies (%)	No pathology (%)
Mathieson (1975)	13	2	2	35	28	20
McMillan *et al* (1987)	n.s.	n.s.	n.s.	60	25	15
Duncan & Sagar (1987)	26	n.s.	n.s.	47	15	12
Bruton (1988)	20[b]	n.s.	n.s.	43	11	26[c]
Estes *et al* (1988)	11	6	6	46	19	n.s.
Wolf *et al* (1993)	35	6	18	72[d]	n.s.	n.s.
Plate *et al* (1993)	56	9	6	22	5	2
Our study[e]	41	11	3	33	2	10

n.s., not specified.
[a]Includes vascular malformations.
[b]Includes vascular malformations and hamartomas.
[c]Includes indefinite (minor) lesions.
[d]This percentage was obtained in a selected subgroup of patients from whom an anatomically well-preserved hippocampal specimen was available for histopathologic evaluation.
[e]Preliminary results (in preparation).

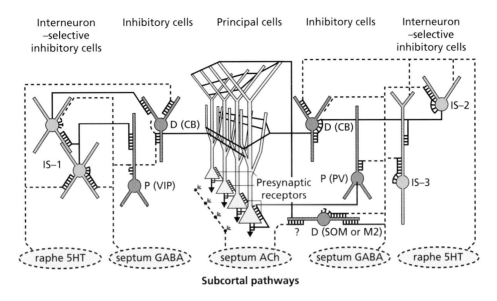

Fig. 11.7 Hippocampal microcircuit involving principal (pyramidal) cells (CA1, CA2, CA3, CA4) and the following interneuron types: 1) D (CB), dendritic inhibitory cells containing calbindin; 1) D (SOM or M2), dendritic inhibitory cells containing somatostatin (SOM) or muscarinic type 2 receptors (M2); P(VIP) and P(PV), perisomatic inhibitory cells containing vasoactive intestinal polypeptide (VIP) or parvalbumin (PV); IS-1, IS-2, IS-3, interneuron-selective inhibitory cells. The selective innervation of different interneuron types by subcortical afferents is indicated by dotted lines. GABAergic septal afferents (labeled by anterograde tracer) form multiple contacts with a perisomatic interneuron in the hippocampus visualized by immunostaining for parvalbumin. Serotonin (5HT)-immunoreactive raphehippocampal afferents form multiple contacts with dendritics interneuron in the hippocampus visualized by immunostaining for calbindin. (From http://muskingum.edu/~biology/hippocp/anatomy/hippintr.htm; Freund 1997.)

window, around 3 months to 5 years of age, during which noxious events are particularly harmful (Spielmeyer 1927; Zimmerman 1940; Corsellis 1957; Ounsted *et al* 1966; Mathieson 1975; Corsellis and Bruton 1983). Newborns presumably have only a few NMDA receptors in the hippocampus (Peterson *et al* 1989).

INVESTIGATIONAL FEATURES

ELECTROENCEPHALOGRAPHY

Certain features of the interictal and ictal EEG are typical of MTLE. Interictally, grouped blunt sharp waves with or without slow waves recur with a frequency of about 1 Hz and show a characteristic maximal predominance in the basal anterior electrodes (such as sphenoidal or true temporal electrodes). They may be unilateral or bilateral, dependent or independent (Wieser 1983a, 1987; Wieser *et al* 1993). Ictal scalp EEG findings typically consist of fairly regular theta rhythms of about 5 Hz with crescendo-like increase of the amplitude paralleled by a slowing of the discharge rhythms. Seizure onset may be characterized by regional or generalized attenuation of background rhythms with disappearance of the interictal 'spikes.' Direct recording from the hippocampal formation often shows a so-called 'hypersynchronous hippocampal discharge pattern' followed by a low-

amplitude high-frequency recruiting rhythm of more than 20 per sec (Engel 1990; Wieser *et al* 1993). The other frequent onset pattern of hippocampal seizures is the low-voltage fast discharge. These two patterns may both predict hippocampal tissue loss, but of different degree and distribution (Townsend and Engel, 1991; Spencer *et al* 1992a, b).

Using stereo-EEG, we have found that amygdala-onset seizures are relatively infrequent, constituting 3–5% of psychomotor seizures (Wieser 1983a). Gotman and Levtova (1996), on the other hand, have reported that in their phase-coherence study there was an amygdala onset in 21% of focal mesial and 53% of regional temporal lobe seizures, and a hippocampal onset in 48.5% of focal mesial and 27% of regional temporal lobe seizures. In the remaining seizures, discharges were synchronous in the two structures.

Contralateral propagation usually occurs and is accompanied by loss of consciousness and the onset of symptoms characteristic of CPS, including disturbance of consciousness. The mean time before the contralateral hippocampus is affected by the discharge is around 15 sec (Wieser and Siegel 1991). A long interhippocampal seizure propagation time is predictive of surgical success (Lieb *et al* 1986; Wieser and Siegel 1991) and has been shown to be inversely correlated with cell counts in CA4 (Spencer *et al* 1992c), supporting the concept that a long interhippocampal propagation time is a characteristic feature of MTLE. Most hippocampal-onset seizures propagate initially to ipsilateral temporal neocortical areas with variable subsequent involvement of frontal and contralateral structures (Lieb *et al* 1986; Wieser 1988a). However, about 30% of hippocampal-onset seizures appear first in the contralateral hippocampus prior to the ipsilateral or contralateral temporal neocortex. Localized hippocampal discharges may occur without any noticeable clinical accompaniments or with 'minor' symptoms only. Isolated hippocampal discharges in the language-dominant hemisphere may express themselves as a marked decline in performance on tachistoscopically presented lexical decision tasks; isolated discharges of the right hippocampus lead to a decline in performance on a tachistoscopic facial expression matching task (Wieser *et al* 1985). Discharges confined to one mesial temporal lobe are usually experienced by the patient as a clearly recognized aura (Wieser 1991a). Scalp EEG ictal discharges may be more widespread in children with MTLE and consist of irregular high-voltage spike-slow-wave patterns (Glaser and Golub 1955).

IMAGING

Magnetic resonance imaging

High-resolution, thin-section, T1-weighted MRI demonstrates hippocampal atrophy in a high percentage of patients with MTLE (Kuzniecky and Jackson 1995), while T2-weighted imaging shows increased signal. Quantitative magnetic resonance volumetry reveals asymmetries. (See Chapter 44 for a detailed discussion of MRI in hippocampal and amygdala sclerosis.)

Magnetic resonance spectroscopy

Magnetic resonance spectroscopy (MRS), in particular ^{1}H-MRS, can indicate neuronal loss and hippocampal sclerosis by measuring reduced *N*-acetyl-L-aspartate and an increased choline/*N*-acetyl-L-aspartate ratio (Matthews *et al* 1990; Laxer *et al* 1993; Wieser *et al* 1996). It may become a valid clinical tool in the future. (See Chapters 44 and 48 for a more detailed discussion of MRS.)

Positron emission tomography

Functional deficits in patients suffering from MTLE can be demonstrated using ^{18}F-fluorodeoxyglucose PET. Interictal hypometabolism is, as a rule, widespread and involves the ipsilateral lateral temporal lobe as well as ipsilateral thalamus and other subcortical structures (Engel *et al* 1991; Hajek *et al* 1993; Henry *et al* 1993). Flumazenil PET has demonstrated reduced benzodiazepine receptor binding (Savic *et al* 1988) and ^{11}C-carfentanil PET upregulation of μ opioid receptor binding mainly in the ipsilateral temporal lobe

(Frost *et al* 1988). On the other hand, ^{18}F-cyclofoxy studies (cyclofoxy binds to μ and κ receptors) and ^{11}C-diprenorphine studies (diprenorphine binds to μ, κ, and δ receptors) did not give conclusive results (Mayberg *et al* 1991; Bartenstein *et al* 1994). (See Chapters 25 and 48 for a more detailed discussion of PET.)

Single-photon emission computed tomography

Interictal SPECT studies have shown reduced blood flow in the temporal lobe ipsilateral to the epileptogenic mesial temporal lobe. With ictal SPECT there is temporal hyperperfusion during MTLE seizures, mesial hyperperfusion and lateral temporal lobe hypoperfusion in the immediate postictal period, and hypoperfusion of the entire temporal lobe in the later postictal phase. ^{99m}Tc-hexamethylpropyleneamineoxime (HMPAO) and ^{99m}Tc-L, L-ethyl cysteinate dimer (ECD) have advantages over ^{123}I-labeled amines (*N-N-N'*-trimethyl-*N'*-[2-hydroxy-3-methyl-5-iodobenzyl]-1,3 propanediamine (HIPDM) and *N*-isopropyl-I-123-*p*-iodoamphetamine [^{123}I-IMP] brain SPECT) because there is no redistribution in the brain. Reduced benzodiazepine receptor binding in the area of the focus can be demonstrated with ^{123}I-lomazenil SPECT (Haldemann *et al* 1992; Wieser 1994). SPECT with inhibitors of monoamine oxidase B (such as Ro 43-0463) may be able to visualize gliosis (Buck *et al* 1998). (See Chapters 26 and 48 for a more detailed discussion of SPECT.)

MEMORY EVALUATION

Animal and human lesion studies have revealed the importance of the hippocampal formation and the amygdala for learning and memory. More precisely, encoding of new information has been associated with the hippocampal formation, in particular with the perirhinal and entorhinal cortices (Squire and Butters 1984; Squire 1986; Squire and Zola-Morgan 1991; Mishkin 1993). Neuropsychologic evaluation of patients with MTLE reveals various degrees of material-specific learning and memory deficits. They tend to be more pronounced with left MTLE and may be associated with subtle speech problems if the dominant hemisphere is predominantly involved (Milner 1975; Ojemann and Dodrill 1985; Gonser *et al* 1986). (See Chapters 30 and 46 for a more detailed discussion of neuropsychologic aspects.)

SELECTIVE TEMPORAL LOBE MEMORY AMOBARBITAL TESTS

The temporary inactivation of the structures that will definitively be resected during surgical treatment is probably the best way to predict the deficits which might possibly follow the resection. The so-called intracarotid amobarbital test was pioneered by Wada (1949) for language lateralization, and then subsequently extended to allow predictions concerning the probability that a patient would develop a severe anterograde amnesic syndrome after surgery for temporal lobe epilepsy. To a certain degree it may be able to predict severe global memory deficits; however, it has considerable limitations when used to assess the risks of material-specific memory deficits developing after mesial temporal lobe excisions. The validity of the amobarbital test has been improved by various selective techniques (Wieser *et al* 1989a, b, 1997), notably:

1. selective inactivation of the territory of the anterior choroidal artery;
2. selective inactivation of the territory of the P2 segment of the posterior cerebral artery in the case of a so-called posterior test;
3. selective inactivation of the territories of the anterior choroidal artery *and* the posterior communicating artery in the case of the technique with temporary balloon occlusion distal to the origin of the anterior choroidal artery.

Nevertheless, problems remain because of the variability of the vascular supply in general and the fact that, as a rule, these arteries supply only a restricted territory of interest (the anterior choroidal artery supplies the amygdala and the anterior part of the hippocampus; the posterior cerebral artery supplies the more posterior hippocampus). Furthermore, the appropriate interpretation of the task performance requires coinjection of a SPECT tracer and concomitant EEG recording from the structures of interest.

Selective temporal lobe memory amobarbital tests in candidates for amygdalohippocampectomy have in general confirmed the material-specific memory role of the anterior mesiotemporal structures. With a dual verbal and nonverbal coding recurrent memory task (so-called DOKO) and nonverbal motor responding (button press), the prediction of postoperative memory performance is rather good for verbal memory but underestimates postoperative nonverbal (figural) memory performance (Wieser *et al* 1997).

EVENT-RELATED POTENTIALS

In patients with temporal lobe epilepsy, intracranial event-related potentials (ERP) show alterations (increase in latency and decrease in amplitude) that correlate well with the Wechsler Memory Scale, while the hippocampal P300 correlates well with neuronal cell density. The recently described N400 recorded from the anterior fusiform gyrus is thought to reflect access to semantic memory, whereas the P300 is thought to reflect rules-based mapping of stimuli on to discrete covert or overt responses, i.e. encoding processes (Nobre *et al* 1994; McCarthy *et al* 1995; Nobre and McCarthy 1995). Paller *et al* (1995) found that late potentials around 500–900 ms account for the subject's engagement in recollection processing, and ERP differentiate priming and recognition to familiar and unfamiliar faces (Begleiter *et al* 1995). Several authors have described limbic correlates of the scalp P300 elicited in visual and auditory odd-ball paradigms using depth electrodes in epileptic patients (Halgren *et al* 1980, 1995; Stapelton and Halgren 1987; Loring *et al* 1988; Grunwald *et al* 1995) and of the scalp N400 in word recognition paradigms (Smith *et al* 1986; Grunwald *et al* 1995). Therefore it can be assumed that the careful study of ERP recorded from mesiobasal temporal structures in patients with temporal lobe epilepsy has the potential to clarify the role of these structures in the various kinds of memory and to quantify preoperative deficits. Indeed, Grunwald *et al* (1995) reported that the amplitude of the intrahippocampal N400 elicited in a word recognition paradigm is an excellent predictor of postoperative memory performance in patients suffering from temporal lobe epilepsy.

ANTIEPILEPTIC DRUG TREATMENT

Carbamazepine is considered to be the treatment of first choice in MTLE and the initial response to it is usually satisfactory. Later, however, a substantial proportion of patients become clearly refractory to antiepileptic drugs, including classic first-line drugs such as carbamazepine, phenytoin, valproate, and barbiturate, and also new drugs such as vigabatrin, lamotrigine, gabapentin, and topiramate.

SURGICAL TREATMENT

Surgery is a highly effective treatment for medically refractory patients with MTLE and renders about 80% seizure-free. Most centers have modified the temporal lobe surgery for MTLE with the aim of resecting mesial temporal lobe structures more radically and minimizing the extent of the lateral temporal lobe resection. Selective amygdalohippocampectomy (SAH) (Wieser and Yasargil 1982; Yasargil *et al* 1985, 1993; Wieser 1986b, 1991b; Yonekawa *et al* 1996) and the so-called Spencer operation (resection of the mesial temporal structures, temporal pole, and only a small amount of anterior lateral temporal cortex) have been strongly advocated (Crandall 1987). There is evidence that sparing the lateral temporal lobe cortex has advantages in terms of neuropsychologic outcome (Wieser 1992), and that preoperatively hypometabolic lateral temporal lobe structures show a trend to normalization of their metabolism postoperatively (Hajek *et al* 1994). No additional clinically relevant deficits occur postoperatively in well-selected candidates for SAH who have preexisting material-specific memory and learning deficits. Furthermore, their contralateral material-specific memory performance usually improves (Wieser 1992). Similar findings were reported with classical anterior temporal lobe resections (Rausch and Crandall 1982). Verbal memory usually deteriorates following left temporal lobe resections in patients without preexisting memory deficits, particularly in those who do not become seizure-free. Selective temporal lobe memory amobarbital tests are used in our unit to predict the likely effect of surgery on the memory and learning of those patients considered to be at risk.

Without surgery the prognosis for patients with medically refractory MTLE is relatively poor. Both the severity and the frequency of their seizures may increase, and their memory may decline, with consequent severe psychosocial disturbances. The best psychosocial outcome is achieved by early surgical intervention, with relief of the disabling seizures before the negative consequences of MTLE interfere critically with vocational and social development (Khan and Wieser 1992). Several groups have reported good surgical results in children with temporal lobe epilepsy (Meyer *et al* 1986; Drake *et al* 1987; Wieser 1988b; Fish *et al* 1991; Munari 1995). The diagnosis of MTLE can often be made without resorting to invasive investigations but EEG recording with 'semi-invasive' foramen ovale electrodes may be very helpful if lateralization is difficult (Wieser and Moser 1988; Wieser and Morris 1997).

ZURICH AMYGDALOHIPPOCAMPECTOMY SERIES

Temporal lobe epilepsy surgery in Zurich was initiated by the neurosurgeon H. Krayenbühl in 1949. At that time, patients suffering from temporal lobe epilepsy received an anterior two-thirds temporal resection. Presurgical evaluation was refined in 1969, with the aim of improving the surgical results, by the introduction of stereo-EEG. Analysis of the stereo-EEG findings resulted in the development of a microsurgical selective operation, i.e. SAH, for MTLE, the main subtype of temporal lobe epilepsy (Wieser 1991b). SAH is intended to be either curative (causal) or palliative. It is a rather standardized type of epilepsy surgery, although it is always to some extent individually tailored according to the preoperative and intraoperative findings.

The criteria for undertaking curative SAH are:

1. unequivocal unilateral mesial temporal focal seizure onset associated with typical clinical symptoms;
2. intact contralateral hippocampal functions, as determined by neuropsychologic testing for learning and memory performance, including the selective memory amobarbital tests;
3. convergent results of the noninvasive tests, such as MRI, PET, SPECT, ^{1}H-MRS, and the electrophysiologic findings.

Palliative operations of this type may be indicated in patients whose primary epileptogenic zone is located in eloquent cortex (posterior temporal neocortex) and cannot be removed without intolerable functional deficits, but only then when the ipsilateral hippocampal formation is rapidly involved by the ictal discharges and acts as a 'secondary pacemaker,' i.e. a seizure-sustaining substrate. Seizure outcome of the Zurich SAH series is given in Table 11.2 and Fig. 11.8.

PREOPERATIVE AND POSTOPERATIVE ANTIEPILEPTIC DRUG TREATMENT IN THE ZURICH SERIES

The number of patients taking one or more antiepileptic drug, both before and in the years after SAH, is shown in Table 11.3 and can be compared with the proportion becoming seizure-free postoperatively shown in Table 11.2. Preoperatively all nontumoral patients were by definition drug resistant. They had taken all the first-line drugs, and most had taken more than two 'new' drugs. At the time of surgery most were taking two or more drugs. Some postoperative outcome data indicate that:

1. 1 year postoperatively 70% were seizure-free, although only 2.4% of the seizure-free patients had discontinued drug treatment;
2. considering all patients of this series (including so-called lesional cases, i.e. tumors and other gross lesions), at 5 year postoperatively 30% were off drugs, 32% were taking one drug, 18% two drugs, and 12% more than two drugs;
3. considering only the so-called non-tumoral cases, at 1 year postoperatively 1% of the seizure-free patients were off drugs; at 2 years postoperatively this figure was 11%, at 5 years postoperatively 35%, and at 10 years postoperatively 65%.

Table 11.2 Year-to-year and last available seizure outcome of the Zurich selective amygdalohippocampectomy series (total number of patients, 405; seizure outcome available for 353 patients; 52 patients missing). Seizure outcome classification is according to Engel et al (1993) into classes I–IV (for definition see Fig. 11.8).

| Outcome categories | Classification | Last available outcome | Year-to-year | | | | | | | | | | | | | | | | | | | | |
			1 years	2 years	3 years	4 years	5 years	6 years	7 years	8 years	9 years	10 years	11 years	12 years	13 years	14 years	15 years	16 years	17 years	18 years	19 years	20 years	21 years
Total			353	301	258	227	198	172	156	136	114	96	81	68	56	44	25	17	10	4	2	1	1
I	NL (%)	70	66	60	60	59	60	63	59	59	55	52	51	55	56	55	54	50	50	100	100	100	100
	L (%)	65	74	69	66	64	65	67	71	73	64	63	62	63	59	64	75	71	75	50	100	100	100
	All (%)	67	70	64	62	61	62	65	66	65	60	57	57	59	57	59	64	59	60	75	50	100	100
II	NL (%)	8	12	14	13	11	9	8	11	12	10	13	10	9	7	9	8	14						
	L (%)	11	8	11	12	12	10	10	9	9	13	13	10	9	7	5	8							
	All (%)	10	9	13	12	11	10	9	10	11	11	13	10	9	7	7	8	6						
III	NL (%)	15	14	16	16	18	18	18	18	18	21	23	23	18	22	23	31	40	50		100			
	L (%)	16	12	13	15	16	16	13	10	8	11	10	12	11	14	14	8	14	25	50				
	All (%)	16	13	15	16	18	18	16	13	13	16	17	17	15	18	18	20	29	40	25	50			
IV	NL (%)	7	9	10	12	12	13	11	12	12	14	13	15	18	15	14	8	10						
	L (%)	8	7	7	8	8	9	9	10	11	13	15	17	17	21	18	8	6						
	All (%)	7	8	8	10	10	11	10	11	11	13	14	16	18	18	16	8	6						

L, 'lesional' cases are defined by the presence of gross structural abnormalities, such as tumors and vascular malformations, on MRI. NL, 'non lesional' cases are defined by the absence of gross structural abnormalities on MRI; this latter category includes cases with hippocampal sclerosis and cases without abnormal findings diagnosed histopathologically or on MRI, but excludes those with dual pathology.

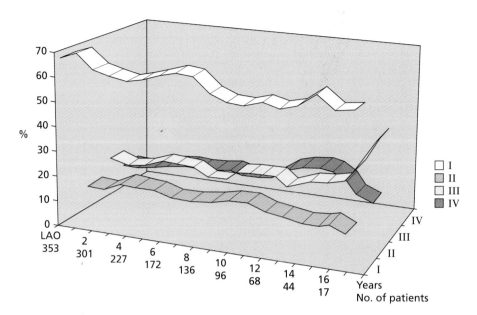

Fig. 11.8 Year-to-year (over 16 years) and last available seizure outcome (LAO) of the Zurich selective amygdalohippocampectomy series (total number of patients, 405; seizure outcome available for 353 patients). Seizure outcome classification is according to Engel (1987): class I, free of disabling seizures (excludes early postoperative seizures in first few weeks); class II, rare disabling seizures ('almost seizure-free'); class III, worthwhile improvement; class IV, no worthwhile improvement (determination of 'worthwhile improvement' in classes III and IV requires quantitative analysis of additional data such as percentage seizure reduction, cognitive function, and quality of life).

Table 11.3 Number of patients administered preoperative and postoperative antiepileptic drugs (AEDs) in the Zurich selective amygdalohippocampectomy series.

No. of AEDs	Preoperative	Years postoperative						
		1	5	7	10	13	16	20
0	4	6	59	54	33	15	6	0
1	149	159	64	44	29	16	4	0
2	111	113	35	22	11	6	3	1
3	66	65	19	17	12	10	4	0
4	16	9	3	2	0	1	0	0
5	1	0	1	0	1	1	0	0
?	38	1	17	17	10	7	0	0
	385	353	198	156	96	56	17	1

NEUROPATHOLOGIC/CLINICAL CORRELATIONS IN PATIENTS WITH HIPPOCAMPAL GLIOSIS

Histopathologic specimens of 81 patients with a diagnosis of hippocampal gliosis from our series of patients with SAH (currently 405) were reevaluated for the purposes of this chapter. The histopathologic evaluation assessed the following hippocampal abnormalities, including a ranking of the degree of the pathology: (a) gliosis; (b) neuronal loss; (c) alteration of the hippocampal CA regions; and (d) granule cell dispersion of the fascia dentata. In order to correlate the clinical data with the histopathology, an additional 32 SAH patients without hippocampal pathology were included in the statistical analyses. The entire population of

113 patients consisted of 71 males and 42 females, 59 with right SAH and 54 left SAH. The demographic data of the patients are given in Table 11.4 and the postoperative seizure outcome in Table 11.5.

Clinical data from both patient groups, along with the results of the *t*-tests, are given in Table 11.6. Patients with

Table 11.4 Demographic data of the 113 patients in the Zurich selective amygdalohippocampectomy series who were histopathologically reevaluated for the purposes of this chapter.

	Age at seizure onset (years)	Duration of illness (years)	Age at surgery (years)	Follow-up (years)
Mean	13.5	20.9	34.3	6.8
Minimum	0.4	2.5	10.3	0.2
Maximum	44.6	46.0	64.4	19

Table 11.5 Seizure outcome data of the 113 patients in the Zurich selective amygdalohippocampectomy series who were histopathologically reevaluated for the purposes of this chapter. Seizure outcome classification is according to Engel (1987) into classes I–IV (for definition see Fig. 11.8).

Outcome categories[a]	No. of patients	%
I	80	71
II	9	8
III	15	13
IV	9	8

[a]Last available outcome classified according to Engel (1987).

Table 11.6 Clinical data of the 113 patients in the Zurich selective amygdalohippocampectomy series who were histopathologically reevaluated for the purposes of this chapter. Comparison of patients with (*n* = 81) and without (*n* = 32) hippocampal pathology.

	No pathology (mean ± SD)	Hippocampal pathology (mean ± SD)	Significance level (t-test)
Age at seizure onset (years)	11.8 ± 9.0	14.2 ± 10.6	P <0.1
Duration of illness (years)	19.3 ± 9.0	21.0 ± 11.1	
Age at surgery (years)	31.1 ± 10.2	35.5 ± 10.8	P <0.05
Outcome (according to Engel I–V [with I seizure-free, II rare seizures, III worthwhile improvement, IV no worthwhile improvement])	2.1 ± 1.3	1.4 ± 0.8	P <0.01
Febrile convulsions			P <0.01
→ Yes	7 (6%)	25 (22%)	
→ No	13 (11%)	35 (31%)	
→ Unknown	12 (11%)	21 (19%)	

Table 11.7 Histopathology of the 81 patients with hippocampal pathology in the Zurich selective amygdalohippocampectomy series reevaluated for the purposes of this chapter.

Degree of pathology	Gliosis	Neuronal loss	CA regions	GC dispersion
Normal		7 (13.5)	31 (38.3)	15 (21.1)
Slight	2 (2.8)	7 (13.5)	11 (13.6)	19 (26.8)
Moderate	32 (45.1)	10 (19.3)	12 (14.8)	18 (25.4)
Severe	37 (52.1)	28 (53.8)	27 (33.3)	19[a] (26.8)
Reevaluation not possible	10	29		10

Numbers in parentheses are percentages.
CA regions, alteration of the architecture of CA regions; GC dispersion, granule cell dispersion of the fascia dentata.
[a]Bilaminar arrangement of the fascia dentata was seen in four patients.

Table 11.8 Correlation coefficients for clinical data and hippocampal pathology of the patients in the Zurich selective amygdalohippocampectomy series who were reevaluated for the purposes of this chapter.

	Gliosis	Neuronal loss	CA regions	GC dispersion	Age at seizure onset	Duration of illness	Age at surgery	Febrile convulsions
Neuronal loss	0.78***							
CA regions	0.51***	0.25***						
GC dispersion	0.66***	0.88***	0.21**					
Age at seizure onset	0.14	−0.15	0.22**	−0.06				
Duration of illness	0.09	0.20**	−0.02	0.16*	−0.45***			
Age at surgery	0.21*	0.02	0.20**	0.10	0.46***	0.55***		
Febrile convulsions	0.10	0.20**	0.01	0.26***	−0.14	−1.06	−0.15	
Outcome	0.33***	0.43***	0.11	0.34***	−0.14	0.11	−0.02	0.18*

CA regions, alteration of the architecture of CA regions; GC dispersion, granule cell dispersion of the fascia dentata.
*P < 0.1; **P < 0.05; ***P < 0.01.

hippocampal pathology differed significantly from those with normal histologic findings with respect to outcome and age at surgery. Patients with hippocampal pathology:

1. had a significantly better seizure outcome;
2. were significantly older at the time of surgery;
3. more often had a history of febrile convulsions;
4. had their seizure onset at an older age;
5. had a longer duration of illness, but not significantly so.

The types and the degree of the histopathologic findings are shown in Table 11.7. Not all the specimens could be evaluated/specified with respect to all the pathologic categories because some hippocampal slices were missing, having been used for other specific studies.

The results of the correlation analysis between the clinical data of all the patients and hippocampal pathology are given in Table 11.8. Apart from significant correlations between the various categories of hippocampal pathology, highly significant correlations were also seen between seizure outcome and gliosis, neuronal loss, and granule cell dispersion of the fascia dentata. Patients with hippocampal pathology had significantly better seizure outcome. Patients with febrile convulsions had a trend towards better seizure outcome and a severe granule cell dispersion. A higher age at seizure onset correlated highly with a severely disrupted architecture of the CA regions.

CONCLUSIONS

Temporal lobe epilepsy is by far the commonest of the localization-related epilepsies, particularly when medically refractory patients are considered. It has also been known for many years that the most common pathologic substrate of temporal lobe epilepsy is hippocampal sclerosis. Data accumulated from surgical series strongly suggest that temporal lobe epilepsy associated with hippocampal sclerosis represents a distinctive epileptic syndrome, i.e. MTLE. Early diagnosis of the condition is important because disabling seizures and their consequences can be prevented in 70–90% of patients by surgical intervention, either limited anterior temporal lobectomy or SAH.

The diagnosis of MTLE is based on etiology, seizure history, clinical presentation, progressive nature, intractability, and special features of the electrophysiologic, neuropsychologic, structural and functional imaging, and histopatho-logic examinations. The *entire* set of clinical and investigational findings must be taken into consideration if the correct diagnosis and treatment are to be achieved. The preoperative diagnosis and recognition of MTLE with hippocampal sclerosis has undoubtedly become much easier since the introduction of special high-resolution MRI techniques, including volumetry and densimetry; most importantly, MRI is noninvasive and therefore is less inconvenient for the patient. However, some experienced centers have noted an increasing number of referrals, with a misdiagnosis or overdiagnosis of MTLE. In our experience this often happens when the diagnosis is based more or less exclusively on MRI findings. In many previously published surgical series, patient data, including histopathology, was mainly evaluated according to the type and localization of gross pathologic findings without considering in detail whether or not the cardinal features of the MTLE syndrome were present. With this in mind, we reevaluated the available histologic specimens of those patients who had an initial diagnosis of hippocampal sclerosis and then correlated various clinical data with various aspects of hippocampal pathology. Highly significant correlations were seen between seizure outcome and gliosis, neuronal loss, and granule cell dispersion of the fascia dentata. Patients with hippocampal pathology had significantly better seizure outcome. Patients with febrile convulsions had a trend towards better seizure outcome and a severe granule cell dispersion. It is interesting that an older age at seizure onset correlated with a more severely disrupted architecture of the CA regions.

KEY POINTS

1. Hippocampal sclerosis consists of a marked neuronal loss with gliosis in the CA1 and hilar regions of the hippocampus, with some loss in CA3/CA4, associated with disorganization of the granule cell layer, mossy fiber sprouting, and selective loss of somatostatin- and neuropeptide Y-containing neurons. The gliosis may extend to other medial temporal lobe structures. The condition is often bilateral but with a marked preponderance on one side.

2. Hippocampal sclerosis is commonly associated with a history of prolonged convulsions during childhood. The neuronal damage is attributed to excessive activation by glutamate and aspartate, which subject postsynaptic neurons to an excessive influx of calcium ions at an age when such a noxious event is particularly harmful.

3. Hippocampal sclerosis may be associated with other pathology (dual pathology), especially a malformation of cortical

development or an indolent tumor such as a dysembryoplastic neuroepithelial tumor.

4. Hippocampal sclerosis is the most common pathologic substrate of MTLE, which is itself probably the most common human epilepsy syndrome.

5. The MTLE syndrome is characterized by simple partial seizures, particularly an epigastric-rising sensation associated with psychic phenomena such as fear, and complex partial seizures, especially

KEY POINTS

oroalimentary and gestural automatisms, sometimes with secondary generalization. The seizures usually commence in childhood or adolescence and the prognosis for achieving adequate control with medication is <60%.

6. Characteristic investigational findings in MTLE with hippocampal sclerosis are:

   (a) EEG (scalp): interictally, blunt sharp waves predominating at the basal anterior electrodes; at seizure onset, a generalized attenuation of background rhythms and disappearance of interictal spikes; and ictally, fairly regular theta rhythms of about 5 Hz with a crescendo-like increase of amplitude and slowing of discharge rhythms. The diagnosis can often be made with noninvasive investigations.

   (b) MRI: hippocampal smallness and increased T2 signal.

   (c) Fluorodeoxyglucose PET: ipsilateral temporal lobe hypometabolism interictally.

   (d) SPECT: ipsilateral temporal lobe hyperperfusion ictally.

   (e) Neuropsychology: various degrees of memory and learning deficit.

7. MTLE is often refractory to medication but resection of medial temporal lobe structures with predominantly unilateral hippocampal sclerosis renders 70–80% seizure-free, or virtually so, without producing additional clinically relevant deficits. The best psychosocial outcome is achieved by surgery soon after it becomes clear that the epilepsy is intractable to medication, including during childhood/early adolescence.

8. The criteria for recommending SAH with a view to cure MTLE are:

   (a) a typical history of MTLE, *with*

   (b) unequivocal evidence of mesial temporal focal seizure onset, as determined by concordance of the electrophysiologic and imaging data, *and with*

   (c) evidence of intact contralateral hippocampus as determined by neuropsychologic and amobarbital (modified Wada) testing.

9. The highest probability that SAH will cure MTLE is among patients with a history of febrile convulsion and/or a marked degree of hippocampal gliosis and neuron loss and dentate granule cell dispersion.

REFERENCES

Abou-Khalil B, Andermann E, Andermann F *et al* (1993) Temporal lobe epilepsy after prolonged febrile convulsions: excellent outcome after surgical treatment. *Epilepsia* **34**:878–883.

Adey WR (1959) Recent studies of the rhinencephalon in relation to temporal lobe epilepsy and behaviour disorders. *International Review of Neurobiology* **1**:1–46.

Ajmone-Marsan C, Ralston BL (1957) *The Epileptic Seizure. Its Functional Morphology and Diagnostic Significance.* Springfield, IL: CC Thomas.

Anderson J (1886) On sensory epilepsy: a case of basal cerebral tumour, affecting the left temporo-sphenoidal lobe, and giving rise to a paroxysmal taste-sensation and dreamy state. *Brain* **9**:385–395.

Annegers JF, Hauser WA, Elveback LR *et al* (1979) The risk of epilepsy following febrile convulsions. *Neurology* **29**:297–303.

Arantius JC (1587) De humano foetu. In: *Ejusdem Anatomicorum Observationum Liber*, pp 44–45. Venetiis.

Armstrong DD, Bruton CJ (1987) Postscript: what terminology is appropriate for tissue pathology? How does it predict outcome? In: Engel J Jr (ed) *Surgical Treatment of the Epilepsies*, pp 541–552. New York: Raven Press.

Babb TL, Brown WJ (1987) Pathological findings in epilepsy. In: Engel J Jr (ed) *Surgical Treatment of the Epilepsies*, pp 511–540. New York: Raven Press.

Bachevalier J, Mishkin M (1994) Effects of selective neonatal temporal lobe lesions on visual recognition memory in rhesus monkeys. *Journal of Neuroscience* **14**:2128–2139.

Baimbridge KG, Mody I, Miller JJ (1985) Reduction of rat hippocampal calcium-binding protein following commissural, amygdala, septal, perforant path, and olfactory bulb kindling. *Epilepsia* **26**:460–465.

Baldwin M, Bailey P (1958) *Temporal Lobe Epilepsy.* Springfield, IL: CC Thomas.

Bancaud J, Talairach J, Bonis A *et al* (1965) *La Stéréo-électroencéphalographie dans l'Épilepsie.* Paris: Masson.

Bartenstein PA, Prevett MP, Duncan JS *et al* (1994) Quantification of opiate receptors in two patients with mesiobasal temporal lobe epilepsy, before and after selective amygdalo-hippocampectomy using positron emission tomography. *Epilepsy Research* **18**:119–125.

Bear DM (1979) Temporal lobe epilepsy. A syndrome of sensory–limbic hyperconnection. *Cortex* **15**:357–384.

Bear DM, Fedio P (1977) Quantitative analysis of interictal behaviour in temporal lobe epilepsy. *Archives of Neurology* **34**:454–467.

Begleiter H, Porjesz B, Wang W *et al* (1995) Event-related brain potentials differentiate priming and recognition to familiar and unfamiliar faces. *Electroencephalography and Clinical Neurophysiology* **94**:41–49.

Bekenstein JW, Bennett JW, Wooten GF *et al* (1990) Autoradiographic evidence that NMDA receptor-coupled channels are located postsynaptically and not presynaptically in the perforant path–dentate gyrus granule cell system of the rat hippocampal formation. *Brain Research* **514**:334–342.

Ben-Ari Y (1981) *The Amygdaloid Complex.* INSERM Symposium 20. Amsterdam: Elsevier/North-Holland Biomedical Press.

Berkovic SF, Howell RA, Hopper JL (1994) Familial temporal epilepsy: a new syndrome with adolescent/adult onset and a benign course. In: Wolf P (ed) *Epileptic Seizures and Syndromes*, pp 257–263. London: John Libbey.

Bickford RG, Dodge HW, Sem-Jacobsen CW (1953) Observations on depth stimulation of the human brain through implanted electrographic leads. *Proceedings of the Mayo Clinic* **22**:333–343.

Bouchet CG, Cazauvieilh G (1825) De l'épilepsie considérée dans ses rapports avec l'aliénation mentale: recherches sur la nature et le siège de ces deux maladies. *Archives Generales de Medicine* **9**:510–542.

Bratz E (1899) Ammonshornbefunde der Epileptischen. *Archiv für Psychiatrie und Nervenkrankheiten* **31**:820–836.

Broca P (1878) Anatomie comparée des circonvolutions cérébrales. Le grand lobe limbique et la scissure limbique dans la série des mammifères. *Revue d'Anthropologie Série* **21**:385–498.

Brown VJ, Desimone R, Mishkin M (1995) Responses of cells in the tail of the caudate nucleus during visual discrimination learning. *Journal of Neurophysiology* **74**:1083–1094.

Bruton CJ (1988) *The Neuropathology of Temporal Lobe Epilepsy*. Oxford: Oxford University Press.

Buck A, Frey LD, Bläuenstein P *et al* (1998) Monoamine oxidase B single-photon emission tomography with [^{123}I] Ro43-0463: imaging in volunteers and patients with temporal lobe epilepsy. *European Journal of Nuclear Medicine* **25**:464–470.

Campbell AW (1905) *Histological Studies in the Localisation of Cerebral Function*. Cambridge: Cambridge University Press.

Cendes F, Andermann F, Dubeau F *et al* (1993a) Early childhood prolonged febrile convulsions, atrophy and sclerosis of mesial structures, and temporal lobe epilepsy: a MRI volumetric study. *Neurology* **43**:1083–1087.

Cendes F, Andermann F, Gloor P *et al* (1993b) Atrophy of mesial structures in patients with temporal lobe epilepsy: cause or consequence of repeated seizures? *Annals of Neurology* **34**:795–801.

Chronister RB, White LE (1975) Fiberarchitecture of the hippocampal formation: anatomy, projections and structural significance. In: Isaacson RL, Pribram KH (eds) *The Hippocampus. I. Structure and Development*, pp 9–39. New York: Plenum Press.

Commission on Classification and Terminology of the International League Against Epilepsy (1969) Clinical and electroencephalographic classification of epileptic seizures. *Epilepsia* **10**(Suppl):2–13.

Commission on Classification and Terminology of the International League Against Epilepsy (1989) Proposal for revised classification of epilepsies and epileptic syndromes. *Epilepsia* **30**:389–399.

Corsellis JAN (1957) The incidence of Ammon's horn sclerosis. *Brain* **80**:193–208.

Corsellis JAN, Bruton CJ (1983) Neuropathology of status epilepticus in humans. *Advances in Neurology* **34**:129–139.

Crandall PH (1987) Cortical resections. In: Engel J Jr (ed) *Surgical Treatment of the Epilepsies*, pp 377–404. New York: Raven Press.

Crandall PH, Walter RD, Rand RW (1963) Clinical applications of studies on stereotactically implanted electrodes in temporal lobe epilepsy. *Journal of Neurosurgery* **21**: 27–840.

Creutzfeldt OD (1983) *Cortex Cerebri: Leistung, Strukturelle und Funktionelle Organisation der Hirnrinde*. Berlin: Springer.

Daly D (1958) Uncinate fits. *Neurology* **8**:250–260.

Davies KG, Hermann BP, Dohan FC Jr (1996) Relationship of hippocampal sclerosis to duration and age of onset of epilepsy, and childhood febrile seizures in temporal lobectomy patients. *Epilepsy Research* **24**:119–126.

De Lanerolle NC, Brines ML, Kim JH (1992) Neurochemical remodeling of the hippocampus in human temporal lobe epilepsy. *Epilepsy Research* Suppl 9:205–220.

Delgado-Escueta AV, Walsh GO (1985) Type I complex partial seizures of hippocampal origin: excellent results of anterior temporal lobectomy. *Neurology* **35**:143–154.

Dragunow M, Robertson HA (1987a) Generalised seizures induce c-fos protein(s) in mammalian neurons. *Neuroscience Letters* **82**:157–161.

Dragunow M, Robertson HA (1987b) Kindling stimulation induces c-fos protein(s) in granule cells of the rat dentate gyrus. *Nature* **329**:441–442.

Drake J, Hoffmann HJ, Kobayashi J *et al* (1987) Surgical management of children with temporal lobe epilepsy and mass lesions. *Neurosurgery* **21**:792–797.

Duncan JS, Sagar HJ (1987) Seizure characteristics, pathology, and outcome after temporal lobectomy. *Neurology* **37**:405–409.

Duvernoy HM (1988) *The Human Hippocampus. An Atlas of Applied Anatomy*. Munich: JF Bergmann.

Earle KM, Baldwin M, Penfield W (1953) Incisural sclerosis and temporal lobe seizure produced by hippocampal herniation at birth. *Archives of Neurology and General Psychiatry* **69**:27–42.

Engel J Jr (1987) Outcome with respect to epileptic seizures. In: Engel J Jr (ed) *Surgical Treatment of the Epilepsies*, pp 553–571. New York: Raven Press.

Engel J Jr (1989) *Seizures and Epilepsy*. Philadelphia: FA Davis.

Engel J Jr (1990) Functional explorations of the human epileptic brain and their therapeutic implications. *Electroencephalography and Clinical Neurophysiology* **76**:296–316.

Engel J Jr (1992) Recent advances in surgical treatment of temporal lobe epilepsy. *Acta Neurologica Scandinavica* Suppl **140**:71–80.

Engel J Jr, Henry TR, Risinger MW (1991) The role of positron emission tomography in presurgical evaluation of temporal lobe epilepsy. In: Lüders H (ed) *Epilepsy Surgery*, pp 231–241. New York: Raven Press.

Engel J Jr, Williamson PD, Wieser HG (1997) Mesial temporal lobe epilepsy. In: Engel J Jr, Pedley J (eds) *Epilepsy: A Comprehensive Textbook*, pp 2417–2426. New York: Raven Press.

Estes ML, Morris HH, Luders H *et al* (1988) Surgery for intractable epilepsy. Clinicopathologic correlates in 60 cases. *Cleveland Clinic Journal of Medicine* **55**:441–447.

Fakhoury T, Abou-Khalil B (1995) Association of ipsilateral head turning and dystonia in temporal lobe seizures. *Epilepsia* **36**:1065–1070.

Falconer MA, Serafetinides EA, Corsellis JAN (1964) Etiology and pathogenesis of temporal lobe epilepsy. *Archives of Neurology* **10**:233–248.

Feindel W (1961) Response patterns elicited from the amygdala and deep temporo-insular cortex. In: Sheer DE (ed) *Electrical Stimulation of the Brain*, pp 519–532. Austin, TX: University Press.

Feindel W, Penfield W (1954) Localisation of discharge in temporal lobe automatism. *Archives of Neurology and Psychiatry* **72**:605–630.

Feindel W, Penfield W, Jasper H (1952) Localization of epileptic discharges in temporal lobe automatism. *Transactions of the American Neurological Society* **77**:14–17.

Ferguson SM, Rayport M (1984) Psychosis and epilepsy. In: Blumer D (ed) *Psychiatric Aspects of Epilepsy*, pp 229–270. Washington, DC: American Psychiatric Press.

Fish DR, Smith SJ, Quesney F (1991) Surgical treatment of children with medically intractable frontal or temporal lobe epilepsy: results and highlights of 40 years experience. *Epilepsia* **34**:244–247.

Flor-Henry P (1969) Psychosis and temporal lobe epilepsy. *Epilepsia* **10**:363–395.

Flor-Henry P (1972) Ictal and interictal psychiatric manifestations of epilepsy. Specific or non-specific? *Epilepsia* **13**:773–783.

Freund TF (1997) Interneurons of the hippocampus. *IBRO News* **25**:6.

Frost JJ, Mayberg HS, Fisher RS *et al* (1988) Mu-opiate receptors measured by positron emission tomography are increased in temporal lobe epilepsy. *Annals of Neurology* **23**:231–237.

Gastaut H (1973) *Dictionary of Epilepsy*. Geneva: World Health Organisation.

Gastaut H, Gastaut Y (1951) Corrélations EEG et cliniques à propos de 100 cas d'épilepsie die 'psychomotrice' avec foyers sur la région temporale du scalp. *Revue d'Oto-Neuro-Ophthalmologie* **23**:257–282.

Geier S, Bancaud J, Talairach J *et al* (1976) Automatisms during frontal lobe epileptic seizures. *Brain* **99**:447–458.

Geier S, Bancaud J, Talairach J *et al* (1977) Ictal tonic postural changes and automatisms during epileptic parietal lobe seizures. *Epilepsia* **18**:517–524.

Gibbs FA, Gibbs EL, Lennox WG (1938) The likeness of the cortical dysrhythmias of schizophrenia and psychomotor epilepsy. *American Journal of Psychiatry* **95**:254–269.

Glaser GH, Golub ML (1955) The electroencephalogram of

psychomotor seizures in children. *Electroencephalography and Clinical Neurophysiology* 7:329–340.

Gloor P (1960) Amygdala. In: Field J, Magnon HW, Hall VE (eds) *Handbook of Physiology. Neurophysiology II*, pp 1395–1420. Washington, DC: American Physiological Society.

Gloor P (1991) Mesial temporal sclerosis: historical background and an overview from modern perspective. In: Lüders H (ed) *Epilepsy Surgery*, pp 689–703. New York: Raven Press.

Gloor P, Feindel W (1963) Affective behaviour and temporal lobe. In: Monnier M (ed) *Physiologie und Pathophysiologie des Vegetativen Nervensystems. Pathophysiologie*, Vol 2, pp 685–716. Stuttgart: Hippokrates.

Gloor P, Olivier A, Quesney LF *et al* (1982) The role of the limbic system in experiential phenomena of temporal lobe epilepsy. *Annals of Neurology* 12:129–144.

Gonser A, Perret E, Wieser HG (1986) Ist der Hippokampus für Lern- und Gedächtnisprozesse notwendig? *Nervenarzt* 57:269–275.

Gotman J, Levtova V (1996) Amygdala–hippocampus relationships in temporal lobe seizures: a phase-coherence study. *Epilepsy Research* 25:51–57.

Gowers WR (1885) (reprinted 1964) *Epilepsy and Other Chronic Convulsive Diseases: Their Causes, Symptoms and Treatment*. New York: Wood, Dover.

Green JD (1964) The hippocampus. *Physiological Reviews* 44:561–608.

Green JR (1967) Temporal lobectomy, with special reference to selection of epileptic patients. *Journal of Neurosurgery* 26:584–593.

Grunwald T, Elger CE, Lehnertz K *et al* (1995) Alterations of intrahippocampal cognitive potentials in temporal lobe epilepsy. *Electroencephalography and Clinical Neurophysiology* 95:53–62.

Hajek M, Antonini A, Leenders KL *et al* (1993) Mesiobasal versus lateral temporal lobe epilepsy: metabolic differences in the temporal lobe shown by interictal ^{18}F-FDG positron emission tomography. *Neurology* 43:79–86.

Hajek M, Wieser HG, Khan N *et al* (1994) Preoperative and postoperative glucose consumption in mesiobasal and lateral temporal lobe epilepsy. *Neurology* 4:2125–2132.

Haldemann RC, Bicik I, Pfeiffer A *et al* (1992) ^{123}I-Iomazenil: a quantitative study of the central benzodiazepine receptor distribution. *Nuclear Medicine* 31:91–97.

Halgren EP, Squires NK, Wilson CL *et al* (1980) Endogenous potentials generated in the human hippocampus formation and amygdala by infrequent events. *Science* 210:803–805.

Halgren EP, Baudena JM, Clarke A *et al* (1995) Intracerebral potentials to a rare target and distractor auditory and visual stimuli. II. Medial, lateral and posterior temporal lobe. *Electroencephalography and Clinical Neurophysiology* 94:229–250.

Haymaker W, Pentschew A, Margoles C *et al* (1958) Occurrence of lesions in the temporal lobe in the absence of convulsive seizures. In: Baldwin M, Bailey P (eds) *Temporal Lobe Epilepsy*, pp166–202. Springfield, IL: CC Thomas.

Hecker A, Andermann F, Rodin E (1972) Spitting automatisms in temporal lobe seizures. *Epilepsia* 13:767–772.

Henry TR, Mazziota JC, Engel J Jr (1993) Interictal metabolic anatomy of limbic temporal lobe epilepsy. *Archives of Neurology* 50:582–589.

Hjorth-Simonsen A, Jeune B (1972) Origin and termination of the hippocampal perforant path in the rat studied by silver impregnation. *Journal of Comparative Neurology* 144:215–232.

Houser CR (1990) Granule cell dispersion in the dentate gyrus of humans with temporal lobe epilepsy. *Brain Research* 535:195–204.

Insausti R, Amaral DG, Cowan WM (1987a) The entorhinal cortex of the monkey: II. Cortical afferents. *Journal of Comparative Neurology* 264:356–395.

Insausti R, Amaral DG, Cowan WM (1987b) The entorhinal cortex of the monkey: III. Subcortical afferents. *Journal of Comparative Neurology* 264:396–408.

Jackson JH (1880) On right- or left-sided spasm at the onset of epileptic paroxysms, and on crude sensation warnings and elaborate mental states. Reprinted in: Taylor J (ed) (1958) *Selected Writings of Jackson JH*, Vol 1, pp 308–317. New York: Basic Books.

Jackson JH (1889) On a particular variety of epilepsy ('intellectual aura'), one case with symptoms of organic brain disease. Reprinted in: Taylor J (ed) (1958) *Selected Writings of Jackson JH*, Vol 1, pp 385–405. New York: Basic Books.

Jackson JH (1931–32) Reprinted in: Taylor J (ed) *Selected Writings of John Hughlings Jackson*. London: Hodder & Stoughton.

Jackson JH, Beevor C (1890) Case of tumour of the right temporo-sphenoidal lobe, bearing on the localisation of the sense of smell and on the interpretation of a particular variety of epilepsy. *Brain* 12:346–357.

Jackson JH, Colman WS (1898) Case of epilepsy with tasting movements and 'dreamy state': very small patch of softening in the left uncinate gyrus. *Brain* 21:580–590.

Jackson JH, Stewart P (1899) Epileptic attacks with a warning of crude sensation of smell and with intellectual aura (dreamy state) in a patient who had symptoms pointing to gross organic disease of the right temporo-sphenoidal lobe. *Brain* 22:334–549.

Jacome DE, Fitzgerald R (1982) Ictus emeticus. *Neurology* 32:209–212.

Jasper HH (1960) Evolution of conceptions of cerebral localisation since Hughlings Jackson. *World Neurology* 1:97–112.

Jasper HH, Kershman J (1941) Electroencephalographic classification of the epilepsies. *Electroencephalography and Clinical Neurophysiology* Suppl 2:123–131.

Jensen I (1976) Temporal lobe epilepsy: etiological factors and surgical results. *Acta Neurologica Scandinavica* 53:103–118.

Johnston D, Hablitz JJ, Wilson WA (1980) Voltage clamp discloses slow inward current in hippocampal burst-firing neurons. *Nature* 386:391–393.

Khan N, Wieser HG (1992) Psychosocial outcome of patients with amygdalo-hippocampectomy. *Journal of Epilepsy* 5:128–134.

Kotagal P (1991) Seizure symptomatology of temporal lobe origin. In: Lüders H (ed) *Epilepsy Surgery*, pp 143–155. New York: Raven Press.

Kotagal P, Lueders HO, Morris HH *et al* (1989) Dystonic posturing in complex partial seizures of temporal lobe onset: a new lateralizing sign. *Neurology* 39:196–201.

Kuks JBM, Cook MJ, Stevens JM *et al* (1993) Hippocampal sclerosis in epilepsy and childhood febrile seizures. *Lancet* 342:1391–1394.

Kuzniecky RI, Jackson GD (1995) *Magnetic Resonance in Epilepsy*. New York: Raven Press.

Laxer KD, Rowley HA, Novotny EJ Jr *et al* (1993) Experimental technologies. In: Engel J Jr (ed) *Surgical Treatment of the Epilepsies*, 2nd edn, pp 291–308. New York: Raven Press.

Lee K, Diaz M, Melchior JC (1981) Temporal lobe epilepsy: not a consequence of childhood febrile convulsions in Denmark. *Acta Neurologica Scandinavica* 63:231–236.

Lennox WG (1960) *Epilepsy and Related Disorders*, Vol 2. Boston: Little, Brown.

Levesque MF, Nakasato N, Vinters HV *et al* (1991) Surgical treatment of limbic epilepsy associated with extrahippocampal lesions: the problem of dual pathology. *Journal of Neurosurgery* 75:364–370.

Lieb JP, Engel J Jr, Babb TL (1986) Interhemispheric propagation time of human hippocampal seizures. I. Relationship to surgical outcome. *Epilepsia* 27:286–293.

Lindsay J, Glass G, Richards P *et al* (1984) Developmental aspects of focal epilepsies of childhood treated by neurosurgery. *Developmental Medicine and Child Neurology* 26:574–587.

Livingston KE, Escobar A (1971) Anatomical bias of the limbic system concept. A proposed reorientation. *Archives of Neurology* 24:17–21.

Loring DW, Meador KJ, King DW *et al* (1988) Relationship of limbic evoked potentials to recent memory performance. *Neurology* 38:45–48.

Lothman EW (1991) Functional anatomy: a challenge for the decade of the brain. *Epilepsia* 32(Suppl 5):S3–S13.

McCarthy G, Nobre AC, Bentin S *et al* (1995) Language-related field potentials in the anterior-medial temporal lobe. *Journal of Neuroscience* **15**:1080–1089.

McLardy T (1962) Zinc enzymes and the hippocampal mossy fibre system. *Nature* **194**:300–302.

MacLean PD (1952) Some psychiatric implications of physiological studies on fronto-temporal portion of limbic system (visceral brain). *Electroencephalography and Clinical Neurophysiology* **4**:407–418.

McMillan TM, Powell GE, Janota I *et al* (1987) Relationships between neuropathology and cognitive functioning in temporal lobectomy patients. *Journal of Neurology, Neurosurgery and Psychiatry* **50**:167–176.

Magnus O, Ponsen L, Van Rijn AJ (1954) Temporal lobe epilepsy. *Folia Psychiatrica Neurologica et Neurochirugica Neerlandica* **59**:264–297.

Malkova L, Mishkin M, Bachevalier J (1995) Long-term effects of selective neonatal temporal lobe lesions on learning and memory in monkeys. *Behavioral Neuroscience* **109**:212–226.

Margerison JH, Corsellis JAN (1966) Epilepsy and the temporal lobes: a clinical electroencephalograophic and neuropathological study of the brain in epilepsy, with particular reference to the temporal lobes. *Brain* **89**:499–530.

Mark VH, Irvine FR (1970) *Violence and the Brain*. New York: Harper and Row.

Mathern GW, Pretorius JK, Babb TL (1995a) Influence of the type of initial precipitating injury and at what age it occurs on course and outcome in patients with temporal lobe seizures. *Journal of Neurosurgery* **82**:220–227.

Mathern GW, Babb TL, Vickrey BG *et al* (1995b) The clinical–pathogenic mechanisms of hippocampal neuron loss and surgical outcomes in temporal lobe epilepsy. *Brain* **118**:105–118.

Mathieson G (1975) Pathology of temporal lobe foci. *Advances in Neurology* **11**:163–185.

Matthews PM, Andermann F, Arnold DL (1990) A proton magnetic resonance spectroscopy study of focal epilepsy in humans. *Neurology* **40**:985–989.

Mayberg HS, Sadzot B, Meltzer CC *et al* (1991) Quantification of mu and non-mu opiate receptors in temporal lobe epilepsy using positron emission tomography. *Annals of Neurology* **30**:3–11.

Meencke HJ, Veith G (1991) Hippocampal sclerosis in epilepsy. In: Lüders H (ed) *Epilepsy Surgery*, pp 705–715. New York: Raven Press.

Meyer FB, Marsh RW, Laws ER *et al* (1986) Temporal lobectomy in children with epilepsy. *Journal of Neurosurgery* **64**:371–376.

Middleton FA, Strick PL (1996) The temporal lobe is a target of output from the basal ganglia. *Proceedings of the National Academy of Sciences of the USA* **93**:8683–8687.

Milner B (1975) Psychological aspects of focal epilepsy and its neurosurgical management. *Advances in Neurology* **8**:299–321.

Mishkin M (1993) Cerebral memory circuits. In: Poggio TA, Glaser DA (eds) *Exploring Brain Function: Models in Neuroscience*, pp 112–125. Chichester: Wiley.

Mody I, Heinemann U (1987) NMDA receptors of dentate gyrus granule cells participate in synaptic transmission following kindling. *Nature* **326**:701–704.

Munari C (1995) Methodologies, results and limits of epilepsy surgery in children. *Gaslini* **27**(Suppl I al N 2):48–53.

Nauta WJH (1958) Hippocampal projections and related neural pathways to the midbrain in the cat. *Brain* **81**:329–341.

Nelson DA, Ray CD (1968) Respiratory arrest from seizure discharges in limbic system. *Archives of Neurology* **19**:199–207.

Newton MR, Berkovic SF, Austin MC *et al* (1992) Dystonia, clinical lateralization, and regional blood flow changes in temporal lobe seizures. *Neurology* **42**:371–377.

Nobre CC, McCarthy G (1995) Language-related field potentials in the anterior-medial temporal lobe: effects of word-type and semantic priming. *Journal of Neuroscience* **15**:1090–1098.

Nobre CC, Allison T, McCarthy G (1994) Word recognition in the human inferior temporal lobe. *Nature* **372**:260–263.

Offen M, Davidoff R, Troost R *et al* (1976) Dacrystic epilepsy. *Journal of Neurology, Neurosurgery and Psychiatry* **34**:829–834.

Ojemann GA, Dodrill CB (1985) Verbal memory deficits after left temporal lobectomy for epilepsy. *Journal of Neurosurgery* **62**:101–107.

Ounsted C, Lindsay J, Norman R (1966) *Biological Factors in Temporal Lobe Epilepsy*, pp 14–49. London: William Heinemann.

Paillas J-E (1958) Aspects cliniques de l'épilepsie temporale. In: Baldwin M, Bailey P (eds) *Temporal Lobe Epilepsy*, pp 411–439. Springfield, IL: CC Thomas.

Paillas J-E, Subirana A (1950) Le lobe temporale en oto-neuro-ophtalmologie. *Revue d'Oto-Neuro-Ophthalmologie* **22**:123–218.

Paillas J-E, Gastaut H, Tamalet J (1949) Les fausses absences d'origine temporale. *Revue Neurologique* **81**:285–287.

Paller KA, Kutas M, Mcisaac HK (1995) Monitoring conscious recollection via the electrical activity of the brain. *Psychological Science* **6**:107–111.

Papez JW (1937) A proposed mechanism of emotion. *Archives of Neurology and Psychiatry* **38**: 725–743.

Papez JW (1958) Visceral brain, its component parts and their connections. *Journal of Nervous and Mental Disease* **126**:40–56.

Penfield W (1952) Memory mechanisms. *Archives of Neurology and Psychiatry* **67**:178–189.

Penfield W (1954) Temporal lobe epilepsy (Hunterian Lecture). *British Journal of Surgery* **41**:337–343.

Penfield W (1959) The interpretive cortex. *Science* **129**:1719–1725.

Penfield W, Erickson T (1941) *Epilepsy and Cerebral Localisation*. Springfield, IL: CC Thomas.

Penfield W, Jasper H (1954) *Epilepsy and the Functional Anatomy of the Human Brain*. Boston: Little, Brown.

Penfield W, Kristiansen K (1951) *Epileptic Seizure Patterns*. Springfield, IL: CC Thomas.

Penfield W, Rasmussen T (1957) *The Cerebral Cortex of Man. A Clinical Study of Localisation of Function*. New York: MacMillan.

Peterson C, Neal JH, Cotman CW (1989) Development of N-methyl-D-aspartate excitotoxicity in cultured hippocampal neurons. *Developmental Brain Research* **48**:187–195.

Plate KH, Wieser HG, Yasargil MG *et al* (1993) Neuropathological findings in 224 patients with temporal lobe epilepsy. *Acta Neuropathologica* **86**:433–438.

Powell EW, Hines G (1975) Septohippocampal interface. In: Isaacson RL, Pribram KH (eds) *The Hippocampus. I: Structure and Development*, pp 41–59. New York: Plenum Press.

Pritchard PB, Wannamaker BB, Sagal J (1983) Endocrine function following complex partial seizures. *Annals of Neurology* **14**:27–32.

Ramon y Cajal S (1909–11) *Histologie du Système Nerveux de l'Homme et des Vertébrés*, Vols I and II. Paris: Maloine.

Rausch R, Crandall PH (1982) Psychological status related to surgical control of temporal lobe seizures. *Epilepsia* **23**:191–192.

Robb P (1965) *Epilepsy: A Review of Basic and Clinical Research*. NINDB Monograph No. 1. US Department of Health, Education, and Welfare, Public Health Service Publication No. 1357.

Rosene DL, Van Hoesen GW (1987) The hippocampal formation of the primate brain. A review of some comparative aspects of cytoarchitecture and connections. In: Jones EG, Peters A (eds) *Cerebral Cortex, Vol 6. Further Aspects of Cortical Function, Including Hippocampus*, pp 345–456. New York: Plenum Press.

Sagar HJ, Oxbury JM (1987) Hippocampal neuronal loss in temporal lobe epilepsy: correlation with early childhood convulsions. *Annals of Neurology* **22**:334–340.

Savic I, Perssen A, Roland P *et al* (1988) In-vivo demonstration of reduced bezodiazepine receptor binding in human epileptic foci. *Lancet* **12**:863–866.

Schaffer K (1892) Beitrag zur Histologie der Ammonshornformation. *Archiv für Mikroskopische Anatomie* **39**:611–632.

Schneider RC, Crosby EC, Calhoun HD (1969) Surgery of convulsive seizures and allied disorders. In: Kahn EA, Crosby EC, Schneider RC, Taren JA (eds) *Correlative Neurosurgery*, pp 279–358. Springfield, IL: CC Thomas.

Siegel AM (1990) *Nachuntersuchungen bei Patienten mit selektiver Amygdala-Hippokampektomie*. Thesis, University of Zurich.

Slater E, Beard AW (1963) The schizophrenia-like psychoses of epilepsy. *British Journal of Psychiatry* **109**:95–150.

Slater E, Beard AW, Glithero E (1965) Schizophrenia-like psychosis of epilepsy. *International Journal of Psychiatry* **1**:6–8.

Smith ME, Stapelton JM, Halgen E (1986) Human medial temporal lobe potentials evoked in memory and language tasks. *Electroencephalography and Clinical Neurophysiology* **63**:145–159.

Smith OA, DeVito JL (1984) Central neural integration for the control of autonomic responses associated with emotion. *Annual Review of Neuroscience* **7**:43–65.

Sommer W (1880) Erkrankung des Ammonshorns als aetiologisches Moment der Epilepsie. *Archiv für Psychiatrie und Nervenkrankheiten* **10**:631–675.

Spencer SS, Guimaraes P, Katz A *et al* (1992a) Morphological patterns of seizures recorded intracranially. *Epilepsia* **33**:537–545.

Spencer SS, Kim J, Spencer DD (1992b) Ictal spikes: a marker of specific hippocampal cell loss. *Electroencephalography and Clinical Neurophysiology* **83**:104–111.

Spencer SS, Marks D, Katz A *et al* (1992c) Anatomical correlates of intrahippocampal seizure propagation time. *Epilepsia* **33**:862–873.

Spielmeyer RW (1927) Die Pathogenese des epileptischen Krampfes. *Zeitschrift für die gesamte Neurologie und Psychiatrie* **109**:501–520.

Squire LR (1986) Mechanisms of memory. *Science* **232**:1612–1619.

Squire LR, Butters N (1984) *Neuropsychology of Memory*. New York: Guilford.

Squire LR, Zola-Morgan SM (1991) The medial temporal lobe memory system. *Science* **253**:1380–1386.

Stapelton JM, Halgren E (1987) Endogenous potentials evoked in simple cognitive tasks: depth components and task correlates. *Electroencephalography and Clinical Neurophysiology* **67**:44–52.

Steward D, Torre E, Tomasulo R *et al* (1991) Neuronal activity upregulates astroglial gene expression. *Proceedings of the National Academy of Sciences of the USA* **88**:6819–6823.

Stodieck SRG, Wieser HG (1986) Autonomic phenomena in temporal lobe epilepsy. *Journal of the Autonomic Nervous System* (Suppl): 611–621.

Stoffels C, Munari C, Bonis A *et al* (1981) Manifestations genitales et 'sexuelles' lors des crises epileptiques partielles chez l'homme. *Revue d'electroencephalographie et de neurophysiologie clinique* **10**:386–392.

Stringer JL, Lothman EW (1990) Use of maximal dentate activation to study the effect of drugs and kindled responses. *Epilepsy Research* **6**:180–186.

Sutula T, He X, Cavazos J *et al* (1988) Synaptic reorganisation in the hippocampus induced by abnormal functional activity. *Science* **239**:1147–1150.

Sutula T, Cascino G, Cavazos J *et al* (1989) Mossy fiber reorganisation in the epileptic human temporal lobe. *Annals of Neurology* **26**:321–330.

Talairach J, David M, Tournoux P (1958) *L'exploration Chirurgicale Stéréotaxique du Lobe Temporale dans l'Épilepsie Temporale. Repérage Anatomique Stéréotaxique et Technique Chirurgicale*. Paris: Masson.

Tauck DL, Nadler JV (1985) Evidence of functional mossy fiber sprouting in hippocampal formation of kainic acid-treated rats. *Journal of Neuroscience* **5**:1016–1022.

Townsend JB, Engel J Jr (1991) Clinicopathological correlations of low voltage fast and high amplitude spike and wave mesial temporal SEEG ictal onsets. *Epilepsia* **32**:21.

Trenerry MR, Jack CR, Sharbrough FW *et al* (1993) Quantitative MRI hippocampal volumes: association with onset and duration of epilepsy, and febrile convulsions in temporal lobectomy patients. *Epilepsy Research* **15**:247–252.

Trimble MR, Bolwig TG (eds) (1992) *The Temporal Lobes and the Limbic System*. Petersfield: Wrightson Biomed.

Van Hoesen GW, Pandya DN (1975) Some connections of the entorhinal (area 28) and perirhinal (area 35) cortices of the rhesus monkey. I. Temporal lobe afferents. *Brain Research* **95**:1–24.

Verdi JM, Birren SJ, Ibanez CF *et al* (1994) P75LNGFR regulates Trk signal transduction and NGF-induced neuronal differentiation in MAH cells. *Neuron* **12**:733–745.

Vogt O (1925) Der Begriff der Pathoclise. *Journal für Psychologie und Neurologie* **31**:245–255.

Vogt C, Vogt O (1937) *Sitz und Wesen der Krankheiten im Lichte der topistischen Hirnforschung und des Variierens der Tiere*, Erster Teil. Leipzig: Barth.

Wada JA (1949) A new method for determination of the side of cerebral speech dominance: a preliminary report on the intracarotid injection of sodium amytal in man. *Igaku Seibutsugaku (Medicine and Biology)* **4**:221–222.

Walsh GO, Delgado-Escueta AV (1984) Type II complex partial seizures: poor results of anterior temporal lobectomy. *Neurology* **34**:1–13.

Waxman SG, Geschwind N (1974) Hypergraphia in temporal lobe epilepsy. *Neurology* **24**:629–638.

Waxman SG, Geschwind N (1975) The interictal behavioural syndrome of temporal lobe epilepsy. *Archives of General Psychiatry* **32**:1580–1586.

Wieser HG (1980) Temporal lobe or psychomotor status epilepticus. A case report. *Electroencephalography and Clinical Neurophysiology* **48**:558–572.

Wieser HG (1983a) *Electroclinical Features of the Psychomotor Seizure. A Stereoelectroencephalographic Study of Ictal Symptoms and Chronotopographical Seizure Patterns Including Clinical Effects of Intracerebral Stimulation*. Stuttgart, New York, London: Fischer, Butterworth.

Wieser HG (1983b) Depth recorded limbic seizures and psychopathology. *Neuroscience and Biobehavioral Reviews* **7**:427–440.

Wieser HG (1986a) Psychomotor seizures of hippocampal–amygdalar origin. In: Pedley TA, Meldrum BS (eds) *Recent Advances in Epilepsy*, Vol 3, pp 57–79. Edinburgh: Churchill Livingstone.

Wieser HG (1986b) Selective amygdalohippocampectomy: indications, investigative technique and results. In: Symon L, Brihaye J, Guidetti B *et al* (eds) *Advances and Technical Standards in Neurosurgery*, Vol 13, pp 39–133. Vienna: Springer.

Wieser HG (1987) The phenomenology of limbic seizures. In: Wieser HG, Speckmann EJ, Engel J Jr (eds) *The Epileptic Focus*, pp 113–136. London: John Libbey.

Wieser HG (1988a) Human limbic seizures: EEG studies, origin, and patterns of spread. In: Meldrum BS, Ferendelli JA, Wieser HG (eds) *Anatomy of Epileptogenesis*, pp 127–138. London: John Libbey.

Wieser HG (1988b) Presurgical evaluation and surgical therapy of children suffering from drug-resistant partial epilepsies. *Electroencephalography and Clinical Neurophysiology* **70**:16.

Wieser HG (1991a) Ictal manifestations of temporal lobe seizures. *Advances in Neurology* **55**:301–315.

Wieser HG (1991b) Selective amygdalohippocampectomy: indications and follow-up. *Canadian Journal of Neurological Sciences* **18**:617–627.

Wieser HG (1992) Behavioural consequences of temporal lobe resections. In: Trimble MR, Bolwig TG (eds) *The Temporal Lobes and the Limbic System*, pp 169–188. Petersfield: Wrightson Biomed.

Wieser HG (1994) PET and SPECT in epilepsy. *European Neurology* **34** (Suppl 1):58–62.

Wieser HG, Morris HH (1997) Foramen ovale and peg electrodes. In:

Engel J Jr, Pedley TA (eds) *Epilepsy: A Comprehensive Textbook*, pp 1707–1717. New York: Raven Press.

Wieser HG, Moser S (1988) Improved multipolar foramen ovale electrode monitoring. *Journal of Epilepsy* **1**:13–22.

Wieser HG, Müller RU (1987) Neocortical temporal seizures. In: Wieser HG, Elger CE (eds) *Presurgical Evaluation of Epileptics*, pp 252–266. Berlin: Springer.

Wieser HG, Siegel AM (1991) Analysis of foramen ovale electrode-recorded seizures and correlation with outcome following amygdalo-hippocampectomy. *Epilepsia* **32**:838–850.

Wieser HG, Williamson PD (1993) Ictal semiology. In: Engel J Jr (ed) *Surgical Treatment of the Epilepsies*, 2nd edn, pp 161–171. New York: Raven Press.

Wieser HG, Yasargil MG (1982) Selective amygdalohippocampectomy as a surgical treatment of mesiobasal limbic epilepsy. *Surgical Neurology* **17**:445–457.

Wieser HG, Hailemariam S, Regard M *et al* (1985) Unilateral limbic epileptic status activity: stereo-EEG, behavioural, and cognitive data. *Epilepsia* **26**:19–29.

Wieser HG, Valavanis A, Roos A *et al* (1989a) 'Selective' and 'superselective' temporal lobe Amytal tests. I. Neuroradiological, neuroanatomical, and electrical data. In: Manelis J, Bental E, Loeber J *et al* (eds) *Advances in Epileptology*, Vol 17, pp 20–27. New York: Raven Press.

Wieser HG, Landis T, Regard M *et al* (1989b) 'Selective' and 'superselective' temporal lobe Amytal tests. II. Neuropsychological test procedure and results. In: Manelis J, Bental E, Loeber J *et al* (eds) *Advances in Epileptology*, Vol 17, pp 28–33. New York: Raven Press.

Wieser HG, Engel J Jr, Williamson PD *et al* (1993) Surgically remediable temporal lobe syndromes. In: Engel J Jr (ed) *Surgical Treatment of the Epilepsies*, 2nd edn, pp 49–63. New York: Raven Press.

Wieser HG, Duc C, Meier D *et al* (1996) Clinical experience with magnetic resonance spectroscopy in epilepsy. In: Pawlik G, Stefan H (eds) *Focus Localization: Multimethodological Assessment of Localization-related Epilepsy*, pp 66–78. Berlin: German Section of ILAE.

Wieser HG, Müller S, Schiess R *et al* (1997) The anterior and posterior selective temporal lobe amobarbital tests: angiographical, clinical, electroencephalographical, PET and SPECT findings, and memory performance. *Brain and Cognition* **33**:71–97.

Williams D (1969) Temporal lobe syndromes. In: Vinken PJ, Bruyn GW (eds) *Handbook of Clinical Neurology, Vol 2. Localization in Clinical Neurology, pp* 700–724. Amsterdam: North Holland.

Winslow JB (1732) *Exposition Anatomique de la Structure du Corps Humain*. Paris.

Wolf HK, Campos MG, Zentner J *et al* (1993) Surgical pathology of temporal lobe epilepsy. Experience with 216 cases. *Journal of Neuropathology and Experimental Neurology* **52**:499–506.

Yakovlev PI (1948) Motility, behavior and the brain. Stereodynamic organization and neural coordinates of behavior. *Journal of Nervous and Mental Disease* **107**:313–335.

Yasargil MG, Teddy PJ, Roth P (1985) Selective amygdalohippocampectomy: operative anatomy and surgical technique. In: Simon L, Brihaye J, Guidetti B *et al* (eds) *Advances and Technical Standards in Neurosurgery*, Vol 12, pp 92–123. Vienna: Springer.

Yasargil MG, Wieser HG, Valavanis A *et al* (1993) Surgery and results of selective amygdala-hippocampectomy in one hundred patients with nonlesional limbic epilepsy. *Neurosurgical Clinics of North America* **4**:1–19.

Yeh GC, Bonhaus DW, Nadler JV *et al* (1989) N-Methyl-D-aspartate receptor plasticity in kindling: quantitative and qualitative alterations in the N-methyl-D-aspartate receptor-channel complex. *Proceedings of the National Academy of Sciences of the USA* **86**:8157–8160.

Yonekawa Y, Leblebicioglou-Könü D, Strommer K *et al* (1996) Selective amygdalohippocampectomy according to Yasargil–Wieser for intractable epilepsy. *Neurosurgeon* **15**:184–191.

Zimmerman HM (1940) The histopathology of convulsive disorders in children. *Journal of Pediatrics* **13**:859–890.

Cerebral vascular disorders in adults

R AL-SHAHI AND P ROTHWELL

It is not very uncommon to find when a patient has recovered or is recovering from hemiplegia, the result of an embolism of the middle cerebral artery, or some branch of this vessel, that he is attacked by convulsion beginning in some part of the paralysed region.

Hughlings Jackson, 1931

John Hughlings Jackson recognized the relationship between cerebrovascular disease (CVD) and seizures in 1864 when he described focal seizures complicating an embolic stroke. Stroke is now the third most common cause of death worldwide and a major cause of lasting physical and psychosocial disability in adults. CVD is a common cause of focal epilepsy in adults, especially in those aged >65 years (Hauser *et al* 1993; Forsgren *et al* 1996). The association between stroke and epilepsy can be viewed from two different perspectives: first, the proportion of late onset, apparently unprovoked, epilepsy in the general adult population that is attributable to CVD; second, the proportion of adults with CVD who go on to develop epilepsy. Studies addressing the first perspective are affected by the methods of detecting the underlying cause, which have

often been poor so that most seizures have been considered to be of unknown etiology, and by the difficulty that arises from assuming that any CVD detected is responsible for the epilepsy. Studies addressing the second perspective are very dependent on design and the length of follow-up, making different studies difficult to compare.

There are relatively few discriminating clinical features of CVD as an underlying cause of epilepsy. Intractable focal epilepsy due to CVD can manifest as any of the localization-related epilepsies, including more unusual types such as musical hallucinations (Couper, 1994), crying seizures (Wang *et al* 1995), and reiterative neologistic speech automatisms (Bell *et al* 1990). Moreover, there are a number of diagnostic pitfalls. For example, cerebral ischemia can cause clonus, limb spasms and shaking (Baquis *et al* 1985;

Ropper, 1988), and repetitive involuntary movements (Yanagihara *et al* 1985). Conversely, seizures, especially those arising from the supplementary motor area causing ictal hemiparesis (Globus *et al* 1982) and speech arrest (Peled *et al* 1984), may mimic transient ischemic attacks (TIA) and strokes (Norris and Hachinski 1982). Moreover, recurrent focal seizures due to underlying CVD can mimic the extension of a stroke. The nature of the association between CVD and epilepsy can be further confused by other coincident causes of seizures following a stroke (Warlow *et al* 1996). Intercurrent CVD can modify the course of epilepsies (Marosi *et al* 1994) to or from an intractable focal type, which may partly explain changing seizure semeiology with age (Tinuper *et al* 1996). Prolonged focal seizures following a stroke may cause a *permanent* exacerbation of a preexisting neurologic deficit as opposed to a transient Todd paresis. This latter may itself be a cerebrovascular phenomenon (Yarnell 1975), possibly due to a direct toxic effect on infarcted brain of excessive excitatory amino acid release (Bogousslavsky *et al* 1992; Hankey 1993).

The quality of the evidence leading to conclusions about CVD and epilepsy must be considered. Prospective, population-based studies with clear inception cohorts are ideal for the assessment of clinical course. Small, retrospective, hospital-based case series are the most subject to bias. Study designs frequently differ with respect to case-mix, duration of follow-up, and the accurate description of seizure semeiology. Hospital-based studies have been subject to many types of selection bias. Patients with severe CVD complicated by epilepsy are more likely to be admitted to hospital, with attendant overestimation of the risk of epilepsy and morbidity attributable to it (Hauser *et al* 1984; Bamford *et al* 1986). Adults with CVD are distributed among a range of specialists and often epilepsy is not recorded as a separate diagnosis. As a result, the external validity of some studies is poor. Internal validity has frequently been affected by lack of specification of diagnostic criteria with respect to the time of seizure onset. Varying proportions of patients have had adequate neuroradiologic investigation, and there has been poor exclusion of other causes of seizures in the setting of CVD, thereby introducing confounding bias.

Focal seizures will be referred to here according to the localization-related categories of the International League Against Epilepsy (ILAE) classification of epilepsies and epileptic syndromes (Commission on Classification and Terminology of the ILAE 1989). Seizures will be referred to as *unprovoked seizures* when there is no obvious precipitant, as *onset seizures* when occurring within 24 hours of a stroke, and as *poststroke seizures* when occurring thereafter. *Early seizures* occur within 2 weeks of the stroke (Annegers

et al 1980) and *poststroke epilepsy* consists of recurrent late seizures or intractable focal epilepsy.

UNPROVOKED SEIZURES ATTRIBUTABLE TO CEREBROVASCULAR DISEASE

A community-based study of people with newly diagnosed epilepsy and apparently unprovoked seizures in Rochester, Minnesota, USA, from 1935 to 1984 found 57% of incident cases to have focal epilepsy alone (Hauser *et al* 1993). The etiology was obscure in two-thirds of them. Most cases of focal epilepsy in those over the age of 35 years with an identifiable antecedent were attributable to CVD, the proportion increasing with age. The authors comment that this finding is at odds with the observed decline in the incidence of stroke in the same community (Broderick *et al* 1989). The increased detection of small, asymptomatic strokes owing to developments in computed tomography (CT) at that time may explain the results (Roberts *et al* 1988).

CVD was the most common identifiable cause of focal seizures in The National General Practice Study of Epilepsy (NGPSE), a prospective study of a population-based cohort of 594 patients with newly diagnosed epileptic seizures (Fig. 12.1) (Manford *et al* 1992). The localization was predominantly extratemporal with rolandic seizures predominating. Frequent focal seizures (defined as > 12 per year) were seen in only 6.9% and only a minority of these cases were accounted for by CVD (Fig 12.2). However, of the 27 patients who died during 3–7 years of follow-up, only cerebral tumors were equal to CVD as an identifiable cause of the seizure disorder.

CVD has been the most common identifiable underlying cause of epilepsy in adults in many of the community-based studies (Hauser *et al* 1991, 1993; Forsgren 1992; Manford *et al* 1992; Cockerell *et al* 1995). Nevertheless, the use of magnetic resonance imaging (MRI) for the investigation of late-onset focal epilepsy (Brooks *et al* 1990; Kilpatrick *et al* 1991; Bergin *et al* 1995) has shown that the frequency of CVD, both symptomatic and asymptomatic, as a cause of chronic focal epilepsy was previously underestimated. In a more recent large, prospective, Swedish population-based study, 68% of apparently unprovoked seizures in adults were partial and stroke was the most common presumed etiology, being detectable in 45% of individuals aged >60 years (Forsgren *et al* 1996).

Seizures attributed to asymptomatic cerebral infarction may precede the development of a stroke. This is a concept

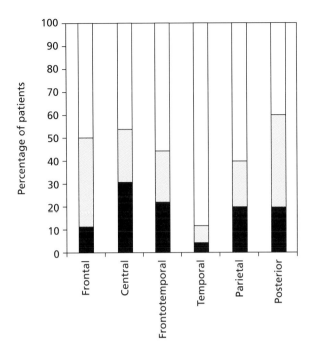

Fig. 12.1 Identifiable causes of localizable focal epilepsies from the National General Practice Study of Epilepsy (NGPSE):cerebro vascular disease (dark shading), unknown (white) and other causes (light shading) are represented as percentages for each type of focal seizure pattern. (Data provided with permission by the authors of the NGPSE.)

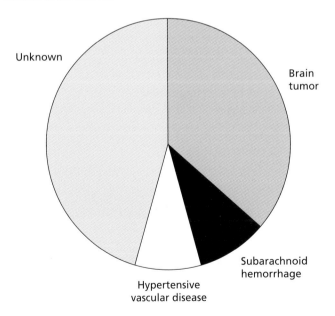

Fig. 12.2 Causes of frequent focal seizures from the NGPSE.

known as *vascular precursor epilepsy* (Barolin *et al* 1971). It appears to be supported by a finding of the Oxfordshire Community Stroke Project that 4 of 7 patients with a first seizure in the year before their stroke had focal motor seizures in the same limb that was subsequently affected by the stroke (Burn *et al* 1997). Furthermore, a relationship has been demonstrated between other cardiovascular risk

factors and late-onset epilepsy (Hesdorffer *et al* 1996), beyond that which is attributable to silent cerebral infarction or stroke (Li *et al* 1997).

CVD may cause focal status epilepticus. A retrospective Dutch study (Scholtes *et al* 1996a) reported 47 cases of simple partial status epilepticus (SPSE), all aged >15 years. Stroke was the 'most prominent' cause in 70% of the 20 patients without previous epilepsy. A second part of the Dutch study covered complex partial status epilepticus (CPSE) (Scholtes *et al* 1996b); CVD was again a prominent cause. A variety of cerebrovascular diseases (cerebral atherosclerosis, systemic lupus erythematosus, cerebral angiitis, cortical vein thrombosis, arteriovenous malformation) accounted for 14% of cases of epilepsia partialis continua (EPC) in a UK study (Cockerell *et al* 1996). Other small studies also describe CVD as a cause of SPSE, CPSE and EPC (Schomer 1993; Krumholz *et al* 1995).

STROKE AS A CAUSE OF FOCAL EPILEPSY

Stroke is 'a clinical syndrome characterized by rapidly developing clinical symptoms and/or signs of focal, and at times global, loss of cerebral function with symptoms lasting more than 24 hours or leading to death with no apparent cause other than that of vascular origin' (Warlow *et al* 1996; WHO Task Force on Stroke and Other Cerebrovascular Disorders 1989). This definition encompasses cerebral infarction, primary intracerebral hemorrhage (PICH), intraventricular hemorrhage, and most cases of subarachnoid hemorrhage (SAH). One of the main studies to examine the occurrence of epileptic seizures *after* stroke has been the Oxfordshire Community Stroke Project (OCSP); in this community-based cohort study, 675 patients with a first-ever stroke were followed for between 2 and 6.5 years (Burn *et al* 1997).

EARLY SEIZURES AFTER STROKE

In the OCSP, a victim of stroke had a relative risk of seizures in comparison to the general population of 35.2 in the first year after stroke and 19.0 in the second year. Two percent of stroke patients had an *onset seizure*; half of these were focal, as in other studies (Gupta *et al* 1988; Giroud *et al* 1994; Norris *et al* 1994). Patients with intracranial hemorrhage were more likely to have an onset seizure than were those with cerebral infarction (Burn *et al* 1997). The Copenhagen Stroke Study (CSS), in a multivariate analysis (Reith *et al* 1997), found that only initial stroke severity correlated with the development of *early seizures*. The authors suggested that the higher frequency of seizures among patients with a primary intracerebral hemorrhage merely indicated their higher initial stroke severity. From hospital-based series, independent predictors of early seizures in first-ever stroke patients are thought to be radiographic evidence of cortical involvement (Lancman *et al* 1993; Arboix *et al* 1997), large (i.e. multilobar) lesions (Lancman *et al* 1993), and hemorrhage (Lancman *et al* 1993). The OCSP and CSS found that patients with onset seizures have an increased risk of further seizures, as did many other series (Hauser *et al* 1984; Gupta *et al* 1988; Sung and Chu, 1989; Kilpatrick *et al* 1992; Heuts-Van Raak *et al* 1993). In contrast to other studies (Arboix *et al* 1996, 1997), they did not find that early seizures had an adverse effect on outcome (Burn *et al* 1997; Reith *et al* 1997).

CHRONIC EPILEPSY AFTER STROKE

The OCSP and other studies (Viitanen *et al* 1988; So *et al* 1996) have found an excess risk in the first year after stroke and a gradual reduction in relative risk thereafter. In the OCSP, 4% of patients who survived the first day had recurrent *poststroke seizures*, and in this group partial seizures occurring alone were less common than at the onset of the stroke. A 5% risk of developing recurrent seizures by 5 years after a stroke has been demonstrated by actuarial analyses (Burn *et al* 1997; Viitanen *et al* 1988). The risk of late seizures is higher after primary intracerebral hemorrhage than after cerebral infarction, although total anterior circulation infarction (TACI) carries a disproportionately high risk (Burn *et al* 1997).

INTRACRANIAL HEMORRHAGE

The best available evidence indicates that of adult cerebrovascular causes of epilepsy, primary intracerebral hemorrhage carries the greatest risk (Burn *et al* 1997). A follow-up study of 222 consecutive patients with CT-documented supratentorial, atraumatic parenchymal brain hemorrhages of heterogeneous etiology, without the use of prophylactic anticonvulsants, found that 3% of patients developed late seizures in 12 months of follow-up, especially when affected by an underlying neoplasm or vascular malformation (Weisberg *et al* 1991). There are few other data on seizure frequency prior to surgery as studies of epilepsy following many types of treatable intracranial hemorrhage are mainly postoperative (Bidzinski *et al* 1992; O'Laoire 1990; Ukkola and Heikkinen 1990).

Primary intracerebral hemorrhage (PICH)

In hospital-based, retrospective case series of patients with PICH followed by epilepsy from Taiwan (Sung and Chu, 1989), Italy (Cervoni *et al* 1994), and the USA (Berger *et al* 1988), most seizures occurred at initial clinical presentation. In the largest of these studies with the longest period of follow-up (Sung and Chu 1989), focal seizures were the commonest type, accounting for 67% of all seizures. Intractable epilepsy developed in 29% of the 38 patients with early seizures, but in 93% of the 26 patients who developed seizures late after the initial hemorrhage. In a retrospective, hospital-based series, a high incidence of early seizures did not predict and infrequently preceded chronic epilepsy, although the prevalence of epilepsy in PICH survivors was much higher than in an age-matched population (Faught *et al* 1989). Epilepsy is more common with lobar than with thalamic or basal ganglia hemorrhages (Berger *et al* 1988; Faught *et al* 1989; Sung and Chu 1989; Weisberg *et al* 1991). This is because lobar bleeds frequently involve the cortex and patients tend to survive longer. Mortality in patients who develop seizures is determined by the deep-seated location of a PICH rather than by the type of seizure (Sung and Chu 1989). Improved CT and MRI have helped recognize the contribution of small lobar hemorrhages as the cause of focal seizures in such cases. Nonetheless, follow-up in all these studies has been too short to allow assessment of the real burden of intractable focal epilepsy.

Subarachnoid hemorrhage (SAH)

Patients with SAH in the OCSP (Burn *et al* 1997) had an excess of onset seizures. Other studies (Hart *et al* 1981; Hasan *et al* 1993) have shown that seizures occur in ~10% of patients in the first 2 weeks after aneurysm rupture, but that one-third of patients did not experience their first seizure until at least 6 months later. Intractable epilepsy may be influenced by initial events such as craniotomy and the volume of cisternal blood (Hasan *et al* 1993), postoperative bleeding, late cerebral infarction, and hypertension (Ohman 1990). Predictive factors for epilepsy have not been identified and focal seizures are often not explicitly described. Intractable focal seizures have been reported in association with unruptured giant cerebral aneurysms of the middle cerebral artery (Kamrin 1966; Whittle *et al* 1985), presumably owing to compression of adjacent temporal lobe structures.

Subdural hematoma (SDH)

There has been considerable variation in the rates of seizures before and after surgery for chronic SDH reported from hospital-based series in which use of prophylactic anti-convulsants has varied (Kotwica and Brzeinski 1991; Ohno *et al* 1993; Rubin and Rappaport 1993; Sabo *et al* 1995). This has led to disagreement about the use of prophylactic anticonvulsants, with some authors arguing for (Sabo *et al* 1995) and others against (Ohno *et al* 1993; Rubin and Rappaport 1993). There appears to be general agreement that the preoperative frequency of seizures is 4–5% (Rubin and Rappaport 1993) with various types of focal seizure reported (Hilt and Alexander 1982; Ohno *et al* 1993).

CEREBRAL INFARCTION

The best evidence on seizure disorders after cerebral infarction comes from the OCSP and from a population-based study from Rochester, Minnesota, USA (So *et al* 1996) that had longer follow-up but inception prior to the modern era of neuroimaging. In the Rochester study, 6% of patients had an early seizure within a week of cerebral infarction, for which the only predictor was total anterior circulation infarction (TACI) as in the OCSP (Burn *et al* 1997). In both studies, 3% of all patients were affected by intractable epilepsy. In the Rochester study, the cumulative probability of developing postinfarction seizures was 7.4% by 5 years and 8.9% by 10 years.

There has been uncertainty about the relative contribution of onset seizures to the development of intractable epilepsy. Few of the 2% with cerebral infarction complicated by onset seizures in the OCSP developed postinfarction epilepsy, although having an onset seizure was associated with an increased risk of developing further seizures. However, 3% of all patients with cerebral infarction were affected by intractable epilepsy, implying that a significant proportion of postinfarction epilepsy is not preceded by onset/early seizures. The Mayo Clinic study found that both early seizures and stroke recurrence were independent predictors of intractable epilepsy and that early seizure occurrence predisposed those with late postinfarction seizures to develop intractable epilepsy (So *et al* 1996).

The Mayo Clinic study incorporated no data concerning seizure localization and the OCSP did not describe the pattern of localization among patients with poststroke seizures. A retrospective evaluation of 100 patients who suffered epileptic seizures following hemispheric cerebral infarction showed that 54% were localization-related and predominantly focal motor (Hornig *et al* 1990). In a series of 118 patients from Taiwan (Sung and Chu 1990), simple focal seizures occurred in 56% of patients and complex focal seizures in 24%.

The mechanism of poststroke epilepsy is not clearly understood. Its preponderance among TACI, however,

may reflect cortical damage (Kilpatrick *et al* 1990; Ryglewicz *et al* 1990; Matsumura *et al* 1993), often to the frontal and temporal cortices, which are known to be the most epileptogenic areas of the brain (French *et al* 1956). There is debate whether infarct size is related to the risk of seizures (Gupta *et al* 1988). Some authors have argued that the size of the ischemic penumbra, epileptogenic in itself, is related to the risk of seizures (Norris *et al* 1994; Reith *et al* 1997). It is uncertain whether seizures are more common with cardioembolic or atherosclerotic stroke (Kilpatrick *et al* 1990; Giroud *et al* 1994; So *et al* 1996; Kraus and Berlit 1998). Involvement of different areas of cortex may predispose to early-onset or late-onset poststroke seizures. A study of 322 patients with CT-proven cortical infarction (Heuts-van Raak *et al* 1996) found that a large infarct involving the supramarginal or superior temporal gyrus carried a fivefold increased risk of late-onset epilepsy. Some studies have found that patients with lacunar syndromes have postinfarction seizures (Giround *et al* 1994; Schreiner *et al* 1995), whereas others have not (Kilpatrick *et al* 1992; Arboix *et al* 1997). Focal motor seizures following lacunar strokes may be attributable to independent cortical infarction and/or ischemia (Heuts-Van Raak *et al* 1993; Giroud and Dumas 1995). Transient ischemic attacks may not only mimic focal seizures but may also be responsible for them. The association has been very hard to prove (Kaplan 1993) but has been reported in small series (Cocito and Loeb, 1986, 1989; Demiati *et al* 1989). A study of a larger prospective Australian series of 1000 patients with CVD reported focal seizures in 3.7% of patients with hemispheric TIA (Kilpatrick *et al* 1990).

INTRACRANIAL VASCULAR MALFORMATIONS (IVM)

There is only one truly population-based IVM study (Brown *et al* 1996) that provides unique data on detection rates, but there are no published data on the risk of epilepsy. With the increasing use of higher-resolution neuroradiology in the investigation of focal seizure disorders (Bronen *et al* 1995), the implications of finding an underlying vascular malformation need to be understood.

ARTERIOVENOUS MALFORMATIONS (AVM)

Epilepsy is the most frequent nonhemorrhagic manifestation of AVM, but relatively few studies have addressed the risk of epilepsy from AVM spared surgical intervention (Murphy 1985). Perceived wisdom is that an hemispheric supratentorial AVM (Fig. 12.3) can cause epilepsy (Itoyama *et al* 1989) and that most intractable epilepsy is focal with or without secondary generalization (Leblanc *et al* 1983). Although unusual, thrombosed AVM are also important in the differential diagnosis of intractable focal seizure disorders (Wharen *et al* 1982).

A study from the Mayo Clinic of untreated AVM without evidence of hemorrhage prior to diagnosis (Brown *et al* 1988) found seizures to be the predominant initial symptom in 66%. Most other studies report a frequency of 20–30% when patients with hemorrhage are included (Fults and Kelly 1984; Murphy 1985; Crawford *et al* 1986; Itoyama *et al* 1989). The Mayo Clinic study provided no follow-up data on the risk of subsequent epilepsy. Prognosis is generally thought to be better for patients presenting with seizures than with hemorrhage (Fults and Kelly 1984).

Perhaps the best data on the risk of epilepsy come from the study of Crawford *et al* (1986). There were 217 patients with unoperated AVM. They were significantly different from the operated group in various ways, such as having larger, deeper AVM (Fig. 12.4) that were more likely to cross the midline. Sixty-one patients (28%) presented with epilepsy. The epilepsy onset was 9 years (mean) before the diagnosis of AVM was made. The patients were followed up for a mean of 10.4 years. Using life survival analyses, allowing for variable or incomplete follow-up, there was an 11% risk of developing *de novo* epilepsy by 10 years after diagnosis. This was not influenced by the size or the depth of the AVM. Risk factors for developing epilepsy were previous hemorrhage (22% risk at 20 years), female sex, younger age at diagnosis and temporal lobe location (perhaps affected by surgical selection bias).

Recent refinements in operative techniques, endovascular embolization, and stereotactic radiotherapy for AVM

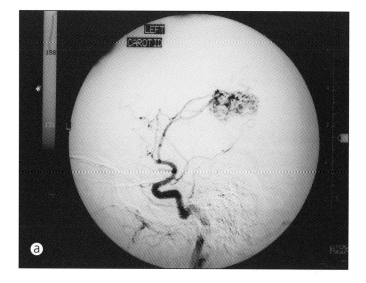

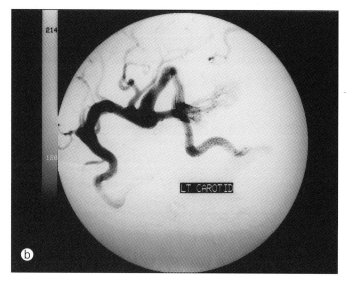

Fig. 12.4 Left carotid angiogram showing a 3 cm AVM lying close to the insula of the left cerebral hemisphere (a) with a large draining vein (b).

Fig. 12.3 MRI of brain showing a left posterior parietal AVM which extended to the cortex, causing intractable focal seizures.

have led to optimism about their aggressive management. However, in the absence of good data on clinical course, and without evidence from randomized controlled clinical trials of the possible interventions, uncertainty will remain about the best management to minimize the frequency of intractable epilepsy.

CAVERNOUS MALFORMATIONS (CM)

Cavernous malformations are not detected by angiography so they have been detected in the noninvasive investigation of epilepsy only since the introduction of MRI (Rigamonti *et al* 1987). CM are multiple in one-fifth of sporadic patients (Fig. 12.5). Familial occurrence has been observed, with a higher frequency of multiple lesions (Rigamonti *et al* 1988a) and the development of new lesions over time (Zabramski *et al* 1994). Most studies have focused on the risks of hemorrhage, which have varied according to radiologic or clinical definition, with annual rates from 0.25% (Del Curling *et al* 1991) to 4.2% (Porter *et al* 1997). The

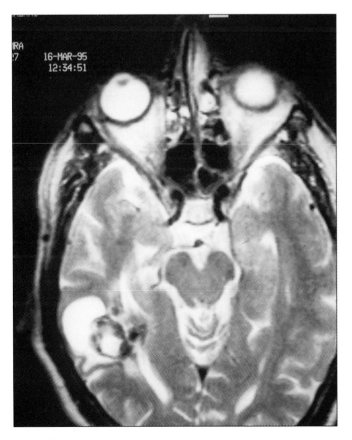

Fig. 12.5 MRI of brain showing a right posterior temporal cavernous malformation with evidence of previous hemorrhage and surrounding cortical atrophy.

occurrence of seizures has not predicted future hemorrhage (Aiba *et al* 1995; Kondziolka *et al* 1995).

Seizures are a presenting symptom of supratentorial CM in 23–36% of patients (Aiba *et al* 1995; Kondziolka *et al* 1995; Porter *et al* 1997). Of 94 seizure-free patients followed prospectively over a mean of 34 months, 4.3% developed new seizures and only one suffered intractable epilepsy (Kondziolka *et al* 1995). Intractable epilepsy occurred in 20% of 84 patients harboring 100 CM. Univariate and multivariate analyses indicated that age <40 years was the only significant factor predisposing to seizure disability (Robinson *et al* 1993).

VENOUS MALFORMATIONS (VM)

As with cavernous malformations, venous malformations have been recognized increasingly since the advent of MRI (Rigamonti *et al* 1988b) but their clinical significance has remained controversial. They are often associated with other vascular malformations (Rigamonti *et al* 1990; Naff *et al* 1998). In a series of 21 patients, 43% had experienced intracerebral hemorrhage and there was one case of intractable focal seizures with headache (Malik *et al* 1988). A prospective series of 63 patients with more than 1 year of prospective follow-up has gone some way to show that the clinical course is benign, although longer follow-up is awaited (Naff *et al* 1998): 30% presented with seizures; the seizure frequency decreased significantly over time; and the risk of hemorrhage was 0.15% per lesion per year.

MISCELLANEOUS CEREBROVASCULAR DISORDERS

CEREBRAL VENOUS SINUS THROMBOSIS (CVST)

CVST is an underdiagnosed condition, which makes it difficult to know the true frequency of focal epilepsy attributable to it. Parasagittal hemorrhage may be preceded by an ischemic phase, often lasting several days, manifested by focal seizures and focal neurological deficits (Warlow *et al* 1996). The combination of headache and focal epilepsy is recognized as one of the four main modes of presentation (Villringer and Einhaupl 1997). A retrospective study of 77 adult patients followed for a mean of 6.5 years found that 14% of the 28 patients with early seizures suffered chronic epilepsy (Preter *et al* 1996). The proportion was higher in a small series of young adults (Partziguian *et al* 1996).

MITOCHONDRIAL ENCEPHALOPATHY, LACTIC ACIDOSIS, AND STROKELIKE EPISODES (MELAS)

MELAS is a rare disorder that usually presents in young adults with recurrent focal cerebral ischemia in an unusual distribution, complicated in the early or later stages by focal and secondary generalized epilepsy (Montagna *et al* 1988; Ciafaloni *et al* 1992). MELAS is associated with a variety of epileptic seizures that may be of increasing severity leading to episodes of epilepsia partialis continua (Andermann *et al* 1986).

VASCULITIDES

The frequency of cerebral vasculitis as a cause of focal seizures remains conjectural in the absence of studies with good histologic evidence (Moore and Richardson 1998). However, cerebral vasculitis should always be considered in younger adults who present with CVD and/or focal seizures in an unusual pattern. Stroke is within the broad spectrum of neuropsychiatric disorders attributable to *systemic lupus erythematosus* (SLE) (Sibley *et al* 1992; Tola *et al* 1992; Moore 1997). Seizures may be the presenting feature in up to 5%. They are seldom intractable. The risk of developing epilepsy in SLE may be related to the titer of anticardiolipin antibodies (Liou *et al* 1996). Most focal seizures in patients with the *primary antiphospholipid antibody syndrome* are related to focal brain infarction caused by small-vessel arterial thrombosis (Rumpl and Rumpl 1979; Leach *et al* 1989; Levine and Brey 1996). Although the small-vessel vasculitis of *Wegener's granulomatosis* predominantly affects the peripheral nervous system, the disease can cause CVD and focal seizures (Nishino *et al* 1993). The neurologic manifestations of *isolated angiitis of the central nervous system* (Cupps *et al* 1983; Moore 1989) are protean and recurrent disease appears to be the rule; strokes may occur, and predominantly focal seizures affect 5% of patients.

AMYLOID ANGIOPATHY

Although the association of an intracerebral hemorrhage with focal seizures suggests an underlying AVM or PICH, amyloid angiopathy should also be borne in mind (Cocito *et al* 1994; Silbert *et al* 1995), even in the absence of lobar hemorrhage (Greenberg *et al* 1993).

CONCLUSIONS

Cerebrovascular disease is a significant cause of focal epilepsy, a small proportion of which goes on to be intractable in adults. There is a need for extensive investigation and careful treatment of patients with poststroke epilepsy, in particular with respect to the underlying disorder. CVD has been the single most common identifiable etiology of apparently unprovoked focal epilepsy and its detection is increasing. The true natural history of poststroke seizures is, of course, unknown as many patients are treated with anticonvulsants, but it is also not known whether anticonvulsants modify the natural history of epilepsy. Onset seizures predict seizure recurrence following stroke and there is a 5% risk of developing epilepsy by 5 years after a stroke.

ACKNOWLEDGMENTS

We would like to thank Tricia Gwynn-Jones of the Chelsea and Westminster Hospital, London for her cheerful assistance with retrieving references for this chapter.

KEY POINTS

1. Cerebrovascular disease is a common cause of focal epilepsy in people aged >65 years, and seizures attributed to asymptomatic cerebral infarction may precede the development of a stroke.
2. The occurrence of a stroke, and especially cerebral hemorrhage, increases the risk of developing epilepsy. The risk of epilepsy is greater after lobar hemorrhage than after thalamic or basal ganglia hemorrhages. Around 3% of people who suffer a cerebral infarction develop intractable epilepsy.
3. Stroke is a prominent cause of epilepsia partialis continua, which may also be caused by a number of other cerebrovascular disorders including MELAS. Stroke may also cause simple and complex partial status epilepticus.
4. Both arteriovenous malformations and cavernous malformations may present with intractable focal epilepsy as the only symptom.

REFERENCES

Aiba T, Tanaka R, Koike T, Kameyama S, Takeda N, Komata T (1995) Natural history of intracranial cavernous malformations. *Journal of Neurosurgery* **83**:56–59.

Andermann F, Lugaresi E, Dvorkin GS, Montagna P (1986) Malignant migraine: the syndrome of prolonged classical migraine, epilepsia partialis continua, and repeated strokes; a clinically characteristic disorder probably due to mitochondrial encephalopathy. *Functional Neurology* **1**:481–486.

Annegers JF, Grabow JD, Groover RV *et al* (1980) Seizures after head trauma: a population study. *Neurology* **30**:683–689.

Arboix A, Comes E, Massons J, Garcia L, Oliveres M (1996) Relevance of early seizures for in-hospital mortality in acute cerebrovascular disease. *Neurology* **47**:1429–1435.

Arboix A, Garcia-Eroles L, Massons JB, Oliveres M, Comes E (1997) Predictive factors of early seizures after acute cerebrovascular disease. *Stroke* **28**:1590–1594.

Bamford J, Sandercock P, Warlow C, Gray M (1986) Why are patients with acute stroke admitted to hospital? *British Medical Journal Clinical Research Edition* **292**:1369–1372.

Baquis GD, Pessin MS, Scott RM (1985) Limb shaking – a carotid TIA. *Stroke* **16**:444–448.

Barolin GS, Scherzer E, Schnaberth G (1971) Epileptic manifestations as precursors of apoplexies. Vascular precursive epilepsy. *Fortschritte der Neurologie, Psychiatrie und Ihrer Grenzgebiete* **39**:199–216.

Bell WL, Horner J, Logue P, Radtke RA (1990) Neologistic speech automatisms during complex partial seizures. *Neurology* **40**:49–52.

Berger AR, Lipton RB, Lesser ML, Lantos G, Portenoy RK (1988) Early seizures following intracerebral hemorrhage: implications for therapy. *Neurology* **38**:1363–1365.

Bergin PS, Fish DR, Shorvon SD, Oatridge A, de Souza NM, Bydder GM (1995) Magnetic resonance imaging in partial epilepsy: additional abnormalities shown with the fluid attenuated inversion recovery (FLAIR) pulse sequence. *Journal of Neurology, Neurosurgery and Psychiatry* **58**:439–443.

Bidzinski J, Marchel A, Sherif A (1992) Risk of epilepsy after aneurysm operations. *Acta Neurochirurgica* **119**:49–52.

Bogousslavsky J, Martin R, Regli F, Despland PA, Bolyn S (1992) Persistent worsening of stroke sequelae after delayed seizures. *Archives of Neurology* **49**:385–388.

Broderick JP, Phillips SJ, Whisnant JP, O'Fallon WMX, Bergstralh EJ (1989) Incidence rates of stroke in the eighties: the end of the decline in stroke? *Stroke* **20**:577–582.

Bronen RA, Fulbright RK, Spencer DD, Spencer SS, Kim JH, Lange RC (1995) MR characteristics of neoplasms and vascular malformations associated with epilepsy. *Magnetic Resonance Imaging* **13**:1153–1162.

Brooks BS, King DW, el Gammal T *et al* (1990) MR imaging in patients with intractable complex partial epileptic seizures. *American Journal of Roentgenology* **154**:577–583.

Brown RD Jr, Wiebers DO, Forbes G *et al* (1988) The natural history of unruptured intracranial arteriovenous malformations. *Journal of Neurosurgery* **68**:352–357.

Brown RD, Jr., Wiebers DO, Torner JC, O'Fallon WM (1996) Incidence and prevalence of intracranial vascular malformations in Olmsted County, Minnesota, 1965 to 1992. *Neurology* **46**:949–952.

Burn J, Dennis M, Bamford J, Sandercock P, Wade D, Warlow C (1997) Epileptic seizures after a first stroke: the Oxfordshire Community Stroke Project. *British Medical Journal* **315**:1582–1587.

Cervoni L, Artico M, Salvati M, Bristot R, Franco C, Delfini R (1994) Epileptic seizures in intracerebral hemorrhage: a clinical and prognostic study of 55 cases. *Neurosurgical Review* **17**:185–188.

Ciafaloni E, Ricci E, Shanske S *et al* (1992) MELAS: clinical features, biochemistry, and molecular genetics. *Annals of Neurology* **31**:391–398.

Cocito L, Loeb C (1986) May focal epileptic seizures be considered a marker of TIAs? *Functional Neurology* **1**:461–465.

Cocito L, Loeb C (1989) Focal epilepsy as a possible sign of transient subclinical ischemia. *European Neurology* **29**:339–344.

Cocito L, Nizzo R, Bisio N, Favale E (1994) Epileptic seizures heralding intracerebral hemorrhage [letter]. *Stroke* **25**:2292–2293.

Cockerell OC, Eckle I, Goodridge DM, Sander JW, Shorvon SD (1995) Epilepsy in a population of 6000 re-examined: secular trends in first attendance rates, prevalence, and prognosis. *Journal of Neurology, Neurosurgery and Psychiatry* **58**:570–576.

Cockerell OC, Rothwell J, Thompson PD, Marsden CD, Shorvon SD (1996) Clinical and physiological features of epilepsia partialis continua. Cases ascertained in the UK. *Brain* **119**:393–407.

Commission on Classification and Terminology of the ILAE (1989) Proposal for revised classification of epilepsies and epileptic syndromes. *Epilepsia* **30**:389–399.

Couper J (1994) Unilateral musical hallucinations and all that jazz. *Australian and New Zealand Journal of Psychiatry* **28**:516–519.

Crawford PM, West CR, Chadwick DW, Shaw MD (1986) Arteriovenous malformations of the brain: natural history in unoperated patients. *Journal of Neurology, Neurosurgery and Psychiatry* **49**:1–10.

Cupps TR, Moore PM, Fauci AS (1983) Isolated angiitis of the central nervous system. Prospective diagnostic and therapeutic experience. *American Journal of Medicine* **74**:97–105.

Del Curling O Jr, Kelly DL Jr, Elster AD, Craven TE (1991) An analysis of the natural history of cavernous angiomas. *Journal of Neurosurgery* **75**:702–708.

Demiati M, Rosa A and Mizon JP (1989) Focal motor crises: a transitory ischemic attack? *Revue Neurologique* **145**:728–731.

Faught E, Peters D, Bartolucci A, Moore L, Miller PC (1989) Seizures after primary intracerebral hemorrhage. *Neurology* **39**:1089–1093.

Forsgren L (1992) Prevalence of epilepsy in adults in northern Sweden. *Epilepsia* **33**:450–458.

Forsgren L, Bucht G, Eriksson S, Bergmark L (1996) Incidence and clinical characterization of unprovoked seizures in adults: a prospective population-based study. *Epilepsia* **37**:224–229.

French JD, Gernandt BE, Livingstone RB (1956) Regional differences in seizure susceptibility in monkey cortex. *Archives of Neurology and Psychiatry* **75**:260–274.

Fults D, Kelly DL Jr (1984) Natural history of arteriovenous malformations of the brain: a clinical study. *Neurosurgery* **15**:658–662.

Giroud M, Dumas R (1995) Role of associated cortical lesions in motor partial seizures and lenticulostriate infarcts. *Epilepsia* **36**:465–470.

Giroud M, Gras P, Fayolle H *et al* (1994) Early seizures after acute stroke: a study of 1,640 cases. *Epilepsia* **35**:959–964.

Globus M, Lavi E, Fich A, Abramsky O (1982) Ictal hemiparesis. *European Neurology* **21**:165–168.

Greenberg SM, Vonsattel JP, Stakes JW, Gruber M, Finklestein SP (1993) The clinical spectrum of cerebral amyloid angiopathy: presentations without lobar hemorrhage. *Neurology* **43**:2073–2079.

Gupta SR, Naheedy MH, Elias D, Rubino FA (1988) Postinfarction seizures. A clinical study. *Stroke* **19**:1477–1481.

Hankey GJ (1993) Prolonged exacerbation of the neurological sequelae of stroke by post-stroke partial epileptic seizures. *Australian and New Zealand Journal of Medicine* **23**:306.

Hart RG, Byer JA, Slaughter JR, Hewett JE, Easton JD (1981) Occurrence and implications of seizures in subarachnoid hemorrhage due to ruptured intracranial aneurysms. *Neurosurgery* **8**:417–421.

Hasan D, Schonck RS, Avezaat CJ, Tanghe HL, van Gijn J, van der Lugt PJ (1993) Epileptic seizures after subarachnoid hemorrhage. *Annals of Neurology* **33**:286–291.

Hauser WA, Ramirez-Lassepas H, Rosenstein R (1984) Risk for seizures and epilepsy following cerebrovascular insults. *Epilepsia* **25**:666 (abstract).

Hauser WA, Annegers JF, Kurland LT (1991) Prevalence of epilepsy in Rochester, Minnesota: 1940–1980. *Epilepsia* **32**:429–445.

Hauser WA, Annegers JF, Kurland LT (1993) Incidence of epilepsy and unprovoked seizures in Rochester, Minnesota: 1935–1984. *Epilepsia* **34**:453–468.

Hesdorffer DC, Hauser WA, Annegers JF, Rocca WA (1996) Severe, uncontrolled hypertension and adult-onset seizures: a case-control study in Rochester, Minnesota. *Epilepsia* **37**:736–741.

Heuts-Van Raak EP, Boellaard A, De Krom MC, Lodder J (1993) Supratentorial brain infarcts in adult-onset seizures; the Masstricht Epilepsy Case Register. *Seizure* **2**:221–227.

Heuts-van Raak L, Lodder J, Kessels F (1996) Late seizures following a first symptomatic brain infarct are related to large infarcts involving the posterior area around the lateral sulcus. *Seizure* **5**:185–194.

Hilt DC, Alexander GE (1982) Jacksonian somatosensory seizures as the sole manifestation of chronic subdural hematoma [letter]. *Archives of Neurology* **39**:786

Hornig CR, Buttner T, Hufnagel A, Schroder-Rosenstock K, Dorndorf W (1990) Epileptic seizures following ischaemic cerebral infarction. Clinical picture, CT findings and prognosis. *European Archives of Psychiatry and Neurological Sciences* **239**:379–383.

Hughlings Jackson J (1931) Epileptiform convulsions from cerebral disease. In: Taylor J, Holmes G, Walshe FMR (eds) *Selected Writings of John Hughlings Jackson on Epilepsy and Epileptiform Convulsion*, pp 330–340. London: Hodder and Stoughton.

Itoyama Y, Uemura S, Ushio Y *et al* (1989) Natural course of unoperated intracranial arteriovenous malformations: study of 50 cases. *Journal of Neurosurgery* **71**:805–809.

Kamrin RP (1966) Temporal lobe epilepsy caused by unruptured middle cerebral artery aneurysms. *Archives of Neurology* **14**:421–427.

Kaplan PW (1993) Focal seizures resembling transient ischaemic attacks due to subclinical ischaemia. *Cerebrovascular Diseases* **3**:241–243.

Kilpatrick CJ, Davis SM, Tress BM, Rossiter SC, Hopper JL, Vandendriesen ML (1990) Epileptic seizures in acute stroke. *Archives of Neurology* **47**:157–160.

Kilpatrick CJ, Tress BM, O'Donnell C, Rossiter SC, Hopper JL (1991) Magnetic resonance imaging and late-onset epilepsy. *Epilepsia* **32**:358–364.

Kilpatrick CJ, Davis SM, Hopper JL, Rossiter SC (1992) Early seizures after acute stroke. Risk of late seizures. *Archives of Neurology* **49**:509–511.

Kondziolka D, Lunsford LD, Kestle JR (1995) The natural history of cerebral cavernous malformations. *Journal of Neurosurgery* **83**:820–824.

Kotwica Z, Brzeinski J (1991) Epilepsy in chronic subdural haematoma. *Acta Neurochirurgica* **113**:118–120.

Kraus JA, Berlit P (1998) Cerebral embolism and epileptic seizures – the role of the embolic source. *Acta Neurologica Scandinavica* **97**:154–159.

Krumholz A, Sung GY, Fisher RS, Barry E, Bergey GK, Grattan LM (1995) Complex partial status epilepticus accompanied by serious morbidity and mortality. *Neurology* **45**:1499–1504.

Lancman ME, Golimstok A, Norscini J, Granillo R (1993) Risk factors for developing seizures after a stroke. *Epilepsia* **34**:141–143.

Leach IH, Lennox G, Jaspan T, Lowe J (1989) Antiphospholipid antibody syndrome presenting with complex partial seizures and transient ischaemic attacks due to widespread small cerebral arterial thrombosis. *Neuropathology and Applied Neurobiology* **15**:579–584.

Leblance R, Feindel W, Ethier R (1983) Epilepsy from cerebral arteriovenous malformations. *Canadian Journal of Neurological Sciences* **10**:91–95.

Levine SR, Brey RL (1996) Neurological aspects of antiphospholipid antibody syndrome. *Lupus* **5**:347–353.

Li X, Breteler MM, de Bruyne MC, Meinardi H, Hauser WA, Hofman A (1997) Vascular determinants of epilepsy: the Rotterdam Study. *Epilepsia* **38**:1216–1220.

Liou HH, Wang CR, Chen CJ *et al* (1996) Elevated levels of anticardiolipin antibodies and epilepsy in lupus patients. *Lupus* **5**:307–312.

Malik GM, Morgan JK, Boulos RS, Ausman JI (1988) Venous angiomas: an underestimated cause of intracranial hemorrhage. *Surgical Neurology* **30**:350–358.

Manford M, Hart YM, Sander JW, Shorvon SD (1992) National General Practice Study of Epilepsy (NGPSE): partial seizure patterns in a general population. *Neurology* **42**:1911–1917.

Marosi M, Luef G, Schett P, Graf M, Sailer U, Bauer G (1994) The effects of brain lesions on the course of chronic epilepsies. *Epilepsy Research* **19**:63–69.

Matsumura T, Kojima S, Shiozawa R (1993) Late onset seizures in cerebral infarction – clinical study of late onset seizures in cortical branch infarction. *Rinsho Shinkeigaku* **33**:95–97.

Montagna P, Gallassi R, Medori R *et al* (1988) MELAS syndrome: characteristic migrainous and epileptic features and maternal transmission. *Neurology* **38**:751–754.

Moore PM (1989) Diagnosis and management of isolated angiitis of the central nervous system. *Neurology* **39**:167–173.

Moore PM (1997) Neuropsychiatric systemic lupus erythematosus. Stress, stroke, and seizures. *Annals of the New York Academy of Sciences* **823**:1–17.

Moore PM Richardson B (1998) Neurology of the vasculitides and connective tissue diseases. *Journal of Neurology, Neurosurgery and Psychiatry* **65**:10–22.

Murphy MJ (1985) Long-term follow-up of seizures associated with cerebral arteriovenous malformations. Results of therapy. *Archives of Neurology* **42**:477–479.

Naff NJ, Wemmer J, Hoenig-Rigamonti K, Rigamonti DR (1998) A longitudinal study of patients with venous malformations: documentation of a negligible hemorrhage risk and benign natural history. *Neurology* **50**:1709–1714.

Nishino H, Rubino FA, DeRemee RA, Swanson JW, Parisi JE (1993) Neurological involvement in Wegener's granulomatosis: an analysis of 324 consecutive patients at the Mayo Clinic. *Annals of Neurology* **33**:4–9.

Norris JW, Hachinski VC (1982) Misdiagnosis of stroke. *Lancet* **1**:328–331.

Norris JW, Bladin CF, Johnston PJ, Alexandrov AV, Smurawska LT (1994) The occurrence of seizures after stroke. *Neurology* **44**:A327 (abstract).

O'Laoire SA (1990) Epilepsy following neurosurgical intervention. *Acta Neurochirurgica, Supplementum* **50**:52–54.

Ohman J (1990) Hypertension as a risk factor for epilepsy after aneurysmal subarachnoid hemorrhage and surgery. *Neurosurgery* **27**:578–581.

Ohno K, Maehara T, Ichimura K, Suzuki R, Hirakawa K, Monma S (1993) Low incidence of seizures in patients with chronic subdural haematoma. *Journal of Neurology, Neurosurgery and Psychiatry* **56**:1231–1233.

Partziguian T, Camerlingo M, Castro L *et al* (1996) Cerebral venous thrombosis in young adults. Experience in a stroke unit, 1988–1994. *Italian Journal of Neurological Sciences* **17**:419–422.

Peled R, Harnes B, Borovich B, Sharf B (1984) Speech arrest and supplementary motor area seizures. *Neurology* **34**:110–111.

Porter PJ, Willinsky RA, Harper W, Wallace MC (1997) Cerebral cavernous malformations: natural history and prognosis after clinical deterioration with or without hemorrhage. *Journal of Neurosurgery* **87**:190–197.

Preter M, Tzourio C, Ameri A, Bousser MG (1996) Long-term prognosis in cerebral venous thrombosis. Follow-up of 77 patients. *Stroke* **27**:243–246.

Reith J, Jorgensen HS, Nakayama H, Raaschou HO, Olsen TS (1997)

Seizures in acute stroke: predictors and prognostic significance. The Copenhagen Stroke Study. *Stroke* **28**:1585–1589.

Rigamonti D, Drayer BP, Johnson PC, Hadley MN, Zabramski J, Spetzler RF (1987) The MRI appearance of cavernous malformations (angiomas). *Journal of Neurosurgery* **67**:518–524.

Rigamonti D, Hadley MN, Drayer BP *et al* (1988a) Cerebral cavernous malformations. Incidence and familial occurrence. *New England Journal of Medicine* **319**:343–347.

Rigamonti D, Spetzler RF, Drayer BP *et al* (1988b) Appearance of venous malformations on magnetic resonance imaging. *Journal of Neurosurgery* **69**:535–539.

Rigamonti D, Spetzler RF, Medina M, Rigamonti K, Geckle DS, Pappas C (1990) Cerebral venous malformations. *Journal of Neurosurgery* **73**:560–564.

Roberts RC, Shorvon SD, Cox TC, Gilliatt RW (1988) Clinically unsuspected cerebral infarction revealed by computed tomography scanning in late onset epilepsy. *Epilepsia* **29**:190–194.

Robinson JR Jr, Awad IA, Magdinec M, Paranandi L (1993) Factors predisposing to clinical disability in patients with cavernous malformations of the brain. *Neurosurgery* **32**:730–736.

Ropper AH (1988) 'Convulsions' in basilar artery occlusion. *Neurology* **38**:1500–1501.

Rubin G, Rappaport ZH (1993) Epilepsy in chronic subdural haematoma. *Acta Neurochirurgica* **123**:39–42.

Rumpl E, Rumpl H (1979) Recurrent transient global amnesia in a case with cerebrovascular lesions and livedo reticularis (Sneddon syndrome). *Journal of Neurology* **221**:127–131.

Ryglewicz D, Baranska-Gieruszczak M, Niedzielska K, Kryst-Widzgowska T (1990) EEG and CT findings in poststroke epilepsy. *Acta Neurologica Scandinavica* **81**:488–490.

Sabo RA, Hanigan WC, Aldag JC (1995) Chronic subdural hematomas and seizures: the role of prophylactic anticonvulsive medication. *Surgical Neurology* **43**:579–582.

Scholtes FB, Renier WO, Meinardi H (1996a) Simple partial status epilepticus: causes, treatment, and outcome in 47 patients. *Journal of Neurology, Neurosurgery and Psychiatry* **61**:90–92.

Scholtes FB, Renier WO, Meinardi H (1996b) Non-convulsive status epilepticus: causes, treatment, and outcome in 65 patients. *Journal of Neurology, Neurosurgery and Psychiatry* **61**:93–95.

Schomer DL (1993) Focal status epilepticus and epilepsia partialis continua in adults and children. *Epilepsia* **34** (Suppl.):S29–S36.

Schreiner A, Pohlmann-Eden B, Schwartz A, Hennerici M. (1995) Epileptic seizures in subcortical vascular encephalopathy. *Journal of the Neurological Sciences* **130**:171–177.

Sibley JT, Olszynski WP, Decoteau WE, Sundaram MB (1992) The incidence and prognosis of central nervous system disease in systemic lupus erythematosus. *Journal of Rheumatology* **19**:47–52.

Silbert PL, Bartleson JD, Miller GM, Parisi JE, Goldman MS, Meyer FB (1995) Cortical petechial hemorrhage, leukoencephalopathy, and subacute dementia associated with seizures due to cerebral amyloid angiopathy. *Mayo Clinic Proceedings* **70**:477–480.

So EL, Annegers JF, Hauser WA, O'Brien PC, Whisnant JP (1996) Population-based study of seizure disorders after cerebral infarction. *Neurology* **46**:350–355.

Sung CY, Chu NS (1989) Epileptic seizures in intracerebral haemorrhage. *Journal of Neurology, Neurosurgery and Psychiatry*, **52**:1273–1276.

Sung CY, Chu NS (1990) Epileptic seizures in thrombotic stroke. *Journal of Neurology* **237**:166–170.

Tinuper P, Provini F, Marini C *et al* (1996) Partial epilepsy of long duration: changing semiology with age. *Epilepsia* **37**:162–164.

Tola MR, Granieri E, Caniatti L *et al* (1992) Systemic lupus erythematosus presenting with neurological disorders. *Journal of Neurology* **239**:61–64.

Ukkola V, Heikkinen ER (1990) Epilepsy after operative treatment of ruptured cerebral aneurysms. *Acta Neurochirurgica* **106**:115–118.

Viitanen M, Eriksson S, Asplund K (1988) Risk of recurrent stroke, myocardial infarction and epilepsy during long-term follow-up after stroke. *European Neurology* **28**:227–231.

Villringer A, Einhaupl KM (1997) Dural sinus and cerebral venous thrombosis. *New Horizons* **5**:332–341.

Wang DZ, Steg RE, Futrell N (1995) Crying seizures after cerebral infarction [letter]. *Journal of Neurology, Neurosurgery and Psychiatry* **58**:380–381.

Warlow CP, Dennis MS, van Gijn J *et al* (1996) *Stroke: A Practical Guide to Management*. Oxford: Blackwell Science.

Weisberg LA, Shamsnia M, Elliott D (1991) Seizures caused by nontraumatic parenchymal brain hemorrhages. *Neurology* **41**:1197–1199.

Wharen RE Jr, Scheithauer BW, Laws ER Jr (1982) Thrombosed arteriovenous malformations of the brain. An important entity in the differential diagnosis of intractable focal seizure disorders. *Journal of Neurosurgery* **57**:520–526.

Whittle IR, Allsop JL, Halmagyi GM (1985) Focal seizures: an unusual presentation of giant intracranial aneurysms. A report of four cases with comments on the natural history and treatment. *Surgical Neurology* **24**:533–540.

WHO Task Force on Stroke and Other Cerebrovascular Disorders (1989) Recommendations on stroke prevention, diagnosis, and therapy. *Stroke* **20**:1407–1431.

Yanagihara T, Piepgras DG, Klass DW (1985) Repetitive involuntary movement associated with episodic cerebral ischemia. *Annals of Neurology* **18**:244–250.

Yarnell PR (1975) Todd's paralysis: a cerebrovascular phenomenon? *Stroke* **6**:301–303.

Zabramski JM, Wascher TM, Spetzler RF *et al* (1994) The natural history of familial cavernous malformations: results of an ongoing study. *Journal of Neurosurgery* **80**:422–432.

Cerebral vascular disorders in children

13

JH CROSS AND FJ KIRKHAM

An understanding of cerebrovascular pathophysiology and clinical manifestations is important for those who manage childhood epilepsy. Surveys of children with partial epilepsies using CT have shown that approximately 6% have a vascular etiology (Fritsch et al 1988; Nair et al 1997). An underlying infarct, sustained prenatally, perinatally, or postnatally, may be revealed in a significant proportion of patients with partial seizures. In one study of individuals presenting with epilepsy, 5% had infarcts and a further 2% had vascular malformations (Young et al 1982).

Epilepsy is a common outcome for stroke and may considerably increase disability. The onset of ischemic or hemorrhagic stroke in childhood is commonly accompanied by seizures and there may be considerable diagnostic confusion between postictal paralysis and vascular stroke presenting with seizures, at least initially. This is particularly true in the conditions that are complicated by both seizures and stroke, e.g. sickle cell disease. As the management of epilepsy improves and prevention and treatment of stroke become realistic possibilities, these issues will gain increasing importance. The diagnosis is not difficult in a child with seizures and a hemiparesis who has an infarct on neuroimaging, but those with intermittent weakness may cause diagnostic diffi-

culty. The differential includes partial epilepsy arising from the frontal lobes, Rasmussen encephalitis, alternating hemiplegia, and hemiplegic migraine. This chapter outlines the relationship between epilepsy and cerebrovascular disease and discusses the common conditions in which both may occur, whether causally linked or not.

INFARCTS/ISCHEMIC LESIONS

CONGENITAL

There are few follow-up studies of children with congenital hemiplegia from which we can determine the prevalence of epilepsy. Studies quote an incidence of 28–45% (Perlstein and Hood 1954; Goutieres et al 1972; Ito et al 1981; Claeys et al 1983; Uvebrant 1988); however, most studies include children with a history of only one seizure, rather than recurring seizures. The incidence of active epilepsy, that is a seizure within the last 5 years, may be considerably less (Uvebrant 1988). Such studies are relatively old, and few include magnetic resonance imaging (MRI) as a mode of investigation. At most, correlative studies have been attempted with CT scan, and it is difficult to determine the relative frequency of ischemic or hemorrhagic lesions, as opposed to developmental disorders, in relation to the occurrence of seizures. Most studies use a classification describing scans as normal, unilateral ventricular enlargement, cortical and/or subcortical cavities, or unclassified (Ito *et al* 1981; Uvebrant 1988; Wiklund and Uvebrant 1991). The only change that could reliably be attributable to ischemia would be cortical and/or subcortical cavities as confirmed by MRI data (Wolff 1998). Unilateral ventricular enlargement could be caused by periventricular hemorrhage in the preterm infant, predominantly a white-matter abnormality in which seizures are seen rarely, but could also include some abnormalities of cortical development.

As a consequence, it is difficult to correlate seizure semeiology with a specific vascular etiology, particularly in those with congenital hemiplegia. Seizure manifestations are likely to reflect the area of brain affected. Most series report simple motor seizures, probably reflecting the frequent involvement of middle cerebral artery territory, or other partial seizures as the most common seizure types (70%) (Goutieres *et al* 1972; Uvebrant 1988). Secondary generalized seizures are the next most common. Hippocampal sclerosis as a cause of mesial temporal seizures may also be seen in association with congenital porencephaly (Ho *et al* 1997). However, in series of 'startle epilepsy,' the presence of hemiplegia associated with a porencephalic cyst on imaging (of likely ischemic etiology) appears to feature prominently (Manford *et al* 1996).

Startle-provoked seizures are defined as those that occur in response to a startle stimulus, whether auditory (natural, particularly if sudden and intense) or somatosensory (tactile or mechanical, most commonly stumbling) but rarely visual (Chauvel *et al* 1992; Manford *et al* 1996). They may demonstrate motor features of a normal startle reaction, but in the majority spontaneous motor seizures are also seen with similar symptomatology. Asymmetrical posturing is due to involvement of the hemiparetic side, which causes increased amplitude and duration of tonic signs. As with the primitive startle reaction seen in the newborn, repetition of the effective stimulus leads to habituation. The startle seizure represents the sensory precipitation of a motor attack of cortical origin. Somatosensory electroencephalography (SEEG) studies using depth electrodes suggest an origin of such seizures within abnormal motor and premotor areas of the frontal lobe (Chauvel *et al* 1992). There is subsequently very rapid spread, usually bilaterally.

ACQUIRED

Neonatal

Congenital hemiplegia is often not clinically evident until some time into the first year of life. It may therefore be difficult on the basis of neuroimaging alone to determine the exact timing of an ischemic lesion leading to such clinical features. However, it has been suggested that neonatal cerebral infarction is the second most common identifiable cause of seizures in full-term infants (second only to hypoxic ischemic encephalopathy) (Estan and Hope 1997). This is unlikely to be a significant cause of congenital hemiplegia as neonates who have presented with seizures secondary to an infarct, when followed prospectively, appear to have a good long-term prognosis with regard to neurodevelopmental outcome, with only a small number of children having a residual hemiplegia or developmental delay in reported series. In addition, although seizures are seen as the presenting feature in the majority, recurring seizures long term – that is, active epilepsy – are rare (Sran and Baumann 1988; Estan and Hope 1997).

Typically, seizures present in term infants, who appear relatively well with no evidence of neurologic disturbance between episodes. Seizures reported are predominantly focal and clonic in nature, or are otherwise generalized or subtle (Estan and Hope 1997). They are relatively easy to control with first-line anticonvulsant medication, which can be withdrawn 3–6 months after presentation (Clancy *et al* 1985; Sran and Baumann 1988; Estan and Hope 1997). A small number at longer-term follow up (3–8 years) have represented with later seizures, but these again have responded promptly to anticonvulsants (Sran and Baumann 1988). EEG may be normal (Estan and Hope 1997) or diffusely abnormal or may demonstrate focal abnormalities (Clancy *et al* 1985; Levy *et al* 1985; Sran and Baumann 1988), whether spikes or slow waves, but does not give any indication of long-term prognosis, with regard either to later seizures or to neurodevelopmental outcome. Cranial ultrasound may also be unrevealing as to the underlying etiology, which is usually diagnosed on serial CT scan (Clancy *et al* 1985; Lien *et al* 1995; Estan and Hope 1997).

The relatively benign course seen in seizures associated with neonatal stroke, in contrast to early-onset seizures in congenital hemiplegia of assumed antenatal origin (Uvebrant 1988; Vargha-Khadem *et al* 1992), could perhaps be explained by the timing of the insult. In the case of those of antenatal origin, the insult is occurring at a time of continuing brain development and could therefore be assumed to have associated malformative lesions. Neonatal ischemic insults occur at a time when brain development is largely complete, and therefore the risk of coexistent malformative brain lesions is considerably less.

Later childhood

Stroke occurs in children with an incidence of 2.6 and 3.1 per 100 000 white and black children, respectively (Broderick *et al* 1993). Approximately half of strokes are hemorrhagic, secondary to arteriovenous malformation or aneurysm (see below) or to bleeding into an ischemic lesion. These children may present with an acute focal neurologic deficit, but commonly present in coma, with or without seizures. Acute hemiparesis, with or without seizures, is the typical presentation of ischemic stroke, which is strongly associated with cerebrovascular disease (Shirane *et al* 1992).

A focal neurologic deficit lasting more than 24 hours is defined as a stroke, while a similar episode lasting for a shorter period of time is considered to be a transient ischemic neurologic deficit. The term 'reversible ischemic neurologic deficit' has been coined to cover those whose deficit lasts more than 24 hours but eventually recovers fully. Modern imaging techniques are challenging these traditional clinical concepts. MRI is more sensitive than CT for the diagnosis of infarction within 24 hours, and is comparable for the diagnosis of hemorrhage (Bryan *et al* 1991). It is now clear that, although the majority of patients with prolonged clinical deficits eventually have infarction on neuroimaging, similar but clinically and radiologically reversible syndromes may occur, for example in severe hemiplegic migraine. On the other hand, patients with short-lasting neurologic syndromes, including seizures, or even with no clinical symptoms at all, may have suffered infarction, sometimes quite extensive, for example in sickle cell disease (Glauser *et al* 1995).

A large number of chronic pediatric conditions, including congenital heart disease and sickle cell anemia, predispose to stroke (Roach and Riela 1995), although at least half of those presenting with stroke have no previous medical history. Venous thrombosis (associated with cyanosis and polycythemia) and embolus are the common mechanisms in cardiac disease, but primary arterial cerebrovascular disease may be more common than has previously been assumed. In previously well children, a history of trauma, however minor, or infection may suggest arterial disease such as dissection or stenosis; the latter has been associated with varicella and human immunodeficiency virus infection as well as with meningitis. Sudden onset may indicate an embolic origin, usually presumed to be cardiogenic in childhood,

while a slowly evolving or stuttering neurologic deficit suggests thrombosis and therefore cerebrovascular disease as the most likely underlying pathology. In children presenting with seizures and/or headache, venous thrombosis should be excluded, whether or not they have a known predisposing condition. These clinical clues to stroke syndromes and subtypes have been worked out in adult populations however (Bogousslavsky and Caplan 1995).

Seizures at the onset of stroke

Before the advent of CT scanning in 1973, the distinction between patients with a cerebral infarct or hemorrhage and those with the onset of a hemiparesis in the context of status epilepticus (hemiseizure–hemiplegia–epilepsy syndrome, HHE (Gastaut *et al* 1960)) was blurred. The series of acute focal neurologic deficits published in this era divided children who had seizures, often unilateral clonic at onset, who were usually young and had a high chance of epilepsy and cognitive deficit as well as hemiparesis at follow-up, from those without seizures, who were generally older and had a somewhat better prognosis (Greer and Waltz 1965; Aicardi *et al* 1969; Aicardi and Chevrie 1970; Tibbles and Brown 1975). About 50% of children had seizures at onset of their focal neurologic deficit (Gastaut *et al* 1960; Bogousslavsky and Caplan 1995; Roach and Riela 1995); the majority were in status or had serial seizures, but a few had 'trivial' seizures in the context of the sudden onset of a hemiparesis.

More recently, authors of papers on childhood stroke have excluded patients with HHE, which is extremely rare nowadays, almost certainly because of improved management of status epilepticus. Neuroimaging studies allow the definition of a group of patients with focal hemorrhage or infarction in the distribution of a vascular territory, separate from those with HHE who usually have hemispheric atrophy. Nevertheless, the incidence of seizures at the onset of ischemic and/or hemorrhagic stroke is much higher in children (20–34%) (Wanifuchi *et al* 1988; Yang *et al* 1995; Mancini *et al* 1997) than in adults (So *et al* 1996), and status epilepticus occurs in 3–8%. In a series of 128 children from Great Ormond Street Hospital (GOSH) with ischemic stroke, mainly in an arterial distribution, 43 (34%) had seizures at presentation, but only 5 (4%) had no other manifestation (V. Ganesan and F.J. Kirkham, unpublished observations). Data from the Canadian Pediatric Ischemic Stroke Registry (CPISR) are very similar: 36% of those with arterial stroke (total *n*=243) and 50% of those with sinovenous thrombosis (total *n*=78) had seizures within the first 24 hours (Meaney *et al* 1997).

The majority of seizures are partial, often focal twitching on the side of the hemiparesis, but generalized seizures occur and may be manifest only on the nonparalyzed side. Seizures may be commoner in young children (Sato *et al* 1991). In the GOSH data, those with seizures at onset were significantly younger (*t*-test, *P*=0.04) (V. Ganesan and F.J. Kirkham, unpublished observations). From the CPISR data, the relative risk in those under 2 years of age for having seizures after stroke was 2.7 for arterial stroke (*P*<0.001) and 2.2 for sinovenous thrombosis (*P*=0.02) (Meaney *et al* 1997).

Early seizures are more likely to occur if there is cortical involvement (Yang *et al* 1995), usually secondary to large-vessel disease in the carotid distribution, but have been reported after basal ganglia infarction (Inagaki *et al* 1992; Mancini *et al* 1997). The latter often occurs apparently idiopathically in previously normal children. From the CPISR, for arterial stroke, the relative risk of developing seizures was 1.7 in those with large artery involvement in carotid territory, compared with those with distal or penetrating small-vessel disease or with vertebrobasilar disease (*P*=0.002) (Meaney *et al* 1997). In the GOSH series, seizures occurred in 14 children with basal ganglia infarction only and in 30 with cortical involvement. There were etiological risk factors in 43, of whom 30 had known medical conditions prior to the stroke (cardiac disease in 17, sickle disease in 8) (F.J. Kirkham and V. Ganesan, unpublished observations): 26 had arterial disease, two had venous thrombosis, 12 had normal vascular imaging, and in four there were no data on cerebral vasculature. Seizures are probably commoner in some forms of cerebrovascular disease – e.g. moyamoya, venous sinus thrombosis – than in others e.g. – dissection – although there are few data available.

Effect of early seizures on stroke outcome

There is considerable controversy about the effects of early seizures on outcome for stroke in adults, with some authors suggesting improved outcome in survivors. There are relatively few data in children, but there is no evidence so far for an adverse effect. The proportion of children with abnormalities on neurologic follow-up 1–197 weeks (median 31 weeks) after arterial stroke was similar whether or not they had seizures at onset in the CPISR study; and, while 66% of those with seizures after venous sinus thrombosis were abnormal compared with 46% of those without (follow up 3–169 (median 59) weeks), this did not reach statistical significance (Meaney *et al* 1997). In the GOSH study, a follow-up parental questionnaire, completed 0.25–13 (median 3) years later by 90/128

parents (an additional 13 patients were known to have died), was used to determine outcome. In a logistic regression examining the effects of age, time since stroke, presence of a previously recognized risk factor, occurrence of seizures at presentation, and infarct location on outcome, only younger age was associated with a poorer outcome (*P*=0.03) (V. Ganesan and F.J. Kirkham, unpublished observations).

Epilepsy as an outcome for stroke in childhood

Figures vary for the incidence of epilepsy after stroke in childhood but they appear to be higher than in adult series. In hospital-based series including both hemorrhage and infarction and grouping all etiologies, approximately 30% appeared to have recurrent seizures (Keidan *et al* 1994; Yang *et al* 1995). The prevalence of epilepsy in the GOSH study was somewhat lower; 13/90 (15%) who responded to the questionnaire were on anticonvulsants for epilepsy and another three of those who had presented with seizures had further seizures (total 16/128; 13%) (F.J. Kirkham and V. Ganesan, unpublished observations). For arterial ischemic stroke and venous sinus thrombosis, the figures for recurrent seizures were 10% and 20%, respectively, in the epidemiologically based CPISR study (Meaney *et al* 1997). The risk is particularly high for those with later onset of seizures after stroke and for those with cortical involvement (Yang *et al* 1995). In a logistic model looking at the effects of age at stroke, etiology, presence of cerebrovascular disease, and presence of cortical involvement on the risk of epilepsy in the 44 GOSH patients with seizures at stroke onset, only cortical involvement was significantly associated (*P*=0.03) (F.J. Kirkham and V. Ganesan, unpublished observations).

Management

The response to anticonvulsant drugs is variable when the underlying pathology is infarction. In Yang's series, of 21 with recurrent seizures, 12 (57%) were seizure-free for 4.5 ± 2.3 years, 5 (24%) had been controlled with anticonvulsant drugs for 7.5 ± 4.7 years, and 4 (19%) were intractable (Yang *et al* 1995). In general, anticonvulsants targeted at focal epilepsy should be tried; vigabatrin has been particularly successful in those with epilepsy associated with hemiplegia. Recent concerns about visual field loss after prolonged use mean that the risk–benefit ratio may prohibit the use of the drug early in the natural history, although a trial is often justified if seizures continue (Eke *et al* 1997; Krauss *et al* 1998). Surgery may be successful in intractable cases (Yang *et al* 1995); hemispherectomy is commonly required (see Chapter 53).

CONDITIONS IN WHICH SEIZURES AND STROKE ARE COMMON

VENOUS SINUS THROMBOSIS

Venous sinus thrombosis was initially described at post-mortem in children with sepsis, dehydration, or conditions predisposing to a hypercoagulable state, such as polycythemia associated with congenital heart disease. Confirmation in life previously required conventional angiography, which was rarely undertaken in sick children, but with the advent of CT and MRI it has become clear that venous sinus thrombosis is a common cause of seizures in premature and term neonates. Some may be diagnosed on CT scan (the empty delta sign), but MR imaging and angiography is more sensitive and may be helpful in defining the extent of thrombosis in those picked up on CT (Medlock *et al* 1992) (Fig. 13.1).

Although these infants can present with other symptoms, such as lethargy (Rivkin *et al* 1992), the majority of cases (50–100% of the reported series) present with focal or generalized seizures (Konishi *et al* 1987; Wong *et al* 1987; Belman *et al* 1990b; Barron *et al* 1992), which are often refractory to anticonvulsant therapy until the thrombosis has resolved. Hemorrhagic infarction in venous sinus thrombosis is particularly likely to be epileptogenic (relative risk 1.6, *P*<0.05) according to the CPISR (Meaney *et al* 1997). Many of these neonates, particularly those who are premature, are already sick; shock, dehydration, and birth asphyxia are recognized associations. Focal or generalized seizures also occur at presentation in about 20% of older children with documented venous sinus thrombosis, although headache is the commonest feature in this group Barron *et al* 1992).

Hematological abnormalities, including polycythemia, iron deficiency anemia, and thrombocytosis (Belman *et al* 1990b), have been documented in children with venous sinus thrombosis. Prothrombotic abnormalities, e.g. antithrombin III deficiency and the factor V Leiden, may play a role in a significant proportion. The available data suggest that the thrombosis resolves with conservative management (rehydration, antibiotics for sepsis) in the majority of infants and children, although there is increasing evidence that anticoagulation is beneficial in adults, but there has been no randomized controlled study in children to date. The majority of children have no sequelae, but

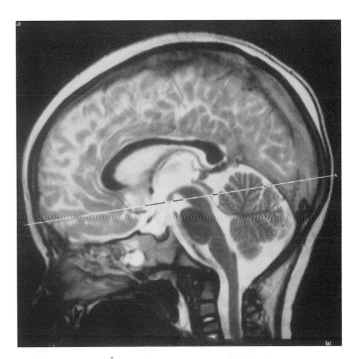

Fig. 13.1 MR venogram from a 3-year-old child with nephrotic syndrome who developed a headache followed by right-sided seizures and a hemiparesis. The EEG showed an excess of slow activity posteriorly and the MR venogram shows sagittal sinus thrombosis.

epilepsy occurs in up to 25% (Medlock *et al* 1992; Andrew *et al* 1997).

MOYAMOYA

The term moyamoya is used to describe the angiographic appearance of the collaterals usually associated with occlusion or very severe stenosis of the terminal internal carotid (Suzuki and Takatu 1969) (Fig. 13.2). The disease is usually, but not always, bilateral, is much commoner in Japan, and is often idiopathic, although cases with sickle cell disease, Down syndrome, Williams syndrome, and various collagen disorders have been described. Typically, infarction occurs in the border zones between the anterior and middle cerebral or the middle and posterior cerebral arteries. Motor recovery is often good, but cognitive deterioration occurs and there may be other manifestations, such as chorea and visual disturbance.

Presentation as a seizure disorder alone has been well documented (Schoenberg *et al* 1977) and may account for up to 10% of cases (Nakase *et al* 1993). Up to 30% present with hemiconvulsions as the main complaint (V. Ganesan and F.J. Kirkham, unpublished observations) and up to 50% may have seizures in addition to transient ischemic episodes (Kurokawa *et al* 1985). Although the condition is rare outside Japan, MR angiography should be considered in cases

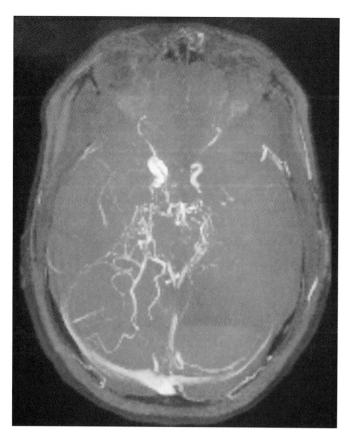

Fig. 13.2 Arteriogram from a child aged 13 years who had had episodes of crying, banging her head on the table, and unresponsiveness from the age of 7 years, treated as epilepsy with anticonvulsant medication. The EEG showed large-amplitude slow activity on overbreathing and the arteriogram shows moyamoya.

of intractable epilepsy, particularly if the seizure semeiology points to a frontal or parietooccipital location or if there is any evidence of infarction on neuroimaging. In those with known moyamoya, it may be very difficult to distinguish partial seizures from transient ischemic episodes (Kurokawa et al 1985) and in many cases a trial of anticonvulsants is worthwhile. Surgical revascularization should certainly be considered in any child with cognitive deterioration or recurrent symptoms and perhaps for all patients (Ishikawa et al 1997).

SICKLE CELL DISEASE

Stroke occurs in all the common sickle genotypes, with an incidence of 0.61/100 patient-years (Ohene-Frempong et al 1998). The peak age for cerebral infarction is around 8 years, and stroke is 280 times more common in those with sickle cell disease than in the rest of the pediatric population. There is pathologic and arteriographic evidence for large-vessel disease in sickle cell disease, with infarction occurring commonly either in the distribution of the middle or anterior cerebral arteries or in the border zones between their territories (Pavlakis et al 1989); subclinical infarction is common and may predict clinical stroke (Kugler et al 1993). Venous thrombosis has also been documented as a cause of stroke in this condition (Ohene-Frempong et al 1988). Risk factors include a low hemoglobin F (Powars et al 1984), a low steady-state hemoglobin concentration (Ohene-Frempong et al 1998), and recent chest crisis (Pavlakis et al 1989), but it has not proved easy to predict stroke in the individual patient from the clinical and hematologic data. The recurrence risk is extremely high, with approximately two-thirds having a further stroke over the subsequent 3 years (Powars et al 1984); most but not all can be prevented by a transfusion program.

Although the majority who experience stroke make a good recovery from the motor point of view, the long-term cognitive outcome is poor (Hariman et al 1991), and there is evidence for frontal lobe dysfunction and poor performance on the Arithmetic subtest of the WISC (Wechsler Intelligence Scale for Children) for those with small subclinical infarcts (Watkins et al 1998). The use of transcranial Doppler sonography (TCD) has been pioneered by Adams, who has shown that high velocities in the middle cerebral or internal carotid arteries predict the majority of infarctive strokes (Adams et al 1992) and that primary prevention is possible if those with very high velocities are transfused prophylactically (Adams et al 1998). Hemorrhagic stroke occurs in childhood, but is much commoner in young adults (Ohene-Frempong et al 1998); a high white cell count and hypertension appear to be risk factors; recognized mechanisms include bleeding into a previous infarct and aneurysmal rupture (Pavlakis et al 1989).

Seizures are considerably more common in the population of patients with homozygous sickle cell disease than in comparable groups, with reported figures of 10–16% in studies covering all age groups (Greer and Schotland 1962; Portnoy and Herion 1972; Adamolekun et al 1993; Liv et al 1994). One study reported a figure of 7% for those with hemoglobin SC disease (Fabian and Peters 1984). Some may occur acutely, in the context of stroke or treatment for crisis with, for example meperidine (Liu et al 1994), but around 11% of adults with sickle cell disease have epilepsy; there are few comparable data for children. In a study based at GOSH of 143 children with sickle cell disease followed from birth for 2–23 (mean 12) years,

15 (10%) had had at least one seizure, but none had intractable epilepsy or required anticonvulsant prophylaxis for more than 2 years.

The majority of seizures in patients with sickle cell disease are generalized tonic–clonic, but partial seizures are also well recognized, and some may be difficult to categorize (Liu *et al* 1994); these may represent manifestations of frontal lobe epilepsy. The prevalence of epilepsy appears to increase with age (Liu *et al* 1994), which is at least in part accounted for by those who have had a clinical stroke. A significant proportion of adults with sickle cell disease and epilepsy have renal failure (Liu *et al* 1994); although renal disease is less common in the pediatric population, hypertensive encephalopathy with seizures may occur. Of the 15 children who had had at least one seizure in the GOSH study, one had neonatal seizures in the context of prematurity and intraventricular hemorrhage, two had febrile seizures in the second year of life, six had cerebrovascular disease, and in the remainder – many of whom had ill-defined single episodes – the etiology was obscure. Age of onset was somewhat higher in those with cerebrovascular disease (11 ± 5 years) than in those without (5 ± 5 years), although this did not achieve statistical significance (*t*-test, *P*=0.08) (F.J. Kirkham, D.K.M. Hewes, and J.E. Evans, unpublished observations).

Seizures are a feature at presentation in at least 16–19% of strokes in the context of sickle cell disease (Powars *et al* 1984; Pavlakis *et al* 1988; Ohene-Frempong 1991; Balkaran *et al* 1992); in the longitudinal GOSH study of 143 children, four (44%) of the nine who had strokes presented with seizures at onset and the numbers were even higher (50%) if our referral population was included (F.J. Kirkham, D.K.M. Hewes, and J.E. Evans, personal communication). All children presenting with their first seizure should therefore have detailed neuroimaging, preferably with MF imaging, arteriography, and venography for optimal delineation of the pathology. Although it has been suggested that epilepsy predicts stroke in sickle cell disease (Mohr *et al* 1982), this remains controversial. Of nine children in the GOSH study who had seizures without cerebrovascular disease, only one has gone on to have a stroke and his case was complicated by hydrocephalus secondary to his neonatal intraventricular hemorrhage (F.J. Kirkham, D.K.M. Hewes, J.E. Evans, personal communication). There is certainly no evidence that an abnormal EEG predicts stroke (Powars *et al* 1984), although very large prospective studies have not been undertaken. After stroke, up to 50% of an untransfused population may have seizures (Powars *et al* 1984). Of 22 children referred to GOSH who have been on long-term transfusion regimes after stroke, 11 had seizures at onset, but only 2 have required anticonvulsants to manage recurrent seizures and both have proved easy to control (F.J. Kirkham, D.K.M. Hewes, J.E. Evans, unpublished observations).

MALIGNANT DISEASE

Neurologic complications are common in children with systemic malignancy, occurring acutely in about 11% (DiMario and Packer 1990). Both the underlying disease and its treatment may contribute. Seizures are most common, but strokes occur in around 1–4% (Packer *et al* 1985; DiMario and Packer 1990) and may present with seizures. Some children have evidence for cerebrovascular disease, usually either small-vessel arterial or venous thrombosis, even if the presentation is with seizures. There is also a long-term risk of epilepsy, stroke, and a syndrome with features of complicated migraine (Shuper *et al* 1995). Some of these patients may have arterial abnormalities such as moyamoya secondary to radiotherapy, but noninvasive investigation with MR is usually preferred initially as there is a risk with arteriography of worsening of the symptoms in those with migrainous episodes (Shuper *et al* 1995).

MENINGITIS

Seizures are common in bacterial meningitis, affecting up to 40% of those with infections due to *Streptococcus pneumoniae*, for example. The underlying mechanisms include vascular involvement. Vasospasm, stenosis, and occlusion of the basal cerebral arteries are important causes of morbidity and may be diagnosed using transcranial Doppler ultrasound (Haring *et al* 1993). Treatment with heparin has been suggested (Haring *et al* 1993), but there is inadequate evidence to support this measure at the present time (Goldman 1994).

HUMAN IMMUNODEFICIENCY VIRUS

Neurologic dysfunction is a particularly distressing component of HIV infection in children. Reports from North America suggest that more than 50% of children with AIDS have evidence of a static or progressive encephalopathy. The advent of seizures and/or focal neurologic signs may indicate a lymphoma, an opportunistic infection, or hemorrhagic or ischemic infarction (Belman 1990a). Infection with *Varicella zoster* may play a part in some cases of stroke associated with the AIDS complex (Frank *et al* 1989).

NEUROCYSTICERCOSIS

Neurocysticercosis is the commonest parasitic disease of the central nervous system, affecting about 50 million people worldwide, with 50 000 deaths (Cantu and Barinagarrementeria 1996). It is an important cause of symptomatic localization-related epilepsy in children as well as in adults (Murthy and Yangala 1998). In young adults, lacunar and large-vessel occlusion stroke syndromes have been recognized increasingly in association with neurocysticercosis and there is evidence for a causal link (Alarcon *et al* 1992). The youngest reported case is 16 years of age, although there is evidence for an association in series of childhood stroke from India and from South Africa (P.D. Singhi and M. Moodley, personal communications). Basal arachnoiditis and cerebral arteritis leading to infarction are found at angiography in many (Barinagarrementaria and Cantu 1998), although the differential diagnosis of acute focal neurologic signs in this condition includes a local effect of an encysted parasite, with or without edema. A small proportion presenting with stroke have seizures at onset.

HEMOLYTIC–UREMIC SYNDROME

Hemolytic–uremic syndrome is not uncommon in childhood and is often associated with *Escherichia coli* O157 gastrointestinal infections (Brandt *et al* 1994); the related thrombotic thrombocytopenic purpura occurs more rarely. Major cerebral vessel thrombosis (Crisp *et al* 1981; Trevathan and Dooling 1987) has been described in association with seizures and stroke. The prognosis may be relatively good even for those with focal infarction demonstrated on CT scan (Crisp *et al* 1981; Steinberg *et al* 1986). Repeated plasma infusions are the mainstay of treatment, but plasma exchange may be beneficial in those with severe disease (Pereira *et al* 1995).

HYPERTENSIVE ENCEPHALOPATHY

Hypertensive encephalopathy may complicate the course of a number of conditions, particularly those involving the kidneys. Cyclosporin, used for immunosuppression in transplantation, may potentiate the effects of minor degrees of hypertension to produce an identical clinical syndrome. The prognosis for hypertensive encephalopathy in childhood is usually good (Trompeter *et al* 1982; Wright and Mathews 1996). Visual symptoms may precede deterioration in consciousness and seizures are a common feature (Wright and Mathews 1996); neuroimaging may show low density in the white matter, particularly in the parietooccipital regions (Kandt *et al* 1995), but may be normal (Wright and Mathews 1996). Border zone infarction may occur if the blood pressure is reduced precipitately (Kandt *et al* 1995), which may be avoided by careful control of the appropriate antihypertensives with immediate infusion of plasma expanders if relative hypotension supervenes. Occasionally, children at risk of hypertensive encephalopathy, e.g. those with poststreptococcal glomerulonephritis, may have a cerebral arteritis as the underlying pathology for their seizures or focal signs (Kaplan *et al* 1993).

ARTERIOVENOUS MALFORMATIONS

Epilepsy as a presenting feature of arteriovenous malformations in childhood is a rare but accepted association. There is very little on this subject within the literature. Epilepsy is the second most frequent presenting symptom, ranging in incidence from 7% to 14% (Mori *et al* 1980; Gerosa *et al* 1981; Hladky *et al* 1994; Humphreys *et al* 1996); some studies report a higher incidence in adults than in children, while others report a similar incidence between the two groups (Waltimo 1973). Hladky *et al* (1994) reviewed the findings in 62 children who had presented with an arteriovenous malformation (AVM) for surgical treatment. They found only five (8%) who had seizures as a presenting symptom, with a further three where seizures occurred in association with the hemorrhage. However Humphreys *et al* (1996) reported seizures in 22/106 (14%).

No patient in Hladky's series who had an AVM revealed by epilepsy suffered an intracranial hemorrhage at a later stage (Hladky *et al* 1994). However, other series have suggested a higher mortality rate in children treated conservatively than in adults (Mori *et al* 1980; Kandt *et al* 1995) as well as a higher rebleed rate (Humphreys *et al* 1996). In part this may be secondary to the degree of bleeding, but also to the higher incidence of position within the posterior fossa (Humphreys *et al* 1996). There is some suggestion that the size of the lesion may influence the type of presentation, small AVMs having a greater tendency to bleed as opposed to larger AVMs, which are more frequently associated with epilepsy and neurologic deficits (Waltimo 1973), possibly caused by a 'blood steal' mechanism from the surrounding parenchyma (Celli *et al* 1984) (Fig. 13.3).

The decision on the most appropriate treatment, particularly with regard to when and whether surgery is appropriate, has to take into account the size of the lesion, the position of the lesion, and type of presentation. For seizures it would appear that a conservative approach could be considered, particularly if the lesion is large and within eloquent cortex, and

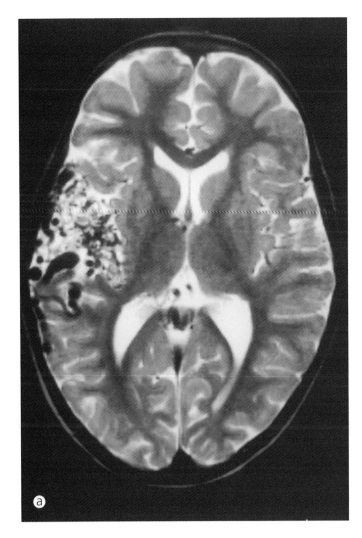

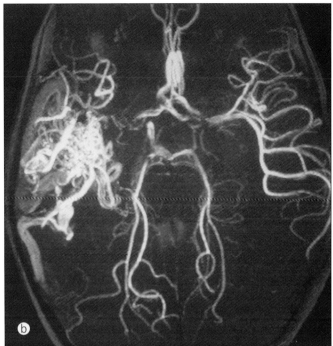

Fig. 13.3 MRI T2-weighted sequence transverse section from a 7-year-old girl with a drug-resistant epilepsy, showing a large arteriovenous malformation in the right cerebral hemisphere (a). The extent is clearly defined on the MR angiogram (b).

rediscussed only if drug resistance becomes apparent. Complete removal is required to eliminate risk of bleeding or seizure recurrence; in Humphreys' series, only 13/22 (59%) who underwent surgical procedures for AVM with epilepsy became seizure-free off anticonvulsant medication (Humphreys *et al* 1996). The presence of a large parenchymal hematoma was a long-term adverse factor for both seizures and persistent neurologic deficit.

Embolization of the AVM is becoming increasingly attractive, but those in children, particularly small malformations, can be difficult to cannulate and with large AVMs the risk of deficit is often greater than possible benefit. In addition, only a small number achieve complete resolution with this technique. Radiosurgery using the gamma knife can also be considered; adult studies suggest complete obliteration in 80% over 3 years. Gerszten *et al* reviewed the success of gamma-knife surgery in children with epilepsy as a presenting symptom: 11 of 15 children became seizure-free off medication, 2 showed significant

improvements but remained on medication and 2 developed seizures after treatment and remained on medication (Gerszten *et al* 1996).

Cavernous angiomas provide a slightly different picture. The majority are angiographically occult and went unrecognized until the advent of magnetic resonance imaging (Figs 13.4 and 13.5). In some series it is difficult to distinguish whether such have been included in the overall discussion of AVMs as a whole, while in others they have been excluded (Mori *et al* 1980). As in adults, epilepsy appears the most common presenting symptom rather than hemorrhage. In one pediatric series, 12/22 (55%) presented with epilepsy (Di Rocco *et al* 1996). As such lesions may lie close to eloquent cortex, and the risk of rebleed is small, surgical resection is reserved for those who demonstrate drug-resistant epilepsy or repeated hemorrhage. However, where resection is performed, in those where seizures are proven to arise from the area of the lesion and not within functionally useful cortex, there is a good prognosis with regard to postoperative seizure outcome (Guilion *et al* 1995; Di Rocco *et al* 1996; Zevgaridis *et al* 1996). However prognosis appears to be related to the duration of epilepsy prior to surgery (Zevgaridis *et al* 1996); therefore, in children with early-onset seizures surgery should perhaps be considered earlier rather than later.

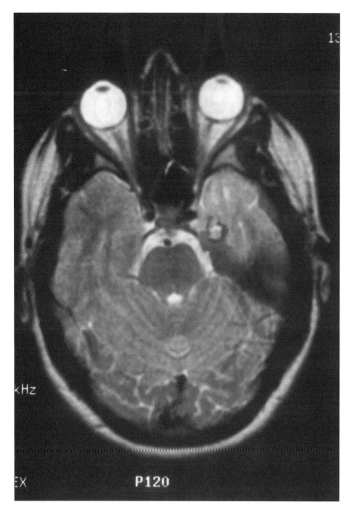

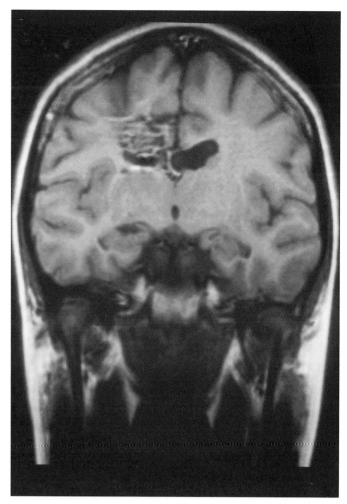

Fig. 13.4 MRI T2-weighted sequence transverse section from a 14-year-old girl who had a history of complex partial seizures of probable temporal lobe origin from the age of 2 years. A small lesion with the characteristics of a cavernous angioma can be seen in the left mesial temporal region.

Fig. 13.5 MRI T1-weighted sequence coronal section from a 15-year-old girl who had presented with left focal motor seizures at the age of 12 years. This shows a larger lesion also consistent with a cavernous angioma in the right parasagittal region, probably abutting motor cortex.

STURGE–WEBER SYNDROME

The cardinal neurologic features of Sturge–Weber syndrome (SWS) are epilepsy, hemiparesis, and learning disability in association with a pial angioma. Neurologic deterioration often occurs with the onset of seizures, commonly partial status epilepticus associated with the development of a transient or permanent hemiplegia (Arzimanoglou and Aicardi 1992).

The unilateral or bilateral angioma lies within the subarachnoid space. There is an abnormality of the cerebral venous system with few superficial cortical veins, enlargement of the deep medullary veins and choroid plexus, and stasis and slowing of the venous circulation (Probst 1986). The hemisphere underlying the angioma shows progressive gliosis, atrophy, and calcification (Marti-Bonmati *et al* 1993; Maria *et al* 1998); these changes are compatible with an ischemic process involving cortical and subcortical brain regions.

The pathogenesis of the ischemia and the cause of the neurologic deterioration in SWS remain controversial. Contralateral seizures and hemiparesis may be related to pathologic events within the angioma. There is some evidence for associated abnormalities of neuronal migration that might account for intractable epilepsy and hemiparesis (Simonati *et al* 1994). Vascular mechanisms could also explain the neurologic and neuropsychologic deterioration. Transient hemiparesis without evidence of ictal activity is well described in SWS and is considered to be related to an abnormal vasomotor response (Arzimanogla and Aicardi 1992). The ictal EEG may show focal slowing rather than spikes, particularly if the seizures are repeated (Aylett *et al* 1999). Interestingly, ictal slowing in association with ictal hypoperfusion on SPECT (single-photon emission computed tomography) is seen occasionally in focal seizures in patients without SWS as well (Cross *et al* 1997). In SWS there is also evidence for a failure of the cerebral blood flow to increase appropriately with vasodilator stimuli, including carbon dioxide (Riela *et al* 1985), acetazolamide (Okudaira *et al* 1997), and seizures (Aylett *et al* 1999). Anticonvulsant treatment is usually indicated if there is clinical and electroencephalographic evidence for epilepsy, and hemispherectomy may improve cognitive outcome compared with allowing the seizures to remain intractable. The use of aspirin appears to be associated with a 65% reduction in the incidence of stroke (Maria *et al* 1998). Use of anticoagulants has been reported anecdotally in a few patients with progressive hemiparesis without epilepsy.

MITOCHONDRIAL ENCEPHALOPATHY, LACTIC ACIDOSIS, AND STROKELIKE EPISODES (MELAS)

Initially the seizures in this condition are infrequent and are easily controlled with anticonvulsant medication. With the onset of the strokelike episodes, the seizures may become more frequent and may evolve into epilepsia partialis continua. A number of mitochondrial DNA mutations have been described as underlying this maternally inherited condition, but there is as yet no specific treatment.

CONDITIONS IN WHICH THE DISTINCTION BETWEEN EPILEPSY AND FOCAL ISCHEMIA MAY BE DIFFICULT

HEMISEIZURE–HEMIPLEGIA–EPILEPSY

This syndrome typically presented as a prolonged, usually febrile, lateralized convulsion with residual hemiparesis and the later development of partial epilepsy (Gastaut *et al* 1960). Findings on neuroimaging revealed initial swelling of the contralateral cerebral hemisphere, followed by global atrophy (Aicardi 1994). This was previously seen as a relatively common phenomenon, but has now considerably reduced in prevalence, probably as a consequence of more aggressive definition and treatment of status epilepticus.

RASMUSSEN ENCEPHALITIS

Rasmussen syndrome (chronic encephalitis and epilepsy) is a progressive condition, usually presenting between the ages of 3 and 10 years with hemiepilepsy (with epilepsia partialis continua in around 50%), progressive hemiplegia, and cognitive deterioration (see Chapter 19). The rate of progression of the disease is highly variable, but even in the

most rapid the evident evolution of the hemiparesis with seizures should be highly suggestive of this disease rather than ischemic injury resulting in seizures. In addition, although imaging may be unhelpful in some, progressive atrophy is seen rather than ischemic lesions.

ALTERNATING HEMIPLEGIA

This is a rare condition of unknown etiology in which there is evidence for an acute reduction of cerebral blood flow during the attacks. Children present in infancy with episodes of eye rolling or of tonic posturing and are often misdiagnosed as having epilepsy. The characteristic hemiplegic episodes do not usually manifest until the second year of life. Flunarizine reduces the number and severity of episodes in a proportion of these children. Many children with this condition also have epilepsy, which is often amenable to anticonvulsant treatment.

HEMIPLEGIC MIGRAINE

This diagnosis is not usually difficult in adults, as headache is a prominent feature. In children, however, hemiparesis, which may be very prolonged, may be the only manifestation, and the child may therefore be considered to have a Todd paresis after an unwitnessed convulsion (Lai *et al* 1982). Prominent unilateral slow-wave activity on EEG is typical and there may be imaging evidence for hemispheric swelling rather than infarction on the opposite side to the weakness (Connelly *et al* 1997).

ICTAL HEMIPARESIS

A phenomenon now well recognized is transient hemiparesis as a manifestation of a focal seizure, so-called ictal hemiparesis. This may be seen in acute presentation and therefore manifest as hemiparesis though in reality it is epilepsia partialis continua (inhibitory motor status) (Hanson and Chodos 1978; Smith *et al* 1997; Dale and Cross 1999), or as intermittent short-lived stereotypic episodes with or without other manifestations suggestive of seizures (Kofman and Tasker 1967; Globus 1982). As investigations may or may not be helpful, such a diagnosis may only be made retrospectively when a response is seen to anticonvulsants.

SUMMARY

Vascular disease is an important underlying etiology in childhood partial epilepsies and should always be considered in the differential diagnosis. The range of conditions that may cause epilepsy and either vascular disease or hemiparesis or both is very wide and, since treatment is often specified by the diagnosis, detailed investigation is mandatory, particularly if the episodes are atypical. Further research is required in this interesting area.

KEY POINTS

1. A vascular etiology underlies around 6% of childhood partial epilepsies. A wide range of conditions may cause epilepsy and vascular disease. They include causes of cerebral embolus and of sinovenous thrombosis, sickle cell disease, moyamoya disease, and MELAS.

2. Neonatal cerebral infarction is second only to hypoxic ischemic encephalopathy as an identifiable cause of seizures in full-term infants. Recurring seizures resulting from neonatal strokes are rare.

3. The incidence of seizures at the onset of ischemic and/or hemorrhagic stroke is higher in children (up to 36%) than in adults. It may be even higher in those with sinovenous thrombosis. Status epilepticus occurs in up to 8%.

4. The incidence of epilepsy following stroke in childhood (up to 30%) is higher than after stroke at an older age. Up to 20% of those who develop epilepsy may be medically intractable.

5. Moyamoya disease may present as a seizure disorder, especially hemiconvulsions, and it may be difficult to distinguish partial seizures from transient ischemic episodes.

6. Early surgery should be considered in children with Sturge-Weber Syndrome, particularly those presenting with seizures in the first few years of life.

7. Up to 14% of children with an arteriovenous malformation present with epilepsy. The epilepsy persists in around 40% after surgical removal of the malformation.

8. Epilepsy is the commonest childhood presentation of a cavernous angioma. Early surgical removal of these angiomas may be important because the chance of achieving complete postoperative seizure relief appears to decrease with increasing duration of the preoperative epilepsy.

REFERENCES

Adamolekun B, Durosinmi MA, Olowu W, Adeniran I (1993) The prevalence and classification of epileptic seizures in Nigerians with sickle cell anaemia. *Journal of Tropical Medicine and Hygeine* **96**:288–290.

Adams R, McKie V, Nichols F *et al* (1992) The use of transcranial ultrasonography to predict stroke in sickle cell disease [see comments]. *New England Journal of Medicine* **326**:605–610.

Adams RJ, Mckie VC, Hsu L *et al* (1998) Prevention of first stroke by transfusion in children with sickle cell anemia and abnormal results on transcranial Doppler ultrasonography. *New England Journal of Medicine* **339**:5–11.

Aicardi J (1994) *Epilepsy in Childhood.* New York: Raven Press.

Aicardi J and Chevrie JJ (1970) Convulsive status epilepticus in infants and children. A study of 239 cases. *Epilepsia* **11**:187–197.

Aicardi J, Amsili J, Chevrie JJ (1969) Acute hemiplegia in infancy and childhood. *Developmental Medicine and Child Neurology* **11**:162.

Alarcon F, Vanormelingen K, Moncayo J, Vinan I (1992) Cerebral cysticercosis as a risk factor for stroke in young and middle-aged people. *Stroke* **23**:1563–1565.

Andrew M, David M, deVeber G, Brooker LA (1997) Arterial thromboembolic complications in paediatric patients. *Thrombosis and Haemostasis* **78**:715–725.

Arzimanoglou A, Aicardi J (1992) The epilepsy of Sturge–Weber syndrome: clinical features and treatment in 23 patients. *Acta Neurologica Scandinavica Supplementum* **140**:18–22.

Aylett SE, Neville BGR, Cross JH, Boyd S, Chong WK, Kirkham FJ (1999) Sturge–Weber syndrome: cerebral haemodynamics during seizure activity. *Developmental Medicine and Child Neurology* **41**: 480–485.

Balkaran B, Char G, Morris JS, Thomas PW, Serjeant BE, Serjeant GR (1992) Stroke in a cohort of patients with homozygous sickle cell disease. *Journal of Pediatrics* **120**:360–366.

Barinagarrementeria F, Cantu C (1998) Frequency of cerebral arteritis in subarachnoid cysticercosis: an angiographic study. *Stroke* **29**:123–125.

Barron MF, Gusnard DA, Zimmerman RA, Clancy RR (1992) Cerebral venous thrombosis in neonates and children. *Pediatric Neurology* **8**:112–116.

Belman AL (1990a) AIDS and pediatric neurology. *Neurologic Clinics* **8**:571–603.

Belman AL, Roque CT, Ancona R, Anand AK, Davis RP (1990b) Cerebral venous thrombosis in a child with iron deficiency anemia and thrombocytosis. *Stroke* **21**:488–493.

Bogousslavsky J, Caplan L (1995) *Stroke Syndromes.* Cambridge: Cambridge University Press.

Brandt JR, Fouser LS, Watkins SL *et al* (1994) *Escherichia coli* O157:H7-associated hemolytic-uremic syndrome after ingestion of contaminated hamburgers. *Journal of Pediatrics* **125**:519–526.

Broderick J, Talbot GT, Prenger E, Leach A, Brott T (1993) Stroke in children within a major metropolitan area: the surprising importance of intracerebral hemorrhage. *Journal of Child Neurology* **8**:250–255.

Bryan RN, Levy LM, Whitlow WD, Killian JM, Preziosi TJ, Rosario JA (1991) Diagnosis of acute cerebral infarction: comparison of CT and MR imaging. *American Journal of Neuroradiology* **12**:611–620.

Cantu C, Barinagarrementeria F (1996) Cerebrovascular complications of neurocysticercosis. Clinical and neuroimaging spectrum. *Archives of Neurology* **53**:233–239.

Celli P, Ferrante L, Palma L, Cavedon G (1984) Cerebral arteriovenous malformations in children. Clinical features and outcome of treatment in children and in adults. *Surgical Neurology* **22**:43–49.

Chauvel P, Trottier S, Vignal JP, Bancaud J (1992) Somatomotor seizures of frontal lobe origin. *Advances in Neurology* **57**:185–232.

Claeys V, Deonna Th, Chrzanowski R (1983) Congenital hemiparesis: the spectrum of lesions. *Helvetica Paediatica Acta* **38**:439–455.

Clancy R, Malin S, Laraque D, Baumgart S, Younkin D (1985) Focal motor seizures heralding stroke in fullterm neonates. *American Journal of Diseases of Children* **139**:601–606.

Connelly A, Chong WK, Johnson CL, Ganesan V, Gadian DG, Kirkham FJ (1997) Diffusion weighted magnetic resonance imaging of compromised tissue in stroke. *Archives of Disease in Childhood* 77:38–41.

Crisp DE, Siegler RL, Bale JF, Thompson JA (1981) Hemorrhagic cerebral infarction in the hemolytic-uremic syndrome. *Journal of Pediatrics* 99:273–276.

Cross JH, Boyd SG, Gordon I, Harper A, Neville BGR (1997) Ictal cerebral perfusion related to EEG in intractable focal epilepsy of childhood. *Journal of Neurology, Neurosurgery and Psychiatry* 62:377–384.

Dale RC, Cross JH (1999) Ictal hemiparesis. *Developmental Medicine and Child Neurology* 41:344–347.

Di Rocco C, Iannelli A, Tamburrini G (1996) Cavernomas of the central nervous system in children. A report of 22 cases. *Acta Neurochirurgica* 138:1267–1274.

DiMario FJ Jr, Packer RJ (1990) Acute mental status changes in children with systemic cancer. *Pediatrics* 85:353–360.

Eke T, Talbot JF, Lawden MC (1997) Severe persistent visual field constriction associated with vigabatrin. *British Medical Journal* 314:1693.

Estan J, Hope P (1997) Unilateral neonatal cerebral infarction in full term infants. *Archives of Disease in Childhood* 76:88–93.

Fabian RH, Peters BH (1984) Neurologic complications of hemoglobin SC disease. *Archives of Neurology* 41:289–292.

Frank Y, Lim W, Kahn E, Farmer P, Gorey M, Pahwa S (1989) Multiple ischemic infarcts in a child with AIDS, *Varicella zoster* infection and cerebral vasculitis. *Pediatric Neurology* 5:64–67.

Fritsch G, Ebner F, Schneider G (1988) Computed tomography in partial epilepsies in childhood. *European Neurology* 28:306–310.

Gastaut H, Poirier F, Payan H, Salomon G, Toga M, Vigouroux M (1960) The HHE syndrome: hemiconvulsions-hemiplegia-epilepsy. *Epilepsia* 1:418–444.

Gerosa MA, Cappellotto P, Licata C, Iraci G, Pordatcher K, Fiore DC (1981) Cerebral artriovenous malformations in children (56 cases). *Child's Brain* 8:356–371.

Gerszten PC, Adelson PD, Kondziolka D, Flickinger JC, Lunsford LD (1996) Seizure outcome in children treated for arteriovenous malformations using gamma knife radiosurgery. *Pediatric Neurosurgery* 24:139–144.

Glauser TA, Siegel MJ, Lee BC, DeBaun MR (1995) Accuracy of neurologic examination and history in detecting evidence of MRI-diagnosed cerebral infarctions in children with sickle cell hemoglobinopathy. *Journal of Child Neurology* 10:88–92.

Globus M (1982) Ictal hemiparesis. *European Neurology* 21:165–168.

Goldman HB (1994) Is heparin really indicated in bacterial meningitis? *Archives of Neurology* 51:13.

Goutieres F, Challamel M-J, Aicardi J, Gilly R (1972) Les hemiplegies congenitales: semiologie, eitiologie et pronostic. *Archives Francaises de Pediatric* 29:839–851.

Greer HD III, Waltz AG (1965) Acute neurologic disorders of infancy and childhood. *Developmental Medicine and Child Neurology* 7:507–17.

Greer M, Schotland D (1962) Abnormal haemoglobin as a cause of neurologic disease. *Neurology* 12:114–123.

Guilion M, Acciarri N, Padovani R, Galassi E (1995) Results of surgery in children with cerebral cavernous angiomas causing epilepsy. *British Journal of Neurosurgery* 9:135–141.

Hanson PA, Chodos R (1978) Hemiparetic seizures. *Neurology* 28:920–923.

Hariman LMF, Griffith ER, Hurtig AL, Keehn MT (1991) Functional outcomes of children with sickle cell disease affected by stroke. *Archives of Physical Medicine and Rehabilitation* 72: 498–502.

Haring HP, Rotzer HK, Reindl H *et al* (1993) Time course of cerebral blood flow velocity in central nervous system infections. A transcranial Doppler sonography study. *Archives of Neurology* 50:98–101.

Hladky JP, Lejeune JP, Blond S, Pruvo JP, Dhellemmes P (1994) Cerebral arteriovenous malformations in children: report on 62 cases. *Child's Nervous System* 10:328–333.

Ho SS, Kuzniecky RI, Gilliam F, Faught E, Bebin M, Morawetz R (1997) Congenital porencephaly and hippocampal sclerosis. Clinical features and epileptic spectrum. *Neurology* 49:1382–1388.

Humphreys RP, Hoffman HJ, Drake JM, Rutka JT (1996) Choices in the 1990s for the management of pediatric cerebral arteriovenous malformations. *Pediatric Neurosurgery* 25:277–285.

Inagaki M, Koeda T, Takeshita K (1992) Prognosis and MRI after ischemic stroke of the basal ganglia. *Pediatric Neurology* 8:104–108.

Ishikawa T, Houkin K, Kamiyama H, Abe H (1997) Effects of surgical revascularization on outcome of patients with pediatric moyamoya disease. *Stroke* 28:1170–1173.

Ito M, Okuno T, Takao T, Konishi Y, Yoshioka M, Mikawa H (1981) Electroencephalographic and cranial computed tomographic findings in children with hemiplegic cerebral palsy. *European Neurology* 20:312–318.

Kandt RS, Caoili AQ, Lorentz WB, Elster AD (1995) Hypertensive encephalopathy in children: neuroimaging and treatment. *Journal of Child Neurology* 10:236–239.

Kaplan RA, Zwick DL, Hellerstein S, Warady BA, Alon U (1993) Cerebral vasculitis in acute post-streptococcal glomerulonephritis. *Pediatric Nephrology* 7:194–195.

Keidan I, Shahar E, Barzilay Z, Passwell J, Brand N (1994) Predictors of outcome of stroke in infants and children based on clinical data and radiologic correlates. *Acta Paediatrica* 83:762–765.

Kofman O, Tasker R (1967) Ipsilateral and focal inhibitory seizures. *Neurology* 17:1082–1086.

Konishi Y, Kuriyama M, Sudo M, Konishi K, Hayakawa K, Ishii Y (1987) Superior sagittal sinus thrombosis in neonates. *Pediatric Neurology* 3:222–225.

Krauss GL, Johnson MA, Miller NR (1998) Vigabatrin-associated retinal cone dysfunction: electroretinogram and ophthalmologic findings. *Neurology* 50:614–618.

Kugler S, Anderson B, Cross D *et al* (1993) Abnormal cranial magnetic resonance imaging scans in sickle cell disease. *Archives of Neurology* 50:629–635.

Kurokawa T, Chen YJ, Tomita S, Kishikawa T, Kitamura K (1985) Cerebrovascular occlusive disease with and without the moyamoya vascular network in children. *Neuropediatrics* 16:29–32.

Lai CW, Ziegler DK, Lansky LL, Torres F (1982) Hemiplegic migraine in childhood: diagnostic and therapeutic aspects. *Journal of Pediatrics* 101:696–699.

Levy SR, Abroms IF, Marshall PC, Rosquete EE (1985) Seizures and cerebral infarction in the full-term newborn. *Annals of Neurology* 17:366–370.

Lien JM, Towers CV, Quillgan EJ, de Veciana M, Toohey JS, Morgan MA (1995) Term early onset neonatal seizures: obstetric characteristics, etiologic classifications and perinatal care. *Obstetrics and Gynecology* 85:163–169.

Liu JE, Gzesh DJ, Ballas SK (1994) The spectrum of epilepsy in sickle cell disease. *Journal of Neurological Science* 123:6–10.

Mancini J, Girard N, Chabrol B *et al* (1997) Ischemic cerebrovascular disease in children: retrospective study of 35 patients. *Journal of Child Neurology* 12:193–199.

Manford MR, Fish DR, Shorvon SD (1996) Startle provoked epileptic seizures: features in 19 patients. *Journal of Neurology, Neurosurgery and Psychiatry* 61:151–156.

Maria BL, Neufeld JA, Rosainz LC *et al* (1998) Central nervous system structure and function in Sturge–Weber syndrome: evidence of neurologic and radiologic progression. *Journal of Child Neurology* 13:606–618.

Marti-Bonmati L, Menor F, Mulas F (1993) The Sturge–Weber syndrome: correlation between the clinical status and radiological CT and MRI findings. *Child's Nervous System* 9:107–109.

Meaney B, Curtis R, deVeber GA (1997) Post-stroke seizures in childhood: experience from the Canadian Pediatric Ischemic Stroke Registry (abstract). *Canadian Journal of Neurological Sciences* Supplement **1**:S45.

Medlock MD, Olivero WC, Hanigan WC, Wright RM, Winek SJ (1992) Children with cerebral venous thrombosis diagnosed with magnetic resonance imaging and magnetic resonance angiography. *Neurosurgery* **31**:870–876.

Mohr JW, Wilson H, Pang EJM (1982) Strokes and their management in sickle cell disease. In: Fried W (ed) *Comparative Clinical Aspects of Sickle Cell Disease*, pp 101–112. Basal: Elsevier North Holland.

Mori K, Murata T, Hashimoto N, Handa H (1980) Clinical analysis of arteriovenous malformations in children. *Child's Brain* **6**:13–25.

Murthy JM, Yangala R (1998) Etiological spectrum of symptomatic localization related epilepsies: a study from South India. *Journal of the Neurological Sciences* **158**:65–70.

Nair KP, Jayakumar PN, Taly AB, Arunodya GR, Swamy HS, Shanmugam V (1997) CT in simple partial seizures in children: a clinical and computed tomography study. *Acta Neurologica Scandinavica* **95**:197–200.

Nakase H, Ohnishi H, Touho H *et al* (1993) Long-term follow-up study of 'epileptic type' moyamoya disease in children. *Neurologia Medico-Chirurgica* **33**:621–624.

Ohene-Frempong K (1991) Stroke in sickle cell disease: demographic, clinical and therapeutic considerations. *Seminars in Hematology* **28**:213–219.

Ohene-Frempong K, Weiner SJ, Sleeper LA *et al* (1988) Cerebrovascular accidents in sickle cell disease: rates and risk factors. *Blood* **91**:288–294.

Okudaira Y, Arai H, Sato K (1997) Hemodynamic compromise as a factor in clinical progression of Sturge–Weber syndrome. *Child's Nervous System* **13**:214–219.

Packer RJ, Rorke LB, Lange BJ, Siegel KR, Evans AE (1985) Cerebrovascular accidents in children with cancer. *Pediatrics* **76**:194–201.

Pavlakis SG, Bello J, Prohovnik I *et al* (1988) Brain infarction in sickle cell anemia: magnetic resonance imaging correlates. *Annals of Neurology* **23**:125–130.

Pavlakis SG, Prohovnik I, Piomelli S, DeVivo DC (1989) Neurologic complications of sickle cell disease. *Advances in Pediatrics* **36**:247–276.

Pereira A, Mazzara R, Monteagudo J *et al* (1995) Thrombotic thrombocytopenic purpura/hemolytic uremic syndrome: a multivariate analysis of factors predicting the response to plasma exchange. *Annals of Hematology* **70**:319–323.

Perlstein MA, Hood PN (1954) Infantile spastic hemiplegia I. Incidence. *Pediatrics* **14**:436–441.

Portnoy BA, Herion JC (1972) Neurologic manifestations in sickle cell disease. *Annals of Internal Medicine* **76**:643–652.

Powars DR, Weiss JN, Chan LS, Schroeder WA (1984) Is there a threshold level of fetal hemoglobin that ameliorates morbidity in sickle cell anemia? *Blood* **63**:921–926.

Probst FP (1986) Vascular morphology and angiographic flow patterns in Sturge–Weber angiomatosis: facts, thoughts and suggestions. *Neuroradiology* **20**:73–78.

Riela A, Stump D, Roach S (1985) Regional cerebral blood flow characteristics of the Sturge–Weber syndrome. *Pediatric Neurology* **1**:85–90.

Rivkin MJ, Anderson ML, Kaye EM (1992) Neonatal idiopathic cerebral venous thrombosis: an unrecognised cause of transient seizures or lethargy. *Annals of Neurology* **32**:51–56.

Roach ES and Riela AR (1995) *Pediatric Cerebrovascular Disorders*, 2nd edn. New York: Futura, Armonk.

Satoh S, Shirane R, Yoshimoto T (1991) Clinical survey of ischemic cerebrovascular disease in children in a district of Japan. *Stroke* **22**:586–589.

Schoenberg BS, Mellinger JF, Schoenberg DG, Barringer FS (1977) Moyamoya disease presenting as a seizure disorder. *Archives of Neurology* **34**:511–512.

Shirane R, Sato S, Yoshimoto T (1992) Angiographic findings of ischemic stroke in children. *Child's Nervous System* **8**:432–436.

Shuper A, Packer RJ, Vezina LG, Nicholson HS, Lafond D (1995) 'Complicated migraine-like episodes' in children following cranial irradiation and chemotherapy. *Neurology* **45**:1837–1840.

Simonati A, Colamaria V, Bricolo A, Dalla Bernardina B, Rizzuto N (1994) Microgyria associated with Sturge–Weber angiomatosis. *Child's Nervous System* **10**:392–395.

Smith RF, Devinsky O, Luciano D (1997) Inhibitory motor status: two new cases and a review of inhibitory motor seizures. *Journal of Epilepsy* **10**:15–20.

So EL, Annegers JF, Hauser WA, O'Brien PC, Whisnant JP (1996) Population-based study of seizure disorders after cerebral infarction. *Neurology* **46**:350–355.

Sran SK, Baumann RJ (1988) Outcome of neonatal strokes *American Journal of Diseases of Children* **142**:1086–1088.

Steinberg A, Ish-Horowitcz, El-Peleg O, Mor J, Branski D (1986) Stroke in a patient with hemolytic-uremic syndrome with a good outcome. *Brain Development* **8**:70–72.

Suzuki J, Takatu A (1969) Cerebrovascular 'moyamoya' disease: disease showing abnormal net-like vessels in base of brain. *Archives of Neurology* **20**:288–299.

Tibbles JAR, Brown BStJ (1975) Acute hemiplegia of childhood. *Canadian Medical Association Journal* **113**:309–314.

Trevathan E, Dooling EC (1987) Large thrombotic strokes in hemolytic-uremic syndrome. *Journal of Pediatrics* **111**:863–866.

Trompeter RS, Smith RL, Hoare RD, Neville BG, Chantler C (1982) Neurological complications of arterial hypertension. *Archives of Disease in Childhood* **57**:913–917.

Uvebrant P (1988) Hemiplegic cerebral palsy aetiology and outcome *Acta Paediatrica Scandinavica* s**345**:65–67.

Vargha-Khadem F, Isaacs E, van der Werf S, Robb S, Wilson J (1992) Development of intelligence and memory in children with hemiplegic cerebral palsy: the deleterious consequences of early seizures. *Brain* **115**:315–329.

Waltimo O (1973) The relationship of size, density and localisation of intracranial arteriovenous malformations to the type of initial symptom. *Journal of Neurological Science* **19**: 13–19.

Wanifuchi H, Kagawa M, Takeshita M, Izawa M, Kitamura K (1988) Ischemic stroke in infancy, childhood and adolescence. *Child's Nervous System* **4**:361–364.

Watkins KE, Hewes DKM, Connelly A, *et al* (1998) Cognitive deficits associated with frontal lobe infarction in children with sickle cell disease. *Developmental Medicine and Child Neurology* **40**:536–543.

Wiklund LM, Uvebrant P (1991) Hemiplegic cerebral palsy: correlation between CT morphology and clinical findings. *Developmental Medicine and Child Neurology* **33**:512–523.

Wolff M (1998) Congenital hemiplegia: correlations between lesion patterns and childhood epilepsies. *Epilepsia* **39**s2:92.

Wong VK, LeMesurier J, Franceschini R, Heikali M, Hanson R (1987) Cerebral venous thrombosis as a cause of neonatal seizures. *Pediatric Neurology* **3**:235–237.

Wright RR, Mathews KD (1996) Hypertensive encephalopathy in childhood. *Journal of Child Neurology* **11**:193–196.

Yang JS, Park YD, Hartlage PL (1995) Seizures associated with stroke in childhood. *Pediatric Neurology* **12**:136–138.

Young AC, Borgcostarzi J, Molir PD, St Clair Forbes W (1982) Is routine computerised axial tomography in epilepsy worthwhile? *Lancet* **2**:1446–1447.

Zevgaridis D, van Velthoven V, Ebeling U, Reulen HJ (1996) Seizure control in supratentorial cavernous malformations: a retrospective study in 77 patients. *Acta Neurochirgica* **138**:672–677.

Posttraumatic seizures and posttraumatic epilepsy

C CHANDLER

The relationship between trauma and seizures has been recognized since the time of Hippocrates (Temkin 1945). Posttraumatic epilepsy is the second most common type of acquired symptomatic epilepsy, accounting for about 20% of cases in a geographical population (Bergamini *et al* 1977; Annegers *et al* 1980). Assessment of risks and determination of incidence are difficult and controversial owing to the difficulty in evaluating published work, much of which is based on speculative studies rather than carefully controlled clinical trials. These limitations have been succinctly analyzed (Deymeer and Leviton 1985). This in turn has led to a lack of consensus among neurosurgeons, neurologists, and other clinicians about the treatment of posttraumatic seizures (PTSz) and posttraumatic epilepsy (PTE) in head-injured patients. Two excellent population studies (one recently extended) of the incidence of posttraumatic seizures and posttraumatic epilepsy have for many years guided clinicians who are not infrequently called upon to quantify these risks (Jennett 1975; Annegers *et al* 1980, 1986). Two other studies (Black *et al* 1972; Hahn *et al* 1988) looked specifically at the risks in head-injured children, and in one of them comparison was made with a control group of siblings who had not suffered head injuries (Black *et al* 1972).

The precise pathophysiology of posttraumatic seizures and posttraumatic epilepsy remains unknown, but an increasing knowledge of the structural and biochemical changes that occur in damaged brain tissue affords a potential understanding of what may initiate and sustain this condition.

The primary treatment of posttraumatic seizures and posttraumatic epilepsy remains medical, but surgery has evolved into an accepted alternative when posttraumatic epilepsy becomes intractable or drug resistant.

DEFINITIONS

Clear definitions are essential for evaluating the range of studies of posttraumatic seizure disorders, yet one of the major impediments in synthesizing all of the work that has been done is the inconsistency in definitions. Seizures are defined as finite events, consisting of an occasional, excessive, disorderly discharge of nerve tissue (Hughlings Jackson 1931), whereas epilepsy is a chronic disorder characterized by recurrent seizures (Gastaut 1973). The etiologies of posttraumatic seizures and posttraumatic epilepsy are almost certainly different, carrying different prognoses and requiring different treatments.

There is now general agreement that posttraumatic seizures are usually subdivided into early seizures, occurring within the first 7 days after the injury, and late seizures, occurring after the first week. Early seizures may also be further subdivided into immediate seizures, defined as those occurring within the first 24 hours, and delayed early seizures, defined as those occurring between 24 hours and 7 days. Posttraumatic epilepsy is more appropriately used to define the situation in which the patient suffers more than two late seizures.

Most studies differentiate between penetrating and nonpenetrating head injuries, as well as defining the severity of the head injury in any one individual. In this chapter, head injury severity will be defined as mild (Glasgow Coma Score (GCS) 14–15), moderate (GCS 9–13), or severe (GCS ≤8), and the chapter will concentrate upon civilian injuries, the majority of which are blunt and nonpenetrating.

The clinician must also bear in mind the important difference between prophylactic anticonvulsant treatment versus treatment in patients who have already suffered a seizure. Prophylaxis refers to the administration of antiepileptic drugs (AED) to prevent the occurrence of seizures in patients following head injury.

INCIDENCE

Clinicians are frequently called upon to quantify the risks of posttraumatic seizures at various times following a head injury or following a neurosurgical procedure. In the published studies it is again difficult to ascertain this owing to large variations in definitions, method of follow-up, and study bias. Those studies in which only the hospital records are used may underestimate the true incidence of posttraumatic seizures. Owing to the high cost of long-term follow-up, some studies have concentrated only on those patients who were considered to be at high risk (Jennett and Lewin 1960; Hendrick and Harris 1968; Jennett 1975). Head-injured patients also represent a difficult group to follow up: they may be poor attenders, poor at complying with treatment, and are at risk of further head injuries that may substantially alter their incidence of posttraumatic seizures.

The incidence of epilepsy in the general population is estimated to be between 0.5% and 2%. Population studies have shown an overall incidence of posttraumatic seizures, including both early-onset and late-onset seizures, of 2–2.5% for all types of civilian head injury (Jennett 1975;

Annegers *et al* 1980), rising to 5% for hospitalized neurosurgical patients (Jennett 1975). These figures underestimate the substantially higher incidence of posttraumatic seizures in severely (GCS ≤8) head-injured patients. In patients sustaining severe head injuries, the overall incidence is 10–15% for adults (Annegers *et al* 1980; Temkin *et al* 1990) and 30–35% for children (Hahn *et al* 1988). In most military series (which contain a substantially higher number of penetrating injuries), the overall incidence is relatively constant at about 30–35%, although the incidence may go as high as 50% in those with penetrating injuries (Salazar *et al* 1985). Again, cogent interpretation of results is marred by wide differences in definitions, inclusion and exclusion criteria, length of follow-up, and treatment.

The incidence of early posttraumatic seizures ranges from 2% to 6%, spread evenly over the first 7 days after injury (Jennett 1975; Annegers *et al* 1980; Temkin *et al* 1995), with a higher rate for children. The ratio of partial to generalized seizures is approximately equal within the first week (Caveness *et al* 1979). An early seizure in an apparently mildly head-injured patient identifies a group of patients whose head injuries must be investigated further, as a significant number will be found to have a more serious underlying brain injury (Lee and Lui 1992).

In comparison, although the incidence of early posttraumatic seizures in children is much higher, the incidence of both late posttraumatic seizures and posttraumatic epilepsy is much lower. The higher incidence of early posttraumatic seizures in children compared with adults can be accounted for by a much higher incidence of immediate (impact) seizures (Black *et al* 1972; Hahn *et al* 1988). The incidence of posttraumatic seizures in children shows considerable variation between studies, ranging from 1.3–15% (early posttraumatic seizures) to 0.2–12% (late posttraumatic seizures); with the overall incidence ranging from 7% to 15% (Hendrick and Harris 1968; Mises *et al* 1970; Black *et al* 1972; Jennett 1975; Hahn *et al* 1988). In common with the experience in adults, the incidence of posttraumatic seizures rises with the severity of the head injury, and the highest incidence of late posttraumatic seizures occurred in those children who had early posttraumatic seizures. Posttraumatic status epilepticus is more common in children, consistent with its increased overall incidence in children.

Within the first year, the incidence of late posttraumatic seizures in head-injured patients exceeds the incidence of epilepsy in the general population by approximately 12% (Caveness 1976). The incidence of late-onset seizures falls with time, with approximately 50% remitting spontaneously, although in patients who have sustained a penetrating injury the seizure risk remains elevated for up to 15 years (Salazar *et al* 1985). Excluding patients who suffer from early posttraumatic seizures, of those who suffer a late posttraumatic seizure 25% will have only one seizure, and 50% or more will have fewer than four seizures (Jennett 1975; Salazar *et al* 1985; Temkin *et al* 1995). Five years after a head injury, the risk of posttraumatic seizures falls to within normal values for the population (Annegers *et al* 1980), penetrating injuries excepted. In a civilian population, 27% had their first seizure within 3 months, 50–66% within 1 year, and 75–85% within 2 years of their head injury (Jennett 1975). Jennett also found that the later the onset of posttraumatic epilepsy (it is important to note that he included patients who had a single seizure) the more likely it was to be persistent (i.e. true posttraumatic epilepsy). Interestingly, similar figures for late seizure onset, 50% within 9 months and 75–80% within 2 years, have been found in military cohorts despite the significantly higher percentages of penetrating injuries (Walker and Erculi 1970; Caveness *et al* 1979). In all studies, civilian and military, the time course for development of late posttraumatic seizures was remarkably constant regardless of the risk factors. In penetrating injury, there did not appear to be any significant relationship between onset latency, seizure frequency, time between first and subsequent seizures, or persistence (Salazar *et al* 1985). In a geographical population study, a significant percentage of those whose first posttraumatic seizures occurred late went on to have posttraumatic epilepsy (Annegers *et al* 1980, 1998).

Although the area of brain affected will determine the semeiology of the seizures, posttraumatic seizures are similar to those occurring in other types of epilepsy. Early posttraumatic seizures tend to become secondarily generalized (Lee and Lui 1992), and although most patients with late posttraumatic seizures have had at least one generalized seizure, partial seizures represent the majority of late posttraumatic seizures particularly when associated with posttraumatic epilepsy (Jennett 1975; Caveness *et al* 1979; Salazar *et al* 1985). Compared with generalized seizures, focal seizures have a greater tendency to be recurrent (Weiss and Careness 1972). These may secondarily generalize, and patients may demonstrate multiple seizure types. In posttraumatic epilepsy the ratio of partial to generalized seizures was about 3:1; focal seizures tended to be more frequent than generalized and to be associated with a longer duration of posttraumatic epilepsy, and patients tended to have a higher overall frequency of seizures (Caveness *et al* 1979).

PATHOPHYSIOLOGY

Head trauma initiates a cascade of structural and biochemical changes that may include disruption of the blood–brain barrier, altered cerebral blood flow, edema, intracranial hypertension, and excitotoxic neurotransmitter release. Though the exact underlying etiology of posttraumatic seizures remains unknown, in many cases a cortical lesion is probably the most important underlying feature in the genesis of seizures. This damage may be caused iatrogenically during an operation or by head trauma, and the macroscopic lesion is almost certainly a hemorrhagic contusion of the brain parenchyma. Immediate and early posttraumatic seizures most probably represent an acute nonspecific response to the physical effects of the head injury and are probably not in themselves epileptogenic. On a microscopic level there may be tearing or stretching of axons, followed later by the formation of retraction balls, collagenous fibrosis, and glial proliferation, with variable destruction of the cortical layers. Focal ischemia, hemorrhage, and necrosis may also occur as secondary injuries. Any of these may exacerbate the primary injury and play a contributory role in the genesis of posttraumatic seizures.

Newer neuroimaging techniques demonstrate some predictive advantages. CT evidence of parenchymal damage or intracerebral hemorrhage within 48 hours of injury correlated well with posttraumatic epilepsy (D'Alessandro *et al* 1982, 1988), and in head-injured children any CT abnormality was associated with a significantly higher likelihood of posttraumatic seizures (Hahn *et al* 1988). Given the higher resolution and specificity of MRI scanning in detecting parenchymal abnormalities, it would seem that this modality may in the future be a more accurate tool for quantifying the risk of posttraumatic epilepsy. Other functional imaging techniques such as PET (positron emission tomography) and SPECT (single-photon emission computed tomography) have not been investigated extensively in the context of posttraumatic seizures or posttraumatic epilepsy, but are widely used in the investigation of patients with intractable epilepsy and may also play a more important role in the future.

The underlying neurophysiologic event is a paroxysmal depolarization shift (PDS), which is an abnormally large prolonged depolarizing postsynaptic potential that can lead to burst firing of neurons and recruitment of other neurons. This results in either focal EEG spikes or ictal activity and clinical evidence of the seizure. Neuronal membrane function, transmitter release, and intracellular ion fluxes may all be altered by head trauma. Any of these factors may alter the firing threshold of a neuron or population of neurons leading to burst firing and seizure initiation.

The concept of kindling (Goddard 1967; Goddard *et al* 1969) has been used as a model for posttraumatic epilepsy. In this model a repeated subthreshold stimulus such as might be initiated by an area of damaged brain leads to lasting changes in brain function. Progressively lower levels of stimulation are able to initiate seizures until eventually seizures occur spontaneously, leading to the establishment of a permanent seizure disorder. The evidence that this occurs in humans is controversial and, if accurate, cannot explain why posttraumatic seizures regress spontaneously in approximately 50% of patients.

Most of the recognized risk factors for posttraumatic seizures or posttraumatic epilepsy involve contact between blood and cortical tissue (Jasper 1970). The association between hemorrhagic intracranial pathology, both spontaneous (hemorrhagic (cerebrovascular accident) –intracerebral hematoma), and traumatic (contusions, intracerebral, subdural, and extradural hematomas), and epilepsy suggests that the liberation of hemoglobin into the parenchyma is an important link in the development of posttraumatic epilepsy (DeCarolis *et al* 1984; Faught *et al* 1989; Kilpatrick *et al* 1990). As the presence of blood in contact with the neuropil appears to define a group at high risk of posttraumatic seizures or posttraumatic epilepsy, the theory that hemorrhage following trauma initiates biochemical or structural changes that may be important in the generation of posttraumatic epilepsy must be given some weight. Human studies have demonstrated that the presence of hemosiderin is, at a microscopic level, a prominent histopathologic feature in the brains of patients with posttraumatic epilepsy (Payan *et al* 1970). Most work has focused upon the iron component as the most important because animal studies have demonstrated the powerful epileptogenic potential of iontophoretically applied iron (Willmore *et al* 1978) as well as the ability of iron salts and those hemoglobin degradation products containing iron to cause focal necrosis, gliosis, and recurrent seizures (Willmore *et al* 1978; Rosen and Frumin 1979). The main theories of how iron deposition leads to seizure activity center on damage to the cell membrane by free radical-mediated lipid peroxidation (Willmore 1990). The free radical-initiated lipid peroxidation of cell membranes is catalyzed by free iron released from hemoglobin, transferrin, or ferritin. Within brain tissue that has been traumatized or rendered ischemic, or both, conditions are favorable for the release of iron from storage proteins – ferritin intracellularly and transferrin extracellularly – in addition to iron from hemorrhage (Hall 1996). Autooxidation of iron is a naturally occurring reaction that leads to the production of free

radicals such as superoxide, hydroxyl, singlet oxygen, and perferryl ions. These free radicals may then react with cell membranes, initiating a vicious circle of lipid peroxidation and the further generation of free radicals. Naturally occurring enzyme systems of limited capacity (superoxide dismutase, catalase, glutathione peroxidase, and peroxidase) exist exclusively within the intracellular space to mop up excess free-radical species and prevent them damaging the cell membrane. Within the extracellular space, protection is mediated by binding of iron, as hemoglobin, to carrier proteins that include transferrin, lactoferrin, ceruloplasmin, and haptoglobins. Once iron is released, it can actively catalyze reactions that produce oxygen free radicals.

Excitotoxicity refers to the toxic accumulation of excitatory neurotransmitters such as glutamate or aspartate, which overexcite the postsynaptic neuron and may, by doing so, damage this neuron. Glutamate is the most widely distributed of these compounds, and has been shown to accumulate following head trauma (Katayama *et al* 1990). Hemorrhage may substantially increase the amount of glutamate, since its concentration in blood is about one thousand times greater than in brain tissue (Duhaime 1994).

Head trauma, through its biochemical and cellular effects, may overwhelm these natural control systems, allowing the production of excess amounts of free radicals, with the consequent damage to the neuronal cell membranes resulting in the generation of an epileptogenic focus. Pretreatment with antioxidants such as α-tocopherol and selenium has been demonstrated to reduce the iron-induced histopathologic damage in animals, lending further weight to the lipid peroxidation theory (Willmore and Rubin 1981).

The study of familial seizures and the idea that levels of heme-binding proteins may be genetically determined have led to the suggestion that an individual's ability to clear free radicals, and hence the individual's susceptibility to posttraumatic seizures, may have a genetic component (Caveness *et al* 1979).

SPECIFIC RISK FACTORS

When the published data are reviewed in perspective, simplistic relationships are not immediately identified, with one exception. There seems to be a consistent relationship between the extent of damage and the incidence of seizures. Immediate seizures (within the first 24 hours) or impact seizures (occurring within 1 hour), particularly, are considered an acute response to trauma, while late posttraumatic seizures are more directly related to an epileptogenic focus and the potential for posttraumatic epilepsy. A summary of the most important risk factors is given in Table 14.1.

The group of patients at greatest and most prolonged risk of both of early and late posttraumatic seizures, as well as posttraumatic epilepsy, are those who have sustained penetrating craniocerebral injuries, an association that has been confirmed in a number of studies, primarily in a military setting (Walker and Yablon 1961; Salazar *et al* 1985). As discussed above, there is a robust association between acute subdural hematoma, intracerebral hematoma, cortical lacerations, hemorrhagic contusions, and posttraumatic epilepsy (Jennett 1975; Annegers *et al* 1980; Desai *et al* 1983), although the relative risk in patients with acute extradural hematomas is low (Jamjoon *et al* 1991). In a civilian population, the strongest risk factors for late posttraumatic seizures were subdural hematoma and brain contusion, both independently and jointly (Annegers *et al* 1998).

The relationship between skull fractures and posttraumatic seizures is not clear-cut. Skull fractures may be complicated by the presence of posttraumatic amnesia, underlying contusions or lacerations, and focal signs, which are themselves independently associated with an increased risk of seizures. Prolonged posttraumatic amnesia and focal signs are more common in patients with depressed skull fractures that tear the dura, and these confounding variables may account for the increased incidence of late posttraumatic seizures in this group of patients. The location of the fracture is also relevant. Those patients whose fractures occur in the region of the central sulcus have the highest incidence of posttraumatic seizures (Caveness *et al* 1979).

Coma (GCS ≤ 8) lasting longer than 24 hours was strongly associated with both early and late posttraumatic seizures (Annegers *et al* 1980). Early posttraumatic seizures are a significant risk factor for late posttraumatic seizures, though less so in children (Jennett and Lewin 1960; Annegers *et al* 1980). Jennett found that 25–35% of adults

who suffered an early seizure went on to develop late seizures, while in a military series more than 50% of those who had early posttraumatic seizures went on to develop late seizures (Caveness *et al* 1979). Although early posttraumatic seizures are a recognized risk factor, the seizure may be only a marker of the severity of the underlying injury (itself the true risk factor). This idea is supported by studies in which the incidence of early posttraumatic seizures was reduced by AED treatment, with no reduction upon the incidence of late posttraumatic seizures (North *et al* 1983; Temkin *et al* 1990).

Intracranial hematomas, especially acute subdural hematomas, are strongly predictive of both early and late posttraumatic seizures and posttraumatic epilepsy. The incidence of early posttraumatic seizures for all types of traumatic intracranial hemorrhage ranges from 19% to 25% in adults (Jennett 1975; Annegers *et al* 1980) and 32% in children (Hahn *et al* 1988). Late posttraumatic seizures occur in 14–35% of adults who sustain a traumatic intracranial hematoma (Jennett 1975; Annegers *et al* 1980).

In children, the major risk factors were found to be any neurologic deficit, and coma lasting more than 1 hour (Black *et al* 1972). In this study the seizure risk was directly proportional to the presence and duration of coma: no coma (7%), coma shorter than 1 hour (15%), coma longer than 1 hour (55%) (Black *et al* 1972). Looking specifically at early posttraumatic seizures, 50% were focal and 50% generalized, although those who sustained generalized early posttraumatic seizures were more likely to have late posttraumatic seizures (Black *et al* 1972). In a much larger study that analyzed 937 children up to 16 years of age who were admitted to hospital after a head injury, the important risk factors were found to be GCS 3–8, diffuse cerebral edema (43% risk), and acute subdural hematoma (32% risk). In this series, seizures were twice as common in children who had abnormal CT scans, and there was no increased incidence in patients who sustained simple skull fractures (Hahn *et al* 1988). The greatly increased incidence of posttraumatic seizures in those children with severe head injuries (35%) compared with those who had minor head injuries (5.1%) was consistent with other studies.

Genetic influences have been postulated to affect an individual's susceptibility to posttraumatic seizures, although this has never been proven. This view is given credence by the remarkably constant overall incidence of posttraumatic epilepsy through a number of wars in spite of significant advances in treatment, and in civilian series, suggesting that the underlying constitutional tendency towards epilepsy is more important than previously believed (Caveness *et al* 1979).

Table 14.1 Specific risk factors for early or late posttraumatic seizures.

Early posttraumatic seizures	Late posttraumatic seizures
Penetrating injuries	
Intracranial hematomas	
Hemorrhagic contusions	
Cortical lacerations	
Linear/depressed skull fracture	Depressed skull fracture
Coma lasting > 24 hours	
Focal neurologic deficit	Early posttraumatic seizures
Children < 5 years old	

TREATMENT

EARLY POSTTRAUMATIC SEIZURES

Aggressive treatment of early posttraumatic seizures in individuals with moderate or severe head injuries is one of the mainstays of modern head-injury management, as the deleterious effects of seizures on a traumatized vulnerable brain are now well recognized. Seizures lead to increased cerebral blood flow leading to raised intracranial pressure; increased cerebral metabolic requirements (glucose utilization, lactate production, cellular/systemic acidosis); release of excitotoxic neurotransmitters; and compromised respiration (hypoxemia, hypercapnia). Any of these may, individually or in combination, cause or exacerbate cerebral edema, cerebral ischemia, and necrosis. The physical movements during a seizure may cause further damage to a patient with multiple injuries, and postictal alterations in the level of consciousness may compromise neurologic assessment. For these reasons, those individuals who are either at high risk or have early posttraumatic seizures should be treated with AED for the first week only or until the acute effects of the head injury have abated and then the AED should be stopped. There is now solid evidence from published studies of the effectiveness of both phenytoin and carbamazepine in controlling early posttraumatic seizures (Glotzner et al 1983; Temkin et al 1990). The conclusions of these studies are summarized in Table 14.2. It was at one time widely believed that prevention of early posttraumatic seizures would reduce the likelihood of developing posttraumatic epilepsy; this idea is discussed in the next section.

Surgical treatment (i.e. evacuation of hematomas, debridement of foreign material, and resection of nonviable brain) in the acute phase of head-injury management is aimed at reducing the pathologic changes in the brain tissue, though the surgery itself may cause some trauma, which might lead to formation of a meningocerebral cicatrix, which is recognised as a potential epileptogenic focus (Penfield and Jasper 1954).

LATE POSTTRAUMATIC SEIZURES AND ANTICONVULSANT PROPHYLAXIS

The use of AED to treat posttraumatic epilepsy may be separated into two issues: (a) are AED indicated in treating patients with late posttraumatic seizures? and (b) do AED, given prophylactically, prevent the onset of posttraumatic epilepsy? Given that individuals who sustain posttraumatic seizures have a higher than average rate of posttraumatic epilepsy and that 75% of individuals who sustain a late posttraumatic seizure will have more than one seizure, the answer to (a) would appear to be yes.

On (b) there is a lack of consensus. Many clinicians would give prophylactic AED to prevent posttraumatic seizures in perceived high-risk patients upon the assumption that late-onset posttraumatic seizures will render the individual more susceptible to further seizures or to posttraumatic epilepsy. There are significant risks to a patient who develops posttraumatic epilepsy, and one must also consider the risk of medicolegal consequences if AED are not given.

When considering the potential adverse effects of posttraumatic epilepsy such as sudden or accidental death, injury, cognitive, behavioral, and psychosocial sequelae, and also loss of livelihood or driver's licence, there seems to be a clear role for its treatment. Balanced against the benefits of stopping or reducing further posttraumatic seizures are the potentially deleterious effects of the treatment itself, which may be significant (Dikmen et al 1991; Foy et al 1992; Smith et al 1994). In 1972, a survey of neurosurgeons demonstrated that more than 60% recommended the use of prophylactic AED to prevent the development of posttraumatic epilepsy (Rapport 1973). Prophylactic AED were initially believed to prevent posttraumatic epilepsy (Wohns 1979) however, well-constructed studies (Table 14.2) have clearly shown that there is no advantage in treating individuals with prophylactic AED to reduce the incidence of late-onset posttraumatic seizures or posttraumatic epilepsy. There are also documented potentially life-threatening adverse effects related to the drugs themselves. Only those who suffer from more than one late posttraumatic seizure or posttraumatic epilepsy should be given AED, and they should continue treatment for as long as is necessary according to known yearly incidences in defined patient groups.

Phenytoin, although it does not affect the underlying cause of the seizures, is the most widely used AED in treating posttraumatic seizures. Its efficacy has been assessed in numerous trials (McQueen et al 1983; Young et al 1983a,b,c; Temkin et al 1990), and it can be given intravenously. Carbamazepine, and sodium valproate are also useful in the treatment of late posttraumatic seizures or posttraumatic epilepsy, and there does not appear to be any particular advantage of one over the other.

Table 14.2 Double-blind controlled studies of the prophylaxis of posttraumatic epilepsy.

Study	Number of cases	Drug	Conclusions
Penry *et al* (1979)	125	Phenytoin+phenobarbital	NSE of AED on late PTSz
Young *et al* (1983a,b)	244	Phenytoin	NSE of AED on early or late PTSz
Temkin *et al* (1990)	404	Phenytoin	Significant reduction in early PTSz by AED NSE of AED on late PTSz
McQueen *et al* (1983)	164	Phenytoin	NSE of AED on late PTSz
Glotzner *et al* (1983)	139	Carbamazepine	Significant reduction in early PTSz by AED NSE of AED on late PTSz
Manaka (1992)	126	Phenobarbital	NSE of AED on late PTSz

AED, antiepileptic drugs; NSE, no significant effect; PTSz, posttraumatic seizures.

POSTOPERATIVE SEIZURES

Patients who have undergone intracranial neurosurgical procedures represent a heterogeneous group with a highly variable incidence of postoperative seizures. Again owing to methodological differences, variable follow-up, and different underlying pathologies, it is difficult to determine precise incidences of postoperative seizures. Foy *et al* studied 1000 patients undergoing a range of neurosurgical procedures and found an overall incidence of 17% (range 12–36%), with a not unexpected higher incidence in those with preoperative seizures (Foy *et al* 1981a). Similar rates of postoperative seizures were found in patients who underwent craniotomy for treatment of either benign or malignant tumors or aneurysms providing they did not have preoperative seizures (Foy 1981a,b). Unsurprisingly, higher incidences were identified in those undergoing craniotomy versus those undergoing burr hole procedures. This supports the idea, which has been confirmed in other studies, that treatment by craniotomy adds to the intrinsic risk of epilepsy from the underlying pathology (Cabral *et al* 1976a,b).

The most important factor influencing the incidence of postoperative seizures after aneurysm surgery relates to the presence of a postoperative neurologic deficit rather than to the site of the aneurysm, although clearly the risk is less with posterior fossa aneurysms (Keranen *et al* 1985; Jennett *et al* 1990).

Shunt operations showed considerable variation with the incidence of postoperative seizures ranging from 9% (Dan and Wade 1986) to 24% (Copeland *et al* 1981). Factors associated with an increased risk of seizures included multiple revisions, a frontal ventricular catheter, and infection (Copeland *et al* 1981; Dan and Wade 1986). It must also be borne in mind that patients with hydrocephalus often have associated underlying or concomitant CNS pathologies which may carry an independent risk of seizures.

SURGERY FOR POSTTRAUMATIC EPILEPSY

If a patient with posttraumatic epilepsy becomes refractory to drug treatment, surgery may offer a viable therapeutic opportunity. Surgical treatment represents an enormous challenge in these patients. The seizure focus is often extratemporal, may be diffuse, and is frequently located within eloquent areas of the brain. The principles of treatment mirror those of the surgical treatment of other types of epilepsy, namely, rigorous identification of the epileptogenic focus by both invasive and non-invasive investigations, establishing the safety of resection, and intraoperative recording both pre and post resection. The results vary widely according to pathology and site.

CONCLUSIONS

Early postraumatic seizures should be treated aggressively to prevent complications and or damage to an acutely traumatized brain. Patients who have posttraumatic seizures should be treated with AED in the same way as other patients with epilepsy. There is evidence that treatment of early posttraumatic seizures is effective at reducing the incidence of seizures in the early period only. There is no evidence that prophylaxis has any effect on the incidence of late posttraumatic seizures or posttraumatic epilepsy.

There does not appear to be any advantage in treating posttraumatic seizures with any particular drug, although most drug studies have focused upon phenytoin, carbamazepine, sodium valproate, and phenobarbital. The treatment should be determined by the nature of the seizures and the individual.

KEY POINTS

1. Head trauma is the second most common cause of acquired symptomatic epilepsy. The incidence of late (>one week posttrauma) posttraumatic seizures (PTSz) exceeds the incidence of epilepsy in the general population by around 12% during the first year after injury. Amongst civilians most injuries are 'blunt' rather than penetrating and the data presented here largely pertain to blunt injuries.

2. Around 80% of first PTSz occur within 2 years of the injury. Five years after injury the incidence falls within the range for the normal population. Around 50% of those who develop late PTSz have no more than 3 and remit spontaneously.

3. Seizures occur in 10–15% adults and 30–35% children after severe head trauma (Glasgow Coma Score <9).

   The risk of late PTSz is increased by penetrating injury, intracranial hematoma (up to 35% in adults), hemorrhagic contusion and cortical laceration, depressed skull fracture, coma lasting >1 hour for children (up to 55%) or >24 hours for adults, and early (first 7 days) PTSz (up to 35% of adults). The risk of the latter (early PTSz) is increased by all the other factors and also by the presence of focal neurological deficit and age <5 years.

4. Early PTSz after moderate/severe head trauma are deleterious because they exacerbate the tendency to cerebral edema, ischemia and necrosis and because the mechanical movements of the seizures may aggravate multiple injuries. Those at high risk or who suffer a PTSz should be treated with phenytoin or carbamazepine for one week or until the acute effects of the head trauma have abated.

5. There is no evidence that prophylactic treatment with an antiepileptic drug will reduce the incidence of late PTSz or posttraumatic epilepsy (PTE). Antiepileptic medication should, however, be given to those who develop PTE. Phenytoin, carbamazepine and sodium valproate are equally efficacious.

6. Neurosurgical procedures carry a risk of postoperative seizures, craniotomy more so than burr holes, thereby adding to the risk from the underlying pathology. Shunt operations also impose a risk that is increased by multiple revisions, the ventricular catheter being frontal, and infection.

REFERENCES

Annegers JF, Grabow JD, Goover RV, Laws AR, Elveback LR, Kurland LT (1980) Seizures after head trauma: a population study. *Neurology* 30:683–689.

Annegers JF, Kennedy CR, Freeman JM (1986) Post traumatic seizures and post traumatic epilepsy in children. *Journal of Head Trauma Rehabilitation* 1:466–73.

Annegers JF, Hauser WA, Coan SP, Rocca WA (1998) A population based study of seizures after traumatic brain injury. *New England Journal of Medicine* 338:20–24.

Bergamini L, Bergamasco B, Benna P, Gilli M (1977) Acquired etiological factors in 1,785 epileptic subjects in clinical-amnestic research. *Epilepsia* 18:437–444.

Black P, Shepard RH, Walker AE (1972) A prospective study of post-traumatic seizures in children. *Transactions of the American Neurology Association* 97:247–250.

Cabral R, King TT, Scott DF (1976a) Incidence of post-operative epilepsy after a transtentorial approach to acoustic nerve tumours. *Journal of Neurology, Neurosurgery and Psychiatry* 39:663–665.

Cabral R, King TT, Scott DF (1976b) Epilepsy after two different neurosurgical approaches to the treatment of ruptured intracranial aneurysms. *Journal of Neurology, Neurosurgery and Psychiatry* 39:1052–1056.

Caveness WF (1976) Epilepsy a product of trauma in our time. *Epilepsia* 17:207–215.

Caveness WF, Meirowsky AM, Rish BL *et al* (1979) The nature of post traumatic epilepsy. *Journal of Neurosurgery* 50:545–553.

Copeland GP, Foy PM, Shaw MDM (1981) The incidence of epilepsy after ventricular shunting operations. *Surgical Neurology* 17:279–281.

D'Alessandro R, Tinuper P, Ferrara R et al (1982) CT scan prediction of late post traumatic epilepsy. *Journal of Neurology, Neurosurgery and Psychiatry* 45:1153–1155.

D'Alessandro R, Ferrara R, Benassi G *et al* (1988) Computed tomographic scans in posttraumatic epilepsy. *Archives of Neurology* 45:42–43.

Dan NQ, Wade MJ (1986) The incidence of epilepsy after ventricular shunting operations. *Journal of Neurosurgery* 65:19–21.

DeCarolis P, D'Allesandro R, Ferrara R, Andreoli A, Sacquegna T, Lugaresi E (1984) Late seizures in patients with internal carotid and middle cerebral artery occlusive disease following ischaemic events. *Journal of Neurology, Neurosurgery and Psychiatry* 47:1345–1347.

Desai BT, Whitman S, Coonley-Hoganson, R *et al* (1983) Seizures and civilian head injuries. *Epilepsia* **24**:289–296.

Deymeer F, Leviton A (1985) Post traumatic seizures: an assessment of the epidemiological literature. *Central Nervous System Trauma* **2**:33–42.

Dikmen SS, Temkin NR, Miller B *et al* (1991) Neurobehavioral effects of phenytoin prophylaxis of post traumatic seizures. *Journal of the American Medical Association* **265**:1271–1277.

Duhaime A-C (1994) Exciting your neurons to death: can we prevent cell loss after brain injury? *Paediatric Neurosurgery* **21**:117–123.

Faught E, Peters D, Bartolucci A, Moore L, Miller PC (1989) Seizures after primary intracerebral haemorrhage. *Neurology* **39**:1089–1093.

Foy PM, Copeland GP, Shaw MDM (1981a) The incidence of post operative seizures. *Acta Neurochirugia* **55**:253–264.

Foy PM, Copeland GP, Shaw MDM (1981b) The natural history of post operative seizures. *Acta Neurochirurgia* **57**:15–22.

Foy PM, Chadwick DW, Rajgopalan N, Johnson AL, Shaw MD (1992) Do prophylactic anticonvulsants alter the pattern of seizures after craniotomy? *Journal of Neurology, Neurosurgery and Psychiatry* **55**:793–797.

Gastaut H (1973) *Dictionary of Epilepsy.* Geneva: World Health Organization.

Glotzner FL, Haubitz I, Miltner F *et al* (1983) Anfallsprophylaze mit carbamazepin nach schweren schadelhirnverletzungen. *Neurochirurgia* **26**:66–79.

Goddard GV (1967) Development of epileptic seizures through brain stimulation at low intensity. *Nature* **214**:1020–1021.

Goddard GV, McIntyre DC, Leech CK (1969) A permanent change in brain function resulting from daily electrical stimulation. *Experimental Neurology* **25**:295–330.

Hahn YS, Fuchs S, Flannery AM, Barthel MJ, McLone DG (1988) Factors influencing post traumatic seizures in children. *Neurosurgery* **22**:864–867.

Hall ED (1996) Mechanisms of secondary CNS injury. In: Palmer J (ed) *Neurosurgery 1996*, pp 505–510. New York: Churchill Livingstone.

Hendrick EB, Harris L (1968) Post traumatic epilepsy in children. *Journal of Trauma* **8**:547–555.

Hughlings Jackson J (1931) *Selected Writings of John Hughlings-Jackson: On Epilepsy and Epileptiform Convulsions*, vol 1. London: Hodder and Staughton.

Jamjoon AB, Kane N, Sandeman DR, Cummins B (1991) Epilepsy related to traumatic extradural haematomas. *British Medical Journal* **302**:448.

Jasper HH (1970) Physiopathological mechanisms of post traumatic epilepsy. *Epilepsia* **11**:73–80.

Jennett WB (1975) *Epilepsy After Non-Missile Injuries*, 2nd edn. London: William Heinemann Medical.

Jennett WB, Lewin W (1960) Traumatic epilepsy after closed head injuries. *Journal of Neurology, Neurosurgery and Psychiatry* **233**:295–301.

Jennett WB, Crandon I, Kay M (1990) Late epilepsy after aneurysm. *Journal of Neurology, Neurosurgery and Psychiatry* **53**:812.

Katayama Y, Becker DP, Tamura T, Hovda DA (1990) Massive increases in extracellular potassium and the indiscriminate release of GLU following concussive brain injury. *Journal of Neurosurgery* **73**:889–890.

Keranen T, Tapaninaho A, Hernesniemi J, Vapalahti M (1985) Late epilepsy after aneurysm operations. *Neurosurgery* **17**:897–890.

Kilpatrick CJ, Davis SM, Tress BM, Rossiter SC, Hopper JL, Vandendriesen ML (1990) Epileptic seizures in acute stroke. *Archives of Neurology* **47**:157–160.

Lee S-T, Lui T-N (1992) Early seizures after mild closed head injury. *Journal Neurosurgery* **76**:435–439.

Manaka S (1992) Cooperative prospective study on post traumatic epilepsy: risk factors and the effect of prophylactic anticonvulsant. *Japanese Journal of Psychiatry and Neurology* **46**:311–315.

McQueen, JK, Blackwood DHR, Harris P *et al* (1983) Low risk of late post traumatic seizures following severe head injury: implications for clinical trials of prophylaxis. *Journal of Neurology, Neurosurgery and Psychiatry* **46**:899–904.

Mises J, Lerique-Koechlin A, Rimbot BP (1970) Post traumatic epilepsy in children. *Epilepsia* **70**:37–39.

North JB, Penhall RK, Harish A *et al* (1983) Phenytoin and postoperative epilepsy: a double blind study. *Journal of Neurosurgery* **58**:672–677.

Payan H, Toga M, Berard-Badier M (1970) The pathology of post traumatic epilepsies. *Epilepsia* **11**:81–94.

Penfield W, Jasper H (1954) *Epilepsy and the Functional Anatomy of the Human Brain*. Boston: Little Brown.

Penry JK, White BG, Brackett CE (1979) A controlled prospective study of the pharmacologic prophylaxis of post traumatic epilepsy. *Neurology* **29**:600–601.

Rapport RL, Penry JK (1973) A survey of attitudes toward the pharmacological prophylaxis of post traumatic epilepsy. *Journal of Neurosurgery* **38**:159–166.

Rosen AD, Frumin NV (1979) Focal epileptogenesis following intracortical haemoglobin injection. *Experimental Neurology* **66**:277–284.

Salazar AM, Jabbari B, Vance SC, Grafman J, Amin D, Dillon JD (1985) Epilepsy after penetrating head injury. I. Clinical correlates: a report of the Vietnam Head Injury Study. *Neurology* **35**:1406–1414.

Smith KR, Goulding PM, Wilderman D, Goldfader PR, Holterman-Hommes P, Wei F (1994) Neurobehavioral effects of phenytoin and carbamazepine in patients recovering from brain trauma: a comparative study. *Archives of Neurology* **51**:653–660.

Temkin O (1945) *The Falling Sickness. A History of Epilepsy from the Greeks to the Beginnings of Modern Neurology*. Baltimore: Johns Hopkins Press.

Temkin NR, Dikmen SS, Wilensky AJ, Kihm J, Chabal S, Winn HR (1990) A randomized double blind study of phenytoin for prevention of post traumatic seizures. *New England Journal of Medicine* **323**:497–502.

Temkin NR, Haglund MM, Winn HR (1995) Causes, prevention and treatment of post traumatic epilepsy. *New Horizons* **3**:518–522.

Walker AE, Erculi F (1970) Post traumatic epilepsy 15 years later. *Epilepsia* **11**:17–26.

Walker AE, Yablon S (1961) A follow-up study of head wounds in World War 2. Washington DC: Veterans Administration.

Weiss GH, Caveness WF (1972) Prognostic factors in the persistence of post traumatic epilepsy. *Journal of Neurosurgery* **37**:164–169.

Willmore LJ (1990) Post traumatic epilepsy: cellular mechanisms and implications for treatment. *Epilepsia* **31**(suppl. 3):S67–73.

Willmore LJ, Rubin JJ (1981) Anti-peroxidant pretreatment and iron induced epileptiform discharge in the rat: EEG and histopathologic study. *Neurology* **31**:63–69.

Willmore LJ, Sypert GW, Munson JB, Hurd RW (1978) Chronic focal epileptiform discharges induced by injection of iron into rat and cat cortex. *Science* **4**:329–336.

Wohns RNW, Wyler AR (1979) Prophylactic phenytoin in severe head injuries. *Journal of Neurosurgery* **51**:507–509.

Young B, Rapp RP, Norton JA, Haack D, Tibbs PA, Bean JR (1983a) Failure of prophylactically administered phenytoin to prevent early post traumatic seizures. *Journal of Neurosurgery* **58**:231–235.

Young B, Rapp RP, Norton JA, Haack D, Tibbs PA, Bean JR (1983b) Failure of prophylactically administered phenytoin to prevent late post traumatic seizures. *Journal of Neurosurgery* **58**:236–241.

Young B, Rapp RP, Norton JA, Haack D, Walsh JW (1983c) Failure of prophylactically administered phenytoin to prevent post traumatic seizures in children. *Child's Brain* **10**:185–192.

Tumors and partial seizures

JJ RIVIELLO JR, M HONAVAR, AND GL HOLMES

Seizures occur frequently with brain tumors, both malignant and benign, and brain tumors may even present with a seizure. Seizures are caused by the tumor because of involvement with the surrounding cortex or more distal areas, and may respond to antiepileptic drugs (AEDs) or produce a chronic, intractable seizure disorder. Seizures may also result from the various treatments of tumors, including surgery, chemotherapy, and radiation therapy. This chapter reviews aspects of epilepsy related to tumors, in both adults and children, including the incidence, presentation, and clinical manifestations, the evaluation, pathology, including dual pathology, and therapy. The controversy about surgical management and seizure control, either with gross total resection alone or resection of both the lesion and the adjacent epileptogenic region, are discussed. Where appropriate, the sections are divided between adults and children.

INCIDENCE

Seizures frequently occur with brain tumors, yet brain tumors are not a frequent cause of seizures. The overall incidence of brain tumors in the population varies from 1 in 20 000 to 1 in 100 000 (Walker *et al* 1985), whereas the incidence of epilepsy is 1% by the age of 20 years, but the cumulative incidence by the age of 75 years is 3%. Recent neuroepidemiologic data reveal an increasing incidence, especially for lymphomas in men (Ahsan *et al* 1995) and for lymphomas and glioblastoma multiforme (GBM) in both sexes, especially the elderly (Werner *et al* 1995).

There have been several large community-based epidemiological studies of epilepsy, most notably from Rochester, Minnesota, and the UK. In a study on the etiology of epilepsy over a span of 40 years in Rochester, brain tumors were responsible for 3.6% (Hauser *et al* 1993). In the National General Practice Study of Epilepsy (NGPSE) in the UK, tumors caused 6% of newly diagnosed cases of epilepsy (Sander *et al* 1990). In both of these studies, the peak incidence of epilepsy caused by tumors is in middle age. In the NGPSE, 30% of adults with newly diagnosed seizures had a brain tumor. In the Rochester study, the incidence of seizures related to tumors was nonexistent in the age group of 0–4 years, increased to about 30% in the age bands 25–44 and 45–64, and decreased after the age of 65 years. In several other recent studies, the incidence of tumors varies from 16% of 221 patients with new-onset seizures after age 25, described by Dam *et al* (1985), through 11% of new-onset adult seizures over a 20-month period in Sweden (Forsgren 1990), to only 0.5% of 1000 consecutive cases of new-onset seizures in adults in Saudi Arabia (al-Rajeh *et al* 1990).

Tumors rarely cause seizures in children. Aicardi (1992) reported an overall incidence of about 0.2–0.3%. The Rochester data showed an incidence of 1% in those less than age 15 years (Hauser *et al* 1993), and the NGPSE had an incidence of 1% in those less than age 30 years (Sander *et al* 1990). There is a lower incidence of seizures in children with brain tumors, partly because posterior fossa tumors (infratentorial) are more common in children and less likely to cause seizures than supratentorial tumors. In an early study from the Mayo Clinic of seizures as a manifestation of tumors in 291 children, infratentorial tumors occurred in 165 (57%) and supratentorial tumors in 126 (43%), and seizures occurred in 50 children (17%) (Backus and Millichap 1962). The Childhood Brain Tumor Consortium database identified 3291 children with brain tumors and seizures (Gilles *et al* 1992). The location was infratentorial in 1421 (51%) and supratentorial in 1339 (49%). Fourteen percent had seizures prior to tumor diagnosis. The overall incidence of epilepsy in those children with supratentorial tumors was 25%. There were a total of 1339 children with supratentorial tumors; 37 children were excluded because there was not sufficient location data. There was an age-dependent variability in supratentorial seizures: seizures occurred in 6% of infratentorial tumors in all age groups, whereas with supratentorial tumors, there were 1196 children aged 0–13 years of whom 22% had seizures, but among 136 patients aged 14–20 seizures occurred in 46% and among those aged 17 years or more it was 68%.

PRESENTATION AND CLINICAL MANIFESTATIONS

Seizures are classified by their site of origin, as either partial seizures (focal, local, localization-related) or generalized seizures (Commission on Classification and Terminology of the International League Against Epilepsy (ILAE) 1989). Partial seizures can be divided into those in which there is no impairment of consciousness (simple partial) and those in which there is some impairment of consciousness (complex partial). Partial seizures may spread and become generalized (secondary generalization). Partial seizures may begin with an aura, which can have localizing significance, although the aura may not be recalled, whereas a generalized seizure has immediate loss of consciousness. But if a seizure begins focally and the discharge spreads rapidly, no overt focal features occur and the outward clinical manifestations are of a generalized process. However, the partial nature of the seizure may subsequently be determined by either focal features on EEG or neuroimaging. The terms primary bilateral synchrony and secondary bilateral synchrony are used: primary bilateral synchrony refers to a generalized discharge, beginning in all areas simultaneously, and secondary bilateral synchrony refers to a seizure that begins in one location and then spreads to all areas.

Two factors are important in regards to the clinical manifestations of a tumor – the location and the tissue type. Tumors are usually solitary, located in one cortical area, and, therefore, seizures associated with tumors have a partial onset, with clinical manifestations dependent on the cortical site of origin. For example, if the discharge begins in motor cortex, the initial clinical manifestations will be motor, whereas if the seizure begins in sensory cortex, the initial manifestations are sensory. In addition, a seizure may begin in one area and then spread to another area, with different patterns evolving with the spread. A seizure may also begin in a silent area (a location not causing any clinical manifestations), and then spread to another area and if clinical manifestations are produced, the seizure will appear to start in the area to which it was propagated, rather than from where it actually started, resulting in false localization.

A focal lesion may present with apparent generalized epilepsy, including a generalized EEG. The responsible lesions include those in the frontal lobes, mesial temporal lobes, the parasagittal areas, and deep midline structures. The EEG pattern of intermittent rhythmic delta activity (IRDA), generated from subcortical structures, may appear generalized and yet result from deep midline lesions. The 3 Hz spike and wave pattern, an EEG pattern seen in absence seizures, occurs in tumors more often than by chance alone (Ajmone-Marsan and Lewis 1960). Ferrie *et al* (1995) recently reviewed absence seizures with focal cerebral pathology, and identified 22 patients with brain tumors and EEG findings suggestive of absence epilepsy. Only 12 of these had clinical absences and most had either clinical or EEG features suggesting secondary bilateral synchrony. The frontal lobes were the most common site of origin, especially the medial surfaces of the intermediate frontal regions, but the cingulate gyrus and the temporal lobe were less common sites of seizure origin.

In general, tumors present in the following ways, dependent upon the location: infratentorial tumors (posterior fossa) present with increased intracranial pressure, headache, vomiting, papilledema, ataxia, and cranial nerve signs, whereas supratentorial tumors have presenting manifestations that vary on tumor location. Seizures are more common with slowly growing supratentorial tumors, whereas rapidly growing tumors, such as a glioblastoma multiforme (GBM), usually present with focal deficits from mass effect or increased intracranial pressure.

In adults, seizures are the most common presentation of low-grade gliomas (Cascino 1990). In a large series from Montreal of 230 patients with gliomas, seizures occurred in 70% of astrocytomas, 92% of oligodendrogliomas, and in 37% of GBMs (Penfield *et al* 1940).

Astrocytomas are classified as either low-grade or high-grade. Low-grade astrocytomas include pilocytic astrocytomas, and high-grade astrocytomas include GBM and anaplastic astrocytoma. In a study of 51 cystic pilocytic astrocytomas of the hemispheres, epilepsy was the most frequent presenting symptom, occurring in 68%, and the most common sign was papilledema, seen in 85% (Palma and Guidetti 1985). In a study of seizure disorders in 65 patients with malignant gliomas, 47 had GBM and 18 had anaplastic astrocytoma. Twenty-nine patients presented with seizures, and 21 had a recurrence of their seizures. Of 36 patients without initial seizures, 10 later developed seizures, and 5 of these 10 had only a single seizure. Thirteen patients had more than one seizure per month, and most recurrent or late-onset seizures occurred despite therapeutic AED levels. Preoperative seizures were a predictor of postoperative seizures, and seizures tended to be refractory. Patients with preoperative seizures tended to continue to have seizures postoperatively and these were likely to be refractory to medication. The median survival time was 18 months (Moots *et al* 1995).

The oligodendroglioma has a high incidence of seizures. The largest clinicopathologic study of oligodendrogliomas, from the Armed Forces Institute of Pathology, identified 323 patients. Headache was the most common symptom, occurring in 170 patients (78%). Seizures were the next frequent symptom, present in 163 (70%) (Ludwig *et al* 1986). In a specific study of seizures in 34 patients with oligodendroglial cell tumors, 25 patients (75%) presented with seizures. The age at diagnosis in those with seizures was much younger than those without (median 36 years versus 57 years). Of nine patients who were initially seizure-free, three developed seizures between 25 and 36 months following treatment. After a mean follow-up period of 30 months, 20 of 25 patients who presented with seizures were alive; 8 of these 20 were seizure-free (40%), and 3 (15%) had experienced less than three postoperative seizures (Whittle and Beaumont 1995).

There was also a significant incidence of epilepsy in patients with meningiomas. In a study of 323 patients with meningiomas, aged between 10 and 79 years, preoperative seizures occurred in 98 (30.3%). Among these 98 patients there were 32 who continued to have seizures postoperatively (32.7%). In the 225 patients without preoperative

seizures, 39 (17.3%) developed seizures after surgery. Postoperative seizures in the first week were caused by edema and hemorrhage at the surgical site, whereas postoperative seizures occurring more than 1 week after surgery were associated with tumor recurrence. Postoperative seizures were more likely if there had been preoperative seizures, and were related to residual tumor, postoperative hemorrhage or edema, and inadequate AED therapy (Chow *et al* 1995). The occurrence of edema is a significant factor in seizures with meningioma. In a specific study of peritumoral edema in 83 patients with meningiomas by Lobato *et al* (1996), the patients were divided into two groups: group A comprised 27 patients who had presented with seizures and group B contained 56 patients who had presented with other symptoms. The area of peritumoral edema was significantly greater in group A, suggesting edema as an epileptogenic factor. Of interest is the fact that generalized seizures were more common with frontal lesions, and partial seizures were more common with a central or parietal lesion (Kawaguchi *et al* 1996).

Seizure control may ultimately occur even with postoperative seizures. In a study of 158 patients with supratentorial meningiomas, 63 patients had preoperative seizures, and of these, 40 (63.5%) had no postoperative seizures. Complete seizure control occurred in 12 of 13 patients (92%) of those with less than three postoperative seizures compared with only four of ten patients with more than three postoperative seizures. Six variables were predictive of postoperative seizures: preoperative seizure history, preoperative language disturbance, extent of tumor removal, parietal location of tumor, postoperative AED status, and postoperative hydrocephalus (Chozick *et al* 1996).

Three recent studies of elderly patients with new-onset seizures show that tumors are a common cause of epilepsy in this age group. In a study of new-onset epilepsy after age 60, stroke was the most frequent cause, seen in 25 patients, and 18 patients had tumors; six had a high-grade glioma, six a meningioma, and six a metastatic lesion (Henny *et al* 1990). In another study, tumors were responsible for epilepsy in 14% of the patients; 15 of their 21 tumors were metastatic lesions, 5 were GBM, and 1 was a meningioma (Luhdorf *et al* 1986). Tumors were the cause of status epilepticus in 8% of those with new-onset seizures after 60 years of age (Sung and Chu 1989).

In children, either headache or seizure is the most frequent presenting symptom. Aicardi (1994) reported the seizure type in 48 children with tumors who presented with a seizure and 28 of these patients had multiple seizure types. Partial motor seizures occurred in 16, unilateral seizures in 7, partial sensory seizures in 8, partial complex seizures in 14, and atypical seizures in 18, generalized attacks in 20, absences in 1, infantile spasms in 1, myotonic and/or atypical absences in 4, and unclassified seizures in 10. In a series of 98 children from the Childrens' Hospital, Boston, with supratentorial astroglial neoplasms and seizures, 50% had seizures as part of their presentation and 30% had seizures as their only presenting complaint (Shady et al 1994). Headaches occurred in 49%, vomiting in 43%, and papilledema in 34%. The seizure could be classified in 43 of 49: complex partial in 58%, simple partial in 30%, secondarily generalized in 23%, generalized tonic–clonic in 2%, tonic in 2%, and atonic in 5%. Tumors involving cerebral cortex significantly correlated with seizures at presentation as compared to noncortical locations; 59% of patients with cortical tumors presented with seizures and only 15% of patients with noncortical tumors experienced seizures. The highest incidence occurred with frontal and temporal lesions.

Several unusual presentations occur in children. Only 2% of children less than 1 year of age with tumors present with a seizure (Rutledge et al 1987). Infantile spasms are rarely caused by tumors (Asanuma et al 1995; Kotagal et al 1995). Landau–Kleffner syndrome, or acquired epileptiform aphasia, has been reported in children with temporal lobe astrocytomas (Nass et al 1993; Solomon et al 1993) and dysembryoplastic neuroepithelial tumors (DNTs) (Raymond et al 1994b), and Lennox–Gastaut syndrome, or childhood epileptiform encephalopathy, with slow-spike wave on EEG, has been reported in a 2-year-old with a temporal lobe astrocytoma, who became seizure-free after resection (Angelini et al 1979).

Patients may have years of intractable epilepsy before a tumor is discovered. This scenario was more frequent prior to modern neuroimaging, with computed axial tomography (CT) scan and magnetic resonance imaging (MRI), when only plain skull radiographs, pneumoencephalography, and angiography were available, but this may still occur with certain tumors. How frequently does this occur? In 190 adults with intractable epilepsy from Yale, 15% had an unsuspected intracranial mass lesion and 10% had a neoplasm (Spencer et al 1984). In 10 450 children evaluated in the Seizure Unit at Children's Hospital, Boston, over a 15-year period, 23 had seizures for 3 years or more prior to tumor detection, with subsequent surgical verification of a glioma (Page et al 1969). This represented only 0.3% of this patient population. In these 23 patients, unilateral or focal EEG abnormalities were not present initially but delta activity developed in 20 of them, 12 patients had a deterioration in their personality or school performance in the 2 years preceding the diagnosis, 14 patients developed a hemiparesis, and papilledema occurred in 12 of the 23 patients described. Therefore, changes in behavior and school

performance, type and frequency of seizures, the neurologic examination, and EEG were considered important factors suggesting a tumor. Of historical interest, this study was done because it was thought that children with chronic epilepsy never had brain tumors. Two decades later, Blume et al (1982) reported that 16 out of 35 patients less than 21 years of age who underwent epilepsy surgery were discovered to have brain tumors (46%). Children with tumors that presented with either progressive neurologic deficit or increased intracranial pressure were excluded. Twelve of these sixteen patients had astrocytomas, two had oligodendrogliomas, one had a GBM, and one a ganglioglioma. Initial CT scans showed the tumor in six, five were discovered on a subsequent scan, and three with normal CT scans had the tumor discovered at surgery. Brain scan and pneuomoencaphalography discovered the other two tumors. Clinical signs of progression occurred in only one patient, in whom progressive dementia developed. Persistent delta activity on EEG was especially helpful: a tumor was found in 10 of 14 patients with persistent delta activity (71%), but in only 6 of the 20 patients without persistent delta activity (30%). A tumor was more likely with normal intelligence and neurologic examinations, and when another reason for the seizures was not present.

Brain tumors may also present with an intracranial hemorrhage as the first manifestation of the tumor, in both adults and children, which may then result in a seizure. The exact mechanism of epileptogenesis with brain tumors is not known. Slowly growing tumors such as astrocytomas, oligodendrogliomas, and gangliogliomas are more likely to cause seizures than more rapidly growing lesions, with seizures occurring in 90% of oligodendrogliomas and gangliogliomas (Pilcher et al 1993). It is postulated that there may be more of an adverse effect on surrounding neurons with a chronic lesion (Penfield et al 1940), related to hypoxic–ischemic changes, and that the mass effect from the tumor results in structural or chemical injury in adjacent neurons (Berger et al 1991). In a study of the cortex surrounding low-grade astrocytomas, Haglund et al (1992) found decreased γ-aminobutyric acid (GABA) and somatostatin neurons in epileptic, nontumor-infiltrated foci, compared to nonepileptic, nontumor cortex from the same patients. These findings implicate hyperexcitable cortex surrounding these lesions. Marco et al (1997), from Spain, studied the cortex surrounding the tumor from a patient with epilepsy and a brain tumor. Immunocytochemistry and quantitative electron microscopy compared the synaptic densities of presumptive excitatory and inhibitory synapses to those in normal cortex. They found a loss of inhibitory synapses on the soma and axon initial segment of pyramidal cells, and numerous excitatory synapses were present on dendrites that would cause a hyperexcitable state. Other postulated reasons include tumor-induced abnormalities of the N-methyl D-aspartate (NMDA)-receptor, axonal calcium or chloride channels, or denervation hypersensitivity (Engel 1989). Hippocampal sclerosis may also be responsible as discussed under Dual Pathology below.

SEIZURES RELATED TO THERAPY

Postoperative seizures may occur, even in those without preoperative seizures. Postoperative seizures have been related to many factors, including the presence of preoperative seizures, surgical manipulation, edema, hemorrhage, stroke, metabolic alterations, including hyponatremia and acidosis, and subtherapeutic AED levels (Table 15.1). In two studies of postoperative seizures after various neurosurgical procedures, the incidence of postoperative seizures was 6% in the first study (Gerstle de Pasquet et al 1976) and 8.9% in the second (Fukamuchi et al 1985). In the first, a study of 600 craniotomies, seizures occurred within 10 days, usually within the first 48 hours, and 78% were partial (Gerstle de Pasquet et al 1976). In the second, postoperative seizures occurred in 44 of 493 craniotomies (8.9%). The postoperative CT scan showed intracranial hemorrhages in nine, cerebral edema in eight, and cerebral infarcts in four (Fukamuchi et al 1985). Michenfelder et al (1990) reported a postoperative seizure in 30 patients among 993 following a supratentorial craniotomy, compared with none in 232 patients with an infratentorial craniotomy. There was also a higher incidence if penicillins were given. However, seizures also occur after posterior fossa surgery, with a reported incidence of 1.8%, related to metabolic acidosis and hyponatremia (Lee et al 1990).

Chemotherapy

Seizures may result from treatment with various chemotherapeutic agents, such as vincristine, L-asparaginase, and cyclosporin. L-Asparaginase has been associated with

Table 15.1 Factors responsible for postoperative seizures.

Preoperative seizures
Surgical manipulation
Edema
Hemorrhage
Stroke
Metabolic alterations
Subtherapeutic AED levels
Incomplete resection
Lesion in eloquent cortex
Dual pathology

seizures, through its tendency to produce hemorrhages secondary to defects in hemostasis, with deficiencies in factors IX and XI, antithrombin, plasminogen, and fibrinogen (Priest et al 1980). However, dural sinus thrombosis (DST), frequently associated with seizures, is more common in patients with cancer, and DST occurs without L-asparaginase therapy (Reddingius et al 1997). High-dose chemotherapy followed by bone marrow transplantation has been used for certain brain tumors, and this therapy may cause a delayed, transient encephalopathy, with seizures and multifocal, predominantly white matter, lesions seen on MRI, but not CT (Tahsildar et al 1996). Cyclosporin A causes an acute encephalopathy with seizures, and neuroimaging reveals typical lesions in the parietooccipital gray–white matter junction (Gleeson et al 1998). Seizures occur following treatment of acute lymphoblastic leukemia in children. In one study of 127 consecutive children with acute lymphatic leukemia (ALL), seizures occurred in 17, and in 8 of these (47%), cerebral lesions were present. The seizures were related to either intrathecal methotrexate or to L-asparaginase therapy (Maytal et al 1995). Busulfan has also been implicated, with dose-related neurotoxicity (Vassal et al 1990), and the use of intracarotid cisplatin and bleomycin (Newton et al 1989). Part of the mechanism for cisplatin toxicity may be hyponatremia secondary to inappropriate antidiuretic hormone (ADH) or hypomagnesemia (Ritch 1988). Vincristine causes encephalopathy, although seizures are rare (Scheithauer et al 1985), and partial seizures have been reported with intravenous vincristine (Dallera et al 1984). Chemotherapy may also lower AED levels. This has been seen with phenytoin (Grossman et al 1989).

Radiation therapy

Seizures are rare after radiation therapy, which may cause a vasculopathy. Cavernous hemangiomas and capillary telangiectasias have occurred after cranial radiation (Humpl et al 1997). However, radiation therapy has also been used to treat refractory seizures in unresectable tumors (Rogers et al 1993).

INVESTIGATION

Neuroimaging is now the procedure of choice for a suspected tumor, although historically, EEG was used prior to modern neuroradiologic techniques. The EEG remains an essential diagnostic tool in patients presenting with seizures.

No EEG pattern is specific for tumor (Table 15.2) (Daly and Markand 1990). The most reliable localizing sign is focal delta activity with suppression of normal background rhythms. Although tumors usually cause suppression of normal EEG rhythms, occasional increases in amplitudes or waveforms may occur, especially with slow-growing lesions. Minimal EEG changes occur with slowly growing extra-axial tumors; rapidly growing tumors produce the greatest EEG change (Daly and Markand 1990). Epileptiform activity may occur first, with focal delta activity seen later (Blume *et al* 1982). When caused by tumor, focal delta activity rarely resolves and may be persistent in sequential records (Daly and Thomas 1958). EEG changes depend on tumor location, size, growth rate, and complications, such as increased intracranial pressure and herniation; a normal EEG occurs in 5–50% of tumors and is location-dependent (Table 15.3) (Fischgold *et al* 1961; Daly and Markand 1990). Hirsch *et al* (1966) investigated the area around tumors with microelectrodes. Three zones of EEG activity were seen around tumors:

1. No EEG activity occurred in the cortical areas involved with tumor.
2. Burst-suppression was seen in the cortex around the tumor.
3. Continuous slowing was seen in more distant areas.

In a study of EEG and clinical manifestations in 25 patients with slowly growing brain tumors (over 25 years), serial EEG recordings localized the lesion in 88%. An increase in slow waves and sharp wave discharges, depression of normal rhythms, a change in the type of seizure, increase in seizure frequency, and a change in neurologic signs and symptoms, especially motor, were seen in these patients (Hughes and Zak 1987).

MRI is now the procedure of choice for epilepsy (ILAE Neuroimaging Commission 1997). Heinz *et al* (1989), from Duke, studied 59 seizure patients with CT, MRI, and EEG. EEG was the most sensitive (67%), MRI the next (53%), and CT was the least sensitive (42%). MRI detected an abnormality in five patients who had a negative CT scan; EEG was positive in all of these patients. CT scan failed to demonstrate a lesion not detected by an MRI. In a specific study of medically refractory partial seizures, Bergen *et al* (1989), from Rush Medical College in Chicago, studied 23 patients with both CT and MRI prior to surgery. Eleven patients had tumors, ten were astrocytomas and one was a ganglioglioma; all of these lesions were detected by MRI but only six of the eleven were visualized on CT scan. However, the CT scan was normal in only one of these, in a patient with an astrocytoma. CT detected focal calcification in three, focal attenuation in three, focal atrophy in two, ventricular asymmetry or compression in one each, and one was normal. Thus CT showed a focal abnormality in 10 of 11 patients but in only 6 of 11 patients were the changes pathognomonic of a tumor. MRI detected all 11 tumors, 10 as focal areas of increased signal on T2-weighted images and one as an area of decreased signal on a T1-weighted image (Bergen *et al* 1989).

There may be abnormalities on CT and MRI following partial seizures, especially if these have been frequent or if status epilepticus occurred. Increased permeability of the blood–brain barrier, with resultant brain edema, is responsible (Yaffe *et al* 1995). MRI is very sensitive in detecting this, so that if signal change is present, a follow-up study is important since this should resolve if it is related to brain edema, whereas it would persist if caused by a tumor. MRI with volumetric assessment of the hippocampus may be useful in the detection of dual pathology (Van Paesschen 1997). If the initial MRI is unremarkable in a patient with refractory seizures, repeat neuroimaging might be useful. MRI also has a higher detection rate of cortical dysplasias.

Table 15.2 EEG abnormalities with tumors.

Polymorphic δ activity or arrhythmic activity
Localized δ activity
Intermittent rhythmic δ activity
Focal attenuation of EEG activity over the tumor
Diffuse or localized theta activity
Spikes, sharp waves, or spike and wave discharges

Table 15.3 Normal EEG with tumors.

Location	% Normal
Cerebral hemispheres	5
Deep midline or basal location	25
Infratentorial tumors	25
Parasagittal parietal region	10–20: normal or nonlocalizing Frontal intermittent rhythmic delta activity (FIRDA)

PATHOLOGY

While virtually any tumor within the cranial cavity may present with seizures, biologically indolent tumors are more likely to be associated with epilepsy. Tumors that are usually associated with chronic pharmacoresistant epilepsy are low-grade intrinsic tumors of the brain. This account concentrates on tumors with a predilection to present with seizures and that are commonly encountered in resected specimens for the surgical treatment of epilepsy.

The frequency with which different tumors are seen in the published series of surgery for epilepsy varies somewhat from center to center, although the types of tumors found are similar. Mathieson (1975), reporting the pathological findings in 857 temporal lobectomies at the Montreal Neurological Institute, found 115 tumors (13.4%), of which 103 were astrocytomas and oligodendrogliomas. The rest were other tumors including ganglioglioma, meningioma, and epidermal cysts. In the series from the Maudsley Hospital, reviewed by Bruton (1988), there were 37 tumors (15%), part of a group referred to as alien tissue lesions (see below) in 249 temporal lobectomies, of which 9 corresponded to astrocytoma, 6 to oligodendroglioma, 13 to oligoastrocytoma – the largest subgroup – and 9 to ganglioglioma. The series of 216 temporal lobectomies from the University of Bonn Medical Center contained 75 tumors (34.7%) of which 34 (45%) were gangliogliomas and 25 (33%) were astrocytomas, comprising of seventeen pilocytic astrocytomas, six fibrillary astrocytomas, one pleomorphic xanthoastrocytoma and one anaplastic tumor (Wolf *et al* 1993a). The remainder comprised nine oligodendrogliomas, one oligoastrocytoma and six DNTs. Their extratemporal resections yielded fewer tumors, 12 in 63 specimens, more than half of which were gangliogliomas (Wolf *et al* 1993b). In a report of 58 temporal lobectomies from the University Hospital of Wales, there were only four tumors (7%), all oligodendrogliomas (Davies and Weeks 1993). In contrast, of 224 amygdalohippocampectomies carried out at the University of Zurich, 126 (56%) had tumors, the great majority of which were intrinsic brain tumors such as low-grade astrocytoma, including pilocytic astrocytoma and pleomorphic xanthoastrocytoma, oligodendroglioma, oligoastrocytoma, and ganglioglioma (Plate *et al* 1993). The series contained 36 high-grade neoplasms of which 15 were glioblastomas. There were three meningiomas, two of which were classified as anaplastic. Tumors rarely encountered in this type of surgical material, such as choroid plexus papilloma, primitive neuroectodermal tumor, osteoma, and lymphoma, were also reported.

The relatively recent recognition of DNT and its subsequent inclusion in the 1993 World Health Organization (WHO) classification of brain tumors (Kleihues *et al* 1993) is reflected in later publications. In the original article by Daumas-Duport *et al* (1988) describing the entity, 20 cases (7.5%) were obtained by reviewing the pathology of 265 cases who had undergone surgery for intractable seizures and a further 19 tumors were found by reviewing the slides of low-grade supratentorial astrocytomas, oligodendrogliomas, and oligoastrocytomas. The review of the pathology of 416 patients who had undergone temporal and extratemporal resections for epilepsy yielded 92 tumors (22%), all low grade, 74 of which were classified as DNT (Honavar *et al* 1999).

The idea has been put forward that irrespective of the histologic diagnosis, tumors associated with chronic epilepsy constitute a distinct clinicopathologic group. This notion has been expressed by many workers in the past, including Bruton (1988) and Cavanagh (1958). Bruton said that while histologically these lesions invited the label of neoplasm, their selection for temporal lobectomy following long periods of seizures and without obvious increase in size made it difficult to be certain. He included them in his group of alien tissue lesions. Cavanagh, in a detailed study of eight tumors in temporal lobectomy specimens, concluded that they were most likely to be hamartomatous formations with a few showing the earliest evidence of neoplastic transformation. A series of 65 patients with intractable seizures and glial tumors, predominantly in the limbic or perilimbic cortex, in which there were low-grade gliomas (61%) and malignant gliomas (17%), shows that as a group these tumors exhibit an indolent biological behavior (Fried *et al* 1994). Postoperative follow-up of more than 1 year showed that a majority of the patients were seizure-free, and that only one patient died as a result of the tumor. Bartolomei *et al* (1997) reported a group of 45 patients with low-grade temporal and nontemporal lobe intrinsic neoplasms: astrocytoma (32); ganglioglioma (7); mixed glioma (4); oligodendroglioma (2); and suggested that these gliomas associated with epilepsy form a subgroup with a much better prognosis compared with similar tumors presenting without seizures. A median postoperative follow-up of 4 years showed that 38 patients were free of seizures, and while none of the patients had received adjuvant radiotherapy, there was no recurrence of tumor. While this series contains no cases of DNT, the authors say that the strikingly similar clinical profiles of their cases to that of DNT raises the possibility that these epilepsy-associated low-grade gliomas of different histologic types may represent variants of DNT.

Tumors of neuroepithelial tissue are thus most frequently associated with chronic epilepsy, and Table 15.4 shows the classification of these tumors from the WHO classification of CNS tumors (Kleihues *et al* 1993).

ASTROCYTIC AND OLIGODENDROGLIAL TUMORS

Astrocytoma: Low-grade astrocytomas are diffusely infiltrative neoplasms, most commonly seen in the cerebral hemispheres of young adults. The tumors are hence poorly

Table 15.4 Tumors of neuroepithelial tissue.

Astrocytic tumors
 Astrocytoma
  Variants: fibrillary, protoplasmic, gemistocytic, or mixed
 Anaplastic (malignant astrocytoma)
 Glioblastoma
  Variants: giant cell glioblastoma, gliosarcoma

Oligodendroglial tumors
 Oligodendroglioma
 Anaplastic (malignant) oligodendroglioma

Mixed gliomas
 Mixed oligoastrocytoma
 Anaplastic (malignant) oligoastrocytoma
 Others

Neuronal and mixed neuronal-glial tumors
 Gangliocytoma
 Dysplastic gangliocytoma of cerebellum (Lhermitte – Duclos)
 Desmoplastic infantile ganglioglioma
 Dysembryoplastic neuroepithelial tumor
 Ganglioglioma
 Anaplastic (malignant) ganglioglioma
 Central neurocytoma
 Olfactory neuroblastoma (esthesioneuroblastoma)
  Variant: olfactory neuroepithelioma

demarcated and expand the affected part of the brain, blurring anatomic landmarks. The tumor may be cystic. *Fibrillary astrocytoma* (WHO grade II) is the most commonly seen variant overall in resections for chronic epilepsy. Mixed forms may be seen. They are tumors of variable cellularity composed of well-differentiated fibrillary astrocytes that consistently express glial fibrillary acidic protein (GFAP). Although histologically indolent tumors, progression to a higher grade of tumor may occur. In a study of low-grade supratentorial astrocytomas, an overall 5-year survival rate of 27% was found, although patients in whom the sole presenting symptom was epilepsy the 5-year survival rate was 63% (van Veelen *et al* 1998). This better prognosis was unaffected by the time interval between the onset of seizures and the treatment by surgery.

The presence of mitotic activity in an astrocytic tumor, however sparse, is the diagnostic criterion for the *anaplastic astrocytoma* (WHO grade III) and is accompanied by increasing cellularity and nuclear atypia. The most malignant astrocytic neoplasm is the *glioblastoma* (WHO grade IV), composed of poorly differentiated cells, sometimes multinucleated tumor giant cells, with vascular endothelial cell proliferation and necrosis.

Pilocytic astrocytoma (WHO grade I) is the commonest glioma in children and is preferentially found in an axial location close to the midline of the CNS in the cerebellum and the region of the third ventricle (Burger *et al* 1997). Though relatively uncommon, it is those arising in the supratentorial cortex, usually in young adults, that present with seizures, associated with headaches, focal neurologic deficits and frequently with evidence of raised intracranial pressure (Clark *et al* 1985; Garcia and Fulling 1985; Palma and Guidetti 1985). The tumor is usually a well-demarcated soft gray mass, occasionally presenting as an intramural nodule of a large cyst, composed of bipolar cells with fine hair-like cytoplasmic processes. The cells are arranged in compact bundles and in loose microcystic areas (Fig. 15.1). Nuclear pleomorphism is common. The presence of brightly eosinophilic Rosenthal fibers, eosinophilic granular bodies and intracellular protein droplets assist in making the diagnosis. Involvement of the leptomeninges, a common feature of this tumor, is not evidence of aggressive behavior. These tumors, classified as WHO grade I gliomas, must be distinguished from the more common fibrillary astrocytoma because of their uniformly better prognosis, with an overall survival of 82% at 10 and 20 years (Forsyth *et al* 1993).

Oligodendroglioma may present in children although it is usually seen in adults with a peak in incidence in the fifth to sixth decades (Mørk *et al* 1985; Shaw *et al* 1992). Seizures are the most frequent presenting complaint, seen in over 50% of patients, and they may be associated with signs of raised intracranial pressure. Patients presenting with seizures are significantly younger than those without (Whittle and Beaumont 1995). The prognosis of these tumors is less favorable than believed; patients with low-grade oligodendrogliomas having 5- and 10-year survival rates of 75% and 46%, respectively (Shaw *et al* 1992). They are soft gray tumors, usually found in the white matter, and although they appear to be well-demarcated masses, infiltration of the adjacent brain parenchyma is common. Calcification is frequent, particularly at the periphery of the

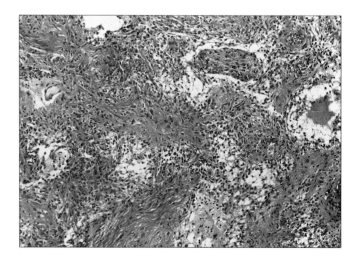

Fig. 15.1 Pilocytic astrocytoma composed of elongated cells in compact bundles and loose areas. Microcystic change is seen in the right and lower edges of the picture. Hematoxylin and eosin.

tumor. Histologically, low-grade oligodendrogliomas are composed of sheets of monomorphic cells with round hyperchromatic nuclei and a small rim of cytoplasm (Fig. 15.2). Perinuclear clearing of the cytoplasm, an artifact of routine processing, produces the characteristic honeycomb appearance in the tumor. The tumors have a striking tendency to invade the cerebral cortex, forming clusters around neurons, referred to as satellitosis. The tumor cells express the markers A2B5, Leu7, and S-100 protein, none of which are specific for oligodendroglioma (Reifenberger *et al* 1997). Most oligodendrogliomas contain a proportion of GFAP-positive cells, reactive astrocytes in some cases, and a neoplastic astrocytic component in others. Some cases contain small round GFAP-positive cells called minigemistocytes or gliofibrillary oligodendrocytes, thought to be a transitional form between oligodendroglial cells and astrocytes. The *anaplastic oligodendroglioma* shows increased cellularity, increasing nuclear atypia, mitotic activity, and necrosis.

A study using a range of neural antigens to distinguish oligodendroglioma from DNT failed to find a distinct pattern of staining to separate the two entities and concluded that the differential diagnosis rested on histologic features (Wolf *et al* 1997). They also found more than 50% of the oligodendrogliomas contained cells that expressed the NR1 subunit of *N*-methyl-D-aspartate receptors, a subtype of ionotropic glutamate receptors that appear to be involved in neuronal excitotoxicity, and suggested that this may contribute to the high epileptogenic potential of these tumors.

The mixed *oligoastrocytoma* is a tumor in which distinct areas of both oligodendroglioma and astrocytoma are clearly identified. These tumors are also seen predominantly in the cerebral hemispheres of adults, and present most commonly with long-standing seizures and other neurologic signs, including those of raised intracranial pressure (Reifenberger *et al* 1997). There are conflicting views about the prognostic significance of the two components of this tumor, but the balance appears to weigh in favor of a good prognosis, like the pure oligodendroglioma, as opposed to that of the fibrillary astrocytoma (Burger and Scheithauer 1994).

NEURONAL-GLIAL TUMORS

Gangliogliomas are solid or cystic, generally well-circumscribed tumors that may occur anywhere in the CNS, although the majority are supratentorial, usually in the temporal lobe, and it is these that are associated with chronic epilepsy (Johannsson *et al* 1981; Wolf *et al* 1994; Prayson *et al* 1995). The tumors are composed of neurons and glia, usually astrocytes (Fig. 15.3). Oligodendroglial cells are rare and are present as small foci along with the predominantly astrocytic glial component. The neurons vary in number and may be found in clusters or distributed unevenly through the neoplasm. They are large and multipolar, with prominent Nissl substance, and binucleate and sometimes multinucleate forms are readily found. The astrocytic component resembles either a pilocytic or a fibrillary astrocytoma. Round eosinophilic granular or hyaline bodies and calcification may be found in the tumor, and a perivascular lymphocytic infiltrate is frequently present. Often a fine reticulin fiber network is seen. Superficial tumors may extend into the leptomeninges, inducing a desmoplastic reaction, and this does not have an adverse prognostic significance. Mitotic figures are rare. The neoplastic neurons express markers such as synaptophysin, neuron-specific

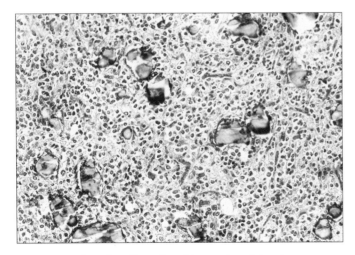

Fig. 15.2 Uniform box-like cells, with round nuclei and characteristic perinuclear clearing in an oligodendroglioma with abundant microcalcification. Hematoxylin and eosin.

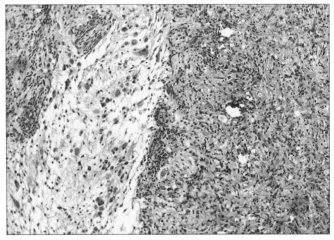

Fig. 15.3 Ganglioglioma with a component resembling fibrillary astrocytoma in which neurons are interspersed, and an area rich in large and small neurons. Hematoxylin and eosin.

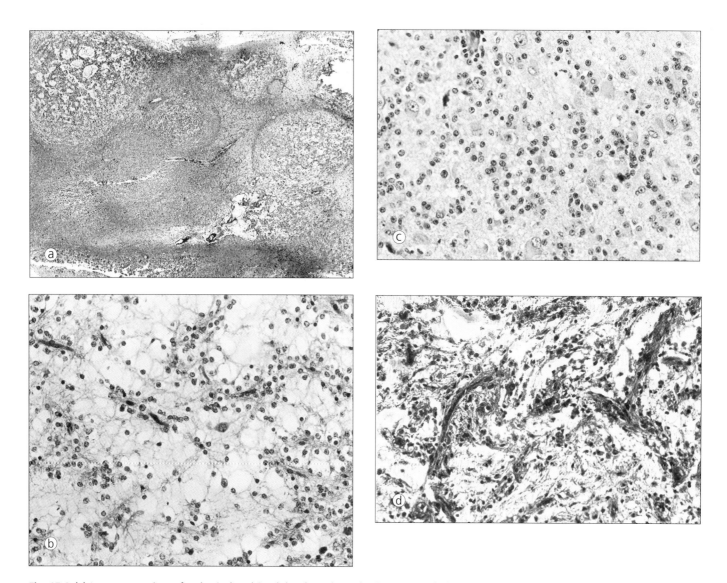

Fig. 15.4 (a) Low-power view of a classical multinodular dysembryoplastic neuroepithelial tumor (DNT). (b) Typical nodule rich in oligodendroglia-like cells (OLC) with clear cytoplasm tending to align themselves along capillaries. Occasional neurons and astrocytes are identified. (c) Solid nodule rich in OLC with tiny flecks of calcification. (d) Nodule resembling an astrocytoma. Hematoxylin and eosin.

enolase, and neurofibrillary protein and the astrocytes are GFAP positive. These studies are of value in identifying both components to establish the diagnosis, particularly when faced with small biopsies. Cell proliferation studies with markers Ki-67 and MIB1 show very low labeling indices in keeping with the indolent biologic behavior of these tumors. Anaplastic gangliogliomas are rare, and in rare instances one that is histologically low grade may progress to a malignant tumor; the anaplastic features are restricted to the astrocytic component.

Dysembryoplastic neuroepithelial tumor

This mixed neuronal-glial tumor often associated with cortical dysplasia appears to be found almost exclusively in the clinical setting of epilepsy resistant to drug therapy

(Daumas-Duport *et al* 1988; Raymond *et al* 1994b; Daumas-Duport and Lantos 1997; Honavar *et al* 1999). It is usually a tumor of childhood, although adult cases are seen, presenting with seizures and unaccompanied by signs of raised intracranial pressure and other focal signs. Predominantly a superficial tumor of the cerebral hemispheres, particularly the temporal lobes, rare cases have been reported affecting the deep gray nuclei, pons and cerebellum.

The tumor is either a well-demarcated nodular mass or a poorly delineated lesion expanding the cortex, up to a couple of centimeters in size, although larger tumors are seen. White matter is frequently involved, and in the temporal lobe, the hippocampus and amygdala are often affected. It may be cystic and calcified. The tumor has a mixed composition, consisting of small oligodendroglia-like cells (OLC), mature neurons and astrocytes with great variation in the relative proportions of the three cell types. The tumors have a much more heterogeneous appearance than was described in early accounts and identification of all three cell types is essential for diagnosis of this lesion. Three histologic subtypes are found: the classical multinodular; the solitary nodular; and the diffuse. The multinodular DNT is composed of nodules of different size, confluent and discrete, in which the OLC, neurons, and astrocytes are dispersed (Fig. 15.4). Often the cells are surrounded by a myxoid matrix which may accumulate to produce a microcystic change. Or, the nodules may be solid. The most characteristic appearance is that of nodules in which OLC predominate, with scattered neurons and astrocytes. Some nodules may consist only of OLC, and other may be composed predominantly of astrocytes and resemble fibrillary or pilocytic astrocytomas. The area between nodules may also be diffusely abnormal, containing a similar mixture of cells. The solitary nodular DNT is composed of a single large nodule, while the diffuse form is a poorly demarcated tumor. They both also contain the same three populations of cells. Involvement of the leptomeninges is not uncommon and is not associated with aggressive behavior, nor is the presence of occasional mitotic figures. Rare tumors show necrosis, also not an adverse prognostic feature. The association of DNT with various forms of cortical dysplasia in the adjacent cortex forms a part of the definition of this neoplasm, and it is found in many cases when adequate, properly orientated cortex is available for examination. Also seen in the adjacent cortex and white matter along with these tumors are tiny microdysgenetic nodules (glioneuronal hamartia) composed of OLC, neurons, and astrocytes. It is speculated these tiny malformations are a precursor lesion for the neoplasm. Immunocytochemical and ultrastructural studies demonstrate that the OLC may show neuronal or oligodendroglial or even astrocytic differentiation, supporting the idea that DNT originates from progenitor cells capable of both neuronal and glial differentiation (Hirose *et al* 1994; Taratuto *et al* 1995; Honavar *et al* 1999). DNT is characterized by its excellent response to surgical treatment, even when tumor excision is incomplete.

DUAL PATHOLOGY

Levesque *et al* (1991), in the first systematic study of dual pathology on specimens obtained from *en bloc* temporal lobectomies done for refractory epilepsy, defined dual pathology as an extrahippocampal lesion associated with hippocampal damage. This type of finding had been reported by Cavanagh (1958) and then by Falconer *et al* (1962) in temporal lobe seizures with distant lesions. Dual pathology actually refers to any two pathologic processes occurring together, not just hippocampal atrophy. There may not be any clinical significance associated with dual pathology when partial seizures are controlled by AEDs, except if a lesion, such as a tumor, is present which needs treatment for other reasons. However, when planning the surgical procedure for a tumor with partial seizures or a cortical resection for intractable partial seizures, the presence of dual pathology is critical since the postoperative outcome for seizures may be dependent on removal of both pathologies and the epileptogenic region.

Levesque *et al* (1991) reviewed the pathology specimens from 178 patients, and did a qualitative assessment of hippocampal sclerosis. Hippocampal sclerosis was considered significant if there was a 30% or greater loss of hippocampal tissue, or mild or minimal if the loss was less than 30%, compared to control values. Of interest, hippocampal cell loss was present in all specimens. Of the 178 specimens, 124 had only hippocampal lesions (no extrahippocampal lesions) and 54 had dual pathology (extrahippocampal lesion with hippocampal damage). Significant hippocampal cell loss was present in 88.7% of those with hippocampal lesions, whereas significant hippocampal cell loss occurred in only 30.3% in those with dual pathology. The degree of cell loss was assessed as either severe or mild in the 54 patients with dual pathology. The cell loss was mild in 12 with only gliomas (defined as ganglioglioma, mixed glioma, low-grade astrocytoma, and high-grade glioma), whereas significant cell loss was always present in the group with heterotopias.

In a follow-up study on the same group of 149 patients followed for 5 years, Nakasato *et al* (1992) evaluated dual pathology and postoperative seizure outcome in two groups: those with worthwhile seizure reduction versus those with residual seizures. There was no statistically significant difference in outcome related to the degree of cell loss in the group with only hippocampal lesions, but in the group with dual pathology, residual seizures occurred in 53% of those with severe cell loss as compared to only 11% of those with mild cell loss. This suggests that in those with dual pathology, epileptogenic tissue extends outside of the boundaries of a standard temporal lobectomy.

Cendes *et al* (1995) studied the frequency and characteristics of dual pathology in 167 patients with temporal or extratemporal partial seizures. Neuronal migration defects (NMD) were found in 48, low-grade tumors in 52, vascular malformations in 34, porencephalic cysts in 16, and gliosis in 17. An atrophic hippocampal formation, determined by MRI volumetric studies, was found in 25 patients (14%). Abnormal volumes were present in 17% of those with temporal and 14% of those with extratemporal lesions. Age of onset and duration of seizures were not significant but febrile seizures in early childhood were found more frequently, but not exclusively, in patients with hippocampal atrophy. The frequency of dual pathology was 2% in tumors, 9% in vascular malformations, but 25% with NMD, 31% with porencephalic cysts, and 23.5% in those with reactive gliosis.

Other disorders in which dual pathology has been reported include congenital porencephaly, Rasmussen's syndrome, NMD, and cortical dysplasias. In a series of 100 patients with hippocampal sclerosis defined by MRI, 15 patients had cortical dysplasia (Raymond *et al* 1994a). Dual pathology has also been noted in childhood refractory seizures. Hwang *et al* (1990), from Toronto, identified mesial temporal sclerosis in the hippocampus in 7 out of 13 children with gangliogliomas and refractory seizures.

What causes the hippocampal damage in patients with dual pathology? Levesque *et al* (1991) found no correlation with duration, severity, or the seizure type, and noted that all seven patients with either anoxia or head trauma had severe hippocampal damage. They postulated that hippocampal sclerosis may have been related to a previous insult. Is there first an epileptic process that predisposes to hippocampal atrophy, has there been some insult, such as anoxia or head trauma, or is there a common predisposing factor, and why is there such a high incidence of hippocampal sclerosis in patients with underlying cortical dysplasia as opposed to tumors? Excititoxic injury or kindling may cause hippocampal damage, explaining why frequent seizures from another area could predispose to this. There may have been prior injury, such as head trauma or anoxia. There does appear to be a difference in the occurrence of dual pathology related to various lesions, less likely with gliomas compared to cortical dysplasias, suggesting that there may be a common pathogenic mechanism during pre- or perinatal development (Li *et al* 1997).

Certain tumors, such as ganglioglioma and DNT, blur the distinction between neoplasia and cortical dysplasia. A study from the Hospital for Sick Children, Toronto, reviewed 1500 brain tumors and determined that 20–25% of tumors demonstrate some neuronal differentiation, with a spectrum ranging from well-defined ganglionic tumors, that may be difficult to differentiate from a cortical dysplasia, to primitive neuroectodermal tumors (Becker 1995). Of the 5% with a definitive ganglionic component, the majority were ganglioglioma or DNT. The subependymal giant cell tumor associated with tuberous sclerosis occasionally has evidence of a cortical dysplasia. The author suggests that a primary induction disorder may involve a combination of a malformative and neoplastic event.

Prayson and Estes (1995), from the Cleveland Clinic, identified a cortical dysplasia in 52 out of 360 patients with partial lobectomy for refractory seizures, an overall incidence of 14%. The temporal lobe was involved in 34, frontal lobe in 18, parietal lobe in 4, occipital lobe in 3, and 3 had involvement of multiple lobes. Three patterns of dysplasia were seen: cortical laminar architectural disorganization or malalignment of neurons in 26 patients, clusters of atypical neurons and glia within the cortex in 28, and a hypercellular molecular layer was seen in 31. Twenty-three had more than one pattern and coexistent tumors were present in 13: these were a ganglioglioma in eight, a DNT in three, and a low-grade astrocytoma in two. Tuberous sclerosis was present in four. In a specific study of tumors and cortical dysplasia in the same group of patients, tumors were identified in 67 patients and cortical dysplasia in 51, with both cortical dysplasia and a tumor in 13, an incidence of 4% (Prayson *et al* 1993).

What explains the occurrence of both tumors and cortical dysplasia, especially with ganglioglioma and DNT? The cytology of the ganglioglioma is similar to a cortical dysplasia, with the cluster ganglioglioma consisting of a disorganized arrangement of atypical neurons and glial cells. There are two main types of ganglioglioma, one an aggressive lesion, but the majority are low-grade neoplasms. Daumas-Duport *et al* (1988) described DNT in 39 cases associated with intractable seizure disorders. These lesions were supratentorial, characterized by an intracortical location, multinodular architecture, heterogeneous cellular composition with astrocytes, oligodendrocytes, and neurons. The location was temporal in the majority, 24 (62%), frontal in 12 (31%), and parietal or occipital in 3 cases. The identification of this lesion is critical since treatment is surgery, while radiation therapy and chemotherapy are not needed. Foci of cortical dysplasia were found in most cases with optimally oriented specimens, and a transition was observed between the specific glioneuronal element and the areas of dysplasia. Since the clinicopathologic features suggested a dysembryoplastic origin, these tumors were called DNTs. The presence of cortical dysplasia suggests that the DNTs arise during formation of the cortex. In another series of DNTs, dysplastic features in the neocortex, white matter, and hippocampus around the glioneuronal tumor mass were found in 12 of 16 specimens and included disarray of cortical lamination, small aggregates of neurons, and neuroblasts in cortex and white matter, and in one case, doubling of the fascia dentata (Raymond *et al* 1994b).

What is the surgical management of dual pathology? Li *et al* (1997) evaluated the surgical treatment of patients with single and dual pathology. The postoperative seizure control in 64 patients with lesional epilepsy was correlated with pathology: 51 patients had a single lesion and 13 had dual pathology, with cortical dysplasia in 7, a contusion in 5, and tumor in only 1. When a single lesion was present,

85% were seizure-free or significantly improved when the lesion was totally removed, compared to only 40% when there was incomplete resection. In those with dual pathology, all three cases in which both the lesion and the hippocampus were removed became seizure-free, whereas only two patients were seizure-free among ten in whom only the lesion or the hippocampus alone were removed. This suggests that when there is dual pathology, both the lesion and the atrophic hippocampus should be resected.

TREATMENT

The treatment of seizures with brain tumors begins with AEDs followed by treatment of the underlying tumor, usually a primary surgical resection, with adjunctive chemotherapy, or radiation therapy, depending on the tumor histology. Tumors might be unresectable, or only partially respectable, depending on location or histology. Radiation therapy could be used for seizure control in that situation. There is current surgical debate about the best operative approach: is gross total resection alone adequate, done without mapping, or is the epilepsy surgery approach preferred, done with electrocorticography (ECoG) to identify the epileptogenic region? The optimal surgical approach may depend on the preoperative seizure frequency, whether there are infrequent seizures, or a refractory seizure disorder, and on the tumor type and location, especially if eloquent cortex is involved.

The goals of surgical therapy for epilepsy associated with brain tumors are similar to those of epilepsy surgery, namely primary resection of the tumor and the reduction of seizure activity without associated neurologic morbidity (Cascino 1990). Early work at the Montreal Neurologic Institute showed that seizure outcome in tumors was the same as the seizure outcome from other lesions, but that surgical removal of the structural lesion alone might not control seizure activity and that reoperation might be necessary to resect the epileptogenic region (Penfield and Jasper 1954). If an epileptic focus is located within an area of eloquent cortex, the morbidity associated with its removal may not be worth the resulting neurologic deficit, especially for language. Haglund et al (1994) studied the cortical localization of language sites in gliomas. In patients with and without temporal lobe gliomas, the superior temporal gyrus (STG) contained significantly more language sites than the middle temporal gyrus. Both groups had language sites anterior to the central sulcus in the STG (12–16%). However, the group without tumors had more language sites in the STG than those with

tumors. Permanent postoperative language deficits were less likely if the distance of the resection margin from the language site was greater than 1 cm.

What is the experience in children with tumors? It is claimed that language dominance may transfer from the left to the right hemisphere if an injury occurs before 6 years of age (Rasmussen and Milner 1977). DeVos et al (1995) studied 12 patients with seizure onset before age 6 with a tumor near potential language areas. Hemisphere dominance, determined by the intracarotid amobarbital procedure (WADA test), showed that it was left in ten patients (83%), right in one patient, and bilateral in two patients. These findings indicate that early low-grade tumors are not associated with language transfer and that mapping of language areas may be needed to prevent postoperative deficits. Duchowny et al (1996) have shown that developmental lesions and early-onset seizures also do not displace language cortex and that displacement occurs only with destruction of the language cortex.

Clearly, excision of the lesion alone may be associated with a good seizure outcome in both children and adults. Goldring et al (1986) analyzed seizure outcome following surgery in 21 patients with chronic epilepsy and tumors who were followed for at least 1 year after surgery: 14 had lesion resection only and seven had resection of lesion and mesial temporal structures. Only three patients had further seizures, one in the lesion-only group and two in the lesion plus mesial structures group. They concluded that mesial resection was not necessary. Schisano et al (1963) reported that tumor removal alone decreased the incidence of seizures from 66.5% preoperatively to 26% postoperatively. Hirsch et al (1989) reported 42 children with benign astrocytic and oligodendrocytic tumors and seizures treated with resection alone with follow-up ranging from 6 months to 17 years. The preoperative seizure incidence was 76%. The postoperative seizure incidence was 19% using lesionectomy alone, although 24% of those without seizures remained on AEDs. There was a longer mean duration of preoperative seizures in the 19% with residual seizures.

In a specific study of postoperative seizure control using lesionectomy alone in children, Packer et al (1994) evaluated 60 children with seizures and low-grade gliomas followed for at least 2 years. Gross total resection was accomplished when all visible tumor had been removed and postoperative neuroimaging (CT and/or MRI) showed no evidence of residual disease. This was achieved in 47 of the 60 children. Seizure outcome was graded as seizure-free (no seizures, other than auras); significantly improved if the patient had fewer than 75% seizures; and not significantly improved if the number was not reduced by 75%. They then divided the patients into two groups, all those with seizures ($n = 60$), and those with more than five seizures prior to therapy (n = 50). However, the majority of these children did have frequent seizures: only 10 had less than five preoperative seizures, 21 had daily seizures, 11 had weekly seizures, 10 had monthly seizures, and 18 had sporadic seizures. Of the total group, 4 of the 60 patients were seizure-free at 2 years. In the 10 with less than five preoperative seizures, 9 were seizure-free. In the 50 with greater than five preoperative seizures, 36 were seizure-free, 2 were significantly improved, and 12 were not significantly improved. Factors associated with poor outcome included a parietal tumor location in the entire group and for those with five or more preoperative seizures, partial tumor resection in both groups; and a history of seizures for greater than 1 year in those with five or more seizures. Seizures that occurred in the first few months following surgery were not predictive of long-term seizure control. Children with the highest postoperative risk for recurrent seizures included those with seizures for longer than 1 year prior to surgery with a partially resected parietal tumor, and a history of seizures for longer than 1 year with more than five preoperative seizures.

In a study done in Montreal by Montes *et al* (1995), lesionectomy alone was evaluated in 18 children presenting with various lesions, mostly tumors. Complete lesionectomy was determined by intraoperative ultrasound and postoperative neuroimaging, and although ECoG was done, it was not used to guide the resection. Sixteen children have been seizure-free, and two have partial seizures, but are improved.

What are the data for lesionectomy alone in adults with tumors? In a study with mixed pathology, Awad *et al* (1991) reported 47 patients with structural lesions in whom 94% of patients with complete lesion resection had good outcome, independent of spike foci resection. In a study involving only tumors, Kirkpatrick *et al* (1993) reported on 31 patients with low-grade temporal tumors and refractory epilepsy who underwent *en bloc* resection. Pathology revealed a high incidence of DNT (27/31). Although ECoG was done both before and after resection, the results were not used to guide the resection. Using the Engel classification, 25 of these 31 cases had achieved a grade 1 outcome (81%) and three patients a grade II outcome (10%), only two patients achieved a grade III outcome (6%), and one a grade IV outcome (3%). Five patients had dual pathology (DNT and mesial temporal sclerosis), four of these achieved a grade I outcome and the other one a grade II outcome. A younger age at the time of resection was associated with a slightly better outcome.

Cascino *et al* (1992) reported on the use of computer-assisted sterotactic lesionectomy in 23 patients. Theoretically, this should best identify the lesion. Seventeen patients (74%) had a greater than 90% reduction in seizures, and 13 (56%) had a grade I outcome. Those with a temporal loca-

tion were less likely to be seizure-free. Boon *et al* (1991), from Yale, studied 50 patients with structural lesions, 38 of which were tumors, who had lesionectomy only, done by obtaining tumor-free margins. Eighty-three percent of the patients were seizure-free, and another 11% had a greater than 90% reduction in seizures. Therefore, in these two studies with excellent results, there were still patients with significant postoperative seizures.

Berger *et al* (1991; 1993), from Seattle, have advocated the use of tumor resection with ECoG for both adults and children with intractable epilepsy. All patients with seizures refractory to medical therapy had ECoG monitoring done during tumor removal. They did not include patients with low-grade gliomas and occasional seizures or those patients who were seizure-free on AEDs. ECoG was done with the following protocol: preresection recordings were taken over 10–20 min, with methohexital (1 mg kg^{-1}) used to induce epileptiform activity if needed (only rarely needed). Postresection ECoG was done in order to ensure that all areas of documented epileptiform activity had been resected prior to ending the procedure. Areas with epileptic activity that were distant from the resection cavity, occasional, or located within functional cortex were not resected. Forty-five patients were reported. The seizure foci were caused by temporal lobe tumors in 29 patients (mesial focus in 26, lateral focus in 15; some had both), frontal lobe tumors in 8, with the focus adjacent to the tumor and in the same lobe, and parietal lobe tumors in 8, and an unidentified focus in 1 patients. The tumor type was astrocytoma in 13, oligodendroglioma in 14, ganglioglioma in 9, and oligoastrocytoma in 9; mild gliosis occurred in the majority, especially in the subpial region. Gross total resection was achieved in 29 (64%), near-total resection in 10 (22%), and subtotal resection in 6 (13%). Forty-one of these 45 patients were seizure-free (91%). When the outcome of these 41 patients classified as seizure-free is examined in detail, 24 no longer take AEDs, 17 are seizure-free but remain on AEDs, 10 have had one or two seizures and subsequently remain seizure-free on AEDs. Four patients continue to have seizures; of these, three had an incomplete resection (in one because the lesion was in functional cortex and two had diffuse tumor infiltration throughout the rolandic cortex). However, Berger *et al* clearly state that mapping techniques are not used if there is either complete seizure control or infrequent seizures with AED treatment, since radical tumor resection alone often controls epilepsy.

Jooma *et al* (1995), from Cincinnati, reported similar findings in 30 patients with complex partial seizures and temporal lobe tumors. Sixteen underwent lesionectomy only and fourteen had lesionectomy with resection of the epileptogenic region identified by ECoG. After lesionectomy with ECoG, 92.8% were seizure-free, whereas only three patients with lesionectomy alone were seizure-free (19%). Five patients from the failed group of eight patients then underwent temporal lobectomy and became seizure-free. They concluded that, at least for temporal lobe tumors, there is a greater chance of becoming seizure-free when the epileptogenic region is removed.

In a specific study of ECoG-guided resection of oligodendrogliomas from Seattle, Pilcher *et al* (1993) reported that optimum resection of the epileptogenic zone usually required that the margins of the resection extend beyond the margins needed for lesionectomy only. ECoG showed nonepileptiform, high-amplitude slow waves over the tumor-involved cortex, whereas the epileptogenic zone had epileptiform spikes over cortex which appeared normal. In those with a temporal lobe lesion, the amygdala, hippocampus, and the parahippocampal gyrus were the actively discharging locations. The pathology specimens were correlated with findings on ECoG; the epileptogenic cortex was free of tumor, whereas no discharges came from tumor-associated cortex.

Therefore in summary, neuroimaging is done in all patients with partial seizures, except those thought to be benign focal epilepsy of childhood, with MRI being the procedure of choice. If tumor is discovered, complete lesionectomy is the surgical goal, if possible. If clinically indicated, such as in patients with many preoperative seizures, neuroimaging may then be repeated, specifically looking for dual pathology. Even when MRI is initially unremarkable, it should be repeated if seizures are refractory. ECoG is done in the operating room after the resection, especially in patients with more than several preoperative seizures, since these are more likely to have a wider epileptogenic area. If the lesion is possibly located within eloquent cortex, invasive monitoring with cortical mapping is done prior to surgery, or an awake craniotomy, with mapping, can be considered. Our current protocol continues AEDs for at least 6 months postoperatively. At that time, a repeat EEG is obtained, and if spike or sharp waves are present, we continue the AEDs. This is similar to the approach with epilepsy surgery in general, in which the presence of spikes or sharp waves on EEG at 6 months following resection was significantly correlated with seizure recurrence (Godoy *et al* 1992).

KEY POINTS

1. Brain tumor is responsible for around 5% of all cases of epilepsy. The peak incidence of tumor, as the cause of epilepsy, is in middle age (around 30%). The incidence in childhood and adolescence is considerably lower (around 1%).

2. Seizures occur more often with slow growing tumors (astrocytoma and oligodendroglioma) than with quick growing glioblastomas. Previously unsuspected tumor (especially oligoastrocytoma, astrocytoma, oligodendroglioma, ganglioglioma, and dysembryoplastic neuroepithelioma) is a common finding in people of all ages undergoing investigation for medically intractable focal epilepsy.

3. Around 30% of patients with a meningioma have seizures preoperatively, and around 35% of them continue to have seizures postoperatively. Seizures develop postoperatively in 15–20% of those who were seizure-free preoperatively.

4. Seizures may develop as a consequence of various measures used to treat tumors, including surgery and chemotherapy.

5. A 63% 5-year survival has been reported when epilepsy is the sole symptom arising from a fibrillary astrocytoma found in resections for chronic epilepsy. A 75% 5-year survival has been reported for oligodendroglioma.

6. Significant hippocampal atrophy is found in association with a small percentage of patients with medically intractable tumoral epilepsy overall. This percentage is considerably lower than in those whose chronic epilepsy is attributed to a neuronal migration defect. The percentage may be considerably higher for those whose tumor is a ganglioglioma or a dysembryoplastic neuroepithelioma of which a considerable proportion have accompanying dysplasia.

7. The best prognosis for seizure relief is when the tumor pathology can be excised completely along with any significant unilateral hippocampal sclerosis, if present. In the absence of significant hippocampal sclerosis, the prognosis may be improved if epileptogenic cortex, as defined by intraoperative electrocorticography, is removed, where possible, in addition to the tumor.

REFERENCES

Ahsan H, Neuget AI, Bruce JN (1995) Trends in incidence of primary malignant brain tumors in USA, 1981–1990. *International Journal of Epidemiology* **24**:1078–1085.

Aicardi J (1992) Tumors of the CNS and other space-occupying lesions. In: *Diseases of the Nervous System in Childhood*, pp 780–849. London: MacKeith Press.

Aicardi J (1994) *Epilepsy in Children*, 2nd edn, pp 334–353. New York: Raven Press.

Ajmone-Marsan C, Lewis WR (1960) Pathologic findings in patients with centrencephalic electroencephalographic patterns. *Neurology* **10**:922–930.

al-Rajeh S, Abomelha A, Awada A, Bademosi O, Ismail H (1990) Epilepsy and other convulsive disorders in Saudi Arabia: a prospective study of 1000 consecutive cases. *Acta Neurologica Scandinavica* **82**:341–345.

Angelini L, Broggi G, Riva D, Lazzaro-Solero C (1979) A case of Lennox–Gastaut syndrome successfully treated by removal of a parietotemporal astrocytoma. *Epilepsia* **20**:665–669.

Asanuma H, Wakai S, Tanaka T, Chiba S (1995) Brain tumors associated with infantile spasms. *Pediatric Neurology* **12**:361–364.

Awad IA, Rosenfield J, Ahl J, Hahn JF, Luders H (1991) Intractable epilepsy and structural lesions of the brain: mapping, resection strategies, and seizure outcome. *Epilepsia* **32**:179–186.

Backus RE, Millichap JG (1962) The seizure as a manifestation of intracranial tumor in childhood. *Pediatrics* **29**:978–984.

Bartolomei JC *et al* (1997) Low-grade gliomas of chronic epilepsy: a distinct clinical and pathological entity. *Journal of Neuro-oncology* **34**:79–84.

Becker LE (1995) Central nervous system tumors in childhood: relationship to dysplasia. *Journal of Neuro-oncology* **24**:13–19.

Bergen D, Bleck T, Ramsey R *et al* (1989) Magnetic resonance imaging as a sensitive and specific predictor of neoplasms removed for intractable epilepsy. *Epilepsia* **30**:318–321.

Berger MS, Ghatan S, Geyer JR, Keles GE, Ojemann GA (1991) Seizure outcome in children with hemispheric tumors and associated intractable epilepsy: the role of tumor removal combined with seizure foci resection. *Pediatric Neurosurgery* **17**:185–191.

Berger MS, Ghatan S, Haglund MH, Dobbins J, Ojemann GA (1993) Low-grade gliomas associated with intractable epilepsy: seizure outcome utilizing electrocorticography during tumor resection. *Journal of Neurosurgery* **79**:62–69.

Blume WT, Girvin JP, Kaufmann JCE (1982) Childhood brain tumors presenting as chronic uncontrolled focal seizure disorders. *Annals of Nerurology* **12**:538–541.

Boon PA, Williamson PD, Fried I *et al* (1991) Intracranial, intra-axial, space-occupying lesions in patients with intractable partial seizures: an anatomoclinical, neuropsychological, and surgical correlation. *Epilepsia* **32**:467–476.

Bruton CJ (1988) *The Neuropathology of Temporal Lobe Epilepsy*. New York: Oxford University Press.

Burger PC, Scheithauer BW (1994) Oligodendroglial neoplasms. In: *Tumours of the Central Nervous System*, pp 107–120. Washington DC: Armed Forces Institute of Pathology.

Burger PC, Paulus W, Kleihues P (1997) Pilocytic astrocytoma. In: Kleihues P, Cavenee WK (eds) *Pathology and Genetics of Tumours of the Nervous System*, pp 29–33. Lyon: International Agency for Research on Cancer.

Cascino GD (1990) Epilepsy and brain tumors: implications for treatment. *Epilepsia* **31** (Suppl 3): S37–S44.

Cascino GD, Kelly PJ, Sharbrough FW, Hulihan JF, Hirschorn KA, Trenerry MR (1992) Long-term follow-up of stereotactic lesionectomy in partial epilepsy: predictive factors and electroencephalographic results. *Epilepsia* **33**:639–644.

Cavanagh JB (1958) On certain small tumors encountered in the temporal lobe. *Brain* **81**:389–405.

Cendes F, Cook MJ, Watson C *et al* (1995) Frequency and characteristics of dual pathology in patients with lesional epilepsy. *Neurology* **45**:2058–2064.

Chow SY, Hsi MS, Tang LM, Fong VH (1995) Epilepsy and intracranial meningiomas. *Chinese Medical Journal* **55**:151–155.

Chozick BS, Reinert SE, Greenblatt SH (1996) Incidence of seizures after surgery for supratentorial meningiomas: a modern analysis. *Journal of Neurosurgery* **84**:382–386.

Clark GB, Henry JM, McKeever PE (1985) Cerebral pilocytic astrocytoma. *Cancer* **56**:1128–1133.

Commission on Classification and Terminology of the International League Against Epilepsy (1989) Proposal for classification of epilepsies and epileptic syndromes. *Epilepsia* **30**:389–399.

Dallera F, Gamoletti R, Costa P (1984) Unilateral seizures following vincristine intravenous injection. *Tumori* **70**:243–244.

Daly DD, Markand ON (1990) Focal brain lesions. In: Daly DD, Pedley TP (eds) *Current Practice of Clinical Electroencephalography*, 2nd edn, pp 335–370. New York: Raven Press.

Daly DD, Thomas JE (1958) Sequential alterations in the electroencephalograms of patients with brain tumors. *EEG in Clinical Neurophysiology* **10**:395–404.

Dam AM, Fuglsang-Frederiksen A, Svarr-Olsen U, Dam M (1985) Late-onset epilepsy: etiologies, types of seizure, and value of clinical investigation, EEG, and computerized tomographic scan. *Epilepsia* **26**:227–231.

Daumas-Duport C, Lantos PL (1997) Dysembryoplastic neuroepithelial tumours. In: Kleihues P, Cavenee WK (eds) *Pathology and Genetics of Tumours of the Nervous System*, pp 73–76 Lyon: International Agency for Research on Cancer.

Daumas-Duport C, Scheithauer BW, Chodkiewicz JP, Laws ER, Vedrenne C (1988) Dysembryoplastic neuroepithelial tumor: a surgically curable tumor of young patients with intractable partial seizures. *Neurosurgery* **23**:545–556.

Davies KG, Weeks RD (1993) Temporal lobectomy for intractable epilepsy: experience with 58 cases over 21 years. *British Journal of Neurosurgery* **7**:23–34.

DeVos KJ, Wyllie E, Geckler G, Kotagal P, Comair Y (1995) Language dominance in patients with early childhood tumors near left hemisphere language areas. *Neurology* **45**:349–356.

Duchowny M, Jayakar P, Harvey AS *et al* (1996) Language cortex representation: effects of developmental versus acquired pathology. *Annals of Neurology* **40**:31–38.

Engel J Jr (1989) Basic mechanisms of epilepsy. In: Engel J Jr (ed.) *Seizures and Epilepsy*, pp 71–111. Philadelphia: FA Davis.

Falconer MA, Driver MV, Serafetinides EA (1962) Temporal lobe epilepsy due to distant lesions: two cases relieved by operation. *Brain* **85**:521–539.

Ferrie CD, Giannakodimos S, Robinson RO, Panayiotopoulos JS (1995) Symptomatic typical absence seizures. In: Duncan JS, Panayiotopoulos CP (eds) *Typical Absences and Related Epileptic Syndromes*, pp 241–252, Edinburgh: Churchill Livingstone.

Fischgold H, Zalis A, Buisson B, Ferey J (1961) Electroencephalography and cerebral tumors. General comments on the use of EEG in the diagnosis and localization of cerebral tumors. *EEG in Clinical Neurophysiology* **19**(Suppl):51–74.

Forsgren L (1990) Prospective incidence study and clinical characterization of seizures in newly referred adults. *Epilepsia* **31**:292–301.

Forsyth PA, Shaw EA, Scheithauer BW, O'Fallon JR, Layton DD, Katzman JA (1993) Supratentorial pilocytic astrocytomas. *Cancer* **72**:1335–1342.

Fried I, Kim JH, Spencer DD (1994) Limbic and neocortical gliomas associated with intractable seizures: a distinct clinicopathological group. *Neurosurgery* **34**(3):815–823.

Fukamuchi A, Koizumi H, Nukui H (1985) Immediate postoperative seizures: incidence and computed tomographic findings. *Surgical Neurology* **24**:671–676.

Garcia DM, Fulling KH (1985) Juvenile pilocytic astrocytoma of the cerebrum in adults. *Journal of Neurosurgery* **63**:382–386.

Gerstle de Pasquet E, Pietra M, Iniquez RA (1976) Epileptic seizures as an early complication of neurosurgery. *Acta Neurologica Latinoamericana* **22**:144–151.

Gilles FH, Sobel E, Leviton A *et al* (1992) Epidemiology of seizures in children with brain tumors. The Childhood Brain Tumor Consortium. *Journal of Neuro-oncology* **12**:53–68.

Gleeson JG, duPlessis AJ, Barnes PD, Riviello JJ Jr (1998) Cyclosporin A acute encephalopathy and seizure syndrome in childhood: clinical features and risk of seizure recurrence. *Journal of Child Neurology* **13**:336–344.

Godoy J, Luders H, Dinner DS, Morris HH, Wyllie E, Murphy D (1992) Significance of sharp waves in routine EEGs after epilepsy surgery. *Epilepsia* **33**:285–288.

Goldring S, Rich KM, Picker S (1986) Experience with gliomas in patients presenting with a chronic seizure disorder. *Clinical Neurosurgery* **33**:15–42.

Grossman SA, Sheidler VR, Gilbert MR (1989) Decreased phenytoin levels in patients receiving chemotherapy. *American Journal of Medicine* **87**:505–510.

Haglund MM, Berger MS, Kunkel DD, Franck JE, Ghatan S, Ojemann GA (1992) Changes in γ-aminobutyric acid and somatostatin in epileptic cortex associated with low-grade gliomas. *Journal of Neurosurgery* **77**:209–216.

Haglund MM, Berger MS, Shamseldin M, Lettich E, Ojemann GA (1994) Cortical localization of temporal lobe language sites in patients with gliomas. *Neurosurgery* **34**:567–576.

Hauser WA, Annegers JF, Kurland LT (1993) Incidence of epilepsy and unprovoked seizures in Rochester, Minnesota: 1935–1984. *Epilepsia* **34**:453–468.

Heinz ER, Heinz TR, Radtke R *et al* (1989) Efficacy of MRI vs CT in epilepsy. *American Journal of Roentgenology* **152**:347–352.

Henny C, Despland PA, Regli F (1990) Initial epileptic crisis after the age of 60: etiology, clinical aspects and EEG. *Journal of Swiss Medicine* **120**:787–792.

Hirose T *et al* (1994) Dysembryoplastic neuroepithelial tumor (DNT): an immunohistochemical and ultrastructural study. *Journal of Neuropathology and Experimental Neurology* **53**(2):184–195.

Hirsch JF, Buisson-Ferey J, Sachs M, Hirsch JC, Scherrer J (1966) Electrocorticogramme et activities unitairs lors de processus expansifs chez l'homme. *EEG in Clinical Neurophysiology* **21**:417–428.

Hirsch JF, Rose CS, Pierre-Kahn A, Pfister A, Hoppe-Hirsch E (1989) Benign astrocytic and oligodendrocytic tumors of the cerebral hemispheres in children. *Journal of Neurosurgery* **70**:568–572.

Honavar M, Janota I, Polkey CE (1999) Histological heterogeneity of dysembryoplastic neuroepithelial tumor: identification and differential diagnosis in a series of 74 cases. *Histopathology* **34**:342–356.

Hughes JR, Zak SM (1987) EEG and clinical changes in patients with chronic seizures. *Archives of Neurology* **44**:540–543.

Humpl T, Bruhl K, Bohl J, Schwarz M, Stoeter P, Gutjahr P (1997) Cerebral hemorrhage in long-term survivors of childhood acute lymphoblastic leukemia. *European Journal of Pediatrics* **156**:367–370.

Hwang PA, Becker LE, Chuang SH (1990) Evaluation, surgical approach and outcome of seizure in patients with gangliogliomas. *Pediatric Neurosurgery* **16**:208–212.

International League Against Epilepsy Neuroimaging Commission (1997) ILAE Neuroimaging Commission recommendations for neuroimaging of patients with epilepsy. *Epilepsia* **38**(Suppl 10):1–2.

Johannsson JH, Rekate HL, Roessmann U (1981) Gangliogliomas:

pathological and clinical correlation. *Journal of Neurosurgery* **54**:58–63.

Jooma R, Yeh H, Privitera MD, Gartner M (1995) Lesionectomy versus electrophysiologically guided resection for temporal lobe tumors manifesting with complex partial seizures. *Journal of Neurosurgery* **83**:231–236.

Kawaguchi T, Kameyama S, Tanaka R (1996) Peritumoral edema and seizures in patients with cerebral convexity and parasagittal meningiomas. *Neurologia Medico-Chirurgica* **36**:568–573.

Kirkpatrick PJ, Honavar M, Janota I, Polkey CE (1993) Control of temporal lobe epilepsy following *en bloc* resection of low-grade tumours. *Journal of Neurosurgery* **78**:19–25.

Kleihues P, Burger PC, Scheithauer BW (1993) *Histologic Typing of Tumours of the Central Nervous System*. New York: Springer Verlag.

Kotagal P, Cohen BH, Hahn JF (1995) Infantile spasms in a child with brain tumor: seizure-free outcome after resection. *Journal of Epilepsy* **8**:57–60.

Lee ST, Lui TN, Chang CN, Cheng WC (1990) Early postoperative seizures after posterior fossa surgery. *Journal of Neurosurgery* **73**:541–544.

Levesque MF, Nakasato N, Vinters HV, Babb TL (1991) Surgical treatment of limbic epilepsy associated with extrahippocampal lesions: the problem of dual pathology. *Journal of Neurosurgery* **75**:364–370.

Li LM, Cendes F, Watson C *et al* (1997) Surgical treatment of patients with single and dual pathology. *Neurology* **48**:437–444.

Lobato RD, Alday R, Gomez PA *et al* (1996) Brain edema in patients with intracranial meningioma. Correlation between clinical, radiological, and histological factors and presence and intensity of edema. *Acta Neurochirurgica* **138**:485–493.

Ludwig CL, Smith MT, Godfrey AD, Armbrustmacher VW (1986) A clinicopathologic study of 323 patients with oligodendroglioma. *Annals of Neurology* **19**:15–21.

Luhdorf K, Jensen LK, Plesner AM (1986) Etiology of epilepsy in the elderly. *Epilepsia* **27**:458–463.

Marco P, Sola RG, Ramon y Cajal S, DeFelipe J (1997) Loss of inhibitory synapses on the soma and axon initial segment of pyramidal cells in human epileptic peritumoral neocortex: implications for epilepsy. *Brain Research Bulletin* **44**:47–66.

Mathieson G (1975) Pathology of temporal foci. In: Penry JK, Daly DD (eds) *Advances in Neurology*, pp 163–181. New York: Raven Press.

Maytal J, Grossman R, Yusuf FH *et al* (1995) Prognosis and treatment of seizures in children with acute lymphoblastic leukemia. *Epilepsia* **36**:831–836.

Michenfelder JD, Cucchiara RF, Sundt TM Jr (1990) Influence of intraoperative antibiotic choice on the incidence of early postcraniotomy seizures. *Journal of Neurosurgery* **72**:703–705.

Montes JL, Rosenblatt B, Farmer JP *et al* (1995) Lesionectomy of MRI-detected lesions in children with epilepsy. *Pediatric Neurosurgery* **22**:167–173.

Moots PL, Maciunas RJ, Eisert DR, Parker RA, Laporte K, Abou-Khalil B (1995) The course of seizures in patients with malignant gliomas. *Archives of Neurology* **52**:717–724.

Mørk SJ, Lindegaard K-F, Halvorsen TB *et al* (1985) Oligodendroglioma: incidence and biologic behavior in a defined population. *Journal of Neurosurgery* **63**:881–889.

Nakasato N, Levesque MF, Babb TL (1992) Seizure outcome following standard temporal lobectomy: correlation with hippocampal neuron loss and extrahippocampal pathology. *Journal of Neurosurgery* **77**:194–200.

Nass R, Heier L, Walket R (1993) Landau–Kleffner syndrome: temporal lobe tumor resection with good results. *Pediatric Neurology* **9**:303–305.

Newton HB, Page MA, Junck L, Greenber HS (1989) Intra-arterial cisplatin for treatment of malignant gliomas. *Journal of Neuro-oncology* **7**:39–45.

Packer RJ, Sutton LN, Patel KM *et al* (1994) Seizure control following tumor surgery for childhood low-grade gliomas. *Journal of Neurosurgery* 80:998–1003.

Page LK, Lombroso CT, Matson DD (1969) Childhood epilepsy with late detection of cerebral glioma. *Journal of Neurosurgery* 31:253–261.

Palma L, Guidetti B (1985) Cystic pilocytic astrocytomas of the cerebral hemispheres. Surgical experience with 51 cases and long-term results. *Journal of Neurosurgery* 62:811–815.

Penfield W, Jasper H (eds) (1954) *Epilepsy and the Functional Anatomy of the Human Brain*, p 774. Boston: Little, Brown.

Penfield W, Erickson TC, Tarlov I (1940) Relation of intracranial tumors and symptomatic epilepsy. *Archives of Neurology and Psychiatry* 44:300–315.

Pilcher WH, Silbergeld DL, Berger MS, Ojemann GA (1993) Intraoperative electrocorticography during tumor resection: impact on seizure outcome in patients with gangliogliomas. *Journal of Neurosurgery* 78:891–902.

Plate KH *et al* (1993) Neuropathological findings in 224 patients with temporal lobe epilepsy. *Acta Neuropathologica* 86:433–438.

Prayson RA, Estes ML (1995) Cortical dysplasia: a histopathologic study of 52 cases of partial lobectomy in patients with epilepsy. *Human Pathology* 26:493–500.

Prayson RA, Estes ML, Morris HH (1993) Coexistence of neoplasia and cortical dysplasia in patients presenting with seizures. *Epilepsia* 34:609–615.

Prayson RA, Khajavi K, Comair YG (1995) Cortical architectural abnormalities and MIB 1 immunoreactivity in gangliogliomas: a study of 60 patients with intracranial tumors. *Journal of Neuropathology and Experimental Neurology* 4:513–520.

Priest JR, Ramsay NK, Latchaw RE *et al* (1980) Thrombotic and hemorrhagic strokes complicating early therapy for childhood acute lymphoblastic leukemia. *Cancer* 46:1548–1554.

Rasmussen T, Milner B (1977) The role of early left-brain injury in determining lateralization of cerebral speech functions. *Annals of the New York Academy of Sciences* 299:355–369.

Raymond AA, Fish DR, Stevens JM, Cook MJ, Sisodiya SM, Shorvon SD (1994a) Association of hippocampal sclerosis with cortical dysgenesis in patients with epilepsy. *Neurology* 44:1841–1845.

Raymond AA, Halpin SFS, Alsanjari N *et al* (1994b) Dysembryoplastic neuroepithelial tumor: features in 16 patients. *Brain* 117:461–475.

Reddingius RE, Patte C, Couanat D, Kalifa C, Lemerle J (1997) Dural sinus thrombosis in children with cancer. *Medical and Pediatric Oncology* 29:296–302.

Reifenberger G (1997) Oligodendroglioma. In: Kleihues P, Cavenee WK (eds) *Pathology and Genetics of Tumours of the Nervous System*, pp 38–42. Lyon: International Agency for Research on Cancer.

Ritch PS (1988) *cis*-Dichlorodiammineplatinum II-induced syndrome of inappropriate secretion of antidiuretic hormone. *Cancer* 61:448–450.

Rogers LR, Morris HH, Lupica K (1993) Effect of cranial irradiation on seizure frequency in adults with low-grade astrocytoma and medically intractable epilepsy. *Neurology* 43:1599–1601.

Rutledge SL, Snead OC III, Morawetz R, Chandra-Sekar B (1987) Brain tumors presenting as a seizure disorder in infants. *Journal of Child Neurology* 2:214–219.

Sander JWAS, Hart YM, Johnson AL, Shorvon SD (1990) National General Practice Study of Epilepsy: newly diagnosed epileptic seizures in the general population. *Lancet* 336:1267–1271.

Scheithauer W, Ludwig H, Maida E (1985) Acute encephalopathy associated with continuous vincristine sulfate combination chemotherapy: case report. *Investigational New Drugs* 3:315–318.

Schisano G, Tovi D, Nordenstam H (1963) Spongioblastoma polare of the cerebral hemisphere. *Journal of Neurosurgery* 20:241–251.

Shady JA, Black PM, Kupsky WJ *et al* (1994) Seizures in children with supratentorial astroglial neoplasms. *Pediatric Neurosurgery* 21:23–30.

Shaw EG, Scheithauer BW, O'Fallon JR, Tazelaar HD, Davis DH (1992) Oligodendrogliomas: the Mayo Clinic experience. *Journal of Neurosurgery* 76:428–434.

Solomon GE, Carson D, Pavlakis S, Fraser R, Labar D (1993) Intracranial EEG monitoring in Landau–Kleffner syndrome associated with left temporal lobe astrocytoma. *Epilepsia* 34: 557–560.

Spencer DD, Spencer SS, Mattson RH *et al* (1984) Intracerebral masses in patients with intractable partial epilepsy. *Neurology* 34:432–436.

Sung CY, Chu NS (1989) Status epilepticus in the elderly: etiology, seizure type, and outcome. *Acta Neurologica Scandinavica* 80:51–56.

Tahsildar HI, Remler BF, Creger RJ *et al* (1996) Delayed, transient encephalopathy after marrow transplantation: case report and MRI findings in four patients. *Journal of Neuro-oncology* 27:241–250.

Taratuto AL *et al* (1995) Dysembryoplastic neuroepithelial tumor: morphological, immunocytochemical, and deoxyribonucleic acid analyses in a pediatric series. *Neurosurgery* 36:474–481.

Vassal G, Deroussent A, Hartmann O *et al* (1990) Dose-dependent neurotoxicity of high-dose busulfan in children: a clinical and pharmacological study. *Cancer Research* 50:6203–6207.

Van Paesschen W (1997) Quantitative MRI of mesial temporal structures in temporal lobe epilepsy. *Epilepsia* 38 (Suppl 10):3–12.

van Veelen ML, Avezaat CJ, Kros JM, van Putten, Vecht C (1998) Supratentorial low-grade astrocytoma: prognostic factors, dedifferentiation, and the issue of early versus late surgery. *Journal of Neurology, Neurosurgery and Psychiatry* 64:581–587.

Walker AE, Robins M, Weinfeld F (1985) Epidemiology of brain tumors: the national survey of intracranial neoplasms. *Neurology* 35:219–226.

Werner MH, Phuphanich S, Lyman GH (1995) The increasing incidence of malignant gliomas and primary central nervous system lymphoma in the elderly. *Cancer* 76:1634–1642.

Whittle IR, Beaumont A (1995) Seizures in patients with supratentorial oligodendroglial tumors. Clincopathological features and management considerations. *Acta Neurochirurgia* 135:19–24.

Wolf HK *et al* (1993a) Surgical pathology of temporal lobe epilepsy. Experience with 216 cases. *Journal of Neuropathology and Experimental Neurology* 52:499–506.

Wolf HK *et al* (1993b) Surgical pathology of chronic epileptic seizure disorders: experience with 63 specimens from extratemporal corticectomies, lobectomies and functional hemispherectomies. *Acta Neuropathologica* (Berlin) 86:466–472.

Wolf HK *et al* (1994) Ganglioglioma. A detailed histopathological and immunohistochemical analysis of 61 cases. *Acta Neuropathologica* 88:166–173.

Wolf HK *et al* (1997) Neural antigens in oligodendrogliomas and dysembryoplastic neuroepithelial tumors. *Acta Neuropathologica* 94:436–443.

Yaffe K, Ferriero D, Barkovich AJ, Rowley H (1995) Reversible MRI abnormalities following seizures. *Neurology* 45:104–108.

Brain infections

JE ADCOCK AND JM OXBURY

Brain infections are implicated as the cause in up to 7% of all cases of epilepsy (Bergamini *et al* 1977; Sander *et al* 1990; Marks *et al* 1992). Bacterial meningitis and viral encephalitis confer at least a sevenfold increased risk of developing epilepsy compared with the normal population (Rantakallio *et al* 1986; Annegers *et al* 1988), the risk being higher after encephalitis (Annegers *et al* 1988; Marks *et al* 1992). There is a particularly strong association with intracranial abscess. Viral meningitis is not associated with an increased risk (Annegers *et al* 1988). The infective organisms were often not identified in the large retrospective series that assessed CNS infection extending back over many years, so that relative risk according to specific infective agents could not be established. Brain infections that cause epilepsy are outlined in Table 16.1. Central nervous system infections are said to be one of the main reasons for the higher incidence of chronic epilepsy in developing countries (Bharucha and Shorvon 1998). Indeed, neurocysticercosis is regarded as the commonest cause of late-onset epilepsy in some Central and South American countries (Medina *et al* 1990).

VIRAL ENCEPHALITIS

There are many forms of viral encephalitis. All are associated to varying degrees with subsequent epilepsy. The risk of developing epilepsy within 20 years of viral encephalitis, regardless of the agent, is around 20% for those who experience early seizures and 10% for those who do not. These rates are 2–10 times higher than for patients with bacterial or aseptic meningitis (Annegers *et al* 1988). Sporadic forms of viral encephalitis include mumps, herpes simplex, rabies, and enteroviral infections. Acute postmeasles encephalopathy and subacute sclerosing panencephalitis are common in some countries and are associated with devastating neurologic sequelae. Arborviruses, such as Japanese encephalitis and dengue, usually present as epidemic outbreaks. Encephalitis due to herpes zoster, mumps, and rubella is well described, and occasional cases of resultant epilepsy do occur, but it is herpes simplex encephalitis that remains the most common sporadic fatal encephalitis with high mortality rates and significant morbidity in survivors.

Table 16.1 Brain infections that cause epilepsy.

Bacterial	
(a) Meningitis	
Acute	*Neisseria meningitidis*
	Streptococcus pneumoniae
	Haemophilus influenzae
	Listeria monocytogenes
	Gram-negative bacilli, e.g., *Escherichia coli,*
	Klebsiella pneumoniae, Pseudomonas
	aeruginosa, Enterobacter
	Staphylococcus aureus and *S. epidermidis*
Chronic	Tuberculosis
(b) Abscess	*Streptococcus,* esp. *S. milleri*
	Bacteroides, esp. *B. fragilis*
	Anaerobes, esp *Clostridium*
	Gram-negative bacilli, e.g. *Proteus,*
	Escherichia coli, Klebsiella pneumoniae,
	Pseudomonas aeruginosa
	Staphylococcus aureus
Viral	
Encephalitis	Herbes simplex
	Epstein–Barr
	Herpes zoster
	Mumps
	Rubella
	Measles
	Japanese encephalitis
	Arborviruses
	Cytomegalovirus
	Postinfectious: subacute sclerosing
	panencephalitis (SSPE)
Parasitic	
Protazoa	*Plasmodium falciparum*
	Toxoplasma gondii
	Entamoeba histolytica
Metazoa	Cysticercosis
	Schistosomosis
	Hydatid
HIV related	
Tumour	Lymphoma
Infective	
Mass lesion	Toxoplasma
	Progressive multifocal leukoencephalopathy
Generalized	Cryptococcal meningitis
	CMV encephalitis
HIV dementia	
Metabolic	Hypomagnesemia
	Hypocalcemia

HERPES SIMPLEX ENCEPHALITIS

Herpes simplex encephalitis (HSE) can occur at any age. Its incidence is considered to be 1:250 00 to 1:500 000 persons per year in the Western world (Skoldenberg 1996). Early epidemiologic studies may misrepresent the true prevalence of postinfective epilepsy in HSE patients since, until recently, it was difficult to calculate accurate morbidity and mortality rates. The diagnosis of HSE previously necessitated brain biopsy. Serological analysis of simultaneously drawn CSF and serum samples now provide a reliable diagnosis of HSE, but significant levels of the virus are not reached until 3–10 days after the onset of neurologic symptoms. Thus, HSE may frequently be misdiagnosed both false positively and false negatively in the early stages. Whitley *et al* (1989), for instance, showed that a range of unsuspected pathologies could be found in the brain biopsies of patients who had been (falsely) given a presumptive diagnosis of HSE. An example of a false negative case is a patient of McGrath *et al* (1997) who presented with brief episodes of unconsciousness and asystole followed by periods of confusion. Her symptoms were attributed to heart disease and a cardiac pacemaker was inserted before it eventually became clear that the attacks were complex partial seizures due to HSE.

A number of studies have shown that the early recognition of HSE and the prompt institution of antiviral therapy, most typically with acyclovir, can significantly reduce the associated mortality and morbidity (Nicholson 1984; Jeffries 1986; Skoldenberg 1991, 1996). If acyclovir can be introduced prior to the loss of consciousness, the mortality rate in HSE can be as low as 17% compared to 70% without therapy (Hanley *et al* 1987). Nevertheless, even when treatment with acyclovir was instituted at 1–30 days after the onset of symptoms, 24% of survivors subsequently developed epilepsy (McGrath *et al* 1997). Chronic epilepsy is more common among survivors who suffered seizures during the acute phase of the illness, but approximately 10% will still develop epilepsy following recovery even if seizures were not present then (Annegers *et al* 1988). In a group of patients with intractable complex partial seizures due to previous CNS infection who underwent presurgical evaluation, somatosensory and auditory auras were frequent in those who had a history of encephalitis compared to those with a history of meningitis.

MEASLES

Measles is still endemic in countries where immunization is limited. Measles encephalitis and the late complication of measles, subacute sclerosing panencephalitis (SSPE), still occur in relatively high numbers in school-age children. Chronic epilepsy is common in the survivors of measles encephalitis. SSPE, the syndrome of severe myoclonic epilepsy, progressive dementia, and motor deficits, which can also be due to other viruses such as rubella and Epstein–Barr virus, is usually fatal (Bharucha *et al* 1996).

EPSTEIN–BARR VIRUS ENCEPHALITIS

The Epstein–Barr virus (EBV) may be the cause in up to 5% of patients with acute viral encephalitis. Nonfebrile seizures are reported as the major presenting sign. They may be focal or generalized. Although sometimes considered a self-limiting illness with few sequelae and complete recovery (Connelly and DeWitt 1994), epilepsy has been reported to occur in up to one-third of survivors of Epstein–Barr virus encephalitis (Domachowske *et al* 1996). Also, SSPE may be associated with EBV. Feorino and Humphrey (1975) described three cases in which the SSPE coincided with primary EBV infection. They suggest that the EBV triggered a latent measles infection by interfering with the normal immunologic mechanism rather than that EBV was the primary cause of SSPE.

CYTOMEGALOVIRUS

An encephalitic illness is rare in nonimmune-compromised adolescent or adult acquired cytomegalovirus (CMV) infection but may occur in association with HIV. Chronic epilepsy can, however, develop in 20–25% of children with symptomatic congenital CMV and may be associated with hearing loss, microcephaly, and learning disability (Stagno 1996). Congenital and/or perinatal CMV is listed as one of the causes of West syndrome (Cassidy and Corbett 1998).

JAPANESE ENCEPHALITIS

Japanese encephalitis (JE) occurs in epidemics in Japan, China, Korea, and India. It is caused by an RNA virus that is transmitted to humans from birds, pigs or cattle by culex mosquitoes and affects children predominantly. The encephalitis is severe, with a mortality of up to 40% and severe neurologic morbidity in up to 45%. Intractable epilepsy occurs in 18%, motor deficits in 30%, and learning disabilities in 20%. Although complete recovery is seen in only about 30% of the pediatric population with JE, some recovery of neurologic function is seen up to 2 years or more post infection. Patients with a prolonged acute illness, or focal neurologic deficits upon presentation of the illness, are more likely to develop chronic epilepsy and other long-term neurologic sequelae (Kumar *et al* 1993; de Bittencourt *et al* 1996).

ARBORVIRUS ENCEPHALITIDES

Arborviruses are usually transmitted to humans by mosquitoes or by ticks. They are a relatively common cause of encephalitis in North America, particularly California encephalitis, Eastern equine encephalitis (EEE), Western equine encephalitis, and St Louis encephalitis (Labar and Harden 1998). EEE accounts for only 1% of cases of encephalitis in North America, but it is a severe encephalitis with a high mortality and morbidity. Patients aged <10 years are highly likely to be left with severe neurologic impairment and intractable epilepsy. Patients over this age either die or recover fully (Przelomski *et al* 1988). Neurologic sequelae, including chronic epilepsy, are less common with the other three arborvirus encephalitides.

HIV

As the number of patients infected with HIV increases, and the average survival increases owing to improved treatment, so the incidence, clinical features, significance, treatment, and outcome of seizures in HIV-infected patients are becoming better understood.

INCIDENCE AND ETIOLOGY

Seizures occur commonly at various stages of the illness, but it is difficult to estimate accurately the exact incidence, particularly as exact rates of HIV positivity are not known. However, it is clear that the incidence is far higher than that in the general population. New-onset seizures are the first symptom of disease in 10–18% of HIV-infected patients (Holtzman *et al* 1989; Wong *et al* 1990). The main causes of seizures are cerebral mass lesions in about 30%, which includes toxoplasmosis, cerebral lymphoma, and progressive multifocal leukoencephalopathy; cryptococcal meningitis in approximately 15%; and HIV dementia in about 30%. Rarer causes include stroke, CMV encephalitis, metabolic abnormalities such as hyponatremia, hypomagnesemia, and hypocalcemia, and thrombotic thrombocytopenic purpura. No apparent cause is found in 30–46% (Holtzman *et al* 1989; Wong *et al* 1990; Bartolomei *et al* 1991; Brew 1992; Guiloff and Fuller 1992; Dore and Brew 1994; Wright *et al* 1996). It is postulated that many of these cases are due to infection of the brain with HIV, per se. (Wong *et al* 1990).

Van Paesschen *et al* (1995) assessed the importance of metabolic abnormalities. Renal impairment and hypomagnesemia were statistically associated with an exacerbation of the seizures. In particular, they seemed to be associated with risk of convulsive status epilepticus. Other contributing factors include concurrent treatment with drugs known to be epileptogenic. Ciprofloxacin, which may be epileptogenic (Fan *et al* 1994), is a commonly used antibiotic in this patient group. Foscarnet is an antiviral agent used in the treatment of CMV infections. Its infusion is known to cause seizures in 12–15% of patients (Dore and Brew 1994; Fan *et al* 1994). Ciprofloxacin interacts with foscarnet to further stimulate seizures (Fan *et al* 1994).

Approximately 70% of seizures in HIV patients are generalized convulsions, with partial seizures occurring in up to 30% (Wong *et al* 1990; Bartolomei *et al* 1991). The underlying etiology is not specifically associated with the seizure type. Partial seizures may occur in patients with meningitis, and generalized convulsions without obvious focal clinical onset may occur in patients with focal mass lesions. Status epilepticus occurs not infrequently, usually in the context of an underlying mass lesion or overt opportunistic infection. Nonconvulsive status has also been reported (Wong *et al* 1990). Any patient with seizures in the context of HIV infection therefore needs to be investigated extensively. All patients routinely require cerebral imaging, preferably with MRI, CSF studies, estimation of cryptococcal antigen levels in blood and CSF, full blood count, liver and renal function tests, and serum magnesium and calcium levels.

MECHANISMS

The mechanisms by which seizures occur in the absence of mass lesions or opportunistic infections is not known specifically. There are various theories as to how HIV causes damage even if the cells themselves are not infected. There is growing support for the existence of HIV or immune-related toxins that directly or indirectly damage neurons via a complex interaction between macrocytes, microglia, astrocytes, and neurons. It is thought that there is probably a final common pathway, involving voltage-dependent Ca^{2+} channels and *N*-methyl-D-aspartate (NMDA) receptor-operated channels, and that this neuronal susceptibility is similar to that observed after non-HIV-related epilepsy, as well as stroke and trauma (Lipton 1992).

One group examined the hippocampi of cats infected with feline immunodeficiency virus (FIV), the animal model of HIV infection (Mitchell *et al* 1998). Gliosis was found within the hilus of the dentate gyrus and granule cell axonal sprouting. More prominent axonal sprouting was seen in cats infected as kittens, suggesting that younger cats may be more susceptible. This suggests that FIV infection causes granule cell axon reorganization in the hippocampus of cats, a process thought to underlie temporal lobe epilepsy in humans.

TREATMENT

Treatment is recommended as up to 70% of patients will have recurrent seizures (Holtzman *et al* 1989; Guiloff and Fuller 1992; Wright *et al* 1996). Seizures are often resistant to standard anticonvulsant therapy (Aronow *et al* 1989). The treatment of epilepsy in the HIV population poses a number of problems: many of the patients are already taking multiple medications, are using homeopathic medicines, are hypoalbuminemic, leukopenic, or thrombocytopenic, and already have abnormal liver function tests.

Anticonvulsants such as phenytoin and sodium valproate are strongly albumin bound and therefore serum free drug concentrations may be elevated, but, even allowing for this, it has been demonstrated that free levels are still higher than in the general population, suggesting additional unknown mechanisms in HIV patients (Dasgupta and McLemore 1998). This may partly explain why a high proportion of adverse drug reactions to phenytoin has been reported in patients with HIV: rash, worsening leukopenia or thrombocytopenia, and worsening liver function. Adverse reactions necessitating discontinuation of phenytoin were experienced by 14% of 87 patients (Holtzman *et al* 1989) and by 26% of 62 patients (Wong *et al* 1990). These are higher incidences of adverse effects than in non-AIDS patients treated with phenytoin. Other drugs may interact with phenytoin to cause additional difficulties. Fluconazole, used frequently for the treatment and prophylaxis of fungal infections, can increase serum phenytoin levels, leading to toxicity. Continuous monitoring of levels is required, especially if short-term high-dose fluconazole is used (Cadle *et al* 1994).

Some groups have suggested the use of sodium valproate (Guiloff and Fuller 1992; Wright *et al* 1996), but it has been demonstrated that valproate inhibits human red blood cell glutathione reductase, which reduces intracellular glutathione, thereby stimulating HIV. Valproate also induces HIV expression in the chronically infected monocytic cell line, which constitutively expresses low levels of the virus (Simon *et al* 1994). Phenobarbital seems to be very well tolerated in this patient group, and is recommended by several authors (Holtzman *et al* 1989; Guiloff and Fuller 1992).

BACTERIAL MENINGITIS

The death rate from bacterial meningitis has fallen from 90% to 10% since the introduction of antibiotics. However, it is unclear whether the incidence of permanent neurologic sequelae, including epilepsy, has also fallen. Certainly, the commonest sequela of sensorineural deafness remains at 10% (Dodge 1986).

ETIOLOGY

The peak incidence of meningitis occurs in children. *Haemophilus influenzae* is the commonest infective organism, followed by *Neisseria meningitidis* and then *Streptococcus pneumoniae*. These cause over 85% of all reported cases in children (Sell 1983). In adults, the commonest causes of community-acquired bacterial meningitis are *Strep. pneumoniae*, *N. meningitidis*, *H. influenzae* and *Listeria monocytogenes*. Other Gram-negative bacilli and *Staphylococcus aureus* infections are seen more commonly in nosocomial infections (Schlech *et al* 1985; Durand *et al* 1993; Sigurdardottir *et al* 1997). Not surprisingly, *H. influenzae* is the most common organism associated with the development of epilepsy.

RISKS OF DEVELOPING EPILEPSY

Up to 31% of patients, particularly children, have seizures acutely in the context of the initial meningitis (Rosman *et al* 1985; Pomeroy *et al* 1990; Durand *et al* 1993; Gomes *et al* 1996). The incidence of subsequent epilepsy requiring treatment is 2–14% (Edwards and Baker 1981; Nielsen *et al* 1983; Sell 1983; Feigin 1987). The main risk factor for developing epilepsy following meningitis is the persistence of focal neurologic deficit (excluding sensorineural deafness). In one series almost all patients who developed epilepsy had persisting neurologic deficits at 1 year post infection (Pomeroy *et al* 1990). Taylor *et al* (1990) also demonstrated that only patients with persisting neurologic deficit developed epilepsy.

Seizures during the acute phase of the illness are also associated with an increased risk of subsequent epilepsy, although this is strongly associated with persisting neurologic deficit. Annegers *et al* (1988) found that 15% of patients with early seizures developed late unprovoked seizures compared to only 2% of those without early seizures. Rosman *et al* (1985) demonstrated that the greatest predictor of early seizures was the presence of high fever and that the likelihood of continuing seizures was 5 times greater if there had been seizures in the acute phase. EEG abnormalities and CSF glucose <1.11 g l^{-1} have been shown to be associated with an increased risk, but these are not independent of neurologic deficit (Pomeroy *et al* 1990). Therefore, even if seizures have occurred during the acute infection, a child has a low risk of developing long-term epilepsy if the neurologic examination is normal on discharge (Pomeroy *et al* 1990; Taylor *et al* 1990).

LATENCY OF THE EPILEPSY

The first late seizure after bacterial meningitis usually occurs within 5 years but can occur up to at least 8 years later (Pomeroy *et al* 1990).

SEIZURE SEMEIOLOGY

The seizure type is usually focal in origin, with or without secondary generalization (Rantakallio *et al* 1986; Annegers *et al* 1988; Pomeroy *et al* 1990; Marks *et al* 1992; Durand *et al* 1993), but the incidence of generalized-onset seizures is also increased threefold (Annegers *et al* 1988). The seizures are often intractable and resistant to treatment (Emerson *et al* 1981; Pomeroy *et al* 1990).

MECHANISMS OF BRAIN INJURY

The mechanisms by which CNS infection causes brain injury and subsequent epilepsy include the direct result of the infection per se, altered cerebral blood flow and subsequent ischemia, secondary venous thrombosis, and cerebral necrosis (Sell 1983; Pomeroy *et al* 1990; Taylor *et al* 1990; Lancman and Morris 1996). Diffuse CNS infection can also cause very localized injury rather than diffuse damage. Epilepsy due to unilateral mesial temporal sclerosis (MTS), bilateral MTS, and focal neocortical abnormality as a consequence of bacterial meningitis and viral encephalitis is well described (Ounsted *et al* 1985; Lancman and Morris 1996). The mechanism by which MTS specifically occurs is less clear, but all of the above factors may play a role. The pyramidal neurons of the CA1 zone of the hippocampus are particularly vulnerable to ischemia. Prolonged febrile seizures unrelated to CNS infection are well known to be associated with MTS, and therefore fever in the context of the acute infection may be a contributing factor.

TREATMENT

As with brain abscess (see below), there is no evidence that one pharmacologic treatment for epilepsy due to bacterial meningitis is better than any other. The issue of surgical treatment for the epilepsy is discussed below.

INTRACRANIAL ABSCESS

An intracranial abscess may be situated extradurally, subdurally (subdural empyema), or intra-axially (cerebral abscess). The last is the most common (Teddy 1996) and may be single or multiple. Both cerebral abscess and subdural empyema may be related to infections of the paranasal sinuses and of the middle ear or to septicemia such that as from bacterial endocarditis and lung abscess. Chronic epilepsy is common in survivors of both cerebral abscess and subdural empyema, with as many as 60% being affected in some series of the latter (Cowie and Williams 1983).

In adults the infective agent of both cerebral abscess and subdural empyema is most often a streptococcus, particularly *Strep. milleri*, a staphylococcus, particularly *Staph. aureus*, or bacteroides. Two or more organisms are cultured in up to 60% of cases. In infants, subdural empyema may be secondary to meningitis caused by *H. influenzae*, *N. meningitidis* or *Strep. pneumoniae*.

CEREBRAL ABSCESS

Seizures may be the first sign of a cerebral abscess in up to one-third of cases (Bell and Britton, 1992; Annegers *et al* 1988). A large number of patients who survive cerebral abscess will suffer chronic and usually medically intractable epilepsy as a result of the residual abscess cavity, the associated infection, or, in some cases, the surgical intevention.

Fortunately, the incidence of cerebral abscess is falling in developed countries as a result of the decline in the prevalence of the associated diseases. In a large epidemiological study conducted in the USA, Nicolosi *et al* (1991) identified an incidence of 0.9 per 100 000 population per year in the period 1965–1981 compared to a rate of 2.7 in the 1930s and 1940s. However, increased incidence has been reported in other parts of the world (Shorvon and Bharucha 1992; Jamjoom *et al* 1994). In regions where parasites are endemic, cerebral abscess can complicate schistosomosis, ambiosis and hydatidosis. The incidence of cerebral abscess is also increased in immunocompromised patients and in those with a predisposing condition such as diabetes, sarcoidosis, and HIV, all of whom are at increased risk from opportunistic organisms. Cerebral abscess is more common in men than in women and ratios of between 2:1 and 3:1 are reported (Nicolosi *et al* 1991; Bell and Britton 1992). Ironically, patients who already have epilepsy may be more at risk of developing a cerebral abscess as a result of implantation with subdural electrodes

in attempts to identify the existing seizure focus (Wyler *et al* 1991).

The mortality has remained considerable, with estimates ranging between 10% and 40% (Legg *et al* 1973; Cowie and Williams, 1983; Nielsen *et al* 1983; Wyler *et al* 1991; Bell and Britton 1992; Koszewski 1991). This is despite improvements in surgical and medical treatments and the invaluable introduction of CT and MRI techniques to facilitate rapid diagnosis. Up to half of the cases may not make a full recovery. Epilepsy remains the most frequent sequel of a supratentorial abscess.

The exact mechanism responsible for the development of epilepsy is uncertain. Northcroft and Wyke (1957) suggested that the fibroglial reactions associated with the formation of a healing cicatrix in the region of the previous inflammatory response, along with vascular disturbances, may form the basis of an epileptic focus by inducing abnormal neuronal activity. This mechanism may explain the considerable latent period before seizures develop in some patients and the apparent lack of an association between early seizures and the subsequent development of epilepsy.

Many of those who survive an intracranial abscess may be left with neurologic or neuropsychologic deficits and epilepsy. Estimates of postinfective epilepsy vary from 0% (Aydin *et al* 1988) to 95% (Bradley *et al* 1984), with most ranging from 40% to 70% (Legg *et al* 1973; Cowie and Williams 1983; Nielsen *et al* 1983; Koszewski 1991). These widely differing figures are due in part to the differences in the populations studied, the follow-up periods used, and other key methodological factors. However, a number of high-risk factors do emerge from the literature as a whole.

GENDER

Cerebral abscess is more prevalent in males than females, and men are also significantly more likely to develop postinfective epilepsy than women (Koszewski 1991).

AGE

It is not clear how age at the time of infection effects the risk of subsequent epilepsy. Legg *et al* (1973) found no significant effect of age in a study of 160 patients followed for up to 30 years; 72% of them developed postinfective seizures. Koszewki (1991) on the other hand, reported that patients aged 15–45 years when they developed the abscess were more prone to subsequent epilepsy than those who were older or younger. Similarly, Cowie and Williams (1983) found the highest incidence of seizures in those who developed an abscess in the second and third decades of life. However, others have found that abscess in childhood is associated with the most serious sequelae, including incapacitating epilepsy and severe learning disability (Nielsen *et al* 1983). The effects of age probably combine with other factors to increase or decrease the risk of subsequent epilepsy.

Szenasy and Nagy (1979) found that epilepsy as a consequence of brain abscess in children was dependent on the length of the catamnestic period and the location of the abscess. They also reported the onset of epilepsy in adulthood, in some cases decades after the acute childhood incident of the abscess, suggesting that the true prevalence of epilepsy following cerebral abscess may be underestimated even by studies that have employed long-term follow-up periods. Renier *et al* (1988), in a unique study of patients who developed a cerebral abscess during the neonatal period, found that the absence of initial seizures, sterile cerebrospinal fluid, normal ventricles, and early aspiration portend a better prognosis in terms of epilepsy and other mental sequelae.

ETIOLOGY

Cerebral abscess is rarely due to the organisms that commonly cause meningitis such as *Strep. pneumoniae, N. meningitidis* and *H. influenzae* (Bharucha *et al* 1996). Nevertheless, Koszewski (1991) reported that abscess following meningitis carries the highest risk of seizures, while lesions of metastatic etiology have the lowest. In the former cases it is difficult to determine whether epilepsy developed as a direct result of abscess or as a complication of the underlying disease involving the rest of the brain tissue. The increased incidence in these patients probably reflects the 'double risk' of abscess and meningitis. Fungal infections have also been associated with a lower risk (Legg *et al* 1973). Culture studies can be difficult because the pus is frequently sterile (Bell and Britton, 1992), but, in those where culture studies yielded results, Koszewski (1991) found no significant relation between the responsible microorganism and the subsequent incidence of epilepsy.

LOCATION

Temporal lobe abscesses are associated with the highest incidence of epilepsy, followed by those in the frontal regions (Legg *et al* 1973; Koszewski 1991). Occipital lobe abscess carries the lowest risk. Scott (1985) found that seizures were more likely to occur following the excision of an abscess from the left hemisphere than from the right. This laterality effect was not confirmed by Koszewski

(1991). As with other etiologies, the localization of the abscess influences the ictal semeiology, although patients with postinfective epilepsy may not experience the 'typical' seizure semeiology associated with focal epilepsy resulting from more common etiologies. For example, Jansen *et al* (1990) report a patient who suffered persistent hiccups and secondary generalized epilepsy following a posttraumatic abscess in the right temporal lobe. Unlike the seizures, the hiccups remained unresponsive to treatment and were associated with left frontal EEG slowing.

CHARACTER AND SIZE

Koszewski (1991) found no differences in the subsequent development of epilepsy between patients who had unilocular, multilocular, and multiple abscesses. However, the number of patients in the latter group was extremely small. Although the size of the abscess did not appear to be proportionally related to the subsequent risk of developing epilepsy, patients with capsules exceeding a threshold of 4 cm in diameter were significantly more likely to develop epilepsy than those with smaller sites.

EARLY SEIZURES

Early seizures, during the treatment phase of the abscess, may occur in up to two-thirds of patients, particularly those with paranasal sepsis (Cowie and Williams 1983). The presence of seizures during this initial period of the disease does not appear to have prognostic value for the later development of chronic seizures, at least in adults (Legg *et al* 1973; Koszewski 1991). The interval between the onset of symptoms and the commencement of treatment does not appear to be a significant factor. Similarly, EEG abnormalities during the acute phase of the abscess do not appear to be related to the subsequent development of epilepsy (Legg *et al* 1973; Koszewski 1991).

LATENCY OF THE EPILEPSY

Severe and medically intractable seizures are likely to develop within 12 months of the acute phase of the abscess (Legg *et al* 1973; Koszewski 1991), particularly in adults aged between 20 and 40 years. Nevertheless, approximately 15% of patients develop epilepsy after this time (Koszewski 1991). In children, the interval between the acute presentation and the onset of the epilepsy may be 15 years or more. Prophylactic anticonvulsant drugs are recommended for at least 2 years for patients who are at high risk of developing seizures, although, as Calliauw *et al* (1984) point out, the risk of seizures in a patient following a supratentorial abscess never returns to baseline levels.

TREATMENT

There have been no randomized control trials investigating the effects of treatment on the risks of subsequent epilepsy. A few patients with small, deep or multiple abscesses have been treated successfully by antibiotics alone, but drainage of pus from whichever intracranial compartment it occupies remains the treatment of choice. At present, surgical treatment varies between total excision and aspiration or drainage via a craniotomy or burr hole, combined with antibiotics and anticonvulsant drugs. A number of studies have reported no significant effects of these different treatments on the subsequent development of epilepsy (Legg *et al* 1973; Cowie and Williams 1983; Koszewski 1991), although small group numbers, particularly in the medically treated groups, preclude any definitive conclusions from these studies.

Overall, supratentorial neurosurgical procedures are associated with a 17% risk of postoperative seizures. The risk (70–90%) is significantly higher for abscess (Foy *et al* 1981), but this figure does not take into account the high base-rates associated with abscess regardless of the treatment. Pellone *et al* (1975) found that in adults excision of the abscess resulted in fewer epileptic complications than did drainage of the abscess cavity. Others have found that children treated by excision of the abscess have an increased risk of subsequent epilepsy than those treated with aspiration/antibiotics (Hirsch *et al* 1983; Aebi *et al* 1991).

OTHER BRAIN INFECTIONS

Many other infections may cause seizures in the acute phase of the illness or as part of an encephalopathy that will lead to death within months at most (e.g. African trypanosomiasis). Discussion here is restricted to those conditions that may lead to chronic epilepsy.

BACTERIAL

Mycobacterium tuberculosis

Tuberculosis is a significant factor in the etiology of chronic epilepsy in countries where tuberculous meningitis is particularly prevalent. The incidence of tuberculosis was falling in developed countries until the mid 1980s but since then there has been some increase, at least partly because of HIV. Approximately 2% of tuberculosis cases are accounted for by tuberculous meningitis (Davies *et al* 1996). Epilepsy develops in around 20% of the survivors of tuberculous

meningitis. It is particularly likely to do so in children and in those who had focal neurologic signs during the acute phase of the illness (Davis and Shih 1999). Around 60% of those who had seizures during the acute phase have recurrent seizures subsequently (Crook *et al* 1996).

A tuberculoma is an avascular mass consisting of a necrotic center surrounded by tuberculous granulation tissue containing epithelioid cells, lymphocytes, and Langhans' giant cells (Traub 1991). Tubercle bacilli can be found in most tuberculosis. Such lesions may be single or multiple within the brain. Their size varies from a few millimeters in diameter to sufficient to fill much of a cerebral hemisphere. Their clinical presentation is typically as an intracranial mass lesion with seizures and with symptoms or signs of focal cerebral or cerebellar dysfunction and raised intracranial pressure. Although currently rare in 'developed' countries they make up a significant proportion of intracranial mass lesions in developing countries, especially India. They effect predominantly those aged <40 years, being situated mainly infratentorially in children and supratentorially in adults. The preferred treatment is with antituberculous drugs, but additional surgery may be necessary in some cases. There is residual chronic epilepsy in at least 10% of cases.

Bordetella pertussis

Encephalopathy is a rare complication of whooping cough causing neurologic features including convulsions, coma, and focal signs. The long-term outcome can be poor, with chronic epilepsy, learning disability, blindness, deafness, and movement disorders.

PROTOZOAL

Amebiosis

Amebic brain abscess is a rare complication of hepatic amebiosis due to *Entamoeba histolytica*. Of other species, *Naegleria fowleri* causes a necrotizing meningoencephalitis and *Acanthamoeba* causes a granulomatous encephalitis. All three conditions usually lead to death within a few weeks (Haddock 1991). It is said, however, that the few survivors are often left with epilepsy among other neurologic sequelae (Davis and Shih 1999).

Malaria

Chronic epilepsy is unusual in adult survivors of cerebral (*Plasmodium falciparum*) malaria. However, it is relatively common in African children who have suffered malaria. The liability to epilepsy in children has been attributed to febrile convulsions and brain swelling during the acute phase of the illness.

Toxoplasma gondii

Congenital toxoplasmosis causes a wide range of symptoms and signs in neonates and infants, and at older ages as a consequence of involvement of the CNS and other body systems (Couvreur and Thulliez 1996). The neurologic features include chronic epilepsy, microcephaly, hydrocephalus, aqueduct stenosis, cerebral calcifications, and learning disability. Toxoplasmosis acquired postnatally is usually subclinical, but at any age it may cause a chronic relapsing meningoencephalitic illness continuing over years. In most cases cerebral toxoplasmosis is associated with systemic disease or immune deficiency as may occur with immunosuppressive drugs, various malignancies, and HIV. The neurologic features include seizures, mental symptoms, focal signs and cranial nerve palsies, symptoms of raised intracranial pressure, a mild CSF pleocytosis and protein elevation, and neuroimaging evidence of a single or multiple mass lesions.

CESTODES (TAPEWORMS)

Hydatid disease

Humans most commonly ingest *Echinococcus granulosus*, the dog tapeworm, by handling contaminated dogs or from contaminated vegetables or water. These tapeworms are widely distributed across Europe and Asia and are also found in parts of Australia, Africa, and South America. Eggs hatch in the duodenum and then penetrate the intestinal wall to gain access to various organs, most often the liver, where cysts are formed (Radford 1996). They can reach the brain, where a small proportion of the cysts is found. Cerebral cysts are usually single and can grow to a large size but they can be multiple. They cause focal epilepsy, symptoms and signs of focal brain dysfunction, and ultimately features of raised intracranial pressure.

Cysticercosis

Cystircercosis arises in eaters of pork from ingestion of the eggs of *Taenia solium*, the pork tapeworm. *T. solium* is common in Mexico and some other South American countries, various parts of Asia including India and China, and in sub-Saharan Africa (Knight 1996; Overbosch 1996). The eggs are digested in the gut, releasing larvae that penetrate the gut wall and are transported via the bloodstream to various tissues. The clinical features are due to encystment

of the larvae, followed by calcification, in the central nervous system (neurocysticercosis), the muscles, and the eye.

Epilepsy is the predominant symptom of neurocysticercosis and neurocysticercosis is one of the commonest causes of epilepsy in various countries of Central and South America and Asia (Medina *et al* 1990; Del-Brutto and Noboa 1991; Senanayake and Roman 1993; Gulati *et al* 1994). Other features of the condition include basal meningitis leading to cranial nerve palsies and communicating hydrocephalus, dementia, and paraplegia due to spinal cord or cauda equina compression. One study of the seizures in neurocysticercosis (Monteiro *et al* 1995) reported that they were most commonly simple partial (46%), followed by generalized tonic–clonic (35%) and then complex partial (19%). The epilepsy was not adequately controlled in around 35% and status epilepticus occurred in around 25% cases. There is evidence that treatment with cysticidal drugs such as albendazole and praziquantel leads to improved seizure control (Vazquez and Sotelo 1992; Medina *et al* 1993; Carpio *et al* 1995).

TREMATODES (FLUKES)

Schistosomosis

Schistosoma japonicum is the species most likely to cause epilepsy (Haddock 1991; Huang 1991). It is confined to the Far East, especially China and the Philippines. Infection of nonimmune persons, and the deposition of eggs by the adult worm, causes an acute illness ('acute schistosomosis,' 'Katayama fever') that can be fatal. Deposition of eggs in the brain is associated with encephalopathic features. The presence of intracranial granulomas resulting from the egg deposition is responsible for a chronic cerebral form of schistosomosis that is characterized by epileptic seizures, features of focal cerebral dysfunction, and raised intracranial pressure. There may be associated hepatic symptoms and signs. *Schistosoma mansoni* (found in Africa, South America, and the Caribbean) and *S. haematobium* (found in Africa) rarely cause epilepsy but may cause a myelopathy (Butterworth and Thomas 1996).

Paragonimosis

There are a number of species of *Paragonimus*. Foci of disease are in Asia, Africa, and Central and South America. Cysts containing young flukes are formed mainly in the lungs, but cysts and granulomata are also formed in other organs including the brain (Vanijanonta 1996) and sometimes in relation to the spinal cord. Chronic cerebral paragonimosis is manifest especially by epilepsy, which may be accompanied by mental disturbance, recurrent eosinophilic meningitis, and symptoms/signs of raised intracranial pressure (Haddock 1991).

SURGICAL TREATMENT OF EPILEPSY DUE TO CNS INFECTION

Up to 14% of patients referred to epilepsy surgery units for assessment have a past history of CNS infection (Lancman and Morris 1996). Patients with epilepsy secondary to CNS infection are generally thought to have diffuse rather than focal brain involvement and thus may not be suitable for epilepsy surgery. However, temporal lobe surgery for mesial temporal lobe epilepsy due to unilateral hippocampal sclerosis associated with previous CNS infection has an excellent outcome, with high rates of Engel class 1 and 2 seizure outcome (Engel *et al* 1993) equivalent to those in patients without such a history. These patients usually have focal MRI abnormalities and characteristic pathologic findings typical of hippocampal sclerosis (Marks *et al* 1992; Lancman and Morris 1996; Lee *et al* 1997).

Surgery for neocortical epilepsy is associated with poor seizure outcome unless there is definite focal pathology detectable on MRI such as a scar from a previous abscess cavity. Otherwise, these patients usually have a poor localization of the seizure onset (Marks *et al* 1992; Lancman and Morris 1996; Lee *et al* 1997). Why some patients develop neocortical epilepsy whereas others develop unilateral or bilateral mesial temporal sclerosis (MTS) is unclear, although there are some predictive factors. Unilateral MTS is more likely to be associated with a history of bacterial meningitis. Bilateral MTS and neocortical epilepsy, particularly from the parietal and temporal lobes, are more likely to be associated with a history of viral encephalitis. The other factors predictive of unilateral MTS due to CNS infection are young age at the time of the infection (<4 years, usually <2 years) and a long latency period between the infection and the development of the intractable epilepsy (Ounsted *et al* 1985; Marks *et al* 1992; Lancman and Morris, 1996; Lee *et al* 1997). Marks *et al* (1992) also found in the few cases of unilateral MTS due to encephalitis that the age at infection in all was <4 years. This supports earlier work suggesting that the critical predictor of MTS is the age of the initial insult.

KEY POINTS

1. Brain infections are implicated as the cause in up to 7% of all cases of epilepsy.
2. The risk of developing epilepsy within 20 years of viral encephalitis is around 20% for those who suffer early seizures and 10% for those who do not. New-onset seizures are the first feature of the disease in 10–18% of HIV-infected patients.
3. Epilepsy develops in >50% of those who survive a cerebral or epidural abscess. Abscesses situated in a temporal or a frontal lobe confer a greater risk of epilepsy than do those situated elsewhere in the brain. The epilepsy usually develops within one year of the acute phase, but may be delayed for several years especially in children.
4. The incidence of epilepsy following meningitis is up to 15% of survivors. Major risk factors are seizures during the acute phase and persisting neurological deficit.
5. Epilepsy develops in 20% of survivors of tuberculous meningitis, including around 60% of those who had seizures during the acute phase and 10% of those treated for a tuberculoma.
6. Neurocysticercosis is one of the commonest causes of epilepsy in various countries of Africa, Central America, South America, and Asia.

REFERENCES

Aebi C, Kaufmann F, Schaad UB (1991) Brain abscess in childhood – long-term experiences. *European Journal of Pediatrics* **150**:282–286.

Annegers JF, Hauser WA, Beghi E, Nicolosi A, Kurland LT (1988) The risk of unprovoked seizures after encephalitis and meningitis. *Neurology* **38**:1407–1410.

Aronow HA, Feraru ER, Lipton RB (1989) New-onset seizures in AIDS patients: etiology, prognosis, and treatment. *Neurology* **39**: (abstract)

Aydin IH, Aladag MA, Kadioglu HH, Onder A (1988) Clinical analysis of cerebral abscesses. *Zentralblatt für Neurochirurgie* **49**:210–219.

Bartolomei F, Pellegrino P, Dhiver C, Quilichini R, Gastaut JA, Gastaut JL (1991) [Epilepsy seizures in HIV infection. 52 cases]. *Presse Medicale* **20**:2135–2138.

Bell BA, Britton JA (1992) Brain abscess. In: Lambert HP (ed) *Infections of the Central Nervous System*, pp 361–373. Philadelphia: B.C. Decker.

Bergamini L, Bergamasco B, Benna P, Gilli M (1977) Acquired etiological factors in 1,785 epileptic subjects: clinical-anamnestic research. *Epilepsia* **18**:437–444.

Bharucha NE, Shorvon SD (1998) Epidemiology in developing countries. In: Engel J and Pedley TA (eds) *Epilepsy: A Comprehensive Textbook*, pp 105–118. Philadelphia: Lippincott-Raven.

Bharucha NE, Bharucha EP, Bhabha SK (1996) Infections of the nervous system. In: Bradley WG, Daroff RB, Fenichel GM, Marsden CD (eds) *Neurology in Clinical Practice*, pp 1181–1243. Boston: Butterworth-Heinemann.

Bradley PJ, Manning KP, Shaw MD (1984) Brain abscess secondary to paranasal sinusitis. *Journal of Laryngology and Otology* **98**:719–725.

Brew BJ (1992) Medical management of AIDS patients. Central and peripheral nervous system abnormalities. *Medical Clinics of North America* **76**:63–81.

Butterworth AE, Thomas JEP (1996) Schistosomiasis. In: Weatherall DJ, Ledingham JGG, Warrell DA (eds) *Oxford Textbook of Medicine*, 3rd edn, vol 1, pp 970–981. Oxford: Oxford University Press.

Cadle RM, Zenon GJ, Rodriguez BM, Hamill RJ (1994) Fluconazole-induced symptomatic phenytoin toxicity. *Annals of Pharmacotherapy* **28**:191–195.

Carpio A, Santillan F, Leon P, Flores C, Hauser WA (1995) Is the course of neurocysticercosis modified by treatment with antihelminthic agents? *Archives of Internal Medicine* **155**:1982–1988.

Calliauw L, De PP, Verbeke L (1984) Postoperative epilepsy in subdural suppurations. *Acta Neurochirurgica Wien* **71**:217–223.

Cassidy G, Corbett J (1998) Learning disorders. In: Engel J, Pedley TA (eds) *Epilepsy: A Comprehensive Textbook*, pp 2053–2063. Philadelphia: Lippincott-Raven.

Connelly KP, DeWitt LD (1994) Neurologic complications of infectious mononucleosis. *Pediatric Neurology* **10**:181–184.

Couvreur J, Thulliez Ph (1996) Toxoplasmosis. In: Weatherall DJ, Ledingham JGG, Warrell DA (eds) *Oxford Textbook of Medicine*, 3rd, edn, vol 1, pp 865–869. Oxford: Oxford University Press.

Cowie R, Williams B (1983) Late seizures and morbidity after subdural empyema. *Journal of Neurosurgery* **58**:569–573.

Crook DWM, Phuapradit P, Warrell DA (1996) Bacterial meningitis. In: Weatherall DJ, Ledingham JGG, Warrell DA (eds) *Oxford Textbook of Medicine*, 3rd edn, vol 3, pp 4050–4064. Oxford: Oxford University Press.

Dasgupta A, McLemore JL (1998) Elevated free phenytoin and free valproic acid concentrations in sera of patients infected with human immunodeficiency virus. *Therapeutic Drug Monitoring* **20**:63–67.

Davies PDO, Girling DJ, Grange JM (1996) Tuberculosis and its problems in developing countries. In: Weatherall DJ, Ledingham JGG, Warrell DA (eds) *Oxford Textbook of Medicine*, 3rd edn, vol 1, pp 638–661. Oxford: Oxford University Press.

Davis LE, Shih JJ (1999) CNS infections and epilepsy. In: Kotagal P, Luders HO (eds) *The Epilepsies: Etiologies and Prevention*, pp 265–275. San Diego: Academic Press.

de Bittencourt PR, Adamolekum B, Bharucha N et al (1996) Epilepsy in the tropics: II. Clinical presentations, pathophysiology, immunologic diagnosis, economics, and therapy. *Epilepsia* **37**:1128–1137.

Del-Brutto OH, Noboa CA (1991) Late-onset epilepsy in Ecuador: aetiology and clinical features in 225 patients. *Journal of Tropical and Geographical Neurology* **1**:31–34.

Dodge PR (1986) Sequelae of bacterial meningitis. *Pediatric Infectious Disease* **5**:618–620.

Domachowske JB, Cunningham CK, Cummings DL, Crosley CJ, Hannan WP, Weiner LB (1996) Acute manifestations and neurologic sequelae of Epstein–Barr virus encephalitis in children [see comments]. *Pediatric Infectious Disease Journal* **15**:871–875.

Dore G, Brew BJ (1994) Prospective analysis of HIV associated seizures. *Sixth Conference of the Australian Society of HIV Medicine, Sydney, Australia* (Abstract) (available from ASHM on request).

Durand ML, Calderwood SB, Weber DJ et al (1993) Acute bacterial meningitis in adults. A review of 493 episodes [see comments]. *New England Journal of Medicine* **328**:21–28.

Edwards MS, Baker CJ (1981) Complications and sequelae of meningococcal infections in children. *Journal of Pediatrics* **99**:540–545.

Emerson R, D'Souza BJ, Vining EP, Holden KR, Mellits ED, Freeman JM (1981) Stopping medication in children with epilepsy: predictors of outcome. *New England Journal of Medicine* **304**:1125–1129.

Engel J Jr, Van Ness PC, Rasmussen TB, Ojemann LM (1993) Outcome with respect to epileptic seizures. In: Engel J Jr (ed) *Surgical Treatment of the Epilepsies*, pp 609–621. New York: Raven Press.

Fan HP, Sanchorawala V, Oh J, Moser EM, Smith SP (1994) Concurrent use of foscarnet and ciprofloxacin may increase the propensity for seizures. *Annals of Pharmacotherapy* **28**:869–872.

Feigin RD (1987) Bacterial meningitis beyond the neonatal period. In: Feigin RD, Cherry JD (eds) *Textbook of Pediatric Infectious Diseases*, pp 439–465. Philadelphia: W.B. Saunders.

Feorino PM, Humphrey D (1975) Mononucleosis-associated subacute sclerosing panencephalitis. *Lancet* **2**:530–532.

Foy PM, Copeland GP, Shaw MD (1981) The incidence of postoperative seizures. *Acta Neurochirurgica Wien* **55**:253–264.

Gomes I, Melo A, Lucena R, et al (1996) Prognosis of bacterial meningitis in children. *Arquivos de Neuro-Psiquiatria* **54**:407–411.

Guiloff RJ, Fuller GN (1992) Other neurological diseases in HIV-1 infection: clinical aspects. *Baillières Clinical Neurology* **1**:175–209.

Gulati P, Jena AN, Tripathi RP, Puri V, Sanchetee PC (1994) MRI (magnetic resonance imaging) spectrum of epilepsy. *Journal of the Indian Medical Association* **92**:110–112.

Haddock DRW (1991) Predominantly tropical and subtropical infections. In: Swash M, Oxbury J (eds) *Clinical Neurology*, vol 1, pp 898–921. Edinburgh: Churchill Livingstone.

Hanley DF, Johnson RT, Whitley RJ (1987) Yes, brain biopsy should be a prerequisite for herpes simplex encephalitis treatment. *Archives of Neurology* **44**:1289–1290.

Hirsch JF, Roux FX, Sainte RC, Renier D, Pierre KA (1983) Brain abscess in childhood. A study of 34 cases treated by puncture and antibiotics. *Child's Brain* **10**:251–265.

Holtzman DM, Kaku DA, So YT (1989) New-onset seizures associated with human immunodeficiency virus infection: causation and clinical features in 100 cases. *American Journal of Medicine* **87**:173–177.

Huang CY (1991) Neurology in Asia. In: Bradley WG, Daroff RB, Fenichel GM, Marsden CD (eds) *Neurology in Clinical Practice*, vol 2, pp 1908–1913. Boston: Butterworth-Heinemann.

Jamjoom A, Jamjoom ZA, Naim UR, Tahan A, Malabarey T, Kambal A (1994) Experience with brain abscess in the central province of Saudi Arabia. *Tropical and Geographical Medicine* **46**:154–156.

Jansen Ph, Joosten EM, Vingerhoets HM (1990) Persistent periodic hiccups following brain abscess: a case report. *Journal of Neurology, Neurosurgery and Psychiatry* **53**:83–84.

Jeffries DJ (1986) Acyclovir update [editorial]. *British Medical Journal, Clinical Research Edition* **293**:1523.

Knight R (1996) Gut cestodes. In: Weatherall DJ, Ledingham JGG, Warrell DA (eds) *Oxford Textbook of Medicine*, 3rd edn, vol 1, pp 959–964. Oxford: Oxford University Press.

Koszewski W (1991) Epilepsy following brain abscess. The evaluation of possible risk factors with emphasis on new concept of epileptic focus formation. *Acta Neurochirurgica Wien* **113**:110–117.

Kumar R, Mathur A, Singh KB, et al (1993) Clinical sequelae of Japanese encephalitis in children. *Indian Journal of Medical Research* **97**:9–13.

Labar DR, Harden C (1998) Infection and inflammatory disease. In: Engel J Jr, Pedley TA (eds) *Epilepsy: A Comprehensive Textbook*, pp 2587–2596. Philadelphia: Lippincott-Raven.

Lancman ME, Morris HH (1996) Epilepsy after central nervous system infection: clinical characteristics and outcome after epilepsy surgery. *Epilepsy Research* **25**:285–290.

Lee JH, Lee BI, Park SC, et al (1997) Experiences of epilepsy surgery in intractable seizures with past history of CNS infection. *Yonsei Medical Journal* **38**:73–78.

Legg NJ, Gupta PC, Scott DF (1973) Epilepsy following cerebral abscess. A clinical and EEG study of 70 patients. *Brain* 96:259–268.

Lipton SA (1992) Models of neuronal injury in AIDS: another role for the NMDA receptor? [see comments]. *Trends in Neurosciences* 15:75–79

Marks DA, Kim J, Spencer DD, Spencer SS (1992) Characteristics of intractable seizures following meningitis and encephalitis [see comments]. *Neurology* 42:1513–1518.

McGrath N, Anderson NE, Croxson MC, Powell KF (1997) Herpes simplex encephalitis treated with acyclovir: diagnosis and long term outcome. *Journal of Neurology, Neurosurgery and Psychiatry* 63:321–326.

Medina MT, Rosas E, Rubio-Donnadieu F, Sotelo J (1990) Neurocysticercosis as the main cause of late-onset epilepsy in Mexico. *Archives of Internal Medicine* 150:325–327.

Medina MT, Genton P, Montoya MC, Cordova S, Dravet C, Sotelo J (1993) Effect of anticysticercal treatment on the prognosis of epilepsy in neurocysticercosis: a pilot trial. *Epilepsia* 34:1024–1027.

Mitchell TW, Buckmaster PS, Hoover EA, Whalen LR, Dudek FE (1998) Axonal sprouting in hippocampus of cats infected with feline immunodeficiency virus (FIV). *Journal of Acquired Immune Deficiency Syndromes and Human Retrovirology* 17:1–8.

Monteiro L, Nunes B, Mendonca D, Lopes J (1995) Spectrum of epilepsy in neurocysticercosis: a long term follow-up of 143 patients. *Acta Neurologica Scandinavica* 92:33–40.

Nicholson KG (1984) Antiviral therapy. Herpes simplex encephalitis, neonatal herpes infections, chronic hepatitis B. *Lancet* 2:736–739.

Nicolosi A, Hauser WA, Musicco M, Kurland LT (1991) Incidence and prognosis of brain abscess in a defined population: Olmsted County, Minnesota, 1935–1981. *Neuroepidemiology* 10:122–131.

Nielsen H, Harmsen A, Gyldensted C (1983) Cerebral abscess. A long-term follow-up. *Acta Neurologica Scandinavica* 67:330–337

Northcroft GB, Wyke BD (1957) Seizures following surgical treatment of intracranial abscesses. *Journal of Neurosurgery* 14:249–263.

Ounsted C, Glaser GH, Lindsay J, Richards P (1985) Focal epilepsy with mesial temporal sclerosis after acute meningitis. *Archives of Neurology* 42:1058–1060.

Overbosch D (1996) Cysticercosis. In: Weatherall DJ, Ledingham JGG, Warrell DA (eds) *Oxford Textbook of Medicine*, 3rd edn, vol 1, pp 964–968. Oxford: Oxford University Press.

Pellone M, Rubini L, Carteri A (1975) Considerations on the results of surgical treatment of cerebral abscesses. *Journal of Neurosurgical Science* 19:152–158.

Pomeroy SL, Holmes SJ, Dodge PR, Feigin RD (1990) Seizures and other neurologic sequelae of bacterial meningitis in children. *New England Journal of Medicine* 323:1651–1657.

Przelomski MM, O'Rourke E, Grady GF, Berardi VP, Markley HG (1988) Eastern equine encephalitis in Massachusetts: a report of 16 cases, 1970–1984. *Neurology* 38:736–739.

Radford AJ (1996) Hydatid disease. In: Weatherall DJ, Ledingham JGG, Warrell DA (eds) *Oxford Textbook of Medicine*, 3rd edn, vol 1, pp. 955–959. Oxford: Oxford University Press.

Rantakallio P, Leskinen M, Von WL (1986) Incidence and prognosis of central nervous system infections in a birth cohort of 12,000 children. *Scandinavian Journal of Infectious Diseases* 18:287–294.

Renier D, Flandin C, Hirsch E, Hirsch JF (1988) Brain abscesses in neonates. A study of 30 cases. *Journal of Neurosurgery* 69:877–882.

Rosman NP, Peterson DB, Kaye EM, Colton T (1985) Seizures in bacterial meningitis: prevalence, patterns, pathogenesis, and prognosis. *Pediatric Neurology* 1:278–285.

Sander JW, Hart YM, Johnson AL, Shorvon SD (1990) National General Practice Study of Epilepsy: newly diagnosed epileptic seizures in a general population. *Lancet* 336:1267–1271.

Schlech WF, Ward JI, Band JD, Hightower A, Fraser DW, Broome CV (1985) Bacterial meningitis in the United States, 1978 through 1981. The National Bacterial Meningitis Surveillance Study. *JAMA* 253:1749–1754.

Scott DF (1985) Left and right cerebral hemisphere differences in the occurrence of epilepsy. *British Journal of Medical Psychology* 58:189–192.

Sell SH (1983) Long term sequelae of bacterial meningitis in children. *Pediatric Infections Disease* 2:90–93.

Senanayake N, Roman GC (1993) Epidemiology of epilepsy in developing coutries. *Bulletin of the World Health Organization* 71:247–258.

Shorvon SD, Bharucha NE (1992) Epilepsy in developing countries: epidemiology, aetiology and healthcare. In: Laidlow J, Richens AL, Chadwick DW (eds) *A Textbook of Epilepsy*, pp 613–636. Edinburgh: Churchill Livingston.

Sigurdardottir B, Bjornsson OM, Jonsdottir KE, Erlendsdottir H, Gudmundsson S (1997) Acute bacterial meningitis in adults. A 20-year overview. *Archives of Internal Medicine* 157:425–430.

Simon G, Moog C, Obert G (1994) Valproic acid reduces the intracellular level of glutathione and stimulates human immunodeficiency virus. *Chemico-Biological Interactions* 91:111–121.

Skoldenberg B (1991) Herpes simplex encephalitis. *Scandinavian Journal of Infectious Diseases Supplement* 80:40–46.

Skoldenberg B (1996) Herpes simplex encephalitis. *Scandinavian Journal of Infectious Diseases Supplement* 100:8–13.

Stagno S (1996) Cytomegalovirus. In: Weatherall DJ, Ledingham JGG, Warrell DA (eds) *Oxford Textbook of Medicine*, 3rd edn, vol 1, pp 359–363. Oxford: Oxford University Press.

Szenasy J, Nagy A (1979) Epilepsy and brain abscess. *Acta Paediatrica Academia Scientifica Hungarica* 20:255–259.

Taylor HG, Mills EL, Ciampi A, *et al* (1990) The sequelae of *Haemophilus influenzae* meningitis in school-age children. *New England Journal of Medicine* 323:1657–1663.

Teddy PJ (1996) Intracranial abscess. In: Weatherall DJ, Ledingham JGG, Warrell DA (eds) *Oxford Textbook of Medicine*, 3rd edn, vol 3, pp 4081–4083. Oxford: Oxford University Press.

Traub M (1991) Tuberculosis of the central nervous system. In: Swash M, Oxbury JM (eds) *Clinical Neurology*, vol 1, pp 872–880. Edinburgh: Churchill Livingstone.

Van Paesschen W, Bodian C, Maker H (1995) Metabolic abnormalities and new-onset seizures in human immunodeficiency virus-seropositive patients. *Epilepsia* 36:146–150.

Vanijanonta S (1996) Lung flukes (paragonimiasis). In: Weatherall DJ, Ledingham JGG, Warrell DA (eds) *Oxford Textbook of Medicine*, 3rd edn, vol 1, pp 988–992. Oxford: Oxford University Press.

Vazquez V, Sotelo J (1992) The course of seizures after treatment for cerebral cysticercosis. *New England Journal of Medicine* 327:696–701.

Whitley RJ, Cobbs CG, Alford-CA J *et al* (1989) Diseases that mimic herpes simplex encephalitis. Diagnosis, presentation, and outcome. NIAD Collaborative Antiviral Study Group. *JAMA* 262:234–239.

Wong MC, Suite ND, Labar DR (1990) Seizures in human immunodeficiency virus infection. *Archives of Neurology* 47:640–642.

Wright EJ, Brew BJ, Currie JN, McArthur JC (1996) Managing HIV. Part 5: Treating secondary outcomes. 5.4 HIV-induced neurological disease. *Medical Journal of Australia* 164: 414–417.

Wyler AR, Walker G, Somes G (1991) The morbidity of long-term seizure monitoring using subdural strip electrodes [see comments]. *Journal of Neurosurgery* 74: 734–737.

Neurocutaneous syndromes

BGR NEVILLE

The disease entities and syndromes that involve skin and brain are several and perhaps have been given prominence because of their obvious diagnostic 'handles'. Whether their separate delineation illuminates pathology, clinical manifestations, and prognosis is more difficult and is explored in this chapter.

The possible questions that could be addressed include:

1. In disorders caused by abnormal neurocutaneous development, are the lesions that are seen in the brain identical to lesions seen in patients without the skin lesions and presumably without the disease?
2. Is there evidence of a more general cerebral cortical dysfunction than can be accounted for by the lesions themselves?
3. Is the epileptogenicity of such lesions in terms of timing, severity, and semeiology subsumed within the expected parameters of size, number, site and thus overall degree of involvement of the cortical gray matter? Or are there disease-specific manifestations that require explanation?
4. Following from question 3, is there any evidence about the effects of the child having more than one lesion except that it is obviously worse than having one lesion?
5. Since the disease is likely to be suspected relatively early and recognized easily because of the skin lesions, it seems likely that these conditions may contain a greater number of asymptomatic children with brain lesions.
6. A neuroectodermal syndrome might be expected to contain some children with noncortical gray matter lesions which may be epileptogenetic.

The propensity for the development of early, including prenatal, onset seizures with a malignant course is high. Thus the children are at a high risk of cognitive arrest, attention deficit, autistic regression, and severe behavior disorder. The severity of these problems justifies early aggressive treatment of epilepsy both medically and surgically which is a common theme in this chapter. This group of children require multidisciplinary assessment and management of these cognitive and behavioral impairments. Many of these issues will be discussed in the chapter on Landau–Kleffner syndrome (see Chapter 22) but need to be emphasized here since they constitute the major concerns of the families and other carers of children with this group of disorders. We shall be looking for syndrome-specific features of such impairments.

LINEAR SEBACEOUS SYNDROME OF JADASSOHN (SOLOMON SYNDROME)

This condition is usually sporadic. The characteristic neuropathologic lesion in this condition is hemimegalencephaly in which there is predominant, but not exclusively, enlargement of one hemisphere (Barth *et al* 1977; Zaremba *et al* 1978). The enlarged abnormal hemisphere is apparent on a magnetic resonance imaging (MRI) scan. The pathologic changes include disturbance of neuronal migration with extensive cortical architectural changes and glial proliferation. The cortex may be thickened with loss of lamination and a chaotic picture of both normal and abnormal neurons (Robain *et al* 1988). The presence of contralateral dysplasia is clearly a critical issue and claims that FDG positron emission tomography (FDG-PET) can identify such lesions in this situation remain uncertain (Chugani *et al* 1996). A range of additional abnormalities including discrete hamartomatous lesions (Levin *et al* 1984; Clancy *et al* 1985), cerebellar abnormalities, and destructive and vascular lesions of brain and spinal cord lesions have been reported (Aicardi 1998). It is not clear that hemimegalencephaly in linear sebaceous nevus syndrome is in any way different to that found in patients without a nevus.

Hemimegalencephaly has been reported with other neurocutaneous syndromes, including Klippel–Trenaunay–Weber, epidermal nevus, Proteus, hypomelanosis of Ito, tuberous sclerosis, incontinentia pigmenti, and neurofibromatosis (Vigevano *et al* 1997). The skin abnormality may consist of a raised yellow linear lesion particularly on the scalp, forehead, or face just to one side of the midline, on the side of the brain abnormality. The nevus may be continuous or broken into a row of papules or verrucous lesions with increased pigmentation. Both types of lesions usually become more obvious with age. The skin lesions, which should probably be more correctly called organoid nevi because of the multiple elements (Barth *et al* 1977), are also reported without neurologic involvement (e.g. 150 cases of Mehregan and Pinkus (1965)). Conjunctival epidemoids and colobomas of the eye may coexist. Facial hypertrophy on the side of the lesion may occur and sometimes more extensive hemihypertrophy. The common clinical presentation is of early, probably intrauterine onset, partial seizures, often with severe cognitive impairment and hemiplegia. The seizures are most commonly partial motor seizures but infantile spasms, often asymmetric, and tonic, atonic, and myoclonic seizures may occur. There is also a report, perhaps not surprisingly, of a case of infantile spasms followed by Lennox–Gaustaut syndrome (Kurokawa *et al* 1981).

MANAGEMENT

Drug treatment of epilepsy in this disease is often very difficult. No specific studies of the efficacy of the usual treatments exist but it is clear that, even if clinical seizure control is good, subclinical hemi-status commonly continues with consequent severe cognitive arrest. If there are continued clinical or subclinical seizures surgical treatment, normally hemispherectomy, is indicated providing the evidence points to an appropriately lateralized seizure source. It is now becoming clear that for many babies with hemimegalencephaly, hemispherectomy is the correct early treatment. When used early it is most groups' experience that cognitive development improves but at a rate at best less than half speed. It is common for there to be a period of difficult behavior because of the increased abilities of the child. The failure to achieve seizure relief in about 40% by surgery in a collaborative series (Holthausen *et al* 1997) remains unexplained – incomplete surgical removal or disconnection or the presence of epileptogenic lesion deep in the affected hemisphere or contralaterally are the likely reasons but have not been investigated rigorously.

PROTEUS SYNDROME

This uncommon, normally sporadic syndrome is one of the most cosmetically deforming diseases of skin and subcutaneous tissues. The components are skin and limb hypertrophy, hyper/hypopigmented streaking of the skin sometimes with lesions resembling shagreen and plantar skin hyperplasia. The thickened subcutaneous tissue contain lymphangiomatous and hemangiomatous elements. A range of occular abnormalities commonly coexist. There may be no neurologic involvement but hemimegalencephaly is the commonest brain malformation. However, it is the author's experience that bilateral involvement is relatively common. The neurologic presentation is very similar to hemimegalencephaly in the linear sebaceous nevus syndrome discussed above, but with the problem that surgery is not usually possible if there is bilateral involvement. The separation of this condition from Klippel–Trenaunay–Weber syndrome is not always clear in the literature (see Vigevano *et al* 1997) and despite the different vascular features the neurologic manifestations are similar.

HYPOMELANOSIS OF ITO

This condition, usually sporadic, has characteristic alternating hyper- and hypopigmented skin lesions, commonly in a whorled or streaked distribution which is usually lateralized. Hemihypertrophy and macrocephaly are common. Although CNS involvement is common there is no typical phenotype. Hemimegalencephaly is described (Pascual-Castoviejo *et al* 1989) which may have bilateral involvement. Probably about half of patients have seizures (Glover *et al* 1989) with a wide range of partial seizures and infantile spasms being reported. MRI scans have shown pachygyria, hemiatrophy, white matter changes, and neuronal heteropia.

No specific epilepsy syndrome emerges to lead to anything more than the general approach to the developmental epilepsies.

INCONTINENTIA PIGMENTI (BLOCH–SULZBERGER SYNDROME)

This condition behaves as an X-linked lethal with the vast majority of those affected being female. The characteristic features are an early or sometimes later blistering rash followed by pigmented lesions which often fade with adult life and may be totally absent. Deficiencies and abnormalities of teeth are very common, and a range of eye defects including retrolental masses with detachment. More than half have neurologic involvement and in some cases the clinical picture and scan findings can suggest an inflammatory disease similar to the early skin lesions. There is no characteristic neurologic syndrome and a range of epilepsies including infantile spasms are reported.

TUBEROUS SCLEROSIS

Tuberous sclerosis is a dominantly inherited disease with a high rate of mutation and a highly variable phenotype. Two genetic loci have been identified. The main lesions are hamartomas, benign tumors of the skin, CNS, retina, kidneys, heart, lungs, spleen, lymph nodes, endocrine organs, pancreas, and gastrointestinal tract. Details of the surveillance and management of nonneurologic manifestations are outside the scope of this chapter. The main neuropathologic changes are cortical tubers, subependymal nodules, and giant cell astrocytomas close to the foramen of Monro.

The tubers, which disrupt normal cortical architecture with large abnormal cells of uncertain origin, are multiple and may be present in the cerebellum. They commonly calcify. Rarely hemimegalencephaly has been reported. The skin lesions include achromic nevi (including depigmented hair), facial adenoma sebaceous, fibrous plaques, shagreen patches, and periungual fibromas.

Cognitive impairment, autistic spectrum features, and attention deficit hyperactivity disorder are common but are confined to those who have epilepsy, particularly seizures in the first 2 years of life (Gomez 1988). Although the number of cerebral lesions is also correlated with cognitive outcome, it appears that this is mainly subsumed within the age of onset of seizures.

Seizures may begin perinatally and are mostly generalized with infantile spasms being the commonest. Tonic, atonic, atypical absences, and complex partial seizures are also commonly seen and the variation in relative frequency in different series probably reflects differing referral criteria. There is a close relationship between early seizures and cognitive impairment and we directly observe regression of responsiveness with early onset seizure disorders, particularly infantile spasms. Observing such regression (epileptic encephalopathy) reinforces the clinical objective of controlling both clinical and subclinical seizures and thus to improve the cognitive and behavioral outcome. The mainstay of treatment of infantile spasms has been corticosteroids, but recent studies have shown both prospectively (Chiron *et al* 1990) and retrospectively (Aicardi *et al* 1996) that vigabatrin is at least as effective and may well be superior in controlling seizures and the prevention of autistic features specifically in children with tuberous sclerosis. It may also be that there is some advantage for vigabatrin in late partial seizures (Curatalo 1994); however, with the concern about visual field defects it seems that the use of vigabatrin will be limited to situations where its effect is critical, and infantile spasms secondary to tuberous sclerosis seems likely to be exactly that.

SURGICAL TREATMENT OF EPILEPSY IN TUBEROUS SCLEROSIS

In the context of a genetic disease that usually produces multiple, potentially epileptogenic, cortical lesions, surgical treatment is difficult and none of the patients will fulfil this criterion for a category A outcome (one in which restoration to normality is likely). They will be at best category B (with the expectation of amelioration and achieving specific, if limited, goals) and several will be category C (more experimental procedures) or in the majority of cases they will be rejected (Taylor *et al* 1997).

Pediatric epilepsy surgical series tend to contain small numbers of children with tuberous sclerosis. Surgery in this situation may have the following specific aims:

1. Resection of apparently isolated tubers in association with a concordant seizure semeiology (to provide a useful period of remission from seizures).
2. A resection in the presence of more than one tuber but with seizures predominantly of one type which are either occurring at a high rate or are intrinsically dangerous (i.e. to reduce the rate of hazardous seizures).
3. Callosotomy for intractable drop attacks (to reduce the rate and severity of drops).
4. Early resective surgery for intractable infantile spasms with focality (to stop infantile spasms and their attendant encephalopathy and allow more normal development).

From the patients reported (see Kotagal and Tuxhorn 1997) and the author's experience it seems that examples of aims 1, 2, and 3 are being performed with some success, but in the main they are reported by a seizure-freedom outcome which makes analysis difficult. From the details available it is clear that these are a widely varying group of patients from the epilepsy point of view despite the common diagnosis of tuberous sclerosis. There has been very little direct approach to aim 4 which could potentially be the most rewarding area.

The need for accurate identification of the seizure source is paramount in the situation of recognized or presumed multiple pathology. Thus seizures must be accurately described and during ictal monitoring and single-photon emission computed tomography (SPECT) one must be clear that it is the habitual seizure that is being studied. In addition to ictal and interictal SPECT, invasive recording may well be necessary to map epileptogenesis and eloquent cortex. The claim that PET specifically identifies the epileptogenic lesion (Chugani *et al* 1996) needs verification.

Despite the possibility of helping some children it is a situation in which the highest investments of resources and effort by child, family, and professionals may reap limited gains. It is essential that aims are agreed before surgery and audited afterwards.

STURGE–WEBER SYNDROME

The Sturge–Weber syndrome consists pathologically of a facial angioma (port-wine stain) and leptomeningeal angioma with anomalous persistence of primitive central draining veins and lack of the mature cortical venous

sinuses. If the facial angioma involves the eyelid margin a choroidal angioma is usually present with a high risk of closed-angle glaucoma. The skin lesions may be wider than the upper face and forehead and the condition may be unilateral or bilateral. A small group of patients have an identical leptomeningeal lesion without a skin lesion (Gomez and Bebin 1987), and there is a similar lesion seen in a small number of patients some of whom have celiac disease (Gobbi *et al* 1988; Tiacci *et al* 1993). Most children with a facial nevus, however, do not have intracranial pathology.

The pathophysiology of the main features of partial epilepsy, progressive cortical atrophy with peripheral calcification, acquired cognitive impairment and episodes of encephalopathy with seizures, loss of cognitive functions and progressive hemiplegia seems to be the failure of the blood supply to the peripheral cortical ribbon due to venous engorgement. There is evidence, using pulsed Doppler ultrasound of the middle cerebral artery and SPECT of failure to mount an appropriate rise in blood flow during a seizure (Aylett *et al* 1999). Also during an encephalopathic episode there is a marked increase in the enhancement normally seen in the region of the leptomeningeal angioma.

Seizures occur in at least 80% of patients (Gomez and Bebin 1987; Sujansky and Conradi 1995) and they usually start in the first few months of life. The commonest attacks are partial motor with a high rate of status epilepticus but all seizure types including infantile spasms are seen. These episodes may amount to an encephalopathy as described earlier which in Sturge–Weber syndrome is associated with a stepwise loss of motor and cognitive function. Cognitive decline is closely related to the severity of the seizure disorder. Episodes of transient hemiplegia either without seizures or as a prelude to seizures are quite common and the latter phenomenon further suggests an ischemic pathogenesis. Treatment with antiepilepsy drugs is variably effective and no definitive studies of efficacy exist or, perhaps, are possible. Aggressive treatment of epilepsy, particularly of episodes of status, is essential. Early onset seizures, status epilepticus, and infantile spasms predict a poor outcome; however, it is possible to have a good response to drug treatment in up to half of those treated (Arzimanoglou and Aicardi 1992). The effect of anticoagulant agents, which has appeared to benefit individual patients, has not been subjected to trial.

Surgical treatment has been used in Sturge–Weber syndrome for more than 40 years and with appropriate selection is very effective (Roach *et al* 1994; Arzimanoglou 1997). The ideal criteria for successful surgical treatment are:

1. Accurate delineation of the extent of the nevus.
2. A seizure/ischemic disorder which has begun early and is predicted to continue.
3. Minimal cognitive damage has already occurred.
4. Surgical resection, e.g. occipital resection or hemispherectomy, could be performed without inflicting an additional deficit.

The surgical approach has been entirely one of resection or disconnection of epileptogenic cerebral cortex with no recognition of the ischemic element to the pathogenesis. Thus if a functional hemispherectomy has been performed much of the cortex in which nonconvulsive seizures occur, with an inadequate vascular system, remains within the head.

The above requirements for successful surgery are not totally achievable.

Criterion 1. MRI with gadolinium enhancement gives an accurate assessment of the extent of the angioma; SPECT and FDG-PET give information on hypoperfusion and hypometabolism, respectively. An interesting observation of relative hyperperfusion of the affected hemisphere in the first year of life needs to be recognized in the interpretation of this functional data (Pinton *et al* 1997).

Criterion 2. The prediction of a poor outcome early has been a major problem. Since it is possible that there may be a long remission following an early group of seizures, one has to balance the chance of a further damaging episode against the risks of surgery. Remission of seizures must be defined to include the absence of nonconvulsive status in sleep and the presence of continued developmental progress.

Criterion 3. Accurate assessment of cognitive function in babies and young children is an essential component of the decision and if surgery is withheld it is essential that development is carefully followed and the decision reviewed.

Criterion 4. The requirement for a focal or lobar, particularly occipital, resection are nonencroachment upon the sensory motor strip and concordant data, and with ideally an established hemianopia in the case of an occipital resection. The accepted justification for the hemispherectomy is purely unilateral involvement with dense hemiplegia and 'intractability'. However, the prediction that further damage will occur is difficult if it hasn't occurred and of course obvious if it has. This has led to a degree of separation of approach between those who feel that they have to accept significant long-term impairment to avoid unnecessary procedures and those who believe that once it is clear that the potential for damage exists surgery should be considered.

The Toronto group experience summarized by Hoffman (1977) reports on 12 hemispherectomies and 11 focal resections between 1971 and 1995. Four of the eight patients having anatomic hemispherectomies became seizure-free, as did all four of those who had the later procedure of hemidecortication. This group advocated early surgery and 10 of the 12 children were young with a mean age of 8.7 months, and 3 of these were 'retarded' as were both of the older children. However, more detailed cognitive and behavioral profiles are not given. Complications were at a low level and finger function is said to be better preserved in the hemidecortication group. In their focal resection group of 11 patients, this was an occipital lesion with variable extension to the parietal and/or temporal lobe. They used electrocorticography to define epileptogenic brain anterior to the angioma. The reported outcome for these is eight seizure-free, two occasional seizures, and one no change with all reported as having normal intellectual function.

Arzimanoglou (1997) reported the combined experience of 20 patients with Sturge–Weber syndrome operated on in Paris and Montreal. Five of these had hemispherectomies and fifteen had focal resections. The indications for hemispherectomy were extensive unilateral pial angioma, progressive atrophy, episodes of increasingly prolonged postictal deficits on the basis of a preexisting hemiparesis (two of five) or an established hemiplegia (three of five). All those having hemispherectomy and seven of those having focal resection were seizure-free, with 'considerable improvement' in all of the 20 patients. Ten had mild to moderate presurgical cognitive impairment and two were severe. Although this series suggests that earlier surgery may be associated with better outcome, the author is conscious of the variation in case-mix which contains early treated occipital lesions, complex angiomas with preserved motor function, and children with a long-term stable course following severe early episodes.

Thus where a resection can be performed without significant penalty surgery is usually indicated, but other cases have to be considered in the usual fashion for surgical resection.

One very interesting surgical outcome from the UK was reported by Vargha-Khadem *et al* (1997) in which hemispherectomy at 8.5 years was followed by the rapid appearance *de novo* of speech. This promotes questions about the mechanisms of such prior learning and the amount of its expression.

The outcome for bilateral Sturge–Weber syndrome is predictably worse than most unilateral disease (Bebin and Gomez 1988). Although surgical treatment is not generally advocated for bilateral disease, several units including the author's report individual cases with minor contralateral involvement who have benefited from hemispherectomy for intractable dangerous seizures.

NEUROFIBROMATOSIS TYPE 1

Neurofibromatosis type 1 (NF1) is a dominantly inherited disorder. The gene is in the pericentric region of the long arm of chromosome 17 (17q11.2) and has a prevalence of 1 in 3000. Its manifestations are protean both within and outside the nervous system and are well covered in general texts (Aicardi 1998). In general, cognitive function is reduced within the group but severe impairment is very uncommon (Ferner and Hughes 1992; Hoffman *et al* 1994; North *et al* 1995). The prevalence of epilepsy has been reported as being between 3.5 and 7.3% (Huson *et al* 1988; North *et al* 1995).

Although specific pathologic associations are reported, for example aqueduct stenosis and meningiomatosis (Huson *et al* 1988), in many cases no lesion is apparent. Generalized tonic–clonic, absence, and partial seizures have been reported. In the Boston series, 22 of 39 patients had epilepsy with a wide range of seizure types but a causative lesion was not apparent on imaging (either CT or MRI). There are several reports of infantile spasms (Korf *et al* 1993; Motte *et al* 1993; Fois *et al* 1994). Motte *et al* (1993) report of 13 children from several centers showing an unusual natural history. Age of onset, spasms, and EEGs were classical but the majority were 'cryptogenic' apart from having NF1; seizure response to corticosteroids was rapid and only one child had definite mental retardation both before and after the seizure disorder. This benign course has not been confirmed. Two children reported with dysembryoplastic neuroepithelial tumors, and severe epilepsy in association with NF1 may indicate a significant association.

In summary, this review of epilepsy in NF1 does not lead us to any specific indication for treatment. Epilepsy should be managed according to normal general rules for the management of childhood epilepsy (Neville 1997).

In returning to the questions that were posed at the beginning of the chapter, some response is possible.

Q1. In disorders caused by abnormal neurocutaneous development, are the lesions that are seen in the brain identical to lesions seen in patients without the skin lesions and presumably without the disease?

The hemimegalencephalies with different cutaneous syndromes and those with no skin lesion appear very similar; likewise, pial angiomas with and without a skin lesion seem to behave in a similar fashion. The tubers of tuberous sclerosis appear, however, to be unique to that condition.

Q2. Is there evidence of a more general cerebral cortical dysfunction than can be accounted for by the lesions themselves?

The best evidence of nonlesional and nonepilepsy-related neural dysfunction is seen in NF1 and incontinentia pigmenti, where cognitive and other impairments may be present without MRI abnormality. The pathology underlying this dysfunction is unknown.

Q3. Is the epileptogenicity of such lesions in terms of timing, severity, and semeiology subsumed within the expected parameters of size, number, site and thus overall degree of involvement of the cortical gray matter? Or are there disease-specific manifestations that require explanation?

Epilepsy in the majority of neurocutaneous syndromes appears to arise in relationship to brain lesions (i.e. with hemimegalencephaly and in Sturge–Weber syndrome and tuberous sclerosis.) However, in NF1 the situation is different, with few identifiable lesions. The general rule is that the earlier the onset of epilepsy the worse the cognitive outcome, with cognitive function appearing to be mainly secondary to the epilepsy. In NF1, by contrast, the general rules of susceptibility to epilepsy appear to apply (i.e. the lower the basic cognitive function the greater the susceptibility to epilepsy). There are no studies that separate these two hypotheses. The additional dimension to epileptogenicity and the acquisition of impairments is the ischemic element of Sturge–Weber syndrome which appears to account for its motor concomitants. The catastrophic nature of the epilepsy associated with hemimegalencephaly is as yet unexplained.

Q4. Following from question 3, is there any evidence about the effects of the child having more than one lesion except that it is obviously worse than having one lesion?

As yet the evidence about any mutual epileptogenicity in the presence of more than one potentially epileptogenic lesion is lacking. It should be possible with modern technology to begin to answer the important question of whether, if one lesion in tuberous sclerosis is the source of discharges, does this lower the threshold for seizures in other lesions or the general seizure threshold for epileptic encephalopathies in the whole brain?

Q5. Since the disease is likely to be suspected relatively early and recognized easily because of the skin lesions, it seems likely that these conditions may contain a greater number of asymptomatic children with brain lesions.

There is no doubt that more people with asymptomatic lesions are recognized as a result of obvious skin lesions, particularly in tuberous sclerosis, and this should allow studies of the risk factors for epilepsy.

Q6. A neuroectodermal syndrome might be expected to contain some children with noncortical gray matter lesions which may be epileptogenetic.

Such lesions have not yet been identified but may be a cause of continuing seizures in surgically treated hemimegalencephaly.

KEY POINTS

1. These conditions impose a high propensity for the development of early seizures, including prenatally, with a malignant course. There is a high risk of cognitive arrest, attention deficit, autistic regression, and severe behavior disorder. Early aggressive treatment of the epilepsy, both medically and surgically if possible, is justified.

2. Tuberous sclerosis is an inherited disorder whose main neuropathologic features are cortical tubers that commonly calcify, subependymal nodules, and giant cell astrocytomas close to the foramen of Munro. Seizures may begin perinatally and are mostly generalized with infantile spasms being commonest. Cognitive impairment, autistic features, and attention deficit/hyperactivity disorder are common, but confined to those who have seizures particularly when aged <2 years. Corticosteroids, and possibly even more so vigabatin, are effective for seizure control and the prevention of autistic features. Surgical treatment of the epilepsy may achieve limited success.

3. The main brain pathology in Sturge–Weber syndrome is a leptomeningeal angioma, usually unilateral but sometimes bilaterally, with anomalous persistence of primitive central draining veins and a lack of mature cortical venous sinuses. Epilepsy (in 80%) that may be medically intractable, with a high rate of status epilepticus, progressive cortical atrophy and calcification, cognitive impairment, hemianopia and progressive hemiplegia are the main neurologic features. Freedom from seizures can sometimes be achieved by focal surgical resection or hemispherectomy.

4. Hemimegalencephaly may occur in isolation or in association with various cutaneous syndromes. These include linear sebaceous naevus (Solomon syndrome), skin/limb hypertrophy +/- altered skin pigmentation and plantar skin hyperplasia (Proteus syndrome), hypermelanosis of Ito, Klippel–Trenaunay–Weber syndrome, tuberous sclerosis, neurofibromatosis, and incontinentia pigmenti. The contralateral hemisphere may be abnormal and there may be other additonal CNS pathology. The epilepsy is often of very early onset, medically intractable, and associated with impaired cognitive development. Hemispherectomy may give relief from the seizures, with improved cognitive development, in around 60% cases.

REFERENCES

Aicardi J (1998) In: Bax M, Poutney M, Davies P (eds) *Diseases of the Nervous System in Childhood*, 2nd edn. London: MacKeith.

Aicardi J, Sabril IS, Investigator and Peer Review Groups *et al* (1996) Vigabatrin as initial therapy for infantile spasms: a European retrospective survey. *Epilepsia* **37**:638–642.

Arzimanoglou A (1997) The surgical treatment of Sturge–Weber syndrome with respect to its clinical spectrum. In: Tuxhorn I, Holthausen H, Boenigk H (eds) *Paediatric Epilepsy Syndromes and Their Surgical Treatment*, pp 353–363. London: John Libbey.

Arzimanoglou A, Aicardi J (1992) The epilepsy of Sturge–Weber syndrome: clinical features and treatments in 23 patients. *Acta Neurologica Scandinavica* **86**(Suppl 140):18–22.

Aylett SE, Neville BG, Cross JH *et al* (1999) Sturge–Weber syndrome: cerebral haemodynamics during seizure activity. *Developmental Medicine and Child Neurology* **41**(7): 480–485.

Barth PG, Valk J, Kalsbeek GL, Blom A (1977) Organoid nevus syndrome (linear nevus sebaceous of Jadassohn). Clinical and radiological study of a case. *Neuropediatrics* **8**:418–428.

Bebin E, Gomez M (1988) Prognosis in Sturge–Weber disease: comparison of unihemispheric and bihemispheric involvement. *Journal of Child Neurology* **3**:181–184.

Chiron C, Dulac O, Luna D *et al* (1990) Vigabatrin in infantile spasms. *Lancet* **335**:363–364.

Chugani H, Kupsky W, Chugani D (1996) Cortical dysplasia: surgical treatment and neuropathological findings in infants and children. In: Guerrini et al (eds) *Dysplasias of Cerebral Cortex and Epilepsy*, pp 427–433. Philadelphia: Lippincott-Raven.

Clancy R, Kurtz M, Baker D, Sladky J, Honig P, Younkin D (1985) Neurologic manifestations of the organoid nevus syndrome. *Archives of Neurology* **42**:36–240.

Curatalo P (1994) Vigabatrin for refractory partial seizures in children with tuberous sclerosis. *Neuropediatrics* **25**:55.

Ferner R, Hughes R (1992) *Intellectual Impairment in NF1*. Proceedings of the International Neurofibromatosis Convention, Vienna.

Fois A, Tine A, Pavone L (1994) Infantile spasms in patients with neurofibromatosis type 1. *Child's Nervous System* **10**:176–179.

Glover M, Brett E, Artherton D (1989) Hypomelanosis of Ito: spectrum of the disease. *Journal of Paediatrics* **115**:75–80.

Gobbi G, Sorrenti G, Santucci M *et al* (1988) Epilepsy with bilateral occipital calcifications: a benign onset with progressive severity. *Neurology* **38**:913–920.

Gomez R (ed.) (1988) *Tuberous Sclerosis*, 2nd edn. New York: Raven Press.

Gomez M, Bebin E (1987) Sturge–Weber syndrome. In: Gomez M (ed.) *Neurocutaneous Diseases: a Practical Approach*, pp 356–367. London:Butterworths.

Hoffman H (1997) Benefits of early surgery in Sturge–Weber syndrome. In: Tuxhorn I, Holthausen H, Boenigk H (eds) *Paediatric Epilepsy Syndromes and Their Surgical Treatment*, pp 364–370. London: John Libbey.

Hoffman K, Harris E, Bryan R, Denckla M (1994) Neurofibromatosis type 1: the cognitive phenotype. *Journal of Paediatrics* **128**:S1–S8.

Holthausen H *et al* (1997) Seizures post hemispherectomy. In: Tuxhorn I, Holthausen H, Boenigk H (eds) *Paediatric Epilepsy Syndromes and Their Surgical Treatment*, pp 377–391. London: John Libbey.

Huson S, Harper P, Compston D (1988) Von Recklinghausen neurofibromatosis: a clinical and population study in south-east Wales. *Brain* **111**:1355–1381.

Korf B, Carrazana E, Holmes G (1993) Patterns of seizures observed in association with neurofibromatosis 1. *Epilepsia* **34**:616–620.

Kotagal P, Tuxhorn I (1997) Epilepsy surgery in tuberous sclerosis and other phakomatoses. In: Tuxhorn I, Holthausen H, Boenigk H (eds) *Paediatric Epilepsy Syndromes and Their Surgical Treatment*, pp 749–773. London: John Libbey.

Kurokawa T, Sasaki K, Hanai T, Goya N, Komaki S (1981) Report of a case with Lennox–Gastaut syndrome following infantile spasms. *Archives of Neurology* **38**:375–377.

Levin S, Robinson R, Aicardi J, Hoare R (1984) Computed tomographic appearance in the linear sebaceous nevus syndrome. *Neuroradiology* **26**:469–472.

Mehregan A, Pinkus H (1965) Life history of organoid nevi. *Archives of Dermatology* **91**:574–587.

Motte J, Billard C, Fejerman N *et al* (1993) Neurofibromatosis type one and West syndrome: a relatively benign association. *Epilepsia* **34**:723–726.

Neville B (1997) Epilepsy in childhood (fortnightly review). *British Medical Journal* **315**:924–930.

North K *et al* (1995) Cognitive function and academic performance in children with neurofibomatosis type 1. *Developmental Medicine and Child Neurology* **37**:427–436.

Pascual-Castoviejo I, Lopez R, De la Cruz M *et al* (1989) Hipomelanosis de Ito. Alteraciones neurologicas en una serie de 48 cases. In: Pascual-Castoviejo I (ed.) *Trastornos Neuroectoridermicos*, pp 127–137. Barcelona: JR Prous.

Pinton F, Chiron C, Enjolras O *et al* (1997) Early single photon emission computed tomography in Sturge–Weber syndrome. *Journal of Neurology, Neurosurgery, and Psychiatry* **63**:616–621.

Roach E, Riela A, Chugani H *et al* (1994) Sturge–Weber syndrome: recommendations for surgery. *Journal of Child Neurology* **9**:190–192.

Robain O, Floquet C, Heldt N, Rozenberg F (1988) Hemimegalencephaly: a clinicopathological study of four cases. *Neuropathology and Applied Biology* **14**:125–135.

Sujansky E, Conradi S (1995) The Sturge–Weber syndrome: age of onset of seizures and glaucoma and the prognosis for affected children. *Journal of Child Neurology* **10**:49–58.

Taylor D, Neville B, Besag F, Cross J (1997) New measures of outcome needed for the surgical treatment of epilepsy. *Epilepsia* **38**:625–630.

Tiacci C, D'Alessandro P, Cantisani T *et al* (1993) Epilepsy with bilateral occipital calcifications: Sturge–Weber variant or a different encephalopathy? *Epilepsia* **34**:528–539.

Vargha–Khadem F, Carr L, Isaacs E *et al* (1997) Onset of speech after left hemispherectomy in a 9-year-old boy. *Brain* **120**:159–182.

Vigevano F, Fusco L, Holthausen H, Lahl R (1997) The morphological spectrum and variable clinical picture in children with hemimegalencephaly. In: Tuxhorn I, Holthausen H, Boenigk H (eds) *Paediatric Epilepsy Syndromes and Their Surgical Treatment*, pp 377–391. London: John Libbey.

Zaremba J, Wislawski J, Bidzinsky J *et al* (1978) Jadassohn's nevus phakomatosis: a report of two cases. *Journal of Mental Defects* **22**:91–102.

Rasmussen syndrome

Y HART AND F ANDERMANN

The syndrome of focal seizures due to chronic localized encephalitis was first reported by Rasmussen and colleagues (Rasmussen *et al* 1958). They described three children aged 18 months to 5 years at the onset of the condition who had in common the development of refractory focal seizures (preceded in two of the patients by a minor infective episode), progressive hemiparesis, and pathologic changes of chronic encephalitis. Cognitive impairment was also a feature of the illness. Two of the patients underwent hemispherectomy with resolution of the seizures and some improvement in mental state, although more limited resection was not helpful. The other child, who underwent frontal lobectomy with little benefit, eventually succumbed to the complications of the seizures (Fig. 18.1). The pathological changes seen included perivascular cuffing, the presence of microglia, spongy degeneration, and gliosis, limited to one cerebral hemisphere in the patient undergoing postmortem examination.

Rasmussen and McCann expanded the description of the clinical features in their publication of 1968, when they described 20 patients operated on for focal epilepsy since 1950 who were found to have pathologic features of chronic encephalitis. Of these, 12 had had a prior inflammatory episode, and in 4 patients a permanent stable hemiparesis developed at the time of the initial febrile illness: in a further 15, a subsequent progressive hemiparesis developed. This paper described abnormalities of the cerebrospinal fluid at some stage of the disease in 11 patients. The EEG showed more or less diffuse slow-wave activity, as well as more localized epileptiform waveforms, with gradual spread of the involved areas of slow-wave abnormality in patients having serial EEGs. The authors' experience from study of these patients was that limited or early surgery was unlikely to produce significant improvement but more radical surgery performed later in the disease process (when progression had slowed down or stopped) was often highly beneficial.

Since the original description of this condition, the story has evolved, with reports of further patients, many with a similar presentation to that of the original children (Gupta *et al* 1974, 1984; Piatt *et al* 1988; Oguni *et al* 1992). More recently a number of patients have been described with atypical features, including a late onset (in adolescence or adulthood) (Gray *et al* 1987; McLachlan *et al* 1993; Hart *et al* 1997), coexistence of the pathologic features with a second pathology in patients with an otherwise typical syndrome (Yacubian *et al* 1996; Hart *et al* 1998), and the occurrence of uveitis in association with the condition (Harvey *et al* 1992; Fukuda *et al* 1994). Although the etiology of Rasmussen encephalitis remains as yet unknown, these reports have led to the hope that the study of such patients may further our understanding of the cause of the

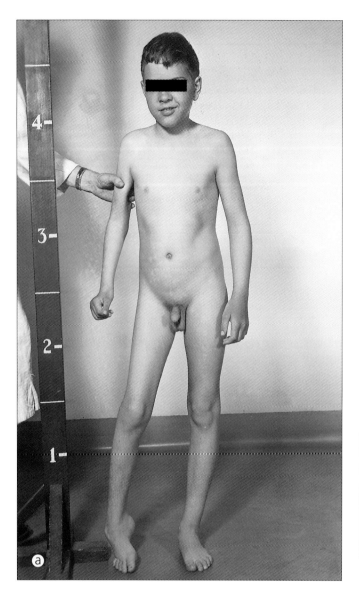

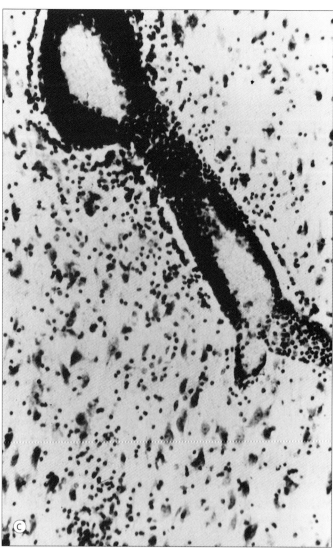

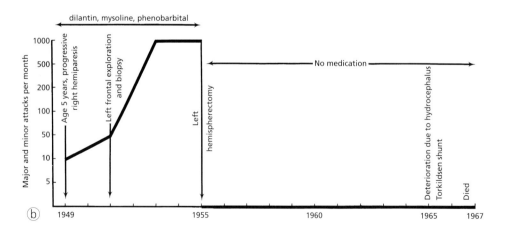

Fig. 18.1 (a) W.G., the first patient in whom a diagnosis of what was later known as Rasmussen syndrome was made. He had a right hemiparesis and asymmetry of growth. Cortical resection did not relieve the seizures. Anatomic hemispherectomy was carried out. He became seizure-free but died several years later due to complications from cerebral hemosiderosis. (b) The clinical course of W.G. (c) The pathologic changes of Rasmussen encephalitis: perivascular infiltrates and microglial nodules.

condition. Perhaps the most important development in our knowledge of Rasmussen syndrome over the last ten years, however, has occurred by serendipity, when in the course of an experiment to generate subtype-specific antibodies to recombinant GluR proteins in which rabbits were immunized with GluR3 fusion protein, it was noted that some of them developed features resembling Rasmussen encephalitis (Rogers *et al* 1994). Attempts to isolate GluR3 antibodies in patients with Rasmussen syndrome have produced variable results, however (Krauss *et al* 1996), and more work remains to be done both to elucidate the cause and to provide an effective treatment.

CLINICAL FEATURES

In the majority of instances, Rasmussen syndrome develops in childhood, most commonly between the ages of 1 and 10 years: in Andermann's series, the median age at onset was 5 years (Andermann *et al* 1990). There is no major difference in incidence between the sexes. In about 50% of patients the onset is preceded by an inflammatory episode (for example, an upper respiratory tract infection, otitis media, or tonsillitis) occurring in the previous 6 months. The first sign of the condition itself in the majority of children is the development of seizures, often generalized tonic–clonic seizures, although simple partial or complex partial seizures occur as the initial seizure type in a significant proportion. Status epilepticus is common, being the presenting feature in about 20% of patients.

Seizures are usually refractory, with little response to standard antiepileptic drugs (Dubeau and Sherwin 1991). It is common for a variety of seizure types to develop over a period of time, and the seizures become increasingly severe and frequent. Focal motor seizures occur in about three-quarters of patients at some time (Fig. 18.2). Epilepsia partialis continua eventually occurs in about 50% of children, usually within 3 years of the onset (Andermann *et al* 1990).

When partial seizures occur, they almost invariably involve the same side of the body. As is not infrequently the case in children, Todd paresis is relatively common, and in the early stages of the illness hemiparesis is postictal and transient, as would be expected. Exceptionally, hemiparesis occurring at this stage may be permanent. With progression of the disease process, however, fixed neurologic deficits, including hemiparesis (usually to the extent of the child losing fine finger movements and developing a hemiparetic gait) and visual field deficits, gradually ensue after a period varying from 3 months to 10 years from the onset of the epilepsy (Oguni *et al* 1991).

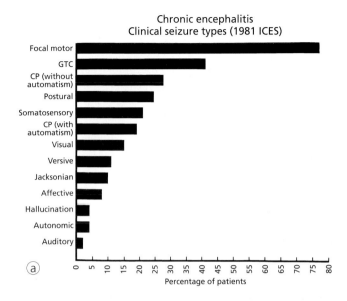

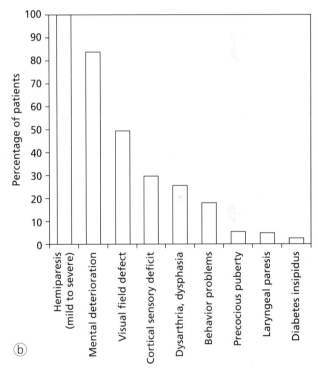

Fig. 18.2 (a) Rasmussen encephalitis in 48 children: clinical seizure types: focal motor seizures are most common, followed by generalized tonic–clonic and complex partial seizures. CP, complex partial; GTC, generalized tonic–clonic. (b) Outcome of chronic encephalitis: all children develop hemiparesis and most develop mental deterioration.

Progressive intellectual impairment is also a feature of the condition, sometimes occurring or worsening in association with a deterioration in seizure control, sometimes apparently independent of seizure activity. As in the case of the focal neurologic deficits, the intellectual deterioration commonly occurs over a number of years, though sometimes over months. Speech deficits (including dysphasia and dysarthria) and cortical sensory loss are also features of the disease, depending on which hemisphere is involved.

Despite the initial course of the illness being generally one of relentless progression, it is relatively unusual for it to cause death. Instead, the disease process eventually appears to burn itself out, usually at a stage at which there is moderate to severe neurologic deficit and intellectual impairment. Further progression of these deficits no longer occurs, and the seizures often revert to being less frequent and severe.

BILATERAL HEMISPHERAL INVOLVEMENT IN RASMUSSEN SYNDROME

The disease continues to affect one hemisphere in the great majority of cases and the reason for this limitation remains unclear. However, over time there is some, usually slight, contralateral ventricular enlargement that may be attributed to the effect of recurrent seizures with anoxia and trauma and to Wallerian changes. Autopsy studies have confirmed that the disorder is usually limited to one hemisphere.

There have been a few exceptions: three of the patients studied by Dulac's group (Chinchilla et al 1994) showed bilateral disease and one of these was treated by high-dose steroids. The patient treated with zidovudine by De Toledo and Smith (1994) also had independent involvement of the opposite hemisphere. Thus it is possible that immunologic therapy may predispose to contralateral spread.

Bilateral disease must be distinguished from secondary epileptogenesis without evidence for inflammatory changes: this tends to occur in patients with long duration of seizures and may persist even after hemispherectomy (F. Andermann, personal observations). These residual seizures are far less frequent or malignant than those arising in the primarily affected hemisphere.

EARLY-ONSET BILATERAL AND FAMILIAL RASMUSSEN SYNDROME

Patients with onset at 1–2 years of age and epilepsia partialis continua involving alternately both sides of the body have been mentioned by Chinchilla et al (1994) and by Takahashi et al (1997). We have studied male siblings with this clinical course (Silver et al 1998), whereas the other patients appeared to be sporadic. Thus, bilateral disease may be more common and more severe in children with infantile onset. Familial onset is unprecedented in children with the classic and other forms of the syndrome and other causes for this subgroup have been excluded as far as possible.

RASMUSSEN SYNDROME DEVELOPING IN ADULTS OR ADOLESCENTS

Although Rasmussen syndrome commonly has its onset in childhood, several authors have now reported the development of seizures associated with a similar pathologic picture starting in adolescence or in adult life (Gray et al 1987; McLachlan et al 1993; Hart et al 1997). In the majority of patients the clinical features have resembled those seen in the childhood form, with the development of intractable (often focal) seizures, progressive neurologic deficit, particularly hemiparesis, and intellectual deterioration. Occipital onset to the seizures has been reported more commonly than in children, and the reports suggest that bilateral disease is more common. One of the patients described by McLachlan et al was unusual in presenting with a slowly progressive hemiparesis several months before seizure onset. Hart et al (1997) reported that the patients fell into three groups. Five of their patients developed seizures in adulthood, but in other respects their condition was similar to the childhood form. Five developed seizures in adolescence, and in this group of patients the course appeared rather more benign than in the younger patients. In three patients the initial features suggested the possibility of an underlying tumor as a cause of the symptoms, with the diagnosis of chronic encephalitis being made at biopsy.

DOUBLE PATHOLOGY IN RASMUSSEN SYNDROME

Several patients (including almost 10% of the Montreal series) have now been described in whom the clinical picture has been typical of Rasmussen syndrome, but the pathology has been surprising in that a second pathology has been present in addition to the typical changes of Rasmussen encephalitis (Robitaille 1991). Yacubian et al (1996) reported a 7-year-old girl presenting with epilepsia partialis continua involving the left side of the body, unresponsive to medical treatment after 1 year and with neuroimaging showing evidence of progressive cerebral atrophy, in whom a frontotemporal resection was performed, the pathologic picture being that of cortical dysgenesis and chronic encephalitis. Hart et al (1998) described five patients, all of whom developed focal onset seizures and progressive hemiparesis, often in association with intellectual deterioration. In one patient the typical pathologic changes of Rasmussen encephalitis occurred in association with cortical dysplasia; in another with the changes of tuberous sclerosis; in a third with tumor; and with vascular abnormalities bearing some resemblance to cavernous angiomata in the other two. These occurrences have led to various suggested explanations: that the two pathologies may have occurred by chance (which seems unlikely, given the rarity of Rasmussen syndrome); that the structural lesion may have caused an alteration in the blood–brain barrier, increasing the chance of viral infection; or that it could have been responsible for the development of a chronic autoimmune response. The correct explanation remains unclear.

RASMUSSEN SYNDROME OCCURRING IN ASSOCIATION WITH UVEITIS

Harvey *et al* (1992) have reported two children who developed uveitis shortly after the onset of seizures, the involvement being on the same side as the cerebral inflammation. In other respects the clinical and pathologic features were typical of Rasmussen syndrome. A further patient developing Rasmussen encephalitis 1 month after surgery for residual cataract due to chronic uveitis was described by Fukuda *et al* (1994). The patient of Gray *et al* (1987) who developed Rasmussen syndrome in adult life also developed choroiditis ipsilateral to the cerebral changes shortly after the development of epilepsy. These associations have led to speculation that a viral infection may have been responsible for both, although it has been recognized that other conditions (for example sarcoidosis, Behçet syndrome, cerebral vasculitis, malignancy, and infection with nonviral organisms) may cause both uveitis and meningoencephalitis.

PATHOLOGY

Rasmussen's original description of chronic localized encephalitis reported an inflammatory process, with marked perivascular cuffing by round cells in both the cortex and white matter. Diffuse patchy inflammatory changes were seen in the cortex and white matter, with prominent microglia in addition to small round cells and occasional polymorphonuclear cells. There was loss of nerve cells, some spongy degeneration, and hypertrophy of the astrocytes, which were also increased in number.

This description has been expanded by Robitaille (1991), who reviewed the pathologic specimens of patients in the Montreal series. He described the features of the disease as the presence of microglial nodules, often displaying neuronophagia (mainly in the medium-size pyramidal cells of the external pyramidal layer), and perivascular cuffs of small lymphocytes and monocytes. In the more active cases he noted that the round cells filled the Virchow–Robin spaces and extended into the neuropil, forming microscopic clusters or larger aggregates. Spongiosis was particularly seen in association with inflammatory changes. He noted the frequent presence of multifocal neuronal loss in the inflamed cortex, especially in the superficial and intermediate cortex. The smaller foci tended to coalesce into large areas of structural collapse, surrounded by inflammatory changes and with sprouting of capillaries resembling granulation tissue. Subarachnoid adhesions were seen not infrequently.

However, in addition Robitaille classified the pathologic specimens into four groups, according to the features of disease activity. Group 1 included those with the most active disease pathologically. The features seen in these specimens were those of an ongoing inflammatory process, with numerous microglial nodules, with or without neuronophagia, perivascular round cells, and glial scarring. Included in group 2 were those with 'active and remote disease,' indicated by the presence of several microglial nodules, cuffs of perivascular round cells, and at least one gyral segment of complete necrosis and cavitation including full-thickness cortex. Group 3 had less active or 'remote' disease, with pathologic appearances of neuronal loss and gliosis, moderately abundant perivascular round cells, and only few microglial nodules. The final group, group 4, consisted of those specimens showing nonspecific changes, with few or no microglial nodules, only mild perivascular inflammation, but various degrees of neuronal loss and glial scarring.

ETIOLOGY

Ever since the original description of Rasmussen encephalitis was published, the underlying cause has been the source of much speculation (Antel and Rasmussen 1996). The most likely mechanisms have been considered to be a chronic viral infection, an acute viral infection leading to a local immune response, and an independent autoimmune process, not linked to infection.

Both the clinical aspects of the disease (with the history of a preceding infective episode in a considerable proportion of patients) and the pathologic features were strongly in favor of an underlying infective cause, as indeed was the close resemblance of the clinical picture to that seen in Russian spring–summer tick-borne encephalitis, described by Kozhevnikov (1991). The patients described by Kozhevnikov, the majority of whom were male and aged between 10 and 20 years, had been previously healthy; they then developed a high temperature, frequently accompanied by delirium and sometimes by seizures and a monoplegia or hemiplegia. This was followed (usually after a few months) by more constant localized epileptic activity. Paralysis was commonly also present in the limbs affected by jerking. The course thereafter was one of chronic seizure activity, although in some patients there was an eventual decrease in seizure frequency. The patients described above, in whom chronic encephalitis was associated with ipsilateral uveitis, also lend support to the viral theory.

Numerous attempts have been made to demonstrate viral particles or genetic evidence of viral material in specimens from patients with Rasmussen encephalitis. Although there have been a number of positive results, it has usually not been possible to reproduce these, and the situation remains unresolved. Friedman *et al* (1977) reported a child of 3 years with hemiplegia, hemiconvulsions, and epilepsy in whom biopsy showed an encephalitic picture with perivascular cuffing with mononuclear cells; viral crystals resembling those of enteroviruses were found in brain cells by electron microscopy. Walter and Renella (1989) reported two patients with chronic encephalitis and epilepsy in whom biopsy showed histologic features of encephalitis; in-situ hybridization showed Epstein–Barr virus (EBV) genome in intranuclear central cores within the encephalitic infiltrations. This raised the possibility of a role for EBV in the pathogenesis of Rasmussen encephalitis. Power *et al* (1990) carried out in-situ hybridization for cytomegalovirus (CMV) on brain biopsy specimens from 10 patients with Rasmussen encephalitis and 46 age-matched control patients with other neurologic diseases. They found CMV genomic material in 7 of the 10 patients with Rasmussen encephalitis and in only 2 of the control patients. Probes for herpes simplex virus and hepatitis B were negative in all patients, although this work has been criticized (Gilden and Lipton 1991; Root-Bernstein 1991). McLachlan *et al* (1993), from the same group, also demonstrated the CMV genome in neurons, glia, and endothelial cells of blood vessels by in-situ hybridization in brain specimens from three patients developing chronic encephalitis and epilepsy in adulthood. Similar assessments for hepatitis B, herpes simplex, and Epstein–Barr virus genome were negative in these patients. Viral antibody titers in the serum and CSF samples were normal, and no viral inclusions or antigens were found in resected brain tissue. Jay *et al* (1995) studied pathologic specimens from 10 patients with chronic encephalitis and intractable seizures by immunohistochemistry for herpes simplex virus (HSV) 1 and 2 and CMV as well as by the polymerase chain reaction (PCR) for viral DNA sequences (HSV1, HSV2, and CMV). They also assessed 8 nonepileptic patients with pathologically demonstrated or clinically suspected encephalitis, and 5 specimens from patients with epilepsy without encephalitis. Using PCR, CMV was present in 6 and HSV1 in 2 of 10 epilepsy patients with chronic encephalitis. CMV was demonstrated by in-situ hybridization in 2 of the 6 patients positive for CMV by PCR. Immunochemistry was negative for viral antigens in all cases. None of the patients without encephalitis was found to have viral sequences by PCR, while 2 of the 8 patients with encephalitis but without epilepsy showed CMV sequences by PCR. The authors suggested that in-situ hybridization might miss some cases.

In contrast to these results, Rasmussen (1978) reported negative standard viral studies (or positive reactions only to herpes simplex and measles virus in low dilution, of doubtful clinical significance). Mizuno *et al* (1985) used immunoperoxidase stains against 10 viral antigens on brain specimens from two patients with Rasmussen syndrome and found all to be negative. Farrell *et al* (1991) were unable to detect CMV using immunostaining with anti-CMV antibodies in their three patients with Rasmussen encephalitis.

Vinters *et al* (1993) studied brain tissue from epileptic children with chronic (usually Rasmussen type) encephalitis. They extracted DNA from specimens of brain tissue and used polymerase chain reaction with primers specific for CMV, varicella zoster, herpes simplex, EBV, and human herpes virus 6 genes. They found evidence of low levels of CMV and EBV genes in most brain specimens from encephalitis patients, and in several brain specimens from patients without encephalitis. The signal strength for both CMV and EBV was much lower in the brains of patients with epilepsy than in the brains of AIDS patients with CMV encephalitis or brain lymphoma. The authors concluded that the small amounts of EBV and CMV genes found suggested that herpes virus infection of the brain did not directly cause Rasmussen encephalitis. Similar nonspecific findings were obtained by Eeg-Olofsson *et al* studying material from our patients (O. Eeg-Olofsson, unpublished observations). Atkins *et al* (1995) studied 10 biopsy and resection specimens from 7 patients using biotinylated double-stranded DNA probes to CMV, HSV, and EBV. Electron microscopy was also carried out on two samples, and one was evaluated using standard immunoperoxidase techniques. However, they were unable to identify any evidence of viral material. The likely role of viruses in the pathogenesis of Rasmussen encephalitis has been reviewed by Asher and Gajdusek (1991).

Andrews *et al* (1990) suggested that immunopathogenetic mechanisms were important in Rasmussen encephalitis. They carried out extensive studies on the hemispherectomy specimen from a child with Rasmussen encephalitis and found widespread cerebral vasculitis with immunofluorescence staining for IgG, IgM, IgA, C3, and C1q. There was also ultrastructural evidence of vascular injury, in addition to severe cortical atrophy with marked neuronal loss. The child had elevated serum antinuclear antibody titers and CSF oligoclonal bands.

Perhaps the most exciting development in our understanding of the etiology of Rasmussen encephalitis in recent years has been the establishment by Rogers *et al* (1994) of a link between circulating antibodies to a ligand-gated ion channel receptor of the central nervous system in rabbits and a progressive encephalopathy with epileptic seizures. These workers reported that 2 out of 4 rabbits immunized with GluR3 fusion protein in order to generate subtype-specific antibodies to recombinant GluR proteins developed seizures, while microscopic examination of their brains demonstrated chronic inflammatory changes consisting of microglial nodules and perivascular lymphocytic infiltration mainly in the cerebral cortex, together with lymphocytic infiltration of the meninges. They reasoned that these changes probably occurred as a result of an autoimmune process directed against GluR3, and went on to look for these antibodies in four patients with pathologically confirmed Rasmussen encephalitis. As controls they used age-matched and sex-matched children with epilepsy, age-matched and sex-matched children without CNS disease, children with active CNS inflammation, other children with epilepsy, and normal children. Immunoreactivity to GluR3 fusion protein was found in sera from two children with Rasmussen encephalitis, one of whom also showed weak immunoreactivity to GluR2 fusion protein. One of the other children with Rasmussen encephalitis also exhibited weak immunoreactivity to GluR2 fusion protein, while the fourth child did not show immunoreactivity to any tested antigen. Only one control showed weak immunoreactivity to GluR3 that was different from the serum GluR immunoreactivity seen in individuals with Rasmussen encephalitis. The GluR immunoreactivity appeared to correlate with disease activity, in that the three children with immunoreactivity had progressive disease or ongoing seizures, while hemispherectomy had been performed several years earlier in the child with no immunoreactivity, resulting in clinical stability and freedom from seizures.

As a result of these findings and the implication that the disease process might be related to circulating antibodies, Rogers *et al* carried out plasma exchange in one of the children with Rasmussen encephalitis showing immunoreactivity who was seriously ill, with resultant decrease in seizures and improvement in neurologic status. However, the improvement was short-lived, with further deterioration over the following 4 weeks. The same team later reported the finding that the antibodies found in Rasmussen encephalitis actually activate the receptor, raising the possibility that the antibodies might directly trigger seizures by

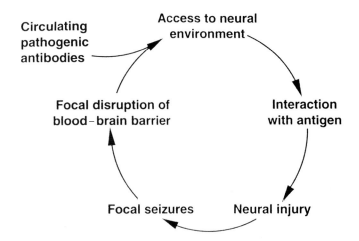

Fig. 18.3 Putative mechanism of Rasmussen syndrome. (From Andrews *et al* (1996) with permission.)

overstimulating the glutamate receptors (Twyman *et al* 1995). The fact that Rasmussen encephalitis not infrequently appears to follow a blow to the head or systemic illness has led these authors to propose a model for the development of Rasmussen encephalitis (Fig. 18.3), namely, that the insult causes a breach in the blood–brain barrier that in individuals with autoantibodies to GluR3 could allow the entry of these antibodies to the brain, with activation of the receptors and subsequent seizures, thus causing a vicious circle in which more rifts would be caused in the blood–brain barrier as a result of seizures. (Alternatively, the GluR3 antibodies may arise as a result of the initial central nervous system damage, thus leading to further damage.)

NATURAL HISTORY

The initial course of Rasmussen encephalitis is frequently characterized by rather nonspecific clinical features, and it may be months or even years before the diagnosis becomes apparent. Andermann *et al* (1990) divided the clinical course into three stages. In the first stage, seizures were mainly simple partial attacks with somatosensory or motor symptoms and complex partial seizures without automatisms (with or without epilepsia partialis continua in each case). They noted that during the later part of stage 1 seizures gradually became more frequent and the hemiparesis, initially postictal and transient, slowly became more permanent. In the second stage, there was a further increase in seizures and the development of more apparent fixed neurologic signs and increasing disability. Eventually there seemed to be a tendency for the disease activity to burn itself out, so that in stage 3 there was a diminution in seizure frequency and severity, without further progression of the neurologic signs (which by this time would commonly include moderate to severe hemiparesis, a visual field defect, and a variable degree of intellectual and language impairment, ranging from mild to severe). (The evolution of radiologic and EEG changes in association with these clinical changes is described below.)

The relentless progression of Rasmussen encephalitis at the onset has led to the introduction of various medical treatments (Dulac *et al* 1991; De Toledo and Smith 1994; Hart *et al* 1994; Andrews *et al* 1996; McLachlan *et al* 1996), none of which has been entirely successful, and to the suggestion that surgical treatment (particularly hemispherectomy, which does appear to halt the disease process in the majority of patients) should be carried out sooner rather than later (Vining *et al* 1993).

OTHER LABORATORY TESTS

Nonspecific abnormalities of the cerebrospinal fluid have been found in about 50% of patients with Rasmussen syndrome. These include minor increases of the white cell count, a modest increase in the protein content of the spinal fluid, and a first-zone or mid-zone abnormality in the colloidal gold curve (Rasmussen and Andermann 1991). Oligoclonal or occasionally monoclonal bands have been found in some patients, but again this finding has not been consistent (Dulac *et al* 1991; Grenier *et al* 1991).

RADIOLOGY

The earliest patients to be reported with focal seizures due to chronic localized encephalitis (Rasmussen *et al* 1958) were studied using pneumoencephalography (PEG) (Fig. 18.4). One of the patients, studied 5 months after the onset, had normal PEG. The second child, who presented with right-sided focal seizures followed by the development of a right hemiparesis, also had normal PEG early in the disease, but by 2 years after the onset there was definite enlargement of the left lateral ventricle. Further PEG performed 3 years later showed more marked evidence of atrophy of the left cerebral hemisphere, while a year later there was marked destruction of the left hemisphere with slight enlargement of the right lateral ventricle. The third patient described in the original paper similarly had normal PEG early in the disease, with

evidence of worsening hemispheric atrophy as the disease progressed.

With the development of more sophisticated methods of imaging the brain, it has become possible to examine the changes in more detail. The advent of computerized tomography (CT) scanning confirmed the development of progressive hemiatrophy, usually beginning in the temporoinsular region, causing enlargement of the temporal horn and sylvian fissure and progressing eventually to involve the remainder of the hemisphere in the majority of patients (Tampieri *et al* 1991). These authors examined the CT scans of 15 patients diagnosed since 1974 and found hemiatrophy of variable severity in 11, diffuse cerebral atrophy in 2, and normal scans in 2 who were examined early in the course of the disease. They noted that the progression of the hemiatrophy could be very rapid, becoming severe in less than 24 months. They also noted that the contralateral ventricle could become enlarged in time. This may be due to Wallerian changes and perhaps to the effect of seizures and trauma. The contralateral atrophy was never comparable to that involving the affected hemisphere.

There have also now been several reports of MRI findings in patients with Rasmussen encephalitis (Fig. 18.5). Tampieri *et al* (1991) reported two patients, both showing hemiatrophy and with abnormal, high-intensity signal on proton density, and with T2-weighted images in keeping with gliosis in one child.

Tien *et al* (1992) reported the results of neuroimaging in four young patients who had had various combinations of CT, xenon CT, and MR scans, and positron emission tomography (PET). Two patients had rather unremarkable CT studies, but had xenon CT scans showing selectively decreased cerebral blood flow to the affected hemisphere. A third patient had CT and MRI scans showing marked atrophy of the affected hemisphere, with decreased FDG tracer uptake in that hemisphere. The fourth patient underwent CT and MR scanning showing severe hemispheric atrophy, with appearances of gliosis in the basal ganglia region and the periventricular area. Zupanc *et al* (1990) reported a patient with typical features of Rasmussen encephalitis in whom repeated MRI scans, with and without gadolinium, were normal, except for one that was carried out approximately 5 months after seizure onset in which MRI demonstrated increased signal intensity in the white and gray matter of the left temporal lobe and a small cortical area of the left parietal lobe on the T2-weighted images, suggestive of edema. Similar findings of hemispheric atrophy and signal change have been reported by other authors (Aguilar *et al* 1996; Yacubian *et al* 1997). Nakasu *et al* (1997) reported serial MRI findings of

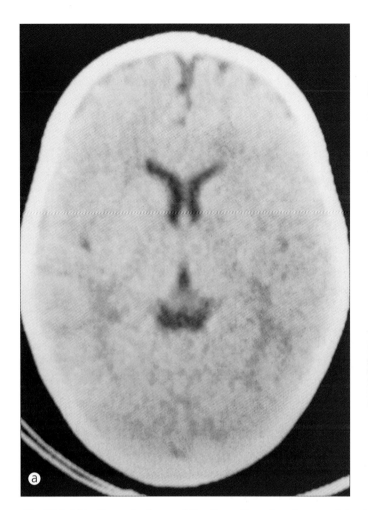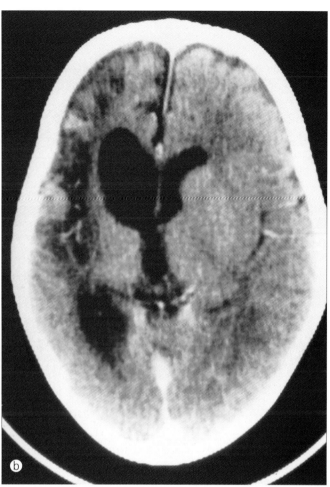

Fig. 18.4 (a) In the early stages of the illness there is only very minimal ventricular asymmetry. (b) Three years later there is severe atrophy of the affected hemisphere, maximal in the frontal region, but there is also slight contralateral atrophy.

Rasmussen encephalitis in a 12-year-old boy who underwent biopsy and treatment with immunoglobulins. No abnormality was seen on the initial scans carried out 1 year after the onset of seizures. Eleven months later, a high-intensity lesion was seen in the left frontal cortex; this lesion rapidly spread into the white matter and then gradually regressed after biopsy and immunoglobulin therapy. Five months after the biopsy, a further high-intensity lesion was seen adjacent to the previous one, despite good seizure control at the time. The signal changes observed in the MRI are often interpreted as due to vascular abnormalities by radiologists who are not aware of the clinical problem. It is thus essential to present the history and findings to the radiologist before the images are analyzed.

Cendes *et al* (1995) performed magnetic resonance spectroscopy (MRS) in three patients with Rasmussen syndrome. They measured the relative resonance intensity of N-acetyl-D-aspartate (NAA) to creatine (NAA:Cr), an index of neuronal loss or damage, for various regions in the brain.

They demonstrated decreased relative NAA signal intensity over the entire affected hemisphere, involving both cortex and white matter and most prominent in the anterior periventricular region. There was a tendency for the changes to be worse in patients with longer duration of disease. Follow-up scans after a year showed progression of the changes. The authors also noted that the changes on MR spectroscopy were more widespread than the structural changes seen on MRI but did not affect the contralateral hemisphere. Two of the patients had epilepsia partialis continua during the follow-up scans only: these patients showed increase in lactate resonance intensity, suggesting that the lactate accumulation resulted from repetitive seizures rather than from the disease process itself. Peeling and Sutherland (1993) carried out MRS on tissue from patients undergoing surgical treatment for Rasmussen encephalitis and found that the metabolite concentrations varied with the severity and extent of the encephalitis, with tissue showing marked abnormalities having decreased

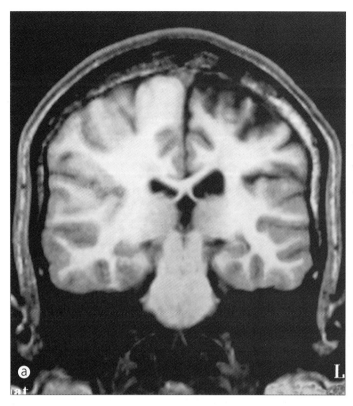
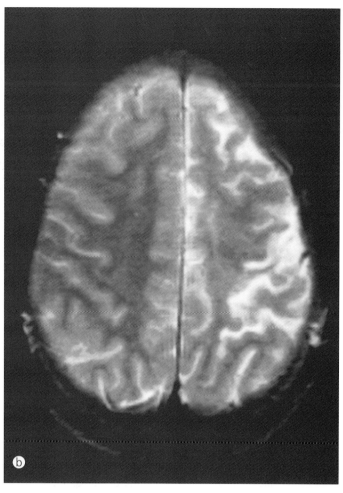

Fig. 18.5 (a) MRI findings in a patient with left hemispheral Rasmussen encephalitis of 6 years' duration. Coronal section showing maximal atrophy in the frontocentral area. (b) Axial section showing the atrophy. The abnormal signal that is often found on MRI is not illustrated here.

NAA, glutamate, cholines, and inositol. The decrease in the levels of NAA and glutamate was greater than in gliotic hippocampal tissue, suggesting the possibility that in-vivo MRS might be helpful in diagnosis and in assessment of results of various forms of immunologic treatment.

Several authors have reported the results of functional imaging in patients with Rasmussen encephalitis. English *et al* (1989) reported five children with this disease: in all, SPECT (single-photon emission computed tomography) imaging demonstrated an area of hypoperfusion or hypometabolism corresponding to the anatomic localization of the epileptogenic foci found by clinical assessment, EEG, and CT. In all cases, the SPECT showed a more extensive area of abnormality than did CT, and in two patients undergoing sequential studies the SPECT reflected the patients' changing clinical condition. Hwang *et al* (1991) reported PET and SPECT studies in patients with Rasmussen encephalitis. One child was studied with ^{99m}Tc-D,1-Hexamethyl-propyleneamine oxime (HMPAO) SPECT, showing an increase in cerebral blood flow in the left temporal lobe ictally and a wider decrease interictally in the left temporal, frontal, and parietal lobes. Five patients

underwent 18-fluoro-2-deoxy-D glucose (FDG) PET scanning, usually showing a regional decrease in the local cerebral metabolic rate in the utilization of glucose, widely distributed over the affected hemisphere and extending beyond the frontal and temporal lobes. However, within the regional hypometabolic zone were one or two more foci of localized increase in metabolic rate that in some cases coincided with focal epileptogenic activity as determined by electrocorticography at surgery. Burke *et al* (1992) described a patient with Rasmussen syndrome in whom ^{99m}Tc-HMPAO SPECT produced grossly abnormal results at a time when the MRI scan showed no structural abnormality: they suggested it might be helpful in the early diagnosis of the condition. Aguilar *et al* (1996) reported an 8-year-old girl with epilepsia partialis continua due to Rasmussen encephalitis involving the left side of the body who underwent ictal and interictal ^{99m}Tc-HMPAO SPECT. In the ictal period this showed increased cerebral blood flow in the right hemisphere, particularly the rolandic area and the temporal lobe, while in the interictal period a decreased flow was seen in the same regions. Yacubian *et al* (1997) also reported a focal increase in regional cerebral blood flow in four patients presenting with epilepsia partialis continua at the time of the HMPAO injection and extensive cortical hypoperfusion in four other patients who received the injection during the interictal state. These authors reported abnormalities of cerebellar function in six patients, two of them with structural damage.

EEG CHANGES

Several authors have studied EEG changes in Rasmussen encephalitis. The largest study to date has been that of So and Gloor (1991), who described the findings in 339 EEGs and 58 electrocorticograms carried out in 49 patients with Rasmussen encephalitis. Analysis of all the preoperative EEGs showed a variety of abnormalities. All but one of the 47 patients for whom preoperative EEGs were available had some abnormality of background activity (either slowing beyond age-adjusted limits or irregularities in the morphology and frequency of waveforms), usually asymmetrical. In the latter EEGs, the majority showed some abnormality bilaterally, but predominantly on one side. All EEGs showed abnormal slow-wave activity, and 44 of the 47 patients had evidence of interictal epileptiform discharges. Frequently there were multiple independent foci lateralized over one hemisphere. Bilateral multiple independent discharges were seen in one-third of patients, but were usually predominant over one side. Almost half of the patients showed bilaterally synchronous spike and wave or sharp- and slow-wave discharges. Clinical or subclinical seizures were recorded in 32 patients, but, although the onset could usually be lateralized to one hemisphere, it was rare for seizures to have a strictly localized electrographic onset. Electrocorticography usually showed widespread regions involved in interictal epileptiform activity, and if several seizures were studied it was common to find multiple independent sites of seizure onset. The evolution of the EEG during the course of the disease process was also studied. Those patients with early disease who had not yet developed hemiparesis were more likely to show unilateral disturbance of background activity. As the disease progressed, bilateral abnormalities became more common. EEG epileptiform abnormalities generally became more widespread with time, and some patients showed the development of independent epileptiform abnormalities over the contralateral hemisphere. Capovilla *et al* (1997) also studied the evolution of the EEG from the onset of the disease in a single patient. They noted focal delta activity over the left temporal region without spikes, at a time when the MRI was normal and ongoing seizure activity was absent. They hypothesized that the presence of such changes in the absence of structural abnormality on imaging should prompt consideration of the diagnosis of Rasmussen encephalitis even before the development of the classical clinical features. Andrews *et al* (1997) studied two patients with pathologically confirmed Rasmussen encephalitis and circulating GluR3 antibodies treated with plasma exchange and immunosuppressive treatment with intravenous immunoglobulins; high-dose steroids were also given in one patient. Repeated EEG monitoring showed that the EEG abnormalities present before plasma exchange, including disturbance of background activity and sleep architecture and frequent epileptiform activity particularly over the affected hemisphere, improved during plasma exchange, only to worsen afterwards, apparently reflecting the change in clinical status.

DIAGNOSIS

The clinical changes of Rasmussen encephalitis, like the pathologic changes, are nonspecific, particularly in the early stages, and several other conditions can present in a rather similar manner. Mitochondrial encephalopathy with lactic acidosis and strokelike episodes (MELAS) (Dvorkin *et al* 1987) is one such condition, the clinical features being episodic vomiting and recurrent strokes, and partial seizures frequently associated with prolonged migrainous manifestations and often developing into epilepsia partialis continua. Cortical dysplasia may cause intractable partial epilepsy (Andermann *et al* 1987; Kuzniecky *et al* 1988), though only occasionally with epilepsia partialis continua. Tuberous sclerosis may cause similar symptoms (Andermann *et al* 1987), as may tumors (Rich *et al* 1985), cerebral vasculitis (Mackworth-Young and Hughes 1985), and Russian spring–summer encephalitis (Kozhevnikov 1991).

In their protocol for treatment of children with Rasmussen encephalitis with high-dose steroids or immunoglobulins, Hart *et al* (1994) suggested the following criteria for diagnosis:

- Children who develop epilepsia partialis continua and meet at least one of the following criteria to suggest the diagnosis of chronic encephalitis:
  (1) progressive neurologic deficit at the beginning or after the onset of epilepsia partialis continua, but before the start of treatment;
  (2) progressive hemispheric atrophy on CT, MRI, or both, with or without density or signal abnormalities;

(3) presence of oligoclonal or monoclonal banding on CSF examination; or

(4) biopsy evidence of chronic encephalitis.

Children not having epilepsia partialis continua but with focal epilepsy and biopsy evidence of chronic encephalitis (who might in addition meet criteria (1), (2), or (3)) were also considered to have the diagnosis.

TREATMENT

The relentless progression of Rasmussen encephalitis in the majority of patients, with the development of intractable seizures, progressive neurologic deficits, and intellectual impairment, and the rarity of the condition, which makes clinical trials difficult, have led clinicians to try a variety of treatments on an empirical basis. Although hemispherectomy appears to be successful in arresting the disease process in the majority of patients, the consequent neurologic deficits mean that there is often reluctance to carry out this procedure until a hemiparesis already exists.

There has long been debate whether the progressive neurologic deficits in Rasmussen encephalitis are secondary to ongoing seizure activity or are an independent effect of the encephalitic process, and initial attempts at treating Rasmussen encephalitis concentrated on the quest for seizure control. The pharmacologic treatment of 25 patients with the condition at the Montreal Neurological Institute was analyzed by Dubeau and Sherwin, who found that all had received polytherapy, often at the expense of significant morbidity as a result of toxic or other adverse effects. Of the seizure types most commonly seen in patients with Rasmussen encephalitis (partial motor, complex partial, and secondarily generalized tonic–clonic seizures), the secondarily generalized tonic–clonic seizures were most likely to respond to treatment.

Most other treatments directed at aborting the disease have relied on the assumption that the cause is either infective, probably viral, or the result of an autoimmune process. Examples of such treatments include antiviral treatments including the use of ganciclovir, zidovudine, high-dose interferon, high-dose steroids and immunoglobulins, and plasma exchange.

De Toledo and Smith (1994) treated a 4-year-old child with epilepsia partialis continua, progressive aphasia, and right hemiparesis with zidovudine (AZT) after the seizures had failed to respond to conventional antiepileptic drugs and adrenocorticotropic hormone (ACTH). Zidovudine was given for 62 days, eventually being discontinued because of granulocytopenia. Seizures stopped and neurologic deterioration was arrested for approximately 21 months within 6 weeks of the onset of treatment. Unfortunately, when the patient relapsed, with seizures affecting the previously uninvolved left hemibody, side-effects prevented further treatment with zidovudine. Zidovudine was also used in three patients by S.D. Shorvon and colleagues (personal communication). There was short-lived and unfortunately unsustained improvement.

Because cytomegalovirus had been implicated in the pathogenesis of Rasmussen syndrome, the effect of ganciclovir was assessed in four patients by McLachlan *et al* (1996). CMV genome was sought in three of these patients, and found in two. One child with very frequent seizures developing over 3 months became seizure-free 5 days after the onset of treatment, with resolution also of focal neurologic signs, cognitive function, and EEG changes. Two other patients treated 34 and 72 months after disease onset showed some improvement, while in the fourth patient there was no benefit.

Early reports of the use of corticosteroids (including dexamethasone, prednisone, and ACTH) in Rasmussen encephalitis (Gupta *et al* 1984; Piatt *et al* 1988) were not encouraging. However, Dulac *et al* (1991), who were among the first to try high-dose steroids in children with Rasmussen encephalitis, produced some promising results. They treated five children with three intravenous infusions of $400\,\mathrm{mg\ m^{-2}}$ of methylprednisolone, one every other day, followed by oral prednisone ($2\,\mathrm{mg\ kg^{-1}\ day^{-1}}$) or hydrocortisone ($10\,\mathrm{mg\ kg^{-1}\ day^{-1}}$) tapered off over 3–24 months. Epilepsia partialis continua ceased in three cases within 1 month of the start of treatment, the EEG improving dramatically in two of these and one other child. Motor and cognitive impairment stopped worsening in all of the children, although only one showed a clear improvement, from a state in which she was bedridden and mute to one in which she could walk and talk. However, two of the patients relapsed within a few months of the cessation of treatment.

As a result of this success, other authors tried this and other immunosuppressive treatment (Walsh 1991; Hart *et al* 1994). Several reports had documented improvement in intractable epilepsy of other etiologies treated with gamma-globulin (Péchadre *et al* 1977; Laffont *et al* 1979; Ariizumi *et al* 1983), and Walsh (1991) reported a 12-year-old boy with Rasmussen syndrome in whom treatment with six infusions ($200\,\mathrm{mg\ kg^{-1}}$) of intravenous immunoglobulin over a period of 3 months showed improvement both in neurologic function and also seizure control during the course of the treatment and for several months afterwards. A second child who had also had a favorable response was briefly mentioned. Hart *et al* (1994) reported 19 patients treated with high-dose steroids, immunoglobulins, or both. Two (both biopsy-proven) had developed Rasmussen syndrome in adulthood; the rest were children. The diagnosis was confirmed by biopsy in all but three of the patients. The treatment protocols varied since the patients were treated at different centers. Seventeen patients received treatment with steroids (usually oral steroids, although six patients received intravenous methylprednisolone at some stage; one child received ACTH injections over 4 weeks). Two patients received intravenous immunoglobulins alone, while seven patients received both high-dose steroids and intravenous immunoglobulins. Seven patients showed no improvement in seizure frequency following treatment with steroids. Two patients showed an improvement of 25% or less, while eight showed at least a 50% reduction in seizure frequency. With the exception of two patients, the frequency of seizures increased within days or weeks of withdrawal of steroids. Side-effects were common and often prominent. Seven of the nine patients treated with intravenous immunoglobulin showed definite improvement in seizure control, at least initially. This was not maintained in three patients. Any improvement in neurologic deficit in these patients was only transient and accompanied by improved seizure control, except in one instance where the hemiparesis improved disproportionately to the improvement in seizure control. It seems likely that treatments such as these might have maximum effect early in the onset of disease. In this study a considerable proportion of the patients had been ill for several years before treatment: 14 already had mild hemiparesis and another four had evidence of intellectual deterioration, and this may be responsible for the rather poor results. Hart *et al* suggested protocols for the treatment of patients with intravenous immunoglobulins or high-dose steroids. With intravenous immunoglobulin, the recommended treatment was 400 mg kg^{-1} day^{-1} by intravenous infusion on three successive days, with a single further infusion of 400 mg kg^{-1} at monthly intervals if improvement occurred. If no improvement was seen, treatment with steroids was recommended, the initial course consisting of intravenous methylprednisolone (400 mg per m^2 of body surface), given as three consecutive infusions on alternate days. Subsequent infusions consisted of single infusions at monthly intervals for the first year, 2-monthly intervals for the second year, and 3-monthly intervals for the third year, unless serious side-effects supervened. The treatment was accompanied by oral prednisolone starting at 2 mg kg^{-1} day^{-1} and reducing very gradually over a period of months depending on clinical response, with the total duration of oral steroid treatment usually being 1–2 years.

A further patient with symptoms highly responsive to repeated courses of immunosuppressant treatment was described by Krauss *et al* (1996). They reported a woman who had developed her first symptoms, partial and secondarily generalized seizures, at the age of 15 years and had gone on to develop typical features of Rasmussen encephalitis. Brain biopsy was also consistent with this diagnosis. Treatment with immunoglobulins at the age of 29 years produced no change in her seizure control or aphasia, but intravenous methylprednisolone brought about a dramatic improvement in her seizures and neurologic deficits. Oral steroids were ineffective. She was also treated with intermittent cyclophosphamide, which was insufficient to contain her symptoms, and with plasmapheresis, though the effect of the latter was unclear. Her serum and CSF were negative for antibodies to GluR3 by both immunoblot and immunocytochemical analysis of cells transfected with GluR3 cDNA, suggesting an alternative immune-mediated process in some patients with chronic encephalitis.

Intraventricular interferon-α (IFN-α) has also been tried in Rasmussen encephalitis (Maria *et al* 1993; Dabbagh *et al* 1997), on the basis that not only do interferons have immunomodulating activity such as enhancement of the phagocytic activity of macrophages and augmentation of the specific cytotoxicity of lymphocytes for target cells, but in addition they inhibit virus replication in virus-infected cells. The 3½-year-old child described by Dabbagh *et al* had epilepsia partialis continua and a right hemiparesis, and was mute at the time of treatment. She was given three doses of 3 000 000 units of IFN-α through an Omaya reservoir in the first week on alternate days, two doses per week in the second and third weeks, and weekly doses for the fourth through sixth weeks. She had a significant reduction in seizures, but relapsed to baseline 3 weeks after stopping treatment: however, she responded to further courses of treatment and, at the time of the report, more than 12 months after the onset of treatment, she remained seizure-free on treatment every third week. The patient reported by Maria *et al* also showed improvement in the control of his epilepsy and neurologic deficit with IFN-α in the short term.

Andrews *et al* (1996) described the use of plasma exchange in four patients (two of them previously described by Rogers *et al* (1994)) with clinical and pathologic features of Rasmussen encephalitis, three of whom had repeated, dramatic, transient clinical improvements shown by reduced seizure frequency, rapid control of status epilepticus, and improved neurologic function. Two of these patients had evidence of active inflammation on pathologic examination; the third had chronic changes (although autoantibodies were present). The fourth patient, who also had pathologic evidence of active inflammation, had a more muted response to repeated plasma exchange. The authors drew attention to the known complications of plasma exchange (infection, anemia, coagulopathy, etc.) and also to its expense, and suggested certain situations in which it might prove particularly helpful – for example, status epilepticus in Rasmussen encephalitis and the evaluation of patients prior to surgery when residual function may be unmasked by the reduction in seizure frequency brought about by the plasma exchange. Andrews *et al* also suggested a protocol, advocating five or six single volumes of plasma exchange initially, with albumin and saline replacement, spread over 10–12 days, with an infusion of $1 g^{-1} kg^{-1}$ of intravenous immunoglobulin given to the patient the day after. They recommended that thereafter subsequent plasma exchange be given on the basis of clinical need for recurrent seizures, perhaps every 2–3 months on average. They considered that interval treatment with immunosuppressive agents might prolong the improvement after each plasma exchange and limit expense.

Despite the promise shown by these treatments in a few patients, at present none has shown itself to reliably affect the course of the disease. Surgical treatment has been tried in a number of patients. Limited focal resection carried out early in the disease appears to be of little lasting benefit (Rasmussen and McCann 1968). There appears to be a consensus of opinion that functional hemispherectomy is a reasonable option when the patient has developed hemiparesis and homonymous hemianopia (Rasmussen 1983). However, some groups believe that, since hemispherectomy is the only procedure that apparently stops progression of the disease, it should be considered an early option, without awaiting the development of maximal hemiparesis (Vining *et al* 1993).

DIRECTION OF FUTURE RESEARCH

The discovery of the GluR3 antibody in some patients with Rasmussen encephalitis has prompted a reexamination of the likely underlying etiology, with a plausible explanation now having been put forward (Antel and Rasmussen 1996). However, despite this exciting advance, the future remains far from clear, and the only treatment that appears to halt disease activity with any consistency remains radical surgery, with its accompanying deficits. Until early diagnosis can be made with certainty, prevention of the underlying process will continue to be problematic. Some patients with apparent Rasmussen encephalitis do not demonstrate the GluR3 antibody, and there is only a limited response in the majority of patients to immunosuppressive treatment and plasma exchange. Nevertheless, it seems likely that future research in the immunologic field will eventually yield results, so that a cure may be found for this distressing disease.

KEY POINTS

1. The characteristic clinical features of Rasmussen syndrome are onset in childhood, refractory focal seizures, progressive hemiparesis, and intellectual impairment.
2. The pathologic features are usually limited to one hemisphere and include perivascular cuffing, the presence of microglia, spongy degeneration, and gliosis.
3. The etiology is unknown, with possible mechanisms including chronic viral infection, acute viral infection leading to a local immune response, and an independent autoimmune process: in some patients circulating antibodies to GluR3 fusion protein are found.
4. Neuroimaging demonstrates progressive atrophy of the affected hemisphere, while EEG usually shows slow wave activity on the affected side, often with multifocal epileptic discharges.
5. Various medical treatments including antiviral agents, intravenous immunoglobulins, high-dose steriods, and plasma exchange have produced limited or short-lived improvement in some patients, but in the longer term usually fail to prevent progression of the disease.
6. Hemispherectomy may be successful in achieving seizure control and preventing further intellectual impairment, but causes hemiparesis if not already present.

REFERENCES

Aguilar RF, Rojas BJC, Villanueva PR, Morales HS (1996) SPECT-99mTc-HMPAO en un caso de epilepsia parcial continua y encefalitis focal. *Revista de Investigacion Clinica* **48**:199–205.

Andermann F, Olivier A, Melanson D, Robitaille Y (1987) Epilepsy due to focal cortical dysplasia with macrogyria and the forme fruste of tuberous sclerosis: a study of 15 patients. In: Wolf P, Dam M, Janz D, Dreifuss F (eds) *Advances in Epileptology: The 16th Epilepsy International Symposium*, pp 35–38. New York: Raven Press.

Andermann F, Oguni H, Rasmussen TB (1990) The syndrome of chronic encephalitis and epilepsy: a study based on the MNI series of 48 cases. *Journal of Epilepsy* **3** (suppl.):325–326.

Andrews JM, Thompson JA, Pysher TJ, Walker ML, Hammond ME (1990) Chronic encephalitis, epilepsy, and cerebrovascular immune complex deposits. *Annals of Neurology* **28**:88–90.

Andrews PI, Dichter MA, Berkovic SF, Newton MR, McNamara JO (1996) Plasmapheresis in Rasmussen's encephalitis. *Neurology* **46**:242–246.

Andrews PI, McNamara JO, Lewis DV (1997) Clinical and electroencephalographic correlates in Rasmussen's encephalitis. *Epilepsia* **38**:189–194.

Antel JP, Rasmussen T (1996) Rasmussen's encephalitis and the new hat. *Neurology* **46**:9–11.

Ariizumi M, Baba K, Shiihara H et al (1983) High dose gamma-globulin for intractable childhood epilepsy. *Lancet* **ii**:162–163.

Asher DM, Gajdusek DC (1991) Virologic studies in chronic encephalitis. In: Andermann F (ed) *Chronic Encephalitis and Epilepsy: Rasmussen's Syndrome*, pp 147–158. Boston: Butterworth-Heinemann.

Atkins MR, Terrell W, Hulette CM (1995) Rasmussen's syndrome: a study of potential viral etiology. *Clinical Neuropathology* **14**:7–12.

Burke GJ, Fifer SA, Yoder J (1992) Early detection of Rasmussen's syndrome by brain SPECT imaging. *Clinical Nuclear Medicine* **17**:730–731.

Capovilla G, Paladin F, Dalla Bernardina B (1997) Rasmussen's syndrome: longitudinal EEG study from the first seizure to epilepsia partialis continua. *Epilepsia* **38**:483–488.

Cendes F, Andermann F, Silver K, Arnold DL (1995) Imaging of axonal damage *in vivo* in Rasmussen's syndrome. *Brain* **118**:753–758.

Chinchilla D, Dulac O, Robain O et al (1994) Reappraisal of Rasmussen's syndrome with special emphasis on treatment with high doses of steroids. *Journal of Neurology, Neurosurgery and Psychiatry* **57**:1325–1333.

Dabbagh O, Gascon G, Crowell J, Bamoggodam F (1997) Intraventricular interferon-α stops seizures in Rasmussen's encephalitis: a case report. *Epilepsia* **38**:1045–1049.

De Toledo JC, Smith DB (1994) Partially successful treatment of Rasmussen's encephalitis with zidovudine: symptomatic improvement followed by involvement of the contralateral hemisphere. *Epilepsia* **35**:352–355.

Dubeau F, Sherwin AL (1991) Pharmacologic principles in the management of chronic encephalitis. In: Andermann F (ed) *Chronic Encephalitis and Epilepsy: Rasmussen's Syndrome*, pp 179–192. Boston: Butterworth-Heinemann.

Dulac O, Robain O, Chiron C et al (1991) High-dose steroid treatment of epilepsia partialis continua due to chronic focal encephalitis. In: Andermann F (ed) *Chronic Encephalitis and Epilepsy: Rasmussen's Syndrome*, pp 79–110. Boston: Butterworth-Heinemann.

Dvorkin GS, Andermann F, Carpenter S et al (1987) Classical migraine, intractable epilepsy and multiple strokes: a syndrome related to mitochondrial encephalomyopathy. In: Andermann F, Lugaresi E (eds) *Migraine and Epilepsy*, pp 202–232. Boston: Butterworths.

English R, Soper N, Shepstone BJ, Hockaday JM, Stores G (1989) Five patients with Rasmussen's syndrome investigated by single-photon-emission computed tomography. *Nuclear Medicine Communications* **10**:5–14.

Farrell M, Cheng L, Cornford ME, Grody WW, Vinters HV (1991) Cytomegalovirus and Rasmussen's encephalitis. *Lancet* **337**:1551–1552.

Friedman H, Ch'ien L, Parham D (1977) Virus in brain of child with hemiplegia, hemiconvulsions, and epilepsy. *Lancet* **ii**:666.

Fukuda T, Oguni H, Yanagaki S et al (1994) Chronic localized encephalitis (Rasmussen's syndrome) preceded by ipsilateral uveitis: a case report. *Epilepsia* **35**:1328–1331.

Gilden DH, Lipton H (1991) Cytomegalovirus and Rasmussen's encephalitis. *Lancet* **337**:239.

Gray F, Serdaru M, Baron H et al (1987) Chronic localised encephalitis (Rasmussen's) in an adult with epilepsia partialis continua. *Journal of Neurology, Neurosurgery and Psychiatry* **50**:747–751.

Grenier Y, Antel JP, Osterland CK (1991) Immunologic studies in chronic encephalitis of Rasmussen. In: Andermann F (ed) *Chronic Encephalitis and Epilepsy: Rasmussen's Syndrome*, pp 125–134. Boston: Butterworth-Heinemann.

Gupta PC, Roy S, Tandon PN (1974) Progressive epilepsy due to chronic persistent encephalitis. Report of four cases. *Journal of Neurological Science* **22**:105–120.

Gupta PC, Rapin I, Houroupian DS, Roy S, Llena JF, Tandon PN (1984) Smouldering encephalitis in children. *Neuropediatrics* **15**:191–197.

Hart YM, Cortez M, Andermann F et al (1994) Medical treatment of Rasmussen's syndrome (chronic encephalitis and epilepsy): effect of high-dose steroids or immunoglobulins in 19 patients. *Neurology* **44**:1030–1036.

Hart YM, Andermann F, Fish DR et al (1997) Chronic encephalitis and epilepsy in adults and adolescents: a variant of Rasmussen's syndrome? *Neurology* **48**:418–424.

Hart YM, Andermann F, Robitaille Y, Laxer KD, Rasmussen T, Davis R (1998) Double pathology in Rasmussen's syndrome: a window on the etiology? *Neurology* **50**:731–735.

Harvey AS, Andermann F, Hopkins IJ, Kirkham TH, Berkovic SF (1992) Chronic encephalitis (Rasmussen's syndrome) and ipsilateral uveitis. *Annals of Neurology* **32**:826–829.

Hwang PA, Gilday DL, Spire J-P et al (1991) Chronic focal encephalitis of Rasmussen: functional neuroimaging studies with positron emission tomography and single-photon emission computed tomography scanning. In: Andermann F (ed) *Chronic Encephalitis and Epilepsy: Rasmussen's Syndrome*, pp 61–72. Boston: Butterworth-Heinemann.

Jay V, Becker LE, Otsubo H, Cortez M, Hwang P, Hoffman HJ, Zielenska M (1995) Chronic encephalitis and epilepsy (Rasmussen's encephalitis): detection of cytomegalovirus and herpes simplex virus 1 by the polymerase chain reaction and in situ hybridization. *Neurology* **45**:108–117.

Kozhevnikov AY (translated by Asher DM) (1991) A particular type of cortical epilepsy (epilepsia corticalis sive partialis continua). In: Andermann F (ed) *Chronic Encephalitis and Epilepsy: Rasmussen's Syndrome*, pp 245–261. Boston: Butterworth-Heinemann.

Krauss GL, Campbell ML, Roche KW, Huganir RL, Niedermeyer E (1996) Chronic steroid-responsive encephalitis without autoantibodies to glutamate receptor GluR3. *Neurology* **46**:247–249.

Kuzniecky R, Berkovic S, Andermann F et al (1988) Focal cortical myoclonus and rolandic cortical dysplasia: clarification by magnetic resonance imaging. *Annals of Neurology* **23**:317–325.

Laffont F, Esnaults S, Gilbert A, Peytour MA, Cathala HP, Eygonnet JP (1979) Effet des gammaglobulines sur des épilepsies rebelles.

Etude préliminaire. *Annales de Médecine Interne (Paris)* **130**:307–312.

Mackworth-Young CG, Hughes GR (1985) Epilepsy: an early symptom of systemic lupus erythematosus (letter). *Journal of Neurology, Neurosurgery and Psychiatry* **48**:185.

Maria BL, Ringdahl DM, Mickle JP *et al* (1993) Intraventricular alpha interferon therapy for Rasmussen's syndrome. *Canadian Journal of Neurological Sciences* **20**:333–336.

McLachlan RS, Girvin JP, Blume WT, Reichman H (1993) Rasmussen's chronic encephalitis in adults. *Archives of Neurology* **50**:269–274.

McLachlan RS, Levin S, Blume WT (1996) Treatment of Rasmussen's syndrome with ganciclovir. *Neurology* **47**:925–928.

Mizuno Y, Chou SM, Estes ML, Erenberg G, Cruse RP, Rothner AD (1985) Chronic localized encephalitis (Rasmussen's) with focal cerebral seizures revisited. *Journal of Neuropathology and Experimental Neurology* **44**:351.

Nakasu S, Isozumi T, Yamamoto A, Okada K, Takano T, Nadasu Y (1997) Serial magnetic resonance imaging findings of Rasmussen's encephalitis: a case report. *Neurologia Medico-Chirurgica (Tokyo)* **37**:924–928.

Oguni H, Andermann F, Rasmussen TB (1991) The natural history of the syndrome of chronic encephalitis and epilepsy: a study of the MNI series of forty-eight cases. In: Andermann F (ed) *Chronic Encephalitis and Epilepsy: Rasmussen's Syndrome*, pp 7–35. Boston: Butterworth-Heinemann.

Oguni H, Andermann F, Rasmussen TB (1992) The syndrome of chronic encephalitis and epilepsy: a study based on the MNI series of 48 cases. *Advances in Neurology* **57**:419–433.

Péchadre JC, Sauvezie B, Osier C, Gibert J (1977) Traitement des encéphalopathies de l'enfant par les gammaglobulines. Résultats préliminaires. *Révue d'Electroéncephalographique et de Neurologie Clinique* **7**:443–447.

Peeling J, Sutherland G (1993) [1]II magnetic resonance spectroscopy of extracts of human epileptic neocortex and hippocampus. *Neurology* **43**:589–594.

Piatt JH, Hwang PA, Armstrong DC, Becker LE, Hoffman HJ (1988) Chronic focal encephalitis (Rasmussen syndrome): six cases. *Epilepsia* **29**:268–279.

Power C, Poland SD, Blume WT, Girvin JP, Rice GPA (1990) Cytomegalovirus and Rasmussen's encephalitis. *Lancet* **336**:1282–1284.

Rasmussen T (1978) Further observations on the syndrome of chronic encephalitis and epilepsy. *Applied Neurophysiology* **41**:1–12.

Rasmussen T (1983) Hemispherectomy for seizures revisited. *Canadian Journal of Neurological Sciences* **10**:71–78.

Rasmussen T, Anderman F (1991) Rasmussen's syndrome: symptomatology of the syndrome of chronic encephalitis and seizures: 35-year experience with 51 cases. In: Luders HO (ed) *Epilepsy Surgery*, pp 173–182. New York. Raven Press.

Rasmussen T, McCann W (1968) Clinical studies of patients with focal epilepsy due to 'chronic encephalitis'. *Transactions of the American Neurological Association* **93**:89–94.

Rasmussen T, Olszewski J, Lloyd-Smith D (1958) Focal seizures due to chronic localized encephalitis. *Neurology* **8**:435–445.

Rich KM, Goldring S, Gado M (1985) Computed tomography in chronic seizure disorder caused by glioma. *Arch Neurol* **42**:26–27.

Robitaille Y (1991) Neuropathologic aspects of chronic encephalitis. In: Andermann F (ed) *Chronic Encephalitis and Epilepsy: Rasmussen's Syndrome*, pp 79–110. Boston: Butterworth-Heinemann.

Rogers SW, Andrews PI, Gahring LC *et al* (1994) Autoantibodies to glutamate receptor GluR3 in Rasmussen's encephalitis. *Science* **265**:648–651.

Root-Bernstein RS (1991) Cytomegalovirus and Rasmussen's encephalitis. *Lancet* **337**:239–240.

Silver K, Meagher Villemure K, Andermann F (1998) Familial alternating epilepsia partialis continua with chronic encephalitis: another variant of Rasmussen's syndrome? *Arch Neurol* **55**:733–736.

So NK, Gloor P (1991) Electroencephalographic and electrocortico-graphic findings in chronic encephalitis of the Rasmussen type. In: Andermann F (ed) *Chronic Encephalitis and Epilepsy: Rasmussen's Syndrome*, pp 37–45. Boston: Butterworth-Heinemann.

Takahashi Y, Kubota H, Fujiwara T, Yagi K, Seino M (1997) Epilepsia partialis continua of childhood involving bilateral brain hemispheres. *Acta Neurol Scand* **96**:345–352.

Tampieri D, Melanson D, Ethier R (1991) Imaging of chronic encephalitis. In: Andermann F (ed) *Chronic Encephalitis and Epilepsy: Rasmussen's Syndrome*, pp 47–60. Boston: Butterworth-Heinemann.

Tien RD, Ashdown BC, Lewis DV, Atkins MR, Burger PC (1992) Rasmussen's encephalitis: neuroimaging findings in four patients. *American Journal of Roentgenology* **158**:1329–1332.

Twyman RE, Gahring LC, Spiess J, Rogers SW (1995) Glutamate receptor antibodies activate a subset of receptors and reveal an agonist binding site. *Neuron* **14**:755–762.

Vining EP, Freeman JM, Brandt J, Carson BS, Uematsu S (1993) Progressive unilateral encephalopathy of childhood (Rasmussen's syndrome): a reappraisal. *Epilepsia* **34**:639–650.

Vinters HV, Wang R, Wiley CA (1993) Herpesviruses in chronic encephalitis associated with intractable childhood epilepsy. *Human Pathology* **24**:871–879.

Walsh PJ (1991) Treatment of Rasmussen's syndrome with intravenous gammaglobulin. In: Andermann F (ed) *Chronic Encephalitis and Epilepsy: Rasmussen's Syndrome*, pp 201–204. Boston: Butterworth-Heinemann.

Walter GF, Renella RR (1989) Epstein–Barr virus in brain and Rasmussen's encephalitis. *Lancet* **i**:279–280.

Yacubian EM, Rosemberg S, Marie SK, Valerio RM, Jorge CL, Cukiert A (1996) Double pathology in Rasmussen's encephalitis: etiologic considerations. *Epilepsia* **37**:495–500.

Yacubian EM, Marie SK, Valerio RM, Jorge CL, Yamaga L, Buchpiguel CA (1997) Neuroimaging findings in Rasmussen's syndrome. *Journal of Neuroimaging* **7**:16–22.

Zupanc ML, Handler EG, Levine RL *et al* (1990) Rasmussen encephalitis: epilepsia partialis continua secondary to chronic encephalitis. *Pediatric Neurology* **6**:397–401.

Nonvascular disorders of early childhood

19

J AICARDI

Most diseases of the central nervous system (CNS) can be responsible for epileptic seizures and many of them can produce recurrent, apparently unprovoked seizures, i.e. epilepsy. Some generalized disorders, especially metabolic diseases, can also generate epilepsy through indirect mechanisms. Nonrecurrent seizures that occur during acute diseases or are regularly precipitated by specific factors, especially febrile convulsions, will not be dealt with. This chapter includes three major categories of causes: (1) chromosomal abnormalities and disorders of brain development; (2) metabolic and degenerative diseases; and (3) acquired brain damage that can produce recurrent seizures through various mechanisms. A complete coverage of all causes is obviously impracticable and only relatively common causes are indicated. However, some very rare disorders (e.g. pyridoxine-dependency) are included because of their therapeutic importance.

CHROMOSOMAL ABNORMALITIES AND BRAIN MALFORMATIONS

This section deals with the chromosomal abnormalities most commonly responsible for epilepsy and, briefly, with a few epileptogenic CNS malformations not described elsewhere in this book, e.g. agenesis of the corpus callosum.

CHROMOSOMAL ABNORMALITIES

Chromosomal abnormalities cause approximately 6% of CNS malformations and increase the risk of epilepsy even though they do not represent a frequent cause of seizure disorders (Guerrini et al 1998). Their diagnosis is important, however, as they often cause intractable seizures and significantly increase the disability of patients already at a disadvantage because of the mental retardation usually associated with these disorders.

Trisomy 21 (Down syndrome)

Trisomy 21 is the most common genetic cause of mental retardation; its approximate incidence is 1/650 births. The incidence of epilepsy in children with Down syndrome has been estimated to be 1.4% but cumulative incidence may increase considerably with maternal age. A high proportion of early seizures result from common medical complications of trisomy 21 such as congenital heart disease or infections. Partial seizures occur mainly in this group (Stafstrom et al 1991). Partial complex seizures may occur, in older patients, although generalized attacks are much more common. Infantile spasms are frequent (Silva *et al* 1996) and usually present as cryptogenic spasms. They may respond well to therapy and only rarely evolve into Lennox–Gastaut syndrome. Reflex precipitation of seizures (more often generalized than partial) is frequent, especially in the form of startle epilepsy (Pueschel and Louis 1993).

Fragile X syndrome

The fragile X syndrome is the most common cause of heritable mental retardation. The condition results from a dynamic mutation with expansion of a repeat CGG trinucleotide within the *FMR1* gene on chromosome Xq27.3. The incidence of epilepsy in the disorder is around 25% (Wisniewski *et al* 1991). Seizures usually appear before age 15 years and tend to remit in adults, indicating a relative benignity in most patients. A majority of seizures are generalized but partial seizures are not rare and all types including infantile spasms have been reported. An EEG pattern of midtemporal spikes has repeatedly been found, although with a variable frequency, and may also be observed in the absence of clinical seizures (Musumeci *et al* 1991). The diagnosis of fragile X syndrome may be difficult as the dysmorphism is often relatively minor. The fragile site is only inconstantly present and the diagnosis currently rests on DNA analysis (Guerrini *et al* 1998).

Angelman syndrome

Angelman syndrome is a peculiar behavioral and dysmorphic syndrome that is associated in 70% of cases with a deletion of maternal origin involving chromosome 15q11–q13. A few cases result from uniparental disomy, both chromosomes 15 being of paternal origin. The remaining cases are due to an abnormality of the imprinting process itself, or associated with a mutation of the *UBE3A* gene.

Epilepsy is present in 84–90% of patients (Matsumoto *et al* 1992). Seizures usually have their onset in infancy or early childhood. Atypical absences, myoclonic seizures, and clonic unilateral seizures are the main ictal patterns (Guerrini *et al* 1998). However, Viani *et al* (1995) thought that complex partial seizures with eye deviation and vomiting, possibly indicating an occipital lobe origin, were frequent. Episodes of myoclonic status epilepticus are a remarkable feature. The myoclonus is often negative and is thought to be of cortical origin (Guerrini *et al* 1996a). Interestingly, the epileptic manifestations of Angelman syndrome seem to be variable with the genotype. Patients with a deletion have severe epilepsy and EEG abnormalities, while those with other genotypic abnormalities, especially

mutation of the *UBE* gene, have much milder epileptic manifestations (Minassian *et al* 1998). This lesser severity is also evident in a milder dysmorphism (Guerrini *et al* 1998).

The clinical diagnosis is often difficult, especially in the first years of life, and complete study of chromosome 15 – including if necessary a methylation test – is recommended for genetic counseling.

Miller–Dieker syndrome

This and other abnormalities of chromosome 17 and of chromosome X responsible for lissencephaly and/or subcortical laminar heterotopias are discussed elsewhere. Although infantile spasms are the most prominent epileptic feature, partial seizures are frequently observed in association with the spasms or, less commonly, in isolation.

Partial monosomy 4p (Wolf–Hirschhorn syndrome)

Partial monosomy 4p is a rare syndrome with a high epileptogenicity (70–100% prevalence) (Sgro *et al* 1995). Seizures have an early onset, usually within the first year of life. Partial seizures are often the first paroxysmal manifestation, but atypical absences seem to be more common after a few years and are associated with a special EEG pattern reminiscent of that observed in patients with Angelman syndrome.

Other chromosomal abnormalities

Other chromosomal abnormalities associated with epilepsy are seldom a cause of partial seizures. Trisomy 12p (Elia *et al* 1995), ring chromosome 20 (Inoue *et al* 1997; Canevini *et al* 1998), and trisomy 9p (Golden and Schoene 1993) are mainly the cause of generalized seizures.

OTHER DEVELOPMENTAL ABNORMALITIES

Multiple brain malformations can be responsible for epilepsies that may feature partial seizures.

Agenesis of the corpus callosum is frequently associated with seizures, often partial, including long-duration unilateral clonic episodes (Nance *et al* 1998). However, the frequency of epilepsy may be more apparent than real as epilepsy is an indication for imaging, which is not necessarily performed in patients with only developmental retardation or no symptoms. The possible inhibitory role of corpus callosum fibers has been suggested as a cause of unilateral attacks. In *Aicardi syndrome*, partial seizures are a very frequent expression of epilepsy, which is also manifested by asymmetrical infantile spasms of likely focal origin (Chevrie and Aicardi 1986). The actual cause of seizures is the presence of abnormalities of cortical development (heterotopias and polymicrogyrias) rather than callosal agenesis. Seizures are very resistant to treatment and are always associated with mental retardation and often with neurologic signs, mostly hemiparesis.

Epilepsy is frequent in cases of *holoprosencephaly*, often in the form of infantile spasms (Watanabe *et al* 1976) but also as focal seizures in the milder cases (Sztriha *et al* 1998). Several mutations of the homeobox gene *Sonic Hedgehog* are found in some cases (Roessler *et al* 1996). Partial simple or complex seizures are a frequent manifestation of *schizencephaly*, also termed 'true' porencephaly (Menezes *et al* 1988). Interestingly, this abnormality can apparently result from mutations in the homeobox gene *EMX2* or from prenatal vascular disturbances (Granata *et al* 1996, 1997), thus illustrating the difficulty of separating malformative from clastic lesions.

Epilepsy is a frequent but indirect complication of *Chiari 2 malformation* resulting from the associated hydrocephalus. All causes of hydrocephalus can produce partial seizures (Saukkonen *et al* 1990), but the role of shunting operation is controversial (Di Rocco *et al* 1985; Bourgeois *et al* 1999).

METABOLIC AND DEGENERATIVE DISORDERS

Metabolic and neurodegenerative disorders are an important cause of seizures and epilepsy especially in childhood as 25% of them are expressed at birth and 90% before the end of puberty (Garcia-Alvarez *et al* 1998). However, the clinical presentation and diagnostic significance of seizures are quite variable and two different groups can be distinguished.

DISORDERS WITH NEUROLOGIC AND SYSTEMIC MANIFESTATIONS

In the first group, which includes mainly neonates and very young infants, epileptic manifestations are accompanied by prominent neurologic and, sometimes systemic symptoms. This is especially the case for newborn infants in whom seizures are often overshadowed by symptoms of acute neurologic distress such as coma, massive hypotonia, and major autonomic disturbances. In such cases, paroxysmal manifestations are often limited to an acute episode in the first days or in the first weeks or months of life and thus do not fulfill the criteria for the diagnosis of epilepsy.

Table 19.1 Metabolic disorders of early infancy in which seizures are part of acute disease with neurologic and/or systemic manifestations.

- Organic acidemias (leucinosis, isovaleric acidemia, propionic and methylmalonic acidemias, β-ketothiolase deficiency): usually acute neonatal distress and sepsis-like features.
- Urea cycle disorders: seizures usually after a few days probably related to development of brain edema.
- Pyruvate dehydrogenase, pyruvate carboxylase deficiency: seizures may persist and be due to prenatal brain damage.
- Nonketotic hyperglycinemia: erratic myoclonus and partial seizures in the first days of life; burst-suppression EEG.
- Molybdenum cofactor and sulfite oxidase deficiency: severe neonatal encephalopathy, multiple seizure types, burst-suppression EEG.
- Glutaric acidemia type 1: postnatal onset; acute encephalopathy with dystonia and partial seizures, often recurrent with infections.
- Hypoglycemia with several disorders of carbohydrate metabolism (fructose-1,6-diphosphatase deficiency, galactosemia, disorders of fatty acid oxidation).

Nevertheless, in some infants, the seizures may continue after the acute episode either because of the persistence of the metabolic disturbance or because of structural lesions resulting from the consequences of abnormal metabolism (e.g. the brain malformations due to pyruvate dehydrogenase deficiency).

The main disorders of this group are listed in Table 19.1. Many of the seizures observed at this age are partial, probably because the immaturity of the neonatal brain rarely allows for the organization of generalized seizures (Aicardi 1994). When the attacks persist, they are often replaced by other types of seizures (e.g. infantile spasms). Epileptic phenomena are particularly prominent in some disorders of this first group.

In *glycine encephalopathy* (nonketotic hyperglycinemia), erratic myoclonus is usually intense and partial seizures with localized discharges of rapid spikes occur on a background of suppression-burst tracing (Seppalainen and Simila 1971). When affected infants survive the first weeks of life, infantile spasms usually appear but partial seizures may also persist (Dalla Bernardina *et al* 1979).

Molybdenum cofactor deficiency is also highly epileptogenic and partial seizures may persist after the neonatal period (Slot *et al* 1993; Van Gennip *et al* 1994).

Glutaric acidemia type 1 presents at a few months of age as an acute encephalitic illness often with unilateral or partial seizures followed by a dystonic syndrome (Hoffmann *et al* 1991, 1996). Correct diagnosis can allow the avoidance of recurrences with a low-protein diet and the administration of carnitine (Hoffmann *et al* 1996).

DISORDERS WITH PREDOMINANT EPILEPTIC MANIFESTATIONS

The second group of metabolic disorders is characterized by the occurrence of repeated epileptic phenomena in a more or less chronic manner, thus corresponding to the definition of epilepsy. The epilepsy may be variably prominent and severe and appear as early as the neonatal period or as late as adolescence or adulthood. Many of the disorders of this group feature neurologic, behavioral, or cognitive abnormalities in addition to seizures (Table 19.2). In some diseases, however, epileptic attacks may be the initial symptom, sometimes for prolonged periods, thus raising a difficult diagnostic problem as these conditions are vastly less common than other causes of epilepsy yet must be recognized, especially as an effective therapy is available for some (e.g., pyridoxine dependency, some cases of biotinidase deficiency, or some mitochondrial diseases). Some of the major features of these disorders are listed in Table 19.2 and more detail is given here for some of them.

Pyridoxine dependency

Pyridoxine dependency (Haenggeli *et al* 1991; Baxter *et al* 1996; Aicardi 1999) is a rare disorder that results from a biochemical defect involving glutamic acid decarboxylase (Gordon 1997), thus reducing brain synthesis and content of γ-aminobutyric acid (GABA), a major inhibitory neurotransmitter. Typically, the disease manifests by repeated neonatal seizures resistant to antiepileptic agents (Haenggeli *et al* 1991).

These seizures are associated with marked irritability, vomiting, hypotonia, and depressed vigilance, thus wrongly suggesting the diagnosis of hypoxic–ischemic encephalopathy. Abdominal distension can wrongly lead to the diagnosis of a surgical condition (Baxter *et al* 1996). In rare cases, seizures appear only weeks or even months after birth. They often present as episodes of unilateral or focal status epilepticus (Goutières and Aicardi 1985), although other types such as infantile spasms may occur. Such seizures may sometimes respond to conventional antiepileptic drugs; although they ultimately recur, this may be only after weeks

Table 19.2 Main metabolic and degenerative disorders with recurrent seizures as a prominent feature.

Disease	Age at onset	Type of seizures	Associated features	EEG	Treatment
Krabbe disease	<6 months	G, Myo, P	Neurologic	Multifocal S	NA
Menkes disease	< 6 months	Myo, IS, P	Neurologic, systemic	Multifocal S	Symptomatic[1]
Hyperphenylalaninemias	0–12 months	IS, G, P	Neurologic	Hypsarrhythmia Multifocal	Dietary, biopterin
Peroxisomal diseases					
Early, recessive	0–12 months	P, G	Neurologic, systemic, dysmorphic	Multifocal S	NA
X-linked		P, G	Neurologic, systemic	Focal or multifocal S	Dietary, bone marrow Transplantation
Biotin disorders					
Holocarboxylase deficiency	0–3 months	G, Myo, P	May be isolated	Suppression burst, multifocal	Biotin
Biotinidase deficiency	3–12 months	G, P	Neurologic and systemic, cutaneous	Focal or multifocal	Biotin
Pyridoxine dependency	0–18 months	P, G, IS, Myo	Often isolated neurologic	SW, multifocal	Pyridoxine
Glucose transporter protein deficiency	1–4 mo	P, G, Myo	Often isolated at onset	Bilateral SW, multifocal	Ketogenic diet
Mitochondrial diseases					
Leigh	>3 months	P, G, IS, more with PDH deficiency	Neurologic	Focal, multifocal	Thiamin, riboflavin, coenzyme Q
MERFF	>4–5 years	Myo, G, P	Neurologic	Bilateral SW, multifocal	Symptomatic
MELAS	>4–5 years	P, G, Myo	Neurologic, systemic	Focal, multifocal, SW	Symptomatic
Alpers' disease	6 month–2 years	P, G, multifocal myoclonus	Neurologic, liver (late)	Small posterior S, multifocal	Symptomatic
Ceroid-lipofuscinoses	6 months–15+ years, depending on type	Myo, G, P	Neurologic	Variable with type	Symptomatic
Carbohydrate-deficient glycoprotein syndromes	<2–3 years	P, G, IS	Neurologic, systemic	Focal, multifocal	Symptomatic

G, generalized; IS, infantile spasms; Myo, myoclonic; P, partial; S, spikes; PDH, pyruvate dehydrogenase; SW, spike–waves; NA, not available.
[1] Copper salts may be partly effective.

or months rather than after the classical 5–10 day period. EEG shows intense paroxysmal activity that disappears – in most cases – upon intravenous administration of 50–150 mg of pyridoxine. Control of clinical seizures is immediate and can be maintained by repetition, probably for a lifetime, of maintenance doses. Cases are often missed because pyridoxine is not thought of and also, especially with status, because it is given after several other drugs, rendering its efficacy difficult to judge. It is thus useful to administer pyridoxine before long-lasting agents. The maintenance dose is not yet defined. It is desirable to obtain a normal GABA level in CSF, but a high glutamate level may still persist and larger doses may be necessary to lower it, although the significance of glutamate levels is still unclear (Baumeister *et al* 1994).

Disorders of biotin metabolism

Disorders of biotin metabolism can be due to a deficiency of holocarboxylase or of biotinidase (Wolff 1995; Garcia-Alvarez *et al* 1998). In the first case, the onset is usually perinatal, whereas it is later in the second. In most cases, neurologic signs such as lethargy and hypotonia and cutaneomucous signs (rashes, alopecia, conjunctivitis) are suggestive, but refractory seizures (partial, generalized, or myoclonic) may be the sole manifestation. Accordingly, systematic administration of biotin should be performed in all convulsive disorders of unknown cause. Administration of biotin does not prevent the biochemical diagnosis of the condition.

Glucose transporter protein deficiency

This is a recently recognized metabolic disease resulting from absence of the GLUT1 protein that actively transports glucose from blood to CSF. Repeated seizures usually appearing at 1–3 months of age are the initial feature; they may be myoclonic or generalized but also partial. Later, microcephaly and neurologic signs may develop. Blood glucose is normal, thus justifying CSF examination despite the rarity of the condition, in the face of refractory, unexplained seizures. The ketogenic diet may permit control of the seizures and normal development (De Vivo *et al* 1991).

Mitochondrial and peroxisomal disorders

Some mitochondrial disorders may also present as isolated seizure disorders. Myoclonic epilepsy with ragged red fibers (MERRF) usually has its onset after 5 years of age, with epilepsy usually with myoclonic seizures (Di Mauro and Moraes 1993; Hirano and Di Mauro 1998). However, partial seizures may be associated. Most patients have growth retardation and deafness is common but may be absent for long periods. EEG usually shows bilateral spike and wave abnormalities rather than focal paroxysms. Mitochondrial encephalomyopathy with lactic acidosis and strokelike episodes (MELAS) causes focal seizures, often of occipital or posterior temporal origin. Partial continuous epilepsy is not infrequently observed (Chevrie *et al* 1987), but generalized attacks and myoclonic seizures are also common. Epilepsy is present in 100% of the cases of MERRF and in 96% of those of MELAS (Hirano and Di Mauro 1998) and is often resistant to drug therapy. The diagnosis of MELAS rests on other clinical features (headaches, vomiting, growth retardation), imaging features (calcification of basal ganglia, strokelike cortical enhancement, or abnormal MR signals), and the lactic acidosis and neurologic features.

Epilepsy is a prominent manifestation of Alpers' disease, which is probably a mitochondrial disease at least in some cases. Seizures are often focal, but myoclonic attacks are also common. The occurrence of prolonged episodes of multifocal myoclonus simulating status epilepticus in children of 1–2 years is highly suggestive (Harding 1990). The presence of focal occipital small spikes has been considered an important diagnostic clue (Aicardi 1998b).

Epilepsy is frequent with peroxisomal disorders. In the most common neonatal forms with absence of detectable peroxisomes (Zellweger syndrome and neonatal adrenoleukodystrophy), seizures occur early, in the neonatal period or the first months of life. They may be partial or present as myoclonic attacks, generalized seizures, or infantile spasms. They are due to the presence of brain migration disorders, especially polymicrogyria (Evrard *et al* 1978). Seizures are uncommon in infantile Refsum disease (Moser *et al* 1993). In classical X-linked adrenoleukodystrophy, seizures, especially partial in type and sometimes severe or repeated in status, may be an early and even a revealing feature, although they are absent in a majority of cases (Mosser *et al* 1995).

Other disorders

Many other degenerative disorders are associated with epilepsy that may include partial seizures. The early types of ceroid-lipofuscinosis occur in infants (early infantile form). The late-infantile forms usually have their onset before 4 years of age. Myoclonic seizures are more frequently seen than partial seizures. The same applies to most progressive myoclonic epilepsies, which include Unverricht–Lundborg disease, type II Gaucher disease, Lafora disease, and other rare disorders that usually manifest only in late childhood and adolescence (Berkovic *et al* 1993; Aicardi 1998b).

EPILEPSY AND ACQUIRED BRAIN DAMAGE

Any acquired brain lesion can be responsible for epilepsy, although the mechanisms whereby a lesion becomes epileptogenic are still imperfectly understood (Aicardi 1980, 1998b). Most destructive lesions are relatively fixed once constituted, but some modifications may occur as a consequence of scarring processes, vascular factors, and epileptic attacks. Acquired factors alone can be responsible for the development of epilepsy. However, genetic factors probably contribute to epileptogenesis and many partial epilepsies are clearly of multifactorial origin (Andermann 1982). First-degree relatives of patients with lesional epilepsy are at increased risk of seizures (Andermann 1982; Berkovic 1998). In one study of children with both epilepsy and cerebral palsy, the risk for epilepsy in relatives was over 7% as opposed to 0.5% in the controls (Curatolo *et al* 1995).

Only the most important causes of lesional epilepsy will be reviewed briefly. For convenience, prenatal, perinatal, and postnatal causes are considered successively, although the distinction may be very difficult and is, to some extent, artificial.

ACQUIRED PRENATAL CAUSES

Acquired causes in the prenatal period may be difficult or even impossible to separate from brain malformations. Indeed, the separation may be somewhat arbitrary: for example, cytomegalovirus infection may cause both necrotic lesions and migration disorders (Barkovich and Lindan 1994), and schizencephaly can probably result both from genetic factors such as mutations in the *EMX2* homeobox gene (Brunelli *et al* 1996; Granata *et al* 1996, 1997) and from vascular factors (Aicardi 1998a).

Cytomegalovirus infection can be responsible for partial epilepsy as well as other types of seizures such as infantile spasms, and this also applies to toxoplasmosis, herpes, and other intrauterine infections.

Circulatory and vascular causes are a frequent cause of acquired prenatal damage resulting in partial epilepsy usually associated with other clinical manifestations. Most lesions of this type are ischemic in nature, resulting either from vascular obstruction, i.e. prenatal stroke (Baumann *et al* 1987; Amato *et al* 1991) or from more generalized vascular insufficiency with diffuse damage or more localized

involvement of border territories (Aicardi 1998a). In fetuses between 28 and 34 weeks gestational age, white-matter lesions, especially periventricular leukomalacias, are predominant and are not usually epileptogenic. In older fetuses, involvement of the gray matter tends to be more severe and is often responsible for epilepsy and cognitive difficulties.

Ischemic lesions may also take the form of porencephaly or schizencephaly. Schizencephaly is probably the result of an early ischemic accident that occurred before the end of neuronal migration and interfered with its completion. Porencephaly is probably of late occurrence after the end of cortical development. Multiple lesions such as multicystic encephalomalacia or hydranencephaly are usually due to late ischemia and occur at the end of gestation. All these lesions are highly epileptogenic and produce focal or multifocal seizures and epileptic EEG paroxysms.

Hemorrhagic lesions are less frequent in the prenatal period (Govaert and De Vries 1997). They may occur as a result of coagulation disorders in the mother, such as thrombopenic purpura producing intraparenchymal lesions of high epileptogenic potential (Burrows and Kelton 1993). Recent work suggests that some of the MR images found postnatally in children with cerebral palsy, especially focal ventricular dilatation, might be the result of prenatal intraventricular hemorrhages and that these lesions may generate focal epilepsy (Krägeloh-Mann *et al* 1995; Aicardi 1998a).

ACQUIRED PERINATAL CAUSES

Perinatal causes of epilepsy are probably less common than prenatal disorders (Nelson and Ellenberg 1986). There is evidence that perinatal adverse events are particularly noxious to the infant's brain when they have been preceded by prenatal abnormalities or supervene on a fragile brain such as that of a preterm neonate (Gaffney *et al* 1994).

Neonatal hypoxic–ischemic encephalopathy is a classical cause of early seizures. There is no doubt that it may result in seizures in the neonatal period (Aicardi 1998b), but these tend to be transient and do not represent 'true' epilepsy. In addition, at least some of these neonatal convulsions are not epileptic in mechanism but may rather represent abnormal nonepileptic movements (Mizrahi and Kellaway 1987). Late seizures following neonatal encephalopathies do occur and may include partial attacks, although infantile spasms are a more common manifestation (Aicardi 1998b). Seizures unassociated with neurologic signs in children who presented signs and symptoms suggestive of hypoxi–ischemic encephalopathy at birth are seldom if ever attributable to the perinatal difficulties.

The most common ischemic lesion in preterm infants is periventricular leukomalacia, usually a lesion of infants born between 28 and 34 weeks and apparently developing during the first days of life. Isolated periventricular leukomalacias are only seldom the cause of later epilepsy.

The situation is different with *hemorrhagic lesions* especially periventricular and intraventricular hemorrhage, a lesion that electively affects preterm infants. A recent study (Amess *et al* 1998) showed that the frequency of epilepsy in very premature preterm infants in whom imaging demonstrated the presence of *hemorrhagic parenchymal infarction*, appearing as markedly increased echodensities within the brain parenchyma extending from the ventricular margin, was much higher than in those with nonhemorrhagic cystic periventricular leukomalacia. The prevalence of epilepsy was 4.3% in such children as against 0% in those with periventricular leukomalacia only. Other perinatal causes such as neonatal CNS infections, neonatal stroke (Bouza *et al* 1994), and venous thrombosis are less commonly encountered.

ACQUIRED POSTNATAL CAUSES

Among the multiple causes of acquired epileptogenic lesions, trauma and infectious diseases deserve a special mention.

Posttraumatic epilepsy is treated in Chapter 14. Suffice it to say that nonaccidental trauma is of special importance in infants and should always be thought of when seizures are associated with intracranial hematoma or cutaneous or eye lesions (Brown and Minns 1993).

Meningitis and encephalitis are common causes of residual epilepsy usually severe and often focal (Marks *et al* 1992).

An unusual but interesting cause is *gluten enteropathy* with intracranial calcification, which can give rise to partial seizures, especially of occipital origin (Gobbi *et al* 1992). The mechanism of the epilepsy is not understood. Calcification is an important diagnostic clue, but diagnosis may be difficult and may require intestinal biopsy.

Postepileptic damage has long been known to occur following status epilepticus (Aicardi and Chevrie 1983). A special type known as hemiconvulsion–hemiplegia–epilepsy syndrome (HHE syndrome) or 'acquired postconvulsive hemiplegia' (Aicardi *et al* 1969) features a long-lasting unilateral, most often clonic, seizure followed by the persistence of hemiplegia, initially flaccid and evolving to spasticity. Partial epilepsy appears after a variable interval (months or years) and is often partial complex in type (mostly of temporal but also of other origins) and refractory to drug therapy. However, other seizures may occur; they

usually belong to those types associated with brain damage, e.g. atypical absences, tonic and astatic seizures, or secondarily generalized seizures, and are probably the expression of diffusion from a focus or from multifocal lesions. Many of these cases are observed in the course of febrile illnesses and there is no doubt that both the seizures and the hemiplegia are often due to a primary brain disease such as meningitis, encephalitis, or vascular disorder (Roger *et al* 1974). However, it appears that hemiplegia and attendant brain damage can be the direct result of the epileptic activity itself, even though the mechanisms remain unclear. The frequency of this syndrome has declined dramatically since the 1970s (Roger *et al* 1982), which suggests that improved emergency treatment of status may have been responsible. In fact, the initial convulsion was often of very long duration and the syndrome is now mainly seen in countries where emergency care is not readily available. The resulting atrophy is remarkable by its diffuse distribution in one hemisphere without any suggestion of vascular distribution. One may speculate that acquired *hippocampal sclerosis* might be a 'modern' form of the HHE syndrome in which damage is localized to the most fragile structures because the reduced duration of status, especially with febrile convulsions, has limited the extent of damage. Long-lasting convulsions are a frequent antecedent of hippocampal sclerosis and there was a good correlation between lateralization of the initial long attack and the side of later partial epilepsy focus (Aicardi and Chevrie 1976). More recent work has shown that atrophy of one hippocampus may appear as a sequel of long febrile seizures (Kuks *et al* 1993, Van Landingham *et al* 1998). Although it must remain speculative, this mechanism clearly deserves further study. A related and no less controversial issue is that of the emergence of increasing damage in a previous epileptogenic focus as a result of its epileptic activity and that of the creation of secondary foci as a result of epileptic 'bombardment' from a distant focus. There is currently no decisive argument in this respect and it will not be considered further.

CLINICAL MANIFESTATIONS OF EPILEPSY DUE TO ACQUIRED BRAIN DAMAGE

Epilepsy from acquired brain lesions is often focal in nature, with or without secondary generalization. However, it can determine virtually any type of epilepsy, including myoclonus, positive or negative, infantile spasms, and rare syndromes such as continuous spike–waves of slow sleep (Guerrini *et al* 1996b).

Lesional epilepsy can remain isolated without any accompanying cognitive behavioral or neurologic abnormality. In such cases, the diagnosis of an epileptogenic lesion, whether acquired or prenatal such as cortical dysplasia, may be very difficult and may require the best methods of imaging for their detection. For this reason, MR imaging is mandatory for all cases that do not rigorously fulfill the criteria for precise idiopathic epilepsy syndromes.

Epilepsies due to structural brain damage often have an early onset and feature several types of seizure (Aicardi 1998b). Some seizure types, e.g. complex partial seizures, atonic attacks, or startle seizures, are usually due to fixed brain lesions. Resistance to treatment should also lead to suspicion of a lesion, but is by no means constant or necessary for diagnosis. Huttenlocher and Hapke (1990) followed 155 children with refractory epilepsy not due to progressive CNS disorder or tuberous sclerosis, 145 of whom were not operated on. Mild to moderate mental retardation was found in 61%, and 39% were of normal intelligence. Among the latter patients, seizure control was found to increase by 4% yearly starting about 4 years after onset of epilepsy and only one-quarter of those followed up for 18 years or more continued to have seizures (usually with drug treatment). Even in mentally retarded patients, 1.5% achieved control during each year of follow-up, but 70% still had seizures after 18 years. Similarly, Goulden et al (1991) found that 13 of 33 children with mental retardation and cerebral palsy achieved remission of their epilepsy. Cases of apparently 'benign' epilepsy syndromes have been reported in association with brain lesions and can either be coincidental or represent an unusual epileptic manifestation of a lesion (Santanelli et al 1989).

In many cases, lesional epilepsies are associated with neurologic signs and/or mental retardation or learning difficulties.

Cerebral palsy is the most common type of neurologic abnormality associated with epilepsy. The term designates 'a disorder of posture and movement due to a static lesion of the developing brain' (Aksu 1990). Some authors exclude lesions acquired after the age of 4 weeks and brain malformations (Goulden et al 1991), but these are usually included.

The frequency of epilepsy varies between 15% and 60% of patients with cerebral palsy (Aksu 1990; Hadjipanayis et al 1997; Stephenson 1998) but is very different with the type. It was present in 50% of children with quadriplegia and 47% of those with hemiplegia, but only in 27% of those with spastic diplegia in one study (Hadjipanayis et al 1997). The incidence of epilepsy in ex-prematures with diplegia was as low as 11% in one series (Amess et al 1998), probably because of the predominance of deep white-matter lesions in such cases. All types of seizures may occur, but partial motor attacks are most common in children with

hemiplegia (73%), whereas generalized seizures predominate in dystonic or quadriplegic cerebral palsy, with only 25% with partial seizures. Infantile spasms were observed in more than 15% of patients (Hadjipanayis et al 1997). Startle epilepsy is mainly observed in children with congenital hemiparesis (Chauvel et al 1987), although it has been reported in patients without previous motor dysfunction (Manford et al 1996). Long hemiclonic seizures may be relatively common (Gastaut et al 1960). Seizure onset is usually in the first year of life in children with quadriplegia but at an average age of 4–5 years in those with hemiplegia. In one series (Hadjipanayis et al 1997), 50% of cases had their onset before 2 years of age.

The course of epilepsy in patients with cerebral palsy is rather severe. In one study (Delgado et al 1996), only 69 of 531 children (12.9%) with both cerebral palsy and epilepsy achieved a remission of 2 years or more. However, almost 60% of those in remission had no relapse following discontinuation of treatment. In other series, the remission rate reached 30–40% (Stephenson 1998) but this result was sometimes obtained only after many years. Epilepsy tends to be more severe in patients with extensive motor involvement and in those with mental retardation. Epilepsy is two to five times more common in children with cerebral palsy with mental retardation than in those without (Hadjipanayis et al 1997).

In a number of children with epilepsy, the neurologic signs do not result in motor or muscular tone abnormalities of a sufficient degree to warrant the diagnosis of cerebral palsy, e.g. microcephaly, ocular motor difficulties, mild ataxia, sensory deficits, clumsiness, or minor movement abnormalities. In some of these patients, the neurologic anomalies may help to localize the origin of partial seizures and/or orientate further investigations. Although such cases have not been studied in detail, the outcome of associated epilepsy seems rather similar to that of cerebral palsy.

Mental retardation and/or learning difficulties often coexist with neurologic signs in children with epilepsy. All degrees of defect are possible, from profound mental retardation to mild specific problems. The presence of mental retardation is clearly an indicator of severity of the associated epilepsy (see above).

In general, epilepsy is an indicator of severity in patients with cerebral palsy and/or mental retardation. Mental retardation was observed in 70% of children with congenital hemiplegia and epilepsy as opposed to 28% of those without epilepsy (Guerrini et al 1998). This is likely to reflect the greater extent of damage. However, in patients with hemiplegia, the presence of epilepsy is associated with greater cognitive and language difficulties, even when only lesions of similar extent are compared (Vargha-Khadem et *al* 1992), thus indicating that epilepsy per se has a noxious influence on brain development and function. This, in turn, would favor early surgical treatment of epileptogenic lesions, the more so as the combination of epilepsy with other impairments has a multiplicative rather than simply additive effect on overall disability.

CONCLUSION

Epilepsy is a frequent but nonspecific manifestation of a very wide spectrum of neurologic and/or general disorders. It may be an early and important diagnostic cue in those diseases in which it is the first symptom, as may be the case with metabolic or degenerative diseases such as biotin deficiency, some cases of adrenoleukodystrophy, or in Alpers' disease. Epilepsy may also be highly significant as far as the prognosis is concerned, especially in cases of nonprogressive brain damage in which it usually indicates a greater severity of the basic lesion and may contribute to make it even more severe through the induction of additional, postepileptic damage.

Epilepsy always requires vigorous therapy, even when it is only a relatively secondary part of the patient's problem, e.g. in degenerative conditions, as it tends to multiply disability and has a major impact on the quality of patients' lives.

KEY POINTS

1. Intractable epilepsy may occur in association with a wide variety of nonvascular disorders presenting in early childhood and not covered in other chapters. An incidence of epilepsy of up to 60% has been reported in cerebral palsy, defined as a disorder of posture and movement due to a static lesion of the developing brain.
2. Intractable epilepsy in children can be due to chromosomal abnormalities including trisomy 21 (Down syndrome), fragile X syndrome, Angelman syndrome, Miller-Dieker syndrome, and partial monosomy 4p (Wolf-Hirschhorn syndrome). It may also be due to multiple brain malformations or metabolic and degenerative disorders.
3. Acquired nonvascular causes of intractable epilepsy in children, not covered in other chapters, include intrauterine infection (e.g. cytomegalovirus), head trauma, postnatal intracranial infection, brain damage consequent upon status epilepticus however caused, and gluten enteropathy with occipital calcification.

REFERENCES

Aicardi J (1980) Epilepsy in brain-injured children. A review. *Developmental Medicine and Child Neurology* **32**:191–202.

Aicardi J (1994) *Epilepsy in Children*, 2nd edn. pp 217–243. New York: Raven Press.

Aicardi J (1998a) Fetal circulatory and vascular disorders. *Diseases of the Nervous System in Childhood*, 2nd edn. pp 12–19. London: Mack Keith Press.

Aicardi J (1998b) *Diseases of the Nervous System in Childhood*, 2nd edn, pp 3–31. London: Mack Keith Press.

Aicardi J (1999) Pyridoxine-responsive seizures. In: Kotagal P (ed) *The Epilepsies* pp 448-448. San Diego: Academic Press.

Aicardi J, Chevrie JJ (1976) Febrile convulsions: neurological sequelae and mental retardation. In: Brasier MA, Coceani F (eds) *Brain Dysfunction in Infantile Febrile Convulsions*, pp 247–257. New York: Raven Press.

Aicardi J, Chevrie JJ (1983) Consequences of status epilepticus in infants and children. *Advances in Neurology* **34**:115–125.

Aicardi J, Amsili J, Chevrie JJ (1969) Acute hemiplegia in infancy and childhood. *Developmental Medicine and Child Neurology* **11**:162–173.

Aksu F (1990) Nature and prognosis of seizures in patients with cerebral palsy. *Developmental Medicine and Child Neurology* **32**:661–668.

Amato M, Hüppi P, Herschkowitz N, Huber P (1991) Prenatal stroke suggested by intrauterine ultrasound and confirmed by magnetic resonance imaging. *Neuropediatrics* **22**:100–102.

Amess PN, Baudin J, Townsend J *et al* (1998) Epilepsy in very preterm infants: neonatal cranial ultrasound reveals a high-risk subcategory. *Developmental Medicine and Child Neurology* **40**:724–730.

Andermann E (1982) Multifactorial inheritance of generalized and focal epilepsy. In: Anderson VE, Hauser WA, Penry JK, Singh CF (eds) *Genetic Basis of the Epilepsies*, pp 355–374. New York. Raven Press.

Barkovich AJ, Lindan CE (1994) Congenital cytomegalovirus infection of the brain: imaging analysis and embryologic considerations. *American Journal of Neuroradiology* **15**:703–715.

Baumann RJ, Carr WA, Shuman RM (1987) Patterns of cerebral arterial injury in children with neurological disabilities. *Journal of Child Neurology* **2**:298–306.

Baumeister EAM, Gsell W, Shin YS, Egger J (1994) Glutamate in pyridoxine-dependent epilepsy: neurotoxic glutamate concentration in the cerebrospinal fluid and its normalization with pyridoxine. *Pediatrics* **94**:318–321.

Baxter P, Griffiths, Kelly T, Gardner-Medwin D (1996) Pyridoxine-dependent seizures: demographic, clinical, MRI and psychometric features and effect of dose on intelligence quotient. *Developmental Medicine and Child Neurology* **38**:998–1006.

Berkovic SF (1998) Genetics of epilepsy syndromes. In: Engel J Jr, Pedley TA (eds) *Epilepsy: A Comprehensive Textbook*, pp 25–37. Philadelphia: Lippincott- Raven.

Berkovic S, Cochius J, Andermann E, Andermann F (1993) Progressive myoclonus epilepsies: clinical and genetic aspects. *Epilepsia* **34** (suppl 3) S19–S30.

Bourgeois M, Sainte-Rose C, Maixner W *et al* (1999) Epilepsy in children with shunted hydrocephalus. *Journal of Neurosurgery*, **90**.

Bouza H, Dubowitz LMS, Rutherford M *et al* (1994) Late magnetic resonance imaging and clinical findings in neonates with unilateral lesions on neonatal ultrasounds. *Developmental Medicine and Child Neurology* **36**:951–964.

Brown JK, Minns RA (1993) Non-accidental head injury with particular reference to whiplash shaking injury and medicolegal aspects. *Developmental Medicine and Child Neurology* **35**:849–869.

Brunelli S, Faiella A, Capra V *et al* (1996) Germline mutations in the homeobox gene *EMX2* in patients with severe schizencephaly. *Nature Genetics* **12**:94–96.

Burrows RE, Kelton JG (1993) Fetal thrombocytopenia and its relation to maternal thrombocytopenia. *New England Journal of Medicine* **329**:1463–1466.

Canevini MP, Sgro V, Zuffardi O *et al* (1998) Chromosome 20 ring: a chromosomal disorder associated with a particular electroclinical pattern. *Epilepsia* **39**:943–950.

Chauvel P, Vignal JP, Liegeois-Chauvel C *et al* (1987) Startle epilepsy with infantile brain damage: the clinical and neurophysiological rationale for surgical therapy. In: Wieser HG, Elger CE (eds) *Presurgical Evaluation of Epileptics*, pp 306–307. Berlin: Springer-Verlag.

Chevrie JJ, Aicardi J (1986) The Aicardi syndrome. In: Pedley TA, Meldrum BS (eds) *Recent Advances in Epilepsy*, vol 3, pp 189–210. Edinburgh: Churchill Livingstone.

Chevrie JJ, Aicardi J, Goutières F (1987) Epilepsy in childhood mitochondrial encephalomyopathies. In: Wolf P, Dam M, Janz D, Dreifuss F (eds) *Advances in Epileptology*, vol 16, pp 181–184. New York: Raven Press.

Curatolo P, Alpino C, Stazi MA, Medda E (1995) Risk factors for the co-occurrence of partial epilepsy, cerebral palsy and mental retardation. *Developmental Medicine and Child Neurology* **37**:776–782.

Dalla Bernardina B, Aicardi J, Goutières F, Plouin P (1979) Glycine encephalopathy. *Neuropaediatrie* **10**:209–225.

Delgado MR, Riela AR, Mills J *et al* (1996) Discontinuation of antiepileptic drug treatment after two seizure-free years in children with cerebral palsy. *Pediatrics* **97**:192–197.

De Vivo DC, Trifiletti RR, Jacobson RI *et al* (1991) Defective glucose transport across the blood-brain barrier as a cause of persistent hypoglycorrhachia, seizures and developmental delay. *New England Journal of Medicine* **325**:705–709.

Di Mauro S, Moraes CT (1993) Mitochondrial encephalomyopathies. *Archives of Neurology* **50**:1187–1208.

Di Rocco C, Ianelli A, Pallini R, Rinaldi A (1985) Epilepsy and its correlation with cerebral ventricular shunting procedures in infantile hydrocephalus. *Journal of Pediatric Neuroscience* **1**:255–263.

Elia M, Musumeci SA, Ferri R *et al* (1995) Trisomy 12p and epilepsy with myoclonic absences: a new case. *Epilepsia* **36** (suppl. 32): 52.

Evrard P, Prats-Vinas J, Lyon G (1978) The mechanism of arrests of neuronal migraiton in the Zellweger malformation and hypothesis based upon cytoarchitectonic analysis. *Acta Neuropathol*, 41, 109–117.

Gaffney G, Sellers S, Flavell V *et al* (1994) Case–control study of intra-partum care, cerebral palsy, and perinatal death. *British Medical Journal* **308**:743–750.

Garcia-Alvarez M, Nordli DR, De Vivo D (1998) Inherited metabolic disorders. In: Engel J Jr, Pedley TA (eds) *Epilepsy: A Comprehensive Textbook*, pp 2547–2562. Philadelphia: Lippincott-Raven.

Gastaut H, Poirier F, Payan *et al* (1960) HHE syndrome: hemiconvulsions-hemiplegia-epilepsy. *Epilepsia* **1**:418–447.

Gobbi G, Ambrosetto P, Zamboni MG *et al* (1992) Celiac disease, posterior cerebral calcification and epilepsy. *Brain Development* **14**:23–29.

Golden JA, Schoene WC (1993) Central nervous system malformations in trisomy 9. *Journal of Neuropathology and Experimental Neurology* **52**:71–77.

Gordon N (1997) Pyridoxine dependency: an update. *Developmental Medicine and Child Neurology* **39**:63–65.

Goulden KJ, Shinnar S, Koller H *et al* (1991) Epilepsy in children with mental retardation: a cohort study. *Epilepsia* **32**:690–697.

Goutières F, Aicardi J (1985) Atypical presentations of pyridoxine-dependent seizures: a treatable cause of intractable epilepsy. *Annals of Neurology* **17**:117–120.

Govaert P, De Vries LS (1997) *An Atlas of Neonatal Brain Sonography*. *Clinics in Developmental Medicine*, No. 141/142. London: Mac Keith Press.

Granata T, Battaglia G, D'Increti I *et al* (1996) Schizencephaly: neuroradiologic and epileptologic findings. *Epilepsia* **37**:1185–1193.

Granata T, Farina L, Fariella A *et al* (1997) Familial schizencephaly associated with EMX2 mutation. *Neurology* **48**:1403–1406.

Guerrini R, DeLorey TM, Bonanni P (1996a) Cortical myoclonus in Angelman syndrome. *Annals of Neurology* **40**:39–48.

Guerrini R, Parmeggiani A, Bureau M *et al* (1996b) Localized cortical dysplasia: good seizure outcome after sleep-related electrical status epilepticus. In: Guerrini R, Andermann F, Canapicchi *et al* (eds) *Dysplasias of the Cerebral Cortex and Epilepsy*, pp 329–335. New York: Lippincott-Raven.

Guerrini R, Gobbi G, Genton P, Bonanni P, Carrozzo R (1998) Chromosomal abnormalities. In: Engel J Jr, Pedley TA (eds) *Epilepsy: A Comprehensive Textbook*, vol. 3, pp 2533–2545. Philadelphia: Lippincott-Raven.

Hadjipanayis A, Hadjichristodoulou C, Youroukos S (1997) Epilepsy in patients with cerebral palsy. *Developmental Medicine and Child Neurology* **39**:659–663.

Haenggeli CA, Girardin E, Paunier L (1991) Pyridoxine-dependent seizures: clinical and therapeutic aspects. *European Journal of Pediatrics* **130**:452–455.

Harding BN (1990) Progressive neuronal degeneration of childhood with liver disease (Alpers–Huttenlocher syndrome). A personal view. *Journal of Child Neurology* **5**:273–287.

Hirano M, Di Mauro S (1998). Primary mitochondrial diseases. In: Engel J Jr, Pedley TA (eds) *Epilepsy: A Comprehensive Textbook*, vol 3. pp 2563–2570. Philadelphia: Lippincott-Raven.

Hoffmann GF, Trefz FK, Barth PG *et al* (1991) Glutaryl coenzyme A dehydrogenase deficiency: a distinct encephalopathy. *Pediatrics* **88**:1194–1203.

Hoffmann GF, Athanassopoulos S, Burlina AB *et al* (1996) Clinical course, early diagnosis, treatment and prevention of disease in glutaryl-CoA dehydrogenase deficiency. *Neuropediatrics* **27**:115–123.

Huttenlocher R, Hapke RJ (1990) A follow-up study of intractable seizures in childhood. *Annals of Neurology* **28**:699–705.

Inoue R, Fujiwara T, Matsuda *et al* (1997) Ring chromosome 20 and nonconvulsive status epilepticus. A new epileptic syndrome. *Brain* **120**:939–953.

Krägeloh-Mann I, Peterson D, Hagberg G *et al* (1995) Bilateral spastic cerebral palsy – MRI pathology and origin. Analysis of a representative series of 56 cases. *Developmental Medicine and Child Neurology* **37**:379–397.

Kuks JBM, Cook MJ, Fish DR *et al* (1993) Hippocampal sclerosis in epilepsy and childhood febrile seizures. *Lancet* **342**:1391–1394.

Manford M, Fish DR, Shorvon SD (1996) Startle-provoked epileptic seizures: features in 19 patients. *Journal of Neurology, Neurosurgery and Psychiatry* **61**:151–156.

Marks DA, Kim J, Spencer DD *et al* (1992) Characteristics of intractable seizures following meningitis and encephalitis. *Neurology* **42**:1513–1518.

Matsumoto A, Kumagai T, Miura K *et al* (1992) Epilepsy in Angelman syndrome associated with 15q deletion. *Epilepsia* **33**:1083–1090.

Menezes L, Aicardi J, Goutières F (1988) Absence of the septum pellucidum with porencephalia: a neuroradiologic syndrome with variable clinical expression. *Archives of Neurology* **45**:542–545.

Minassian BA, DeLorey TM, Olsen RW *et al* (1998) Angelman syndrome: correlations between epilepsy phenotypes and genotypes. *Annals of Neurology* **43**:485–493.

Mizrahi EM, Kellaway P (1987) Characterization and classification of neonatal seizures. *Neurology* **37**:1837–1844.

Moser AB, Rasmussen M, Naidu S *et al* (1993) Phenotype of patients with peroxisomal disorders subdivided into sixteen complementation groups. *Journal of Pediatrics* **127**:13–22.

Mosser HW, Smith KD, Moser AB (1995) X-linked adrenoleukodystrophy. In: Scriver CR, Beaudet AL, Sly W, Valle D (eds) *The Metabolic and Molecular Bases of Inherited Disease,* 7th edn, pp 2325–2349. New York: McGraw-Hill.

Musumeci SA, Ferri R, Elia M, Cologna RM, Bergonzi P, Tassinari CA (1991) Epilepsy and fragile X syndrome: a follow-up study. *American Journal of Medical Genetics* **38**:511–513.

Nance MA, Hauser WA, Anderson VE (1998) Genetic disease associated with epilepsy. In: Engel J Jr, Pedley TA (eds) *Epilepsy: A Comprehensive Textbook*, vol 1, pp 197–209. Philadelphia: Lippincott-Raven.

Nelson KB, Ellenberg JH (1986) Antecedents of cerebral palsy. Multivariate analysis of risks. *New England Journal of Medicine* **315**:81–86.

Pueschel SM, Louis S (1993) Reflex seizures in Down syndrome. *Child's Nervous System* **9**:23–24.

Roessler E, Belloni E, Gaudenz K *et al* (1996) Mutations in the human Sonic Hedgehog gene cause holoprosencephaly. *Nature Genetics* **14**:357–360.

Roger J, Lob H, Tassinari CA (1974) Status epilepticus. In: Vinken PJ, Bruyn GW (eds) *Handbook of Neurology*, vol 15, *The Epilepsies*, pp. 145–188. Amsterdam: North-Holland.

Roger J, Dravet C, Bureau M (1982) Unilateral seizures (hemiconvulsion-hemiplegia syndrome and hemiconvulsion-hemiplegia-epilepsy syndrome). *Electroencephalography and Clinical Neurophysiology* suppl.**35**:211–221.

Santanelli P, Bureau M, Magaudda A *et al* (1989) Benign partial epilepsy with centrotemporal (or rolandic) spikes and brain lesion. *Epilepsia* **30**:182–188.

Saukkonen AL, Serlo W, Von Wendt L (1990) Epilepsy in hydrocephalic children. *Acta Paediatrica Scandinavica* **79**:212–218.

Seppalainen AM, Simila S (1971) Electroencephalographic findings in three patients with nonketotic hyperglycinemia. *Epilepsia* **12**:101–107.

Sgro X, Riva E, Canevini MP *et al* (1995) 4p-Syndrome: a chromosomal disorder associated with a particular EEG pattern. *Epilepsia* **36**:1206–1214.

Silva MI, Cienta C, Guerrini R, Plouin P, Livet MO, Dulac O (1996) Early clinical and EEG features of infantile spasms in Down syndrome. *Epilepsia* **37**:977–982.

Slot HMJ, Overweg-Plandsoen WCG, Bakker HD *et al* (1993) Molybdenum-cofactor deficiency: an easily missed cause of neonatal convulsions. *Neuropediatrics* **24**:139–142.

Stafstrom CE, Patxot CE, Gilmore HE, Wisniewski KE (1991) Seizures in children with Down syndrome: etiology, characteristics and outcome. *Developmental Medicine and Child Neurology* **33**:191–200.

Stephenson JBP (1998) Cerebral palsy. In: Engel J Jr, Pedley TA (eds) *Epilepsy: A Comprehensive Textbook*, vol. 3, pp 2571–2577. Philadelphia: Lippincott-Raven.

Sztriha L, Varady E, Hertecaut J, Nork M (1998) Mediobasal and mantle defect of the prosencephalon: lobar holoprosencephaly, schizencephaly and diabetes insipidus. *Neuropediatrics* **29**:272–275.

Van Landingham KE, Heinz ER, Cavazos JE, Lewis DV (1998) Magnetic resonance imaging evidence of hippocampal injury after prolonged focal febrile convulsions. *Annals of Neurology* **43**:413–426.

Van Gennip AH, Abeling NGGM, Strommer AEM *et al* (1994) The detection of molybdenum-cofactor deficiency: clinical symptomatology and urinary metabolite profile. *Journal of Inherited Metabolic Disease* **17**:142–145.

Vargha-Khadem F, Isaacs E, van der Werf S *et al* (1992) Development of intelligence and memory in children with cerebral palsy. The deleterious consequences of early seizures. *Brain* **115**:315–329.

Viani F, Romeo A, Viri M *et al* (1995) Seizures and EEG patterns in Angelman's syndrome. *Journal of Child Neurology* **10**:467–471.

Watanabe K, Hara K, Iwane K (1976) The evolution of neurophysiological features in holoprosencephaly. *Neuropediatrics* **7**:19–41.

Wisniewski KE, Segan SM, Miejejeski EA, Sersen EA, Rudelli RD (1991) The Fra(X) syndrome: neurological, electrophysiological and neuropathological abnormalities. *American Journal of Medical Genetics* **38**:476–480.

Wolf B (1995) Disorders of biotin metabolism. In: Scriver CR, Beaudet AL, Sly WS, Valle D (eds) *The Metabolic and Molecular Bases of Inherited Disease* 7th edn, pp 3151–3177. New York: McGraw-Hill.

Idiopathic focal epilepsies of childhood

AS HARVEY

The idiopathic focal or partial epilepsies are defined by the International League Against Epilepsy (ILAE) revised classification of epilepsies and epileptic syndromes as seizure disorders manifest by partial seizures in which there is no underlying cause other than a possible hereditary predisposition (Commission on Classification and Terminology of the International League Against Epilepsy 1989). Idiopathic focal epilepsies account for approximately one-quarter of childhood seizure disorders and as a group share the following features: age-dependent onset of partial seizures, absence of neurologic and psychologic deficits, stereotyped focal epileptiform patterns on interictal EEG, normal neuroimaging, frequent family history of seizures, and excellent prognosis with seizures remitting spontaneously in later childhood or adolescence.

The ILAE classification recognizes three specific syndromes of idiopathic focal epilepsy, namely benign childhood epilepsy with centrotemporal spikes (benign rolandic epilepsy), childhood epilepsy with occipital paroxysms (benign occipital epilepsy), and primary reading epilepsy (Commission on Classification and Terminology of the International League Against Epilepsy, 1989). The word 'benign' implies that the seizures are usually brief, infrequent, and uncomplicated, and that there is an excellent prognosis for seizure remission and neurologic development. However, some atypical forms of idiopathic focal epilepsy do not conform to this use of the word benign (Duchowny and Harvey 1996).

The spectrum of idiopathic focal epilepsy in childhood has been broadened in recent years with the recognition of atypical varieties of benign rolandic epilepsy, the delineation of several types of idiopathic occipital epilepsy, and the description of several familial syndromes of partial epilepsy in infants, children, and adults.

BENIGN FOCAL EPILEPSY OF CHILDHOOD WITH CENTROTEMPORAL SPIKES

Benign focal epilepsy of childhood with centrotemporal spikes (BFEC-CTS) or benign rolandic epilepsy is the most common epilepsy syndrome in childhood (Sidenvall et al 1993), representing 10–25% of childhood epilepsies between 5 and 15 years of age and three-quarters of the idiopathic focal epilepsies of childhood (Loiseau and Duché 1989; Panayiotopoulos 1993). BFEC-CTS occurs with a slightly greater incidence in boys, with onset between 3 and 13 years of age (peak 9 years). Seizures in BFEC-CTS have highly characteristic orofaciobrachial manifestations (Beaussart 1972; Loiseau and Beaussart 1973; Beaumanoir et al

1974). Seizures manifest as either simple partial attacks with sensorimotor symptoms involving the mouth, tongue, and face, with or without arm involvement, or as hemiconvulsive or secondarily generalized seizures (25%) with impairment of consciousness. Sialorrhea and anarthria are common ictal manifestations. Seizures characteristically (>75%) occur on going to sleep or on waking from sleep. Seizures are usually brief in duration, rarely manifest with convulsive status, but may be associated with postictal hemiparesis or speech disturbance (Beaussart 1972; Loiseau and Beaussart 1973; Beaumanoir *et al* 1974).

The interictal EEG (Figs 20.1 and 20.2) shows a stereotypic focal epileptiform pattern, with monomorphic, sharp, and sharp–slow wave discharges in the centrotemporal

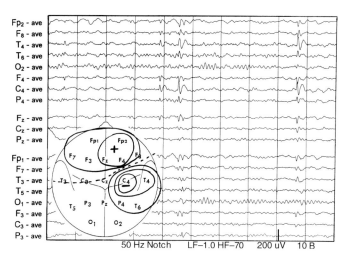

Fig. 20.2 Interictal awake EEG (average reference montage) of a 9-year-old boy with benign focal epilepsy of childhood with centrotemporal spikes. A tangential dipole is apparent with high-amplitude negative sharp waves in the right central and temporal regions and synchronous low-amplitude positive sharp waves in the frontal regions.

regions on one (70%) or both (30%) sides (Beaussart 1972; Loiseau and Beaussart 1973; Beaumanoir *et al* 1974). Bilateral discharges are usually independent, although delayed corticocortical conduction to the contralateral midtemporal electrode may be seen. Some authors stress that the broad sharp–slow morphology, rather than the precise location of discharges, is more important in diagnosing BFEC-CTS (Drury and Beydoun 1991; Frost *et al* 1992). The maximal field of the negative sharp wave is usually in the mid central (C3, C4) or low central (C5, C6) region, the latter often giving the impression of a midtemporal focus when extra electrodes are not employed (Legarda *et al* 1994). A tangential dipole is invariably present, with diffuse low-amplitude positivity recorded synchronously over the frontal regions, best seen on referential recordings (Gregory and Wong 1984, 1992). Discharges with a similar morphology are sometimes recorded at the vertex, across the sylvian fissure, and in the occipital region, and about 10% of patients have additional generalized spike–wave discharges. Drowsiness and slow-wave sleep cause dramatic activation of epileptiform activity, often unmasking the contralateral focus and sometimes leading to periods of continuous focal epileptiform activity. In fact, the sleep activation and dipolar field of bilateral CTS may give the appearance of generalized electrical status in sleep. Ictal recordings are rare but when captured show unilateral or bilateral central sharp–slow or fast activity, with polarity reversal of the tangential dipole (Gutierrez *et al* 1990; Harvey *et al* 1995). Thus, the clinical and EEG features of BFEC-CTS suggest a focus in the low central (rolandic) fissure. Brain imaging in typical BFEC-CTS does not reveal causative lesions.

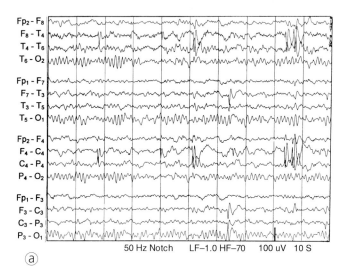

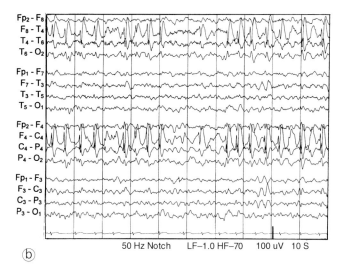

Fig. 20.1 Interictal EEG (longitudinal bipolar montage) of a 7-year-old boy with benign focal epilepsy of childhood with centrotemporal spikes. The awake EEG (a) shows independent left and right centrotemporal spikes. The asleep EEG (b) shows continuous right centrotemporal spikes.

A family history of seizures is present in 20–30% of children and clinical genetic studies favor autosomal dominant inheritance with incomplete penetrance. The clinical course of typical BFEC-CTS is invariably excellent, with more than 95% children outgrowing seizures before their adult years (Bouma *et al* 1997), most before their teen years. The EEG normalizes in the teen years, following seizure remission. Most children have relatively few seizures (13–20% have only a single seizure) and treatment with antiepileptic medication is not always necessary. Those who are treated with medication usually respond to small doses of carbamazepine, often given as a nighttime dose, and can be considered for drug withdrawal after 12 months of seizure freedom. The benign nature of typical BFEC-CTS, with infrequent seizures and absence of neurologic and psychologic comorbidity, has prompted one author to substitute the phrase 'seizure susceptibility syndrome' for 'epilepsy' in order to avoid stigmatizing children (Panayiotopoulos 1993).

ATYPICAL MANIFESTATIONS OF BENIGN FOCAL EPILEPSY OF CHILDHOOD WITH CENTROTEMPORAL SPIKES

Given the prevalence of BFEC and CTS, it is not surprising that atypical seizure manifestations and associations are described.

A younger presentation with different ictal manifestations is described as 'atypical BFEC' (Aicardi and Chevrie 1982). These children present between 2 and 6 years of age with atonic falls, atypical absences, and focal or generalized convulsive seizures, persisting over several years despite antiepileptic treatment but ultimately remitting in later childhood without developmental consequences. The EEG shows frequent CTS that become bilaterally synchronous and continuous during sleep. The occurrence of drop attacks with CTS in apparent BFEC has been characterized as a negative myoclonus manifestation of repetitive epileptiform activity in the motor and/or premotor areas on one or both sides (Kanazawa and Kawai 1990; Cirignotta and Lugaresi 1991; Oguni *et al* 1992; Harvey *et al* 1994). This seizure type is often refractory to treatment with carbamazepine, due to persistence of epileptiform activity, although benzodiazepines may be effective and long-term outcome is still favorable.

A syndrome of oromotor apraxia with speech and swallowing disturbance is reported as a manifestation of continuous, bilateral epileptiform activity in rare patients with BFEC-CTS, sometimes termed the epileptic opercular syndrome (Fejerman and Di Blasi 1997 Roulet *et al* 1989; Colamaria *et al* 1991). These children have a history of typical nocturnal orofacial seizures or exhibit subtle orofacial myoclonias. The presence of continuous, bilateral CTS in these patients presumably leads to a functional pseudobulbar palsy, similar to the auditory agnosia of Landau–Kleffner syndrome that apparently results from continuous bilateral epileptiform activity localizing to the superior temporal gyri (Morrell *et al* 1995). As with atypical BFEC presenting with atonic falls, 'spike-suppressant' treatment with benzodiazepines may be of benefit and long-term outcome is favorable. A family with rolandic epilepsy and speech dyspraxia affecting several generations has been reported, the inheritance in this family suggesting autosomal dominant transmission with anticipation (Scheffer *et al* 1995a).

BFEC-CTS is reported with a variety of cerebral lesions and insults (Santanelli *et al* 1989; Ambrosetto 1992; Shevell *et al* 1996; Sheth *et al* 1997; Wohlrab *et al* 1997). Interestingly, not all the reported lesions were located in the rolandic fissure, suggesting that the cerebral lesion was a coincidental finding or that the CTS were a relatively nonspecific marker of abnormal brain development. Furthermore, the course of the seizures in these cases was benign, suggesting that the seizures were not symptomatic of the lesions.

CTS are the most common focal EEG pattern recorded in pediatric EEG laboratories and are seen in 2% of normal children (Eeg-Olofsson *et al* 1971; Cavazzuti *et al* 1980; Autret *et al* 1992a). CTS are not infrequently identified in children with nonepileptic neurologic problems who are referred for EEG (Lerman and Kivity-Ephraim 1981; Van der Meij *et al* 1992a), especially in children with developmental disorders such as language delay and attentional or learning problems. The significance of such findings is uncertain, especially in the absence of controlled clinical studies. It is possible that the coexistence is simply coincidental or, more likely, that the CTS are a nonspecific marker of cerebral immaturity or dysfunction (Doose and Baier 1989; Doose *et al* 1996). Antiepileptic medication is rarely beneficial and the CTS remit in later childhood, regardless of the developmental outcome. This association of CTS with developmental problems, and the electroclinical similarities between BFEC-CTS and the epileptic aphasias, remains controversial. Controversy also exists as to the ability to distinguish 'epileptic' from 'functional' CTS by EEG morphology and field topography (Gregory and Wong 1992; Van der Meij *et al* 1992b, 1993).

IDIOPATHIC FOCAL EPILEPSIES WITH OCCIPITAL SEIZURES AND OCCIPITAL PAROXYSMS

In recent years there has been greater delineation of the syndromes of occipital epilepsy occurring in childhood and adulthood, both idiopathic and symptomatic. Partial seizures of occipital lobe origin vary greatly in their clinical manifestations but characteristic features include elementary visual hallucinations (e.g. phosphenes), visual distortions (e.g. micropsia, macropsia, metamorphopsia), negative visual phenomena (e.g. scotoma, blindness, hemianopia), tonic or clonic head and eye movements, axial tonic posturing, hemiconvulsions, impaired consciousness, and headache (Blume *et al* 1991; Williamson *et al* 1992; Palmini *et al* 1993). Differentiation of occipital seizures from migraine can be difficult due to common clinical features, posterior EEG abnormalities, and response to antiepileptic medications. Idiopathic occipital epilepsies account for 20–25% of benign partial epilepsies in childhood (Panayiotopoulos 1989) and three syndromes are distinguished by their typical clinical and EEG manifestations.

BENIGN OCCIPITAL EPILEPSY: LATE OR CLASSIC VARIANT

The syndrome of benign childhood epilepsy with occipital paroxysms, as initially described by Gastaut (1982), is the most well known of the idiopathic occipital epilepsies and is recognized by the ILAE. It is sometimes referred to as the late variant of benign occipital epilepsy (Panayiotopoulos 1993, 1998). Onset is typically in mid-late childhood or adolescence with diurnal seizures characterized by visual symptomatology (e.g. hallucinations, metamorphopsia, blindness), often with associated eye deviation, clonic jerking of the limbs, altered consciousness, and postictal 'migrainous' headache and vomiting. Seizures are usually brief. There is frequently a family history of seizures or migraine. Neurologic examination and brain imaging are normal. The interictal awake EEG (Fig. 20.3) shows a characteristic pattern with bilateral occipital sharp–slow activity on eye closure or fixation-off. Photic sensitivity is not normally present. Some patients have frequent brief seizures and require antiepileptic medication, carbamazepine being the treatment of choice. The syndrome has a good prognosis but some patients have persistent seizures or migraine attacks over several years.

BENIGN OCCIPITAL EPILEPSY: EARLY CHILDHOOD VARIANT

A quite distinct early childhood variant of benign occipital epilepsy is well described but underdiagnosed. This syndrome has a female preponderance and peak onset between 2 and 5 years of age. Nocturnal seizures are characteristic, with prominent vomiting, retching, tonic eye deviation, altered consciousness, and unilateral or bilateral clonic jerking. Seizures may be of short duration or quite prolonged, with catastrophic presentations in complex partial or convulsive status occurring in almost one-half of patients (Panayiotopoulos 1989, 1998; Panayiotopoulos and Igoe 1992; Ferrie *et al* 1997). There is often a family history of seizures. The children are neurologically and developmentally normal and brain imaging is unremarkable. The interictal EEG in this syndrome (Fig. 20.4) shows unilateral or bilateral occipital spike–wave discharges, usually activated by sleep and suppressed by eye opening. Photic sensitivity is not present. Some patients have associated CTS. Some young patients do not show occipital epileptic activity at presentation (Guerrini *et al* 1997). The syndrome has an excellent prognosis, with 30% of patients having only one seizure and the mean period of active seizures being 1 year (Ferrie *et al* 1997). Prescription of rectal diazepam should be considered for children presenting with status epilepticus. Treatment with carbamazepine for 1–2 years is indicated in children with recurrent seizures.

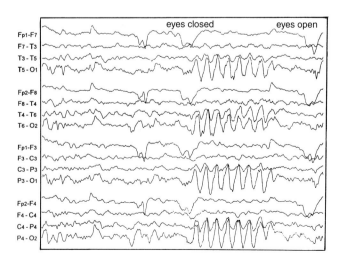

Fig. 20.3 Interictal awake EEG (longitudinal bipolar montage) of an 8-year-old girl with recurrent simple partial seizures characterized by amaurosis and oculoclonic jerks. Paroxysms of monomorphic rhythmic delta activity at 3.5 Hz were seen in the occipital regions on eye closure. The electroclinical picture is typical of the classic or late variant of benign occipital epilepsy.

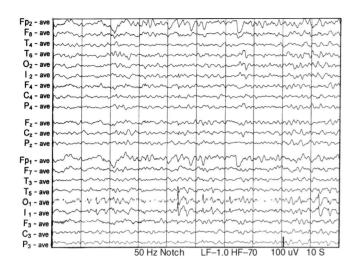

Fig. 20.4 Interictal asleep EEG (average reference montage) of a 4-year-old girl who presented 3 weeks earlier with a prolonged complex partial seizure characterized by waking from sleep, staring, tonic head and eye deviation to the right, and vomiting. The EEG shows brief runs of left occipital sharp–slow wave activity, the maximum field being in the left occipital (O1) and suboccipital (I1) electrodes. Computerized tomography of the brain was normal. The electroclinical picture is typical of the early variant of benign occipital epilepsy.

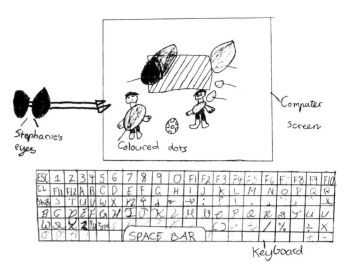

Fig. 20.5 Drawing by an 11-year-old girl who experienced colored blotches in her field of vision followed by bilateral clonic jerks of the upper limbs while playing a computer soccer game. Her interictal EEG showed irregular spike–wave discharges during photic stimulation, maximal in the posterior regions. The electroclinical picture is typical of the syndrome of idiopathic photosensitive occipital epilepsy.

IDIOPATHIC PHOTOSENSITIVE OCCIPITAL EPILEPSY

Idiopathic photosensitive occipital lobe epilepsy is a recently described entity that starts typically in late childhood or adolescence with visual seizures, complex partial seizures, and secondarily generalized seizures, characteristically occurring while the patient is watching television, playing a video game, or working on a computer (Guerrini et al 1995) (Fig. 20.5). Neurologic examination and brain imaging are normal. In this syndrome, the interictal EEG shows generalized or biposterior spike–wave activity at rest and with photic sensitivity. Distinction from photosensitive (generalized) epilepsy is based on recognition of the focal seizure symptomatology. Avoidance of precipitating stimuli and treatment with sodium valproate is indicated in children with recurrent seizures.

Symptomatic varieties of occipital lobe epilepsy should be suspected when the presentation does not conform to one of the above syndromes, the stereotypic interictal EEG patterns are not present, and when there is associated visual dysfunction or developmental delay. However, it should be recognized that reactive occipital epileptiform EEG patterns and photic-induced partial seizures are not specific for the idiopathic occipital epilepsies, as they can occur in symptomatic occipital epilepsies, idiopathic generalized epilepsies, and other idiopathic partial epilepsies of childhood (Cooper and Lee 1991; Riviello and Foley 1992; Talwar et al 1992; Guerrini et al 1994; Maher et al 1995).

OTHER IDIOPATHIC FOCAL EPILEPSIES OF CHILDHOOD

The ILAE classification does not recognise formally idiopathic partial epilepsies which are not of rolandic or occipital origin. Nevertheless, there are many neurologically normal children who present with partial seizures, have normal brain imaging and ultimately outgrow their seizures, without neurologic or psychologic sequelae, yet do not fulfill criteria for BFEC-CTS or one of the idiopathic occipital epilepsies. A clue to idiopathic focal epilepsy in a neurologically normal child with infrequent partial seizures is the presence of frequent, monomorphic, bilaterally independent, focal epileptiform discharges on a normal background, especially when associated with tangential dipoles across major fissures and when activated by sleep. However, such paradoxically dramatic focal epileptiform patterns on EEG are not always present in benign and familial partial epilepsies.

IDIOPATHIC TEMPORAL LOBE EPILEPSY

It has long been recognized that approximately one-third of children with temporal lobe epilepsy (TLE) have no underlying temporal lobe lesion, no associated psychologic deficits, and show ultimate remission of seizures in later childhood (Ounsted *et al* 1987; Dalla Bernardina *et al* 1992). Although many patients in older studies of childhood TLE undoubtedly had unrecognized BFEC-CTS, recent clinical studies employing high-resolution magnetic resonance imaging (MRI) suggest that a proportion of children with cryptogenic TLE may have truly idiopathic seizures (Harvey *et al* 1997a,b). A syndrome of familial TLE with a benign course is described (Berkovic *et al* 1996; Cendes *et al* 1998), affected individuals typically manifesting simple partial seizures with psychic and autonomic symptomatology in adolescence or young adult life, with minimal abnormalities on EEG and normal brain imaging. Autosomal dominant inheritance with incomplete penetrance is postulated.

IDIOPATHIC FRONTAL LOBE EPILEPSY

Partial epilepsy with frontal lobe semeiology, showing onset in childhood, a strong family history, and a benign course, is also recognized (Lerman and Kivity 1991; Vigevano and Fusco 1993). Of great interest in this regard is the recent characterization of the syndrome of autosomal dominant nocturnal frontal lobe epilepsy, which probably accounts for many reported children with 'benign frontal epilepsy' and familial parasomnias. This syndrome is characterized by brief nocturnal seizures with hyperkinetic or tonic motor manifestations, sometimes associated with an aura, which invariably occur on going to sleep or on awakening from sleep. Seizures typically begin in childhood and persist into adulthood, with varying severity within families. Interictal EEG may be normal, although ictal recordings have confirmed the epileptic nature and frontal origin of the seizures. MRI is normal (Scheffer *et al* 1995b). Linkage to chromosome 20q is reported in some families (Phillips *et al* 1995), with the genetic basis in these being a missense mutation of the neuronal nicotinic acetylcholine receptor α_4 subunit (Steinlein *et al* 1995).

BENIGN FOCAL EPILEPSIES OF INFANCY

Just as many epilepsies with onset of seizures in childhood are known to have a benign course, it has long been recognized that many neurologically normal infants presenting with complex partial seizures or poorly characterized convulsive seizures outgrow their seizures and develop normally. Watanabe and colleagues reported infants with complex partial seizures and secondarily generalized seizures in whom seizure onset was in the first 6 months, neurologic development was normal, interictal EEG and brain imaging were normal, and prolonged seizure remission followed (Watanabe *et al* 1987, 1993; Okumura *et al* 1996).

The existence of a benign partial epilepsy syndrome of infancy was a major controversy in the literature (Dulac *et al* 1989) until the characterization of the syndrome of benign infantile familial convulsions. Onset in this syndrome is typically between 3 and 12 months with a cluster of convulsive seizures in which lateralized tonic or versive manifestations may be appreciated (Vigevano *et al* 1992; Echenne *et al* 1994). Interictal EEG is usually normal and brain imaging shows no abnormality. Fortuitous ictal EEG recordings have shown focal onset in the central and posterior regions. Seizures respond promptly to antiepileptic medication, with rare recurrences after infancy and normal subsequent neurologic development. A similar history is obtained in a parent or other relative. Linkage has been shown to chromosome 19q, distinct from the reported linkage of benign familial neonatal convulsions (Malafosse *et al* 1994; Guipponi *et al* 1997).

CONCLUSIONS

The idiopathic focal epilepsies of childhood are some of the most common and well-described seizure disorders of childhood but remain somewhat poorly understood in terms of their pathogenesis and nosology. How do the nonrolandic varieties of idiopathic focal epilepsy relate to each other and to BFEC-CTS? What is the relationship between the idiopathic focal and generalized epilepsies? What is the mechanism by which genetically determined epilepsies manifest with focal seizures and focal epileptiform EEG patterns? What is the significance of CTS and other idiopathic focal epileptiform EEG patterns in nonepileptic children with developmental problems? With increasing awareness of the idiopathic focal epilepsies by clinicians, further improvements in MRI, and continued advances in the molecular genetics of the epilepsies, it is likely that these nosologic and pathogenetic uncertainties will be understood.

Clinicians should consider idiopathic focal epilepsy when assessing children with intractable focal epilepsy in whom partial seizures begin in midchildhood, there is a family history of seizures, MRI is normal, or the interictal epileptiform activity is extremely frequent and stereotyped. It should also be remembered that poorly controlled seizures, associated developmental disabilities, and lesions on brain imaging do not necessarily indicate a symptomatic etiology.

KEY POINTS

1. Idiopathic focal epilepsies account for approximately one-quarter of childhood seizure disorders.
2. Idiopathic focal epilepsies share the following features:
   (a) age-dependent onset of partial seizures;
   (b) absence of neurologic and psychologic deficits;
   (c) stereotyped focal epileptiform patterns on interictal EEG;
   (d) normal neuroimaging;
   (e) frequent family history of seizures;
   (f) excellent prognosis with remission of seizures in later childhood or adolescence.
3. The most well-characterized varieties of idiopathic focal epilepsy are:
   (a) benign childhood epilepsy with centrotemporal spikes (benign rolandic epilepsy);
   (b) several syndromes of childhood epilepsy with occipital paroxysms (benign occipital epilepsies).

REFERENCES

Aicardi J, Chevrie JJ (1982) Atypical benign partial epilepsy of childhood. *Developmental Medicine and Child Neurology* 24:281–292.

Ambrosetto G (1992) Unilateral opercular macrogyria and benign childhood epilepsy with centrotemporal (rolandic) spikes: report of a case. *Epilepsia* 33:499–503.

Autret A, Lucas B, Degiovanni E, de Toffol B, Billard C (1992) A note on the occurrence of unusual electroencephalographic sleep patterns in selected normal children. *Journal of Child Neurology* 7:422–426.

Beaumanoir A, Ballis T, Varfis G, Ansari K (1974) Benign epilepsy of childhood with rolandic spikes. *Epilepsia* 15:301–315.

Beaussart M (1972) Benign epilepsy of children with rolandic (centrotemporal) paroxysmal foci. *Epilepsia* 13:795–811.

Berkovic SF, McIntosh A, Howell RA *et al* (1996) Familial temporal lobe epilepsy: a common disorder identified in twins. *Annals of Neurology* 40:227–235.

Blume WT, Whiting SE, Girvin JP (1991) Epilepsy surgery in the posterior cortex. *Annals of Neurology* 29:638–645.

Bouma PA, Bovenkerk AC, Westendorp RG, Brouwer OF (1997) The clinical course of benign partial epilepsy of childhood with centrotemporal spikes: a meta-analysis. *Neurology* 48:430–437.

Cavazzuti GB, Cappella L, Nalin A (1980) Longitudinal study of epileptiform EEG patterns in normal children. *Epilepsia* 21:43–55.

Cendes F, Lopes-Cendes I, Andermann E, Andermann F (1998) Familial temporal lobe epilepsy: a clinically heterogeneous syndrome. *Neurology* 50:554–557.

Cirignotta F, Lugaresi E (1991) Partial motor epilepsy with 'negative myoclonus'. *Epilepsia* 32:54–58.

Colamaria V, Sgrò V, Caraballo R *et al* (1991) Status epilepticus in benign rolandic epilepsy manifesting as anterior operculum syndrome. *Epilepsia* 32:329–334.

Commission on Classification and Terminology of the International League Against Epilepsy (1989) Proposal for revised classification of epilepsies and epileptic syndromes. *Epilepsia* 30:389–399.

Cooper GW, Lee SI (1991) Reactive occipital epileptiform activity: is it benign? *Epilepsia* 32:63–68.

Dalla Bernardina B, Colamaria V, Chiamenti C *et al* (1992) Benign partial epilepsy with affective symptoms ('benign psychomotor epilepsy'). In: Roger J, Bureau M, Dravet C, Dreifuss FE, Perret A, Wolf P (eds) *Epileptic Syndromes in Infancy, Childhood and Adolescence*, 2nd edn, pp 219–223. London: John Libbey.

Doose H, Baier WK (1989) Benign partial epilepsy and related conditions: multifactorial pathogenesis with hereditary impairment of brain maturation. *European Journal of Pediatrics* 149:152–158.

Doose H, Neubauer B, Carlsson G (1996) Children with benign focal sharp waves in the EEG: developmental disorders and epilepsy. *Neuropediatrics* 27:227–241.

Drury I, Beydoun A (1991) Benign partial epilepsy of childhood with monomorphic sharp waves in centrotemporal and other locations. *Epilepsia* 32:662–667.

Duchowny M, Harvey AS (1996) Pediatric epilepsy syndromes: an update and critical review. *Epilepsia* 37(Suppl 1):S26–S40.

Dulac O, Cusmai R, De Oliveira K (1989) Is there a partial benign epilepsy in infancy? *Epilepsia* 30:798–801.

Echenne B, Humbertclaude V, Rivier F, Malafosse A, Cheminal R (1994) Benign infantile epilepsy with autosomal dominant inheritance. *Brain and Development* 16:108–111.

Eeg-Olofsson O, Petersén I, Selldén U (1971) The development of the electroencephalogram in normal children from the age 1 through 15 years. *Neuropediatrics* 2:375–404.

Fejerman N, Di Blasi M (1987) Status epilepticus of benign partial epilepsies in children: report of two cases. *Epilepsia* 28:351–355.

Ferrie CD, Beaumanoir A, Guerrini R *et al* (1997) Early-onset benign occipital seizure susceptibility syndrome. *Epilepsia* 38:285–293.

Frost Jr JD, Hrachovy RA, Glaze DG (1992) Spike morphology in childhood focal epilepsy: relationship to syndromic classification. *Epilepsia* 33:531–536.

Gastaut H (1982) A new type of epilepsy: benign partial epilepsy of childhood with occipital spike-waves. *Clinical Electroencephalography* 13:13–22.

Gregory DL, & Wong PK (1984) Topographical analysis of the centrotemporal discharges in benign rolandic epilepsy of childhood. *Epilepsia* 25:705–711.

Gregory DL, Wong PKH (1992) Clinical relevance of a dipole field in rolandic spikes. *Epilepsia* 33:36–44.

Guerrini R, Ferrari AR, Battaglia A, Salvadori P, Bonanni P (1994) Occipitotemporal seizures with ictus emeticus induced by intermittent photic stimulation. *Neurology* 44:253–259.

Guerrini R, Dravet C, Genton P *et al* (1995) Idiopathic photosensitive occipital lobe epilepsy. *Epilepsia* 36:883–891.

Guerrini R, Belmonte A, Veggiotti P, Mattia D, Bonanni P (1997) Delayed appearance of interictal EEG abnormalities in early onset childhood epilepsy with occipital paroxysms. *Brain and Development* 19:343–346.

Guipponi M, Rivier F, Vigevano F *et al* (1997) Linkage mapping of benign familial infantile convulsions (BFIC) to chromosome 19q. *Human Molecular Genetics* 6:473–477.

Gutierrez AR, Brick JF, Bodensteiner J (1990) Dipole reversal: an ictal feature of benign partial epilepsy with centrotemporal spikes. *Epilepsia* 31:544–548.

Harvey AS, Jayakar P, Resnick TR *et al* (1994) 'Rolandic drop attacks'. partial onset atonic seizures of axial musculature. *Epilepsia* **35**(Suppl 8):14.

Harvey AS, Jayakar P, Duchowny MS *et al* (1995) Ictal recordings in benign partial epilepsy of childhood with centrotemporal spikes. *Electroencephalography and Clinical Neurophysiology* **95**:36p.

Harvey AS, Berkovic SF, Wrennall JA, Hopkins IJ (1997a) Temporal lobe epilepsy in childhood: clinical, EEG and neuroimaging findings and syndrome classification in a cohort with new-onset seizures. *Neurology* **49**:960–968.

Harvey AS, Hopkins IJ, Wrennall JA, Berkovic SF (1997b) Etiology predicts seizure outcome in new-onset temporal lobe epilepsy in childhood. *Annals of Neurology* **42**:505.

Kanazawa O, Kawai I (1990) Status epilepticus characterized by repetitive asymmetrical atonia: two cases accompanied by partial seizures. *Epilepsia* **31**:536–543.

Legarda S, Jayakar P, Duchowny M, Alvarez L, Resnick T (1994) Benign rolandic epilepsy: high central and low central subgroups. *Epilepsia* **35**:1125–1129.

Lerman P, Kivity S (1991) The benign partial nonrolandic epilepsies. *Journal of Clinical Neurophysiology* **8**:275–287.

Lerman P, Kivity-Ephraim S (1981) Focal epileptic EEG discharges in children not suffering from clinical epilepsy: etiology, clinical significance, and management. *Epilepsia* **22**:551–558.

Loiseau P, Beaussart M (1973) The seizures of benign childhood epilepsy with rolandic paroxysmal discharges. *Epilepsia* **14**:381–389.

Loiseau P, Duché B (1989) Benign childhood epilepsy with centrotemporal spikes. *Cleveland Clinic Journal of Medicine* **56**(Suppl 1):S17–S22.

Maher J, Ronen GM, Ogunyemi AO, Goulden KJ (1995) Occipital paroxysmal discharges suppressed by eye opening: variability in clinical and seizure manifestations in childhood. *Epilepsia* **36**:52–57.

Malafosse A, Beck C, Bellet H *et al* (1994) Benign infantile familial convulsions are not an allelic form of the benign familial neonatal convulsions gene. *Annals of Neurology* **35**:479–482.

Morrell F, Whisler WW, Smith MC *et al* (1995) Landau–Kleffner syndrome. Treatment with subpial intracortical transection. *Brain* **118**:1529–1546.

Oguni H, Sato F, Hayashi K, Wang PJ, Fukuyama Y (1992) A study of unilateral brief focal atonia in childhood partial epilepsy. *Epilepsia* **33**:75–83.

Okumura A, Hayakawa F, Kuno K, Watanabe K (1996) Benign partial epilepsy in infancy. *Archives of Disease in Childhood* **74**:19–21.

Ounsted C, Lindsay J, Richards P (1987) Temporal lobe epilepsy 1948–1986. A biographical study. *Clinics in Developmental Medicine* **103**:6–33.

Palmini A, Andermann F, Dubeau F *et al* (1993) Occipitotemporal epilepsies: evaluation of selected patients requiring depth electrodes studies and rationale for surgical approaches. *Epilepsia* **34**:84–96.

Panayiotopoulos CP (1989) Benign childhood epilepsy with occipital paroxysms: a 15-year prospective study. *Annals of Neurology* **26**:51–56.

Panayiotopoulos CP (1993) Benign childhood partial epilepsies: benign childhood seizure susceptibility syndromes. *Journal of Neurology, Neurosurgery and Psychiatry* **56**:2–5.

Panayiotopoulos CP (1998) Benign childhood occipital seizures. *Archives of Disease in Childhood* **78**:3–4.

Panayiotopoulos CP, Igoe DM (1992) Cerebral insult-like partial status epilepticus in the early-onset variant of benign childhood epilepsy with occipital paroxysms. *Seizure* **1**:99–102.

Phillips HA, Scheffer IE, Berkovic SF *et al* (1995) Localization of a gene for autosomal dominant nocturnal frontal lobe epilepsy to chromosome 20q13.2. *Nature Genetics* **10**:4–6.

Riviello JJ, Foley CM (1992) The epileptiform significance of intermittent rhythmic delta activity in childhood. *Journal of Child Neurology* **7**:156–160.

Roulet E, Deonna T, Despland PA (1989) Prolonged intermittent drooling and oromotor dyspraxia in benign childhood epilepsy with centrotemporal spikes. *Epilepsia* **30**:564–568.

Santanelli P, Bureau M, Magaudda A, Gobbi G, Roger J (1989) Benign partial epilepsy with centrotemporal (or rolandic) spikes and brain lesion. *Epilepsia* **30**:182–188.

Scheffer IE, Jones L, Pozzebon M *et al* (1995a) Autosomal dominant rolandic epilepsy and speech dyspraxia: a new syndrome with anticipation. *Annals of Neurology* **38**:633–642.

Scheffer IE, Bhatia KP, Lopes-Cendes I *et al* (1995b) Autosomal dominant nocturnal frontal lobe epilepsy. A distinctive clinical disorder. *Brain* **118**:61–73.

Sheth RD, Gutierrez AR, Riggs JE (1997) Rolandic epilepsy and cortical dysplasia: MRI correlation of epileptiform discharges. *Pediatric Neurology* **17**:177–179.

Shevell MI, Rosenblatt B, Watters GV, O'Gorman AM, Montes JL (1996) 'Pseudo-BECRS'. intracranial focal lesions suggestive of a primary partial epilepsy syndrome. *Pediatric Neurology* **14**:31–35.

Sidenvall R, Forsgren L, Blomquist HK, Heijbel J (1993) A community-based prospective incidence study of epileptic seizures in children. *Acta Paediatrica Scandinavica* **82**:60–65.

Steinlein OK, Mulley JC, Propping P *et al* (1995) A missense mutation in the neuronal nicotinic acetylcholine receptor alpha 4 subunit is associated with autosomal dominant nocturnal frontal lobe epilepsy. *Nature Genetics* **11**:201–203.

Talwar D, Rask CA, Torres F (1992) Clinical manifestations in children with occipital spike–wave paroxysms. *Epilepsia* **33**:667–674.

Van der Meij W, Van Huffelen AC, Willemse J, Schenk-Rootlieb AJF, Meiners LC (1992a) Rolandic spikes in the inter-ictal EEG of children: contribution to diagnosis, classification and prognosis of epilepsy. *Developmental Medicine and Child Neurology* **34**:893–903.

Van der Meij W, Van Huffelen AC, Wieneke GH, Willemse J (1992b) Sequential EEG mapping may differentiate 'epileptic' from 'non-epileptic' rolandic spikes. *Electroencephalography and Clinical Neurophysiology* **82**:408–414.

Van der Meij W, Wieneke GH, Van Huffelen AC, Schenk-Rootlieb AJF, Willemse J (1993) Identical morphology of the rolandic spike-and-wave complex in different clinical entities. *Epilepsia* **34**:540–550.

Vigevano F, Fusco L (1993) Hypnic tonic postural seizures in healthy children provide evidence for a partial epileptic syndrome of frontal lobe origin. *Epilepsia* **39**:110–119.

Vigevano F, Fusco L, DiCapua M *et al* (1992) Benign infantile familial convulsions. *European Journal of Pediatrics* **151**:608–612.

Watanabe K, Yamamoto N, Negoro T *et al* (1987) Benign complex partial epilepsies in infancy. *Pediatric Neurology* **3**:208–211.

Watanabe K, Negoro T, Aso K (1993) Benign partial epilepsy with secondarily generalized seizures in infancy. *Epilepsia* **34**:635–638.

Williamson PD, Thadani VM, Darcey TM *et al* (1992) Occipital lobe epilepsy: clinical characteristics, seizure spread patterns, and results of surgery. *Annals of Neurology* **31**:3–13.

Wohlrab G, Schmitt B, Boltshauser E (1997) Benign focal epileptiform discharges in children after severe head trauma: prognostic value and clinical course. *Epilepsia* **38**:275–278.

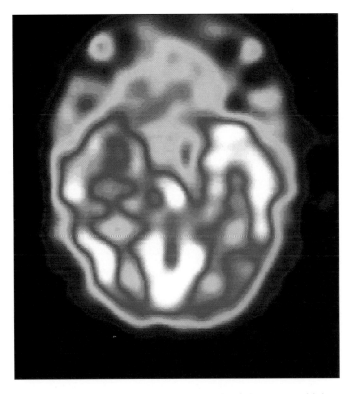

Plate 1 SPECT dataset sliced in the long axis of the temporal lobes, in a patient with a left mesial temporal seizure source. HMPAO injection was carried out during a complex partial seizure. The image shows hypeperfusion of the left temporal lobe, with mild hypoperfusion of the posterior temporal cortex.

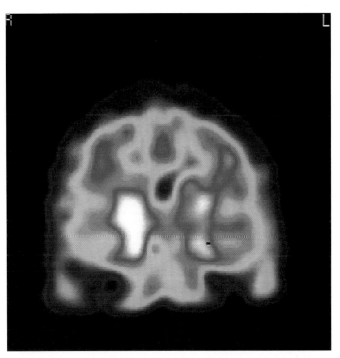

Plate 2 SPECT dataset sliced coronally, in a patient with a right mesial temporal seizure source. HMPAO injection was carried out during the clonic phase of a secondary generalized seizure. The image shows generalized hypoperfusion of the cortical mantle, most evident in the lateral temporal cortex, with hyperperfusion of the mesial temporal areas and basal ganglia, more marked on the right.

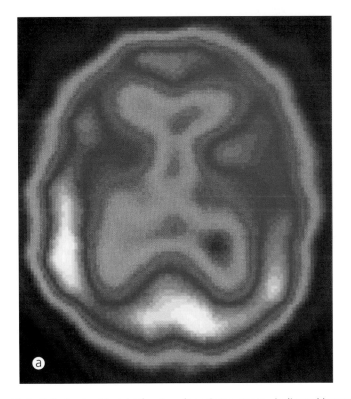

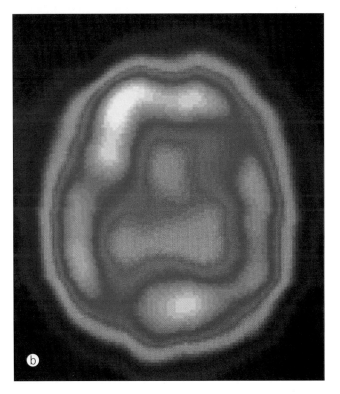

Plate 3 Patient with right frontopolar seizure source, indicated by stereotactic EEG and confirmed by successful resection. The acquisitions were carried out using a single-head gamma camera at the Centre Eugene Marquis, Rennes, France. HMPAO injection and localizing investigations were carried out at the Unité Van Gogh, CHRU Pontchaillou, Rennes, France, under the auspices of Dr A Biraben. (a) Interictal phase. Orbitomeatal slice through the frontal lobes, showing normal perfusion pattern. (b) Ictal phase. Equivalent slice to (a), showing hyperperfusion of the right frontal lobe, most marked in the polar area. A degree of hyperperfusion is also seen on the left.

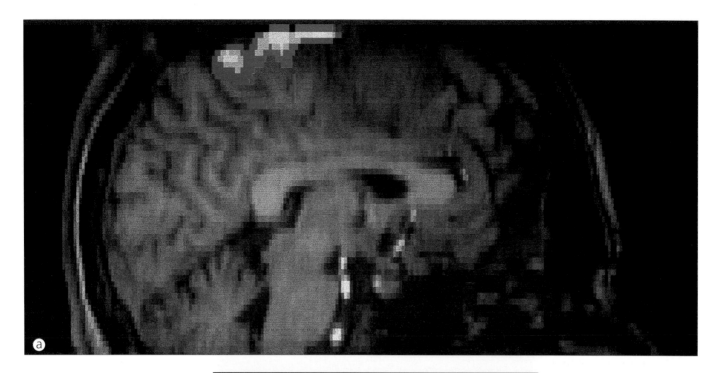

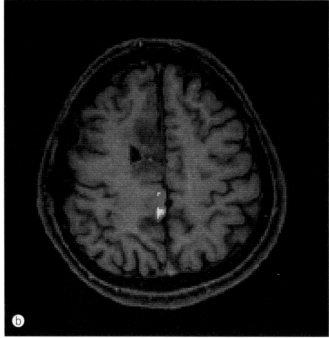

Plate 4 Figures showing axial and sagittal slices of an anatomic and functional MRI study of a patient with a right frontal tumor causing epilepsy. The task was a motor block designed paradigm performed with the left foot at 1Hz. The study was acquired at 3T using a gradient echo EPI sequence (TR 3000ms, TE 30ms, matrix 64 × 64 × 21, FOV 256 × 256 covering the whole brain). The structural images were acquired using a turbo FLASH inversion recovery sequence. Pixels activated by the paradigm (corrected p < 0.01) are shown in color. The functional activation corresponds with the anatomic right foot area (see Chapter 48). Courtesy of R Piniero and JE Adcock, FMRIB Center, Oxford, UK.

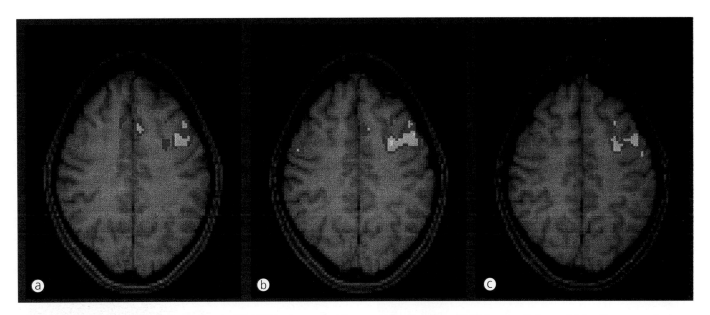

Plate 5 Language dominance determined with FMRI using verbal fluency tasks. Functional MRI is potentially useful for the presurgical localization of language areas in patients with epilepsy. Verbal fluency tasks were performed covertly to generate (a) words from letters, (b) verbal exemplars from categories (e.g. plants, animals), and (c) verbs from nouns. The three maps, from a single subject, show significant activation of left Broca's area and anterior cingulate gyrus (see Chapter 48). Courtesy of JE Adcock, FMRIB Centre, Oxford, UK.

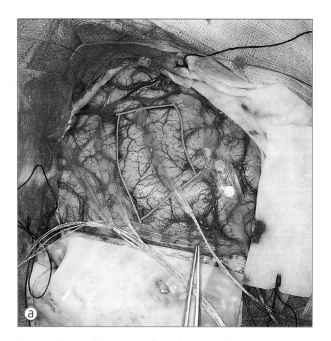

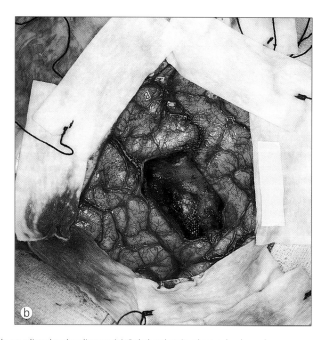

Plate 6 Case 1. Photographs from the exposed Broca area of a patient with an oligodendroglioma: (a) Subdural strip electrodes have been placed on and adjacent to the tumor. (b) Postexcision photography (see Chapter 52).

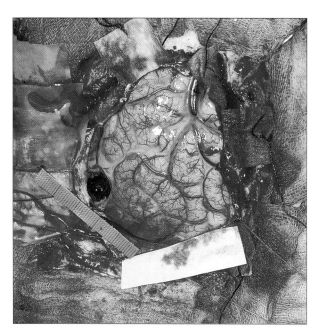

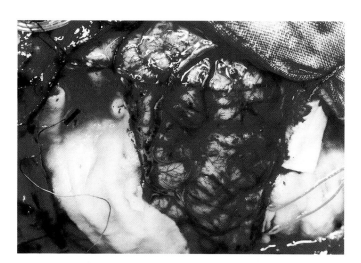

Plate 8 Appearance of the cortex in a patient with Rasmussen encephalitis who has undergone a frontal resection combined with multiple subdued transection of the central cortex posterior to the resection (see Chapter 54).

Plate 7 Case 4. A postexcision photograph of the exposed right occipital lobe after removal of a small mesioparasagittal astrocytoma. (Figures 52.3b,c show the preoperative (narrow lines) and postoperative (thick line) visual fields).

Adult idiopathic and cryptogenic focal epilepsies

RC ROBERTS

21

The original international classification of epilepsies and epilepsy syndromes included just two groups of localization-related (focal) epilepsies, *idiopathic with age-related onset* and *symptomatic* (Commission on Classification and Terminology of the International League Against Epilepsy 1985). The revised classification added a third group, *cryptogenic* (Commission on Classification and Terminology of the International League Against Epilepsy 1989). It was recommended that the term 'idiopathic' should be used when there is 'no underlying cause other than a possible hereditary predisposition' and a 'presumed genetic aetiology,' and that the term 'cryptogenic' should be used when the epilepsy is 'presumed to be symptomatic, but the aetiology is unknown.' Whereas in the past 'idiopathic' has been more loosely used to describe any epilepsy of unknown etiology, it is now recommended that it should be confined to well-defined, genetically determined epilepsy syndromes in which epilepsy is the only manifestation of the disorder. Nevertheless the distinctions between idiopathic, cryptogenic, and symptomatic epilepsy syndromes are blurred and the terminology is unsatisfactory. For instance, many symptomatic and cryptogenic focal epilepsies will occur partly on account of a genetic predisposition (and therefore be partly idiopathic?). When an epilepsy is primarily genetically determined, the gene defect might cause a structural brain abnormality such as a malformation of cortical development, leading to uncertainty as to whether the epilepsy should be considered idiopathic or symptomatic. The international classification of the epilepsies and epilepsy syndromes so far includes only three idiopathic with age-related onset focal epilepsy syndromes: benign childhood epilepsy with centrotemporal spikes, childhood epilepsy with occipital paroxysms, and primary reading epilepsy. Only primary reading epilepsy can have an onset in adult life; its inclusion in the classification as an idiopathic focal epilepsy is controversial as is that of the other so-called reflex epilepsies.

IDIOPATHIC FOCAL EPILEPSY SYNDROMES

These are focal epilepsies without any definable underlying structural pathology, such as a malformation of cortical development, that have a genetic etiology or are presumed to have such an etiology.

FAMILIAL TEMPORAL LOBE EPILEPSY

Familial temporal lobe epilepsy (TLE) was identified by a large Australian twin study, in which 55 twin pairs with symptomatic or apparently cryptogenic partial epilepsies were identified (Berkovic *et al* 1996). Concordance was found for 5 of 13 monozygotic pairs with cryptogenic partial epilepsy (38%), but for none of the dizygotic pairs or those with symptomatic partial epilepsies. The five concordant pairs all had seizures suggestive of a temporal lobe origin. Seven additional nontwin families were identified, each with two or more individuals with cryptogenic TLE, from one neurologist's practice. The twin and nontwin families contained 38 individuals with probable familial TLE. There was no history of prenatal or perinatal insult, febrile convulsions, meningitis or encephalitis, and no history of head injury thought to be relevant to the epilepsy. Onset was usually in adolescence or early adult life (age range, 10–63 years; mean, 24 years). Simple partial seizures occurred in 89%, complex partial seizures in 66%, and tonic–clonic seizures in 66%. The simple partial seizure onsets exhibited mainly psychic (particularly *déjà vu*), autonomic, or special sensory symptoms, suggesting a medial temporal origin. EEG showed focal temporal epileptiform abnormalities in only 22% of cases. Magnetic resonance imaging (MRI) of the brain was normal.

It was concluded that autosomal dominant inheritance with age-related penetrance was most likely. Overall the severity of the epilepsy was mild, with apparent response to carbamazepine, phenytoin, and sodium valproate. One-quarter of the affected individuals were diagnosed as a result of the study. Although one-third of the subjects had tonic–clonic seizures after starting treatment, at the time of the study only five individuals had poorly controlled epilepsy and only one of these was severe enough for surgical treatment to be considered. Familial TLE thus probably accounts for a very significant proportion of mild apparently cryptogenic focal epilepsy but only a small proportion of more severe intractable cryptogenic focal epilepsy.

A single family has been described with partial seizures suggestive of a lateral temporal lobe onset and linkage to chromosome 10q (Ottman *et al* 1995).

AUTOSOMAL DOMINANT NOCTURNAL FRONTAL LOBE EPILEPSY

Autosomal dominant nocturnal frontal lobe epilepsy has only recently been recognized but is now a well-defined epilepsy syndrome (Scheffer *et al* 1995; Oldani *et al* 1998). Seizures usually start in childhood or the teens, although about 12% of cases begin over the age of 20 years and onset at up to 52 years has been reported. Most attacks occur during sleep, although about one-quarter of patients report infrequent awake attacks. The sleep attacks tend to occur in clusters with typically four to eleven attacks per night, most often during dozing soon after falling asleep or shortly before awakening. The semeiology of the seizures is characteristic of a frontal origin. An aura (somatosensory, special sensory, psychic, or autonomic) has been described in

70% of patients. The attacks tend to be brief, beginning with a gasp, grunt, or vocalization. The motor features vary from thrashing hyperkinetic activity to tonic stiffening with or without clonic jerking. About 70% of patients say that they retain awareness during most of their attacks, and many report a sensation of breathing difficulty or choking. Although most seizures are partial, secondary generalization can occur. The severity of the disorder varies widely. Some patients are well controlled on carbamazepine, but sodium valproate has been reported as 'generally not effective' (Scheffer *et al* 1995). Interictal EEG epileptiform activity has been present in only a minority of patients, usually frontally; ictal EEG recordings do not always show any definite ictal discharges. A mutation of the α_4 subunit of the neuronal nicotinic acetylcholine receptor has been found in a minority of families, although other families have shown no linkage to this chromosomal region (Steinlein *et al* 1995, 1997; Oldani *et al* 1998). It is important that the possibility of autosomal dominant nocturnal frontal lobe epilepsy be considered in patients presenting with attacks predominantly occurring in sleep, as misdiagnosis of nonepileptic disorders has been common. These latter disorders include benign nocturnal parasomnias, psychiatric disorders, sleep paralysis, startle disease, asthma, and enuresis. The attacks in autosomal dominant frontal lobe epilepsy are indistinguishable from those previously described in nocturnal paroxysmal dystonia (Lugaresi *et al* 1986), and the term 'nocturnal paroxysmal dystonia', which implies a nonepileptic disorder, should not be used in this context. Although autosomal dominant nocturnal frontal lobe epilepsy accounts for only a very small proportion of adult intractable focal epilepsy, it is important that it is accurately diagnosed in view of the therapeutic implications.

READING EPILEPSY

Reading epilepsy is a rare type of reflex epilepsy in which seizures are triggered by reading, especially aloud; spontaneous seizures do not usually occur (Bickford *et al* 1956; Saenz-Lope *et al* 1985; Wolf 1992; Radhakrishnan *et al* 1995; Koutroumanidis *et al* 1998). The content of the material read is irrelevant. In many patients seizures may also be provoked by other language-related activities. The most common type of reading epilepsy is the primary reading epilepsy of Bickford *et al* (1956). Koutroumanidis *et al* (1998) have suggested that this type should be called myoclonic reading epilepsy on account of the characteristic features of the seizures. These begin with myoclonic jerks involving the jaw, mouth, and throat, which may spread to the arms. If the subject continues to read, they may undergo secondary generalization. The age of onset is usually in the teens but can be later. During reading, the EEG shows a variety of brief epileptiform discharges, which can be either bilaterally synchronous or focal (most often on the left). An ictal positron emission tomography (PET) study has shown areas of bifrontal and bitemporal activation during the myoclonic seizures (Koepp *et al* 1998). Control of the seizures can usually be achieved with sodium valproate or clonazepam, and patients may learn to avoid attacks. Most cases are idiopathic, with only rare symptomatic cases reported. About 25% of patients with primary reading epilepsy have a first-degree relative with epilepsy, which is most often also reading epilepsy (Wolf 1992). This suggests a strong genetic factor, although the mode of inheritance has not been established.

Small numbers of patients have been reported with reading epilepsy and other types of attack that do not involve jaw myoclonus. Koutroumanidis *et al* (1998) have emphasized the existence of patients having partial reading epilepsy, with partial seizures manifesting as prolonged alexia and varying degrees of aphasia. These attacks have been associated with unilateral focal ictal EEG changes over the language-dominant posterior temporoparietooccipital region. Both idiopathic and symptomatic cases have been described. In contrast, Singh *et al* (1995) have described a patient with reading-induced absence seizures.

The place of reading epilepsy in the international classification of epilepsies and epilepsy syndromes is controversial, despite the inclusion of primary reading epilepsy as an idiopathic localization-related epilepsy (Radhakrishnan *et al* 1995; Koutroumanidis *et al* 1998; Ramani 1998). There are cases which are clearly localization-related (partial reading epilepsy), and cases which are generalized (reading-induced absence seizures). The classification of the most frequent variety, myoclonic reading epilepsy, is more difficult. Brain activation is focal but the initial seizure manifestation is myoclonus. EEG changes can be either focal or generalized. The attacks respond best to clonazepam and valproate, rather than drugs more specifically active against partial seizures. The current classification does not easily encompass this type of epilepsy that is provoked by a specific mode of activation.

HOT WATER EPILEPSY

Hot water epilepsy is a common form of reflex epilepsy in southern India. The seizures are usually triggered by pouring mugs of hot water over the head in quick succession (Satischandra *et al* 1988, 1998). Occasional cases have been described from other parts of the world. Although the onset is usually in childhood, adult-onset cases have been reported. Most cases have complex partial seizures with infrequent secondary generalization. A small number of families have been described with more than two affected members, and it seems appropriate to include hot water epilepsy as an idiopathic focal epilepsy.

OTHER REFLEX EPILEPSIES WITH PARTIAL SEIZURES

There are various other types of rare reflex epilepsy with partial seizures, including musicogenic epilepsy, eating epilepsy, and epilepsy with seizures induced by thinking. The seizures of musicogenic epilepsy are triggered by listening to music, and sometimes by thinking about music (Wieser *et al* 1997; Zifkin and Zatorre 1998). They are usually complex partial with infrequent secondary generalization, and their onset is usually after the age of 20 years. The interval between beginning to listen to music and a seizure may be several minutes, leading to controversy as to whether these subjects should be classified as having a 'reflex' epilepsy. Most reported cases also have spontaneous seizures, so that musicogenic epilepsy has not been generally recognized as an epilepsy syndrome. EEG abnormalities are usually temporal but without consistent lateralization. Some cases are symptomatic and others cryptogenic.

The seizures of eating epilepsy usually occur in relation to eating and are usually partial, sometimes with secondary generalization (Remillard *et al* 1998). The relationship with particular aspects of eating is variable, both between patients and sometimes within individual patients. Seizures may occur with the sight or smell of food, at different times during a meal, and sometimes with particular foods. Patients have been divided into those with temporolimbic seizure onset and those with extralimbic, perirolandic, suprasylvian onset. The latter are more likely to have spontaneous seizures in addition to those induced by eating. Many cases have a symptomatic epilepsy, but some are cryptogenic.

There is little evidence at present that these types of complex reflex epilepsy (musicogenic, eating, thinking) will emerge as idiopathic focal epilepsy syndromes.

CRYPTOGENIC FOCAL EPILEPSY

These epilepsies are presumed to be symptomatic but the underlying structural pathology cannot be defined.

PREVALENCE AND DIAGNOSIS

The prevalence of cryptogenic focal epilepsy depends on the patient sample (community, hospital, etc.) and on the extent to which investigations are performed in an attempt to detect underlying pathology. In a large prospective community-based study of patients presenting with epilepsy and investigated routinely, 24.6% were assigned to the cryptogenic localization-related epilepsy category if febrile seizures were excluded (Manford *et al* 1992). These represented the majority (58%) of those with focal epilepsies, over 60% of the total group falling into the undetermined and the acute symptomatic categories. The prevalence of cryptogenic focal epilepsy has decreased as brain imaging techniques to detect underlying focal pathology have improved. Epilepsy was cryptogenic in most adult patients with focal epilepsy prior to the advent of CT. CT brain scanning detects focal pathology in up to one-third of adults with epileptic seizures, although a higher proportion of those with medically intractable focal epilepsy are positive (Gastaut and Gastaut 1976; Young *et al* 1982; Ramirez-Lassepas *et al* 1984; Hopkins *et al* 1988; Roberts *et al* 1988; Schoenenberger and Heim 1994). Since the advent of MRI, focal pathology has been detected in most patients with localization-related epilepsies (Duncan 1997). MRI techniques that can be applied routinely detect focal pathology in up to 80% of those with intractable focal epilepsy (Cook and Stevens 1995; Duncan 1997; Duncan and Fish 1998). A few of the remaining 20% have one of the idiopathic focal epilepsies discussed above, but most fall into the cryptogenic focal epilepsy category. However, in those presenting for the first time with partial epilepsies, many of which do not become intractable, the proportion of cryptogenic focal epilepsy may be higher; the results of large prospective studies of high-quality MRI in new patients are awaited. The proportion of patients with cryptogenic focal epilepsy is lowest in those with a seizure origin in a temporal lobe and higher in those with seizure origins elsewhere.

All patients with intractable focal epilepsy should undergo MRI if there is no contraindication. The Neuroimaging Commission of the International League Against Epilepsy has produced recommendations concerning the MRI sequences that may be considered adequate to detect relevant focal pathology (International League Against Epilepsy Neuroimaging Commission 1997). Imaging should include T1 and T2 weighted sequences to cover the whole brain in at least two orthogonal planes, with the minimum slice thickness possible. Gadolinium enhancement is not indicated except to clarify abnormalities. Ideally the protocol should include volumetric acquisition with a slice thickness of 1.5 mm or less in order to permit reformatting in any plane, volume measurements, and the possibility of three-dimensional reconstruction. A label of cryptogenic focal epilepsy should only be applied if the patient has

undergone such an MRI protocol and no evidence of relevant brain pathology has been found. Evidence that the epilepsy is focal will, of course, come from the clinical history and/or EEG findings. When evidence of focal pathology is found on MRI, the epilepsy should only be considered symptomatic if the abnormality is of a type that might be epileptogenic (e.g. this would be in doubt with a small arachnoid cyst) and is at a site in keeping with the clinical features of the epilepsy.

In particular, MRI has enabled detection of mesial temporal sclerosis, many cases with cortical dysgenesis, and a small number of cases with other structural lesions, including tumors, dysembryoplastic neuroepitheliomas, gangliogliomas, cavernous hemangiomas, and gliosis, that would not be detected by CT (Li *et al* 1995; Duncan 1997). With malformations of cortical development, 68% of cases in one MRI series had normal CT scans (Raymond *et al* 1995). Twenty years ago most temporal lobe epilepsy was cryptogenic, and in those undergoing temporal lobectomy the underlying pathology was often only identified by pathologic examination of the resection specimen (Bruton 1988). Now the majority of cases of intractable temporal lobe epilepsy can be labeled symptomatic following MRI, and there would be reservations about epilepsy surgery unless the underlying pathology had been identified preoperatively. In contrast, a relatively high proportion of patients with frontal lobe seizures can still only be labeled cryptogenic and surgical outcomes are less favorable.

Difficulty can arise when there is dual pathology, particularly when there is a combination of hippocampal sclerosis and another focal extrahippocampal lesion. This arises in 5–30% of patients with refractory focal epilepsy (Levesque *et al* 1991; Cascino *et al* 1993; Raymond *et al* 1994; Cendes *et al* 1995; Li *et al* 1995). Dual pathology occurs most commonly in patients with neuronal migration defects and cortical dysplasia; in particular, there is an association between hippocampal sclerosis and subependymal heterotopia (Cendes *et al* 1995; Li *et al* 1995). The epilepsy can be labeled symptomatic because of the presence of relevant pathology, but it also remains to an extent cryptogenic. This is because there is often uncertainty as to which of the lesions is epileptogenic, or whether both might be. The results of surgery in patients with dual pathology, where one of the lesions is hippocampal sclerosis, suggest that often both lesions are epileptogenic. Good results are obtained if both the atrophic hippocampus and the extrahippocampal lesion are removed; the chances of seizure freedom are less good if just one of the lesions is resected (Cascino *et al* 1993; Li *et al* 1997).

Another difficulty arises when epilepsy surgery fails and seizures persist, despite confirmation on MRI of the adequacy of resection and removal of the presumed epileptogenic lesion. Epilepsy confidently labeled symptomatic then becomes cryptogenic. In patients with hippocampal sclerosis who undergo surgery, this occurs in up to 30% (Bruton 1988; Engel 1996) and suggests that there may be undetected dual pathology. Contralateral temporal seizures and operative complications account for only a small proportion of the failures. A common cause, however, may be subtle extrahippocampal structural cortical abnormalities not detected on visual inspection of magnetic resonance images but revealed by quantitative postprocessing 'block analysis.' This has demonstrated widespread quantitative abnormalities not visible on visual inspection of magnetic resonance images in patients with cortical dysgenesis, suggesting that mild additional underlying malformation of cortical development is being detected (Sisodiya et al 1995). When quantitative postprocessing was performed on preoperative MRI scans of patients who had temporal lobe surgery and pathologically proven hippocampal sclerosis, extrahippocampal abnormalities were found in a much higher proportion of those who continued to have seizures than in those who became seizure-free (Sisodiya et al 1997). This suggests that mild malformations of cortical development may be present in a significant minority of patients with hippocampal sclerosis and could account for much of the cryptogenic epilepsy that emerges after unsuccessful temporal lobe surgery.

In some patients with dual pathology, hippocampal sclerosis has probably arisen as a consequence of the epileptic seizures and, indirectly, as a consequence of the second pathology. This is more likely when the degree of volume loss is relatively small. The association between prolonged febrile convulsions in early childhood and later temporal lobe epilepsy with underlying hippocampal sclerosis is well established. In infants MRI evidence has been obtained of acute hippocampal pathology arising during, or as an immediate consequence of status epilepticus or complex febrile convulsions, and of the subsequent development of hippocampal atrophy (DeLong and Heinz 1997; Van Landingham et al 1998). There are also a few reports of hippocampal atrophy emerging in adult patients after status epilepticus or generalized tonic–clonic seizures (Oxbury et al 1997; Wieshmann et al 1997). The results of long-term follow-up studies with MRI will determine how often, and to what extent, hippocampal atrophy emerges secondarily after the onset of chronic epilepsy.

Routine postprocessing of MRI in epilepsy, employing three-dimensional reconstruction with surface rendering, block analysis, and other techniques, would reduce the proportion of patients with cryptogenic focal epilepsy further. (Three-dimensional reformatting may allow detection of focal abnormalities of the gyral patterns not apparent on two-dimensional imaging.) At present these techniques are time-consuming, complex, and not routinely available. It is not necessary to apply them just to determine whether an epilepsy is symptomatic or cryptogenic. However, if a patient is a potential candidate for epilepsy surgery, it is likely that they will become mandatory. Nevertheless, even when all these techniques to detect structural brain abnormalities are applied, a small but significant proportion of patients with intractable focal epilepsy remains cryptogenic.

MANIFESTATIONS AND SPECULATION ON ETIOLOGY

The remaining patients with cryptogenic focal epilepsies have partial seizures, with or without secondary generalization, that may be either easily controlled or drug resistant. There are no specific EEG findings. There may be focal, multifocal, or bilateral epileptiform abnormalities or the EEG may be normal. In some patients the seizure semeiology and EEG findings indicate a consistent focal origin. In others the origin of the seizures remains uncertain. Patients with temporal lobe epilepsy are now less likely to be cryptogenic than those with frontal, parietal, or occipital lobe epilepsies.

Given that cryptogenic focal epilepsy is what remains after investigations to identify an etiology, it is likely to include patients with a variety of underlying disorders that are difficult to define with the currently available technology. There will be various genetic and acquired predisposing factors present in different proportions in different patients. These genetic factors may be predominant in some patients and additional idiopathic focal epilepsies may possibly emerge, as have familial temporal lobe epilepsy and autosomal dominant nocturnal frontal lobe epilepsy. It is probable that malformations of cortical development make a major contribution to cryptogenic focal epilepsy. The quantitative postprocessing of MRI discussed above has indicated that significant structural cortical abnormalities may be present despite normal visual analysis. Nevertheless, it is possible that some minor malformations (e.g. some neuronal migration disorders) may not be detectable by any current imaging techniques. There is likely to be a significant genetic contribution to many of these disorders.

Acquired factors that may underlie adult-onset cryptogenic focal epilepsies include prenatal and perinatal trauma (Bergamasco et al 1987), minor head injury, and cerebrovascular disease, the degree of associated brain injury not being detectable by current routine brain imaging techniques. The extent of the contribution of these acquired factors is uncertain. Cerebrovascular disease is likely to play a significant role in patients over the age of 60 years, when seizures may be the only manifestation. An increased incidence of silent infarcts has been found by CT scanning in patients presenting over the age of 40 years with epileptic seizures compared with age- and sex-matched controls (Roberts *et al* 1988). These patients had no history of symptoms suggestive of transient ischemic attacks or stroke. Infarcts were present in 15 of 132 patients presenting with epilepsy and in only 2 of 132 controls. Many of the infarcts were deep lacunes, which were presumably an indication of undetected cortical infarcts responsible for the epilepsy. Since the advent of MRI, which is more sensitive than CT, it is common to detect evidence of asymptomatic cerebrovascular disease in older subjects. In an individual older patient presenting with epilepsy it can sometimes be difficult to be certain about the relevance of mild ischemic changes on MRI, although in the absence of other causes for the epilepsy they are often likely to be significant. In a series of 176 cases presenting with a first stroke, 4.5% had a history of previous epileptic seizures, many of which were likely to have been the initial manifestation of the cerebrovascular disease (Shinton *et al* 1987).

There may still be a very small proportion of patients with hippocampal sclerosis not detected by MRI (Kuzniecky *et al* 1997), but this accounts for very few cases of cryptogenic focal epilepsy. Pathology in the amygdala is likely to be responsible for some cases, but at present they are not well recognized (Van Paesschen *et al* 1996).

Neuropathologic examination of post-mortem and epilepsy surgery specimens sometimes reveals previously unidentified abnormalities, such as neuronal migration disorders, and leads to reclassification of a focal epilepsy from cryptogenic to symptomatic. However, in some cryptogenic focal epilepsies the histopathology is normal. Standard neuropathologic examination may not detect any abnormality in focal epilepsies due to an alteration in the function of synapses and/or ion channels without structural abnormality. A challenge for the future is the identification of these functional changes. Molecular genetic techniques may be productive, as in familial frontal lobe epilepsy, with the emergence from the cryptogenic group of idiopathic focal epilepsy syndromes with a defined genetic cause. The increasing sophistication of PET and single-photon emission computed tomography (SPECT) and of magnetic resonance spectroscopy could play a role, but they face the difficulty of distinguishing between the abnormalities causing the seizures and those that are a consequence of them (Duncan 1997).

CONCLUSION

The proportion of patients labeled as having cryptogenic focal epilepsy will decrease as structural and functional imaging techniques improve and identify focal pathology better. There is likely to be improvement in our ability to identify patients with the idiopathic epilepsy syndromes as more of these syndromes are recognized and the underlying genetic causes are elucidated. We may perhaps look forward to the day when cryptogenic focal epilepsy will disappear.

KEY POINTS

1. By definition, idiopathic focal epilepsy syndromes are genetically determined and not due to definable structural brain pathology. The syndromes affecting adults include familial temporal lobe epilepsy (TLE), autosomal dominant nocturnal frontal lobe epilepsy, reading epilepsy, and hot water epilepsy.

2. The term 'cryptogenic focal epilepsy' is applied when the epilepsy is presumed to be symptomatic but underlying structural pathology cannot be defined. The prevalence of such cases decreases as the sophistication of investigation techniques increases. The diagnosis should only be considered after investigation with an appropriate MRI protocol has excluded the presence of relevant pathology.

3. Familial TLE may account for a considerable proportion of the cases of mild TLE that have previously been considered to be cryptogenic, but it can only account for a small proportion of cases with intractable TLE.

4. With currently available investigation techniques approximately 20% of cases of intractable focal epilepsy fall into the cryptogenic group.

5. A considerable proportion of the cases of 'cryptogenic' focal epilepsy presenting in adolescence and early adulthood may in reality be due to as yet undetermined genetic syndromes or to areas of cortical maldevelopment too small to be detected by visual inspection of MRI data. Cerebrovascular changes may be a major factor in those presenting in middle age and thereafter.

REFERENCES

Bergamasco B, Benna P, Ferrero P *et al* (1987) Neonatal hypoxia and epileptic risk. *Epilepsia* **25**:131–136.

Berkovic SF, McIntosh A, Howell RA *et al* (1996) Familial temporal lobe epilepsy: a common disorder identified in twins. *Annals of Neurology* **40**:227–235.

Bickford RG, Whelan JL, Klass DW *et al* (1956) Reading epilepsy: clinical and electroencephalographic studies of a new syndrome. *Transactions of the American Neurological Association* **81**:100–102.

Bruton CJ (1988) *The Neuropathology of Temporal Lobe Epilepsy*. Oxford: Oxford University Press.

Cascino GD, Jack CR Jr, Parisi JE *et al* (1993) Operative strategy in patients with MRI-identified dual pathology and temporal lobe epilepsy. *Epilepsy Research* **14**:175–182.

Cendes F, Cook MJ, Watson C *et al* (1995) Frequency and characteristics of dual pathology in patients with lesional epilepsy. *Neurology* **45**:2058–2064.

Commission on Classification and Terminology of the International League Against Epilepsy (1985) Proposal for classification of epilepsy and epileptic syndromes. *Epilepsia* **26**:268–278.

Commission on Classification and Terminology of the International League Against Epilepsy (1989) Proposal for revised classification of epilepsies and epileptic syndromes. *Epilepsia* **30**:389–399.

Cook M, Stevens JM (1995) Imaging in epilepsy. In: Hopkins A, Shorvon S, Cascino G (eds) *Epilepsy*, 2nd edn, pp 143–169. London: Chapman & Hall.

DeLong GR, Heinz ER (1997) The clinical syndrome of early-life bilateral hippocampal sclerosis. *Annals of Neurology* **42**:11–17.

Duncan JS (1997) Imaging and epilepsy. *Brain* **120**:339–377.

Duncan JS, Fish DR (1998) Seizure disorders: integration of structural and functional data. *Current Opinion in Neurology* **11**:119–122.

Engel J Jr (1996) Surgery for seizures. *New England Journal of Medicine* **334**:647–652.

Gastaut H, Gastaut JL (1976) Computerised axial transverse tomography in epilepsy. *Epilepsia* **17**:325–336.

Hopkins A, Garman A, Clarke C (1988) The first seizure in adult life. Value of clinical features, electroencephalography and computerised tomographic scanning in prediction of seizure recurrence. *Lancet* **i**:721–726.

International League Against Epilepsy Neuroimaging Commission (1997) ILAE Neuroimaging Commission recommendations for neuro-imaging of patients with epilepsy. *Epilepsia* **38**(Suppl 10):1–2.

Koepp MJ, Hansen M, Pressler RM *et al* (1998) Comparison of EEG, MRI and PET in reading epilepsy: a case report. *Epilepsy Research* **29**:251–257.

Koutroumanidis M, Koepp MJ, Richardson MP *et al* (1998) The variants of reading epilepsy. A clinical and video-EEG study of 17 patients with reading-induced seizures. *Brain* **121**:1409–1427.

Kuzniecky RI, Jackson G, Morawetz R *et al* (1997) Multimodality MRI in mesial temporal sclerosis: relative sensitivity and specificity. *Neurology* **49**:774–778.

Levesque MS, Nakasato N, Vinters HV *et al* (1991) Surgical treatment of limbic epilepsy associated with extrahippocampal lesions: the problem of dual pathology. *Journal of Neurosurgery* **75**:364–370.

Li LM, Fish DR, Sisodiya SM *et al* (1995) High resolution magnetic resonance imaging in adults with partial or secondary generalised epilepsy attending a tertiary referral unit. *Journal of Neurology, Neurosurgery and Psychiatry* **59**:384–387.

Li LM, Cendes MD, Watson MD *et al* (1997) Surgical treatment of patients with single and dual pathology: relevance of lesion and of hippocampal atrophy to seizure outcome. *Neurology* **48**:437–444.

Lugaresi E, Cirignotta F, Montagna P (1986) Nocturnal paroxysmal dystonia. *Journal of Neurology, Neurosurgery and Psychiatry* **49**:375–380.

Manford M, Hart YM, Sander JWAS *et al* (1992) National General Practice Study of Epilepsy (NGPSE). The syndromic classification of the International League against Epilepsy applied to epilepsy in a general population. *Archives of Neurology* **49**:801–808.

Oldani A, Zucconi M, Asselta R *et al* (1998) Autosomal dominant nocturnal frontal lobe epilepsy: a video-polysomnographic and genetic appraisal of 40 patients and delineation of the epileptic syndrome. *Brain* **121**:205–223.

Ottman R, Risch N, Hauser WA *et al* (1995) Localization of a gene for partial epilepsy to chromosome 10q. *Nature Genetics* **10**:56–60.

Oxbury S, Oxbury J, Renowden S *et al* (1997) Severe amnesia: an unusual late complication after temporal lobectomy. *Neuropsychologia* **35**:975–988.

Radhakrishnan K, Silbert PL, Klass DW (1995) Reading epilepsy. An appraisal of 20 patients diagnosed at the Mayo Clinic, Rochester, Minnesota, between 1949 and 1989, and delineation of the epileptic syndrome. *Brain* **118**:75–89.

Ramani V (1998) Reading epilepsy. *Advances in Neurology* **75**:241–262.

Ramirez-Lassepas M, Cipolle RJ, Morillo LR *et al* (1984) Value of computed tomographic scan in the evaluation of adult patients after their first seizure. *Annals of Neurology* **15**:536–543.

Raymond AA, Fish DR, Stevens JM *et al* (1994) Association of hippocampal sclerosis with cortical dysgenesis in patients with epilepsy. *Neurology* **44**:1841–1845.

Raymond AA, Fish DR, Sisodiya SM *et al* (1995) Abnormalities of gyration, heterotopias, tuberous sclerosis, focal cortical dysplasia, microdysgenesis, dysembryoplastic neuroepithelial tumour and dysgenesis of the archicortex in epilepsy. Clinical, EEG and neuroimaging features in 100 adult patients. *Brain* **118**:629–660.

Remillard GM, Zifkin BG, Andermann F (1998) Seizures induced by eating. *Advances in Neurology* **75**:227–240.

Roberts RC, Shorvon SD, Cox TC *et al* (1988) Clinically unsuspected cerebral infarction revealed by computed tomography scanning in late onset epilepsy. *Epilepsia* **29**:190–194.

Saenz-Lope E, Herranz-Tanarro FJ, Masdeu JC (1985) Primary reading epilepsy. *Epilepsia* **26**:649–656.

Satishchandra P, Shivaramakrishana A, Kaliaperumal VG *et al* (1988) Hot water epilepsy: a variant of reflex epilepsy in Southern India. *Epilepsia* **29**:52–56.

Satishchandra P, Ullal GR, Shankar SK (1998) Hot water epilepsy. *Advances in Neurology* **75**:285–293.

Scheffer IE, Bhatia KP, Lopes-Cendes I *et al* (1995) Autosomal dominant nocturnal frontal lobe epilepsy: a distinctive clinical disorder. *Brain* **118**:61–73.

Schoenenberger RA, Heim SM (1994) Indication for computed tomography of the brain in patients with first uncomplicated generalised seizure. *British Medical Journal* **309**:986–989.

Shinton RA, Gill JS, Zezulka AV *et al* (1987) The frequency of epilepsy preceding stroke. *Lancet* **i**:11–13.

Singh B, Anderson L, al Gashlan M *et al* (1995) Reading induced absence seizures. *Neurology* **45**:1623–1624.

Sisodiya SM, Free SL, Stevens JM *et al* (1995) Widespread cerebral structural changes in patients with cortical dysgenesis and epilepsy. *Brain* **118**:1039–1050.

Sisodiya SM, Moran N, Free SL *et al* (1997) Correlation of widespread preoperative magnetic resonance imaging changes with unsuccessful surgery for hippocampal sclerosis. *Annals of Neurology* **41**:490–496.

Steinlein OK, Mulley JC, Propping P *et al* (1995) A missense mutation in the neuronal nicotinic acetylcholine receptor alpha4 subunit is associated with autosomal dominant frontal lobe epilepsy. *Nature Genetics* **11**:201–203.

Steinlein OK, Magnussen A, Stoodt J *et al* (1997) An insertion mutation of the CHRNA4 gene in a family with autosomal dominant frontal lobe epilepsy. *Human Molecular Genetics* **6**:943–947.

Van Landingham KE, Heinz ER, Cavazos JE *et al* (1998) Magnetic resonance imaging evidence of hippocampal injury after prolonged focal febrile convulsions. *Annals of Neurology* **43**:413–426.

Van Paesschen W, Connelly A, Johnson CL *et al* (1996) The amygdala and intractable temporal lobe epilepsy: a quantitative magnetic resonance imaging study. *Neurology* **47**:1021–1031.

Wieser HG, Hungerbuhler H, Siegel AM *et al* (1997) Musicogenic epilepsy: review of the literature and case report with ictal single photon emission computed tomography. *Epilepsia* **38**:200–207.

Wieshmann UC, Woermann FG, Lemieux L *et al* (1997) Development of hippocampal atrophy: a serial magnetic resonance imaging study in a patient who developed epilepsy after generalised status epilepticus. *Epilepsia* **38**:1238–1241.

Wolf P (1992) Reading epilepsy. In: Roger J, Bureau M, Dravet C *et al* (eds) *Epileptic Syndromes in Infancy, Childhood and Adolescence*, 2nd edn, pp 281–298. London: John Libbey.

Young AC, Costanzi JB, Mohr PD *et al* (1982) Is routine axial tomography in epilepsy worthwhile? *Lancet* **ii**:1446–1447.

Zifkin BG, Zatorre RJ (1998) Musicogenic epilepsy. *Advances in Neurology* **75**:273–281.

Landau-Kleffner syndrome

BGR NEVILLE, V BURCH, H CASS, AND J LEES

Landau–Kleffner syndrome (LKS) is an uncommon and poorly understood form of childhood epilepsy. In this chapter we suggest that the definition commonly used may be broadened to inform treatment approaches, discuss the need for appropriate outcome measures to demonstrate response to treatment, and review previous treatment studies and their generally inadequate outcome measures. We also illustrate the benefits of a focused multidisciplinary clinical and research team in the management of children with LKS.

DEFINITION

Classically this condition manifests as normal development in a child up to the age of 2 years or more with subsequent loss of language comprehension and speech but with preservation of nonlanguage cognitive functions. The context is one of seizures, usually complex partial and often severe, with a proportion of children (20–30%) having no clinical seizures but all demonstrating interictal centrotemporal discharges that increase in slow-wave sleep. No lesion is apparent on magnetic resonance imaging (MRI). The condition may show a dramatic response to antiepileptic drugs, particularly corticosteroids, or may leave the child with long-term impairments of compre-

hension. In a chapter devoted to treatment it is necessary to examine the appropriateness of this classical definition. A restricted definition based upon theoretic constructs could exclude children with a much wider range of impairments who do however have the core features of the syndrome and could be potentially treatable. The grounds for widening the spectrum of LKS-like disorders are discussed but bring a wider range of treatment problems into the argument. There are several effects of widening the definition to include children who, in addition to acquired aphasia, have attention deficit, hyperactivity sometimes amounting to mania, motor organizational problems, features within the autistic spectrum, and global regression. Assessment tools have to be able to assess each of these important domains of function. The measures have to be sensitive to change and able to be repeated fairly frequently. The assessment team has to possess skills in developmental neurology, speech and language, developmental psychology, and behavioral disorder and be able to work with a group of children with markedly fluctuating levels of function.

One danger is that by attempting to be inclusive we run the risk of using potentially hazardous treatments, particularly corticosteroids and surgery, on an *ad hoc* basis without any clear ability to document the results of treatment. However, our experience suggests that a wide definition is appropriate for treatment and management purposes. Thus our operational definition has the following elements.

1. There is a clear acquired loss of language function that is not explained by a defined degenerative disorder; this is an early presenting feature of the condition. Language may be affected at any level: a verbal auditory agnosia (Cooper and Ferry 1978), word finding difficulty and reading difficulties (Dugas *et al* 1976), paraphasias (Van der Sandt-Koenderman *et al* 1984), and defects of prosody (Deonna *et al* 1987).
2. There is a typical centrotemporal EEG abnormality, enhanced by slow-wave sleep.
3. The language disorder may be accompanied by a behavioral disorder, typically attention deficit and hyperactivity that may be severe, lack of impulse control, apathy sometimes amounting to catatonia-like lack of activity, and obsessional behavior.
4. There may be all degrees of loss of social functioning, often with marked autistic features.
5. There may be a degree of global loss of cognitive function.
6. There are motor impairments, particularly bulbar and global apraxia.

Two further groups of children should be mentioned but kept as subgroups since a similar picture of regression may be seen: (i) children with early mild or moderate developmental delay, and (ii) children with lesions that may require different treatment.

This consensus has developed within our multidisciplinary group, which has been managing a large group of children with acquired epilepsy-related aphasia. Interestingly, in the original publication of Landau and Kleffner (1957) the children were reported to have, in addition to aphasia, a range of other problems including situational rigidity, attention difficulties, hyperkinesis, negativism, being hard to manage, behavior suggestive of psychogenic regression, and enuresis. This association is repeated in other reports (Dugas *et al* 1976). The lack of behavioral problems seen by Worster-Drought (1971), an astute clinical observer, probably reflects the selection criteria for the special school that the children in his study attended.

Our purpose has been to provide objective measures of treatment within this very difficult group of children. Reports of treatment outcomes in the literature are weak with regard to numbers, objective measures, case definition, and planned studies; no controlled studies are currently available.

MODELS OF PATHOGENESIS

NEUROPHYSIOLOGIC MODEL

LKS is an example of a relatively selective 'epileptic encephalopathy.' This term is used to describe situations in which there is a loss of cerebral function in association with epilepsy, particularly subclinical epilepsy. The lack of any change on MRI or in rate of head growth supports the notion that this is a direct functional effect of seizures inhibiting specific cortical function rather than a progressive neurologic disease. Although the clinical features fluctuate, they are relatively much more stable than the paroxysmal events typical of epilepsy. The mechanisms of this process are not known, although selective temporal lobe hypoperfusion (McKinney and McGreal 1974; O'Tuara *et al* 1992) and hypometabolism (Deuel and Lenn 1977; Rintahaka *et al* 1995) are reported in some patients. However, the evidence is not consistent regarding localization or even lateralization and several reports of hypermetabolism exist in sedated children in which the scans are presumed to be ictal (Morell *et al* 1995). One of the main factors that any discussion on pathogenesis has to engage is the potential reversibility of all aspects of the disorder.

A subgroup of developmental epilepsies that have been designated as malignant (infantile polymorphic, West syndrome, Lennox–Gastaut syndrome) share two features of their natural history, developmental arrest and regression, with LKS. Measures of 'intractability' and outcome in all these syndromes have to include cognitive and behavioral assessments as well as seizure frequency. Most treatments have aimed at terminating seizures using drugs, and although some notable successes have been achieved we are still uncertain if this will remain the first line of therapy in the future. It tends to be assumed that the drugs act by stopping seizures even though these medications, particularly corticosteroids, have a wide range of other effects.

Single cases do not make good evidence for the general application of treatments; however, the phenomena observed in individuals have to be explained by our hypotheses. The occasional total recovery of all language, motor, and behavioral impairments has to be regarded as strong evidence against an acquired structural lesion and in favor of some mechanism like epileptic seizures, be they clinical or subclinical, that can be switched off with suitable treatment. The secondary hypothesis is that centrotemporal subclinical seizures, particularly in sleep, though focal in origin can severely disrupt function bilaterally in the cortical regions that subsume language.

LINGUISTIC MODEL

The level at which language processing is blocked in LKS is of interest. The finding of habituation to the same phoneme and 'recognition' of a new phoneme by cortical auditory-coded responses in a child with maximal communication regression (Boyd *et al* 1996) and the assertion by one girl that she could understand but not react to speech (Neville and Boyd 1995) suggests a new language defect, i.e. inability to respond to processed speech.

There are interesting analogies with benign epilepsy with centrotemporal (rolandic) spikes. The similarities include seizure semeiology, EEG abnormality, the occurrence of bulbar apraxia (Deonna 1993; Scheffer *et al* 1995), and of a mild but significant language processing disorder in over half of one series (Staden *et al* 1998). However, these impairments do not appear to be a continuous spectrum but are bimodally distributed between mild and severe impairments. They help to focus the question of what is the pathogenic mechanism that throws the cognitive switch in LKS.

LESIONAL MODELS

The lesional cases, particularly those with dysembryoplastic neuroepithelial tumors, provide some important clues to pathogenesis that are important in planning new treatments.

1. The lesions tend to be developmental masses of the temporal lobe.
2. They may affect the right or left temporal lobe.
3. There is a specifically highly regressive presentation that we have observed in five children with onset of epilepsy in the first year who suffered severe arrest and regression of cognitive and communication function.

LKS is an epilepsy syndrome dominated by subclinical seizure activity in one or both centrotemporal regions. Although usually nonlesional, it may be related to developmental lesions of the temporal lobes, in which the seizure activity far from being a stimulus to relocation of function appears to prevent any further language development. The impairments are potentially reversible if seizure activity can be prevented from affecting the other temporal lobe (assuming that the seizures arise unilaterally). Clinical seizure control is largely irrelevant and cognitive, psychiatric, and behavioral outcome measures are essential.

TREATMENT

Logically these arguments lead to a hierarchy of treatment aims. Can the seizure activity be stopped by either drugs or surgical resection of a lesion? Can the spread of seizure activity be limited by drugs or a functional surgical disconnection procedure? Can the behavioral components of the syndrome be directly treated if they persist despite primary vigorous treatment of the epilepsy? The regular reporting of spontaneous recovery of individual cases has to be remembered in assessing the reports of therapeutic 'cure'.

MEASUREMENT OF TREATMENT RESPONSES

The problems previously encountered with assessment have been the difficulties with compliance for severely regressed children, the wide range of performance levels, including some children with very low levels of function, the need to repeat testing at short intervals to measure treatment responses, and the importance of documenting changes in behavior, all of which allow longitudinal studies to be conducted. Because of the lack of appropriate methods for monitoring treatment responses we have developed a test battery of both formal and criterion-referenced assessments (Cass *et al* in preparation). The elements of this test battery are measures of attention level, formal language, constructive play, cognitive ability, behavior, social communication, social interaction, and spontaneous activity. This schedule has been used on a series of 20 children in an ABA controlled study on the use of antiepileptic drugs, particularly corticosteroids (Lees *et al* 1998).

ANTIEPILEPTIC DRUGS

All the antiepileptic drugs have been used in LKS. Usually the clinical seizures respond easily, although a small minority are much more difficult to control and may occasionally not even respond to corticosteroids. Improvements of cognitive impairment in single cases have been reported but have not led to a consistent message about management.

CORTICOSTEROIDS

Evidence for the efficacy of corticosteroids has been found in small series and single cases, which tend to lack consistency in case definition, steroid dosage and length of treatment, measures of efficacy, and longitudinal information. These studies are shown in Table 22.1 and the small size and scientific weakness of the evidence is apparent. All that one can say is that sufficient children have

Table 22.1 Corticosteroids in Landau–Kleffner syndrome.

Reference	No. of patients	Corticosteroid regimen	Outcome	Outcome measures
McKinney and McGreal (1974)	3	ACTH/prednisolone ACTH ACTH/gammaglobulin	Normal speech Complete recovery 'Normal'	'Clinical'
Lerman et al (1991)	4	ACTH 80 U > 0.3 y ×2 Prednisolone 60 mg > 0.5 y Prednisolone 60 mg > 0.3 y Dexamethasone 4 mg > 0.3 y	All five episodes recovered	'Clinical'
Kellerman (1978)	1	Prednisolone ×2	Three episodes without recovery	'Clinical'
Van der Sandt-Koenderman et al (1984)	1	Prednisolone ×2	Partial improvements	
Zardini et al (1995)	1	ACTH 100 U > 0.10 y	Significant improvement	WISC/language assessment
White and Sreenivasa (1987) Deuel and Lenn (1977)	1	Prednisolone	No improvement	'Clinical'
Vance (1991)	1	'Steroids'	Continuing problems (report not really used to study steroid response)	Language assessment
Marescaux et al (1990)	3	Hydrocortisone 12 mg kg^{-1} day^{-1} Prednisolone 2 mg kg^{-1} day^{-1}	Significant and useful improvements	'Clinical'
Perez et al (1993)	3	Prednisolone 2 mg kg^{-1} day^{-1}	Child 1: progressive improvement incomplete and relapsed Child 2: behavioral improvement but significant cognitive deficits persisted Child 3: improved behavior and performance	Standardized established tests but problems with low functioning children and behavioral questionnaire
Lanzi et al (1994)	1	Methylprednisolone 1 mg kg^{-1} ×2, 8 mg kg^{-1} ×1	Improvement in language	Language assessment
Nevismalova et al (1992)	4	Not given	Three of four improved	'Clinical'
Papagano and Basso (1993)	1	ACTH	Aphasia unchanged, seizures stopped	Language and neuropsychologic tests
Paquier et al (1992)	1	Prednisolone	Partial response	'Clinical'
Aykut-Bingoleta et al (1996)	1	Methylprednisolone 500 mg day^{-1} i.v. for 5 days then 250 mg monthly	Significant improvement	WISC and language tests
Carabello et al (in press)	2	Prednisolone 1 mg kg^{-1} day^{-1} for 6–8 months	Near full recovery	'Clinical'
Chamlin et al (1992)	2	Prednisolone 2 and 3 mg kg^{-1} day^{-1} for 4–6 weeks	Dramatic speech recovery and speech improvement	'Clinical'
Genton et al (1992)	1	Prednisolone 2 mg kg^{-1} day^{-1}	Marked slow recovery of speech	'Clinical'
Genton et al (1995)	1	Prednisolone	Rapid improvement and relapse	'Clinical'

ACTH, adrenocorticotropic hormone; WISC, Wechsler Intelligence Scale for Children.

shown improvement in language at a time closely related to use of corticosteroids that it seems likely that some children with LKS respond to corticosteroids. The need is for studies that use appropriate measures, sufficient numbers, consistent treatment regimens, and some element of control in the data. In our series of children treated with 2 mg kg^{-1} day^{-1} prednisolone for 6 weeks, followed by a 6-week weaning period, more than half showed useful improvement using formal and criterion-referenced developmental assessments (Lees et al 1998).

MULTIPLE SUBPIAL TRANSECTION

Evaluation of multiple subpial transection, pioneered by the late Frank Morell and colleagues in Chicago (Morell et al 1995), needs more cases than the 18 currently reported (Table 22.2). The Chicago group were very selective, particularly excluding children with autism and other evidence of widespread cognitive deficit. They used mainly the methohexital suppression test to identify a 'driving' hemisphere, although other techniques to identify lateralization and localization, including carotid amobarbital and

Table 22.2 Multiple subpial transection in Landau–Kleffner syndrome.

Reference	No. of patients	Stage of syndrome (years)	Age (years)	Outcome	Outcome measures
Morell et al (1995)	14	2+	5–13	Six recovered age-appropriate speech Five showed marked improvement	Not given

Sawkney et al (1995)	3
	(1 pres)
		5
		3
			10
			14
				Mute: sentences after treatment
				Substantial improvement
				  Mute: useful speech
				  Recovery of social functioning
					Not given

		4	8	Mute: single words after treatment	
Neville et al (1997)	1	2	7	Recovery of social communication but language delay persists	Informal developmental measures

Table 22.3 Resective surgery in Landau–Kleffner syndrome.

Reference	No. of patients	Procedure	Outcome	Outcome measures
Cole et al (1987)	2 (nonlesional)	Temporal lobectomy	Rapid improvement in speech	WISC
		Temporal lobectomy	No change in language	Language tests and dictative listening
McKinney and McGreal (1974)	1	Temporal lobectomy	Almost normal speech and improved understanding	Not given
Deonna (1993)	1	Removal of lesion from foramen of Monro for tuberous sclerosis	Possible lessening of autistic features	Autism scales and WISC
Neville et al (1997)	1	Right temporal resection for dysembryoplastic neuroepichelioma	Improvement in autistic features	Informal developmental measures

WISC, Wechsler Intelligence Scale for Children.

magnetic source imaging, were also employed. Their data suggest that those with selective language deficits ('true LKS') have discharges limited to the parietotemporal regions, with a sylvian dipole with frontal negativity in a group of 13 children and temporal positivity. Magnetic source imaging supports the more localized abnormality in these children and the presence of multiple generator sites in those with wider cognitive and behavioral phenotypes (Morell *et al* 1997). They categorize these patients as 'LKS look-alikes' and 'electrographic imposters'. This may not be appropriate if one is using the categories as a method of choosing those who may respond to treatment, based upon the primary hypothesis that nonconvulsive status is interfering with higher cortical function. Of the 14 procedures carried out by Morell and colleagues, four were performed on the right hemisphere; only a mild morbidity was reported.

As far as the evidence goes it suggests that multiple subpial transection planned in the manner described can be followed by major improvement. However the variables of initial lateralization, extent of surgery (i.e. cortex transected and details of these transections, e.g. into the sylvian

fissure), and the patchy nature of the outcome measures leave doubt about the individual components of the procedure. Clearly more cases are needed, with full details of the assessment used to judge the efficacy and indications for this procedure. The physiologic basis for the procedure, i.e prevention of lateral spread of seizure activity in the cortex whilst allowing the long neuronal connections at right angles to the cortex to function, remains a hypothesis. However, Morell's results have encouraged several centers to perform this procedure and their findings are awaited.

RESECTIVE SURGERY

The results of resective surgery, both nonlesional and lesional, are too sparse for any conclusions except that, on general principles, regression associated with complex partial seizures and a resectable lesion should be urgently considered for surgery (Table 22.3). The earliest operation, a temporal resection at 12 months, was followed by some recovery (Neville *et al* 1997).

MANAGEMENT

The comprehensive management of LKS is a complex and difficult subject. It is essential that if speech is severely impaired an alternative system of communication should be offered. The sophistication of the system, which will depend on cognitive level, continuing communicative intent, and the functions that survive, may range from simple picture communication boards through simple and complex signing systems to the use of writing. The use of such techniques may be dependent on effective management of behavior problems. Attention deficit and hyperactivity are very common and require assessment, careful planning of the structure of the child's life, and family support. Methylphenidate or dexamphetamine may be very effective in some children, sometimes revealing cognitive skills that may not be evident until attention control is improved. Not infrequently the level of activity and lack of

impulse control may produce a condition of dangerous mania that requires high levels of additional care and support, sometimes best provided in a residential setting. Specific interventions and education for autistic spectrum disorder may be required. Thus a multidisciplinary team with neurologic, developmental, behavioral, cognitive, and speech and language skills are needed for assessment and management; it is absolutely essential that there is liaison between the team and the home, school, and local medical services (Neville *et al* 1997).

The management of LKS therefore has most of the problems that characterize pediatric epilepsy practice. None of these are unique to LKS and are seen in other syndromes of childhood epilepsy. However their concentration and severity in LKS provide a formidable test of our ability to help and a clear message about the importance of nonmedical agencies. Family support groups are an important source of education and encouragement and help to focus the efforts of professionals.

KEY POINTS

1. Landau–Kleffner syndrome (LKS) is a relatively selective epileptic encephalopathy manifest by loss of language function in a child who has previously developed normally in association with seizures in 70–80% cases and with a centro-temporal EEG abnormality enhanced by slow-wave sleep. Non-language cognitive functions are relatively preserved. There may be behavior disorder, bulbar and global apraxia, and a loss of social functioning with autistic features.

2. The EEG abnormality may be unilateral or bilateral. Brain MRI is usually normal but focal pathology such as a dysembryoplastic neuroepithelial tumor is found in some cases, most often in a temporal lobe (left or right).

3. Clinical seizures usually respond easily to antiepileptic drug treatment but the aphasia rarely does so. Language function improvement may be brought about by treatment with corticosteroids or by multiple subpial transection in the parietotemporal region on the side driving the EEG abnormality (usually left), if that can be established.

REFERENCES

Aykut-Bingoleta C, Arman A, Tokol O *et al* (1996) Pulse methylprednisolone therapy in Landau–Kleffner syndrome. *Journal of Epilepsy* 9:189–191.

Boyd SG, Rivera-Gaxiolo M, Towell AD *et al* (1996) Discrimination of speech sounds in a boy with Landau–Kleffner syndrome: an intraoperative event-related potential study. *Neuropediatrics* 27:211–215.

Carabello RH *et al* (in press) Long-term steroid treatment in two patients with acquired epileptic aphasia. *Pediatric Neurology* 8:364.

Cass HD, Lees JA, Waring M, Burch V, Neville BGR Developmental correlates of centro-temporal epilepsy: a review of the literature and model for assessment (in preparation).

Chamlin SL, Chez M, Heydemann P, Van Slyke P (1992) Prednisone therapy in Landau–Kleffner syndrome: improved speech performance and correlating EEG changes. *Annals of Neurology* 32:476.

Cooper JA, Ferry PC (1978) Acquired auditory verbal agnosia and

seizures in childhood. *Journal of Speech and Hearing Disorders* XLIII:176–184.

Deonna T (1993) Cognitive and behavioural correlates of epileptic activity in children. *Journal of Child Psychology and Psychiatry and Allied Disciplines* 34:611–620.

Deonna T, Cheurie C, Hornung E (1987) Childhood epileptic speech disorder: prolonged isolated deficit of prosodic features. *Developmental Medicine and Child Neurology* 29:96–109.

Deuel RK, Lenn NJ (1977) Treatment of acquired epileptic aphasia. *Journal of Pediatrics* 90:959–961.

Dugas M, Grenet P, Masson M, Mialet JP, Jaquet G (1976) Childhood aphasia with epilepsy remission with antiepileptic treatment. *Revue Neurologique* 132:489–493.

Genton P, Maton B, Ogihara M *et al* (1992) Continuous focal spikes during REM sleep in a case of acquired aphasia (Landau–Kleffner syndrome). *Sleep* 15:454–460.

Genton P, Guerrini R, Bureau M, Dravet C (1995) Continuous focal discharges during REM sleep in a case of Landau–Kleffner syndrome: a 3 year follow-up. In: *Continuous Spikes and Waves during Slow Sleep*, pp 155–159.

Kellerman K (1978) Recurrent aphasia with subclinical bioelectric status epilepticus during sleep. *European Journal of Pediatrics* **128**:207–212.

Landau WM, Kleffner FR (1957) Syndrome of acquired aphasia with convulsive disorder in children. *Neurology* 7:523–531.

Lanzi G *et al* (1994) A correlated fluctuation of language and EEG abnormalities in a case of the Landau–Kleffner. **16**:329–334.

Lees JA, Cass H, Waring M, Burch VM, Neville BGR (1998) Measuring response to pharmacological treatment in children with epilepsy related aphasias (Landau–Kleffner syndrome) (Abstract). *Developmental Medicine and Child Neurology* 77:9.

Lerman P, Lerman-Sagie T (1989) Early steroid therapy in Landau–Kleffner syndrome. *Advances in Epileptology* 17:330–360.

Lerman P, Lerman-Sagie T, Kivity S (1991) Effect of early corticosteroid therapy for Landau–Kleffner syndrome. *Developmental Medicine and Child Neurology* 33:257–266.

McKinney W, McGreal DA (1974) An aphasic syndrome in children. *Medical Association Journal* 110:636–639.

Marescaux C, Hirsh E, Finck S *et al* (1990) Landau–Kleffner syndrome: a pharmacologic study of five cases. *Epilepsia* 31:768–777.

Morell F, Whisler WW, Smith MC *et al* (1995) Landau–Kleffner syndrome: treatment with subpial intracortical transection. *Brain* **118**:1529–1546.

Morell F, Kanner AM, Hoeppner TJ, Detoledo-Morrell L, Whisler WW (1997) Surgical treatment of Landau-Kleffner syndrome. In: *Paediatric Epilepsy Syndromes and their Surgical Treatment*. London: John Libbey.

Neville BGR, Boyd SG (1995) Selective epileptic gait disorder. *Journal of Neurology, Neurosurgery and Psychiatry* **58**:371–373.

Neville BGR, Harkness WJF, Cross JH *et al* (1997) Surgical treatment of severe autistic regression in childhood epilepsy. *Pediatric Neurology* **16**:137–140.

Nevsimalova S, Tauberova A, Doutlik S, Kucera V, Dlouha O (1992) A role of autoimmunity in the etiopathogenesis of Landau–Kleffner syndrome. *Brain and Development* 14:342–345.

O'Tuara LA, Urion DK, Janicek MJ, Treves ST, Bjornson B, Moriarty JM (1992) Regional cerebral perfusion in Landau–Kleffner syndrome and related childhood aphasias. *Journal of Nuclear Medicine* **33**:1758–1765.

Papagano C, Basso A (1993) Impairment of written language and mathematical skills in a case of Landau–Kleffner syndrome. *Aphasiology* 7:451–461.

Paquier PF, Van Dongen H, Loonen C (1992) The Landau–Kleffner syndrome of 'acquired aphasia with convulsive disorder'. *Archives of Neurology* 49:354–359.

Perez *et al* (1993).

Rintahaka PJ, Chugani HT, Sankar R (1995) Landau–Kleffner syndrome with continuous spikes and waves during slow-wave sleep. *Journal of Child Neurology* **10**:127–133.

Scheffer IE, Jones L, Pozzebon M, Howell RA, Saling MM, Berkovic SF (1995) Autosomal dominant rolandic epilepsy and speech dyspraxia: a new syndrome with anticipation. *Annals of Neurology* **38**:633–642.

Staden U, Isaacs E, Boyd SG, Brandl U, Neville BGR (1998) Language dysfunction in children with Rolandic epilepsy. *Neuropediatrics* (in press).

Vance M (1991) Educational and therapeutic used with a child presenting with acquired aphasia with convulsive disorder (Landau–Kleffner syndrome). *Child Language Teaching and Therapy* **XX**:41–60.

Van der Sandt-Koenderman WME, Smit IAC, van Dongen, van Hest JBC (1984) A case of acquired aphasia and convulsive disorder: some linguistic aspects of recovery and breakdown. *Brain and Language* 21:174–183.

White H, Sreenivasa V (1987) Epilepsy–aphasia syndrome in children: an unusual presentation to psychiatry. *Canadian Journal of Psychiatry* **32**:509–601.

Worster-Drought C (1971) An unusual form of acquired aphasia in children. *Developmental Medicine and Child Neurology* 13:563–571.

Zardini G, Molteni B, Nardocci N, Sarti D, Avanzini G, Granata T (1995) Linguistic development in a patient with Landau–Kleffner syndrome: a nine-year follow-up. *Neuropediatrics* **26**:19–25.

Partial seizures in West syndrome 23

S WEISS AND OC SNEAD

West syndrome is defined as the clinical triad of infantile spasms, arrest of psychomotor development, and the typical EEG pattern of hypsarrhythmia (Commission on Classification and Terminology of the International League Against Epilepsy 1989), and is the most important member of the catastrophic seizure disorders that occur in childhood (Shields *et al* 1992). The first clinical description of infantile spasms was made in 1841 by West in a letter to *Lancet*, in which he described a mysterious malady afflicting his son characterized by 'bobbings of the head' and 'bowings and relaxings' in clusters of 'from ten to twenty or more times at each attack' and a progressive deterioration of intellect such that '[he] never smiles or takes any notice, but looks placid and pitiful.' The clinical presentation of infantile spasms, so lucidly described by West, has been further characterized by continuous monitoring with EEG-videotelemetry (Kellaway *et al* 1979). The spasms may be divided into flexor, extensor, and mixed, with mixed spasms being the most common and extensor spasms the least common. Flexor spasms consist of flexion of the neck, trunk, arms, and legs. Abdominal flexion may be massive, giving rise to the 'jack-knife' or 'salaam' seizures that are the hallmark of infantile spasms. During extensor spasms, there is abrupt extension of the neck, trunk, and legs. The mixed flexor–extensor spasms are characterized by flexion of the neck, trunk, and arms, and extension of the legs. Infantile spasms usually occur in clusters many times daily but particularly upon awakening, and are often associated with a cry. Infantile spasms are associated with a mortality of 10–20% and a morbidity of 75–90% (Jeavons and Bower 1964; Jeavons *et al* 1973; Lacy and Penry 1976) that consists of moderate to severe mental retardation. Infantile spasms are quite age-specific, usually occurring within the first 6 months of life. The incidence declines rapidly after 12 months, and the spasms seldom occur after the age of 4 years (Holmes 1987).

The EEG abnormality classically associated with infantile spasms was described as 'hypsarrhythmic' by Gibbs and Gibbs (1952). This term refers to high-voltage chaotic slowing, multifocal spikes, and marked asynchrony. Since the 1950s the definition of hypsarrhythmia has been broadened to include areas of focal abnormality, focal asynchrony, asymmetrical hypsarrhythmia, and/or burst suppression (Hrachovy *et al* 1984).

CLASSIFICATION OF WEST SYNDROME: A GENERALIZED OR LOCALIZATION-RELATED EPILEPSY SYNDROME?

West syndrome may be classified etiologically as either symptomatic or cryptogenic. Infantile spasms in symptomatic West syndrome result from a clearly delineated structural brain abnormality or well-defined metabolic cause in a child who usually has a preexisting neurologic and/or developmental abnormality. Cryptogenic spasms occur in a child who may or may not have a preexisting developmental or neurologic abnormality, but in whom all neuroimaging and metabolic studies are normal. Recently, it has been proposed that a third group, idiopathic spasms, be added to this group. The idiopathic group of West syndrome may be defined by normal development before the onset of symmetric spasms without any other kind of seizure, normal clinical examination, normal neuroimaging studies, recurrence of hypsarrhythmia between consecutive spasms of a cluster, and a lack of any focal interictal or ictal EEG abnormality (Dreifuss *et al* 1991). Over the past 20 years the numbers of children in the symptomatic category of West syndrome has steadily increased because of the advent of sophisticated neuroimaging techniques that has allowed the detection of subtle neuronal migrational abnormalities which give rise to infantile spasms (Jellinger 1987; Chiron *et al* 1993; Otsubo *et al* 1993; van Bogaert *et al* 1993; Vinters *et al* 1993; Chugani 1994; Miyazaki *et al* 1994a; Hwang *et al* 1996; Watanabe 1998). The use of positron emission tomography (PET) in the diagnostic evaluation of infantile spasms has been reported to increase the percentage of children in the symptomatic group of West syndrome from 30 to 96% (Chugani and Conti 1996).

Advances in molecular biology also have increased the number of children with West syndrome classified as symptomatic by revealing a variety of mitochondrial abnormalities that may underlie infantile spasms (Boor *et al* 1992; Makela-Benzs *et al* 1995; Otero *et al* 1995). These advances have improved our understanding of the pathologic substrate of infantile spasms to a certain extent, although the basic mechanisms that underlie the pathogenesis of infantile spasms remain unknown.

The etiologic classification of West syndrome is relatively straightforward, but the clinical and electrographic classification remains controversial. Correct classification is crucial in designing surgical treatment strategies for children with partial seizures and West syndrome. Currently West syndrome is classified as an age-related cryptogenic or symptomatic generalized epilepsy syndrome (Commission on Classification and Terminology of the International League Against Epilepsy 1989). However, the literature (see below) suggests that the EEG and clinical manifestations of infantile spasms in West syndrome are not always generalized. Hence, the official classification of this disorder as a generalized epilepsy syndrome often may be inaccurate.

Shortly after the first description of hypsarrhythmia by Gibbs and Gibbs (1952), it became clear that generalized hypsarrhythmia may not occur in all patients with infantile spasms (Hess and Neuhaus 1952; Bower and Jeavons 1959; Kramer *et al* 1997a). Otohara (1965) was the first to describe asymmetric hypsarrhythmia in West syndrome, a pattern now well recognized (Tjam *et al* 1978; Dulac *et al* 1987; Fusco and Vigevano 1993; Plouin *et al* 1993; Tachibana and Shimizu 1993; Donat and Lo 1994; Drury *et al* 1995; Gaily *et al* 1995). Further, Hrachovy *et al* (1984) have described hypsarrhythmia with a consistent focus of abnormal discharge. In addition to focal EEG abnormalities, up to 30% of children with infantile spasms may have clinical evidence of partial seizure activity (Donat and Lo 1994; Donat and Wright 1996). This number exceeds 50% in children with symptomatic West syndrome (Plouin *et al* 1993). Focal cortical lesions may underlie infantile spasms in many children with symptomatic West syndrome (Branch and Dyken 1979; Dolman *et al* 1981; Mimaki *et al* 1983; Alvarez *et al* 1987; Palm *et al* 1988; Ruggieri *et al* 1989; Askenasi and Snead 1991; Cusmai *et al* 1993; Ohtahara *et al* 1993; Otsubo *et al* 1993; Vinters *et al* 1993; Miyazaki *et al* 1994b; Viani *et al* 1994; Koo and Hwang 1996; Kuwahara *et al* 1996). Therefore, it appears that the combination of asymmetric infantile spasms and/or asymmetric and/or focally asynchronous hypsarrhythymia, contralateral central region pathology, and typical onset in infancy may represent a subset of children with infantile spasms who have a symptomatic, age-specific, localization-related epilepsy. Therefore the classification of West syndrome may need revision as a special syndrome to reflect the fact that it may be a manifestation of either a localization-related or a generalized epilepsy syndrome (Dreifuss *et al* 1991).

PARTIAL SEIZURES AND WEST SYNDROME

Focal components of infantile spasms, such as eye deviation (Lombroso 1983; Carrazana *et al* 1990; Donat and Wright 1996), laughter (Druckman and Chao 1957), and focal myoclonus (Jeavons and Bower 1964), and localizing findings on the EEG with hypsarrhythmia (Branch and Dyken

1979; Alvarez *et al* 1987; Ruggieri *et al* 1989) are known to occur in West syndrome. In addition, partial seizures have been reported to trigger, or precede, infantile spasms in West syndrome, co-occur with this disorder, or appear after the onset of the spasms. Children with West syndrome characterized by infantile spasms and partial seizures are more likely to have asymmetric spasms, hemiparesis, asymmetric hypsarrhythmia, and a significantly less favorable seizure prognosis than those children with infantile spasms without partial seizures (Donat and Lo 1994; Gaily *et al* 1995; Haga *et al* 1995; Ohtsuka *et al* 1996). Although partial seizures and West syndrome certainly is not a new association, interest in this subgroup of children with West syndrome has intensified greatly since the report by Chugani *et al* (1990) of a small group of four children with infantile spasms and partial seizures and/or focally abnormal EEG who had a successful outcome from epilepsy surgery guided by interictal PET and electrocorticography.

Branch and Dyken (1979) were the first to report a child with infantile spasms whose spasms disappeared after surgical resection of a lesion. However, the initial report of partial seizures that clearly preceded infantile spasms was made by Yamamoto *et al* (1988) who reported that the clinical manifestations of the partial seizures which preceded the spasms included staring, flushing, automatisms, and increased limb tone and laughter. Carrazana *et al* (1990, 1993) have reported an additional group of patients in whom the onset of clusters of infantile spasms appeared to be triggered by partial seizures; 75% of this group had a focal cerebral lesion and all children had partial seizures with EEG localization; the spasms however were bilateral. Ohtsuka *et al* (1996) reported another group of patients in whom partial seizures appeared before the spasms. After the onset of spasms in this group of patients all the EEGs showed hypsarrhythmia.

Partial seizures that precede infantile spasms emanate mainly from the temporal and rolandic areas and, to a lesser degree, from occipital and frontal regions. Children in whom partial seizures occur prior to infantile spasms may account for as many as 19% of patients with West syndrome who undergo long-term monitoring (Plouin *et al* 1993; Kramer *et al* 1997b)

The coexistence of infantile spasms and partial seizures also has been long recognized and has been shown to herald a worse outcome (Lacy and Penry 1976; Riikonen 1982; Lombroso 1983; Hrachovy *et al* 1984; Jeavons 1985; Koo *et al* 1993; Plouin *et al* 1993; Donat and Wright 1996; Ohtsuka *et al* 1996; Kramer *et al* 1997b; Watanabe 1998). In the majority of children with West syndrome and coexisting partial seizures, the partial seizures appear at the same time as the spasms, but usually immediately precede

the onset of the cluster of spasms (Ohtsuka *et al* 1996). The most common ictal manifestations of partial seizures that co-occur with spasms in children with West syndrome are focal clonic seizures, which involve the face and hands, and eye deviation (Ohtsuka *et al* 1996).

Infantile spasms in West syndrome may evolve into partial seizures (Riikonen 1982; Askenasi and Snead 1991; Ohtsuka *et al* 1996; Watanabe 1998), often with a frontal lobe focus (Askenasi and Snead 1991; Koo and Hwang 1996; Ohtsuka *et al* 1996). This is in contradistinction to the posterior origin of partial seizures that precede or co-occur with West syndrome. (Wenzel 1987; Chugani *et al* 1990; Jambaque *et al* 1993; Koo and Hwang 1996). The clinical manifestations of partial seizures that occur after the cessation of infantile spasms in children with West syndrome are more stereotyped than those that co-occur with or precede infantile spasms.

ETIOLOGY OF PARTIAL SEIZURES IN WEST SYNDROME

An extensive diagnostic evaluation of children with West syndrome that includes careful neuroimaging with magnetic resonance imaging (MRI), PET, and single-photon emission computed tomography (SPECT), as well as an extensive search for metabolic and chromosomal abnormalities, will provide evidence for an etiology of the spasms, and thus support for classification of the West syndrome as symptomatic, in 60–70% of cases (Shields *et al* 1992). The causes of partial seizures in infantile spasms include tuberous sclerosis (Riikonen and Simell 1990), Sturge–Weber syndrome (Millichap *et al* 1962), brain tumors (Branch and Dyken 1979; Mimaki *et al* 1983; Ruggieri *et al* 1989; Askenasi and Snead 1991; Viani *et al* 1994), brain abscess (Lombroso 1983), perinatal brain injury (Cusmai *et al* 1993; Ohtahara *et al* 1993; Watanabe 1998), cerebral infarction (Alvarez *et al* 1987) and grossly dysmorphic anomalies of the brain such as lissencephaly (Plouin *et al* 1993; Kramer *et al* 1997b), porencephaly (Palm *et al* 1988; Uthman *et al* 1991; Cusmai *et al* 1993; Ohtahara *et al* 1993; Miyazaki *et al* 1994b), large heterotopias (Palm *et al* 1986; Kuwahara *et al* 1996), and hemimegalencephaly (Tjam *et al* 1978; Jellinger 1987; Robain *et al* 1989). More recently, with increasing use of sophisticated neuroimaging techniques, it has become apparent that neuronal migration abnormalities, such as focal cortical dysplasias of varying degrees of size and severity, probably account for the majority of children with West syndrome and partial seizures (Jeavons 1985; Chugani *et al* 1990; Otsubo *et al* 1993;

Vinters *et al* 1993; Miyazaki *et al* 1994b; Sankar *et al* 1995; Hwang *et al* 1996).

MEDICAL TREATMENT OF PARTIAL SEIZURES AND WEST SYNDROME

The medical treatment of infantile spasms remains empirical at best since it is based on no theoretic underpinning. This empiricism is reflected by the fact that the clinical observation that corticosteroids and adrenocorticotropic hormone (ACTH) are of therapeutic value in infantile spasms, made 40 years ago (Sorel and Dusaucy-Bauloye 1958), remains one of the defining characteristics of this disorder.

The effect of oral steroids on the convulsive state was reported in 1942 when McQuarrie *et al* observed that deoxycorticosterone made seizures worse. Hoefer and Glaser (1950) demonstrated subsequently that both ACTH and cortisone were associated clinically with EEG slowing. There was some debate in the late 1940s and early 1950s concerning the effect of these compounds on cerebral excitability, with some authors (Dorfman *et al* 1951; Wayne 1954) expressing concern that ACTH might be proconvulsant in adult seizure patients, while others (Friedlander and Rottgers 1951; Pine *et al* 1951) reached the opposite conclusion, namely that ACTH and cortisone treatment were associated with improvement of the EEG towards normal.

The initial report of therapeutic efficacy of ACTH therapy in childhood seizures appeared in 1950, when Klein and Livingston described a beneficial effect of ACTH treatment in four of six children ranging in age from 4.5 to 16 years who were suffering from a variety of seizure types intractable to standard medical therapy. Eight years later Sorel and Dusaucy-Bauloye (1958) reported a dramatic response to ACTH therapy in a series of children with infantile spasms. These patients showed normalization of behavior, control of seizures, and an improvement in the EEG after treatment with the drug. This finding was confirmed the following year (Dumermuth 1959; Gastaut *et al* 1959; Stamps *et al* 1959) and the benefit of oral steroids in this condition was also established (Low 1958; Dumermuth 1959). From the time of those reports in the late 1950s, there has been little agreement about many aspects of the treatment and outcome of infantile spasms; however, there is a consensus that the only drugs effective against infantile spasms are either oral corticosteroids or parenteral ACTH and that standard antiepileptic drugs such as phenytoin, phenobarbital, and carbamazepine appear to have little effect against infantile spasms. Since the 1980s

benzodiazepines (Dreifuss *et al* 1986), valproic acid (Dyken *et al* 1985), vitamin B$_6$ (Blennow and Starck 1986), and vigabatrin (Snead 1994; Vigevano and Cilio 1997) have been added to the list of effective compounds. Although there is disagreement as to whether ACTH or oral corticosteroids are superior in the treatment of infantile spasms (Hrachovy *et al* 1983, 1994; Snead *et al* 1983, 1989), the data would suggest that currently the drug of choice for the treatment of the child with West syndrome is either ACTH or vigabatrin (Snead *et al* 1983, 1989; Baram *et al* 1996; Heiskala *et al* 1996; Vigevano and Cilio 1997).

There are few reports in the literature that have specifically addressed the medical treatment of that subset of children with West syndrome and partial seizures. Antiepileptic drugs used against partial seizures are not considered useful in the treatment of infantile spasms (Snead 1994). Further, ACTH may be of benefit in some children with infantile spasms that originate from a focal lesion (Kuwahara *et al* 1996). However, there are some data that suggest carbamazepine may be useful in the treatment of children with West syndrome with partial seizures, focal neurologic abnormalities, radiologic evidence of a structural lesion of the brain, and/or lateralizing or focal EEG abnormalities (Tatzer *et al* 1987; Yamamoto *et al* 1988; Miyazaki *et al* 1994b). Those children who fit this subgroup of patients with West syndrome and partial seizures who prove intractable to ACTH and/or vigabatrin should be given a trial of carbamazepine therapy.

SURGICAL TREATMENT OF PARTIAL SEIZURES AND WEST SYNDROME

Branch and Dyken (1979) first reported the successful treatment of a 7-month-old infant with West syndrome by surgical excision of a lesion. Following removal of a choroid plexus papilloma of the left lateral ventricle, the infantile spasms resolved and the child resumed normal development. From 1979 to 1990 there were a number of individual case reports of children with symptomatic West syndrome secondary to a variety of etiologies who underwent surgical resection of a lesion (Gabriel 1980; Dolman *et al* 1981; Mimaki *et al* 1983; Palm *et al* 1988; Ruggieri *et al* 1989) (Table 23.1). Most of these children have had a successful outcome, at least in terms of resolution of the spasms. In 1990, Chugani *et al* reported a series of 13 children with cryptogenic infantile spasms who had 2-deoxy-[^{18}F]fluoro-D-glucose PET. Of these, five children showed focal areas of decreased cerebral glucose metabolism without corresponding structural abnormalities on CT or MRI

Table 23.1 Children with West syndrome and partial seizures who had surgery for infantile spasms.

Reference	Pathology	No. of children
Branch and Dyken (1979)	Choroid plexus papilloma	1
Gabriel (1980)	Ganglioglioma	1
Dolman et al (1981)	Fibromatosis of dura	1
Mimaki et al (1983)	Temporal lobe astrocytoma	1
Palm et al (1988)	Porencephalic cyst	9
Ruggieri et al (1989)	Anaplastic ependymoma	1
Askenasi and Snead (1991)	Ganglioglioma	1
Uthman et al (1991)	Porencephalic cyst	1
Chugani et al (1993)	Focal cortical dysplasia	14
	Gliosis	4
	Glial cysts	2
	Tuberous sclerosis	1
	Neuronal heterotopia	1
	Normal	1
Ozek et al (1995)	Multiple pineal cysts	1
Wyllie et al (1996)	Ganglioglioma	1
	Cortical dysplasia (in patient with periventricular leukomalacia)	1
Kramer et al (1997b)	Hemimegalencephaly	2
	Tuberous sclerosis	1
	Neonatal stroke	1
	Pachygyria	2
	Cortical dysplasia	3

scan. Four of these five children underwent electrocorticographic-guided resection of the hypometabolic cortical regions. The pathology of resected tissue showed focal cortical dysplasia. All children in this series who had surgery had some focal component to their seizures. Two had partial seizures at the time of surgery. The others had focal components to the spasms, focal findings on neurologic examination, or focal features on the EEG. In other words, no patient in this initial surgical series of children with West syndrome as reported by Chugani et al (1990) had classical bilateral spasms without focality, an EEG that was hypsarrhythmic with no focal features, and/or a normal neurologic examination. Similarly, in a follow-up report from the same group (Chugani et al 1993) (Table 23.1), all children with West syndrome who had surgery based on a focal area of hypometabolism as shown by PET had some focal characteristic to their seizure, partial seizures that coexisted with the spasms, focal features on EEG, and/or a focally abnormal neurologic examination. Since the report by Chugani et al (1990), others have reported beneficial results from surgery in children with West syndrome with focal cerebral abnormalities (Kramer et al 1997b, Uthman et al 1991) (Table 23.1)

The value of interictal PET scanning in identifying surgical candidates among children with West syndrome, first reported by Chugani et al (1990), has been validated by

other authors (Ferrie et al 1996; Kramer et al 1997b). However, one should bear two things in mind concerning the use of PET as a diagnostic modality in West syndrome. First, PET should be reserved for those children who appear to fit into the subset of West syndrome and partial seizures, i.e. those with focal characteristics to their seizure, partial seizures that coexist with the spasms, focal features on EEG, and/or a focally abnormal neurologic examination. Kramer et al (1997b) have suggested that PET be done in this group only when MRI is normal. Second, when contemplating the surgical candidacy of a child with West syndrome the PET data should be considered in the context of other neuroimaging studies, the neurologic examination, the semiology of the seizures, and the video-EEG data, rather than in isolation (Snead and Nelson 1993; Snead et al 1996). One should use great caution in making a surgical decision in infantile spasms based on PET data that are discordant with other neuroimaging, electrophysiologic, and clinical data.

When considering the surgical candidacy of a child with West syndrome, it is important to remember that partial seizures that coexist with infantile spasms, or hemispasms, may be the result of diffuse or multifocal cerebral pathology and therefore may not always indicate the presence of a surgically accessible lesion (Ohtsuka et al 1996). However, any child with West syndrome with partial seizures, focal neurologic abnormalities, and/or lateralizing or focal EEG

Table 23.2 Diagnostic findings in children with West syndrome and partial seizures suggestive of an indication for epilepsy surgery.

History and/or observation of asymmetric infantile spasms
  Unilateral spasms with one side predominantly involved
  Bilateral spasm more pronounced on one side, either stronger on one side or asynchronous with one side typically involved initially
  Spasm with persistent unilateral deviation of head and/or eyes
Focal findings on neurologic examination
  Hemiatrophy
  Asymmetric quadriplegia
  Hemiparesis
  Reflex asymmetry
Partial seizures
  Before presentation of infantile spasms
  During infantile spasms, either independently or preceding the spasms
  After the spasms
EEG demonstrating lateralized or focal features
  Hemihypsarrhythmia
  Asymmetry or asynchrony
  Persistently focal slowing, focal sharp waves, or focal spikes
Radiologic evidence of a focal structural abnormality
  CT/MRI
  Functional imaging with interictal PET, interictal/ictal SPECT

MRI, magnetic resonance imaging; PET, positron emission tomography; SPECT, single-photon emission computed tomography.

abnormalities, whose seizures are intractable to ACTH and vigabatrin, should be considered a potential candidate for epilepsy surgery. This is especially true if there is radiologic evidence of a structural lesion of the brain. If MRI of such a child is normal, one should proceed to PET scanning.

INVESTIGATION OF CHILDREN WITH WEST SYNDROME AND PARTIAL SEIZURES

The critical question that must be answered by the diagnostic evaluation of the child who presents with West syndrome concerns not only the etiology, and therefore classification, of the spasms but also whether the child is a candidate for epilepsy surgery. The prerequisite for undergoing epilepsy surgery is focality: focal components to the seizure, focal findings on neurologic examination, focal features to the EEG, or evidence of a focal lesion on neuroimaging. Rarely is there a single diagnostic modality or physical finding that provides a definitive answer to the question of whether a child with West syndrome is a candidate for epilepsy surgery. The best candidate would be a child with a stereotypic partial seizure that occurred either before or during the infantile spasms with lateralizing physical findings and *concordant* radiologic data (MRI, PET, SPECT) and EEG localizing data. The least optimal candidate would be a child with partial seizures, not stereotypical, associated with bilateral infantile spasms, generalized and/or multifocal hypsarrhythmia along with shifting asymmetries of the EEG, no lateralizing physical findings, and normal neuroimaging studies. Therefore, the diagnostic work-up of the child with West syndrome and partial seizures should be designed to accrue as much evidence as possible that might point to a single, surgically excisable focus as an etiology for the infantile spasms (Table 23.2).

The diagnostic evaluation of the child with West syndrome should include a thorough history followed by a careful physical and neurologic examination. The physical examination should always include scrutiny of the skin for depigmented or hyperpigmented lesions, since tuberous sclerosis may be a cause of infantile spasms (Riikonen and Simell 1990; Hwang *et al* 1996; Snead *et al* 1996). Surgery may be of benefit in children with tuberous sclerosis and West syndrome (Chugani *et al* 1993; Kramer *et al* 1997b). A careful description of the spasms and any attendant seizure types should be obtained and reinforced with EEG-video monitoring during waking and sleep. MRI is the preferred initial neuroimaging procedure since it is much more sensitive than CT (van Bogaert *et al* 1993). An initial

negative MRI early in life should be repeated later if there is suspicion of a neuronal migration disorder because cortical dysplasias may not be apparent until myelination is complete or nearly complete (Sankar *et al* 1995).

If the child has EEG, semeiologic, or objective physical findings suggestive of focality but the MRI is negative, one should progress to functional imaging, i.e. PET and/or SPECT (Chugani 1994; Kramer *et al* 1997b), to determine if there are areas of aberrant blood flow (Chiron *et al* 1993; Miyazaki *et al* 1994a; Hwang *et al* 1996) or metabolism (Commission on Classification and Terminology of the International League Against Epilepsy 1989; Chugani *et al* 1990; Chugani 1994; Sankar *et al* 1995; Ferrie *et al* 1996; Kramer *et al* 1997b), which might be concordant with the physical, EEG, or semeiologic findings and thus supportive of a surgical treatment option.

OUTCOME OF PARTIAL SEIZURES AND WEST SYNDROME

The major predictor of outcome in West syndrome is the underlying pathologic process (Riikonen 1982; Lombroso 1983). Adverse prognostic indicators in West syndrome include an onset of infantile spasms at less than 3 months of age, the presence of a preexisting neurologic impairment and/or significant developmental delay at the onset of the spasms, an atypical EEG (Lombroso 1983), unilateral features to the seizures such as asymmetric spasms (Dulac *et al* 1996), occurrence of other seizure types, and failure to respond to ACTH therapy (Riikonen 1982; Koo *et al* 1993; Asarnow *et al* 1997). Conversely, in patients with cryptogenic West syndrome the most sensitive predictive factors for favorable outcome appear to be the absence of significant mental regression with preserved visual function combined with the lack of a persistent interictal EEG focus; however, even in cryptogenic West syndrome, evidence of focality carries adverse prognostic implications (Dulac *et al* 1993).

There are several reports of beneficial outcome following surgery for infantile spasms. However, only one developmental outcome study in a group of children who had resective surgery for medically intractable infantile spasms has been published (Asarnow *et al* 1997). This study indicates a significant increase in the developmental level 2 years after surgery compared with developmental levels before surgery; however, there was no control group matched for age and similar seizure characteristics. Another finding of this outcome study was that children who were younger at the time of surgery seemed to have better outcomes than children who were older. Although this finding appeared to be independent of length of follow-up interval, the region of brain removed, medications, or gender, no analysis was made of the relation of the finding to the clinical characteristics of the seizures. This is important because children with West syndrome who have *clear* evidence of partial seizures might go to surgery earlier than those in whom the early manifestations of partial seizures are more subtle and likely to be missed, or in whom the partial seizures occur after the spasms.

In summary, children with West syndrome and partial seizures have a less favorable seizure prognosis than those without partial seizures (Ohtsuka *et al* 1996). This statement may seem to be at odds with an older study that deals indirectly with the prognosis of infantile spasms and partial seizures. In 1978, Chevrie and Aicardi reported prognostic outcome data on 313 infants with onset of seizures in the first year of life who were followed for 1 year and longer. The prognosis in this series of patients was found to be universally poor, even in those who had seizure types other than infantile spasms. The highest incidence of neurologic abnormalities occurred in children with symptomatic partial seizures and in those with status epilepticus. This series was published before the ability to characterize seizure semeiology precisely with video-EEG recording became commonplace and prior to the development of sophisticated neuroimaging. Therefore, many children in this series characterized as 'other-partial' may have had asymmetric spasms or the combination of infantile spasms and partial seizures.

It is not known whether children with West syndrome with partial seizures that precede, co-occur, or follow infantile spasms and which are associated with focal cortical abnormalities have a superior outcome following surgery compared with children with similar pathology who respond to medical therapy (Kuwahara *et al* 1996). Although there are preliminary data (Asarnow *et al* 1997) to suggest that the timing of surgery is important, i.e. the earlier the better, not all potential confounding variables have been examined to confirm that impression.

PARTIAL SEIZURES AND WEST SYNDROME: CLUES TO PATHOPHYSIOLOGY?

The basic pathogenesis of West syndrome is unknown. One of the major reasons for this lack of knowledge is that there is no known animal model for this epilepsy syndrome. Until such a model is found, the underlying abnormality can only be speculated upon. Any proposed theory of pathogenesis

of infantile spasms should reconcile a number of clinical observations.

1. *Clinical and electrographic features*: infantile spasms are characterized by massive myoclonus and there is frequent association with a hypsarrhythmic EEG.
2. *Time course*: infantile spasms clearly are age-related, with a narrow window of age of onset of 4–7 months. Moreover they appear to be self-limited in time, disappearing within 1–2 years of onset by either spontaneously resolving or evolving into other types of seizures.
3. *Sleep characteristics*: there is a marked decrease in REM sleep in children with infantile spasms, yet the EEG abnormalities disappear during REM sleep (Fukuyama *et al* 1979; Hrachovy *et al* 1981).
4. *Etiology*: there is no common etiology; in addition, West syndrome may occur in some children with a specific neurologic disorder but not all, e.g. tuberous sclerosis.
5. *Outcome*: West syndrome carries a high morbidity in terms of subsequent cognitive delay and intractable epilepsy.
6. *Disorder-specific therapies*: infantile spasms respond only to corticosteroid and ACTH therapy, and to those antiepileptic drugs (e.g. vigabatrin and benzodiazepines) that appear to act via γ-aminobutyric acid.
7. *Serotonin abnormalities*: there is some evidence that serotonin precursors may induce infantile spasms in susceptible patients (Coleman 1971) and in some species of animals (Klawans *et al* 1973); however, serotonin antagonists appear to have no demonstrable therapeutic effect against spasms (Hrachovy *et al* 1988, 1989).

In the past much of the speculation about the pathophysiology of infantile spasms derived from postulated mechanisms of actions of ACTH and corticosteroids in this disorder, since these drugs appear to be uniquely effective against infantile spasms. For example, it has been postulated that since the serotonergic raphe striatal projection is tonically regulated by corticosteroids this system is perturbed in infantile spasms (Silverstein and Johnston 1984). Alternatively, corticotropin releasing factor (CRF), a peptide that is quite epileptogenic, has been hypothesized to play a role in the pathogenesis of infantile spasms (Baram 1993). Both ACTH and cortisol could owe their effectiveness against infantile spasms to their ability to inhibit CRF release.

Although a critical role of the brainstem in the pathogenesis of infantile spasms has long been hypothesized (Fukuyama *et al* 1979; Hrachovy *et al* 1981; Saroh *et al* 1986; Miyazaki *et al* 1993), Yamamoto *et al* (1988) were the first to postulate that clusters of infantile spasms might be triggered in children with partial seizures and West syndrome by focal cortical discharges that descend into the brainstem. This hypothesis was further developed in 1990 by Carrazana *et al* in a case report of a child with West syndrome and agenesis of the corpus callosum in whom the infantile spasms were persistently preceded by a partial seizure. These authors suggested that the absence of normal interhemispheric communication through the corpus callosum excluded rapid secondary generalization, thereby validating the hypothesis of Yamamoto *et al*. Since that report a number of other patients with partial seizures, West syndrome, and agenesis of the corpus callosum have been reported (Carrazana *et al* 1993; Pinard *et al* 1993). However, routes of secondary generalization other than the brainstem might be operative in these children, i.e. anterior and posterior commissure, hippocampal commissure, and/or thalamus.

The idea of a brainstem-mediated mechanism for infantile spasms in children with West syndrome and partial seizures was developed further by the work of Chugani *et al* (1992), who demonstrated a symmetrical hypermetabolism in the lenticular nuclei in 32 of 42 children with infantile spasms who received a PET scan. This abnormality occurred regardless of whether the spasms were cryptogenic or symptomatic, and was associated with focal cortical hypometabolism in 22 of the 32 patients in whom it was found and with focal cortical hypermetabolism in five children. The activation of the lenticular nuclei occurred in 16 children who had no focal abnormalities on PET. There are no clinical data provided in this report that would allow one to correlate the PET findings with the clinical characteristics of the spasms, their relation to partial seizures, focal EEG abnormalities, or neurologic examination of the patients. In any event, based on these data Chugani and colleagues have proposed a hypothetical model of infantile spasms in which a cortical lesion, either diffuse or focal, may induce abnormal functional interactions with brainstem serotonergic raphe nuclei at a critical stage of brain maturation. The raphe nuclei, thus activated by aberrant cortical

discharges, are postulated to mediate hypsarrhythmic changes on EEG and myoclonic seizures via a raphe–striatal pathway. Clinical myoclonus is postulated to involve projections from the raphe to the spinal cord. However, in this model there is no hypothesized 'final common pathway' from striatum back to cortex by which the hypsarrhythmic EEG changes might be mediated. Also, this theory of pathogenesis of infantile spasms makes no attempt to differentiate between the mechanisms of spasms in children with cryptogenic West syndrome with generalized hypsarrhythmia vs those with symptomatic West Syndrome and partial seizures.

Finally, additional support for a role of focal cortical abnormalities in the generation of infantile spasms in West syndrome is provided by a study of 93 patients with focal cortical lesions, which demonstrates that the localization of the lesion in the cortex influences the age of onset of infantile spasms. Occipital lesions were found to be associated with the earliest onset of spasms and frontal lesions with later age of onset. This age distribution is closely connected with the normal sequence of brain myelination (Koo and Hwang 1996).

CONCLUSION

West syndrome is a catastrophic childhood seizure disorder characterized by a poor developmental and neurologic outcome that is made even worse by the presence of partial seizures. Careful evaluation for evidence of focality is crucial in the evaluation of patients with infantile spasms and partial seizures because some children with specific unifocal lesions may have a more favorable outcome if epilepsy surgery is performed. Presently many issues regarding surgery in these patients are unknown, including the optimal timing and precise surgical indications. Further clinical and animal research studies are required to answer the question of the optimum treatment of children with West syndrome and partial seizures.

KEY POINTS

1. West syndrome is defined as the clinical triad of infantile spasms, arrest of psychomotor development, and the typical EEG pattern of hypsarrythmia.

2. Although West syndrome is classified as an age-related cryptogenic or symptomatic generalized epilepsy, the EEG and clinical manifestations are not always generalized.

3. The classification of West syndrome may need revision as a special syndrome to reflect that it may be

KEY POINTS

a manifestation of either a localization-related or a generalized epilepsy syndrome.

4. Children with West syndrome and partial seizures are more likely to have asymmetric spasms, hemiparesis, asymmetric hypsarrythmia and a significantly less favorable seizure prognosis than those without partial seizures.

5. It has been recently reported that neuronal migration or abnormalities such as focal cortical dysplasias probably account for the majority of children with West syndrome and partial seizures although there may be other

structural lesions which are discussed in this chapter.

6. The current opinion regarding medical therapy for children with West syndrome is to use either ACTH or vigabatrin.

7. Children with partial seizures, focal abnormalities, lateralized or focal EEG findings and West syndrome should be considered for surgery if seizures are intractable to medical therapy.

8. Beneficial outcome following surgery in this group of children has been reported, but it is not yet known if the outcome in these children following surgery will be superior compared to children with

similar pathology who respond to medical therapy.

9. Although the basic pathogenesis of West syndrome is not known, in this chapter it is discussed that the clues gained from the coexistence of partial seizures in West syndrome will further our understanding of this disease.

10. In summary, careful evaluation for evidence of focality in children with West syndrome is crucial as some children with specific unifocal lesions may have a more favorable outcome if epilepsy surgery is performed.

REFERENCES

Alvarez LA, Shinnar S, Moshe SL (1987) Infantile spasms due to unilateral cerebral infarcts. *Pediatrics* **79**:1024–1026.

Asarnow RF, Lo Presti C, Guthrie D *et al* (1997) Developmental outcomes in children receiving resection surgery for medically intractable infantile spasms. *Developmental Medicine and Child Neurology* **39**:430–440.

Askenasi A, Snead OC (1991) Infantile spasms secondary to a brain tumor. *Journal of Child Neurology* **6**:180–182.

Baram TZ (1993) Pathophysiology of massive infantile spasms: perspective on the putative role of the brain adrenal axis. *Annals of Neurology* **33**:231–236.

Baram TZ, Mitchell WG, Hanson RA *et al* (1996) High dose corticotropin (ACTH) vs prednisone for infantile spasms: a prospective, randomized blinded study. *Pediatrics* **97**:375–379.

Blennow G, Starck L (1986) High dose B$_6$ treatment in infantile spasms. *Neuropediatrics* **17**:7–10.

Boor R, Rachels R, Walther B *et al* (1992) Aplasia of the retinal vessels combined with optic nerve hypoplasia, neonatal epileptic seizures, and lactic acidosis due to mitochondrial complex I deficiency. *European Journal of Pediatrics* **151**:519–521.

Bower BD, Jeavons PM (1959) Infantile spasms and hypsarrhythmia. *Lancet* i:605–609.

Branch CE, Dyken PR (1979) Choroid plexus papilloma and infantile spasms. *Annals of Neurology* **5**:302–304.

Carrazana EJ, Barlow JK, Holmes GL (1990) Infantile spasms provoked by partial seizures. *Journal of Epilepsy* **3**:97–100.

Carrazana E, Lombroso CT, Mikati M *et al* (1993) Facilitation of infantile spasms by partial seizures. *Epilepsia* **34**:97–100.

Chevrie JJ, Aicardi J (1978) Convulsive disorders in the first year of life: neurological and mental outcome and mortality. *Epilepsia* **19**:67–74.

Chiron C, Dulac O, Bulteau C *et al* (1993) Study of regional cerebral blood flow in West syndrome. *Epilepsia* **34**:707–715.

Chugani HT (1994) The role of PET in childhood epilepsy. *Journal of Child Neurology* **9**(Suppl):S82–S88.

Chugani HT, Conti JR (1996) Etiologic classification of infantile spasms in 140 cases: role of positron emission tomography. *Journal of Child Neurology* **11**:44–48.

Chugani HT, Shields WD, Shewmon DA *et al* (1990) Infantile spasms: I. PET identifies focal cortical dysgenesis in cryptogenic cases for surgical treatment. *Annals of Neurology* **27**:406–413.

Chugani HT, Shewmon DA, Sankar R *et al* (1992) Infantile spasms: II. Lenticular nuclei and brain stem activation on positron emission tomography. *Annals of Neurology* **31**:212–219.

Chugani HT, Shewmon DA, Shields WD *et al* (1993) Surgery for intractable infantile spasms: neuroimaging perspectives. *Epilepsia* **34**:764–771.

Coleman M (1971) Infantile spasms associated with 5-hydroxytryptophan administration in patients with Downs' syndrome. *Neurology* **21**:911–919.

Commission on Classification and Terminology of the International League Against Epilepsy (1989) Proposal for revised classification of epilepsies and epileptic syndromes. *Epilepsia* **30**:389–399.

Cusmai R, Ricci S, Pinard JM *et al* (1993) West syndrome due to perinatal insults. *Epilepsia* **34**:738–742.

Dolman CL, Crichton JU, Jones EA *et al* (1981) Fibromatosis of dura presenting as infantile spasms. *Journal of the Neurological Sciences* **49**:31–39.

Donat JF, Lo WD (1994) Asymmetric hypsarrhythmia and infantile spasms in West syndrome. *Journal of Child Neurology* **9**:290–296.

Donat JF, Wright FS (1996) Unusual variants of infantile spasms. *Journal of Child Neurology* **6**:313–318.

Dorfman A, Apter NS, Smull K *et al* (1951) Status epilepticus coincident with the use of pituitary adrenocorticotrophic hormone: report of three cases. *Journal of the American Medical Association* **146**:25–29.

Dreifuss F, Farwell J, Holmes G *et al* (1986) Infantile spasms. Comparative trial of nitrazepam and corticotropin. *Archives of Neurology* **43**:1107–1110.

Dreifuss F, Roger J, Chugani H *et al* (1991) Workshop on infantile spasms. *Epilepsia* **33**:195.

Druckman R, Chao D (1957) Laughter in epilepsy. *Neurology* 7:26–36.

Drury I, Beydoun A, Garofalo EA *et al* (1995) Asymmetric hypsarrhythmia: clinical electroencephalographic and radiologic findings. *Epilepsia* **36**:41–47.

Dulac O, Chiron C, Jambaque I *et al* (1987) Infantile spasms. *Progress in Clinical Neuroscience* 2:97–100.

Dulac O, Plouin P, Jambaque I (1993) Predicting favourable outcome in idiopathic West syndrome. *Epilepsia* **34**:747–756.

Dulac O, Plouin P, Schlumberger E (1996) Infantile spasms. In: Wyllie E (ed) *The Treatment of Epilepsy: Principles and Practice*, 2nd edn, pp 540–572. Baltimore: Williams and Wilkins.

Dumermuth G (1959) Über die Blitz-Nick-Salaam-Krämpfe und ihre Behandlung mit ACTH und Hydrocortison. *Helvetica Pediatrica Acta* **14**:250–270.

Dyken PR, Durant RH, Minden DB *et al* (1985) Short term effects of valproate on infantile spasms. *Pediatric Neurology* 1:34–37.

Ferrie CD, Maisey M, Cox T *et al* (1996) Focal abnormalities detected by [18]FDG PET in epileptic encephalopathies. *Archives of Disease in Childhood* **75**:102–107.

Friedlander WJ, Rottgers E (1951) The effects of cortisone on the electroencephalograph. *Electroencephalography and Clinical Neurophysiology* **3**:311–320.

Fukuyama Y, Shionaga A, Iida Y (1979) Polygraphic study during whole night sleep in infantile spasms. *European Neurology* **18**:302–311.

Fusco L, Vigevano F (1993) Ictal clinical electroencephalographic findings of spasms in West syndrome. *Epilepsia* **34**:671–678.

Gabriel YH (1980) Unilateral hemispheric ganglio-glioma with infantile spasms. *Annals of Neurology* 7:287–288.

Gaily EK, Shewmon DA, Chugani HT *et al* (1995) Asymmetric and asynchronous infantile spasms. *Epilepsia* **36**:873–882.

Gastaut H, Salfiel J, Raybaud C *et al* (1959) A propos du traitement par l'ACTH des encéphalites myoclonique de la premiére enfance avec majeure (hypsarrythmia). *Pediatrie* **14**:35–45.

Gibbs FA, Gibbs EL (1952) *Atlas of Electroencephalography, Vol 2: Epilepsy.* Cambridge, MA: Addison-Wesley.

Haga Y, Watanabe K, Negoro T *et al* (1995) Asymmetric spasms in West syndrome. *Journal of Epilepsy* **8**:61–67.

Heiskala H, Riikonen R, Santavuori P *et al* (1996) West syndrome: individualized ACTH therapy. *Brain and Development* **18**:456–460.

Hess R, Neuhaus T (1952) Das elektrencephalogramm, Les Blitz, Nick and Salaamkrampfer und bein andern Anfallsformer des Kindezalters. *Arch Psychiatr Zeitschr Neurol* **89**:37–58.

Hoefer PFA, Glaser GH (1950) Effects of pituitary adrenocorticotrophic hormone therapy: electroencephalographic and neuropsychiatric changes in 15 patients. *Journal of the American Medical Association* **143**:620–624.

Holmes GL (1987) *Diagnosis and Management of Seizures in Children*, pp 212–225. Philadelphia: WB Saunders.

Hrachovy RA, Frost JD, Kellaway P (1981) Sleep characteristics in infantile spasms. *Neurology* **31**:688–694.

Hrachovy RA, Frost JD, Kellaway PR *et al* (1983) Double-blind study of ACTH vs. prednisone therapy in infantile spasms. *Journal of Pediatrics* **103**:641–645.

Hrachovy RA, Frost JD, Kellaway P (1984) Hypsarrhythmia: variations on the theme. *Epilepsia* **25**:317–325.

Hrachovy RA, Frost JD, Glaze DG (1988) Treatment of infantile spasms with tetrabenazine. *Epilepsia* **29**:561–563.

Hrachovy RA, Frost JD, Glaze DG *et al* (1989) Treatment of infantile spasms with methyscrgide and alpha-methylparatyrosine. *Epilepsia* **30**:607–610.

Hrachovy RA, Frost JD, Glaze DG (1994) High-dose, long duration versus low-dose, short duration corticotropin therapy for infantile spasms. *Journal of Pediatric* **124**:803–806.

Hwang PA, Otsubo H, Koo BKK *et al* (1996) Infantile spasms: cerebral blood flow abnormalities correlate with EEG, neuroimaging, and pathologic findings. *Pediatric Neurology* **14**:220–225.

Jambaque I, Chiron C, Dulac O *et al* (1993) Visual inattention in West syndrome: a neuropsychological and neurofunctional study. *Epilepsia* **34**:692–700.

Jeavons PM (1985) West syndrome: infantile spasms. In: Roger J, Dravet C, Bureau M *et al* (eds) *Epileptic Syndromes in Infancy, Childhood, and Adolescence*, pp. 42–50. London: John Libbey Eurotext.

Jeavons PM, Bower BD (1964) *Infantile Spasms: A Review of the Literature and a Study of 112 Cases.* London: Heineman.

Jeavons PM, Bower BD, Dimitrakoudi M (1973) Long term prognosis of 150 cases of 'West syndrome'. *Epilepsia* **14**:153–164.

Jellinger K (1987) Neuropathological aspects of infantile spasms. *Brain and Development* **9**:349–357.

Kellaway P, Hrachovy RA, Frost JD *et al* (1979) Precise characterization and quantification of infantile spasms. *Annals of Neurology* 6:214–218.

Klawans HL Jr, Goetz C, Weiner WJ (1973) 5-Hydroxytryptophan-induced myoclonus in guinea pigs and the possible role of serotonin in infantile myoclonus. *Neurology* **23**:1234–1240.

Klein R, Livingston S (1950) The effect of adrenocorticotrophic hormone in epilepsy. *Journal of Pediatrics* **37**:733–742.

Koo B, Hwang P (1996) Localization of focal cortical lesions influences age of onset of infantile spasms. *Epilepsia* **37**:1968–1971.

Koo B, Hwang PA, Logan WJ (1993) Infantile spasms: outcome and prognostic factors of cryptogenic and symptomatic groups. *Neurology* **43**:2322–2327.

Kramer U, Sue WC, Mikati MA (1997a) Hypsarrhythmia: frequency of variant patterns and correlation with etiology and outcome. *Neurology* **48**:197–203.

Kramer U, Sue WC, Mikati MA (1997b) Focal features in West syndrome indicating candidacy for surgery. *Pediatric Neurology* **16**:213–217.

Kuwahara M, Shima M, Nakai H *et al* (1996) A case of West syndrome with atypical massive gray matter heterotopia that is well controlled by ACTH therapy. *Acta Paediatrica Japonica* **38**:274–277.

Lacy JR, Penry JK (1976) *Infantile Spasms.* New York: Raven Press.

Lombroso CT (1983) A prospective study of infantile spasms: clinical and therapeutic correlation. *Epilepsia* **24**:135–158.

Low NL (1958) Infantile spasms with mental retardation: I. Treatment with cortisone and adrenocorticotropin. *Pediatrics* **22**:1165–1169.

McQuarrie I, Anderson JA, Ziegler RR (1942) Observations on the antagonistic effects of posterior pituitary and cortico-adrenal hormones in the epileptic subject. *Journal of Clinical Endocrinology* 2:406–410.

Makela-Benzs P, Somalainen A, Majander A *et al* (1995) Correlation between the clinical syndromes and proportion of mitochondrial DNA carrying the 8993 point mutation in the NARP syndrome. *Pediatric Research* **37**:634–639.

Millichap JG, Bickford RG, Klass RB *et al* (1962) Infantile spasms, hypsarrhythmia, and mental retardation. A study of etiology in 61 patients. *Epilepsia* 3:188–197.

Mimaki T, Ono J, Yabuchi H (1983) Temporal lobe astrocytoma with infantile spasms. *Annals of Neurology* **14**:695–696.

Miyazaki M, Hashimoto T, Tayama M, Kuroda Y (1993) Brainstem involvement in infantile spasms: a study employing brainstem evoked potentials and magnetic resonance imaging. *Neuropediatrics* **24**:126–130.

Miyazaki M, Hashimoto T, Fujii E *et al* (1994a) Infantile spasms: localized cerebral lesions on SPECT. *Epilepsia* **35**:988–992.

Miyazaki M, Hashimoto T, Omura H *et al* (1994b) Infantile spasms with predominantly unilateral cerebral abnormalities. *Neuropediatrics* **25**:325–330.

Ohtahara S (1965) Electroencephalographic studies in infantile spasms. *Developmental Medicine and Child Neurology* 7:707.

Ohtahara S, Ohtsuka Y, Yamatogi Y *et al* (1993) Prenatal etiologies of West syndrome. *Epilepsia* **34**:716–722.

Ohtsuka Y, Murashima I, Asano T *et al* (1996) Partial seizures in West syndrome. *Epilepsia* **37**:1060–1067.

Otero LJ, Brown GK, Silver K *et al* (1995) Association of cerebral dysgenesis and lactic acidemia with X-linked PDH E1 α subunit mutations in females. *Pediatric Neurology* **13**:327–332.

Otsubo H, Hwang PA, Jay V *et al* (1993) Focal cortical dysplasia in children with localization-related epilepsy: EEG, MRI, and SPECT findings. *Pediatric Neurology* **9**:101–107.

Ozek E, Ozek MM, Caliskan M *et al* (1995) Multiple pineal cysts associated with an ependymal cyst presenting with infantile spasms. *Child's Nervous System* **11**:246–249.

Palm L, Blennow G, Brun A (1986) Infantile spasms and neuronal heterotopias. *Acta Paediatrica Scandinavica* **75**:855–859.

Palm DG, Brant M, Korinthenberg R *et al* (1988) West syndrome and Lennox–Gastaut syndrome in children with porencephalic cysts. In: Niedermeyere E, Degen R (eds) *The Lennox–Gastaut Syndrome*, pp 419–426. New York: Alan R Liss.

Pinard JM, Delalande O, Plouin P *et al* (1993) Callosotomy in West syndrome suggests a cortical origin of hypsarrhythmia. *Epilepsia* **34**:780–787.

Pine I, Engle L, Schwartz TB (1951) The electroencephalogram in ACTH and cortisone treated patients. *Electroencephalography and Clinical Neurophysiology* **3**:301–310.

Plouin P, Dulac O, Jalin C *et al* (1993) Twenty-four-hour ambulatory EEG monitoring in infantile spasms. *Epilepsia* **34**:686–691.

Riikonen R (1982) A long-term follow-up study of 21 children with the syndrome of infantile spasms. *Neuropediatrics* **13**:14–23.

Riikonen R, Simell O (1990) Tuberous sclerosis and infantile spasms. *Developmental Medicine and Child Neurology* **32**:203–209.

Robain O, Chiron C, Dulac O (1989) Electron microscopic and Golgi study in a case of hemimegalencephaly. *Acta Neuropathologica* **77**:664–666.

Ruggieri V, Carvallo R, Fejerman N (1989) Intracranial tumors and West syndrome. *Pediatric Neurology* **5**:327–329.

Sankar R, Curran JG, Rintahaka PJ *et al* (1995) Microscopic cortical dysplasia in infantile spasms: evolution of white matter abnormalities. *American Journal of Neuroradiology* **16**:1265–1272.

Saroh J, Mizutani T, Morimatsu Y (1986) Neuropathology of the brainstem in age-dependent epileptic encephalopathy: especially of cases with infantile spasms. *Brain and Development* **8**:443–449.

Shields WD, Shewmon DA, Chugani HT *et al* (1992) Treatment of infantile spasms: medical or surgical? *Epilepsia* **33**(Suppl 4):S26–S31.

Silverstein F, Johnston MV (1984) Cerebrospinal fluid monoamine metabolites in patients with infantile spasms. *Neurology* **34**:102–105.

Snead OC (1994) Medical treatment of infantile spasms. In: Dulac O, Chugani HT, Della Bernadina B (eds) *Infantile Spasms and West Syndrome*, pp 244–256. London: WB Saunders.

Snead OC, Nelson MD (1993) PET does not eliminate the need for extraoperative intracranial monitoring in pediatric epilepsy surgery. *Pediatric Neurology* **9**:405–411.

Snead OC, Benton JW, Myers GJ (1983) ACTH and prednisone in childhood seizure disorders. *Neurology* **33**:966–970.

Snead OC, Benton JW, Hosey LC *et al* (1989) Treatment of infantile spasms with high dose ACTH: efficacy and plasma levels of ACTH and cortisol. *Neurology* **39**:1027–1030.

Snead OC, Chen LS, Mitchell WG *et al* (1996) Usefulness of [18F]fluorodeoxyglucose positron emission tomography in pediatric epilepsy surgery. *Pediatric Neurology* **14**:98–107.

Sorel L, Dusaucy-Bauloye A (1958) A propos de cas d'hypsarrhythmia de Gibbs: son traitement spectaculaire par l'ACTH. *Acta Neurologica Belgica* **58**:130–141.

Stamps FW, Gibbs EL, Rosenthal IM *et al* (1959) Treatment of hypsarrhythmia with ACTH. *Journal of the American Medical Association* **171**:408–411.

Tachibana Y, Shimizu A (1993) Clinical and electroencephalographic study of unilateral or predominantly unilateral seizures. *Japanese Journal of Psychiatry and Neurology* **47**:207–210.

Tatzer E, Groh C, Muller R *et al* (1987) Carbamazepine and benzodiazepines in combination: a possibility to improve the efficacy of treatment of patients with 'intractable' infantile spasms? *Brain and Development* **9**:415–417.

Tjam AT, Stefanko S, Schenk VMD *et al* (1978) Infantile spasms associated with hypsarrhythmia and hemimegalencephaly. *Developmental Medicine and Child Neurology* **20**:779–798.

Uthman BM, Reid SA, Wilder BJ *et al* (1991) Outcome for West syndrome following surgical treatment. *Epilepsia* **32**:668–671.

van Bogaert P, Chiron C, Adamsbaum C *et al* (1993) Value of magnetic resonance imaging in West syndrome of unknown etiology. *Epilepsia* **34**:701–706.

Viani F, Romeo A, Mastrangelo M *et al* (1994) Infantile spasms secondary to the surgical excision of a brain tumor. *Journal of Child Neurology* **9**:103–104.

Vigevano F, Cilio MR (1997) Vigabatrin versus ACTH as first-line treatment for infantile spasms: a randomized, prospective study. *Epilepsia* **38**:1270–1274.

Vinters HV, De Rosa MJ, Farrell MA (1993) Neuropathologic study of resected cerebral tissue from patients with infantile spasms. *Epilepsia* **34**:772–779.

Watanabe K (1998) West syndrome: etiological and prognostic aspects. *Brain and Development* **20**:1–8.

Wayne HS (1954) Convulsive seizures complicating cortisone and ACTH therapy: clinical and electroencephalographic observations. *Journal of Clinical Endocrinology and Metabolism* **14**:1039–1045.

Wenzel D (1987) Evoked potentials in infantile spasms. *Brain and Development* **9**:365–368.

West WJ (1841) On a peculiar form of infantile convulsions. *Lancet* i:724–725.

Wyllie E, Comair YG, Kotagal P *et al* (1996) Epilepsy surgery in infants. *Epilepsia* **37**:625–637.

Yamamoto N, Watanabe K, Negoro T *et al* (1988) Partial seizures evolving to infantile spasms. *Epilepsia* **29**:34–40.

Investigation of intractable focal epilepsy

Diagnostic neuroradiology

P ANSLOW AND J OXBURY

24

Developments in computerized brain imaging during the last quarter century, initially X-ray CT and then magnetic resonance imaging (MRI), have established that structural brain pathology underlies intractable focal epilepsy in most cases. Developments in structural imaging have been accompanied by a parallel development of functional imaging techniques such as position emission tomography (PET), single-photon emission computed tomography (SPECT), MR spectroscopy, and functional MRI (fMRI). These are considered in other chapters. The concern here is entirely with structural imaging. MRI is superior to CT in that it is more sensitive for detecting the presence and specifying the nature of pathology. All patients with intractable focal epilepsy merit examination with MRI in a search for pathology and to assist in an accurate diagnosis of their epilepsy syndrome so that an appropriate treatment plan can be established (Commission on Neuroimaging of the International League Against Epilepsy 1997; Duncan 1997). CT should be reserved for special circumstances such as when there is a need to search for calcium (see below).

The pathology underlying intractable focal epilepsy may be either static/nonprogressive, such as Ammon's horn sclerosis, or progressive such as a glioma that is growing, all be it slowly. An MRI study of 146 patients with chronic partial epilepsy (Cook and Stevens 1995) revealed pathol-ogy in 85%. Hippocampal atrophy was the most common (34%), followed by a malformation of cortical development (16%), tumor including dysembryoplastic neuroepithe-lioma (16%), and vascular malformation (10%). Pathology was detected more often in those with temporal lobe epilepsy (TLE) (>90%) than in those with an extratemporal epilepsy (65%). The proportion of patients in whom no pathology is defined may well fall even lower with the application of increasingly sophisticated techniques such as quantitative MRI block analysis (Sisodiya *et al* 1995).

The pathologic substrates to intractable focal epilepsy may be divided into five categories (Friedland and Bronen 1996): mesial temporal sclerosis/hippocampal sclerosis, malformations of cortical development, neoplasms, vascular abnormalities, and miscellaneous including the manifesta-tions of infection such as cysticercal cysts and tuberculo-mata, traumatic lesions and nonspecific gliosis. The neuroradiology of the first two of these pathologies is detailed in Chapters 10, 11 and 44 and is not considered specifically here. The purpose of neuroradiologic investiga-tion is not only to establish the presence of the pathology and its nature, but also to specify its precise anatomic loca-tion. This latter is of paramount importance given the increasing availability of surgery as a viable treatment. It is essential, therefore, that the strategy should be to apply the best possible practicable imaging technology.

METHODS OF INVESTIGATION

MRI and CT form the basis for cross-sectional imaging of epilepsy patients. There can be no doubt, however, that MRI should be offered to all patients with intractable focal epilepsy.

X-RAY COMPUTED TOMOGRAPHY

Even high-quality CT is less sensitive than MRI. It has little value as a first-line imaging modality for intractable epilepsy. It does, however, have a particular value in the detection of calcification and in the assessment of vascularity.

Calcification

Calcification is a prominent feature of several pathological processes (Table 24.1). MRI may well detect the soft tissue matrix of a calcified lesion but if the lesion is made of calcium predominantly it may be completely 'invisible' to MRI. CT, on the other hand, detects such lesions without difficulty and furthermore may help to clarify the nature of an abnormality initially detected on MRI.

Vascularity

Both gadolinium-enhanced MRI and contrast-enhanced CT image disturbances of the blood–brain barrier. Contrast leaks from the intravascular space into the extracellular spaces where it accumulates and is imaged. The degree of enhancement depends on a number of factors including the concentration of the contrast, the degree of the blood–brain barrier breakdown and the vascularity of the lesion. It should be realized that whereas contrast CT consistently enhances the vascular component of a lesion, the vascular enhancement with MRI is less consistent due to flow-related effects.

MAGNETIC RESONANCE IMAGING

Machines vary in their technical capability and spatial and contrast resolution, but as a simple guide, scans of the whole brain should be obtained in three planes (sagittal, axial, and coronal), employing three different pulse sequences, for example T1, T2 and proton density. This minimum set of sequences can usually be obtained in a tolerable time frame (5–15 min, depending on field strength). The combination gives a very reliable and comprehensive assessment of the epilepsy patient. There are, however, a number of pulse sequences that offer specific advantages to patients with chronic epilepsy.

Fluid attenuated inversion recovery (FLAIR)

This is a valuable pulse sequence for supratentorial lesions. It increases the conspicuity of pathologic processes where increased tissue water is a feature. The image itself is a relatively low contrast, mid-gray. Lesions are of high signal and stand out clearly from the background (Fig. 24.1).

Table 24.1 Conditions associated with cerebral calcification which also cause intractable focal epilepsy.

Low-grade glioma/oligodendroglioma, astrocytoma grade 2
Dysembryoplastic neuroepithelioma
Cortical dysplasia, malformation of cortical development
Tuberous sclerosis
Sturge–Weber syndrome
Cavernous angioma
Calcified aneurysm
Neonatal cerebral hemorrhage
Congenital brain infection including cytomegalovirus and toxoplasmosis
Postnatal infection including cysticercosis and tuberculoma
Calcified abscess cavity
Celiac disease with epilepsy and cerebral calcifications

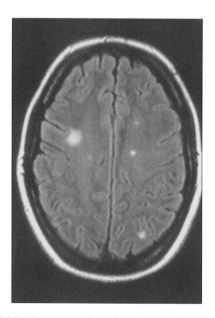

Fig. 24.1 Axial FLAIR sequence through brain at a level above the lateral ventricles. The high signal lesions are characteristic of multiple sclerosis.

T1 volume acquisitions

These are known by a number of different acronyms depending on the manufacturer (e.g. SPGR – International General Electric; MPRAGE–Siemens Medical Systems). The pulse sequences typically produce 128 contiguous 1 mm thick images, usually in the coronal plane. The voxels are almost cubic and it is possible, therefore, to submit the data set to multiplanar reconstruction with very little loss of spatial resolution. The pulse sequence is particularly valuable in the assessment of hippocampal atrophy (see Chapters 11 and 44). It has a particular value also in the assessment of malformations of cortical development since there is usually high gray/white discrimination. The assessment of the image set for subtle malformations of cortical development requires a considerable amount of radiologic expertise and time since all 128 images must be specifically examined both individually and as part of a sequence and in multiple planes (Barkovich 1995). In children aged <2 years there may be poor contrast between white and gray matter, because of incomplete myelination, so that it may be difficult to detect cortical abnormalities. Consequently, MRI in young children may need to be repeated at an older age.

Diffusion-weighted imaging

Essentially this is an echo-planar pulse sequence designed to image axoplasmic flow. Scans are therefore performed in all three axes (x, y, and z). Areas of signal change represent flow change in differing areas of brain.

Gadolinium enhancement

This is rarely of value in the *detection* of lesions responsible for epilepsy but is of value in their subsequent *characterization*. As stated above, gadolinium accumulates at areas in the brain where the blood–brain barrier has been disturbed. It is valuable, therefore, in detecting areas of neoplasia or inflammatory change.

Once a good-quality CT or MRI scan has been performed, two assessments have to be made. Firstly, any lesion must be detected. The likelihood of that happening is influenced by the intrinsic contrast of the lesion, by the spatial resolution of the scan, and by the observer's knowledge of deviations from normal anatomy. The second part of the process is lesion characterization.

THE RADIOLOGIC DIAGNOSTIC PROCESS

The radiologic process involves the detection of focal abnormalities in cerebral architecture. Subtle lesions require a considerable amount of effort from both the radiographer, who must produce excellent-quality images, and the radiologist who must spend much time examining in great detail what may in the end turn out to be hundreds of images. Having detected a focal abnormality the radiologic process involves detailed descriptions of the morphology of the lesion under a number of headings (Table 24.2) and of the precise location.

A diagnosis, that is a statement of the most likely pathology, is based on the morphologic characteristics in conjunction with the features of the clinical presentation. The latter aspect is of great importance. The increased availability of surgical treatment for intractable epilepsy has created a need for extreme accuracy of diagnosis of the nature of the pathology and of localization of its precise position. This is because the prognosis for good outcome after surgery is better with some forms of pathology than with others (Bruton 1988) and if a complete rather than a partial excision can be achieved (Montes *et al* 1995).

MORPHOLOGY

The structural imaging features of hippocampal sclerosis and of malformations of cortical development are described in the chapters on those conditions and are not considered here. Brief descriptions are, however, given of the structural imaging characteristics of various other conditions commonly underlying intractable focal epilepsy.

Table 24.2 Aspects of lesion morphology.

Location
Morphology
  Size
  Definition of edge
  Presence of cysts
  Presence of necrosis or cavitation
  Presence of edema
  Homogeneity
  Enhancement characteristics

TUMORS

Indolent glioma–oligodendroglioma, grade 2 astrocytoma

Such tumors are appreciated by changes of signal – usually of increased signal on T2-weighted images. The lesions may exhibit mass effect but some low-grade gliomas do not do so and do not have associated edema. So, great care must be taken to distinguish them from areas of infarction or cerebral damage. Calcification is a common but not invariable feature of oligodendrogliomas. Cyst formation is frequently seen in astrocytomas. Contrast enhancement is rarely a prominent feature of these lesions and reflects their benign nature. Necrosis within such tumors and vasogenic-type edema around them indicates that they may be undergoing malignant transformation. Calvarial erosion may be detected.

The MRI abnormality indicative of a low-grade glioma may be very extensive, in contrast to the virtual absence of abnormal neurologic signs, particularly in a patient with a long history of epilepsy (Fig. 24.2).

Dysembryoplastic neuroepithelioma and ganglioglioma

These two tumor types have a very variable scan morphology that reflects their variable histopathology. It seems to be generally agreed that they may be indistinguishable. Both are situated more commonly in a temporal lobe than in other parts of a cerebral hemisphere and around 25% of each type show calcification. Both tend to be hypo-intense on T1-weighted images with increased signal on T2. They may have some mass effect and gangliogliomas may show slight enhancement. There may be concomitant hippocampal atrophy (dual pathology), especially in a patient with a history of a prolonged convulsion in early childhood, and calvarial erosion may be seen. Dysembryoplastic neuroepitheliomas usually have a cortical location and there may be clear evidence of associated cortical dysplasia that can be remote from the tumor itself. There should not be edema, and the presence of this feature should suggest a different diagnosis (Fig. 24.3).

Dermoid and epidermoid

These epithelial tumors are most often situated in the middle and posterior fossae, or in the midline in the anterior fossa. They are usually extra-axial, but occasionally parenchymal. Their density on CT is almost always low, whereas on MRI the signal characteristics vary according to the relative proportions of fat, soft tissue, and water within them. Occasionally a dermoid ruptures spontaneously into the subarachnoid space, giving a flurry of seizures and a syndrome of chemical meningitis. More often these indolent, benign tumors cause occasional seizure disorders, including chronic epilepsy, and symptoms related to their mass effect (Fig. 24.4).

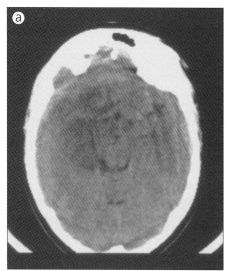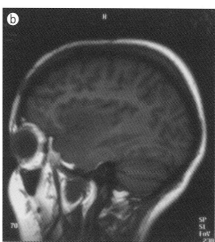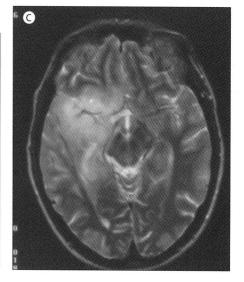

Fig. 24.2 Proven grade II astrocytoma. (a) Axial CT scan. A faint area of low density can just be appreciated in the medial aspect of the right temporal lobe. (b) Sagittal T1-weighted scan. An area of low signal intensity is seen involving both the superficial aspect of the temporal lobe and the insular cortex. (c) Axial T2-weighted MRI scan. This scan illustrates the huge increase in sensitivity of MRI over CT. Whereas the CT lesion is subtle, the MRI lesion is obvious and involves temporal and inferior frontal cortex as well as insular cortex.

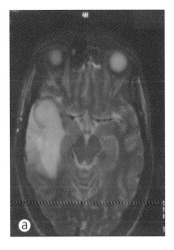
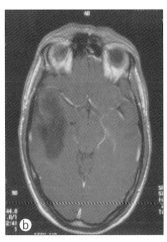

Fig. 24.3 Disembryoplastic neuroepithelioma. (a) Axial T2-weighted scan showing large lesion in right temporal lobe. (b) Axial T1-weighted scan after the administration of gadolinium. Note the lack of contrast enhancement. This was a young patient with habitual epilepsy. These tumours are morphologically diverse, but should not have edema or enhance. This lesion is unusual in that there is both an intrinsic and exophytic component.

Tuberous sclerosis

CT and/or MRI abnormalities are said to be present in >90% of people with tuberous sclerosis (Houser and Nixon 1988). Indeed the detection of cortical tubers is one of the prime diagnostic features of the condition. A number of abnormalities may be seen on CT including multiple calcified subependymal nodules and multiple hypodense foci, more often in the cerebral hemispheres than in the cerebellum, which may become hyperintense due to calcification and are indicative of tubers. A subependymal nodule may undergo gliomatous change, then appearing as an enhancing mass lesion, that may be calcified, particularly in the region of the foramen of Munro. There may be ventricular dilatation. On MRI, the calcification may be easily missed. The subependymal nodules may be isointense with white matter on both T1- and T2-weighted images but appear as soft tissue masses projecting into the ventricles. Tubers appear as foci of increased T2 signal especially in the immediate subcortical plane. While most lesions are easily identified, these lesions may be very subtle and the scans need to be very closely inspected (Fig. 24.5).

VASCULAR ABNORMALITIES

Cerebral arteriovenous malformations, cavernous angiomas, and the pial angiomatosis of Sturge–Weber syndrome are vascular abnormalities with intractable epilepsy as one of their common manifestations. The radiologic appearances consequent upon the prenatal and perinatal vascular accidents that underlie the syndrome of infantile hemiplegia with epilepsy are also considered here. Venous malformations, dural arteriovenous malformations, and capillary telangiectasia are not considered because their relationship to intractable focal epilepsy is more tenuous.

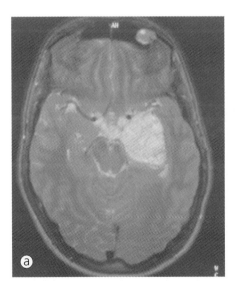
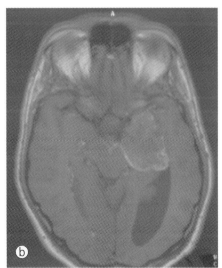
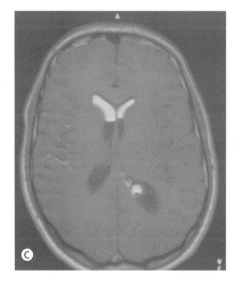

Fig. 24.4 Dermoid. (a) Axial T2-weighted scan. Complex high signal lesion in medial temporal lobe. (b) Same slice, axial T1-weighted scan. The lesion contains high signal consistent with fat. (c) Axial T1-weighted scan at level of ventricles. There is a fat/fluid interface within the lateral ventricles and some globules of fat are seen in the trigone region. This young patient had occasional seizures and then presented acutely with a flurry of seizures at the point when his dermoid spontaneously ruptured into his ventricular system.

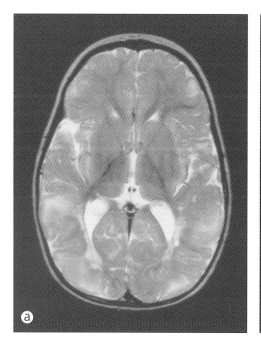
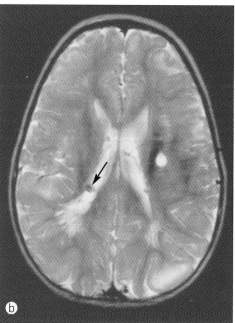

Fig. 24.5 Tuberous sclerosis. (a) Axial T2-weighted MRI scan reveals areas of subcortical high signal indicative of the hamartomatous malformation of tuberous sclerosis. (b) Axial T2-weighted scan showing a small lesion arising from the right ventricular wall. The lesion is of low signal on this T2-weighted scan and represents a calcified tuber (arrow). This scan was obtained in an 18-month-old child with severe epilepsy and characteristic skin lesions. It is unusual to see such a high lesion load in a child of this age. Note also the dilated Virchow–Robin spaces (a nonspecific feature of tuberous sclerosis).

Cerebral arteriovenous malformation (AVM)

An AVM consists of a central nidus of tangled malformed vessels, consisting of arteries connecting to veins without an interposed capillary bed, supplied by one or more arteries and draining into one or more major veins. Secondary changes such as thrombosis, fibrosis, and calcification occur, and there may be hemosiderin deposits. The lesions vary in size from very small to a size that involves a whole hemisphere.

Small lesions cannot be identified on CT unless they are calcified or unless contrast is given and enhancement is seen. Larger lesions can be appreciated on noncontrast scans since their feeding and draining vessels are serpiginous in outline and of slightly greater density than brain. MRI reveals the serpiginous mass of even small malformations without contrast administration. Vessels that contain flowing blood are of low signal intensity on T2-weighted scans and are readily seen against the relatively neutral intensity of the brain (Fig. 24.6). The huge advantage of MRI in the assessment of AVM lies in the technique's capacity to localize the pathology precisely so that rational decisions can be made about surgical approaches, resectibility, and endovascular therapy.

Conventional angiography and/or magnetic resonance angiography is necessary to achieve a more precise definition of the arterial supply and venous drainage.

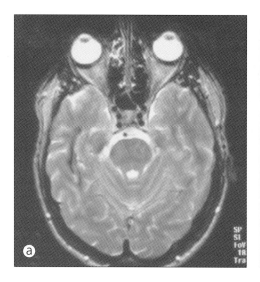
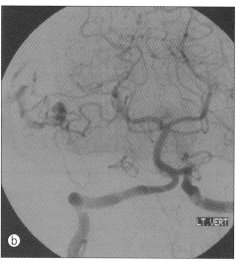

Fig. 24.6 Temporal lobe AVM. (a) Axial T2-weighted scan shows linear slit of low signal intensity consistent with hemosiderin deposition in the wall of a subacute hematoma. Complex small flow voids are seen medial to the hemosiderin suggestive of an arteriovenous malformation. (b) Contrast angiogram via the left vertebral artery shows an enlarged branch of the right posterior cerebral artery supplying the malformation and an early draining vein. This patient presented with seizures: there was no history of an ictus related to the presumed hematoma.

Cavernous angioma (CA)

These lesions consist of vascular spaces, not truly arterial or venous, usually containing hemosiderin and thrombus and/or calcification but not neural tissue. They bleed repetitively but not usually sufficiently to cause clinical symptoms. The bleeds lead to hemosiderin deposition and a gliotic reaction. CAs are of variable size. They may be single or multiple and in the case of the latter particularly they may be familial. They were rarely diagnosed in the CT era, 'popcorn' calcification usually being their only CT feature, although occasionally a soft tissue mass lesion is seen. They are frequently diagnosed with MRI.

The MRI features of CA are dominated by hemosiderin. On T2-weighted scans, dark complex shapes of successive generations of hemosiderin are outlined by high-signal gliosis, making the lesions very conspicuous. T1-weighted scans may reveal the high signal of methemoglobin if a recent bleed has occurred. Contrast enhancement does not occur within the vascular pools of these lesions, since they are effectively isolated from the circulation (Fig. 24.7).

Sturge–Weber syndrome (SWS)

The radiologic features of SWS are usually very characteristic. They include cerebral hemisphere atrophy and ipsilateral 'tramline' calcification of the cerebral cortex that are usually unilateral and most prominent in the occipital and parietal regions, and enhancement of the pial angiomatosis. Both CT and MRI may demonstrate the focal atrophy induced by the pial vascular malformation. CT demon-

strates the fine curvilinear cortical calcification when it is present. Otherwise the only other feature of the disorder on CT is an enlarged choroid plexus ipsilateral to the pial angiomatosis. Contrast enhancement does occur on CT, but is difficult to identify against the high density of the inner table of the skull. MRI does not demonstrate the cortical calcification, but does reveal the cortical atrophy associated with the calcification and the pial malformation. The enlarged choroid plexus is easily seen. Gadolinium enhancement frequently produces dramatic pial enhancement and demonstrates enlarged veins related to the choroid plexus and the cerebral surface (Fig. 24.8).

Pre- and perinatal cerebral infarction

Intrauterine and perinatal strokes are relatively frequent events that are increasingly recognized. The territory most frequently involved is that supplied by the middle cerebral artery, that is much of the lateral aspect of the hemisphere and the basal ganglia. Consequently, hemiplegic cerebral palsy is a frequent outcome and intractable focal epilepsy may develop.

Both CT and MRI demonstrate the typical appearances of a classical middle cerebral artery territory distribution of infarction. The cerebral tissue is usually completely resorbed in the damaged area leaving only a localized area of cystic encephalomalacia. Close inspection of the affected hemisphere frequently reveals it to be much smaller than is its companion, even after the volume of the infarcted tissue is subtracted. Equally frequently, the volume of the contralateral hemisphere appears larger than normal, possibly reflecting true hypertrophy in response to an early life event (Fig. 24.9).

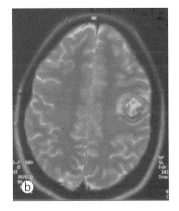

Fig. 24.7 Cavernoma. (a) Sagittal T1-weighted scan showing complex high and low signal lesion in posterior aspect of frontal lobe. The high signal is methemoglobin and probably represents a subacute bleed. (b) Axial T2-weighted scan showing classical 'popcorn' appearance with low signal hemosiderin deposition indicative of previous bleeds. Note the surrounding edema suggesting a recent event.

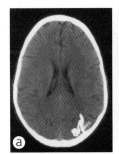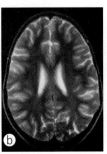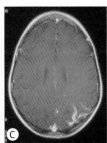

Fig. 24.8 Sturge–Weber syndrome. (a) Axial CT scan showing gyral calcification in left parietal region. (b) Axial T2-weighted MRI scan at exactly the same level does not show any easily detectable lesion. (c) Axial T1-weighted MRI scan after contrast administration shows pial enhancement at the site of calcification.

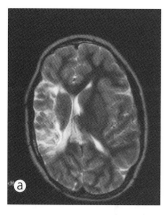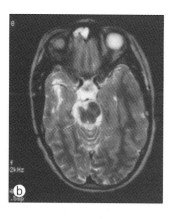

Fig. 24.9 Congenital hemiplegia. (a) Axial T2-weighted scan showing a very small right hemisphere and atrophic cortex. Note ulegyria of the cortex supplied by the right middle cerebral artery. (b) Note the very small cerebral peduncle secondary to Wallerian degeneration of the corticospinal tract. This child presented in infancy with mild hemiparesis and seizures.

INFECTIONS AND OTHER ENCEPHALITIDES

Rasmussen encephalitis

All imaging may be normal in the early stages of this severe illness. Atrophy of the affected hemisphere, possibly with mild contralateral atrophy, is seen later (Fig. 24.10).

Neurocysticercosis and tuberculoma

The acute lesions of neurocysticercosis are seen, on both MRI and CT, as small solitary or multiple, solid or ring-enhancing areas scattered throughout the white matter. There are no specific features and the differential diagnosis for this appearance consists of multiple metastases, abscesses or other granulomata including tuberculomata. Later the lesions may heal and calcify resulting in tiny specks of dense

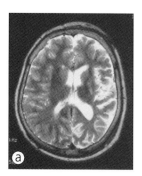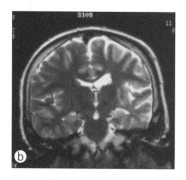

Fig. 24.10 Rasmussen encephalitis. (a) Axial T2-weighted scan showing atrophy of the left hemisphere. (b) Coronal T2-weighted scan showing atrophy of the left hemisphere. Five years previously an MRI scan had been normal, at the start of the seizure disorder. The focal atrophic changes had evolved over this time. The diagnosis was confirmed at pathology following hemispherectomy.

calcification best demonstrated on CT. Diagnosis is assisted by a geographic history and by the potential for exposure to the parasite (Fig. 24.11).

Tuberculoma arises in the differential diagnosis of single or multiple enhancing lesions demonstrated either on CT or MRI. Although tuberculomata may be multiple it is unusual to see more than three to four lesions in an affected individual. Lesions may reach 2–3 cm in diameter before cavitation occurs. Chronic lesions may calcify, but this is a relatively infrequent event if effective chemotherapy is offered (Fig. 24.12).

Both tuberculoma and neurocysticercosis are prevalent in the same regions of the world and both are treatable by medication. So, it is important that if possible the two should be differentiated radiologically, thereby preventing the need for excision biopsy. Most tuberculomata are larger than 20 mm diameter whereas most cysticercal granulomata are below that size (Rajshekhar *et al* 1993). A single small enhancing lesion due to cysticercosis seen on CT may resolve spontaneously (Rajshekhar 1991). Conversely, a solitary cysticercal granuloma may enlarge and so be mistaken for a tuberculoma (Rajshekhar and Chandy 1994).

Congenital cytomegalovirus (CMV) and toxoplasmosis infection

These two organisms are capable of causing an intrauterine infection and inflicting damage on the developing fetal brain. Children infected *in utero* may be microcephalic. Calcification may be present. If so it is best demonstrated by CT. Whereas in CMV infection the calcifications are numerous and tend to be clustered around the (dilated) ventricular surfaces, the calcifications of toxoplasmosis are less numerous and likely to be larger and coarser (Fig. 24.13). This difference in morphology is reasonably discriminatory. Cerebral malformations varying from lissencephaly to polymicrogyria may be seen depending on the timing of the infection.

Abscess cavity

Late-stage calcification of the residual abscess cavity is uncommon in the era of early surgical drainage and effective antimicrobial chemotherapy. An abscess cavity may resolve and heal so that all radiologically detectable abnormality disappears. More often, however, some detectable damage persists. This may vary from simple areas of gliosis (high signal on T2-weighted scans), to more gross damage resembling areas of frank infarction (Fig. 24.14).

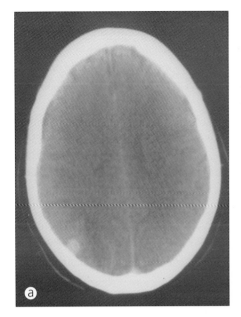
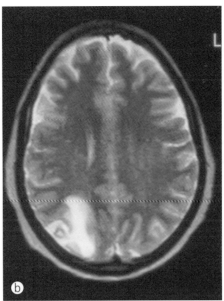

Fig. 24.11 Cerebral cysticercosis. (a) CT scan with contrast shows a small area of enhancement located superficially in the right parietal lobe. There is a little edema associated with it. (b) Axial T2-weighted MRI scan at the same level shows a small irregular ring of low signal surrounded by high-signal edema in the adjacent cortex and white matter. This patient developed habitual epilepsy after a period of service in Africa; the lesion evolved despite thorough antiparasitic chemotherapy.

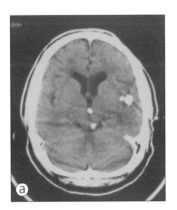
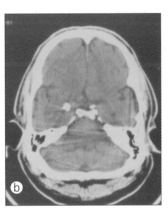
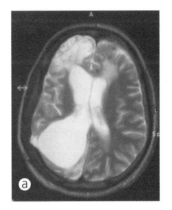
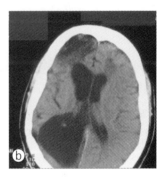

Fig. 24.12 Tuberculoma. CT scans showing dense calcification in temporal lobe and sylvian fissures following tuberculous meningitis and abscess formation. (Images courtesy of G. Quaghebeur.)

Fig. 24.14 (a) Axial T2 MRI shows focal damage in the right frontal lobe in addition to general volume loss in the right hemisphere (patient convalescing after subdural empyema and multiple cerebral abscesses). (b) Axial CT.

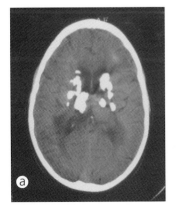
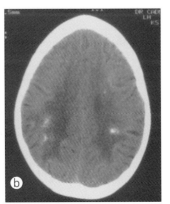

Fig. 24.13 Cerebral toxoplasmosis. (a) CT brain scan. Coarse basal calcifications demonstrated. (b) CT brain scan. Note the subcortical calcifications.

TRAUMA

Epilepsy is a common sequel of cerebral trauma, especially if there has been a penetrating injury, depressed skull fracture, or intracranial hemorrhage. Forms of damage that may be relevant to the development of epilepsy include:

1. Cerebral contusion related to penetrating injury or depressed fracture.
2. Coup and contre-coup injuries.
3. Shear hemorrhages (as part of a diffuse axonal injury).
4. Shear/split hemorrhages (as part of a shaking injury in infancy).

It should also be remembered that surgical intervention, both in terms of brain cutting and retraction injury, may cause epilepsy.

MRI is the radiologic technique of choice for the investigation of late posttraumatic epilepsy. In this circumstance, gradient echo sequences are of great value due to their ability to detect iron deposition following old hemorrhage. Volume acquisitions are able to detect very subtle areas of cortical damage (Fig. 24.15).

LOCALIZATION

Methods for establishing the precise location of pathology in relation to the cortical areas subserving major functions such as speech and limb movement have become very important in recent years following the great expansion in the surgical treatment of epilepsy. Surgery must as far as possible spare functionally eloquent areas to prevent postoperative deficits. So, the surgeon must be briefed about these anatomic considerations prior to surgical planning, even if there is an intention to carry out functional mapping, and the patient must be given a realistic statement of the risks based on the plan.

The location of a lesion clearly is of paramount importance:

1. It is a major factor determining the natural history of the epilepsy and the seizure semeiology.

2. It may limit the resectibility. Thus, a lesion close to the motor strip may be benign but unresectable without a high risk of subsequent contralateral limb weakness.
3. It has an influence on the likely pathology in that some lesions are seen with greater frequency in certain regions of brain.

Since the advent of good-quality MRI images, it has become possible to definitively localize several gyri of particular importance in the surgical treatment of epilepsy. These include:

1. The pre- and postcentral gyri (primary motor and sensory cortex).
2. Heschl's gyrus (primary auditory cortex situated anterior to Wernicke's area).

More difficulty is experienced with Broca's area on the inferolateral aspect of the frontal lobe.

THE PRE- AND POSTCENTRAL GYRI, THE PARACENTRAL LOBULE, AND THE CENTRAL SULCUS

The central sulcus extends from the sylvian fissure to the vertex and marks the boundary on the lateral surface between the frontal and parietal lobes.

The central sulcus does not reach as far as the midline. Instead the two parallel gyri, the pre- and postcentral gyri, fuse like the two limbs of a hairpin to form the paracentral lobule just before they reach the midline.

In Figure 24.16, the cingulate gyrus is a very obvious structure parallel to the corpus callosum. Above it the cingulate sulcus meanders to the vertex of the brain, continuing as its marginal branch.

The paracentral lobule on the medial surface of the hemisphere is bounded:

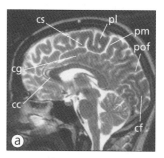
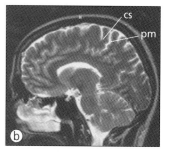

Fig. 24.16 Anatomy of medial hemisphere. (a) Sagittal T2-weighted scan close to midline to show corpus callosum (cc), cingulate gyrus (cg), cingulate sulcus (cs), pars marginalis (pm), and paracentral lobule (pl). Note also the parieto-occipital fissure (pof) and calcarine fissures (cf). (b) Parasagittal T2-weighted scan showing the central sulcus just anterior to the pars marginalis.

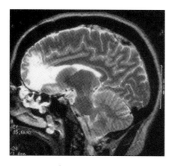

Fig. 24.15 Sagittal T2-weighted scan showing frontal and subfrontal cortical and white matter damage resulting in chronic epilepsy (patient was damaged during functional sinus surgery).

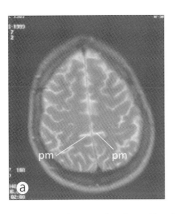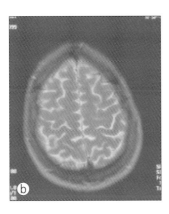

Fig. 24.17 The 'Pars bracket'. (a) Axial T2-weighted MRI scan close to vertex. Note the horizontal line made up by symmetrical pars marginalis (pm) sulci on either side of the midline. (b) Slightly higher slice than (a) showing the central sulci approaching the midline, but 'prevented' from doing so by the paracentral lobule.

1. anteriorly by the paracentral sulcus;
2. inferiorly by the cingulate sulcus;
3. posteriorly by the marginal branch of the cingulate sulcus, the pars marginalis.

It follows from this account that whereas the central sulcus fails to reach the midline, being 'prevented' from doing so

by the paracentral lobule, the pars marginalis does form a midline sulcus readily visible on midline sagittal and axial scans. On midline sagittal images the pars marginalis is a constant posterior relation of the paracentral lobule; on axial scans the central sulcus and the pars marginalis form an easily recognizable pattern, the 'pars bracket' (Figs 24.17 and 24.18).

Once the pars bracket is identified, other gyri and sulci become identifiable as a consequence:

1. Pre- and postcentral gyrae – axial images (Fig. 24.18)
2. Superior and middle frontal gyri – axial images (Fig. 24.18)
3. Superior parietal lobule – sagittal images (Fig. 24.18)
4. Precuneus – sagittal images (Fig. 24.19)

HESCHL'S GYRUS AND WERNICKE'S AREA

Parasagittal images of the brain at approximately the plane of the globe of the eye demonstrate the sylvian fissure, insular cortex, and frontal and temporal lobes to best advantage (Fig. 24.20).

From a series of images, the superior surface of the temporal lobe can be readily identified as a gently undulating

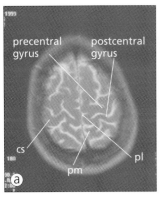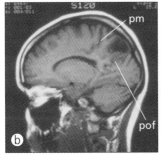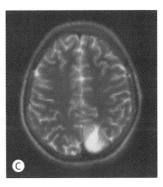

Fig. 24.18 Pre- and postcentral gyrae. (a) High axial slice showing arrangement of pars marginalis (pm), paracentral lobule (pl), central sulcus (cs), and pre- and postcental sulci. (b) Sagittal T1-weighted scan of a patient with dysembryoplastic neuroepithelioma. Note the relationship between the pars marginalis, the parietooccipital fissure (pof) and the low-density lesion indicating the lesion lies in the parietal lobe. (c) Axial T2-weighted scan showing lesion in medial surface of hemisphere. From this image it is not possible to be certain what relationship this lesion has to the motor cortex. It is the *combination* of sagittal and axial slices which is so powerful.

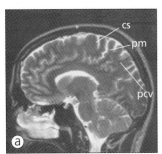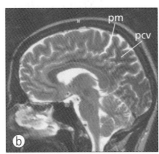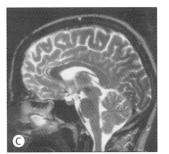

Fig. 24.19 Three consecutive images showing relationship of pars marginalis (pm), central sulcus (cs) and precuneus (pcu).

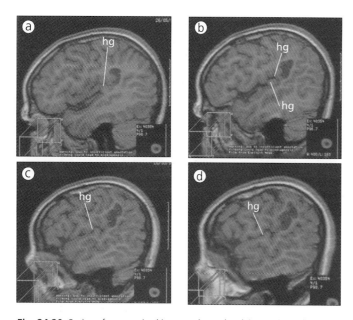

Fig. 24.20 Series of parasagittal images through sylvian region. The low-signal lesion is a presumed dysembryoplastic neuroepitheliana within the angular gyrus; (a) and b) also show Heschl's gyrus (hg) to good effect. Note its proximity to the angular gyrus.

margin. Heschl's gyrus is an inconstantly shaped discontinuity in that margin more posteriorly. The gyrus can be omega or heart shaped. Occasionally an extra sulcus (Beck's sulcus) cleaves the 'heart' in twain. In coronal scans, Heschl's gyrus is best identified on an image situated close to the level of fusion of the two fornices in the midline. Here, the sylvian fissure appears as a letter 'T' lying on its side, and Heschl's gyrus lies between the horizontal and vertical parts of the 'T' inferiorly (Fig. 24.21).

In the axial plane, the gyri are best demonstrated on an image running close to the upper aspect of the third ventricle at the level of the massa intermedia or the internal cerebral veins (Fig. 24.22).

As stated earlier, location of a pathologic process is of prime importance in focal epilepsy, not only from the perspective of the epilepsy itself but also when resection is being considered. At this point, functional studies such as fMRI may be considered to confirm, for example, that what has been identified from its structure as the precentral gyrus does indeed harbor motor function.

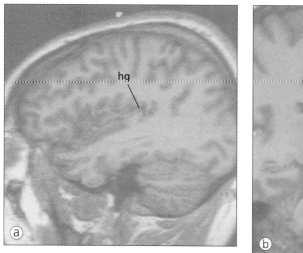

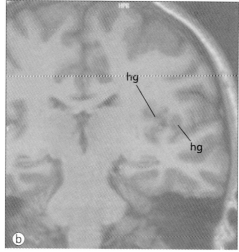

Fig. 24.21 (a) Sagittal and (b) coronal MPR showing Heschl's gyrus (hg) close to the posterior aspect of the sylvian fissure.

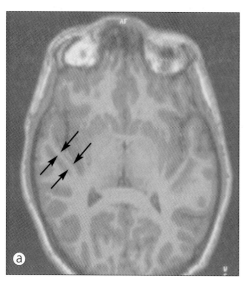

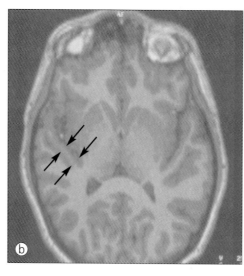

Fig. 24.22 Axial images through Heschl's gyrus (arrows) from an MPR study.

KEY POINTS

1. Structural brain pathology underlies intractable focal epilepsy in most cases and all patients with the condition merit examination with MRI. CT should be reserved for special circumstances such as when there is a need to search for calcium or assess the extent of vascularity. The purpose of neuroradiologic investigation is not only to establish the presence and nature of pathology, but also its precise anatomic location.

2. MRI scans of the whole brain should be obtained in the sagittal, coronal, and axial planes using three different pulse sequences, including T1 and T2, with a third such as proton density. Diagnosis, that is a statement of the most likely pathology, is based on the morphologic characteristics, established by the neuroradiologic investigation, in conjunction with the features of the clinical presentation.

3. T1 volume acquisitions are particularly valuable for the assessment of hippocampal atrophy and malformations of cortical development. The fluid attenuation inversion recovery (FLAIR) pulse sequence inceases the conspicuity of pathologic processes where increased tissue water is a feature. Gadolinium enhancement is rarely of value in the detection of pathology responsible for intractable epilepsy, but it may help in the subsequent characterization of pathology.

4. Brief descriptions are given of the structural imaging characteristics of indolent glioma, dysembryoplastic neuroepithelioma and ganglioglioma, dermoid and epidermoid, tuberous sclerosis, arteriovenous malformation, cavernous angioma, Sturge–Weber syndrome, pre- and perinatal cerebral infarction, Rasmussen encephalitis, neurocysticerosis and tuberculoma, congenital cytomegalovirus and toxoplasmosis, abcess cavity, and brain trauma.

5. The position of the central sulcus can be reliably established by locating the paracentral lobule that prevents the sulcus reaching the midline. On midline sagittal images the paracentral lobule constantly has the pars marginalis (the marginal branch of the cingulate sulcus) as its posterior relation. On axial images the pars marginalis and the central sulcus form an easily recognizable pattern known as the pars bracket enabling the central sulcus to be clearly located.

REFERENCES

Barkovitch AJ (1995) *Pediatric Neuroimaging*, 2nd edn.: Lippincott-Raven.

Bruton CJ (1988) *The Neuropathology of Temporal Lobe Epilepsy*. Oxford: Oxford University Press.

Commission on Neuroimaging of the International League Against Epilepsy (1997) Recommendations for neuroimaging of patients with epilepsy. *Epilepsia* **38**:1255–1256.

Cook M, Stevens JM (1995) Imaging in epilepsy. In: Hopkins A, Shorvon S, Cascino G (eds) *Epilepsy*, pp 143–169. London: Chapman & Hall.

Duncan JS (1997) Imaging and epilepsy. *Brain* **120**:339–377.

Friedland RJ, Bronen RA (1996) Magnetic resonance imaging of neoplastic, vascular, and indeterminate substrates. In: Cascino GD, Jack CR Jr (eds) *Neuroimaging in Epilepsy: Principles and Practice*, pp 29–50. Boston: Butterworth-Heinemann.

Houser OW, Nixon JR (1988) Central nervous system imaging. In: Gomez MR (ed.) *Tuberous Sclerosis*, 2nd edn, pp 51–62. New York: Raven Press.

Montes JL, Rosenblatt B, Farmer JP *et al* (1995) Lesionectomy of MRI-detected lesions in children with epilepsy. *Pediatric Neurosurgery* **22**:167–173.

Naidich T, Brightbill TC Systems for localizing frontoparietal gyri and sulci on axial CT and MRI. *International Journal of Neuroradiology* **2**(4):313–338.

Naidich T, Brightbill TC (1996) The pars marginalis: Part 1. *International Journal of Neuroradiology* **2**(1):3–19.

Rajshekhar V (1991) Etiology and management of single small CT lesions in patients with seizures: understanding a controversy. *Acta Neurologica Scandinavica* **84**:465–470.

Rajshekhar V, Chandy MJ (1994) Enlarging solitary cysticercus granulomas. *Journal of Neurosurgery* **80**:840–843.

Rajshekhar V, Haran RP, Prakash GS, Chandy MJ (1993) Differentiating solitary small cysticercus granulomas and tuberculomas in patients with epilepsy. *Journal of Neurosurgery* **78**:402–407.

Sisodiya SM, Free SL, Stevens JM, Fish DR, Shorvon SD (1995) Widespread cerebral structural changes in patients with cortical dysgenesis and epilepsy. *Brain* **118**:1039–1050.

Yousry TA, Fesl G, Buttner A, Noachtar S, Schmid UD (1997) Heschl's gyrus. *International Journal of Neuroradiology* **3**(1):2–12.

Diagnostic positron emission tomography

25

JR SHAH, DC CHUGANI, AND HT CHUGANI

Positron emission tomography (PET) is a noninvasive functional imaging tool that can be used to measure local uptake/affinity of a metabolic substrate or chemical in the brain and other organs. The application of PET in the evaluation of patients with intractable epilepsy has proved to be extremely useful in some circumstances and is now being implemented in a number of epilepsy surgery programs.

The most basic principle underlying the surgical treatment of intractable partial epilepsy is to identify a discrete epileptogenic focus lateralized and/or localized to one hemisphere. Not uncommonly, the surface EEG fails to provide the necessary localization or even the lateralization of the epileptogenic foci. Structural brain imaging with CT and magnetic resonance imaging (MRI) may also fail to identify discrete lesions associated with the epilepsy. As a result, many of these patients are labeled as nonsurgical candidates and some are subjected to invasive monitoring with numerous intracranial electrodes as a diagnostic procedure rather than as a means to address specific questions related to 'eloquent' cortex. In such patients, noninvasive localization of the epileptogenic focus by PET with the tracer 2-deoxy-2[^{18}F]fluoro-D-glucose (FDG) allows a metabolic focus to be defined and, depending upon its concordance with other data, might even eliminate the need for chronic invasive EEG monitoring. The purpose of this chapter is to review how PET is used as a noninvasive *diagnostic* test in

selected patients being evaluated for epilepsy surgery. Although PET is used also as a research tool in the study of the pathophysiology of epilepsy, this application is beyond the scope of the present chapter but is discussed in other reviews (Chugani *et al* 1997; Henry and Chugani 1997).

POSITRON EMISSION TOMOGRAPHY: THE METHOD

Positrons emitted from positron-emitting isotopes collide with surrounding electrons, resulting in annihilation of both particles and the release of paired high-energy (511 keV) photons. These photons travel in opposite directions and can be recorded by multiple pairs of oppositely situated detectors that constitute the PET camera (Hoffman and Phelps 1986; Ter-Pogossian 1995). Furthermore, by using tracer kinetic models that mathematically describe various physiologic or biochemical reaction sequences of compounds labeled with positron-emitting isotopes, the kinetics of biologic processes can be characterized (Huang and Phelps 1986). Thus, PET is a quantitative technique that allows not only imaging but also measurement of the rates of chemical reaction and various physiologic processes. Because PET isotopes have short half-lives (minutes to hours), the cyclotron used to generate these isotopes must be situated either on-site or within several hours travel distance from the PET scanning facility (Fowler and Wolf 1986).

GLUCOSE METABOLISM PET

TEMPORAL LOBE EPILEPSY

In adults and children with temporal lobe epilepsy (TLE), FDG-PET studies performed during the interictal period have identified areas of decreased glucose utilization; these regions of 'hypometabolism' (Fig. 25.1a) correspond anatomically with pathologic and invasive EEG localization of epileptogenic lesions (Henry *et al* 1993a; Henry and Chugani 1997). At times, focal 'interictal' hypermetabolism may be seen on the PET scan in the presence of an active focal epileptiform discharge on the EEG and results in false lateralization (Chugani *et al* 1993a; Sperling *et al* 1995). For this reason, EEG monitoring is important during the PET scan and should be routinely performed. When this is not practical, at least those patients known to have active epileptiform EEGs should have EEG monitoring during PET.

The sensitivity of PET in identifying the epileptogenic focus in patients with TLE is almost equivalent to that of depth electrode recording (Engel *et al* 1990). However, since PET is a noninvasive tool and is performed in the outpatient setting, it does not have the morbidity associated with depth electrode recordings. When PET is available, either on-site or within reasonable travel distance, it is far more cost-effective than the use of depth electrodes and, when given the choice, patients almost invariably choose to travel to have a PET scan in order to avoid having to undergo invasive monitoring.

The presence of temporal lobe hypometabolism may be of prognostic significance for the success of temporal lobectomy. Radtke *et al* (1993) found that the degree and extent of temporal lobe hypometabolism correlated positively with a favorable surgical outcome. However, at least two other studies have not found any significant differences in outcome between patients with temporal lobe hypometabolism and patients with either normal or nonlocalizing PET findings (Engel *et al* 1987; Theodore *et al* 1990). Salanova *et al* (1992) correlated memory function during intracarotid amobarbital procedure with PET hypometabolism in patients undergoing evaluation for intractable TLE; they found that memory impairment was never present contralateral to the side of hypometabolism and was ipsilateral to the hypometabolism in as many as 65% of patients.

The glucose metabolism patterns differ somewhat between patients with neocortical TLE and those with medial TLE. In patients with hippocampal sclerosis, glucose metabolism of the entire temporal lobe (both medial and lateral aspects) was found to be much lower than in patients with neocortical TLE, who showed hypometabolism primarily in the temporal neocortex (Hajek *et al* 1993). The hypometabolism on FDG-PET usually reflects underlying medial temporal lobe sclerosis and neuronal loss. Engel *et al* (1982) found a statistically significant correlation between the degree of sclerosis and degree of hypometabolism,

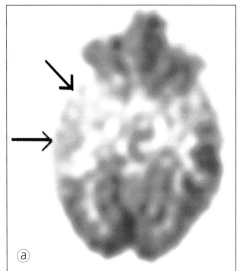 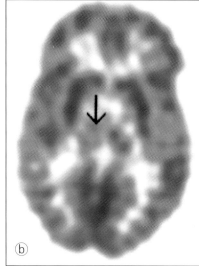 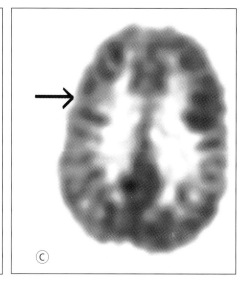

Fig. 25.1 Glucose metabolism PET image of an adult patient with right temporal lobe epilepsy based on seizure semeiology and EEG findings. Hypometabolism is seen in (a) right temporal lobe (arrows), (b) right thalamus (arrow), and (c) right frontal cortex (arrow).

although subsequent studies found this relationship to be less strong (Sackellares *et al* 1990; Henry *et al* 1994; O'Brien *et al* 1997). Theodore *et al* (1992) reported that quantitative measurements of asymmetry (> 15%) of lateral temporal lobe hypometabolism was predictive of seizure-free outcome.

Chee *et al* (1993) found that FDG-PET provides corroborative lateralizing information to the interictal temporal spikes in as many as 70% of patients with TLE. More recently, Knowlton *et al* (1997), in a multimodality comparison including FDG-PET, hippocampal volumetry, T2 relaxometry, and proton magnetic resonance spectroscopic imaging, reported that FDG-PET remains the most sensitive neuroimaging method for depicting the epileptic focus in EEG-lateralized TLE. In patients with nonlocalizing surface ictal EEG, FDG-PET provides valuable localization data and can reduce the number of subjects who require invasive EEG monitoring (Theodore *et al* 1997).

Common findings in FDG-PET of patients with TLE include hypometabolism of the ipsilateral thalamus (Fig. 25.1b) and basal ganglia, and parietal and frontal cortex (Fig. 25.1c); less frequently, occipital cortex may also show hypometabolism (Henry *et al* 1993a). These may represent diaschisis, seizure propagation sites, or secondary epileptogenic foci. One study found that patients with extratemporal hypometabolism had a worse surgical outcome compared with those with hypometabolism restricted to the temporal lobe (Swartz *et al* 1992a). Henry *et al* (1990) postulated that thalamic nuclei may participate in initiation and propagation of amygdalohippocampal ictal discharges and are possible anatomic substrates of the interictal behavioral and cognitive dysfunction seen in TLE patients. Widespread metabolic dysfunction on FDG-PET in TLE patients might also be related to behavioral and neuropsychologic abnormalities (Arnold *et al* 1996). From a practical standpoint, extratemporal cortical hypometabolism in patients suspected of having TLE requires careful electrographic correlation in order to exclude the possibility that it may represent additional independent epileptic foci.

FRONTAL LOBE EPILEPSY

Although patients with frontal lobe epilepsy constitute the second largest group undergoing epilepsy surgery, postoperative outcome remains unsatisfactory compared with temporal lobectomy. The outcome is better in patients with a lesion on MRI compared with those with nonlesional frontal lobe epilepsy. Thus, frontal cortical resection guided solely by seizure semeiology, scalp EEG, and intracranial recordings without the benefit of neuroimaging localization

is associated with only modest success. This is illustrated in the review of Van Ness (1991), who reevaluated the outcome of 983 patients following extratemporal (mostly frontal) cortical resections at 10 prominent epilepsy surgery centers; only 30.1% of the patients were seizure-free or had occasional seizures.

Swartz *et al* (1992b) studied 22 patients with frontal lobe epilepsy using FDG-PET; 32% of these patients exhibited abnormalities on CT and 45% showed abnormalities on MRI. Focal, regional, or hemispheric hypometabolism was observed in 64% of patients and correlated well with ictal EEG localization. In a more recent study from our center using a higher spatial resolution scanner, FDG-PET was 92% sensitive in identifying frontal lobe hypometabolism in children with nonlesional frontal lobe epilepsy (daSilva *et al* 1997a) (Fig. 25.2). However, glucose hypometabolism also was observed outside the frontal lobes in a significant number of patients, and these regions may represent diaschisis, seizure propagation sites, or secondary epileptic foci as mentioned earlier. Our current policy is to address with corticography, either intraoperatively or chronically, all cortical areas that show a metabolic abnormality and that are within reasonable surgical approach from the suspected primary focus. In the future, PET tracers capable of differentiating between areas of epileptogenicity and areas of diaschisis, seizure propagation and secondary epileptogenicity may reduce or eliminate the need for chronic invasive EEG monitoring and further improve surgical outcome.

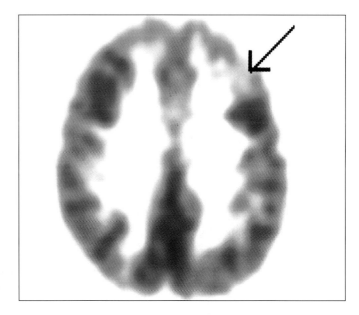

Fig. 25.2 PET image showing left frontal cortex glucose hypometabolism (arrow) in a child with frontal lobe epilepsy, normal MRI, and epileptiform activity localized to the left frontal lobe on interictal and ictal EEG.

EPILEPSY SYNDROMES OF INFANCY AND CHILDHOOD

NEONATAL SEIZURES

When onset of medically refractory partial seizures occurs during the neonatal period or early infancy, a structural lesion (often dysplastic) is typically present. Such lesions may be difficult to define with MRI at this early age because of the relatively high water content of neonatal brain and paucity of myelin (Sankar *et al* 1995). In these patients, FDG-PET can be quite helpful in defining an area of decreased or increased glucose metabolism to guide potential surgical treatment (Fig. 25.3). Even so, when focal hypometabolism is the predominant finding, the extent of frontal lobe involvement can be difficult to ascertain since this brain region is physiologically 'hypometabolic' before about 8–12 months of age (Chugani *et al* 1987a).

INFANTILE SPASMS

PET studies of cerebral glucose utilization have altered significantly the management of infants with intractable spasms and have introduced new concepts regarding the pathophysiology of infantile spasms. It is now generally accepted that most infants diagnosed with 'cryptogenic' spasms have, in fact, focal cortical regions of decreased (less commonly, increased) glucose utilization on FDG-PET (Chugani *et al* 1990, 1993b; Chugani and Conti 1996) (Fig. 25.4). These metabolic foci generally are concordant with the location of interictal and/or ictal

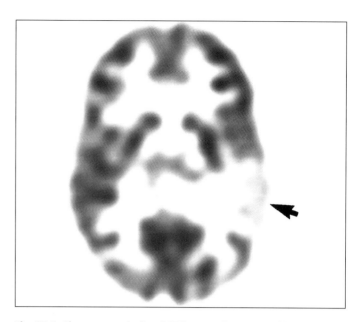

Fig. 25.4 Glucose metabolism PET image of a 2-year-old girl with medically refractory infantile spasms. The MRI scan was normal, but EEG abnormalities corresponded well with the PET focus in the left temporal lobe (arrow). Following cortical resection she is seizure-free. Pathologic examination of resected tissue revealed cortical dysplasia.

EEG abnormalities, which may either precede or follow the presence of hypsarrhythmia during the clinical course.

In about 20% of infants with cryptogenic spasms, FDG-PET shows a single metabolic focus in the cerebral cortex involving one or more lobes; these infants are the ideal candidates for cortical resection if the spasms remain intractable (Chugani and Conti 1996). Surgery is effective in not only controlling the seizures but also providing the potential for normal cognitive development (Chugani *et al* 1993b; Asarnow and Lopresti 1997; Shewmon *et al* 1997). The surgically resected brain tissue typically reveals a previously unsuspected area of cortical dysplasia (Vinters *et al* 1992).

Unfortunately, the majority of infants with cryptogenic spasms harbor more than one cortical metabolic focus of presumed dysplasia. In some of these infants, resection of the predominant seizure focus can still be of benefit but rarely leads to dramatic cognitive gains. Evaluating such infants for surgery should follow an approach similar to that for some children with tuberous sclerosis and multiple tubers, in whom resection of the offending tuber can result in significant seizure control with some cognitive improvement (see below). The common finding of cortical lesions with MRI and PET in patients with infantile spasms, as well as alleviation of spasms following cortical resection, supports the concept that infantile spasms originate from a

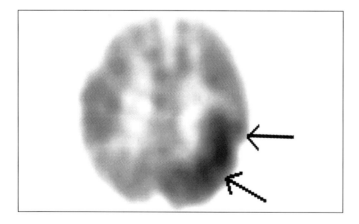

Fig. 25.3 Glucose metabolism PET image of an infant with neonatal seizures associated with closed-lip schizencephaly of the left parietal lobe. The EEG showed continuous epileptiform activity from the left parietal cortex. Note the increased glucose metabolism (arrows) outlining the epileptogenic zone as confirmed with intraoperative electrocorticography.

cortical focus and are secondarily generalized in a manner that is age specific (Chugani *et al* 1992).

LENNOX–GASTAUT SYNDROME

In children with Lennox–Gastaut syndrome, four metabolic patterns have been identified with FDG-PET: unilateral focal, unilateral diffuse, bilateral diffuse, and normal pattern of metabolism (Chugani *et al* 1987b; Iinuma *et al* 1987; Theodore *et al* 1987). These glucose metabolic patterns may serve as a guide in determining the type of surgical intervention in patients with intractable seizures.

STURGE–WEBER SYNDROME

In children and adults with advanced calcification in Sturge–Weber syndrome, FDG-PET typically reveals widespread unilateral hypometabolism (Fig. 25.5b) ipsilateral to the facial nevus in a distribution that extends beyond the abnormalities seen on CT. In contrast, infants (< 1 year) with Sturge–Weber syndrome may show an unusual interictal pattern of increased glucose utilization in the cerebral cortex of the anatomically affected hemisphere (Chugani *et al* 1989) (Fig. 25.5a).

FDG-PET is clinically useful in the early detection of cerebral involvement in infants with port-wine stain and in monitoring disease progression. When the seizures are refractory to medication or if increasing cognitive delay is present, FDG-PET is useful in guiding the extent of focal resection, evaluating the functional integrity of the opposite hemisphere, and in assessing candidacy for early hemispherectomy. Contralateral abnormalities (usually hypometabolism) are of concern and consist of two types. When contralateral hypometabolism involves prefrontal cortex, it is typically mild and symmetric and is not due to an underlying lesion. Symmetric prefrontal cortex hypometabolism occurs on a functional basis and is a nonspecific finding seen in patients with various types of chronic encephalopathy, whether epilepsy is present or not. It is suspected that some medications might also cause symmetric prefrontal cortex hypometabolism. These patients may still be candidates for focal resection or hemispherectomy since the prefrontal cortex of the contralateral side is, as a rule, not associated with electrographic abnormalities. On the other hand, severe *asymmetric* contralateral hypometabolism may occur anywhere in the cortex of the less affected hemisphere and usually indicates the presence of an additional leptomeningeal angioma. Patients with Sturge–Weber syndrome having bilateral leptomeningeal angiomas are seldom candidates for surgical resection.

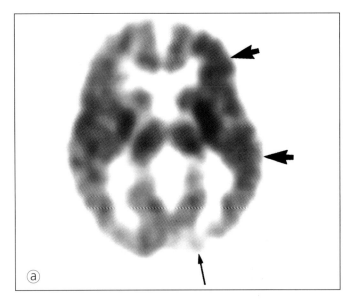

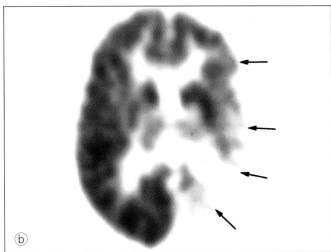

Fig. 25.5 Glucose metabolism PET image of an infant with Sturge–Weber syndrome. (a) At 5 months of age, both increased (thick arrows) and decreased (thin arrow) metabolism is seen in the left hemisphere during an *interictal* study. (b) At 14 months, hypermetabolism is no longer present; instead, there is widespread left cortical hypometabolism (thin arrows) and left thalamic hypometabolism.

TUBEROUS SCLEROSIS

Cortical tubers in tuberous sclerosis appear as hypometabolic areas interictally on FDG-PET scanning, presumably due to simplified dendritic arborization within the tubers (Szelies *et al* 1983; Rintahaka and Chugani 1997). In the rare instance of a prolonged seizure occurring early in the FDG uptake period, the epileptogenic tuber may show increased metabolism. There has been recent interest in surgical removal of the epileptogenic tuber(s) in children with intractable epilepsy associated with tuberous sclerosis. As a result, efforts have intensified in differentiating between epileptogenic and nonepileptogenic tubers preoperatively. The interictal EEG usually shows multifocal abnormalities and the ictal EEG may or may not show localized or lateralized onset of seizures. Although the usefulness of FDG-PET in this regard is limited, recent studies using PET imaging of brain serotonin synthesis have been very promising (see below).

HEMIMEGALENCEPHALY

Hemimegalencephaly is a rare developmental malformation characterized by congenital hypertrophy of one cerebral hemisphere and ipsilateral ventriculomegaly. Intractable epilepsy is frequent in these infants, in which case hemispherectomy is recommended. However, it is interesting that compared with other children who undergo hemispherectomy, such as those with Sturge–Weber syndrome or chronic focal encephalitis of Rasmussen, children with hemimegalencephaly tend to have a less favorable cognitive outcome even when the hemispherectomy has been successful in terms of seizure control. At least in part, this can be explained by FDG-PET findings showing the frequent presence of bilateral metabolic abnormalities in children with hemimegalencephaly, suggesting some degree of dysplastic lesion in the better hemisphere (Rintahaka *et al* 1993). Therefore, the preoperative assessment of the less affected hemisphere with FDG-PET may provide important prognostic information.

LANDAU–KLEFFNER SYNDROME

Landau–Kleffner syndrome (acquired epileptic aphasia) is characterized by language regression following normal acquisition of language skills, accompanied by epileptiform abnormalities on EEG with or without clinical seizures. Structural neuroimaging with CT and MRI is usually normal. Unilateral or bilateral temporal lobe hypometabolism, less commonly hypermetabolism, during sleep or wakefulness was observed in all patients with Landau–Kleffner syndrome in one large study (daSilva *et al* 1997b) (Fig. 25.6). These findings suggest that temporal lobe structures play an integral part in the pathophysiology of this syndrome. Because the temporal lobe metabolic abnormalities are frequently asymmetric, FDG-PET is being used at some centers to guide surgical treatment with multiple subpial transections on the more affected side. At present, there are no published data to judge whether this approach is beneficial.

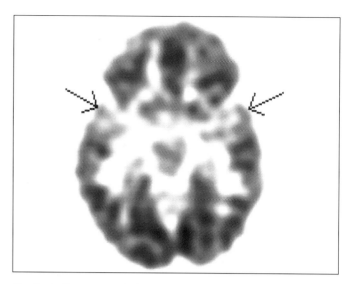

Fig. 25.6 Glucose metabolism PET image of a child with Landau–Kleffner syndrome showing bilateral temporal cortex hypometabolism (arrows).

NEUROTRANSMITTER RECEPTOR PET

As illustrated above, the application of FDG-PET has had significant impact in the management of some patients with intractable epilepsy. However, the imaging of glucose metabolism has limitations. For example, in addition to depicting the epileptogenic cortex, FDG-PET often shows widespread metabolic abnormalities outside the primary epileptogenic focus. Thus, patients with TLE often show hypometabolism in the ipsilateral thalamus, parietal cortex, and frontal cortex (Henry *et al* 1990, 1993a). In such cases, unless the ictal EEG is strongly localizing, it may be difficult to distinguish between epileptogenicity and dysfunction (resulting from diaschisis, seizure propagation, or secondary epileptic foci) in the parietal and frontal cortex. When there is not strong concordance among the various localization modalities, these patients may be subject to invasive EEG monitoring. Therefore, there has been considerable interest in developing PET probes more specific for demarcating epileptogenic cortex than is capable with FDG.

OPIATE RECEPTOR PET

A number of studies have shown that postictal phenomena in epilepsy are mediated by opioid mechanisms. The application of PET using ^{11}C-carfentanil, a ligand with high affinity for μ opiate receptors, in patients with TLE has shown increased binding in the temporal neocortex ipsilateral to seizure onset compared with the contralateral temporal neocortex; this lateralization corresponded with temporal lobe hypometabolism on FDG-PET in the same subjects (Frost *et al* 1988). Medial temporal structures did not show any asymmetry in receptor binding. These findings suggest that ^{11}C-carfentanil PET may be an indicator of tonic inhibition surrounding epileptogenic regions.

HISTAMINE RECEPTOR PET

Using PET with ^{11}C-doxepin, an antidepressant with high affinity for histamine H_1 receptors, Iinuma *et al* (1993) studied patients with complex partial seizures of temporal or frontal lobe origin. Within the same subjects, these investigators found increased H_1-receptor binding in cortical regions that showed hypometabolism on FDG-PET. Since histamine is involved in termination of seizures and may function as an endogenous anticonvulsant, ^{11}C-doxepin PET may be an indicator of the defensive mechanism restricting the spread of epileptic discharges.

BENZODIAZEPINE RECEPTOR PET

Benzodiazepine receptors are closely linked to γ-aminobutyric acid receptors and are located in the same macromolecular receptor complex, which governs ionic movement through chloride channels. The efficacy of benzodiazepines as anticonvulsants is well established. PET studies of benzodiazepine receptors using the antagonist ^{11}C-flumazenil are now available in a number of centers (Savic *et al* 1988). Henry *et al* (1993b) demonstrated that ^{11}C-flumazenil PET shows a more restricted distribution of abnormality (usually decreased binding) in the epileptogenic brain region when compared with the hypometabolism seen on FDG-PET, suggesting that ^{11}C-flumazenil binding is more specific than glucose metabolism in identifying epileptogenic cortex.

In further studies, Savic *et al* (1996) reported that the degree of benzodiazepine receptor reduction correlated positively with seizure frequency. In particular, ^{11}C-flumazenil PET is very sensitive in detecting medial temporal sclerosis (Burdette *et al* 1995) (Fig. 25.7). In one study comparing ^{11}C-flumazenil PET with MRI hippocampal volume measurements, there was 100% correlation between the two methods (Koepp *et al* 1997). A recent study found that ^{11}C-flumazenil PET also may depict the epileptogenic cortex in patients with frontal lobe epilepsy (Savic *et al* 1995). We have found ^{11}C-flumazenil PET to be very useful in patients being evaluated for reoperation after initial unsuccessful surgery. In these patients, FDG-PET is of limited value because the typically large areas of

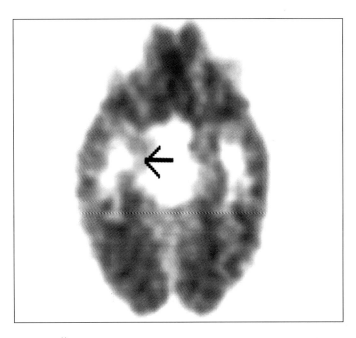

Fig. 25.7 ^{11}C-Flumazenil PET image of an adult patient with right temporal lobe epilepsy with medial onset of seizures. Note the dramatic reduction of benzodiazepine receptor binding in the right medial temporal lobe structures (arrow), with a lesser degree of binding reduction in the temporal neocortex compared with the left side.

hypometabolism seen include not only remaining epileptogenic cortex but also diaschisis resulting from the prior resection. Decreased ^{11}C-flumazenil binding, on the other hand, appears to be more specific for unresected epileptogenic cortex.

SEROTONIN SYNTHESIS PET

There are several lines of evidence which suggest that serotonergic mechanisms play a role in epileptogenesis, and these have been reviewed (Chugani *et al* 1998). In general, pharmacologic treatments that facilitate serotonergic neurotransmission have an anticonvulsant effect, whereas the lowering of brain serotonin concentrations leads to increased susceptibility to seizures in animal models of epilepsy as well as in humans. In human brain tissue surgically removed for seizure control, levels of the serotonin metabolite 5-hydroxyindoleacetic acid were found to be higher in actively spiking cortex compared with nonspiking cortex (Louw *et al* 1989; Pintor *et al* 1990).

The recent development of ^{11}C-α-methyl-L-tryptophan (^{11}C-AMT) as a PET tracer for the measurement of

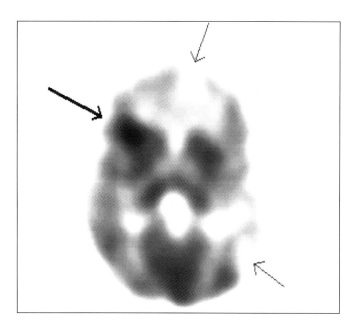

Fig. 25.8 Serotonin synthesis PET image in a 2-year-old child with tuberous sclerosis and right frontal onset seizures. Glucose metabolism PET showed multiple tubers, all appearing hypometabolic. The serotonin PET scan showed increased uptake in a right frontal tuber (thick arrow), with other tubers showing decreased uptake (thin arrows)

serotonin synthesis *in vivo* is an excellent example of the potential specificity for epileptogenic cortex that can be achieved through the development of PET chemistry. In patients with tuberous sclerosis, ^{11}C-AMT-PET performed interictally is able to differentiate between epileptogenic tubers (which show increased ^{11}C-AMT uptake) and nonepileptogenic tubers (which show decreased ^{11}C-AMT uptake) (Chugani *et al* 1998) (Fig. 25.8). This is in contrast to interictal FDG-PET, which shows decreased glucose utilization in all tubers with no specificity for epileptogenic tubers. Needless to say, the availability of ^{11}C-AMT-PET will have significant clinical impact on the many children with tuberous sclerosis who suffer from intractable epilepsy but whose offending tuber is difficult to localize.

FUNCTIONAL BRAIN MAPPING

Changes in regional cerebral blood flow are known to be closely linked to regional neuronal activation due to increased synaptic function. PET using $H_2^{15}O$ as an indicator of cerebral blood flow is an established technique for detecting regional brain activation related to cognitive and sensorimotor tasks. In this method, the tracer $H_2^{15}O$ contained in saline is injected into the patient's vein. Task per-

formance and corresponding brain activation are associated with increased regional cerebral blood flow and relatively high radioisotope uptake compared with baseline or control conditions. The very short half-life (122 s) of ^{15}O permits the acquisition of many separate scans per patient and session. Regional tracer uptake can then be compared between task and control conditions by means of a subtraction technique.

Functional MRI is also being developed to achieve the same goals. Both techniques have advantages and disadvantages. A disadvantage of PET is that it requires exposure to a small dose of radiation (Silbersweig *et al* 1993), which is not an issue with MRI. However, MRI is exquisitely sensitive to movement artifact and there is a risk of obtaining uninterpretable data after a long session. With PET, movement can be corrected using a number of programs designed to address this problem.

In patients with intractable epilepsy whose seizure foci (shown on interictal baseline FDG-PET) lie near language or primary sensorimotor cortex (eloquent cortex), presurgical functional mapping of these eloquent regions is extremely useful and can play an important role in surgical planning. Studies on motor and language reorganization after early brain injury in an epileptic population suggest that the tendency for interhemispheric reorganization during maturation is somewhat stronger for language than for motor functions. Not uncommonly, these issues need to be addressed during evaluation for epilepsy surgery in patients with one or more lesions acquired at various ages during development.

Using $H_2^{15}O$-PET, Müller *et al* (1997a, 1998a,b) demonstrated that functional brain mapping is possible with epilepsy patients as young as 5 years of age. Functional mapping during task performance has shown activation of those regions with severe resting hypometabolism on FDG-PET (Müller *et al* 1997b). Following hemispherectomy, the rolandic region is not the primary locus of functional reorganization for motor control. Motor reorganization occurs in the supplementary motor area, the inferior frontal and premotor cortex, and the bilateral cerebellum. Language reorganization also occurs in the remaining hemisphere (Müller *et al* 1997a).

Noninvasive functional brain mapping using neuroimaging is an important advance because other techniques for language lateralization and localization, such as the intracarotid amobarbital procedure and cortical stimulation, are expensive, uncomfortable, and associated with considerable morbidity and mortality particularly in children. Bookheimer *et al* (1997) compared language localization using $H_2^{15}O$-PET and electrocortical stimulation and found good concordance between the two approaches. In studies on adult subjects, Pardo and Fox (1993) reported good concordance between language lateralization using $H_2^{15}O$-PET and the intracarotid amobarbital procedure.

CONCLUSION

It is clear that the application of PET in selected patients with intractable epilepsy can have significant impact in the diagnostic evaluation and surgical planning. PET is particularly useful in patients who fail to show a lesion on structural neuroimaging such as CT and MRI. In such situations, the metabolic focus shown on PET often provides the necessary neuroimaging localization for correlation with electrographic data in evaluation for surgery. When there is good correspondence between the PET focus and ictal EEG, invasive intracranial EEG monitoring may not be required in some patients, unless eloquent areas are involved and further mapping of these regions is required. With further research in functional brain mapping, such as $H_2^{15}O$-PET and functional MRI, the need for intracarotid amobarbital may also be reduced or even eliminated. Neurotransmitter and receptor probes being developed will further refine the delineation of epileptogenic brain regions.

KEY POINTS

1. PET is a functional imaging tool that can measure local uptake and affinity of a metabolic substrate or chemical in the brain. As such, it may be used as a noninvasive diagnostic test in selected patients being evaluated for epilepsy surgery.

2. Interictal deoxy-2 [^{18}F] fluoro-D-glucose positron emission tomography (FDG-PET) studies on patients with temporal lobe epilepsy (TLE) show temporal lobe hypometabolism. Those with hippocampal sclerosis have hypometabolism throughout the temporal lobe whereas those with neocortical foci have hypometabolism primarily in temporal neocortex. The sensitivity of FDG-PET for identifying temporal lobe epileptogenic cortex may render intracranial EEG monitoring unnecessary, but if extratemporal hypometabolism is seen, very careful EEG assessment is essential to exclude additional independent epileptic foci.

3. Interictal FDG-PET shows frontal lobe hypometabolism in a high proportion of children with non-lesional frontal lobe epilepsy, but hypometabolism is also seen outside the frontal lobes in a significant proportion of them.

4. Most children with cryptogenic infantile spasms have focal areas of hypometabolism with FDG-PET. There is a single focus in around 20% of these children. They may be amenable to surgical treatments.

5. FDG-PET may be useful for assessing the integrity of the opposite hemisphere in children with presumed unilateral Sturge-Weber pathology. It often shows bilateral abnormalities in children with hemimegalencephaly.

6. PET studies of benzodiazepine receptors using the antagonist ^{11}C-flumazenil may be more specific than FDG-PET for localizing epileptogenic cortex especially mesial temporal sclerosis. ^{11}C-flumazenil PET may also delineate epileptogenic frontal cortex, and it may be useful in patients being evaluated for reoperation.

7. ^{11}C-methyl-L-tryptophan PET may be able to distinguish between epileptogenic and non-epileptogenic tubers in tuberous sclerosis.

8. Functional brain mapping using $H_2^{15}O$-PET is possible in epileptic children as young as 5 years of age.

REFERENCES

Arnold S, Schlaug G, Neimann H *et al* (1996) Topography of interictal glucose hypometabolism in unilateral mesiotemporal epilepsy. *Neurology* **46**:1422–1430.

Asarnow RF, Lopresti C (1997) Adaptive functioning in children receiving resective surgery for medically intractable infantile spasms. In: Tuxhorn I, Holthausen H, Boenigk H (eds) *Paediatric Epilepsy Syndromes and Their Surgical Treatment*, pp 526–536. London: John Libby.

Bookheimer SY, Zeffiro TA, Blaxton T *et al* (1997) A direct comparison of PET activation and electrocortical stimulation mapping for language localization. *Neurology* **48**:1056–1065.

Burdette DE, Sakurai SY, Henry TR *et al* (1995) Temporal lobe central benzodiazepine binding in unilateral mesial temporal lobe epilepsy. *Neurology* **45**:934–941.

Chee MW, Morris III HH, Antar MA *et al* (1993) Presurgical evaluation of temporal lobe epilepsy using interictal temporal spikes and positron emission tomography. *Archives of Neurology* **50**:45–48.

Chugani HT, Conti JC (1996) Etiological classification of infantile spasms in 140 cases: role of positron emission tomography. *Journal of Child Neurology* 11:44–48.

Chugani HT, Phelps ME, Mazziotta JC (1987a) Positron emission tomography study of human brain functional development. *Annals of Neurology* 22:487–497.

Chugani HT, Mazziotta JC, Engel J Jr et al (1987b) The Lennox–Gastaut syndrome: metabolic subtypes determined by 2-deoxy-2 [^{18}F]fluoro-D-glucose positron emission tomography. *Annals of Neurology* 21:4–13.

Chugani HT, Mazziotta JC, Phelps ME (1989) Sturge–Weber syndrome: a study of cerebral glucose utilization with positron emission tomography. *Journal of Pediatrics* 114:244–253.

Chugani HT, Shields WD, Shewmon DA et al (1990) Infantile spasms: I. PET identifies focal cortical dysgenesis in cryptogenic cases for surgical treatment. *Annals of Neurology* 27:406–413.

Chugani HT, Shewmon DA, Sankar R et al (1992) Infantile spasms: II. Lenticular nuclei and brain stem activation on positron emission tomography. *Annals of Neurology* 31:212–219.

Chugani HT, Shewmon DA, Khanna S, et al (1993a) Interictal and postictal focal hypermetabolism on positron emission tomography. *Pediatric Neurology* 9:10–15.

Chugani HT, Shields WD, Shewmon DA et al (1993b) Surgery for intractable infantile spasms: neuroimaging perspectives. *Epilepsia* 34:764–771.

Chugani HT, daSilva E, Chugani DC et al (1997) PET in the diagnostic evaluation of children with focal epilepsy. In: Tuxhorn I, Holthausen H, Boengik H (eds) *Paediatric Epilepsy Syndromes and Their Surgical Treatment*, pp 592–606. London: John Libby.

Chugani DC, Chugani HT, Muzik O et al (1998) Imaging epileptogenic tubers in children with tuberous sclerosis complex using alpha [C-11]methyl-L-tryptophan PET. *Annals of Neurology* 44:858–866.

daSilva EA, Chugani DC, Muzik O et al (1997a) Identification of frontal lobe epileptic foci in children using positron emission tomography. *Epilepsia* 38:1198–1208.

daSilva EA, Chugani DC, Muzik O et al (1997b) Landau–Kleffner syndrome: metabolic abnormalities in temporal lobes are a common feature. *Journal of Child Neurology* 12:489–495.

Engel J Jr, Kuhl DE, Phelps ME et al (1982) Comparative localization of epileptic foci in partial epilepsy by PCT and EEG. *Annals of Neurology* 12:529–537.

Engel J Jr, Babb TL, Phelps ME (1987) Contributions of positron emission tomography to understanding mechanisms of epilepsy. In: Engel J Jr, Ojemann GA, Luders HO, Williamson PD (eds) *Fundamental Mechanisms of Human Brain Function*, pp 209–218. New York: Raven Press.

Engel J Jr, Henry TR, Risinger MW et al (1990) Presurgical evaluation for partial epilepsy: relative contribution of chronic depth-electrode recordings versus FDG-PET and scalp-sphenoidal ictal EEG. *Neurology* 40:1670–1677.

Fowler JS, Wolf AP (1986) Positron emitting compounds: priorities and problems. In: Phelps ME, Mazziotta JC, Schelbert HR (eds) *Positron Emission Tomography and Autoradiography: Principles and Applications for the Brain and Heart*, pp 391–450. New York: Raven Press.

Frost JJ, Mayberg HS, Fisher RS et al (1988) Mu-opiate receptors measured by positron emission tomography are increased in temporal lobe epilepsy. *Annals of Neurology* 23:231–237.

Hajek M, Antonini A, Leenders KL et al (1993) Mesiobasal versus lateral temporal lobe epilepsy: metabolic differences in the temporal lobe shown by interictal cerebral ^{18}F-FDG positron emission tomography *Neurology* 43:79–86.

Henry TR, Chugani HT (1997) Positron emission tomography. In: Engel J Jr, Pedley TA (eds) *Epilepsy: A Comprehensive Textbook*, pp 947–968. Philadelphia: Lippincott-Raven.

Henry TR, Mazziotta JC, Engel J Jr et al (1990) Quantifying interictal metabolic activity in human temporal lobe epilepsy. *Journal of Cerebral Blood Flow and Metabolism* 10:748–757.

Henry TR, Mazziotta JC, Engel J Jr (1993a) Interictal metabolic anatomy of mesial temporal lobe epilepsy. *Archives of Neurology* 50:582–589.

Henry TR, Frey KA, Sackellares JC et al (1993b) *In vivo* cerebral metabolism and central benzodiazepine-receptor binding in temporal lobe epilepsy. *Neurology* 43:1998–2006.

Henry TR, Babb TL, Engel J Jr et al (1994) Hippocampal neuronal loss and regional hypometabolism in temporal lobe epilepsy. *Annals of Neurology* 36:925–927.

Hoffman EJ, Phelps ME (1986) Positron emission tomography: principles and quantitation. In: Phelps ME, Mazziotta JC, Schelbert HR (eds) *Positron Emission Tomography and Autoradiography: Principles and Applications for the Brain and Heart*, pp 237–286. New York: Raven Press.

Huang SC, Phelps ME (1986) Principles of tracer kinetic modeling in positron emission tomography and autoradiography. In: Phelps ME, Mazziotta JC, Schelbert HR (eds) *Positron Emission Tomography and Autoradiography: Principles and Applications for the Brain and Heart*, pp 287–346. New York: Raven Press

Iinuma K, Yanai K, Yanagisawa T et al (1987) Cerebral glucose metabolism in five patients with Lennox–Gastaut syndrome. *Pediatric Neurology* 3:12–18.

Iinuma K, Yokoyama H, Otsuki T et al (1993) Histamine H$_1$ receptors in complex partial seizures. *Lancet* 341:238.

Knowlton RC, Laxer KD, Ende G et al (1997) Presurgical multimodality neuroimaging in electroencephalographically lateralized temporal lobe epilepsy. *Annals of Neurology* 42:829–837.

Koepp MJ, Richardson MP, Labbe C et al (1997) [^{11}C]Flumazenil PET: volumetric MRI and quantitative pathology in mesial temporal lobe epilepsy. *Neurology* 49:764–773.

Louw WD, Sutherland GR, Glavin GB et al (1989) A study of monoamine metabolism in human epilepsy. *Canadian Journal of Neurological Sciences* 16:394–397.

Müller R-A, Rothermel RD, Muzik O et al (1997a) Plasticity of motor organization in children and adults. *Neuroreport* 8:3103–3108.

Müller R-A, Chugani HT, Muzik O et al (1997b) Language and motor functions activate calcified hemisphere in patients with Sturge–Weber syndrome: a PET study. *Journal of Child Neurology* 12:431–437.

Müller R-A, Rothermel RD, Muzik O et al (1998a) Determination of language dominance by [^{15}O]-water PET in children and adolescents: a comparison with the WADA test. *Journal of Epilepsy* 11:152–161.

Müller R-A, Rothermel RD, Behen ME et al (1998b) Brain organization of language after early unilateral lesion: a PET study. *Brain and Language* 62:422–451.

O'Brien TJ, Newton MR, Cook MJ et al (1997) Hippocampal atrophy is not a major determinant of regional hypometabolism in temporal lobe epilepsy. *Epilepsia* 38:74–80.

Pardo JV, Fox PT (1993) Preoperative assessment of the cerebral hemispheric dominance for language with CBF PET. *Human Brain Mapping* 1:57–68.

Pintor M, Mefford IN, Hutter I et al (1990) The levels of biogenic amines, their metabolites and tyrosine hydroxylase in the human epileptic temporal cortex. *Synapse* 5:152–156.

Radtke RA, Hanson MW, Hoffman JM et al (1993) Temporal lobe hypometabolism on PET: predictor of seizure control after temporal lobectomy *Neurology* 43:1088–1092.

Rintahaka PJ, Chugani HT (1997) Clinical role of positron emission tomography in children with tuberous sclerosis complex. *Journal of Child Neurology* 12:42–52.

Rintahaka PJ, Chugani HT, Messa C et al (1993) Hemimegalencephaly: evaluation with positron emission tomography. *Pediatric Neurology* 9:21–28.

Sackellares JC, Siegel GJ, Abou-Khalil BW et al (1990) Differences between lateral and mesial temporal metabolism interictally in epilepsy of mesial temporal origin. *Neurology* **40**:1420–1426.

Salanova V, Morris III HH, Rehm P *et al* (1992) Comparison of intracartoid amobarbital procedure and interictal cerebral 18-fluorodeoxyglucose positron emission tomography scans in refractory temporal lobe epilepsy. *Epilepsia* **33**:635–638.

Sankar R, Curren JG, Kevill JW *et al* (1995) Microscopic cortical dysplasia in infantile spasms: evolution of white matter abnormalities. *American Journal of Neuroradiology* **16**:1265–1272.

Savic I, Ronald P, Sedvall G *et al* (1988) *In vivo* demonstration of BZ receptor binding in human epileptic foci. *Lancet* **ii**:863–866.

Savic I, Thorell JO, Roland P (1995) [^{11}C]Flumazenil positron emission tomography visualizes frontal epileptogenic regions. *Epilepsia* **36**:1225–1232.

Savic I, Svanborg E, Thorell JO (1996) Cortical benzodiazepine receptor changes are related to frequency of partial seizures: a positron emission tomography study. *Epilepsia* **37**:236–244.

Shewmon DA, Shields WD, Sankar R *et al* (1997) Follow-up on infants with surgery for catastrophic epilepsy. In: Tuxhorn I, Holthausen H, Boenigk H (eds) *Paediatric Epilepsy Syndromes and Their Surgical Treatment*, pp 513–525. London: John Libby.

Silbersweig DA, Stern E, Frith CD *et al* (1993) Detection of thirty-second cognitive activations in single subjects with positron emission tomography: a new low dose H$_2$^{15}O regional cerebral blood flow three dimensional imaging technique. *Journal of Cerebral Blood Flow and Metabolism* **13**:617–629.

Sperling MR, Alavi A, Reivich M *et al* (1995) False lateralization of temporal lobe epilepsy with positron emission tomography. *Epilepsia* **36**:722–727.

Swartz BE, Tomiyasu U, Delgado-Escueta AV *et al* (1992a) Neuroimaging in temporal lobe epilepsy, test sensitivity and relationships to pathology and postoperative outcome. *Epilepsia* **33**:624–634.

Swartz BE, Theodore WH, Sanabria E *et al* (1992b) Positron emission tomography and single photon emission computed tomographic studies in the frontal lobe with emphasis on the relationship to seizure foci. In: Chauvel P, Delgado-Escueta AV, Halgren E, Bancaud J (eds) *Frontal Lobe Seizures and Epilepsies*, pp 487–497. New York: Raven Press.

Szelies B, Herholz K, Heiss WD *et al* (1983) Hypometabolic cortical lesions in tuberous sclerosis with epilepsy: demonstration by positron emission tomography. *Journal of Computer Assisted Tomography* **7**:946–53.

Ter-Pogossian MM (1995) Positron emission tomography. In: Wagner HN, Szabo Z, Buchanan JW (eds) *Principles of Nuclear Medicine*, pp 342–346. London: WB Saunders.

Theodore WH, Rose D, Patronas N *et al* (1987) Cerebral glucose metabolism in the Lennox–Gastaut syndrome. *Annals of Neurology* **21**:14–21.

Theodore WH, Katz D, Kufta C *et al* (1990) Pathology of temporal lobe foci: correlation with CT, MRI, and PET. *Neurology* **40**:797–803.

Theodore WH, Sato S, Kufta C *et al* (1992) Temporal lobectomy for uncontrolled seizures: the role of positron emission tomography. *Annals of Neurology* **32**:789–794.

Theodore WH, Sato S, Kufta CV *et al* (1997) FDG positron emission tomography and invasive EEG: seizure focus detection and surgical outcome. *Epilepsia* **38**:81–86.

Van Ness PC (1991) Surgical outcome for neocortical (extra-hippocampal) focal epilepsy. In: Luders HO (ed) *Epilepsy Surgery*, pp 613–624. New York: Raven Press.

Vinters HV, Fisher RS, Cornford ME *et al* (1992) Morphological substrates of infantile spasms on surgically resected brain tissue. *Child's Nervous System* **8**:8–17.

Single-photon emission computed tomography in focal epilepsies

R DUNCAN

Single-photon emission computed tomography (SPECT) has been applied to focal epilepsies for nearly two decades. It was used at first to image interictal regional cerebral perfusion (rCP), and early studies (Bonte *et al* 1983; Devous *et al* 1990) showed focal hypoperfusion. Sensitivity and specificity turned out to be lower than in interictal PET (positron emission tomography) studies of metabolism (Kuhl *et al* 1980; Engel *et al* 1982; Theodore *et al* 1983), but the advent of the tracer hexamethyl-propyleneamine oxime (HMPAO), with its novel trapping paradigm, made SPECT a practical tool for studying the local and regional peri-ictal changes in rCP that had first been observed by Penfield and Gibbs 50 years earlier (Gibbs *et al* 1934; Penfield 1937; Penfield *et al* 1939). To date, this has turned out to be the most useful and interesting application of SPECT in epilepsy, and there exists a large and growing body of literature on the use of peri-ictal rCP SPECT for localizing seizures.

This chapter focuses on peri-ictal rCP SPECT, the practicalities of its use, the rCP patterns associated with different focal seizures, and the interpretation of those patterns in the context of presurgical investigation.

SPECT STUDIES OF FOCAL EPILEPSY

THE INTERICTAL PHASE

The pathophysiologic basis of interictal hypoperfusion in mesial temporal epilepsies is unknown. It appears to be most strongly associated with epilepsy of early onset (Duncan *et al* 1996a), although other associations have been found, (Valmier *et al* 1987; Duncan *et al* 1992). It is often, though not always, congruent with mesial temporal sclerosis (Ryvlin *et al* 1992). There appears to be a relationship with interictal spiking (Guillon *et al* 1998).

Abnormalities of rCP have been found in approximately 50–80% of patients without gross anatomic lesions (Bonte *et al* 1983; Podreka *et al* 1988; Ryding *et al* 1988; Devous *et al* 1990; Duncan *et al* 1990a,b,c; Rowe *et al* 1991a; Cruickshank 1997). Later studies tend toward the lower end of this range, possibly because of better methodology (e.g., the use of normative data). The hypoperfusion usually involves all of the temporal lobe (Fig. 26.1), and is usually predominant laterally, although isolated medial hypoperfusion is seen. The ipsilateral frontal lobe, and occasionally the ipsilateral

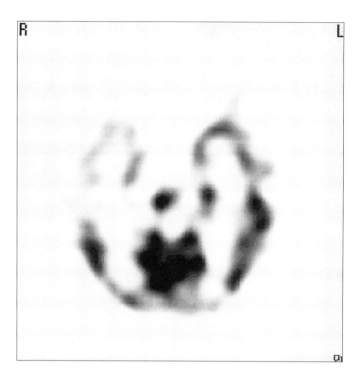

Fig. 26.1 SPECT dataset sliced in the long axis of the temporal lobes, in a patient with a right mesial temporal seizure source. Injection of HMPAO was carried out in the interictal phase. The image shows hypoperfusion of the right temporal lobe.

hemisphere may also be hypoperfused. The hypoperfusion is most often predominant in the lateral temporal cortex. Bilateral temporal hypoperfusion may occur.

A minority of patients have focal interictal hyperperperfusion, without clinical or surface EEG evidence of a seizure at the time of injection (Duncan *et al* 1990c). This may be associated with some tumors and vascular malformations that have high HMPAO uptake (Cruickshank 1997), or related to postictal hyperperfusion, which can occasionally persists for some days (Lang *et al* 1988). A repeat scan should differentiate the two.

Relatively little information is available in the literature, but the sensitivity of rCP SPECT appears to be 10% or less in nonlesional extratemporal epilepsies (Harvey *et al* 1993; Duncan *et al* 1997a).

Interictal hypoperfusion reflects functional changes associated with seizures, and is not a specific marker for epileptogenicity. As a localizing test, it has limitations in sensitivity and specificity (Duncan *et al* 1990b), and its best use is as a baseline to assess peri-ictal or ictal changes in rCP. Persistent unilateral temporal hypoperfusion probably does have significant cognitive implications, in principle posing a contraindication to excision of contralateral temporal lobe structures.

THE ICTAL AND POSTICTAL PHASES

Choice of tracer and other practical aspects of peri-ictal rCP SPECT

Interictal localizing tests such as MRI are becoming more sensitive and specific but, until we can directly detect and localize the abnormal excitability that gives rise to seizures, the most confident localization of an epileptogenic zone will depend on demonstrating a localized physiologic change that takes place in temporal association with the clinical event to be treated. Currently, the only practicable methods for recording peri-ictal pathophysiologic changes are EEG and SPECT. However rCP SPECT has a different temporal and spatial resolution and a different sampling error compared to EEG techniques, differences that must constantly be borne in mind when interpreting results.

The main sampling error of ictal EEG is in space. Recordings are taken from a series of points, which may be on the scalp, on the surface of the brain, or in the brain. The recording gives limited information on what occurs distant from those points, but the recording is continuous in time. In contrast, the SPECT image of rCP is complete in space, and is (usually) of the whole brain, but is based on limited sampling in time: tracer uptake does not begin until the tracer reaches the brain and then carries on for approximately 40 seconds (Andersen *et al* 1988; Friberg *et al* 1994) (Fig. 26.2). Therefore the image will not be affected by changes that take place outside this period and will only reflect changes that have taken place during it that are of sufficient magnitude, extent, and duration.

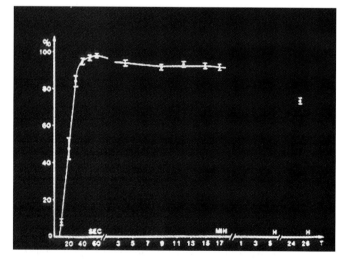

Fig. 26.2 Graph showing rate of uptake of HMPAO into the brain following intravenous injection. Note that uptake begins 10–15 seconds after injection and is effectively complete at 40 seconds. Even at 26 hours post injection, retention is 80%. (Adapted from Andersen *et al* 1988.)

Both the spatial resolution and the temporal resolution of the image need to be considered. The spatial resolution will depend mainly on which scanner is used and on what collimator(s) and reconstruction parameters are used. The temporal resolution is determined by the tracer: the image is of rCP roughly averaged over the uptake period, and its temporal resolution is of the order of 40 seconds, no better (this probably applies to both HMPAO and Bicisate [ECD – see below]).

The time course of rCP changes relative to other aspects of seizure pathophysiology also needs to be considered. The onset of ictal changes in rCP is usually within seconds of the electrical onset, but may well outlast the electrical discharge if the seizure has been relatively long; the obvious example of this is the persistence of mesial temporal hyperperfusion after the end of mesial temporal lobe seizures. Ictal hyperperfusion may persist after shorter seizures, but probably for a shorter time (Gibbs *et al* 1934; Penfield 1937; Penfield *et al* 1939; Dymond and Crandall 1976). At the lower limit, changes in rCP are sometimes seen when tracer has been injected at the end of a seizure lasting 20 seconds; but with seizures any shorter than this, the injection has to be given at or near the seizure onset. This will only be possible if the seizure can be provoked, or if a premixed tracer is used, with the syringe connected to the cannula ready for the injection. Given the transit time from arm to brain, it is probably not worth trying to capture single seizures lasting less than 15 seconds.

One disadvantage of the original rCP SPECT tracer, HMPAO, is that once mixed with ^{99m}Tc it is usable only for 30 minutes. It can, however, be rendered stable by mixing with cobalt chloride (a ready-made product will soon be available). The newer tracer, ^{99m}Tc ECD (Bicisate-Neurolite, Dupont Pharma (Friberg *et al* 1994)) is stable for several hours.

The stability or otherwise of the tracer will affect the choice of tracer. In adults, the majority of seizures arise in the mesial temporal lobe. These seizures tend to be relatively long (e.g. ictal phase 1–2 minutes) but relatively infrequent (typically 1–5 per week in patients in hospital with withdrawal of medication). HMPAO and ^{99m}Tc pertechnetate can be mixed in approximately 15 seconds. This period of time is seldom significant with respect to the long timescale of the seizure and little is gained by using a premixed stable tracer. ECD requires 30 minutes or so to combine with technetium, and so must be used premixed. Premixed doses may be wasted unless they can be used for other patients before the compound degrades or the ^{99m}Tc decays.

However, in patients with short and frequent seizures there is good likelihood of seeing a seizure within a given working day. The few seconds spent mixing the compound become important in the context of the short duration of these seizures, and stable tracers can then improve the chances of capturing rCP changes. Stable compounds can also allow the use of rCP SPECT where local regulations prevent the mixing of isotopes and markers on the ward or monitoring unit, a factor that is important in some countries in continental Europe.

Whatever the choice of tracer, it is important that the same tracer be used for the ictal as for the interictal injection. HMPAO and ECD have different trapping mechanisms, and their distributions in normal brain are not the same: differences are seen mainly in the mesial temporal lobe and the occipital lobe. Differences are also seen in some pathologic situations, e.g. luxury perfusion after stroke (Sperling and Lassen 1993; Lassen and Sperling 1994). HMPAO has been validated at high flows in the rat (Duncan *et al* 1996b), and shows a relative slowing of uptake as flow increases. Although it is clear that ECD does show high uptake on ictal SPECT scans (Grunwald *et al* 1994), the relationship between its uptake and flow at high flow rates has not been defined, as its trapping mechanism works only in primates. ECD gives slightly better gray–white-matter contrast than does HMPAO.

The practicalities of carrying out ictal SPECT depend mainly on the local situation, and factors such as radiation protection procedures tend to define how and where the investigation is carried out. Ideally, tracer injection is carried out in a monitoring unit, so that blood flow changes can be temporally related to clinical and electrical manifestations of seizures. With good clinical seizure observation, the investigation can be carried out without EEG monitoring. This requires thorough knowledge of the patient's usual seizure semeiology and its relation to the ictal discharge, and is not advised where experience is limited.

PERI-ICTAL CHANGES IN rCP

Penfield made the first observations of rCP changes associated with seizures, observing them directly in patients who had seizures induced intraoperatively. He noted both hyperperfusion and hypoperfusion. He eventually thought that ictal hyperperfusion was simply a consequence of increased energy demand, a conclusion that most evidence supports today. He noted areas of ictal hypoperfusion, usually surrounding the hyperperfused area. This is of course seen in ictal SPECT images and has its counterpart in animal models of epilepsy (Collins *et al* 1976), where it has been related to electrical inhibition (Prince and Wilder 1967) and termed 'surround inhibition'.

Mesial temporal lobe seizures

There is now considerable experience of rCP changes associated with mesial temporal lobe seizures. If injection is carried out during the seizure discharge or up to 15 seconds after its termination, SPECT will usually find marked hyperperfusion of the whole temporal lobe (see Plate 1). This may be accompanied by hypoperfusion of surrounding cortical structures, most often the adjacent orbital cortex, the ipsilateral frontal lobe, or the ipsilateral hemisphere (Lee *et al* 1988; Shen *et al* 1990; Newton *et al* 1992a,b; Berkovic *et al* 1993; Duncan *et al* 1993; Harvey *et al* 1993a).

Ictal hyperperfusion of the lateral temporal cortex is thought to be due to secondary activation by the seizure discharge. The ipsilateral orbital cortex, the ipsilateral motor cortex, and the basal ganglia are also commonly hyperperfused. Hyperperfusion of the basal ganglia has been associated with contralateral tonic posturing during the seizure (Newton *et al* 1992b). In some patients, hyperperfusion extends posteriorly into the lateral temporal cortex, often basally, and in a minority of patients bilateral changes are seen (Ho *et al* 1996).

Patterns of perfusion seen during temporal lobe seizures have been related to eventual operative outcome (Ho *et al* 1997). The typical pattern described above, a bilateral pattern, and the typical pattern with posterior extension of hyperperfusion were all associated with good outcome, whereas atypical patterns were associated with lack of pathology and poor outcome (presumably because atypical rCP patterns were associated with epileptogenesis outside the field of the excision).

Injection during secondary generalized seizures may show localizing rCP changes, particularly if the seizure has had a clear focal onset. Injection must be early, if it is carried out in the clonic phase, it is the author's experience that a bilateral postictal pattern (see below) is usually seen, giving localizing, but not lateralizing, information. Ictal SPECT seems to show similar findings in mesial temporal lobe seizures in children (Harvey *et al* 1993a; Cross *et al* 1997) as in adults.

In the immediate postictal period (0–4 minutes after the end of the ictal discharge), the lateral temporal cortex rapidly becomes markedly hypoperfused. As in the ictal phase, this often extends into the ipsilateral frontal lobe, or hemisphere (Rowe *et al* 1989, 1991b; Duncan *et al* 1993). Occasionally, areas of hypoperfusion may be seen in the contralateral hemisphere, causing difficulty in interpretation, particularly if the exact temporal relation of the injection to the seizure discharge is not known. During this early postictal period, the mesial temporal cortex remains hyperperfused, becoming isoperfused relative to the contralateral mesial temporal cortex later (4–15 minutes). As time goes on, it too becomes hypoperfused, but even relatively late into the postictal period there is usually some preservation of mesial perfusion relative to the lateral cortex.

Approximately 20% of patients injected in the postictal period will show bilateral and more or less symmetric changes (Rowe *et al* 1989; Duncan *et al* 1993) (see Plate 2). This provides evidence of mesial temporal lobe origin for the seizure, but does not then help in lateralization. Where bilateral and asymmetric changes are seen, it is sometimes tempting to decide that the side with the most marked change is the side of onset, but the author would regard the reliability of such a judgement as suspect. Similarly, if a unilateral postictal perfusion pattern is anything other than typical, it should be interpreted cautiously. Two examples (author's unpublished data) of postictal SPECT have initially been interpreted as showing atypical postictal temporal lobe rCP patterns, mainly because persistent mesial temporal hyperperfusion was seen: examination of seizure semeiology, EEG studies, and true ictal SPECT subsequently indicated origin at the temporo-parieto-occipital junction (TPOJ).

The sensitivity of peri-ictal SPECT in mesial temporal epilepsies depends mostly on the timing of the injection. Ictal injections show changes in almost all cases, although bilateral changes occasionally prevent confident lateralization. Postictal injections give a sensitivity of 70–90%, depending on the time between the end of the seizure and the injection (Rowe *et al* 1989, 1991b). With true ictal injection, the specificity appears to be close to 100%, *provided the perfusion pattern is typical*. In the postictal phase, there have been reports of occasional false-localizing studies (Berkovic *et al* 1993) when changes are subtle.

Whatever the timing of the injection, it must be remembered that the localizing information obtained from an rCP SPECT study pertains *only* to that seizure during which the patient was injected. A minority of patients do turn out to have bilateral or even multiple seizure foci.

Seizures originating outside the mesial temporal lobe

In recent years a number of series describing rCP during seizures originating outside mesial temporal structures have been published (Marks *et al* 1992; Harvey *et al* 1993b; Ho *et al* 1993; Newton *et al* 1995; Duncan *et al* 1996c; Duncan 1997a). Nonetheless, ictal rCP changes associated with these seizures are less well defined than those of mesial temporal seizures, and postictal patterns are not described. The work that has been published so far shows patterns of perfusion clearly different from those seen during mesial temporal seizures.

Temporo-parieto-occipital junction (TPOJ) seizures

TPOJ seizures are not widely recognized as an entity, but seizures originating in this area have clinical and electrographic characteristics that suggest origin in the posterolateral cortex plus variable propagation usually into the ipsilateral temporal lobe. Such seizures do appear to be distinct in terms of ictal SPECT findings. Only two series have been published (Duncan *et al* 1995,1996c). TPOJ seizures are associated with marked increases of ictal perfusion in the area of seizure onset (Fig. 26.3). This may occur as an isolated finding, but there may also be variable degrees of hyperperfusion of the ipsilateral anterolateral temporal lobe structures, with mesial temporal structures being hyperperfused to a lesser degree, or even hypoperfused. There may be a small area of hyperperfusion in the contralateral parietal lobe, which may correlate with bilateralization of the seizure discharge.

Frontal lobe seizures

The use of SPECT in frontal lobe epilepsies may present technical problems, mainly owing to the brevity of the seizures. The use of a premixed tracer will be necessary to capture seizures lasting less than 30 seconds, even when the person injecting is standing over the patient waiting for a seizure. Where the seizure semeiology allows, raising the arm immediately after injection can shorten the tracer transit time by a few seconds, but even then seizures lasting less that 15 seconds will probably not be captured. Postictal injection is usually of no value.

Frontal lobe seizures appear to be associated with a variety of ictal changes (Marks *et al* 1992; Harvey *et al* 1993b; Newton *et al* 1995; Duncan 1997a; Duncan *et al* 1997a), offering limited scope for a generalized description. The patterns recorded seem to be quite distinct from those seen in mesial temporal seizures, although information on orbital frontal seizures is scant. One or two cases do suggest that rCP changes in orbital frontal seizures are distinct from those in mesial temporal lobe seizures, but this has yet to be confirmed in patients who have appropriate invasive EEG data and good surgical outcome.

In cases published so far, ictal perfusion changes appear to be consistent with the site of origin of the seizure within the frontal lobe (Plate 3) where this is known (Harvey *et al* 1993b; Duncan *et al* 1997a), although in one case changes were seen distant from the site of origin indicated by EEG, albeit within the 'correct' frontal lobe. However, hyperperfusion may involve the whole frontal lobe or may be bilateral, limiting the localizing information gained (Duncan *et al* 1997a). Associated hyperperfusion of subcortical structures such as the basal ganglia, thalamus, and cerebellum seems to be more common than in mesial temporal seizures (Harvey *et al* 1993b; Duncan *et al* 1997a).

Ictal hypoperfusion is commonly seen in frontal lobe

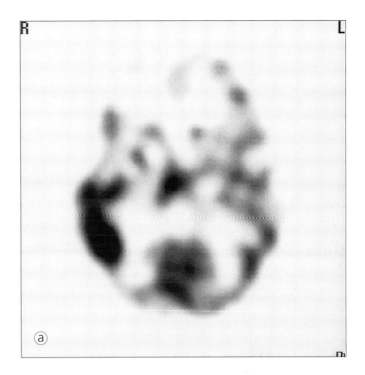

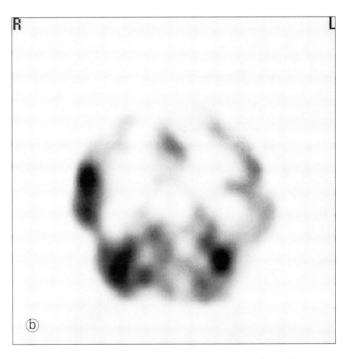

Fig. 26.3 Patient with surface EEG seizure onset in the right posterolateral leads. Interictal HMPAO SPECT showed focal hypoperfusion of the right temporo-parieto-occipital junction (TPOJ). MRI was normal. HMPAO injection was carried out during a complex partial seizure. (a) Orbitomeatal slice, showing marked hyperperfusion of the right TPOJ. The rest of the right hemisphere is hypoperfused. (b) Coronal slice through the TPOJ, showing the vertical extent of the ictal hyperperfusion.

seizures, and is highly variable in pattern and location. Hemispheric hypoperfusion may be either ipsilateral or contralateral to ictal hyperperfusion (Duncan 1997a; Duncan *et al* 1997a), and is often prominent in the posterior part of the hemisphere. Smaller areas of hypoperfusion may be seen within the frontal lobes.

From all this it is clear that perfusion patterns in frontal lobe seizures can be complex, requiring careful interpretation.

Parietal lobe seizures

Little has been published, but pure parietal lobe seizures seem to be associated simply with localized hyperperfusion in the parietal lobe (Fig. 26.4), if any changes are seen at all (Ho *et al* 1993).

Occipital lobe seizures

One small series is available in the literature (Duncan *et al* 1997b). Occipital lobe seizures seem to be in some senses similar to TPOJ seizures, in that some examples show hyperperfusion of one occipital lobe (Fig. 26.5) while others also show changes in the ipsilateral temporal lobe. In the examples published, the temporal lobe changes have consisted of hyperperfusion of mesial structures, with lateral hypoperfusion. The few cases described furnished limited

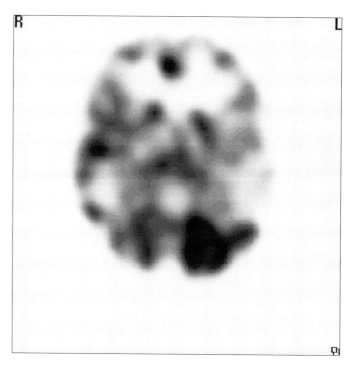

Fig. 26.5 Patient with complex partial seizures beginning with a right-sided elemental visual aura, associated with a surface EEG onset in the occipital leads. Ictal HMPAO SPECT dataset. Horizontal slice through the occipital lobes showing marked hyperperfusion of the right occipital lobe. There is also a degree of hyperperfusion of the right lateral temporal cortex.

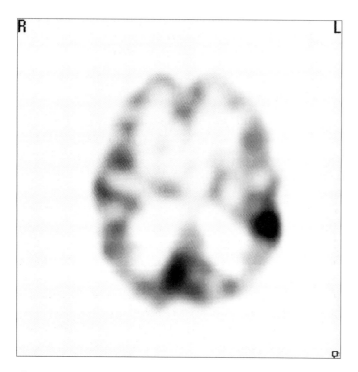

Fig. 26.4 Patient with complex partial seizures beginning with right sensory aura. Ictal HMPAO SPECT dataset. Horizontal slice through the parietal lobes showing localized hyperperfusion in the left parietal lobe.

evidence that the difference between these two patterns of change was determined by analogous differences in the electrical propagation pattern of the seizures recorded, i.e. that patients with evidence of anterior propagation electrically also had temporal lobe changes on ictal SPECT.

INTERPRETATION AND ANALYSIS OF PERI-ICTAL rCP IMAGES

Image interpretation presents particular problems in the context of peri-ictal rCP changes. These may be complex, and can only be properly assessed by formal comparison of peri-ictal with interictal datasets. Where the ictal change is simply a localized area of hyperperfusion, interpretation is relatively straightforward, but where changes involve a number of brain structures it may not be a simple case of deciding that the seizure originates at a 'bright spot' on the scan. For this reason, the process of interpretation may be usefully divided into a number of stages:

1. Determination of the interictal perfusion pattern
2. Determination of the peri-ictal perfusion pattern

3. Determination of the change that has taken place between the two
4. Explaining the rCP change by means of a hypothesis of seizure origin and spread.

The first three stages primarily require expertise in imaging. It is strongly recommended that the practice of independent reporting by at least two individuals be adopted as a clinical routine, and that blinding to other localizing data be as complete as possible within the context of an integrated surgical program.

The fourth stage requires the input of someone who has experience in epileptology, and in particular who understands the pathophysiology of seizure genesis and spread. When perfusion patterns are complex or unusual, one should be ready to consider more than one hypothesis of seizure localization and spread to explain ictal rCP changes. This part of the process does require knowledge of other localizing test results, as the localization process seeks a hypothesis that explains all the available data.

NUMERIC ANALYSIS OF ICTAL SPECT IMAGES

Most recent research work on ictal rCP changes has featured some attempt at numeric analysis of images. SPECT is not quantitative, so any image-based measurement that is made has to be related to some reference (Duncan 1997b). At the simplest, this can be a contralateral homotopic region of interest, producing a simple asymmetry index (AI), and a change in AI from the interictal to the ictal scan can be measured. However, this is insensitive to bilateral changes, however. The count density in one particular region that is of interest can be referred to a reference region, the assumption being that the perfusion level in the reference region does not change. However, any brain region may show perfusion changes during a seizure, and the use of a single reference structure as a standard for measuring ictal changes is not recommended. The total count for the whole brain represents a more stable standard, but hemispheric hypoperfusion is common on ictal datasets and may change whole-brain counts to a degree that will significantly distort any comparison with an interictal image. Statistical parametric mapping and similar techniques (Friston et al 1990) can statistically compare patterns of perfusion to the average pattern of a database of normal datasets. Such techniques overcome many of the disadvantages of the techniques mentioned above, and their use is becoming more widespread. Coregistration of ictal and interictal datasets, and with MRI is desirable for the use of numeric techniques (note that coregistration with anatomic images can also improve the anatomic precision of visual analysis of SPECT datasets). Some centers have overlaid SPECT onto coregistrered MRI images. This usually causes confusion in terms of color scale, and it is probably much clearer to (say) draw a region of interest (ROI) round an area of hyperperfusion seen on the SPECT dataset, and then project that ROI onto the corresponding slice of a pure anatomic image.

Formal coregistration and subtraction of images (Zubla et al 1996) can be useful in defining ictal hyperperfusion that takes place at the margin of an area that is hypoperfused interictally, but its application and interpretation requires care and experience.

The above techniques are useful in a research setting, but it should be emphasized that visual analysis remains the primary technique for determination of ictal rCP changes.

SPECT IMAGING OF NEUROTRANSMITTER RECEPTOR FUNCTION IN EPILEPSY

PET has been more widely used than SPECT for imaging receptors in epilepsy, mainly because of its better spatial resolution and because of a wider choice of markers. However, a number of SPECT neuroreceptor ligands are available, two of which have been applied to epilepsy.

BENZODIAZEPINE RECEPTORS

As the main inhibitory system in the brain, the GABA (γ-aminobutyric acid) system has been of considerable interest to epileptologists. There is currently no SPECT ligand for the GABA receptor itself, but the associated benzodiazepine (BZ) site can be imaged with SPECT using ^{123}I iomazenil. Iomazenil is a partial inverse BZ agonist that binds to central-type BZ receptors. Several small-scale studies have been carried out in epilepsy, showing focal reductions of central-type BZ receptor binding. These studies have found such focal reductions in relatively high proportions of patients (compared to HMPAO SPECT), although there is preliminary evidence that false localizations occur: for example, one study (van Huffelen et al 1990) found correct localization in 11/13 patients, with one false localization. There is evidence that reduction in BZ binding correlates with cell loss in the mesial temporal lobe (McDonald et al 1991; Koepp et al 1996) and may simply be a sensitive marker for it.

MUSCARINIC RECEPTORS

Some work is being carried out using a muscarinic agent, ^{123}I-dexetamide and shows localized reductions in binding in mesial temporal cortex in mesial temporal lobe epilepsies (Muller *et al* 1993; Rowe *et al* 1997).

THE USE OF rCP SPECT IN A PROGRAM FOR THE SURGICAL TREATMENT OF EPILEPSY

Peri-ictal rCP SPECT is now a routine part of presurgical evaluation at a number of centers, particularly in Australia, continental Europe, and the USA. In most cases, it is carried out at the same time as ictal surface EEG monitoring. This effectively means that most patients who have peri-ictal SPECT will also have had specialized MRI studies and ictal EEG recordings. In many patients with mesial temporal lobe epilepsies, this combination of noninvasive investi-

gations will give sufficient information either to proceed to surgery or to determine that the patient is not a surgical candidate. If there is doubt as to where in the hemisphere an epilepsy originates (e.g. in patients with mesial temporal sclerosis who have atypical seizure semeiology or atypically distributed but ipsilateral ictal EEG discharges), ictal SPECT can often settle that doubt. Increasing weight is being given to MRI findings in presurgical investigation, but it does appear that MRI-negative patients who have good localization on ictal rCP SPECT can have good surgical outcomes (Ho *et al* 1997).

Where initial data suggest an extratemporal epilepsy, then ictal SPECT data may be most usefully deployed in deciding on the placement of electrodes for intracranial EEG monitoring, and may be particularly useful in this regard if no lesion is detected on MRI.

However peri-ictal SPECT is used the data should be regarded no differently from those obtained using any other technique, that is, with due regard to its strengths and weaknesses and to its relation to other localizing data.

KEY POINTS

1. Interictal rCP SPECT lacks sensitivity and specificity, but can help localization as an ancillary investigation.
2. Ictal SPECT: changes in rCP usually begin within seconds of the electrical onset of the seizure, but may outlast the electrical discharge if the seizure is relatively long.
3. Mesial temporal lobe onset seizures: Ictal SPECT shows a well-established pattern of change in rCP with

hyperperfusion of the whole temporal lobe as its central feature. The specificity for the seizure focus seems to be near 100%, with the proviso that the pattern is typical.

4. Some frontal lobe seizures may be too brief to capture using ictal SPECT. Perfusion patterns associated with frontal seizures may be complex, requiring careful interpretation.

5. Ictal SPECT can be used to confirm surface ictal EEG localization in MRI-negative patients, and can usually determine whether seizures are temporal or extratemporal. A routine package of MRI with ictal SPECT and ictal surface EEG will provide noninvasive localization that will allow a surgical decision in many patients.

REFERENCES

Andersen AR, Friberg H, Schmidt JF, Hasselbalch SG (1988) Quantitative measurements of cerebral blood flow using SPECT and Tc99m D,L-HMPAO compared to xenon-133. *Journal of Cerebral Blood Flow and Metabolism* **8** (suppl. 1):S69–81.

Berkovic SF, Newton MR, Chiron C, Dulac O (1993) Single photon emission computed tomography. In: Engel JR (ed) *Surgical Treatment of the Epilepsies*, pp 233–243. New York: Raven Press

Bonte FJ, Devous MD, Stokely EM, Homan RW (1983) Single photon tomographic determination of regional cerebral blood flow in epilepsy. *American Journal of Neuroradiology* **4**:544–546.

Collins RC, Kennedy C, Sokoloff L, Plum F (1976) Metabolic anatomy of focal motor seizures. *Archives of Neurology* **33**:536–542

Cross JH, Boyd SG, Gordon I, Harper A, Neville BG (1997) Ictal

cerebral perfusion related to EEG in drug resistant focal epilepsy of childhood. *Journal of Neurology, Neurosurgery and Psychiatry* **62**:377–384

Cruickshank GS (1997) In: Duncan R (ed) *SPECT Imaging of the Brain*, pp 161–178. Kluwer: Dordrecht.

Devous MD, Leroy RF, Homan RW (1990) Single photon emission computed tomography in epilepsy. *Seminars in Nuclear Medicine* **10**:349–356.

Duncan R (1997a) In: Duncan R (ed) *SPECT Imaging of the Brain*, p 57. Dordrecht: Kluwer.

Duncan R (1997b) In: Duncan R (ed) *SPECT Imaging of the Brain*, pp 31–34. Dordrecht: Kluwer.

Duncan R, Patterson J, Hadley DM, Bone I, Wyper D (1990a) SPECT in temporal lobe epilepsy: ictal and interictal studies. In: Baldy Moulinier M, Lassen NA, Engel J, Askienazy S (eds) *Current Problems in Epilepsy*, vol 6, pp 79–93. London: Libbey.

Duncan R, Patterson J, Hadley DM *et al* (1990b) CT, MR and SPECT imaging in temporal lobe epilepsy. *Journal of Neurology, Neurosurgery and Psychiatry* **53**:11–15.

Duncan R, Patterson J, Bone I, Wyper DJ, McGeorge AP (1990c) Tc99m HMPAO single photon emission computed tomography in temporal lobe epilepsy *Acta Neurologica Scandinavica* **81**:287–293.

Duncan S, Gillan J, Duncan R, Brodie M (1992) Interictal HMPAO SPECT: a routine investigation in medically intractable complex partial epilepsy? *Epilepsy Research* **13**:83–87.

Duncan R, Patterson J, Roberts R, Hadley DM, Bone I (1993) Ictal/postictal SPECT in the pre-surgical localisation of complex partial seizures. *Journal of Neurology, Neurosurgery and Psychiatry* **56**:141–148.

Duncan R, Patterson J, Roberts R Hadley D (1995) Regional cerebral blood flow during posterior seizures: an HMPAO SPECT study. *Journal of Neurology, Neurosurgery and Psychiatry* **59**:203.

Duncan R, Patterson J, Hadley DM, Roberts R, Bone I (1996a) Interictal temporal hypoperfusion is related to early onset temporal lobe epilepsy. *Epilepsia* **37**:134–140.

Duncan R, Patterson J, Macrae IM (1996b) HMPAO as a regional cerebral blood flow tracer at high flow levels. *Journal of Nuclear Medicine* **37**:661–664.

Duncan R, Rahi S, Bernard AM *et al* (1996c) Ictal cerebral blood flow in seizures originating in the posterolateral cortex. *Journal of Nuclear Medicine* **37**:1946–1951.

Duncan R, Patterson J, Hadley DM, Roberts R (1997a) Ictal regional cerebral blood flow in frontal lobe seizures. *Seizure* **6**:393–401.

Duncan R, Patterson J, Hadley D *et al* (1997b) Ictal SPECT in occipital lobe seizures. *Epilepsia* **38**:839–843.

Dymond AM, Crandall PH (1976) Oxygen availability and blood flow in the temporal lobes during spontaneous epileptic seizures in man. *Brain Research* **102**:191–196.

Engel J, Brown WJ, Kuhl DE, Phelps ME, Mazziotta JC, Crandall PH (1982) Pathological findings underlying focal temporal lobe hypometabolism in partial epilepsy. *Annals of Neurology* **12**:518–528.

Friberg L, Andersen AR, Lassen NA, Holm S, Dam M (1994) Retention of 99mTc bicisate in the human brain after intracarotid injection. *Journal of Cerebral Blood Flow and Metabolism* **14**(suppl. 1):S19–27.

Friston JJ, Frith CD, Liddee PF, Dola RJ, Lammrtsma AA, Frackoviack RSJ (1990) The relationship between global and local changes in PET scans. *Journal of Cerebral Blood Flow and Metabolism* **10**:458–466.

Gibbs FA, Lennox WG, Gibbs EL (1934) Cerebral blood flow preceding and accompanying seizures in man. *Archives of Neurology and Psychiatry* **32**:257–272.

Grunwald F, Menzel C, Pavics L *et al* (1994) Ictal and interictal brain SPECT imaging in epilepsy using technetium 99m ECD. *Journal of Nuclear Medicine* **35**:1896–1901

Guillon B, Duncan R, Biraben A, Bernard AM, Vignal JP, Chauvel P (1998) Correlation between interictal regional cerebral blood flow and depth recorded interictal spiking in temporal lobe epilepsy. *Epilepsia* **39**:67–76.

Harvey AS, Bowe JM, Hopkins IJ, Shield LK, Cook DJ, Berkovic SF (1993a) Ictal 99mTc HMPAO single photon emission computed tomography in children with temporal lobe epilepsy. *Epilepsia* **34**:869–877

Harvey AS, Hopkins IJ, Bowe JM, Cook DJ, Shield LK, Berkovic SF (1993b) Frontal lobe epilepsy: clinical seizure characteristics and localisation with ictal ^{99m}Tc HMPAO SPECT. *Neurology* **43**:1966–1980

Ho SS, Berkovic SF, Newton MR, Austin MC, McKay WJ, Bladin PF (1993) Ictal 99mTc HMPAO SPECT findings in parietal lobe epilepsy. *Epilepsia* **34** (suppl. 2):112.

Ho SS, Berkovic SF, Ms Kay WJ, Kalnins RM, Bladin PF (1996) Temporal lobe epilepsy subtypes: differential patterns of cerebral perfusion seen on ictal SPECT. *Epilepsia* **37**:788–795.

Ho SS, Newton MR, McIntosh AM *et al* (1997) Perfusion patterns during temporal lobe seizures: relationship to surgical outcome. *Brain* **120**:1921–1928

Koepp MJ, Richardson MP, Brooks DJ *et al* (1996) Central benzodiazepine receptors in hippocampal sclerosis: an objective in vivo analysis. *Brain* **119**:1677–1687.

Kuhl DE, Engel J, Phelps ME, Selin C (1980) Epileptic patterns of local cerebral metabolism and perfusion in humans determined by emission computed tomography of 18FDG and 13NH3. *Annals of Neurology* **8**:348–360.

Lang W, Podreka I, Suess E, Muller C, Deecke L (1988) Single photon emission computed tomography during and between seizures. *Journal of Neurology* **235**:277–284.

Lassen NA, Sperling BK (1994) 99mTc Bicisate reliably images chronic brain disease but fails to show reflow hyperemia in acute stroke: report of a multicentre trial of 105 cases comparing 133Xe and 99mTc bicisate (ECD-Neurolite) measured by SPECT on same day. *Journal of Cerebral Blood Flow and Metabolism* **14**:S44.

Lee BI, Markand ON, Wellman HN *et al* (1988) HIPDM SPECT in patients with medically intractable complex partial seizures. *Archives of Neurology* **45**:397–402

Marks DA, Katz A, Hoffer P, Spencer SS (1992) Localisation of extratemporal epileptic foci during ictal single photon emission computed tomography. *Annals of Neurology* **31**:250–253.

McDonald JW, Garofalo EA, Hood T *et al* (1991) Altered excitatory and inhibitory amino acid receptor binding in hippocampus of patients with temporal lobe epilepsy. *Annals of Neurology* **29**:529–541.

Muller Gartner HW, Links JM, Prince JL, *et al* (1993) Decreased hippocampal muscarinic choline receptor binding measured by 132I iododexetimide and single photon emission computed tomography in epilepsy *Annals of Neurology* **34**:235–238.

Newton MR, Bercovik SF, Austin MC, Rowe CC, McKay WJ, Bladin PF (1992a) Postictal switch in blood flow distribution and temporal lobe seizures. *Journal of Neurology, Neurosurgery and Psychiatry* **55**:891–894

Newton MR, Berkovic SF, Austen MC (1992b) Dystonia, clinical lateralisation and regional blood flow changes in temporal lobe seizures. *Neurology* **42**:371–377

Newton MR, Berkovic SF, Austin MC, Rowe CC, McKay WJ, Bladin PF (1995) SPECT in the localisation of extratemporal and temporal seizure foci. *Journal of Neurology, Neurosurgery and Psychiatry* **59**:26–30

Penfield W (1937) The circulation of the epileptic brain. *Research Publications of the Association of Nervous and Mental Disorders* **18**:605–737.

Penfield W, von Santha K, Cipriani A (1939) Cerebral blood flow during induced epileptiform seizures in animals and man. *Journal of Neurophysiology* **2**:257–267.

Podreka I, Lang W, Suess E *et al* (1988) Hexamethyl-propylene-amine-oxime (HMPAO) single photon emission computed tomography (SPECT) in epilepsy. *Brain Topography* **1**:55–60.

Prince DA, Wilder BJ (1967) Control mechanisms in cortical epileptogenic foci, 'surround' inhibition. *Archives of Neurology* **16**:194–202.

Rowe CC, Bercovic SF, Sia STB *et al* (1989) Localisation of epileptic foci with postictal single photon emission computed tomography. *Annals of Neurology* **26**:660–668.

Rowe CC, Berkovic SF, Austin MC *et al* (1991a) Visual and quantitative analysis of interictal SPECT with Tc99m HMPAO in temporal lobe epilepsy. *Journal of Nuclear Medicine* **32**:1688–1694.

Rowe CC, Berkovic SF, Sia STB, Bladin PF (1991b) Patterns of postictal blood flow in temporal lobe epilepsy: qualitative and quantitative findings. *Neurology* **41**:1096–1103.

Rowe CC, Boundy KL, Kitchener L *et al* (1997) Ictal 99mTc

HMPAO SPECT and 123I-iododexetimide SPECT in temporal lobe epilepsy In: DeDeyn P, Dierckx RA, Alavi A, Pickut BA (eds) *SPECT in Neurology and Psychiatry*, pp 219–224. London: Libbey.

Ryding E, Rosen I, Elmqvist D, Ingvar DH (1988) SPECT measurements with 99Tc HMPAO in focal epilepsy. *Journal of Cerebral Blood Flow and Metabolism* **8**:S95–S100.

Ryvlin P, Garcia-Larrea L, Phillipon B *et al* (1992) High signal intensity on T2 weighted MRI correlates with hypoperfusion in temporal lobe epilepsy. *Epilepsia* **33**:28–35.

Shen W, Lee BI, Park HM *et al* (1990) HIPDM-SPECT brain imaging in the presurgical evaluation of patients with intractable seizures. *Journal of Nuclear Medicine* **31**:1280–1284.

Sperling B, Lassen NA (1993) Hyperfixation of HMPAO in subacute ischaemic stroke leading to spuriously high estimates of cerebral blood flow by SPECT. *Stroke* **24**:193–194.

Theodore WH, Newmark ME, Sato S (1983) [18F]Fluorodeoxyglucose positron emission tomography in refractory complex partial seizures. *Annals of Neurology* **14**:429–437.

Valmier J, Touchon J, Daures P, Zanca M, Baldy Moulinier M (1987) Correlations between cerebral blood flow variations and clinical parameters in temporal lobe epilepsy: an interictal study. *Journal of Neurology, Neurosurgery and Psychiatry* **50**:1306–1311.

van Huffelen AC, van Isselt JW, van Veelen CW (1990) Identification of the side of the epileptic focus with 123I Iomazenil SPECT: a comparison with 18FDG and ictal EEG findings in patients with medically intractable complex partial seizures. *Acta Neurochirurgia Wien* **50** (suppl. 1):95–99.

Zubla IG, Spencer SS, Imam K *et al* (1996) Difference image calculated from ictal and interictal technetium-99m-HMPAO SPECT scans of epilepsy. *Journal of Nuclear Medicine* **37**:1080–1083.

Neurophysiologic investigation of adults

27

RP KENNETT

The extracranially recorded EEG has passed through cycles of importance in the investigation of patients with suspected partial seizures. For many years it was the only available noninvasive investigation, but popularity declined with the advent of modern imaging procedures that were soon shown to be far more sensitive in detecting the pathologic basis of partial seizures. Other unfavorable factors were (a) the observation that less than 50% of patients with established epilepsy show diagnostic abnormalities on a single recording, making the investigation of limited value as a screening tool; (b) the perceived difficulty in visual identification of abnormalities, leading to overinterpretation or underinterpretation; (c) the reported high rate of false localization of the epileptic focus in patients being assessed for surgical treatment, resulting in a reliance on intracranial recording; and (d) the development of functional neuroimaging techniques to define areas of disturbed cortical metabolism. None the less, the EEG remains the most widely available and simplest method of assessing brain function and recently there has been renewed interest in its use, particularly when the information obtained is combined with other readily available tests with the aim of avoiding invasive techniques, which are expensive and carry their own inherent risks.

This chapter is divided into four sections. The first deals with the theoretic basis of identifying epileptic EEG abnormalities, including the cellular basis and origin of the electrical abnormalities occurring in partial epilepsy, the appearance of these changes on extracranial EEG recordings and how they can be separated from activity unrelated to epilepsy, the principles of localization of electrical abnormalities, and the way computers may assist in EEG analysis. The second section is concerned with practical aspects of recording interictal and ictal phenomena. The third and fourth sections describe the extracranial EEG abnormalities that may be seen in temporal and extratemporal lobe epilepsies respectively.

THEORETIC BASIS OF EPILEPTIC EEG ABNORMALITIES

This section starts with some useful definitions and proceeds to describe the cellular basis of EEG activity and epileptic abnormalities. The aim is to provide a conceptual framework upon which correct interpretation of observed phenomena can be based. Electrical discharges recorded on the scalp must be divided into those related to an epileptic pathophysiology and those which are innocent biophysical events or artifacts. This area of EEG interpretation is often subjective and leads to difficulties of overinterpretation or underinterpretation. The discussion on the differentiation of nonepileptic transient activity that follows is intended to help reduce these difficulties. When a transient potential has been identified as having an epileptic origin, the next step is to decide its location on the scalp and the likely source of the cerebral generator. This is covered under the heading of source localization. This section concludes with a brief discussion on the role of computers and the way in which they have been used to increase the objectivity and sensitivity of EEG analysis.

DEFINITIONS

The EEG hallmark of partial epilepsy is a transient electrical potential: the *interictal epileptic discharge*. This is isolated from the background EEG activity, and to be clearly different from ongoing rhythms should preferably have an amplitude twice that of the preceding 5 s of recording and should not be the result of superimposition of existing waves. It usually has a characteristic triangular waveform, rapidly rising to a point followed by a slower falling phase, and may be associated with a slow wave. By definition, a transient discharge having these characteristics and with a duration <70 ms is called a *spike*, whereas a *sharp wave* has a duration of 80–200 ms. These two terms are often used loosely and interchangeably. Interictal epileptic discharges are closely associated with the presence of epilepsy but have to be differentiated from similar looking potentials that do not have an epileptic basis. These 'epileptiform' transients may be cerebral biologic discharges or artifacts, as discussed below.

The area of brain producing interictal epileptic discharges is termed the *irritative zone*, as it is assumed that this region of cortex has abnormal excitability. The irritative zone is often large and usually, but not always, contains the area of brain in which the patient's seizures are initially generated: the *ictal onset zone*. Defining the irritative and ictal onset zones is one of the main roles of the EEG evaluation of partial epilepsy. Further terms useful conceptually are the *epileptogenic zone* and the *epileptogenic pathology*. The epileptogenic zone is that area of brain necessary for the generation of habitual seizures and whose removal, or disconnection, produces a cure. This usually contains the identifiable pathologic abnormality causing the epilepsy and the ictal onset zone; however, it is important to remember that the irritative zone is larger and may be separate, especially in extratemporal epilepsies.

PRINCIPLES OF EEG GENERATORS

Although the rhythmic activity seen in the EEG is not fully understood, the columnar organization of the cerebral

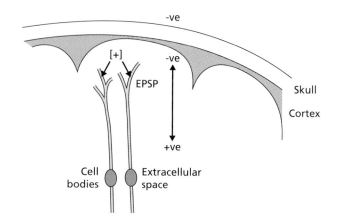

Fig. 27.1 Cellular events producing EEG signals recorded on the scalp. Synchronous excitatory potentials in the apical dendrites (EPSP) due to influx of cations leaves the extracellular space and adjacent area of scalp negatively charged relative to deeper layers of brain or distant regions of the scalp. The dipole in this example is orientated radial to the skull.

cortex is thought to be the basis (Figure 27.1). The large output neuron cell bodies lie in the deeper layers of the cortex, with their dendritic arborizations extending to the surface and the axon leading perpendicularly in the opposite direction. Synaptic connections from input neurons, local interneurons, and feedback collateral sprouts from the cell itself are formed either on the outer dendrites or closer to the cell body. At both sites the synapses are either excitatory or inhibitory. Excitatory synapses act via *N*-methyl-D-aspartate (NMDA) or glutamate receptors that open membrane channels to allow influx of Na^+ or Ca^{2+}, producing transient depolarization: the excitatory postsynaptic potential (EPSP). Inhibitory synapses act predominantly through γ-amino butyric acid (GABA) receptors that activate channels permitting an inward chloride current, producing hyperpolarization of the cell: the inhibitory postsynaptic potential (IPSP). These receptors are affected by a number of modifying influences, and the ion channels are voltage and time dependent. Synapses further from the cell body have a smaller influence on the output discharge than those close to it. These factors increase the complexity of neuronal activity.

The EEG detects electrical potential changes occurring in the extracellular space of the cerebral cortex at a distance from the site of generation by a process known as volume conduction. If an EPSP occurs at the surface of the cortex, the influx of positively charged ions into cells leaves the extracellular space relatively electrically negative. To restore equilibrium, a current flows from the deeper layers of the cortex. Simply from Ohm's law, it follows that because the electrical resistance of the extracellular space is low, even large flows of charge from deep cortical layers only generate small voltages. One feature of a volume conductor is that the potential decays in proportion to the square of the distance from the source, so that the already small voltage generated by a single EPSP declines rapidly as recordings are made further from the cortical surface. From this it is deduced that many thousands of EPSPs have to occur synchronously to generate an extracellular voltage large enough to be recorded on the scalp. Because of the decay of voltage with distance and because volume conduction through brain tissue is thought not to occur (Cooper *et al* 1965), only activity in the most superficial layers of the cortex is detected on the scalp.

The EPSPs described above have the effect of making the extracellular space near the cortical surface negatively charged with respect to a positive area around the cell body. This is analogous to a bar magnet with a negative and positive pole (dipole); in the case we have been considering the negative pole is at the surface and the positive pole is orientated perpendicularly (radially), facing towards the center of the brain. A similarly orientated dipole is generated by an IPSP near the cell body, as the inward chloride current has the effect of making the extracellular space positive compared with the cortical surface. Radial dipoles in the opposite direction, with the positive pole at the surface, are generated by either an IPSP occurring in the outer cortical layers of the dendritic arborization or an EPSP at a deeper level.

Two further properties have an important influence on the interpretation of scalp EEG recordings. Firstly, there is attenuation of voltage by the electrical resistance of the skull and scalp tissue. Simultaneous recordings of spontaneous potentials by intracranial and surface electrodes and measurements of signals generated by electrodes implanted into the brain have shown a reduction of voltage in the region of 2000–5000 times from the cerebral substance to the surface (Cooper *et al* 1965; Alarcon *et al* 1994). The implication is that scalp-recorded EEG signals are generated in the cortex adjacent to the skull and not from deeper sources. Furthermore, early experiments suggested that an area of cortex in the region of $6\,cm^2$ has to be active synchronously in order to generate a potential that can be recorded on the scalp (Cooper *et al* 1965). This is in good agreement with more recent magnetoencephalographic experiments measuring the magnetic field around a spike discharge, which estimated that the smallest area of active cortex measurable on the scalp is in the region of 10–$12\,cm^2$ (Sutherling *et al* 1988). Secondly, bone and connective tissue impose a filtering effect on cerebral activity, resulting in attenuation of high-frequency activity and relative preservation of lower frequencies. The result of this is that biologically important high-frequency activity may be difficult to record from the surface EEG.

Interictal activity

The pathophysiology of interictal epileptic activity in humans is still to be fully elucidated. Spontaneous field potentials are rarely observed in neocortical tissue slices obtained during resective surgery for epilepsy, but may be evoked by electrical stimulation of white matter tracts or various pharmacologic manipulations of the bathing medium. This has led to the conclusion that interictal spikes are derived by the same mechanism as paroxysmal depolarizing shifts (PDS), seen in experimental animal models of epilepsy. In these models, large afferent inputs to the cortex cause depolarization of cortical neurons sufficient to generate repetitive action potentials from the cortical output neurons. This is followed by a period when the cell is hyperpolarized. The precise cellular mechanisms underlying PDS are complex, although the depolarization is thought to be mainly due to a calcium excitatory current that is partly synaptic and voltage-dependent, and the hyperpolarization to a voltage-dependent potassium current with a contribution from calcium currents and receptor-mediated inhibitory synaptic currents (Dichter 1989, 1993; Swanson 1995). From the earlier discussion, it will be appreciated that PDS have to occur synchronously in a large population of cortical neurons for a spike to be detected by scalp EEG, implying that recurrent neurons and interneurons are vital to the process of neural synchronization. The epileptic spike is thought to result from the summation of either synchronous output cell action potentials or dendritic EPSPs, and the following slow wave from either cellular hyperpolarization or dendritic IPSPs. The negative end of the dipole created in this way would orientate towards the cortical surface and explain the virtually universal surface negativity of interictal epileptic spikes.

Despite these theoretic considerations, little is fully established about the pathophysiology of interictal epileptiform activity in humans. Recordings on temporal tissue slices, obtained during resection at the time of surgery, have shown that field potentials are less prominent than in control tissue, probably because pyramidal cells in the sclerotic hippocampus are reduced in number. Inhibitory mechanisms have been shown to be impaired, with IPSPs less likely to be evoked by stimulation, and pyramidal cells are more likely to fire in bursts (Knowles *et al* 1992). Blockade of GABA receptors may also cause burst firing at levels that would be subthreshold for this phenomenon in control tissue, again indicating impaired synaptic inhibition (Franck *et al* 1995). In contrast, the excitatory synaptic input to remaining pyramidal cells in sclerotic hippocampi appears to be normal (Urban *et al* 1993). Understanding the relationship between interictal spiking and the epileptogenic pathology or ictal onset zone is vital if this information is to be used rationally in clinical decision-making. In the past it was assumed that spiking reflects an abnormal state of cortical hyperexcitability central to the process of epileptogenesis, and that surgical excision of the cortex generating these spikes was essential for the successful surgical treatment of epilepsy (Luders *et al* 1989). Subsequent studies have shown that this is not the case and residual spiking, albeit less frequent, is the norm after resections that are subsequently shown to render the patient seizure-free (Fiol *et al* 1991; McBride *et al* 1991; Godoy *et al* 1992; Tuunainen *et al* 1994; Alarcon *et al* 1997). Indeed, in hippocampal sclerosis spikes are usually recorded from pathologically normal neocortex and resection of only the mesial temporal lobe structures is required for a surgical cure; in occipital epilepsy it is usual to find spike foci away from the epileptogenic pathology. Thus, a complex interaction between distinct anatomic areas of cortex underlies interictal spike discharges. Dipole modeling has helped to clarify this interaction. Early dipole models suggested that spikes in mesial temporal lobe epilepsy (MTLE) are orientated between the medial and lateral temporal structures (Ebersole and Wade 1991), implying that both are involved simultaneously in the generation of the discharge. More advanced modeling, using the average from spike-triggered sweeps and devising solutions to the dipole generator vectors sequentially, has suggested propagation of electrical activity from the mesial to lateral temporal neocortex (Baumgartner *et al* 1995; Merlet *et al* 1996). The concept arising from these studies is of mesial temporal activity driving a response from the lateral temporal cortex. Although there are theoretic arguments against these observations from advanced dipole modeling (i.e. the electrical potentials of activity in the hippocampus are too small to be measured on the surface, questioning the inverse solution of relating surface recordings back to the hippocampus; Alarcon *et al* 1994), the main evidence against this concept is provided by observations of interictal spikes using a combination of depth, subdural, and scalp electrodes.

It is recognized that spikes may be localized to a small number of intracerebral electrodes, with discharges appearing at some points but not at others only a few millimeters away (Privitera *et al* 1990), and not propagating from one site to another. Simultaneous recordings of interictal spikes from scalp, sphenoidal, depth, and subdural electrodes have given new insights into the possible intracranial generators (Marks *et al* 1992). When surface spikes could be recorded there was usually simultaneous activity in a large mesiobasal region that included the hippocampus and parahippocampal, fusiform, and inferior temporal gyri. It is unlikely that a single source from within the hippocampus could produce such a large and widespread depolarization, given that brain substance inhibits volume conduction of electrical activity (Cooper *et al* 1965), although this conclusion is drawn to explain dipole reconstructions (Lantz *et al* 1996). The precise mechanism for synchronization of activity at all these sites is unknown, but it is possible that they are all driven by activity in the entorhinal cortex, stimulation of which is known to activate hippocampal spikes. Extracranial recordings from mesial and lateral temporal areas may show some mesial discharges preceding the lateral ones by 30–35 ms, consistent with oligosynaptic propagation from mesial to lateral temporal structures (Sutherling and Barth 1989). However, propagation from the hippocampus to the neocortex is an infrequent finding (Spencer *et al* 1987), and lateral temporal discharges often appear independently of mesial activity (Marks *et al* 1992; Tsai *et al* 1993), suggesting that the neocortical activity is independent of the main site of epileptic pathology in MTLE. Another survey of over 600 spikes found five distinct patterns of discharges (Alarcon *et al* 1994):

1. recorded only from electrodes near the hippocampus;
2. recorded synchronously at deep and surface electrodes with no latency difference;
3. recorded at deep and surface electrodes with a short latency difference (< 50 ms);
4. recorded at deep and surface electrodes with a long latency difference (> 50 ms);
5. recorded only at surface electrodes.

When discharges could be recorded synchronously at both depth and surface electrodes, 88% were from the same hemisphere and < 1% were exclusively at contralateral deep and surface electrodes. The remaining activity was recorded from unilateral deep and bilateral surface electrodes or vice versa.

From these observations it would appear that there is a complex relationship between the ictal onset zone (and epileptogenic pathology) and interictal spike discharges. While some discharges at the neocortex appear as a result of propagation from deeper sites, either by fast-conducting axons or by slower spread along the cortex, other discharges occur independently. When an interconnection occurs, excision of the primary 'leading' region is required for a good surgical outcome (Alarcon *et al* 1997). Presumably, this indicates that cortical areas away from the epileptogenic pathology have abnormal excitability, and explains why the irritative zone is larger than the ictal onset zone and may not even include it. The cause of this increased cortical excitability is not understood, although in the past it was concluded that these areas represent 'mirror foci' as seen in the kindling model of experimental epilepsy. However, observations that the extent of spiking are unrelated to the duration or severity of epilepsy in humans cast doubt on this hypothesis (Lieb *et al* 1981a; Niediek *et al* 1990; Lim *et al* 1991; Morris *et al* 1993; Gilmore *et al* 1994).

Ictal conversion

The mechanisms underlying the development of seizures are even less well understood. Some theories suggest that the hyperpolarization phase of the PDS is replaced by depolarization, perhaps because of accumulation of extracellular K^+ or a fall in Ca^{2+} (Dichter 1989). This theory is not supported by intracranial recordings from the human hippocampus, which show seizure onset most often associated with the abrupt appearance of fast activity not preceded by interictal spiking (Spencer and Spencer 1994). Other theories suggest that dendritic bursts are driven by sustained depolarization or by increased axonal or presynaptic terminal excitability (Traub *et al* 1996). However, in human tissue slices, the absence of dentate cell burst firing appears to correlate with low-voltage fast activity at seizure onset (Williamson *et al* 1995), and preictal spiking, when seen, correlates with loss of IPSPs, indicating a different cellular mechanism for this activity and PDS (which is caused by GABA-mediated inhibition). Sustained synaptic activity is probably involved in the generation of seizures since frequency potentiation is known to increase the size of EPSPs and reduce IPSPs, sometimes called dual synaptic modulation (Dichter 1993). Presumably the alterations in the synaptic connections or modulatory influences resulting from hippocampal cell loss, including inhibitory interneurons (Marco *et al* 1996), enhance this process. Spread of seizure activity then probably proceeds to more distant areas via neuronal pathways, the high-frequency activity recruiting more cells because of dual synaptic modulation. Although the cell loss and secondary changes in the hippocampus appear to be at the heart of this process in MTLE, it is not clear whether the events triggering seizure onset start here or in the entorhinal area of basal temporal neocortex. This region has a major input into the hippocampus and afferent stimulation may evoke hippocampal spikes (Rutecki *et al* 1989). Furthermore, intracranial recordings have shown that ictal onsets may occur in the entorhinal cortex, hippocampus, or at both sites simultaneously in the same patient with pathologically proven hippocampal sclerosis (Spencer and Spencer 1994).

IDENTIFICATION OF TRANSIENT EEG ACTIVITY

The aim of EEG analysis is to identify transient electrical activity associated with the presence of epilepsy or the lesion causing it. This requires analysis of background rhythms and the differentiation of epileptic from nonepileptic cerebral transient potentials or artifacts. A more detailed description of normal EEG activity can be found in standard textbooks (Niedermeyer and Lopes da Silva 1993).

Background rhythms

Alpha rhythm

The *alpha rhythm* is abnormal if there is a persistent asymmetry of amplitude greater than 50% or in frequency of more than 1 Hz. The abnormality is on the side with the lower amplitude or slower frequency.

Slow rhythms

Slow rhythms require considerable judgment. Most EEG recordings contain some posterior slow waves and rhythmic centrotemporal theta activity, especially during drowsiness. Asymmetric theta rhythms may occur as a normal variant, especially subclinical rhythmic EEG discharges of adults, seen mainly in the temporal or parietal regions of awake elderly patients and consisting of a repetitive sinusoidal pattern at 4–7 Hz with abrupt termination. About one-third of runs are independent and may last 40–80 s. This activity resembles an ictal rhythm but there is no alteration of consciousness, even during long trains, and repeated episodes are seen in subsequent recordings from the same individuals. Focal posterior delta slow waves, especially on the right, are a feature of immature EEG recordings. In the elderly, left temporal theta activity may be seen in 60% of individuals. Abnormal slow wave activity is either continuous or intermittent, persistently localized, and may be in the theta or delta ranges (polymorphic slow waves).

Fast activity

Fast activity is abnormal if it is persistently asymmetric or localized, except over a defect in the skull vault (breach rhythm). Reduced barbiturate-induced fast activity may occur on the side of hippocampal sclerosis.

Epileptic discharges

Spike and slow wave complexes are easily identified by their characteristic appearance (see Fig. 27.5) although difficulties arise if the waveform is distorted. For instance, discharges arising in deep locations may have attenuation of the spike component, leaving only an ill-defined slow wave discharge at the surface. Unusual waveforms, such as triangular or notched slow waves, can also be difficult to identify.

Cerebral nonepileptic transient activity

Mu rhythm

Mu rhythm (previously called wicket, comb, or arceau rhythm) consists of arch-shaped trains at 7–11 Hz in the central and parietal areas. It is often asynchronous, blocked by contralateral limb movement, and abnormal when persistently unilateral.

Lambda waves

Lambda waves are saw-toothed, positive, occipital discharges occurring during visual inspection and may be associated with an eye-movement artifact (see Fig. 27.3).

Transient activity during sleep

Positive occipital sharp transient (discharges) of sleep (POSTS) have a similar appearance to lambda waves. Other normal transient activity occurring during sleep includes vertex sharp waves, which are negative about the central midline, and benign epileptiform transient discharges of sleep (BETS). The latter are of low amplitude and short duration and, although widespread, are maximal in the temporal regions. They have horizontal dipoles, which makes them difficult to localize with bipolar montages, and are best demonstrated on referential recordings (Molaie *et al* 1991).

Kappa rhythm

Kappa rhythm refers to low-amplitude temporal alpha or theta activity appearing during mental exertion.

Wicket spikes

Wicket spikes are negative discharges of greater than 200 mV amplitude appearing in any head region, especially when there is fast, sharply contoured activity in the background. They look similar to components of mu rhythm and are seen mainly in the elderly.

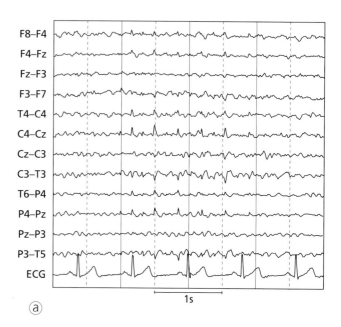

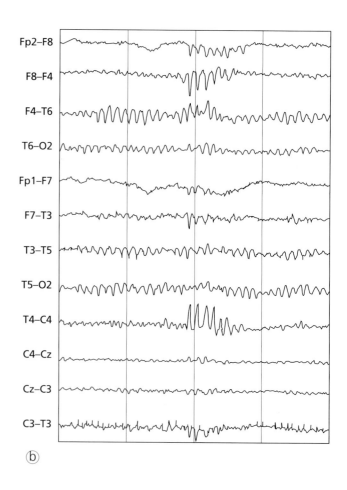

Fig. 27.2 Examples of cerebral nonepileptic transient activity: (a) burst of low-amplitude 6-Hz spike and slow wave complexes in the centrotemporal regions; (b) run of right midtemporal, sharply contoured, focal theta activity (psychomotor variant).

Six per second spike–wave or phantom spike–wave

These repetitive spike–wave complexes at 4–7 Hz usually contain spikes of low amplitude and short duration (less than 40 mV and 30 ms) (Fig. 27.2a). Paroxysms are usually bilaterally synchronous, last less than 1 s, and occur during drowsiness or eye closure. Posterior activity is benign, but anterior activity may overlap with true epileptic discharges.

Positive spikes

Isolated positive spikes at 14 and 6 Hz (ctenoids) are mostly seen during sleep in adolescents. They are maximal in the posterior temporal areas, either independently or bisynchronously, and are best seen in referential montages or bipolar arrays with long interelectrode distances.

Rhythmic midtemporal discharges

Rhythmic midtemporal discharges (psychomotor variant) (Fig. 27.2b). appear in bursts at 4–7 Hz and are maximal in young adults during drowsiness or sleep. They may be independent or bisynchronous and show a tendency to vary in amplitude during the train.

Extracerebral or artifactual transient activity

Blink artifact

Blink artifact or lateral eye movements produce a characteristic deflection at frontal electrodes, probably because movement of the charged retinal cell layer creates an electrical field. Eye flutter artifact can occur rhythmically at fast rates and thus may be confused with paroxysmal frontal lobe activity; careful observation of the patient is needed to confirm the nature of this artifact. Lateral eye movements may be associated with a single sharp potential referable to the F7,8 electrodes (the lateral rectus spike). If this occurs in conjunction with an eye movement artifact, a complex that may be confused with an epileptic spike and slow wave results (Fig. 27.3).

Muscle spikes

Muscle spikes are usually easily identified as they are very brief and occur in short bursts over temporal or frontal electrodes. Repetitive movements from chewing or tremor may give rise to muscle spikes and slow wave artifacts, superficially resembling epileptic discharges. These are most difficult to identify correctly when the patient cannot be

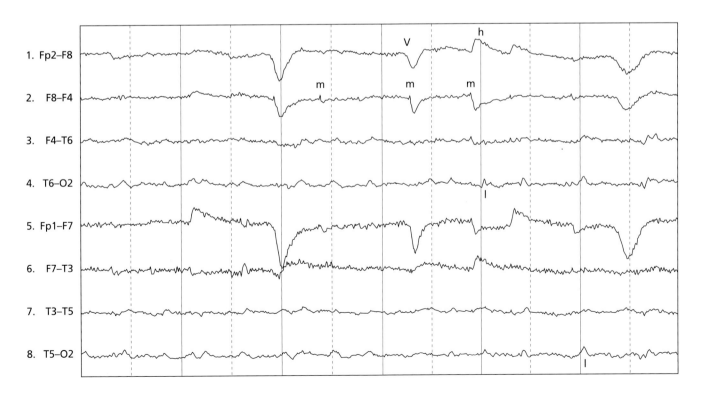

Fig. 27.3 Examples of extracerebral nonepileptic transient activity. Vertical (v) and horizontal (h) eye movements and lateral rectus muscle spikes (m) are often seen in standard EEG recordings. Cerebral lambda waves (l) are also present.

observed, as during ambulatory cassette EEG recording. Other movements, such as breathing, restlessness, tremors, tics, myoclonic jerks, and the balistocardiographic effect, can produce slow wave artifacts. If suspected, these can be positively identified by the use of accelerometers, respiration monitors, or other biologic recordings.

ECG

The ECG may often be recorded on the scalp, especially in people with short necks. The orientation of the R wave causes scalp positivity maximal in the region of the T5 electrode. Use of a single-lead ECG channel should allow identification of this artifact; if this is not used problems can arise, particularly if the patient has ectopic beats as these appear as intermittent transient discharges on the scalp. Pulse artifact, a smooth or triangular slow wave due to electrode movement caused by arterial pulsation, may also be detected by using an ECG channel.

Electrode popping

Electrode popping is a brief positive deflection caused by transient movement or change in electrical contact at the recording site. It is recognized by the characteristic waveform and, as with other electrode artifacts, occurs only at one electrode.

Glossokinetic artifact

The glossokinetic artifact is mainly seen at frontal channels and is due to movement of the tongue (whose tip is negatively charged relative to the base) when chewing, swallowing, or talking. As with other movement artifacts, this mainly causes difficulties in interpretation when the patient cannot be closely observed.

PRINCIPLES OF EEG SOURCE LOCALIZATION

Of paramount importance in the interpretation of EEG data is the ability to accurately determine the location of an electrical potential on the scalp. This requires analysis of the size of the electrical signal at each electrode followed by a mental or graphic plot on to the outline of a head. The site of the cerebral generator can then be estimated using knowledge of electrode positions relative to underlying cortical structures (Homan *et al* 1987). As discussed above, cerebral potentials have an electrical field with negative and positive poles, between which there are equipotential lines, usually represented as circles. Potential differences have to be recorded between a pair of electrodes and, by EEG

convention, negativity at the first electrode relative to the second is registered as an upward deflection on the recording. Consequently, negativity at the second electrode renders the first relatively positive and a downward deflection on the print-out is registered. In bipolar recording montages, the pairs of electrodes are usually adjacent sites in the 10–20 international system. In referential montages, either the first electrode is one of the scalp sites and the second scalp site common to all channels, or the potential recorded at each electrode is referred to an average electrical potential generated from all the participating recording sites.

Figure 27.4 shows spike discharges with a localization commonly seen in MTLE; in Fig. 27.4a a negative transient discharge has occurred under the F8 electrode. The potential at this point is maximal relative to the whole head and the average reference montage shows the largest deflection from this channel. The potential gradient is also registered at the Fp2 and T4 electrodes but to a lesser extent. The bipolar recording shows a downward deflection in channel 1 since the Fp2 electrode is relatively positive compared with the F8 electrode, but this is negative compared with the T4 electrode, giving an upward deflection in channel 2. This appearance of 'phase reversal' between two recording channels in a bipolar montage localizes the greatest area of electrical negativity to the shared electrode in the same way that the highest amplitude of deflection localizes it in the referential montage. In Fig. 27.4b the maximum negativity occurs between the F8 and T4 electrodes. Now the referential montage shows a similar amplitude of deflection from these two electrodes since they lie on an equipotential line. On the bipolar montage, there is no potential difference between the F8 and T4 electrodes and so no deflection occurs in channel 2 but phase reversal is seen between channels 1 and 3.

These illustrations demonstrate how restricted potentials generated by radial dipoles can be localized. More widespread lateralized electrical fields are more difficult to detect using these methods, although such transients are unlikely to have an epileptic basis. It should also be appreciated that bipolar montages are most useful if:

1. rows of adjacent electrodes are linked;
2. both horizontal and vertical arrays are used;
3. montages do not have single channels alternating from one side of the head to the other (which makes recognition of phase reversal difficult);
4. wide or double spacing is avoided as the chance of having electrodes on equipotential lines is increased (conversely if the discharge fortuitously occurs under an electrode the deflection is larger as the potential gradient between electrodes is greater).

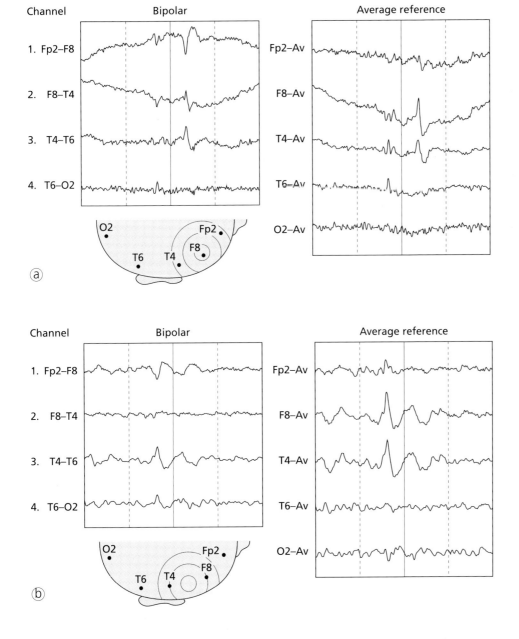

Fig. 27.4 Principles for localizing the source of interictal epileptic discharges recorded from patients with mesial temporal lobe epilepsy. Isopotential lines are represented as circles on the skull diagram. (a) The maximum negativity is under the F8 electrode. The bipolar montage shows reversal of polarity between channels 1 and 2; the average reference montage shows the largest amplitude deflection at the F8-Av channel. (b) The maximum negativity is between the F8 and T4 electrodes. No deflection is recorded on the bipolar montage at channel 2 as both the F8 and T4 electrodes are on equipotential lines. These electrodes show a similar amplitude of deflection on the average reference montage. (See text for further details.)

When a potential is analyzed in this way it is possible to draw a map of the negativity and equipotential lines to demonstrate the position of the discharge. In the past this was mainly a mental process performed when reviewing the EEG, but the advent of digital EEG recorders has allowed simple potential maps to be plotted (Koszer *et al* 1996).

More advanced computerized dipole potential mapping has received considerable interest recently. The first difficulty is to determine the orientation of the potential dipole. In most cases the EEG-recorded dipole has a vertical (also termed radial) orientation where the negative pole is at the surface and the positive pole is at 180° to the scalp, located in the center of the brain and not recorded at the surface.

The vector producing the scalp recording can be modeled (the reverse solution) but this relies upon estimates of the potential gradient at points not actually measured, allowance for the shape and thickness of the skull, and a judgment of the dipoles contributing to the final vector. The latter is imponderable because it is likely that many generators with variable orientation around the curved and convoluted cortex contribute to the final summated vector. Infrequently, both negative and positive poles appear on the scalp simultaneously at different locations. These horizontal or tangential dipoles produce electrical fields not readily detected by scalp electrodes, although the associated magnetic field can be localized by magnetoencephalography.

COMPUTER-ASSISTED EEG ANALYSIS

Use of computers to detect specified electrical events is discussed in relation to video-EEG telemetry (see also Gotman 1985). Another use of computers is to quantitatively analyze the EEG signal, allowing statistical evaluation and topographic mapping. The first step is to transform the EEG signal to produce a numerical value. This is easily done by digital EEG acquisition systems that perform analog to digital conversion during recording. Modern converters have a sufficient sampling rate and number of 'bits' to avoid problems of aliasing and distortion of the EEG signal to any significant extent during the quantitation process. The resulting numerical data have the advantage of being displayed in a number of different formats and statistical analysis should eliminate reader variability, possibly by detecting changes that are not easily seen. Despite these theoretic advantages and attempts to use quantitative EEG over the years, it is still to be fully incorporated into clinical practice. This is mainly because in the process of quantitation data are lost from the raw signal and the approximations that have to be made can cause errors. Furthermore, there is a belief that little if any further useful information is obtained over visual inspection by an experienced interpreter (Koszer *et al* 1996).

Spectral analysis based on fast Fourier transformation is the type of quantitative evaluation most used. This is based on the principle that a continuous signal can be described by a combination of sine and cosine waves of various phases, frequencies, and amplitudes. The resulting data can be expressed either in the time domain by an amplitude vs. time plot, or in the frequency domain by an amplitude (or phase) vs. frequency plot (the power spectrum). In the process, the morphology of the original tracing is lost and large amounts of data are summarized by a few descriptors, although the relationship between the selected features is determined more precisely than by visual inspection. The characteristics usually assessed are the absolute and relative band power, and the spectral edge and absolute peak frequencies. The absolute band is the approximate area under the curve of the power spectrum plot between arbitrarily chosen frequencies. The relative band is this area expressed as a proportion of the whole spectrum or another arbitrary bandwidth. The spectral edge is a preselected frequency that separates a chosen percentage of the absolute band (for instance, 50 or 90%). The absolute peak frequency is that frequency with the greatest power in a selected band. All these values may be plotted across the head in order to observe asymmetries, or sequentially (as a compressed spectral array) to look for changes with time, for instance during operative or intensive-care monitoring. There is currently only a limited role

for spectral EEG analysis in epileptic patients, although studies in temporal lobe epilepsy have suggested that subtle focal slow wave changes may be detected for long periods postictally (Tuunainen *et al* 1995) and fluctuations in the spectral edge frequency may be less on the side of ictal onset (Wang and Wieser 1994). Spectral analysis of intracranial recordings can be useful for the detection of subtle electrodecremental events consisting of low-amplitude high-frequency activity (Alarcon *et al* 1995).

In topographic mapping, the distribution of recorded activity across the scalp may be used to emphasize change with time. A special feature is usually chosen for analysis (such as a spike discharge) and the voltage, frequency, or a statistical value is plotted at points over the skull. Spike analysis in this way may make it possible to differentiate medial from lateral temporal lobe epilepsy when no differences are apparent by visual inspection of the EEG (Ebersole 1994). The mathematics required for dipole modeling have become sophisticated, and despite the theoretic difficulties it is now possible to map both interictal and ictal epileptic activity. Dipole analysis studies have shown different source patterns in mesial and lateral temporal lobe epilepsy (Boon *et al* 1996; Assaf and Ebersole 1997), suggesting that this technique may be used in the selection of patients for surgical treatment even though it is not yet clear how this would compare with other established noninvasive protocols.

PRACTICAL ASPECTS OF RECORDING INTERICTAL AND ICTAL PHENOMENA

This section reviews the ways that epileptic activity can be recorded from the patients. The standard procedure is a short EEG recording lasting less than 1 hour, which detects interictal epileptic discharges in about 30% of patients with partial epilepsy (Doppelbauer *et al* 1993); the detection rate is increased to about 80% if the seizures are frequent and if repeated recordings are made (Doppelbauer *et al* 1993). Other methods to enhance the sensitivity of detection of epileptic discharges using additional electrodes are also discussed. One of the most significant advances in clinical EEG is the ability to perform long-term recordings in order to observe ictal phenomena. These techniques are described in the last part of this section.

STANDARD EEG RECORDING APPARATUS

To be able to record the electrical activity generated by a charge moving within the brain, a circuit has to be established from the head via electrodes and cables to the recording machine amplifiers and back again. The patient–electrode interface is a vulnerable point at which the circuit may break down, and it is therefore important to establish good electrical contact at this site. Local abrasion of the skin helps remove oils and dead skin which, containing few electrolytes, would impede the flow of electrical charge. The interface between scalp tissue and the metal electrode is made with an electrolyte solution or jelly, preferably containing the anion of the metal in the electrode. This malleable interface allows movement at the same time as maximizing contact for low-resistance recording. A paste has the advantage of keeping the electrode in place for a short period, although for long-term recordings it is necessary to attach the electrode with collodion glue and squirt jelly underneath at regular intervals. The electrode and solute interface should preferably allow charge to flow equally in both directions. However, most electrodes are 'polarizable' to some extent, having a preferential charge flow in one direction that causes a build-up of charged ions at the metal–solute junction. This can impair current flow, especially at low frequencies. Consequently, the electrodes themselves have an influence on the recorded cerebral activity because of their low-frequency filtering characteristics. Most electrodes in use for EEG recording do not attenuate activity at frequencies between 0.5 and 70 Hz, and the high-input impedancies of modern amplifiers reduce the current flowing through the circuit and further limit the risk of electrode polarization. However, problems may arise if electrodes of different materials are used in the same circuit: the different junctional potentials produce varying biases and variable low-frequency filtering effects. Thus, a spike and slow wave complex appears differently when recorded with stainless steel or silver chloride electrodes because the former attenuates low frequencies to a greater extent.

Use of the 10–20 international system of electrode placements is now almost universal because it allows standardized positioning of electrodes relative to underlying cerebral structures irrespective of head size or shape (Homan *et al* 1987). Thus, the Fp electrodes cover the frontal lobe poles, F3,z,4 the frontal convexities, F7,8 the temporal poles, T3,4,5,6 the lateral temporal lobes, and P3,z,4, O1,2 the parietal and occipital lobes. Additional electrodes can be added to the system, either at halfway intervals or at a lower level, to increase the specificity of recordings. Electrodes set in a rubber cap are much less satisfactory because recording positions cannot be controlled.

Recording machines should have at least 16 channels to record sufficient EEG data from both hemispheres for accurate topographic assessment and for simultaneous recording of biological variables such as ECG, respiration, and eye movements, which may be necessary for the identification of artifacts. The availability and falling cost of high-performance microcomputers has made digital EEG possible. These systems have the great advantage of being able to reformat montages during playback so that a single potential can be inspected in bipolar or referential form. This is particularly useful in recordings with a low incidence of abnormality. Other advantages over paper recordings are the reduced storage requirements and the higher resolution of screen displays without the loss of detail incurred by the mechanical effects of pen movements. Digital data can be transmitted over long distances without loss of signal quality. Finally, digital data can be easily subjected to quantitative analysis. For these reasons, digital electronic EEG recorders are rapidly replacing mechanical machines.

Recording strategies

A standard EEG recording performed in a quiet environment should allow assessment of the background cerebral EEG activity in awake and drowsy states, and possibly in sleep. It is customary to also perform the activating procedures of hyperventilation and intermittent photic stimulation. Incorporation of all these procedures results in a standard recording of 30–60 min duration. Longer recordings are required when the aim is to obtain a sample from sleep or when special electrodes are being used. Anticonvulsant medication has little influence on the prevalence of interictal epileptic abnormalities and should not be withdrawn for standard recordings.

Activating procedures

The standard procedures of hyperventilation and intermittent photic stimulation are most useful for eliminating patients with primary generalized epilepsy. Widespread paroxysms of 3-Hz spike and slow wave complexes are activated in this condition. It should be remembered that paroxysms of epileptic discharges in the resting recording may be asymmetric in primary generalized epilepsy (Aliberti *et al* 1994; Lancman *et al* 1994; Lombroso 1997), sometimes leading to difficulty of interpretation. Occasionally a focal slow wave abnormality related to a structural brain lesion in patients with partial epilepsy appears during hyperventilation. Generalized paroxysms of spike and slow wave activity provoked by intermittent photic stimulation are very rare in partial epilepsy, but may be seen in some occipital epilepsies.

It is well recognized that epileptic EEG abnormalities may be seen only in sleep. This is particularly true in non-REM sleep of patients with temporal lobe epilepsy. Controversy has surrounded the relative merits of sleep deprivation, natural sleep, and drug induction of sleep, and there are advocates of all these methods of obtaining the EEG during this state. Despite the long debate, it is generally agreed that there are no particular advantages of any method. If possible the deeper stages of sleep including REM sleep should be obtained. This is because spikes occur more often in slow-wave sleep (stages 3 and 4) and a spike focus in REM sleep is more likely to be lateralized to the side of ictal onset (Sammaritano *et al* 1991). However, spikes are of higher amplitude in early sleep and there is a greater likelihood of an increased spike distribution in slow-wave sleep (Frost *et al* 1991; Sammaritano *et al* 1991).

Drug activation

Barbiturate drugs have been used to activate interictal epileptiform activity for over 40 years. Published data confirm that the activated focus correlates with the abnormal temporal lobe determined by other means (Hufnagel *et al* 1992). In our method, recordings are made in an operating theater. Methohexital is infused at a rate of 10 mg min^{-1} until a light level of surgical anesthesia is reached. This increases the rate of interictal epileptiform activity in the majority of patients with presumed temporal lobe complex partial seizures, and it is unusual for no spikes to be recorded. As with other investigators (see below), we have found that activation of a spike focus with maximum negativity at the sphenoidal electrodes and lateralization >90% correlates well with other investigations that indicate an ipsilateral disorder of hippocampal function and with a good outcome from surgical resection. As with other state-dependent epileptiform discharges, the distribution of spiking tends to be regional rather than focal at one electrode. We have observed some patients with a drug-activated focus at midtemporal rather than anterior temporal electrodes who, following further investigation, subsequently had a good outcome after hippocampal excision; however, multifocal spiking outside the temporal lobe, as with spontaneous epileptiform activity, indicates disease beyond the hippocampus. It has been suggested that oral barbiturates induce more epileptiform activity than when given intravenously, although in this study the drug was delivered as a single bolus rather than a slow infusion (Jennum *et al* 1993). The short-acting hypnotic etomidate, which is chemically unrelated to the barbiturates, also enhances interictal epileptiform activity (Gancher *et al* 1984).

Nasopharyngeal and sphenoidal electrodes

A concern about extracranial EEG recording is that discharges arising from the basal brain structures, rather than the cerebral convexity, may not be recorded from the standard 10–20 electrode positions. This has prompted the use of additional special electrodes that can be placed more closely adjacent to the base of the brain. The nasopharyngeal electrode consists of a conducting wire embedded in plastic with an uninsulated 25-mm diameter ball at the end for recording. It is inserted via the nostril and is pushed backwards and outwards so that the ball lies near the skull base in the region of the middle cranial fossa. Discomfort from the electrode and the insertion technique, the frequent development of artifact, and the fact that it is no more sensitive than appropriately placed anterior temporal scalp electrodes have limited the popularity of the nasopharyngeal electrode (Sperling and Engel 1985).

The sphenoidal electrode consists of multistranded braided silver or stainless steel wire insulated, except at the tip, with Teflon. It is inserted percutaneously via the mandibular notch to lie below the middle cranial fossa in the region of the foramen ovale. During insertion, discomfort can be reduced by applying a topical anesthetic cream to the preauricular area under an occlusive dressing (Bazil and Walczak 1996). It is probably best to avoid injected local anesthetic as this can cause a transient facial palsy (Iriarte *et al* 1996). The electrode is introduced by threading it through a 22-gauge, 4-cm spinal needle with a Luer connector and the bare tip is bent over the point. The needle is inserted under the zygoma at a point 2.5 cm anterior to the tragus on a line leading to the bottom of the nose. The mandibular notch is enlarged by having the patient's mouth slightly open and the needle is inserted up to the lock aiming towards the outer canthus of the opposite eye, i.e. in an upward and forward direction. The needle is then rotated and withdrawn, leaving the wire in place. It is secured with tape for subsequent recording and at the end of the session is removed simply by pulling it out. Bleeding at the point of insertion is stopped by local pressure and a hematoma is unusual. Lacrimation or a deep pain felt in the upper teeth settles quickly and infection at the site of entry is a rare complication. Occasionally a piece of the wire may break off, but this can be left in place without problem.

Controversy has surrounded the need for sphenoidal electrodes in extracranial EEG evaluation of partial epilepsy. Studies comparing the sphenoidal electrode with scalp electrodes showed it to be superior to both ear and nasopharyngeal electrodes in the detection of interictal discharges

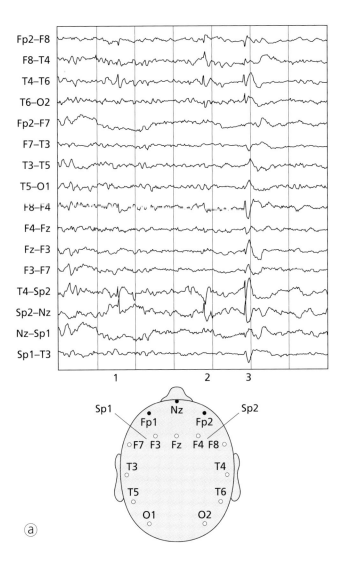

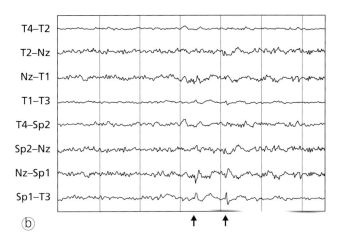

Fig. 27.5 Interictal epileptic discharges recorded from patients with mesial temporal lobe epilepsy using sphenoidal and scalp surface electrodes. (a) The majority of discharges have the distribution shown in (1) and (2), maximal at the sphenoidal and anterior temporal–inferior frontal electrodes, although there may be a second independent lateral temporal focus; (3) recorded from the same patient. (b) Some sharp-wave discharges can be identified at the left sphenoidal electrode (arrows) that would escape detection at scalp electrodes, including at extra positions (here T_1 and T_2).

(Sperling *et al* 1986) (Fig. 27.5). However, the sensitivity of detection can be improved by the use of additional scalp electrodes in the anterior temporal region (T1,2) or below the zygoma (Homan *et al* 1988; Binnie *et al* 1989; Goodin *et al* 1990), and most investigators agree that for routine EEG in the diagnosis of partial epilepsy the sphenoidal electrode gives little added value over scalp electrodes in these positions. When patients are being investigated for surgical treatment, the sphenoidal electrode is more usually included in the extracranial evaluation. This is because discharges with negativity maximal at the sphenoidal electrode have been shown by intracranial recordings to arise predominantly from the mesiobasal temporal neocortex, a pattern characteristic of MTLE associated with hippocampal disease (Morris *et al* 1989; Marks *et al* 1992). Similarly, for ictal recordings, some authors describe increased accuracy of prediction of the epileptogenic zone using strict criteria and sphenoidal electrodes (Risinger *et al* 1989; Ives *et al* 1996), although others assert that the anterior cheek

surface electrodes provide equivalent information about the side and site of rhythmic EEG activity at seizure onset (Krauss *et al* 1992).

The increased sensitivity of sphenoidal over scalp electrodes in the detection of interictal epileptiform discharges is partly technical. If bipolar montages are used, the consequent wide spacing of electrodes enhances the potential gradient and increases the amplitude of discharges recorded at the sphenoidal electrode. However, even if average reference montages are used the spikes recorded at the sphenoidal electrode have a greater negativity than at the scalp in the majority of patients with suspected MTLE (Binnie *et al* 1989). The implication is that the sphenoidal electrode preferentially records discharges arising in the mesiobasal temporal lobe structures. Recordings using multiple-contact sphenoidal electrodes showed the interictal potentials to be maximal at the most medial recording site (Binnie *et al* 1989), and to record with maximum sensitivity it may be necessary to position the sphenoidal electrode as close as possible to the foramen ovale (Kanner *et al* 1995). In most cases, however, the exact position of the electrode tip appears to be unimportant as no significant changes in recording can be observed when the tip drifts laterally over time (Wilkus and Thompson 1985). For this reason insertion under fluoroscopic guidance or subsequent X-rays to check the electrode position are not necessary. Furthermore, only inferior-vertical dipoles with positivity in the hippocampus and negativity at the basal temporal structures appear at the sphenoidal electrode (Marks *et al* 1992), implying that the orientation of the spike generator is as important as the position of the recording electrode for spike detection.

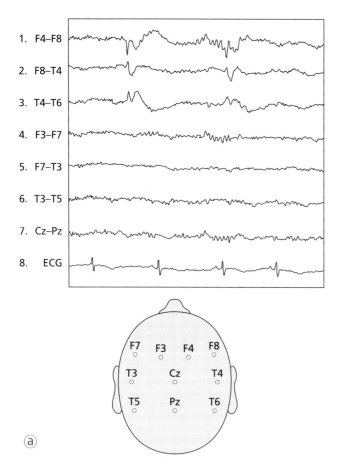

(a)

ICTAL RECORDINGS

The apparatus for long-term EEG monitoring aimed at recording ictal events falls into two main categories, ambulatory cassette and video-telemetry systems, both of which are now readily available commercially. Technical standards for recording have been set (Engel *et al* 1993).

Ambulatory cassette

In this system, slow recording speeds are used to enable 24 hours of EEG data to be captured on a standard audio cassette. The data are then analyzed at fast replay speeds. Early recorders were limited to three or four EEG channels but modern systems employ 8 or 16 channels, each with a solid-state preamplifier inside the cassette recorder or attached to the patient's head. One channel is usually devoted to ECG recording and an additional channel is used for a time signal or for marking events.

Montage design is an important consideration for ambulatory cassette EEG recording because of the limited number of channels and the need to detect electrical abnormalities visually at high replay speeds. Computer-assisted replay can make the review process easier (Morris *et al* 1994). For routine work, the best design is a frontotemporal bipolar montage with channels on the same side of the head viewed together, which allows over 85% of interictal activity to be captured (Leroy and Ebersole 1983). Recordings over 10–24 hours detect interictal activity in 85% of patients, even with a very limited number of recording channels (Bridgers and Ebersole 1985; Tuunainen *et al* 1990). Examples of interictal and ictal

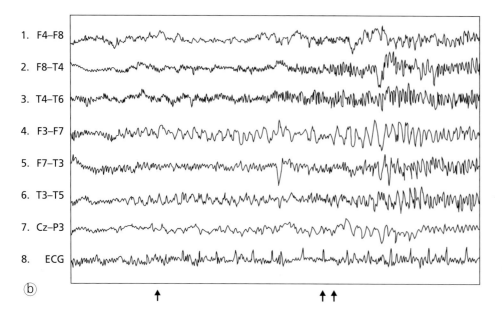

(b)

Fig. 27.6 Recordings made by ambulatory cassette. (a) Interictal spike and slow wave discharge in the right anterior temporal–inferior frontal region. (b) Ictal recording from a different patient with mesial temporal lobe epilepsy. The first change is left-sided frontotemporal theta activity at 4–5 Hz (single arrow) that increases in amplitude and later appears bilaterally (double arrow).

epileptic activity from patients with temporal lobe epilepsy are shown in Fig. 27.6. Ambulatory cassette recording is also used to record subclinical events and seizures in particular settings, such as the classroom or at work. Quantifying seizures for anticonvulsant drug trials is another application.

The main disadvantage of cassette EEG recording is the lack of clinical and EEG correlation. Extracranial EEG artifacts can be extremely difficult to identify when the patient's movements are unknown, especially if a limited number of recording channels is used. Rhythmic artifact can appear very much like seizure activity, leading to the possible misdiagnosis of nonepileptic seizures. Attempts are being made to overcome this problem by linking a portable videocamera film of the patient with the cassette apparatus.

Video-EEG telemetry

The disadvantage of ambulatory cassette EEG recording is the main advantage of video-EEG telemetry: it allows very close clinical and EEG correlation of events at the expense of placing patients in a confined unnatural environment. The system consists of a closed-circuit television that is usually recorded on to standard videotape. A camera able to record at low light levels is essential for nighttime recordings, when 37% of frontal and 26% of temporal lobe seizures occur (Bazil and Walczak 1997). EEG may be obtained from up to 128 channels, allowing a variety of standard and additional 10–20 electrode positions to be selected. For long-term recording, the electrodes are attached with collodion glue and the leads fitted to a preamplifier box carried by the patient. The amplified EEG signal is then multiplexed into short segments from each channel, which can then be transmitted by cable (or, less satisfactorily, by radio) to the main recording system. The signal is decoded and reformatted so that it can be displayed on a monitor. The EEG data are recorded on to the sound channels of the videotape or electronically on computer disk for long-term storage. Additional computer software generates a time signal that allows exact synchronization of EEG and video data in real time. The standard set-up should include an audio channel and a second monitor at the nurses' station for patient observation. Special effects can be used to enhance this basic set-up, including splitting the screen to incorporate wide-angle and close-up views and a tracking device to allow the camera to follow the patient around the recording room. Two-way audio communication permits an observer to assess whether the patient is able to speak or understand during an attack and is especially useful if a warning system is used to alert observers that an attack is occurring (Qu and Gotman 1995).

In the analysis of partial seizures, recordings over a long period are often needed before a sufficient sample of the patient's seizures can be obtained. Although it is theoretically possible to continue recording over several weeks, discomfort from the electrodes and confinement to one area usually tax the patient's cooperation after more than 7 days. Monitoring for this length of time generates a huge amount of video and EEG data. As it is not feasible to review all this manually, another vital component of the system is a means of detecting and recording events as it is well recognized that patients or their observers fail to register about one-fifth of seizures (Pauri et al 1992; Salinsky 1997). A computer-based system that continuously examines the EEG for changes in rhythmic activity markedly increases the number of seizure detections (Gotman 1982). The sensitivity of these seizure-detection algorithms may be improved by artificial neural networks, which 'learn' about the nature of ictal rhythms or biologic artifacts in an individual patient (Gabor and Seyal 1992; Qu and Gotman 1993; Gabor et al 1996; Webber et al 1996). A similar computer-based EEG sampling system may be used to detect interictal spikes and a number of algorithms for this purpose have been tested and validated (Gotman et al 1979; Hostetler et al 1992). These programs should have appropriate sensitivity so that real spikes are infrequently missed, while detection of artifact or extracranial discharges is kept to a minimum. The sensitivity can be improved if allowance is made for the state of the patient, e.g. vertex sharp waves are not falsely detected as spikes when the subject is asleep (Gotman and Wang 1991, 1992). The continuous computer review consequently reduces the EEG data considerably and the technician's role is to reject false spike or seizure detections rather than having to go through the laborious process of visually assessing all the original recording (Spatt et al 1997).

The two main uses of video-EEG telemetry in partial epilepsy are the classification of clinical events, with the aim of determining the site of origin of habitual seizures, and the selection of candidates for surgical treatment. Accurate clinical observation and close EEG correlation help improve seizure semeiology (Morrell et al 1991; Saygi et al 1994; Theodore et al 1994; Gil-Nagel and Risinger 1997), but perhaps are most useful in defining non-epileptic seizures (Meierkord et al 1991; Ozkara and Dreifuss 1993; Thacker et al 1993; DeToledo and Ramsay 1996; Henry and Drury 1997). An example of the way video-EEG telemetry has improved diagnosis is nocturnal paroxysmal movement disorders. When initially described, these were thought to represent a form of dystonia (Lugaresi et al 1986) but further video-EEG telemetry studies indicated that the short-duration attacks are more likely to be frontal lobe partial seizures (Tinuper *et al* 1990; Meierkord *et al* 1992; Sforza *et al* 1993).

In presurgical evaluation, review of the videotape helps classify the seizures clinically; however, the main information to be derived from the EEG is whether the changes at ictal onset are entirely unilateral, mostly unilateral, or bilateral, and if unilateral whether they are consistent with a mesial temporal or neocortical epilepsy. The aim of this evaluation is to help predict the outcome from surgery. Many centers advocate video recording of all patients for this purpose before surgery, although, as discussed below, some features of the history and the results of other investigations may give similar or better prognostic information. We thus confine the test to patients whose seizure history is ill defined or apparently at variance with the suspected anatomic location. If all seizures appear to originate unilaterally, the chances of eradicating the seizures should be good. If more than 90% start unilaterally, a worthwhile improvement could be achieved. If less than 90% of attacks are unilateral, the expectation would be that an unacceptable number of seizures would remain after surgery, giving a poor outcome, although outcome in this group can be good if patients are carefully selected on the basis of magnetic resonance imaging (MRI) and intracarotid amobarbital testing (Sirven *et al* 1997a).

An important consideration is how many seizures to record in order to provide this prognostic information with certainty. One solution is to use binomial statistical theory (Bland 1995). This assumes that the probability of a seizure starting in either hemisphere is the same, and thus the chances of ipsilateral seizure onset appearing sequentially can be calculated. Five attacks in a row with the same side of onset would be expected with a probability of $< 0.05\%$. However, if some seizures are contralateral, the sample size required to give the same level of probability, i.e. that 90% or more of attacks start on the same side, increases to 17–20. Retrospective studies have shown that it takes 2.9–3.7 days to capture one seizure, 4.5–5.5 days to capture three and 6.1–7.6 days to record five (Todorov *et al* 1994) but up to 12 days to be sure of obtaining a sample of five attacks in all patients. The binomial theory therefore becomes impracticable if the first five seizures are not unilateral. An alternative approach to decide the number of seizures to record is to use Bayes' theorem, which states that the predictive value of a positive test result depends on the probability of a given outcome before the test (prior probability). For ictal monitoring of patients with MTLE, retrospective studies have shown bilateral seizure onsets in 14–23% of patients (So *et al* 1989a; Hirsch *et al* 1991a). Using this ~80% prior probability, it can be calculated that five seizures arising from the same side are required to give a 95% probability that this is the side of ictal onset in at least 90% of attacks (Blum 1994). Unilateral interictal spiking increases the prior probability of concordant seizure onset and, if present, the number of attacks that have to be recorded falls to four. These calculations have been validated with patient data. The same has not been done for other features which would increase the prior probability that $> 90\%$ of seizures start from one side. However, a history of a childhood complicated convulsion, ipsilateral hippocampal atrophy on MRI, a concordant neuropsychologic deficit, and appropriate abnormality of positron emission tomography (PET) would all influence the prior probability of unilateral ictal onset. When the prior probability reaches a high level, the recording of EEG ictal onset becomes of limited value because the probability after the test is unaffected whatever the result.

Neither of these two approaches takes into consideration extracranial ictal recordings which do not have lateralizing features. It may be impossible to determine the side of onset because of artifact or because ictal changes are generalized, as is the case in up to 25% of temporal lobe and 50% of extratemporal seizures (Walczak *et al* 1992). If the first recorded seizure is uninformative, it is likely that further attacks will also be nonlocalizing (Sum and Morrell 1995). It is also important to decide how to deal with seizures that occur within a short time of each other, as these may be clustered to the same side of onset (Haut *et al* 1997). Nevertheless, these theoretical approaches have allowed a consensus to develop: to decide if seizures are sufficiently unilateral to allow surgical treatment, video-EEG telemetry should capture five of the patient's habitual seizures (Haut *et al* 1997; Sirven *et al* 1997b).

Because inpatient video-EEG telemetry is an expensive procedure and often a limited resource, most centers attempt to capture the required sample of habitual seizures in the shortest possible time. This often requires a reduction in anticonvulsant medication, especially for patients with medial temporal lobe seizures due to hippocampal atrophy (Swick *et al* 1996). As seizures occur more frequently when serum anticonvulsant levels are low (So and Gotman 1990), drug reduction may need to be started before the scheduled monitoring period. A number of studies have shown that drug reduction in patients with small ictal onset zones does not affect the electrographic pattern at the start of attacks or induce new seizure types, although secondary generalized convulsions become more frequent (Marciani *et al* 1985; So and Gotman 1990; Marks *et al* 1991). Studies that have suggested 'false' localization of ictal onset after drug reduction contain patients with either structural cerebral disease, in whom it is known that the ictal onset may appear at a distance from the lesion (Engel and Crandall 1983; Sammaritano *et al* 1987), or multifocal ictal onsets or rapid propagation from a single focus (Spencer *et al* 1981; Binnie *et al* 1994). Patients with these characteristics usually fare badly from surgical treatment, and the further information obtained from anticonvulsant withdrawal, indicating widespread cerebral hyperexcitability, is therefore useful before advocating surgery rather than a 'negative' finding. A final word of caution about anticonvulsant withdrawal in order to record seizures: the risk of sudden death due to epilepsy is increased, although the extent of the risk is unknown at present.

EXTRACRANIAL EEG ABNORMALITIES IN TEMPORAL LOBE EPILEPSY

Earlier descriptions of the use, sensitivity, and significance of the EEG in partial epilepsy suffered from the inclusion of patients with unspecified or unknown epileptogenic pathology, or because the site of the epileptogenic lesion had not been verified by the eradication of seizures following its surgical resection. Although the majority of patients in these earlier reports had seizures related to atrophy or sclerosis of the hippocampus, as this is the most common epileptogenic pathology treated surgically, it was not until the general acceptance of MTLE syndrome with its characteristic clinical, radiologic, and neuropsychologic features that the EEG features of temporal lobe epilepsy became fully defined. Retrospective studies of defined patient populations with a good outcome from resection of pathologically proven hippocampal sclerosis have been used to describe the EEG changes in MTLE and these may be used in the prospective selection of patients for surgery. It is clear that patients with neocortical temporal lobe epilepsy have a different outcome from surgical treatment than those with MTLE and require a different presurgical evaluation, often including expensive ictal recordings using intracranial electrodes. The extracranial EEG features indicating neocortical rather than mesial temporal lobe epilepsy are therefore important considerations when selecting patients for surgery. This section describes the extracranial features of MTLE, shows how they may be used in presurgical evaluation, and concludes with differences between the findings in MTLE and neocortical temporal lobe epilepsy.

INTERICTAL FINDINGS IN MTLE

It is accepted that MTLE is a disease continuum, ranging from purely unilateral seizures to both sides being equally affected. Similarly, the extracranial EEG findings range from being highly lateralized to being bilaterally symmetric. Patients with unilateral seizures and concordant, lateralized EEG changes may expect a good outcome from surgical treatment without the need for EEG recording with intracranial electrodes. The simplest EEG investigation is the standard recording to observe the distribution and nature of interictal epileptiform abnormalities. This may be modified by the use of closely spaced scalp electrodes, the addition of sphenoidal or nasopharyngeal electrodes, or by recording in different states of arousal including during drug activation.

Interictal epileptiform activity in MTLE usually takes the form of spike or sharp wave discharges, often with an accompanying slow wave, showing maximum negativity at the sphenoidal or anterior temporal (F7,8) electrodes (Engel *et al* 1975; Williamson *et al* 1993; Ebner and Hoppe 1995; Gambardella *et al* 1995a). Some patients may have a second focus with maximal negativity at the mid or posterior temporal electrodes (T3,4, T5,6), but the major focus should be anteriorly (Kanner *et al* 1993). Spiking beyond this distribution is a marker of less good surgical outcome (Barry *et al* 1992), probably because it indicates widespread cortical hyperexcitability (Engel *et al* 1975). Examples of interictal discharges recorded from patients with MTLE are shown in Fig. 27.5.

Focal delta activity in the temporal regions is also commonly seen in patients with medial temporal atrophy (Panet-Raymond and Gotman 1990; Gambardella *et al* 1995b); some authors consider this activity, when paroxysmal, to have the same localizing significance as epileptic spikes (Gambardella *et al* 1995b; Cascino *et al* 1996). Although temporal intermittent delta activity can occur in isolation, it is usual for focal spike discharges to appear at the same site during the recording (Normand *et al* 1995). Barbiturate-induced fast activity has been reported to be reduced in about one-third of patients with hippocampal atrophy (Engel *et al* 1975), although this finding is less often used in localization than the distribution of paroxysmal activity.

Interictal epileptiform activity may be present bilaterally; even in patients with proven unilateral hippocampal atrophy bilateral spikes can be expected in about 30–50% of patients (Hirsch *et al* 1991a; Williamson *et al* 1993; Gambardella *et al* 1995a). In one series this was not significantly different from patients with bilateral hippocampal disease (Gambardella *et al* 1995a). When bilateral spikes occur in unilateral hippocampal atrophy the contralateral activity should be at, and not beyond, the homologous anterior temporal or sphenoidal electrodes (Engel *et al* 1975; Ebner and Hoppe 1995). Unilateral interictal spikes correlate well with ipsilateral hippocampal seizure onset and a good outcome from surgical excision on that side (Hirsch *et al* 1991a; Blume *et al* 1993; Kanner *et al* 1993; Cascino *et al* 1996; Holmes *et al* 1996a,b). However, the definition of unilateral varies among authors. Earlier studies suggested that a ratio of 5:1 of spike discharges indicated lateralization (Engel *et al* 1975), while others require more than 80% (Spencer *et al* 1982) or 90% (Kanner *et al* 1993) of spikes or paroxysmal discharges to be on one side. In one study the best surgical outcome was observed when the interictal spikes showed >90% predominance in the ipsilateral temporal lobe (Chung *et al* 1991); this degree of lateralization would appear to be the most useful for practical purposes. The number of spikes that have to be counted to give a statistically significant 90% lateralization can be estimated from the binomial distribution. As with estimating the number of seizures, it is assumed that spikes are equally likely to occur in each hemisphere. This may not be true and spiking may have a left-sided dominance (Dean *et al* 1997). To obtain a lateralization of >90% of interictal discharges with a probability of >0.95 requires a sample of about 20 spikes. A sample of at least 20 interictal spikes may be easily obtained in patients with vigorous spike activity, although some patients have very low rates of paroxysmal discharges and may show little epileptiform activity even after four standard recordings (Salinsky *et al* 1987) or prolonged telemetric recording. In about 5% of patients spontaneously occurring interictal epileptiform discharges cannot be recorded (Williamson *et al* 1993; Cascino *et al* 1996). In these patients drug activation may be valuable. Some reports have suggested that even >90% predominance of unilateral temporal spikes may not be universally associated with a good outcome from ipsilateral temporal lobe surgery (Spencer *et al* 1982; Hirsch *et al* 1991a). The patients in these series generally did not have the benefit of MRI or functional imaging to help identify the epileptogenic pathology; additionally, some of the poor results from surgery may have been due to pathology other than hippocampal sclerosis. The reasons why some patients with unilateral hippocampal atrophy have a poor surgical outcome are unresolved (Kilpatrick *et al* 1997). Our own data from patients with histologically proven hippocampal sclerosis show that the best outcome is achieved if there is a history of complicated early childhood convulsion. If this is not present, the outlook is less good whether or not the interictal spikes are lateralized. Finally, it is recognized that up to 10% of patients with hippocampal atrophy show bilaterally synchronous interictal spike and slow wave complexes (Sadler and Blume 1989). This phenomenon may be more common in patients with a high frequency of generalized convulsion, although it does not appear to affect the outcome of surgical resection assuming there is a dominant anterior temporal spike focus.

ICTAL FINDINGS IN MTLE

Intracranial recordings of seizure onset using depth electrodes implanted in the mesial temporal lobe structures have identified a number of characteristic features in MTLE. The most commonly observed pattern is for background activity to be suddenly replaced by rhythmic discharges faster than 13 Hz (Spencer *et al* 1992a). This may be preceded by periodic low-frequency spikes, particularly when hippocampal cell loss is pronounced (Spencer *et al* 1992b; Park *et al* 1996). There is usually no electrodecremental change at seizure onset in the hippocampus (King and Spencer 1995). To be of good localizing significance, the rhythmic activity should be simultaneous with the clinical onset or precede it (Gotman *et al* 1995). High-frequency activity appears to correlate with small epileptogenic zones, as seen in MTLE, rather than the wider zones typical of neocortical epilepsy; maximum frequency may not be reached until about 10 s after the ictal onset (Gotman *et al* 1995). Ictal activity usually propagates first to the ipsilateral temporal neocortical structures (Gotman 1987; Lieb *et al* 1987; Spencer *et al* 1987, 1990; Luders *et al* 1989; Weinand *et al* 1992). About 25% of seizures remain confined to the ipsilateral temporal lobe (Adam *et al* 1994), with the remainder propagating usually to the ipsilateral frontal lobe. Propagation to the other hemisphere occurs in about 25–30% of patients (Spencer *et al* 1987, 1992c), usually to the opposite hippocampus before the contralateral temporal or frontal neocortex (Spencer *et al* 1987; Lieb *et al* 1991). Propagation to the contralateral hippocampus is slower if the cell density in the CA4 layer is reduced on the side of seizure onset (Spencer *et al* 1992c) and these patients have a better outcome from surgical treatment than those whose seizures propagate rapidly from the ipsilateral temporal lobe to the frontal or contralateral temporal lobes (Lieb *et al* 1986; Adam *et al* 1994; Cascino *et al* 1995).

Subdural recordings from the temporal and frontal neocortex have shown that the initial fast rhythms in the hippocampus may be associated with a desynchronized, low-amplitude pattern at mesiobasal cortical electrodes (Weinand *et al* 1992). Simple partial seizures can be confined to the hippocampus, with limited spread of rhythmic activity to the adjacent neocortex (Sperling and O'Connor 1989, 1990; Spencer *et al* 1990).

These intracranial observations help explain the ictal patterns seen with scalp and sphenoidal electrodes. Because extracranial electrodes only detect activity in the neocortex and not within brain substance (Cooper *et al* 1965), it is not surprising that the first scalp EEG changes occur after clinical onset in 80–95% of patients (Delgado-Escueta and Walsh 1985; Williamson *et al* 1993). Early studies on unspecified or a variety of different types of epilepsy showed that partial seizures are associated with an initial localized reduction in amplitude (an electrodecremental response) in 11% of patients and with a mixture of sinusoidal or repetitive epileptiform potentials in 86% of patients (Blume *et al* 1984). Because these were undoubtedly lateralized in only about 50% of patients and localized to one lobe in only 40%, it was concluded that scalp ictal onsets were of poor localizing value (Spencer *et al* 1985). This prompted attempts to define more clearly the extracranial ictal patterns in definite MTLE. Retrospective studies of patients with this condition showed the extracranial change to consist of rhythmic delta, theta, or alpha activity lateralized or localized with maximal amplitude at sphenoidal, anterior temporal, or midtemporal electrodes (Delgado-Escueta and Walsh 1985; Ebner and Hoppe 1995; Sirven *et al* 1997b). The rhythmical activity may fluctuate in amplitude and frequency as the seizure progresses (Atalla *et al* 1996). Attenuation or repetitive spiking are seen at ictal onset in <10% of seizures (Steinhoff *et al* 1995). The most detailed description of the early extracranial EEG patterns during temporal lobe partial seizures defined seven groups (Ebersole and Pacia 1996). The patterns typical of MTLE were an initial 5–9 Hz inferotemporal rhythm and, less commonly, a vertex/parasagittal positive rhythm, or a combination of the two (Pacia and Ebersole 1997). Intracranial recordings showed the former pattern to be associated with recruitment of inferolateral temporal neocortex and the latter with discharges confined to the mesiobasal temporal neocortex. Discharges confined to the hippocampus produced no scalp rhythms and this no doubt explains why extracranial ictal changes cannot be detected in over 60% of patients with simple partial temporal lobe seizures (Bare *et al* 1994; Sirven *et al* 1996). When extracranial EEG changes occur in simple partial temporal lobe seizures they have the same localizing significance as complex partial seizures; both are more highly predictive of an ipsilateral hippocampal ictal onset zone if the interictal epileptiform activity is lateralized to the same side (Sperling and O'Connor 1990; Sirven *et al* 1996). Examples of different ictal recording patterns in patients with MTLE are shown in Figs 27.6–27.8.

The strict criterion of the presence of 5-Hz fast rhythmic activity maximal at one sphenoidal or temporal location at some stage during the seizure was found to predict an ipsilateral temporal depth onset correctly in 82% of patients (Risinger *et al* 1989). This pattern was found in about 52% of consecutive patients with complex partial seizures of

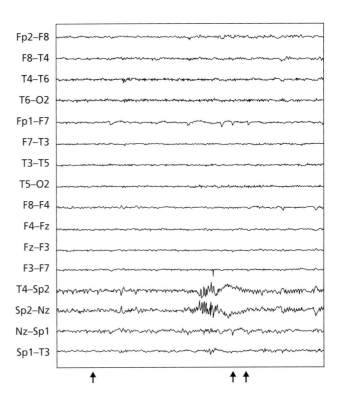

Fig. 27.7 Recording of a simple partial seizure in a patient with mesial temporal lobe epilepsy. There is rhythmic spiking at the right sphenoidal electrode (single arrow), followed by 7-Hz theta activity that can also be seen at temporal scalp electrodes (double arrow).

unknown pathologic basis, although in patients with proven hippocampal sclerosis a lateralized pattern of rhythmic activity at 5–10 Hz has been reported in 50–80% of patients (Kuzniecky *et al* 1991; Williamson *et al* 1993).

Postictal abnormalities are seen in about 70% of patients and consist of localized delta activity, attenuation of background rhythms, or activation of focal spiking (Kaibara and Blume 1988). When these changes occur they are always maximal on the side of seizure origin (Williamson *et al* 1993).

Significantly more scalp recordings lateralize to one side if the interictal spikes are strongly ipsilateral; in this circumstance over 90% of ictal onsets have been reported to be lateralized to one side, with virtually 100% predictive value of a good surgical outcome from an operation on the concordant side (Steinhoff *et al* 1995). Bilateral interictal epileptiform activity is a marker of more diffuse cortical excitability and, when present, ictal onsets are less likely to be localized or predictive of the side of surgery (Steinhoff *et al* 1995; Sirven *et al* 1997b). In a retrospective study of proven hippocampal sclerosis, only 3% of lateralized scalp ictal onsets were contralateral to the pathologic side (Ebner and Hoppe 1995).

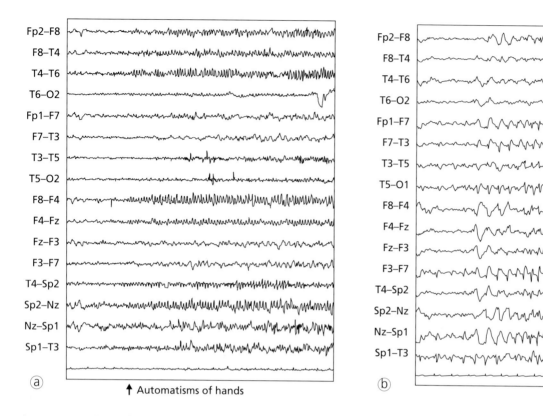

Fig. 27.8 Recordings of complex partial seizures in mesial temporal lobe epilepsy. (a) The most commonly seen pattern of sharply contoured theta activity appears at the right frontotemporal and sphenoidal electrodes simultaneously with automatisms of the hands. (b) A less common pattern of synchronized 2-Hz spike and slow wave complexes; here, maximal at the left midtemporal scalp electrodes. Intracranial recordings confirmed a mesial temporal ictal onset in this patient.

SURGICAL EVALUATION OF MTLE

Retrospective studies have shown that the convergence of unilateral interictal and ictal scalp EEG patterns, MRI, PET, and neuropsychologic deficit (including intracarotid amobarbital testing) indicating a localized abnormality in one temporal lobe results in a favorable outcome from surgery (Engel *et al* 1990; Jack *et al* 1992; Thadani *et al* 1995; Kilpatrick *et al* 1997). These criteria can be used prospectively to select patients for surgery without the need for intracranial ictal EEG recordings in 50–90% of patients in different centers with different patient population characteristics (Sperling *et al* 1992; Murro *et al* 1993; Cendes *et al* 1997). Use of strict criteria to define unilateral interictal temporal spikes and scalp ictal EEG onset result in a good outcome from surgical treatment (Blume *et al* 1993). Patients with bitemporal interictal activity and nonlocalizing scalp ictal onsets may have a unilateral ictal onset discovered by intracranial recordings and become surgical candidates (So *et al* 1989a,b). Good outcomes can be achieved if all intracranially recorded ictal onsets are unilateral (Holmes *et al* 1997), although generally the outcome of surgical treatment is less good than in the patients who could be selected without the need for invasive recordings

(Spencer *et al* 1982; Chung *et al* 1991; Hirsch *et al* 1991b; Cascino *et al* 1995; Holmes *et al* 1996a; Gilliam *et al* 1995). Patients who continue to have seizures after surgery usually show interictal epileptiform activity on standard EEG recordings, whereas this activity usually disappears from patients who are seizure-free (Tuunainen *et al* 1994; Patrick *et al* 1995).

EEG PATTERNS IN LATERAL TEMPORAL LOBE EPILEPSY

It is recognized that temporal tumors are associated with bilateral interictal spikes in 30–70% of patients. This is not related to the duration of epilepsy, the number of seizures, or the outcome from surgical treatment (Lieb *et al* 1981a,b; Lim *et al* 1991; Morris *et al* 1993; Gilmore *et al* 1994). The characteristics of interictal spikes in patients with temporal tumors are not significantly different from those seen in patients with hippocampal atrophy (O'Brien *et al* 1996).

The scalp-recorded ictal onsets in patients with temporal lobe tumors may contain faster frequencies than those seen in patients with hippocampal atrophy (Lieb *et al* 1981b).

The ictal onsets are more often bilateral and bilateral changes develop more frequently during progression of the seizure. Bilateral propagation is also more rapid in patients with temporal lobe tumors (O'Brien *et al* 1996).

Electrographic differences between hippocampal and neocortical temporal lobe epilepsy mainly relate to ictal findings. No significant differences can be detected in the scalp state-dependent spikes, frequency of spiking, distribution or lateralization of spikes or slow waves (Burgerman *et al* 1995). Intracranial recordings of neocortical seizures have shown low-frequency periodic spikes and rhythms faster than 13 Hz at ictal onset to be associated with normal histologic appearances (Spencer *et al* 1992a). Lower frequency activity is associated with pathologic abnormalities of the neocortex and is also a marker of a large epileptic zone (Gotman *et al* 1995). Extracranial recordings may show an electrodecremental change at seizure origin if the epileptogenic zone is large (Arroyo *et al* 1994). Rhythmic activity in temporal neocortical seizures most often consists of polymorphic 2–5 Hz lateralized discharges or periodic sharp waves, which may be followed by faster inferotemporal or parasagittal rhythms (Ebersole and Pacia 1996). These changes also appear bilaterally more often in seizures of neocortical origin, sometimes because of rapid propagation from one temporal lobe to the other (Pacia and Ebersole 1997).

EXTRACRANIAL EEG ABNORMALITIES IN EXTRATEMPORAL EPILEPSY

Although it has been reported that the site of scalp-recorded interictal spikes correlates well with the origin of seizures (Holmes *et al* 1996a), most observers consider that extracranial interictal and ictal EEG has poor localizing value in neocortical epilepsies outside the temporal lobe. This section examines the extracranial EEG findings in neocortical epilepsy arising in the frontal, parietal, and occipital lobes.

FRONTAL LOBE EPILEPSY

The interictal EEG in patients with frontal lobe epilepsy may fail to show specific epileptiform activity in 20–40% of patients (Salanova *et al* 1993; Laskowitz *et al* 1995). When present, the spikes are restricted to the abnormal lobe in only about 25% of patients, and generalized spike–wave paroxysms and bilateral frontal, temporal, or multilobar spikes commonly occur (Laskowitz *et al* 1995). However, the principal spike focus, when present, usually localizes the epileptogenic zone (Salanova *et al* 1993; Manford *et al* 1996), slightly more often for complex partial seizures than

for focal motor or supplementary motor seizures (Salanova *et al* 1995).

In keeping with other neocortical epilepsies, intracranial recordings often show the epileptogenic zone to be wide (Salanova *et al* 1994). Although focal ictal patterns may be recorded near lesions the onset is often regional (Williamson and Spencer 1986; Sutherling *et al* 1990), propagating rapidly or associated with widespread very high-frequency low-amplitude activity (Allen *et al* 1992). On the scalp this latter pattern produces a reduction in amplitude that may be bilateral, despite lateralized clinical manifestations (Arroyo *et al* 1994). About one-third of frontal lobe seizures either show no extracranial EEG change or are obscured by artifact; in another third the ictal rhythms are bilateral or widespread at onset (Laskowitz *et al* 1995). A localized frontal onset may be seen in the remaining third but this is often contralateral to the ictal onset zone determined by other means. Scalp ictal recordings in focal motor seizures are usually of greater localizing value than in supplementary motor or complex partial seizures (Salanova *et al* 1995). When ictal onsets are localized on scalp recordings there is a poor correlation with the extent of the epileptogenic zone recorded intracranially (Salanova *et al* 1993). An example of interictal and ictal recordings in a patient with frontal lobe epilepsy is shown in Fig. 27.9.

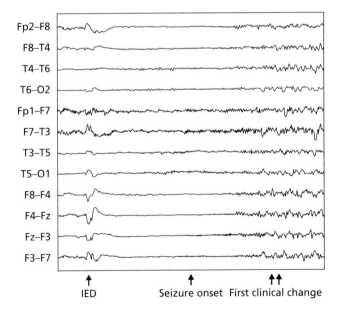

Fig. 27.9 Recordings from a patient with frontal lobe epilepsy. The interictal epileptic discharges (IED) consist of left frontal spike and slow wave complexes. The electrographic seizure onset consists of 40-Hz fast activity at the F3 and F7 electrodes that increases in amplitude and decreases in frequency. The first clinical change is head and eye deviation to the left, with clonic movements of the right side of the face.

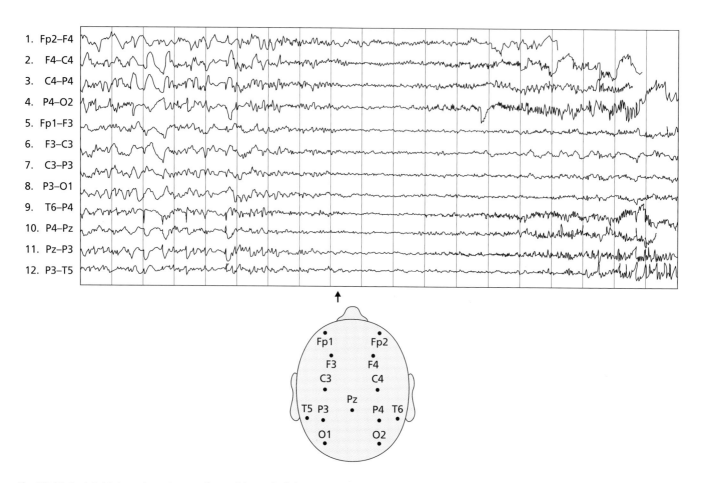

Fig. 27.10 Parietal lobe seizure in a patient with cortical dysgenesis. Profuse interictal spike discharges occur in the right parietal region, leading to a seizure with initial suppression of ongoing activity (arrow) followed by fast rhythms of increasing amplitude and decreasing frequency, maximal in the region of the P4 electrode.

PARIETAL LOBE EPILEPSY

No interictal activity can be detected in about one-fifth of patients with parietal epilepsies and, when seen, the spikes are rarely confined to the parietal lobe (Williamson *et al* 1992a). Bifrontal, frontotemporal, temporal, and contralateral parietal and temporal independent spike activity is often encountered (Williamson *et al* 1992a; Cascino *et al* 1993a). Scalp-recorded ictal changes are absent in 10% and are poorly localizing in the remainder. The usual ictal pattern is a bilateral abnormality with or without attenuation; a lateralized rhythmic build-up is seen in less than one-third of patients that is rarely confined to the parietal lobe (Williamson *et al* 1992a; Cascino *et al* 1993a). Scalp ictal recordings from a patient with parietal lobe seizures are shown in Fig. 27.10.

OCCIPITAL LOBE EPILEPSY

The presence of longitudinal white matter tracts from the occipital lobes (Williamson and Spencer 1986) probably explains why epileptiform activity in occipital seizures is often widespread. Bilaterally synchronous frontal, temporal, or diffuse paroxysms are seen interictally in about one-third of patients (Williamson *et al* 1992b); anterior, mid, or posterior temporal foci are particularly common, being found in 40–60% (Salanova *et al* 1992; Williamson *et al* 1992b; Palmini *et al* 1993). The spike focus is confined to the occipital lobe in less than 10% of patients. A midline Oz electrode may be essential for the detection of the occipital focus (Guerrini *et al* 1995). However, a retrospective study of patients with a good outcome following posterior corticectomy showed that the principal focus correlated well with the epileptogenic lobe in this selected group (Blume *et al* 1991). Similarly, scalp-recorded seizures identified the abnormal occipital lobe in 63% of this series. Other reports of patients not treated surgically have stressed the multilobar, temporal, hemispheric, or generalized change at ictal onset, with no seizures starting solely at the occipital electrodes (Palmini *et al* 1993). Examples of interictal recordings from a patient with

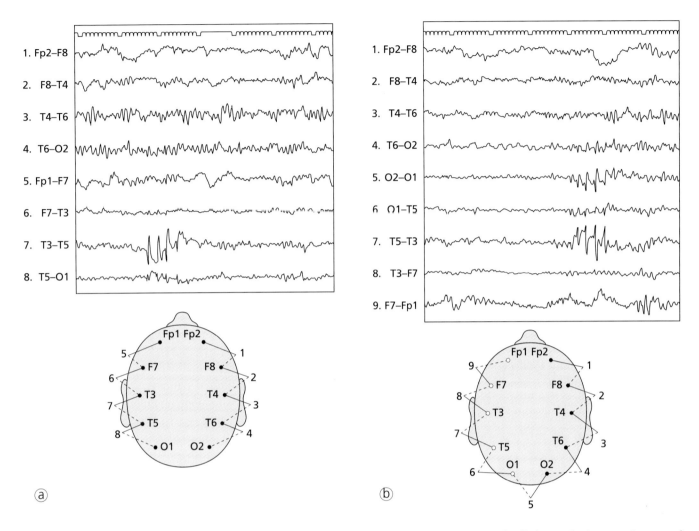

Fig. 27.11 Interictal discharges in a patient with occipital cortical dysgenesis. (a) Runs of occipital spike discharges in the posterior part of the left hemisphere recorded on a longitudinal montage. Note the reduction in the alpha rhythm on the affected side. (b) Use of a bipolar montage linking the O1 and O2 electrodes helps confirm the occipital location.

occipital epilepsy secondary to cortical dysplasia are shown in Fig. 27.11.

EEG FINDINGS IN NEOCORTICAL EPILEPSY WITH DEFINED PATHOLOGY

Some studies have indicated a high incidence of a second pathology in patients with intractable epilepsy shown to have hippocampal atrophy on MRI (Raymond *et al* 1994a; Cendes *et al* 1995). The surgical outcome in these patients is often poor unless both pathologic lesions are treated (Li *et al* 1997). Teams performing preoperative evaluation for temporal lobe surgery should be aware of the possibility of dual pathology, especially when the interictal epileptiform activity is widespread, beyond the anterior temporal electrodes, or when scalp ictal onsets are not localized or are extratemporal (Hirabayashi *et al* 1993; Li *et al* 1997).

Tumors

Differences between tumoral and nonlesional temporal lobe epilepsy have already been described. About one-third of patients with chronic low-grade tumors show polymorphic delta slow wave activity. This is usually localized to the affected lobe but may extend to the adjacent lobe or become generalized (Britton *et al* 1994). Interictal epileptiform activity is localized to the lobe of the tumor or adjacent lobe in 60–75% of patients, whereas this activity is generalized or independent over the contralateral hemisphere in up to 15% of patients (Boon *et al* 1991; Britton *et al* 1994). Scalp-recorded ictal onsets localize to the affected lobe in 60–90% of patients (Boon *et al* 1991; Britton *et al* 1994), although false lateralization of ictal onset may occur with gross cerebral lesion developing in early life (Sammaritano *et al* 1987). As with other causes of neocortical epilepsy, the extent of the distribution of interictal epileptiform activity does not correlate with the outcome from surgical lesionectomy (Cascino *et al* 1992), although interictal activity disappears in those who are seizure-free postoperatively (Patrick *et al* 1995). Intracranial EEG recording has confirmed that twice as many patients have an epileptogenic zone that extends beyond the tumor or is remote from it as patients having an epileptogenic zone confined to the lesion. None the less surgical outcome only correlates with the completeness of the resection of the pathology (Awad *et al* 1991).

A study of patients with dysembryoplastic neuroepithelial tumors confirmed that these show a high incidence of slow-wave activity localized over the lesion, with focal spikes that are often more extensive and distant from the lesion (Raymond *et al* 1994b). Epilepsy secondary to neurocystercosis is usually associated with generalized EEG abnormalities, with focal changes being present only in patients with a single cyst (Del Brutto *et al* 1992). Hypothalamic hamartomas are associated with the syndrome of gelastic epilepsy, which often shows a poor response to surgery even when the ictal recordings are apparently localized to one temporal lobe, probably because the tumors have intrinsic epileptogenicity (Kuzniecky *et al* 1997). Because of the midline site of the lesion, interictal epileptiform changes are often bihemispheric (Cascino *et al* 1993b).

Neuronal migration disorders

Improvements in imaging have increasingly shown that neuronal migration disorders are an important cause of intractable partial epilepsy. In the heterotopias, especially if subependymal, the interictal activity is usually widespread and may take the form of generalized 3-Hz spike and slow wave complexes, wrongly suggesting primary generalized epilepsy (Raymond *et al* 1994c). Many patients show unilateral or bitemporal spikes, although interictal epileptiform activity is multilobar in one-third (Dubeau *et al* 1995). Periventricular nodular heterotopia may be bilateral or unilateral when focal interictal abnormalities correlate with the site of pathology (Battaglia *et al* 1997). Neuronal migration disorders have epileptogenic areas extending beyond the lesion identified by MRI in more than 70% of patients, explaining the widespread nature of interictal epileptiform activity (Palmini *et al* 1991b). Focal rhythmic epileptiform discharges may localize the epileptogenic area more accurately than isolated spikes in these patients with focal cortical dysplasia (Gambardella *et al* 1996) (see Fig. 27.11). Diffuse scalp EEG abnormalities do not necessarily indicate a poor outcome from surgical treatment (Palmini *et al* 1991a). The same is true for tuberous sclerosis and forme frustes of it, where despite multifocal interictal epileptiform activity the scalp-recorded ictal onset is usually localized to a prominent imaging abnormality that may be resected, with favorable outcome (Bebin *et al* 1993).

Cerebrovascular accidents

Hospital-based studies of patients with epilepsy after cerebrovascular accidents (strokes) usually demonstrate a high incidence of focal slow-wave abnormalities with persistent focal changes in three-fifths of patients and paroxysmal discharges in half. Generalized abnormalities are also common and normal EEGs are seen in less than 5% of patients (Ryglewicz *et al* 1990). However, community-based studies show the EEG to be abnormal much less often and to have poor localizing value, probably because the partial seizures and strokes in these patients are less severe (Manford *et al* 1992).

Hydrocephalus

In hydrocephalus abnormal EEGs may be expected in about 50% of nonshunted patients, with focal paroxysmal discharges in about 10% (Graebner and Celesia 1973). The rate of abnormality increases to 85–95% of patients who have ventricular shunts inserted, with focal paroxysmal discharges frequently occurring in the region of the shunt (Graebner and Celesia 1973; Ines and Markland 1977).

Head injury

After severe head injury focal slow-wave abnormalities correlate with neurologic deficits and an anterior temporal or central spike focus is closely related with the presence of posttraumatic epileptic seizures (Jabbari *et al* 1986). A more extensive presurgical evaluation showed mesial temporal ictal onsets in patients suffering head injuries before the age of 5, although when the injury was later in life the epileptogenic focus was likely to be neocortical and difficult to localize (Marks *et al* 1995).

Multiple sclerosis

Seizures in patients with multiple sclerosis are often associated with regional spike and slow wave activity, although diffuse slowing or bitemporal spike and slow waves may also be present (Thompson *et al* 1993).

Alcoholism

In chronic alcoholism, withdrawal seizures are usually generalized, even in patients with focal EEG abnormalities.

When focal changes occur they correlate with head injuries or structural brain lesions. The majority of patients with alcohol-withdrawal seizures have have normal or low-amplitude EEG recordings (Krauss and Niedermeyer 1991).

Dementia

There has been little recent interest in the EEG associations in patients with dementia and epilepsy. It is recognized that multifocal epileptiform discharges may be seen in the EEG recordings of patients with Alzheimer's disease, although this does not correlate well with the presence of epilepsy.

CONCLUSIONS

The extracranial EEG has a well-established and continuing role in the accurate diagnosis and classification of epilepsy.

This requires correct identification and localization of epileptic discharges and an understanding of the pathophysiology of the cellular generators of these electrical potentials: these have been the main themes of this chapter. For patients who are not candidates for surgical treatment the standard EEG remains one of the mainstays of investigation, although ictal recordings are likely to be used more as the technology becomes widely available. For surgical candidates, standard EEG recordings are inexpensive in comparison with functional imaging and without the risks associated with intracranial evaluations. For these reasons attention is being increasingly directed to the ways that a good outcome can be achieved using extracranial EEG in conjunction with other investigations. Advanced computer-based EEG analysis, including dipole modeling and coregistration of EEG and imaging, is likely to contribute to this process in the future.

KEY POINTS

1. Pathophysiologic changes in partial epilepsy lead to specific electrical abnormalities, i.e. interictal epileptic discharges and ictal rhythms, that can be recorded by the scalp EEG.
2. Brief standard EEG recordings have a low sensitivity but high specificity and are most useful when interictal epileptic discharges are present.
3. Interictal epileptic discharges and ictal rhythms must be differentiated from biologic and technical artifacts and from innocent normal variations.

4. In surgical candidates, interictal epileptic discharges can be further defined by using nonstandard electrodes and pharmacologic activation to increase their occurrence.
5. Technical advances in ambulatory cassette recorders and cable telemetry linked to videos have made prolonged EEGs to capture seizures possible.
6. The localization of interictal epileptic discharges and ictal rhythms helps delineate partial epilepsy syndromes.

7. In MTLE, the syndrome can be defined by combining extracranial interictal and ictal EEG abnormalities with clinical and imaging findings, and a good surgical outcome achieved without the need for intracranial recording.
8. Extracranial EEG recordings are less successful in defining epileptogenic zones in patients with neocortical epilepsy.
9. Methods for automated, computerized analysis of the EEG are becoming available but are of unproven clinical benefit.

REFERENCES

Adam C, Saint-Hilaire J-M, Richer F (1994) Temporal and spatial characteristics of intracerebral seizure propagation: predictive value in surgery for temporal lobe epilepsy. *Epilepsia* **35**:1065–1072.

Alarcon G, Guy CN, Binnie CD, Walker SR, Elwes RDC, Polkey CE (1994) Intracerebral propagation of interictal activity in partial epilepsy: implications for source localisation. *Journal of Neurology, Neurosurgery and Psychiatry* **57**:435–449.

Alarcon G, Binnie CD, Elwes RDC, Polkey CE (1995) Power spectrum and intracranial EEG patterns at seizure onset in partial epilepsy. *Electroencephalography and Clinical Neurophysiology* **94**:326–337.

Alarcon G, Garcia Seoane JJ, Binnie CD *et al* (1997) Origin and propagation of interictal discharges in the acute electrocorticogram: implications for pathophysiology and surgical treatment of temporal lobe epilepsy. *Brain* **120**:2259–2282.

Aliberti V, Grunewald RA, Panayiotopoulos CP, Chroni E (1994) Focal electroencephalographic abnormalities in juvenile myoclonic epilepsy. *Epilepsia* **35**:297–301.

Allen PJ, Fish DR, Smith SJM (1992) Very high-frequency rhythmic activity during SEEG suppression in frontal lobe epilepsy. *Electroencephalography and Clinical Neurophysiology* **82**:155–159.

Arroyo S, Lesser RP, Fisher RS *et al* (1994) Clinical and electroencephalographic evidence for sites of origin of seizures with diffuse electrodecremental pattern. *Epilepsia* **35**:974–987.

Assaf BA, Ebersole JS (1997) Continuous source imaging of scalp ictal rhythms in temporal lobe epilepsy. *Epilepsia* **38**:1114–1123.

Atalla N, Abou-Khalil B, Fakhoury T (1996) The stop-start phenomenon in scalp–sphenoidal ictal recordings. *Electroencephalography and Clinical Neurophysiology* **98**:9–13.

Awad IA, Rosenfeld J, Ahl J, Hahn JF, Luders H (1991) Intractable epilepsy and structural lesions of the brain: mapping, resection strategies, and seizure outcome. *Epilepsia* **32**:179–186.

Bare MA, Burnstine TH, Fisher RS, Lesser RP (1994) Electroencephalographic changes during simple partial seizures. *Epilepsia* **35**:715–720.

Barry E, Sussman NM, O'Connor MJ, Harner RN (1992) Presurgical electroencephalographic patterns and outcome from anterior temporal lobectomy. *Archives of Neurology* **49**:21–27.

Battaglia G, Granata T, Farina L, D'Incerti L, Franceschetti S, Avanzini G (1997) Periventricular nodular heterotopia: epileptogenic findings. *Epilepsia* **38**:1173–1182.

Baumgartner C, Lindinger G, Ebner A *et al* (1995) Propagation of interictal epileptic activity in temporal lobe epilepsy. *Neurology* **45**:118–122.

Bazil CW, Walczak TS (1996) Sphenoidal electrode insertion using topical anesthesia. *Epilepsia* **37**:102–103.

Bazil CW, Walczak TS (1997) Effects of sleep and sleep stage on epileptic and nonepileptic seizures. *Epilepsia* **38**:56–62.

Bebin EM, Kelly PJ, Gomez MR (1993) Surgical treatment for epilepsy in cerebral tuberous sclerosis. *Epilepsia* **34**:651–657.

Binnie CD, Marston D, Polkey CE, Amin D (1989) Distribution of temporal spikes in relation to the sphenoidal electrode. *Electroencephalography and Clinical Neurophysiology* **73**:403–409.

Binnie CD, Elwes RDC, Polkey CE, Volans A (1994) Utility of stereoelectroencephalography in preoperative assessment of temporal lobe epilepsy *Journal of Neurology, Neurosurgery and Psychiatry* **57**:58–65.

Bland M (1995) *An Introduction to Medical Statistics*, 2nd edn. Oxford: Oxford University Press.

Blum D (1994) Prevalence of bilateral partial seizure foci and implications for electroencephalographic telemetry monitoring and epilepsy surgery. *Electroencephalography and Clinical Neurophysiology* **91**:329–336.

Blume WT, Young GB, Lemieux JF (1984) EEG morphology of partial epileptic seizures. *Electroencephalography and Clinical Neurophysiology* **57**:295–302.

Blume WT, Whiting SE, Girvin JP (1991) Epilepsy surgery in the posterior cortex. *Annals of Neurology* **29**:638–645.

Blume WT, Borghesi JL, Lemieux JF (1993) Interictal indices of temporal lobe seizure origin. *Annals of Neurology* **34**:703–709.

Boon P, Have MD, Adam C *et al* (1996) Dipole modeling in epilepsy surgery candidates. *Epilepsia* **38**:208–218.

Boon PA, Williamson PD, Fried I *et al* (1991) Intracranial, intraaxial, space-occupying lesions in patients with intractable partial seizures: anatomicoclinical, neuropsychological, and surgical correlation. *Epilepsia* **32**:467–476.

Bridgers SL, Ebersole JS (1985) The clinical utility of ambulatory cassette EEG. *Neurology* **35**:166–173.

Britton JW, Cascino GD, Sharbrough FW, Kelly PJ (1994) Low-grade glial neoplasms and intractable partial epilepsy: efficacy of surgical treatment. *Epilepsia* **35**:1130–1135.

Burgerman RS, Sperling MR, French JA, Saykin AJ, O'Connor MJ (1995) Comparison of mesial versus neocortical onset temporal lobe seizures: neurodiagnostic findings and surgical outcome. *Epilepsia* **36**:662–670.

Cascino GD, Kelly PJ, Sharbrough FW, Hulihan JF, Hirschorn KA, Trenerry MR (1992) Long-term follow-up of stereotactic lesionectomy in partial epilepsy: predictive factors and electroencephalographic results. *Epilepsia* **33**:639–644.

Cascino GD, Hulihan JF, Sharbrough FW, Kelly PJ (1993a) Parietal lobe lesional epilepsy: electroclinical correlation and operative outcome. *Epilepsia* **34**:522–527.

Cascino GD, Andermann F, Berkovic SF *et al* (1993b) Gelastic seizures and hypothalamic hamartomas: evaluation of patients undergoing chronic intracranial EEG monitoring and outcome of surgical treatment. *Neurology* **43**:747–750.

Cascino GD, Trenerry MR, Sharbrough FW, So EL, Marsh WR, Strelow DC (1995) Depth electrode studies in temporal lobe epilepsy: relation to quantitative magnetic resonance imaging and operative outcome. *Epilepsia* **36**:230–235.

Cascino GD, Trenerry MR, So EL *et al* (1996) Routine EEG and temporal lobe epilepsy: relation to long-term EEG monitoring, quantitative MRI, and operative outcome. *Epilepsia* **37**:651–656.

Cendes F, Cook MJ, Watson C *et al* (1995) Frequency and characteristics of dual pathology in patients with lesional epilepsy. *Neurology* **45**:2058–2064.

Cendes F, Caramanos Z, Andermann F, Dubeau F, Arnold DL (1997) Proton magnetic resonance spectroscopic imaging and magnetic resonance imaging volumetry in the lateralization of temporal lobe epilepsy: a series of 100 patients. *Annals of Neurology* **42**:737–746.

Chung MY, Walczak TS, Lewis DV, Dawson DV, Radtke R (1991) Temporal lobectomy and independent bitemporal interictal activity: what degree of lateralization is sufficient? *Epilepsia* **32**:195–201.

Cooper R, Winter AL, Walter WG (1965) Comparison of subcortical, cortical and scalp activity using chronically indwelling electrodes in man. *Electroencephalography and Clinical Neurophysiology* **18**:217–228.

Dean AC, Solomon G, Harden C, Papakostas G, Labar DR (1997) Left hemisphere dominance of epileptiform discharges. *Epilepsia* **38**:503–505.

Del Brutto OH, Santibanez R, Noboa CA, Aguirre R, Diaz E, Alarcon TA (1992) Epilepsy due to neurocysticercosis: analysis of 203 patients. *Neurology* **42**:389–392.

Delgado-Escueta AV, Walsh GO (1985) Type 1 complex partial seizures of hippocampal origin: excellent results of anterior temporal lobectomy. *Neurology* **35**:143–154.

DeToledo JC, Ramsay RE (1996) Patterns of involvement of facial muscles during epileptic and nonepileptic events: review of 654 events. *Neurology* **47**:621–625.

Dichter MA (1989) Cellular mechanisms of epilepsy and potential new treatment strategies. *Epilepsia* **30**:S3–S12.

Dichter MA (1993) The premise, the promise, and the problems with basic research in epilepsy. *Epilepsia* **34**:791–799.

Doppelbauer A, Zeithofer J, Zifko U, Baumgartner C, Mayr N, Deecke L (1993) Occurrence of epileptiform activity in the routine EEG of epileptic patients. *Acta Neurologica Scandinavica* **87**:345–352.

Dubeau F, Tampieri D, Lee N *et al* (1995) Periventricular and subcortical nodular heterotopia: a study of 33 patients. *Brain* **118**:1273–1287.

Ebersole JS (1994) Non-invasive localization of the epileptogenic focus by EEG dipole modeling. *Acta Neurologica Scandinavica* Suppl **152**:20–28.

Ebersole JS, Pacia SV (1996) Localization of temporal lobe foci by ictal EEG patterns. *Epilepsia* **37**:386–399.

Ebersole JS, Wade PB (1991) Spike voltage topography identifies two types of frontotemporal epileptic foci. *Neurology* **41**:1425–1433.

Ebner A, Hoppe M (1995) Noninvasive electroencephalography and mesial temporal sclerosis. *Journal of Clinical Neurophysiology* **12**:23–31.

Engel J, Crandall PH (1983) Falsely localizing ictal onsets with depth EEG telemetry during anticonvulsant withdrawal. *Epilepsia* **24**:344–355.

Engel J, Driver MV, Falconer MA (1975) Electrophysiological correlates of pathology and surgical results in temporal lobe epilepsy. *Brain* **98**:129–156.

Engel J, Henry TR, Risinger MW *et al* (1990) Presurgical evaluation for partial epilepsy: relative contributions of chronic depth-electrode recordings versus FDG-PET and scalp–sphenoidal ictal EEG. *Neurology* **40**:1670–1677.

Engel J, Burchfiel J, Ebersole J *et al* (1993) Long-term monitoring for epilepsy. Report of an IFCN committee. *Electroencephalography and Clinical Neurophysiology* **87**:437–458.

Fiol ME, Gates JR, Torres F, Maxwell RE (1991) The prognostic value of residual spikes in the postexcision electrocorticogram after temporal lobectomy. *Neurology* **41**:512–516.

Franck JE, Pokorny J, Kunkel DD, Schwartzkroin PA (1995) Physiologic and morphologic characteristics of granule cell circuitry in human epileptic hippocampus. *Epilepsia* **36**.543–558.

Frost JD, Hrachovy RA, Glaze DG, McCully MI (1991) Sleep modulation of interictal spike configuration in untreated children with partial seizures. *Epilepsia* **32**:341–346.

Gabor AJ, Seyal M (1992) Automated interictal EEG spike detection using artificial neural networks. *Electroencephalography and Clinical Neurophysiology* **83**:271–280.

Gabor AJ, Leach RR, Dowla FU (1996) Automated seizure detection using a self-organizing neural network. *Electroencephalography and Clinical Neurophysiology* **99**:257–266.

Gambardella A, Gotman J, Cendes F, Andermann F (1995a) The relation of spike foci and clinical seizure characteristics to different patterns of mesial temporal atrophy. *Archives of Neurology* **52**:287–293.

Gambardella A, Gotman J, Cendes F, Andermann F (1995b) Focal intermittent delta activity in patients with mesiotemporal atrophy: a reliable marker of the epileptogenic focus. *Epilepsia* **36**:122–129.

Gambardella A, Palmini A, Andermann F *et al* (1996) Usefulness of focal rhythmic discharges on scalp EEG of patients with focal cortical dysplasia and intractable epilepsy. *Electroencephalography and Clinical Neurophysiology* **98**:243–249.

Gancher S, Laxer KD, Krieger W (1984) Activation of epileptogenic activity by etomidate. *Anesthesiology* **61**:616–618.

Gilliam F, Bowling S, Bilir E *et al* (1995) Association of combined MFI, interictal EEG, and ictal EEG results with outcome and pathology after temporal lobectomy. *Epilepsia* **38**:1315–1320.

Gilmore R, Morris H, Van Ness PC, Gilmore-Pollak W, Estes M (1994) Mirror focus: function of seizure frequency and influence on outcome after surgery. *Epilepsia* **35**:258–263.

Gil-Nagel A, Risinger MW (1997) Ictal semiology in hippocampal versus extrahippocampal temporal lobe epilepsy. *Brain* **120**:183–192.

Godoy J, Luders H, Dinner DS, Morris HH, Wyllie E, Murphy D (1992) Significance of sharp waves in routine EEGs after epilepsy surgery. *Epilepsia* **33**:285–288.

Goodin DS, Aminoff MJ, Laxer KD (1990) Detection of epileptiform activity by different noninvasive EEG methods in complex partial epilepsy. *Annals of Neurology* **27**:330–334.

Gotman J (1982) Automatic recognition of epileptic seizures in the EEG. *Electroencephalography and Clinical Neurophysiology* **54**:530–540.

Gotman J (1985) Practical use of computer-assisted EEG interpretation in epilepsy. *Journal of Clinical Neurophysiology* **2**:251–265.

Gotman J (1987) Interhemispheric interactions in seizures of focal onset: data from human intracranial recordings. *Electroencephalography and Clinical Neurophysiology* **67**:120–133.

Gotman J, Wang LY (1991) State-dependent spike detection: concepts and preliminary results. *Electroencephalography and Clinical Neurophysiology* **79**:11–19.

Gotman J, Wang L-Y (1992) State-dependent spike detection: validation. *Electroencephalography and Clinical Neurophysiology* **83**:12–18.

Gotman J, Ives JR, Gloor P (1979) Automatic recognition of inter-ictal epileptic activity in prolonged EEG recordings. *Electroencephalography and Clinical Neurophysiology* **46**:510–520.

Gotman J, Levtova V, Olivier A (1995) Frequency of the electroencephalographic discharge in seizures of focal and widespread onset in intracerebral recordings. *Epilepsia* **36**:697–703.

Graebner RW, Celesia GG (1973) EEG findings in hydrocephalus and their relation to shunting procedures. *Electroencephalography and Clinical Neurophysiology* **35**:517–521.

Guerrini R, Dravet C, Genton P *et al* (1995) Idiopathic photosensitive occipital lobe epilepsy. *Epilepsia* **36**:883–891.

Haut SR, Legatt AD, O'Dell C, Moshe SL, Shinnar S (1997) Seizure lateralization during EEG monitoring in patients with bilateral foci: the cluster effect. *Epilepsia* **38**:937–940.

Henry TR, Drury I (1997) Non-epileptic seizures in temporal lobectomy candidates with medically refractory seizures. *Neurology* **48**:1374–1382.

Hirabayashi S, Binnie CD, Janota I, Polkey CE (1993) Surgical treatment of epilepsy due to cortical dysplasia: clinical and EEG findings. *Journal of Neurology, Neurosurgery and Psychiatry* **56**:765–770.

Hirsch LJ, Spencer SS, Williamson PD, Spencer DD, Mattson RH (1991a) Comparison of bitemporal and unitemporal epilepsy defined by depth electroencephalography. *Annals of Neurology* **30**:340–346.

Hirsch LJ, Spencer SS, Spencer DD, Williamson PD, Mattson RH (1991b) Temporal lobectomy in patients with bitemporal epilepsy defined by depth electroencephalography. *Annals of Neurology* **30**:347–356.

Holmes MD, Dodrill CB, Ojemann LM, Ojemann GA (1996a) Five-year outcome after epilepsy surgery in nonmonitored and monitored surgical candidates. *Epilepsia* **37**:748–752.

Holmes MD, Dodrill CB, Wilensky AJ, Ojemann LM, Ojemann GA (1996b) Unilateral focal preponderance of interictal epileptiform discharges as a predictor of seizure origin. *Archives of Neurology* **53**:228–232.

Holmes MD, Dodrill CB, Ojemann GA, Wilensky AJ, Ojemann LK (1997) Outcome following surgery in patients with bitemporal interictal epileptiform patterns. *Neurology* **48**:1037–1040.

Homan RW, Herman J, Purdy P (1987) Cerebral location of international 10–20 system electrode placement. *Electroencephalography and Clinical Neurophysiology* **66**:376–382.

Homan RW, Jones MC, Rawat S (1988) Anterior temporal electrodes in complex partial seizures. *Electroencephalography and Clinical Neurophysiology* **70**:105–109.

Hostetler WE, Doller HJ, Homan RW (1992) Assessment of a computer program to detect epileptiform spikes. *Electroencephalography and Clinical Neurophysiology* **83**:1–11.

Hufnagel A, Burr W, Elger CE, Nadstawek J, Hefner G (1992) Localization of the epileptic focus during methohexital-induced anesthesia. *Epilepsia* **33**:271–284.

Ines DF, Markland ON (1977) Epileptic seizures and abnormal electroencephalographic findings in hydrocephalus and their relation to the shunting procedures. *Electroencephalography and Clinical Neurophysiology* **42**:761–768.

Iriarte J, Parra J, Kanner AM (1996) Transient facial palsy in sphenoidal electrode placement. *Epilepsia* **37**:1239–1241.

Ives JR, Drislane FW, Schachter SC *et al* (1996) Comparison of coronal sphenoidal versus standard anteroposterior temporal montage in the EEG recording of temporal lobe seizures. *Electroencephalography and Clinical Neurophysiology* **98**:417–421.

Jabbari B, Vengrow MI, Salazar AM, Harper MG, Smutok MA, Amin D (1986) Clinical and radiological correlates of EEG in the late phase of head injury: a study of 515 Vietnam veterans. *Electroencephalography and Clinical Neurophysiology* **64**:285–293.

Jack CR, Sharbrough FW, Cascino GD, Hirschorn KA, O'Brien PC, Marsh ER (1992) Mangetic resonance image-based hippocampal volumetry: correlation with outcome after temporal lobectomy. *Annals of Neurology* **31**:138–146.

Jennum P, Dam M, Fuglsang-Frederiksen A (1993) Effect of barbiturate on epileptiform activity: comparison between intravenous and oral administration. *Acta Neurologica Scandinavica* **88**:284–288.

Kaibara M, Blume WT (1988) The postictal electroencephalogram. *Electroencephalography and Clinical Neurophysiology* **70**:99–104.

Kanner AM, Morris HH, Luders H, Dinner DS, Van Ness P, Wyllie E (1993) Usefulness of unilateral interictal sharp waves of temporal lobe origin in prolonged video-EEG monitoring studies. *Epilepsia* **34**:884–889.

Kanner AM, Ramirez L, Jones JC (1995) The utility of placing sphenoidal electrodes under the foramen ovale with fluoroscopic guidance. *Journal of Clinical Neurophysiology* **12**:72–81.

Kilpatrick C, Cook M, Kaye A, Murphy M, Matkovic Z (1997) Non-invasive investigations successfully select patients for temporal lobe surgery. *Journal of Neurology, Neurosurgery and Psychiatry* **63**:327–333.

King D, Spencer S (1995) Invasive electroencephalography in mesial temporal lobe epilepsy. *Journal of Clinical Neurophysiology* **12**:32–45.

Knowles WD, Awad IA, Nayel MH (1992) Differences of *in vitro* electrophysiology of hippocampal neurons from epileptic patients with mesiotemporal sclerosis versus structural lesions. *Epilepsia* **33**:601–609.

Koszer S, Moshe SL, Legatt AD, Shinnar S, Goldensohn ES (1996) Surface mapping of spike potential fields: experienced EEGers vs. computerized analysis. *Electroencephalography and Clinical Neurophysiology* **98**:199–205.

Krauss GL, Niedermeyer E (1991) Electroencephalogram and seizures in chronic alcoholism. *Electroencephalography and Clinical Neurophysiology* **78**:97–104.

Krauss GL, Lesser RP, Fisher RS, Arroyo S (1992) Anterior 'cheek' electrodes are comparable to sphenoidal electrodes for the identification of ictal activity. *Electroencephalography and Clinical Neurophysiology* **83**:333–338.

Kuzniecky R, Faught E, Morawetz R (1991) Electroencephalographic correlations of extracranial and epidural electrodes in temporal lobe epilepsy. *Epilepsia* **32**:335–340.

Kuzniecky R, Guthrie B, Mountz J *et al* (1997) Intrinsic epileptogenesis of hypothalamic hamartomas in gelastic epilepsy. *Annals of Neurology* **42**:60–67.

Lancman ME, Asconape JJ, Penry JK (1994) Clinical and EEG asymmetries in juvenile myoclonic epilepsy. *Epilepsia* **35**:302–306.

Lantz G, Holub M, Ryding E, Rosen I (1996) Simultaneous intracranial and extracranial recording of interictal epileptiform activity in patients with drug resistant partial epilepsy: patterns of conduction and results from dipole reconstructions. *Electroencephalography and Clinical Neurophysiology* **99**:69–78.

Laskowitz DT, Sperling MR, French JA, O'Connor MJ (1995) The syndrome of frontal lobe epilepsy: characteristics and surgical management. *Neurology* **45**:780–787.

Leroy RF, Ebersole JS (1983) An evaluation of ambulatory, cassette EEG monitoring. 1. Montage design. *Neurology* **33**:1–7.

Li LM, Cendes F, Watson C *et al* (1997) Surgical treatment of patients with single and dual pathology. *Neurology* **48**:437–444.

Lieb JP, Engel J, Gevins A, Crandall PH (1981a) Surface and deep EEG correlates of surgical outcome in temporal lobe epilepsy. *Epilepsia* **22**:515–538.

Lieb JP, Engel J, Brown WJ, Gevins AS, Crandall PH (1981b) Neuropathological findings following temporal lobectomy related to surface and deep EEG patterns. *Epilepsia* **22**:539–549.

Lieb JP, Engel J, Babb TL (1986) Interhemispheric propagation time of hippocampal seizures. 1. Relationship to surgical outcome. *Epilepsia* **27**:286–293.

Lieb JP, Hoque K, Skomer CE, Song X-W (1987) Inter-hemispheric propagation of human mesial temporal lobe seizures: a coherence/phase analysis. *Electroencephalography and Clinical Neurophysiology* **67**:101–119.

Lieb JP, Dasheiff RM, Engel J (1991) Role of the frontal lobe in the propagation of mesial temporal lobe seizures. *Epilepsia* **32**:822–837.

Lim SH, So NK, Luders H, Morris HH, Turnbull J (1991) Etiologic factors for unitemporal vs bitemporal epileptiform discharges. *Archives of Neurology* **48**:1225–1228.

Lombroso CT (1997) Consistent EEG focalities detected in subjects with primary generalized epilepsies monitored for two decades. *Epilepsia* **38**:797–812.

Luders H, Hahn J, Lesser RP *et al* (1989) Basal temporal subdural electrodes in the evaluation of patients with intractable epilepsy. *Epilepsia* **30**:131–142.

Lugaresi E, Cirignotta F, Montagna P (1986) Nocturnal paroxysmal dystonia. *Journal of Neurology, Neurosurgery and Psychiatry* **49**:375–380.

McBride MC, Binnie CD, Janota I, Polkey CE (1991) Predictive value of intraoperative electrocorticograms in resective epilepsy surgery. *Annals of Neurology* **30**:526–532.

Manford M, Hart YM, Sander JWAS, Shorvon SD (1992) National General Practice Study of Epilepsy (NGPSE): partial seizure patterns in a general population. *Neurology* **42**:1911–1917.

Manford M, Fish DR, Shorvon SD (1996) An analysis of clinical seizure patterns and their localizing value in frontal and temporal lobe epilepsies. *Brain* **119**:17–40.

Marciani MG, Gotman J, Andermann F, Olivier A (1985) Patterns of seizure activation after withdrawal of antiepileptic medication. *Neurology* **35**:1537–1543.

Marco P, Sola RG, Pulido P *et al* (1996) Inhibitory neurons in the human epileptogenic temporal neocortex: an immunocytochemical study. *Brain* **119**:1327–1347.

Marks DA, Katz A, Scheyer R, Spencer SS (1991) Clinical and electrographic effects of acute anticonvulsant withdrawal in epileptic patients. *Neurology* **41**:508–512.

Marks DA, Katz A, Booke J, Spencer DD, Spencer SS (1992) Comparisons and correlation of surface and sphenoidal electrodes with simultaneous intracranial recording: an interictal study. *Electroencephalography and Clinical Neurophysiology* **82**:23–29.

Marks DA, Kim J, Spencer DS, Spencer SS (1995) Seizure localization and pathology following head injury in patients with uncontrolled epilepsy. *Neurology* **45**:2051–2057.

Meierkord H, Will B, Fish D, Shorvon S (1991) The clinical features and prognosis of pseudoseizures diagnosed using video-EEG telemetry. *Neurology* **41**:1643–1646.

Meierkord H, Fish DR, Smith SJM, Scott CA, Shorvon SD, Marsden CD (1992) Is noctural paroxysmal dystonia a form of frontal lobe epilepsy? *Movement Disorders* **7**:38–42.

Merlet I, Garcia-Larrea L, Gregoire MC, Lavenne F, Mauguiere F (1996) Source propagation of interictal spikes in temporal lobe epilepsy: correlations between spike dipole modelling and [^{18}F]fluorodeoxyglucose PET data. *Brain* **119**:377–392.

Molaie M, Santana HB, Otero C, Cavanaugh WA (1991) Effect of epilepsy and sleep deprivation on the rate of benign epileptiform transients of sleep. *Epilepsia* **32**:44–50.

Morrell MJ, Phillips CA, O'Connor MJ, Sperling MR (1991) Speech during partial seizures: intracranial EEG correlates. *Epilepsia* **32**:886–889.

Morris GL, Galezowska J, Leroy R, North R (1994) The results of computer-assisted ambulatory 16-channel EEG. *Electroencephalography and Clinical Neurophysiology* **91**:229–231.

Morris HH, Kanner A, Luders H *et al* (1989) Can sharp waves localized at the sphenoidal electrode accurately identify a mesio-temporal epileptogenic focus? *Epilepsia* **30**:532–539.

Morris HH, Estes ML, Gilmore R, Van Ness PC, Barnett GH, Turnbull J (1993) Chronic intractable epilepsy as the only symptom of primary brain tumor. *Epilepsia* **34**:1038–1043.

Murro AM, Park YD, King DW et al (1993) Seizure localization in temporal lobe epilepsy: a comparison of scalp–sphenoidal EEG and volumetric MRI. *Neurology* 43:2531–2533.

Niedermeyer E, Lopes da Silva F (1993) *Electroencephalography: Basic Principles, Clinical Applications, and Related Fields*, 3rd edn. Baltimore: Williams & Wilkins.

Niediek T, Franke HG, Degen R, Ettlinger G (1990) The development of independent foci in epileptic patients. *Archives of Neurology* 47:406–411.

Normand MM, Wszolek ZK, Klass DW (1995) Temporal intermittent rhythmic delta activity in electroencephalograms. *Journal of Clinical Neurophysiology* 12:280–284.

O'Brien TJ, Kilpatrick C, Murrie V, Vogrin S, Morris K, Cook MJ (1996) Temporal lobe epilepsy caused by mesial temporal sclerosis and temporal neocortical lesions: a clinical and electroencephalographic study of 46 pathologically proven cases. *Brain* 119:2133–2141.

Ozkara C, Dreifuss FE (1993) Differential diagnosis in pseudoepileptic seizures. *Epilepsia* 34:294–298.

Pacia SV, Ebersole JS (1997) Intracranial EEG substrates of scalp ictal patterns from temporal lobe foci. *Epilepsia* 38:642–654.

Palmini A, Andermann F, Olivier A et al (1991a) Focal neuronal migration disorders and intractable partial epilepsy: a study of 30 patients. *Annals of Neurology* 30:741–749.

Palmini A, Andermann F, Olivier A, Tampieri D, Robitaille Y (1991b) Focal neuronal migration disorders and intractable partial epilepsy: results of surgical treatment. *Annals of Neurology* 30:750–757.

Palmini A, Andermann F, Debeau F et al (1993) Occipitotemporal epilepsies: evaluation of selected patients requiring depth electrodes studies and rationale for surgical approaches. *Epilepsia* 34:84–96.

Panet-Raymond D, Gotman J (1990) Asymmetry in delta activity in patients with focal epilepsy. *Electroencephalography and Clinical Neurophysiology* 75:474–481.

Park YD, Murro AM, King DW, Gallagher BB, Smith JR, Yaghmai F (1996) The significance of ictal depth EEG patterns in patients with temporal lobe epilepsy. *Electroencephalography and Clinical Neurophysiology* 99:412–415.

Patrick S, Berg A, Spencer SS (1995) EEG and seizure outcome after epilepsy surgery. *Epilepsia* 36:236–240.

Pauri F, Pierelli F, Chatrian G-E, Erdly WW (1992) Long-term EEG-video-audio monitoring: computer detection of focal EEG seizure patterns. *Electroencephalography and Clinical Neurophysiology* 82:1–9.

Privitera MD, Quinlan JG, Yeh H-S (1990) Interictal spike detection comparing subdural and depth electrodes during electrocorticography. *Electroencephalography and Clinical Neurophysiology* 76:379–387.

Qu H, Gotman J (1993) Improvements in seizure detection performance by automatic adaptation to the EEG of each patient. *Electroencephalography and Clinical Neurophysiology* 86:79–87.

Qu H, Gotman J (1995) A seizure warning system for long-term epilepsy monitoring. *Neurology* 45:2250–2254.

Raymond AA, Fish DR, Stevens JM, Cook MJ, Sisodiya SM, Shorvon SD (1994a) Association of hippocampal sclerosis with cortical dysgenesis in patients with epilepsy. *Neurology* 44:1841–1845.

Raymond AA, Halpin SFS, Alsanjari N et al (1994b) Dysembryoplastic neuroepithelial tumour features in 16 patients. *Brain* 117:461–475.

Raymond AA, Fish DR, Stevens JM, Sisodiya SM, Alsanjari N, Shorvon SD (1994c) Subependymal heterotopias: a distinct neuronal migration disorder associated with epilepsy. *Journal of Neurology, Neurosurgery and Psychiatry* 57:1195–1202.

Risinger MW, Engel J, Van Ness PC, Henry TR, Crandall PH (1989) Ictal localization of temporal lobe seizures with scalp/sphenoidal recordings. *Neurology* 39:1288–1293.

Rutecki PA, Grossman RG, Armstrong D, Irish-Loewen S (1989) Electrophysiological connections between the hippocampus and entorhinal cortex in patients with complex partial seizures. *Journal of Neurosurgery* 70:667–675.

Ryglewicz D, Baranska-Gieruszczak M, Niedzielska K, Kryst-Widzgowska T (1990) EEG and CT findings in poststroke epilepsy. *Acta Neurologica Scandinavica* 81:488–490.

Sadler RM, Blume WT (1989) Significance of bisynchronous spike-waves in patients with temporal lobe spikes. *Epilepsia* 30:143–146.

Salanova V, Andermann F, Olivier A, Rasmussen T, Quesney LF (1992) Occipital lobe epilepsy: electroclinical manifestations, electrocorticography, cortical stimulation and outcome in 42 patients treated between 1930 and 1991. *Brain* 115:1655–1680.

Salanova V, Morris HH, Van Ness PC, Luders H, Dinner D, Wyllie E (1993) Comparison of scalp electroencephalogram with subdural recordings and functional mapping in frontal lobe epilepsy. *Archives of Neurology* 50:294–299.

Salanova V, Quesney LF, Rasmussen T, Andermann F, Olivier A (1994) Reevaluation of surgical failures and the role of reoperation in 39 patients with frontal lobe epilepsy. *Epilepsia* 35:70–80.

Salanova V, Morris HH, Van Ness P, Kotagal P, Wyllie E, Luders H (1995) Frontal lobe seizures: electroclinical syndromes. *Epilepsia* 36:16–24.

Salinsky MC (1997) A practical analysis of computer based detection during continuous video-EEG monitoring. *Electroencephalography and Clinical Neurophysiology* 103:445–449.

Salinsky M, Kanter R, Dasheiff RM (1987) Effectiveness of multiple EEGs in supporting the diagnosis of epilepsy: an operational curve. *Epilepsia* 28:331–334.

Sammaritano M, de Lotbiniere A, Andermann F, Olivier A, Gloor P, Quesney LF (1987) False lateralization by surface EEG of seizure onset in patients with temporal lobe epilepsy and gross focal cerebral lesions. *Annals of Neurology* 21:361–369.

Sammaritano M, Gigli GL, Gotman J (1991) Interictal spiking during wakefulness and sleep and the localization of foci in temporal lobe epilepsy. *Neurology* 41:290–297.

Saygi S, Spencer SS, Scheyer R, Katz A, Mattson R, Spencer DD (1994) Differentiation of temporal lobe ictal behavior associated with hippocampal sclerosis and tumors of temporal lobe. *Epilepsia* 35:737–742.

Sforza E, Montagna P, Rinaldi R et al (1993) Paroxysmal periodic motor attacks during sleep: clinical and polygraphic features. *Electroencephalography and Clinical Neurophysiology* 86:161–166.

Sirven JI, Sperling MR, French JA, O'Connor MJ (1996) Significance of simple partial seizures in temporal lobe epilepsy. *Epilepsia* 37:450–454.

Sirven JI, Malamut BL, Liporace JD, O'Connor MJ, Sperling MR (1997a) Outcome after temporal lobectomy in bilateral temporal lobe epilepsy. *Annals of Neurology* 42:873–878.

Sirven JI, Liporace JD, French JA, O'Connor MJ, Sperling MR (1997b) Seizures in temporal lobe epilepsy. 1. Reliability of scalp/sphenoidal ictal recording. *Neurology* 48:1041–1046.

So N, Gotman J (1990) Changes in seizure activity following anticonvulsant drug withdrawal. *Neurology* 40:407–413.

So N, Gloor P, Quesney LF, Jones-Gotman M, Olivier A, Andermann F (1989a) Depth electrode investigations in patients with bitemporal epileptiform abnormalities. *Annals of Neurology* 25:423–431.

So N, Olivier A, Andermann F, Gloor P, Quesney LF (1989b) Results of surgical treatment in patients with bitemporal epileptiform abnormalities. *Annals of Neurology* 25:432–439.

Spatt J, Pelzl G, Mamoli B (1997) Reliability of automatic and visual analysis of interictal spikes in lateralising an epileptic focus during video-EEG monitoring. *Electroencephalography and Clinical Neurophysiology* 103:421–425.

Spencer SS, Spencer DD (1994) Entorhinal-hippocampal interactions in medial temporal lobe epilepsy. *Epilepsia* 35:721–727.

Spencer SS, Spencer DD, Williamson PD, Mattson RH (1981) Ictal effects of anticonvulsant medication withdrawal in epileptic patients. *Epilepsia* 22:297–307.

Spencer SS, Spencer DD, Williamson PD, Mattson RH (1982) The localizing value of depth electroencephalography in 32 patients with refractory epilepsy. *Annals of Neurology* 12:248–253.

Spencer SS, Williamson PD, Bridgers SL, Mattson RH, Cicchetti DV, Spencer DD (1985) Reliability and accuracy of localization by scalp ictal EEG. *Neurology* 35:1567–1575.

Spencer SS, Williamson PD, Spencer DD, Mattson RH (1987) Human hippocampal seizure spread studied by depth and subdural recording: the hippocampal commissure. *Epilepsia* 28:479–489.

Spencer SS, Spencer DD, Williamson PD, Mattson R (1990) Combined depth and subdural electrode investigation in uncontrolled epilepsy. *Neurology* 40:74–79.

Spencer SS, Guimaraes P, Katz A, Kim J, Spencer D (1992a) Morphological patterns of seizures recorded intracranially. *Epilepsia* 33:537–545.

Spencer SS, Kim J, Spencer DD (1992b) Ictal spikes: a marker of specific hippocampal cell loss. *Electroencephalography and Clinical Neurophysiology* 83:104–111.

Spencer SS, Marks DD, Katz A, Kim J, Spencer DD (1992c) Anatomic correlates of interhippocampal seizure propagation time. *Epilepsia* 33:862–873.

Sperling MR, Engel J (1985) Electroencephalographic recording from the temporal lobes: a comparison of ear, anterior temporal, and nasopharyngeal electrodes. *Annals of Neurology* 17:510–513.

Sperling MR, O'Connor MJ (1989) Comparison of depth and subdural electrodes in recording temporal lobe seizures. *Neurology* 39:1497–1504.

Sperling MR, O'Connor MJ (1990) Auras and subclinical seizures: characteristics and prognostic significance. *Annals of Neurology* 28:320–328.

Sperling MR, Mendius JR, Engel J (1986) Mesial temporal spikes: a simultaneous comparison of sphenoidal, nasopharyngeal, and ear electrodes. *Epilepsia* 27:81–86.

Sperling MR, O'Connor MJ, Saykin AJ et al (1992) A noninvasive protocol for anterior temporal lobectomy. *Neurology* 42:416–422.

Steinhoff BJ, So NK, Lim S, Luders HO (1995) Ictal scalp EEG in temporal lobe epilepsy with unitemporal versus bitemporal interictal epileptiform discharges. *Neurology* 45:889–896.

Sum JM, Morrell MJ (1995) Predictive value of the first ictal recording in determining localization of the epileptogenic region by scalp/sphenoidal EEG. *Epilepsia* 36:1033–1040.

Sutherling WW, Barth DS (1989) Neocortical propagation in temporal lobe spike foci on magnetoencephalography and electroencephalography. *Annals of Neurology* 25:373–381.

Sutherling WW, Crandall PH, Cahan LD, Barth DS (1988) The magnetic field of epileptic spikes agrees with intracranial localizations in complex partial epilepsy. *Neurology* 38:778–786.

Sutherling WW, Risinger MW, Crandall PH et al (1990) Focal functional anatomy of dorsolateral frontocentral seizures. *Neurology* 40:87–98.

Swanson TH (1995) The pathophysiology of human mesial temporal lobe epilepsy. *Journal of Clinical Neurophysiology* 12:2–22.

Swick CT, Bouthillier A, Spencer SS (1996) Seizure occurrence during long-term monitoring. *Epilepsia* 37:927–930.

Thacker K, Devinsky O, Perrine K, Alper K, Luciano D (1993) Nonepileptic seizures during apparent sleep. *Annals of Neurology* 33:414–418.

Thadani VM, Williamson PD, Berger R, et al (1995) Successful epilepsy surgery without intracranial EEG recording: criteria for patient selection. *Epilepsia* 36:7–15.

Theodore WH, Porter RJ, Albert P et al (1994) The secondarily generalized tonic–clonic seizure: a videotape analysis. *Neurology* 44:1403–1407.

Thompson AJ, Kermode AG, Moseley IF, MacManus DG, McDonald WI (1993) Seizures due to multiple sclerosis: seven patients with MRI correlations. *Journal of Neurology, Neurosurgery and Psychiatry* 56:1317–1320.

Tinuper P, Cerullo A, Cirignotta F, Cortelli P, Lugaresi E, Montagna P (1990) Noctural paroxysmal dystonia with short-lasting attacks: three cases with evidence for an epileptic frontal lobe origin of seizures. *Epilepsia* 31:549–556.

Todorov AB, Lesser RP, Uematsu SS, Yankov YA, Todorov AA (1994) Distribution in time of seizures during presurgical EEG monitoring. *Neurology* 44:1060–1064.

Traub RD, Borck C, Colling SB, Jeffreys JGR (1996) On the structure of ictal events *in vitro*. *Epilepsia* 37:879–891.

Tsai M-L, Chatrian G-E, Pauri F et al (1993) Electrocorticography in patients with medically intractable temporal lobe seizures. 1. Quantification of epileptiform discharges prior to resective surgery. *Electroencephalography and Clinical Neurophysiology* 87:10–24.

Tuunainen A, Nousiainen U, Mervaala E, Riekkinen P (1990) Efficacy of a 1- to 3-day ambulatory electroencephalogram in recording epileptic seizures. *Archives of Neurology* 47:799–800.

Tuunainen A, Nousiainen U, Mervaala E et al (1994) Postoperative EEG and electrocorticography: relation to clinical outcome in patients with temporal lobe surgery. *Epilepsia* 35:1165–1173.

Tuunainen A, Nousiainen U, Pilke A, Mervaala E, Partanen J, Riekkinen P (1995) Spectral EEG during short-term discontinuation of antiepileptic medication. *Epilepsia* 36:817–823.

Urban L, Aitken PG, Crain BJ, Friedman AH, Somjen GG (1993) Correlation between function and structure in 'epileptic' human hippocampal tissue maintained *in vitro*. *Epilepsia* 34:54–60.

Walczak TS, Radtke RA, Lewis DV (1992) Accuracy and interobserver reliability of scalp ictal EEG. *Neurology* 42:2279–2285.

Wang J, Wieser HG (1994) Regional 'rigidity' of background EEG activity in the epileptogenic zone. *Epilepsia* 35:495–504.

Webber WRS, Lesser RP, Richardson RT, Wilson K (1996) An approach to seizure detection using an artificial neural network (ANN). *Electroencephalography and Clinical Neurophysiology* 98:250–272.

Weinand ME, Wyler AR, Richey ET, Phillips BA, Somes GW (1992) Long-term ictal monitoring with subdural strip electrodes: prognostic factors for selecting temporal lobectomy candidates. *Journal of Neurosurgery* 77:20–28.

Wilkus RJ, Thompson PM (1985) Sphenoidal electrode positions and basal EEG during long term monitoring. *Epilepsia* 26:137–142.

Williamson A, Spencer SS, Spencer DD (1995) Depth electrode studies and intracellular dentate granule cell recordings in temporal lobe epilepsy. *Annals of Neurology* 38:778–787.

Williamson PD, Spencer SS (1986) Clinical and EEG features of complex partial seizures of extratemporal origin. *Epilepsia* 27(Suppl 2):S46–S63.

Williamson PD, Boon PA, Thadani VM et al (1992a) Parietal lobe epilepsy: diagnostic considerations and results of surgery. *Annals of Neurology* 31:193–201.

Williamson PD, Thadani VM, Darcey TM, Spencer DD, Spencer SS, Mattson RH (1992b) Occipital lobe epilepsy: characteristics, seizure spread patterns, and results of surgery. *Annals of Neurology* 31:3–13.

Williamson PD, French JA, Thadani VM et al (1993) Characteristics of medial temporal lobe epilepsy. II. Interictal and ictal scalp electroencephalography, neuropsychological testing, neuroimaging, surgical results, and pathology. *Annals of Neurology* 34:781–787.

Invasive neurophysiologic evaluation of partial epilepsy in children

P JAYAKAR AND M DUCHOWNY

INTRODUCTION

Surgical excision of the epileptogenic region is now an established therapeutic option for children with medically resistant seizures. The primary goal of the preoperative evaluation is to define accurately the region that needs to be resected in order to ameliorate all seizures. All cortical regions revealing significant epileptogenicity must be excised as residual epileptogenic tissue increases the risk of postoperative seizures. In most adults where mesial temporal sclerosis is the prime pathology, the anatomic limits of the temporal lobectomy have been standardized and the causal side can usually be identified on the basis of clinical data, scalp EEG, and neuroimaging information. Chronic epilepsy in childhood, on the other hand, generally presents with developmental pathology as the most frequent underlying substrate. Typically, the epileptogenic regions are variable and often involve functionally related regions extensively transgressing known anatomic boundaries. Seizures commonly arise extratemporally and even temporal lobe seizures are rarely of pure limbic origin, with wider posterobasal or orbitofrontal involvement being common (Duchowny et al 1992; 1994).

With the advances in structural and functional neuroimaging, presurgical evaluation in many children can be adequately achieved through noninvasive means and the need for a two-stage chronic invasive monitoring protocol has diminished. Yet noninvasive assessment remains imprecise in a significant subgroup of medically refractory children, and accurate localization of seizure foci is only achieved through intracranial EEG monitoring. This review discusses the continuing role of invasive monitoring in the evaluation of childhood epilepsy.

METHODOLOGY

While the intracranial EEG evaluation of the child is generally similar to adults (Luders et al 1987; Ajmone-Marsan 1990; Spencer 1991), the stress of invasive EEG monitoring on young children is considerable and should be addressed preoperatively through proper counseling. A child life or clinical nurse specialist can help to introduce the intracranial monitoring procedure to the child and educate the family prior to hospitalization.

The number and location of electrode placement is determined by comprehensive preoperative evaluation which generally includes scalp video-EEG, CT/magnetic resonance imaging (MRI) scans with functional imaging such as positron emission tomography or single-photon emission computed topography (PET/SPECT) offering complementary localizing information. When epileptogenic regions encroach upon critical cortex, additional coverage must be provided in order to perform functional mapping.

Subdural electrodes provide coverage of large areas of the neocortical surface and also allow functional mapping of critical cortex (Wyllie *et al* 1988; Duchowny *et al* 1993). When seizures arise from deep-seated lesions, strategically placed depth electrodes are often used in conjunction with subdural electrodes to provide comprehensive coverage. Electrodes are generally implanted under direct observation following craniotomy although stereotactic depth placement or subdural strips via burr holes may occasionally be performed (Luders *et al* 1987; Wyler *et al* 1988; Wyllie *et al* 1988; Nespeca *et al* 1990). Electrode location can be confirmed extraoperatively on plain X-ray or CT scan. While platinum and nichrome electrodes offer MRI compatibility, they are more expensive.

INDICATIONS FOR SUBDURAL RECORDING

There are no standard criteria for the use of invasive EEG monitoring in pediatric patients and implantation protocols vary widely between centers. Recognizing that each child must be evaluated on an individualized basis, the main goals of invasive monitoring are to define accurately the extent of resection that is necessary to achieve seizure freedom and to define eloquent cortical regions so that critical neurologic functions are not jeopardized.

DEFINING THE EPILEPTOGENIC REGION

With advances in MRI and the introduction of PET and SPECT scans, there has been in general a reduction in the number of patients requiring subdural implantation. Specific subgroups of patients can now be identified where a generous resection of a lesion evident on MRI scans with additional guidance from intraoperative electrocorticography (ECoG) results in a satisfactory outcome. Functional imaging such as PET, SPECT, or MR spectroscopy have a high degree of sensitivity and are likewise advocated as being adequate for surgical planning. However, the variability of their findings, lack of specificity, and pitfalls of interpretation are being increasingly recognized. Although promising, functional imaging thus needs further validation before being widely used as the primary tool for surgical planning in intractable childhood epilepsy.

Although the epileptogenic region can be defined by intraoperative ECoG (Gloor 1975; Ajmone-Marsan 1990), reliance solely on interictal data may not always be adequate. Furthermore, general anesthesia often suppresses

spiking or may occasionally paradoxically activate it, creating a misleading picture of the epileptogenic zone (Jayakar *et al* 1992c). Within this context, the following case scenarios may be considered the most likely indications for invasive monitoring:

Normal or nonspecific CT or MRI scans

The localization of the epileptogenic region in nonlesional cases is more challenging than those with lesions and many pediatric epilepsy centers tend to exclude them from surgical consideration. In children with infantile spasms, resections are guided by interictal PET data in conjunction with intraoperative ECoG monitoring (Chugani *et al* 1990). It is tempting to contemplate a similar approach in older children with partial seizures especially if the scalp EEG and PET or ictal SPECT data are all congruent. Pending further validity studies, functional imaging currently serves as an important tool to optimize accurate placement of intracranial electrodes for a chronic study and minimizes the risk of erroneous or undersampling.

In nonlesional cases where functional studies are not definitive or where there is a likelihood of involvement of critical cortex, invasive EEG recording will, however, continue to play a decisive role. In the authors' experience, nonlesional epilepsy patients achieve seizure freedom only if zones of ictal onset and significant interictal abnormalities are completely resected. In the authors' series of 116 children with normal or nonspecific imaging studies (Table 28.1), seizure-freedom was achieved in 75% of patients who had complete resection. By contrast, only 13% of patients were seizure-free when involvement of critical cortex precluded removal of the entire ictal and interictal epileptogenic region (Jayakar *et al* 1992a, 1997).

Epileptogenic regions wider than the structural lesion

Identification of a discrete structural abnormality on imaging studies biases the presurgical evaluation against invasive studies but there are many documented failures following lesionectomy, indicating that the epileptogenic zone is more extensive than the lesion (Palmini *et al* 1991).

In a series of 75 children with lesional epilepsy at Miami Children's Hospital (Table 28.1), 80% who underwent excision of the lesion and the entire epileptogenic region were seizure-free. Outcome was comparably good in patients with developmental tumors and dysplastic lesions following complete resections. However, whereas over half of the children with developmental tumors were seizure-free following lesion removal, the dysplastic lesions fared poorly when proximity of

Table 28.1 Outcome of resectional surgery in 191 children. (Complete: the entire epileptogenic region was removed; incomplete: critical cortex prevented complete resection.)

Group	Number of cases	Seizure-free (%)	Improved	Unchanged
a. Lesional				
Developmental tumors				
Complete	21	18 (86)	1	2
Incomplete	10	6 (60)	2	2
Cortical dysplasia				
Complete	24	19 (79)	3	2
Incomplete	20	3 (15)	7	10
b. Nonlesional				
Complete	68	51 (75)	10	7
Incomplete	48	6 (13)	16	26

critical cortex prevented complete resection of the electrophysiologically abnormal region (Jayakar *et al* 1997).

It is thus becoming increasingly apparent that lesional epilepsy in childhood is not homogeneous and mandates a type-specific approach based on the underlying pathology. As a general rule, if the imaging characteristics are indicative of a noninfiltrative developmental tumor or low-flow vascular lesion, a one-stage lesion resection tailored to ECoG is adequate. By contrast, in children with low-grade dysplastic lesions, while the need to perform invasive EEG may at first appear less compelling, the epileptogenic boundaries are often deceptive and a two-stage evaluation may be the only means to guarantee completeness of resection (Jayakar *et al* 1997). It is in the latter category that the evolving role of functional imaging will be crucial to define.

Noncongruent preoperative data

When clinical seizure semeiology, interictal or ictal EEG, and functional and structural imaging data are noncongruent, localization of the epileptogenic zone almost always requires invasive EEG recording. However, care must be taken to ensure adequate sampling, since noncongruence frequently results from rapid and complex spread patterns and interactions between regions (Jayakar *et al* 1991). A combined use of subdural and strategically placed depth electrodes may be particularly indicated to minimize the risk of false localization.

Multiple lesions and/or multifocal interictal epileptiform activity

Children with multiple structural lesions and/or multifocal interictal spike discharges were once regarded as unsuitable candidates for resective procedures. This view has changed, particularly in children with tuberous sclerosis who have benefited from the resection of a single epileptogenic tuber.

Ictal SPECT provides important corroborating evidence in about half the number of cases and reveals a penumbra of increased blood flow surrounding a candidate lesion (Koh *et al* 1998). When the SPECT findings are convergent with the scalp EEG and clinical semeiology, surgical success is likely following a one-stage resection. However, intraictal activation of secondary foci is common in the presence of multiple lesions and represents a potential pitfall for SPECT interpretation (Jayakar *et al* 1994). Invasive EEG clarifies ambiguities of seizure origin and facilitates surgery in many of these difficult cases.

Defining seizure onset in subcortical lesions

While patients with deep-seated subcortical lesions are a distinct minority of all epileptics, their seizures are often medically resistant. A particularly compelling example is the clinical syndrome of gelastic seizures and hypothalamic hamartoma. If an ictal SPECT during gelastic seizures fails to demonstrate hyperperfusion in the hamartoma, definitive confirmation can be achieved by stereotactic EEG recording directly from the hamartoma (Kahane *et al* 1997) or by reproducing gelastic seizures by electrical stimulation (Kuzniecky *et al* 1995). Other subcortical lesions such as heterotropic nodules or the rare syndrome of cerebellar ganglioglioma in infants (Harvey *et al* 1996) may also require invasive EEG recording when the epileptic nature of candidate lesions cannot be established through noninvasive means.

FUNCTIONAL MAPPING

Epileptogenic regions in children are often widespread or contiguous with eloquent cortex. Children with developmental pathology may reveal anomalous representation of sensory-motor homunculi which impact on surgical planning. Furthermore, unlike destructive acquired lesions, developmental pathology does not force language cortex to transfer to the opposite hemisphere even when it involves the left hemisphere extensively (Duchowny *et al* 1996). Occasionally, language cortex may develop over the right hemisphere even if the patient is right-hand dominant for motor functions (Fig. 28.1). Defining critical sensory-motor or language regions is therefore indispensable even in the young child and constitutes an important part of the presurgical evaluation.

Language cortex in the child can only be mapped extra-operatively via subdurally implanted electrodes. The sensory cortex can be defined intraoperatively by evoking responses to median nerve stimulation, but motor responses to direct cortical stimulation may be difficult to elicit under general anesthesia. The adult stimulation paradigm needs to be modified when mapping infants or young children with sequentially increasing current intensity and

pulse duration in a stepwise fashion (Jayakar *et al* 1992b). Of practical note is the fact that clinical responses in children often occur at or above after-discharge threshold (Jayakar and Duchowny 1997). Thus, the lack of a clinical response during an after-discharge does not necessarily exclude the presence of eloquent cortex.

INTERPRETATION OF INVASIVE EEG

Intracranially recorded EEG presents voluminous amounts of data fraught with difficulties in interpretation. Although the pitfalls and limitations of intracranial EEG are well recognized (Gloor 1975; Lieb *et al* 1980; Luders *et al* 1987; Ajmone-Marsan 1990; Jayakar *et al* 1991), guidelines for

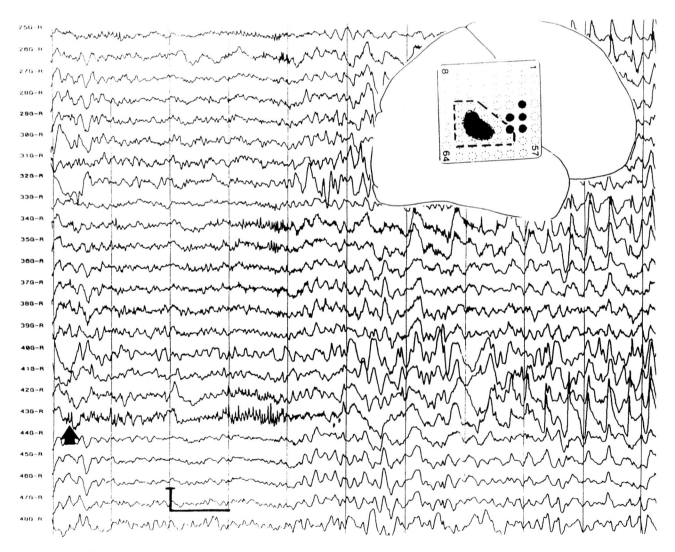

Fig. 28.1 Subdural EEG recording in a right-handed individual showing seizure onset over the right temporoparietal convexity (shaded area). Functional mapping demonstrated language cortex anteriorly (solid circles).

its use in defining the epileptogenic region are not fully established.

Abnormalities of the background activity show considerable temporal variability and may reflect nonspecific changes in reaction to anesthesia and subdural electrode implantation. Thus, polymorphic slowing is often multifocal and may evolve over the course of monitoring. By contrast, focal attenuation of fast activity remains consistent over time and in the authors' experience is the most reliable background abnormality in patients with focal epilepsy. Occasionally, however, fast activity may be focally accentuated and occur either continuously or in brief runs over the epileptic focus. Severely damaged cortex may exhibit chronic 'burst suppression' activity which may persist during a seizure.

Interictal spikes and sharp waves vary in their duration, morphology, field, phase, and polarity (Gloor 1975; Ajmone-Marsan 1990) and may also be state dependent. Given such marked variability, the role of interictal discharges towards defining epileptogenic regions is questionable (Lieb *et al* 1978; Marks *et al* 1992). As a general policy, we do not attribute much significance to interictal discharges remote from the ictal onset zone unless they occur in rhythmic runs or are associated with patterns of intraictal activation.

The area of seizure onset and early propagation is considered to be the most reliable means of defining the epileptogenic region (Fig. 28.2). Patterns of ictal onset include focal low-amplitude fast activity, burst of spike or polyspikes, run of repetitive spike or sharp waves, or a phase of marked electrodecrement. Onsets revealing rhythmic slow frequencies in the theta range generally reflect propagated patterns, implying that the true focus is distant from the recording electrodes.

Patients with well-localized ictal onset may occasionally develop independent electroencephalographic sequences in adjacent cortex during the course of their seizure (Jayakar *et al* 1994). Such secondarily activated neocortical foci are capable of independent epileptogenesis and should be resected whenever possible. Subclinical electrographic

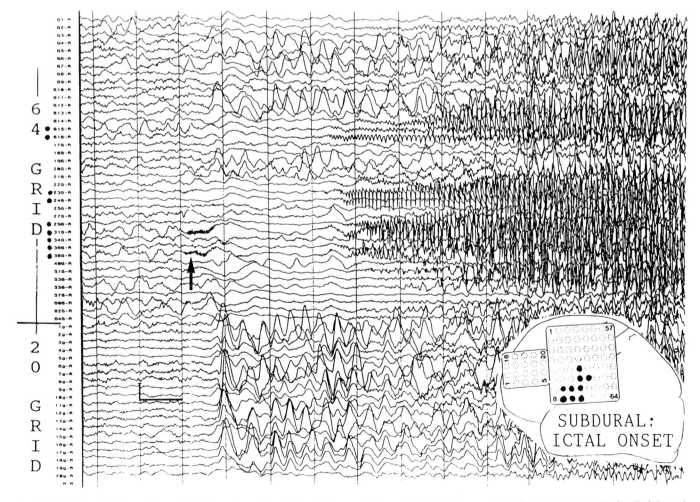

Fig. 28.2 Subdural EEG recording with ictal onset over the left frontal convexity (arrow). Note the low-amplitude fast activity occurring focally followed by electrodecrement (solid circles).

seizures are common during subdural recording and are thought to arise from cortical regions which do not subserve critical functions. Subclinical seizure foci are resected when they coincide with the patient's symptomatic seizure focus but they create a management dilemma when they are distant to the symptomatic focus.

In conclusion, while the role of invasive EEG recording in the evaluation of children for resectional surgery is evolving, the technique will undoubtedly continue to provide a valuable means to localize neocortical seizure foci and map eloquent cortex. Future efforts should be directed towards correlating the results of recording and stimulation with anatomic and functional imaging data.

KEY POINTS

1. The primary goal of the preoperative evaluation in pediatric patients is to accurately define the extent of resection necessary to achieve seizure freedom. Invasive neurophysiologic investigations are often indicated in nonlesional cases, and when there is reason to believe that the epileptogenic region is wider than or noncongruent to the structural lesion.

2. Lesional epilepsy in childhood is not homogeneous and mandates a type-specific approach based on underlying pathology. Malformations of cortical development are more likely to require invasive electrodes, as their epileptogenic boundaries are often unclear and more likely to remain outside the margin of resection.

3. Focal attenuation of fast frequencies remains consistent over time, and is the most reliable background abnormality in patients being monitored for epilepsy. The region of seizure onset and early propagation is considered to be the most reliable means of defining the epileptogenic region.

REFERENCES

Ajmone-Marsan C (1990) Chronic intracranial recording and electrocorticography. In: Daly DD, Pedley TA (eds) *Current Practice of Clinical Electroencephalography*, pp 535–560. New York: Raven Press.

Chugani HT, Shields DW, Shewmon DA, Olson D, Phelps M, Peacock W (1990) Infantile spasms: I. PET identifies focal cortical dysgenesis in cryptogenic cases for surgical treatment. *Annals of Neurology* 27:406–413.

Duchowny M, Levin B, Jayakar P *et al* (1992) Temporal lobectomy in early childhood. *Epilepsia* 33:298–303.

Duchowny M, Shewmon A, Wyllie E, Andermann F, Mizrahi E (1993) Special considerations for preoperative evaluation in childhood. In: Engel J Jr (ed) *Surgical Treatment of the Epilepsies*, pp. 415–427. New York: Raven Press.

Duchowny M, Levin B, Jayakar P, Resnick T, Alvarez L (1994) Posterior temporal epilepsy: electroclinical features. *Annals of Neurology* 35:427–431.

Duchowny MS, Jayakar P, Harvey AS, Levin B, Resnick TJ, Alvarez LA (1996) Language cortex representation: effects of developmental vs. acquired pathology. *Annals of Neurology* 40:31–38.

Gloor P (1975) Contributions of electroencephalography and electrocorticography to the neurosurgical treatment of the epilepsies. In: Purpura DP, Penry JK, Walter RD (eds) *Neurosurgical Management of the Epilepsies. Advances in Neurology*, Vol 8, pp 59–105. New York: Raven Press.

Harvey AS, Jayakar P, Duchowny MS *et al* (1996) Hemifacial seizures and cerebellar ganglioglioma in infancy: an epilepsy syndrome with seizures of cerebellar origin. *Annals of Neurology* 40:91–98.

Jayakar P, Duchowny MS (1997) Invasive EEG recording and functional mapping in children. In: Tuxhorn I, Holthausen H, Boenik HE (eds) *Pediatric Epilepsy Syndromes and Their Surgical Treatment*. London: John Libbeyt.

Jayakar P, Resnick TJ, Duchowny MS, Alvarez LA (1991) Pitfalls and caveats of localizing seizure foci. *Journal of Clinical Neurophysiology* 8:414–431.

Jayakar P, Resnick TJ, Duchowny MS, Alvarez LA (1992a) Outcome of excisional surgery in children with nonlesional frontal/parietal seizure foci (Abstract). *Epilepsia* 33(suppl 3):91.

Jayakar P, Resnick TJ, Duchowny MS, Alvarez LA (1992b) A safe and effective paradigm to functionally map the cortex in childhood. *Journal of Clinical Neurophysiology* 9:288–293.

Jayakar P, Resnick TJ, Duchowny MS, Alvarez LA (1992c) The epileptic region determined by electrocorticography: comparison with extraoperative subdural EEG (Abstract). *Electroenphalography and Clinical Neurophysiology* 83:69.

Jayakar P, Resnick TJ, Duchowny MS, Alvarez LA (1994) Intra-ictal activation in the neocortex: a marker of the epileptogenic region. *Epilepsia* 35(3):489–494.

Jayakar P, Udani PM, Resnick T *et al* (1997) Surgical treatment of cortical dysplasias. American Epilepsy Society Proceedings. *Epilepsia* 38(8):53.

Kahane P, Munari C, Minotti L *et al* (1997) The role of hypothalamic hamartoma in the genesis of gelastic and dacrystic seizures. In: Tuxhorn I, Holthausen H, Boenik HE (eds) *Pediatric Epilepsy Syndromes and Their Surgical Treatment*. London: John Libbeyt.

Koh S, Jayakar P, Resnick T, Duchowny M, Alvarez LA (1998) Role of ictal SPECT in defining seizure origin in children with tuberous sclerosis. American Epilepsy Society Proceedings. *Epilepsia* 39(6):105.

Kuzniecky R, Guthrie B, Mountz J, Gilliam F, Faught E (1995) Hypothalamic hamartomas and gelastic seizures: evidence for subcortical seizure generation by ictal SPECT and cerebral stimulation. *Epilepsia* **36**(3):S266.

Lieb JP, Woods SC, Siccardi A, Crandall PH, Walter DO, Leake B (1978) Quantitative analysis of depth spiking in relation to seizure foci in patients with temporal lobe epilespy. *Electroencephalography and Clinical Neurophysiology* **44**:641–663.

Lieb JP, Joseph JP, Engel J Jr, Walker J, Crandall PH (1980) Sleep state and seizure foci related to depth spike activity in patients with temporal lobe epilepsy. *Electroencephalography and Clinical Neurophysiology* **49**:538–557.

Luders H, Lesser RP, Dinner DS (1987) Commentary: chronic intracranial recording and stimulation with subdural electrodes. In: Engel J Jr (ed) *Surgical Treatment of the Epilepsies*, pp 297–321. New York: Raven Press.

Marks DA, Katz A, Booke J, Spencer DD, Spencer SS (1992) Correlation of surface and sphenoidal electrodes with simultaneous intracranial recording: an interictal study. *Electroencephalography and Clinical Neurophysiology* **82**:23–29.

Nespeca M, Wyllie E, Luders H *et al* (1990) EEG recording and functional localization studies with subdural electrodes in infants and young children. *Journal of Epilepsy* **3**:107–124.

Palmini A, Andermann F, Olivier A *et al* (1991) Focal neuronal migration disorders and intractable partial epilepsy: a study of 30 patients. *Annals of Neurology* **30**:741–749.

Spencer SS (1991) Intracranial recording. In: Spencer SS, Spencer DD (eds) *Surgery for Epilepsy*, pp 54–65. Cambridge, MA: Blackwell Scientific.

Wyler AR, Walker G, Richet T, Hermann BP (1988) Chronic subdural strip electrode recordings for difficult epileptic problems. *Journal of Epilepsy* **1**:71–78.

Wyllie E, Luders H, Morris HH *et al* (1988) Subdural electrodes in the evaluation for epilepsy surgery in children and adults. *Neuropediatrics* **19**:80–86.

Magnetoencephalography in intractable focal epilepsies

H STEFAN

In the presurgical evaluation of focal pharmacoresistant epilepsies, functionally important areas have to be correlated with the localization of the epileptogenic area. Since neurosurgical approaches have become routine procedures in the treatment of pharmacoresistant focal epilepsies, the diagnostic challenge culminates in determining the site and extent of epileptogenic tissue to be removed without risk of functional deficit. To this purpose, the combined findings of diagnostic methods may contribute anatomic (CT, MRI) blood flow (SPECT; single-photon emission computed tomography), and electrophysiologic information, the last comprising long-established noninvasive surface EEG and invasive EEG recordings, and, as a comparatively new method, magnetoencephalography (MEG). MEG, being a noninvasive method with high temporal and spatial resolution and offering data on electrophysiologic phenomena from a point of view somewhat different from the EEG, has been found to be a potentially useful addition to the pool of techniques applied in preoperative focus localization of pharmacologically intractable epilepsies. As the standard procedure for MEG processing includes corecording with MRI, activity localized from MEG data is usually displayed in the corresponding anatomic images. This particularly advantageous combined technique is called magnetic source imaging (MSI) (Stefan *et al* 1988; Gallen *et al* 1993).

METHOD

For details of the different methodological aspects of basic mechanisms, modeling instrumentation, and coregistration with MRI, the reader is referred to our review (Stefan and Hummel 1999). In most investigations, an equivalent dipole (multiple dipoles or current density) in an homogeneous sphere, or a realistically shaped head model, is used for source analysis.

APPLICATIONS OF MSI IN EPILEPTIC PATIENTS

EVOKED ACTIVITY

In cases where neurosurgery remains the only therapeutic hope for epileptic patients, it is essential not only that the site of the epileptogenic region be known (see below) but also to determine whether removal of the tissue in question may cause functional deficits.

More recently, an additional functional validation of MSI has been obtained with various sensory modalities. Source localization is based upon evoked magnetic responses to repeated stimulation, in accordance with the well-established technique for evoked potentials, averaged over a number of stimulus-related EEG epochs (Hari 1990).

So far, evoked magnetic responses to acoustic (AEF), visual (VEF), somatosensory (SEF), and olfactory (OEF) stimulation has been obtained (Baumgartner 1993; Hari 1994; Paetau *et al* 1995; Kettenmann *et al* 1996). Magnetic fields representing motor activity generated by voluntary finger and limb movements have been reported (Deecke *et al* 1985; Cheyne *et al* 1991). Thus, localization of cortical generators calculated from magnetic evoked activity could become an established tool to provide information about functionally significant areas, and particularly so if MSI and neurosurgery have access to compatible systems of space coordinates ('neuronavigation' systems are already being established in operating rooms). Using a variety of stimulating sites, SEF localizations illustrate the 'homuncular' organization and its variations in the somatosensory cortex (Ganslandt *et al* 1997; Stefan and Hummel 1999). It is also possible to locate functional regions for language (Papanicolaou *et al* 1998).

SPONTANEOUS ACTIVITY

The sources of spontaneous epileptic activity are often located less superficially than the cortical generators of evoked responses. With increasing depth of the source, the signals recorded at the surface decline as the square of the distance from the source, so that deep sources are more difficult to locate than superficial ones (Baumgartner *et al* 1992). A crucial question in the management of drug-resistant epilepsy is the ability of magnetic field recordings of spontaneous brain activity to localize deep sources in the mesial structures of the temporal lobe. Initial attempts have been made to approach this issue in temporal lobe epilepsy. In a study where experimental dipoles were established at the tips of foramen ovale electrodes, we found that these dipoles were localized in deeper parts of the temporal brain regions in the range of 8 to 22 mm distant to the experimental dipole generator. This result gives some encouragement for the use of MSI localizations for presumed deep epileptic foci. However, the arrangement of cell layers, e.g. in the amygdala, may cause partial cancelation of magnetic fields, thus jeopardizing detection of the signals. An unfavorable sensor configuration may also impair results. The possiblity of recording from deeper sources depends on the use of sensors (axial versus planar gradiometer, magnetometer).

Owing to the distribution of focal origins of seizure disorders, clinical MSI studies in epileptic patients mostly include the temporal lobe (Rose *et al* 1987; Sutherling *et al* 1988; Stefan *et al* 1990, 1994; Ebersole *et al* 1993, 1995). Nevertheless, presurgical evaluation of patients with frontal lobe epilepsies has, sporadically, also been reported to benefit from MSI (Hari *et al* 1993; Stefan *et al* 1995; Stefan and Hummel 1999).

The newer generations of biomagnetic systems, allowing for simultaneous examination of large fields of interest, or even both hemispheres, are particularly welcome in the investigation of epileptic spikes (Stefan *et al* 1991; Paetau *et al* 1992), as they offer the opportunity to investigate temporal relationships of events with extended spatial distribution, for example mirror foci (Hari *et al* 1993).

In small children the limited cooperation and the small head size can impose limitations on recording and analysis modeling. Because of the relatively short recording time, spikes are not detected in all patients with focal epilepsy. In these cases, spike activation using methohexital and/or clondine can be used (Kirchberger *et al* 1998).

In frontal and other extratemporal epilepsies, intralobar localizations (predominantly lateral and frontobasal) can be confirmed by invasive recordings but to date the number of investigated patients is rather small (Stefan *et al* 1995; Fukao *et al* 1998). The rate of spike detection in focal epilepsies varies between 70% and 90% if spontaneous spikes are considered. Neocortical frontal epilepsies tend to show more

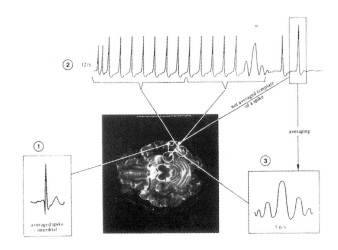

Fig. 29.1 Interictal and ictal localization in a patient with temporal lobe epilepsy (MRI): hippocampal and discrete temporal neocortical atrophy on the right. (1) Interictal spike (average): lateral temporal (small circle). (2) Ictal recording (lateral to mesial) indicated by means of large circles. (3) After using the last spike for definition of a template and averaging identical templates, 5–6 s⁻¹ theta activity is recognized. The localization of theta activity is shown in the square. The interictal center of dipolar activity is closely related to the ictal centers of epileptic activity. (From H. Stefan *et al.* (1992)). Multichannel MEG and EEG recordings of interictal and ictal epileptic activity in temporal lobe epilepsy. In: K. Bachmann, H. Stefan, J. Vieth (eds) *Biomagnetism: Principles, Models and Clinical Research.* Erlangen: Palm und Enke Verlag.

spikes during a 30-minute recording than mesial temporal epilepsies.

INTERICTAL RECORDING

Thus, recording sessions are typically hardly longer than 45 minutes and, owing to these rather short registration times (compared with long-term EEG monitoring), most recordings miss ictal activity, even in inpatients whose antiepileptic medication is reduced for presurgical evaluation purposes. The restricted access to ictal recording presently remains one of the basic problems of MSI.

SPECIFIC EPILEPTIC SIGNALS

As spikes often have large amplitudes, unaveraged signals may be used for dipole localization, but averaging of epochs with identical spike patterns can be useful to improve signal-to-noise ratio (SNR) (Sutherling *et al* 1988; Stefan *et al* 1990), thus facilitating localization of small spikes or those detected from simultaneous EEG recordings.

Validation of source locations with respect to the 'true' source is necessary. MEG findings on epileptogenic foci need to be compared with the results of other diagnostic techniques considered as most reliably detecting the epileptogenic brain tissue. Whether ictal video-EEG, which is generally regarded as the 'gold standard' (Engel *et al* 1993), invasive EEG monitoring, or intraoperative electrocorticography (ECoG) need to be used to check correctness of MEG focus localization has to be decided in each

individual case, depending on other clinical findings. Initial results indicate that MEG indeed yields fairly good accuracy, even though the activity investigated is mostly interictal (Sutherling *et al* 1987; Nakasato *et al* 1994; Smith *et al* 1994; Stefan *et al* 1994; Ebersole *et al* 1995; Knowlton *et al* 1997). There are, however, cases where MEG spike localization does not result in focal source findings (Seino *et al* 1995). Spikes recorded in the MEG could be localized in 70 to 80% congruent with other findings of presurgical evaluation (Eliashiv *et al* 1998). In 72% of patients with successfully operated temporal lobe epilepsy, a spatial correlation between predominant focal epileptic activity in MEG and other localization methods of presurgical evaluation and intraoperative ECoG was found (Stefan *et al* 1993a,b). Anteroposterior orientation may favor a temporomesial and oblique or radial orientation neocortical generators (Ebersole *et al* 1995). In children, only a limited number of recordings exist, predominantly investigations of neocortical focal epilepsies and functionally important areas such as in Landau–Kleffner syndrome where MST leads to a reduction of epileptic activity and an improvement in language function (Morrell *et al* 1995).

In many cases, cerebral MRI of epileptic patients shows abnormal morphology, varying from subtle alterations to extensive mass lesions. However, abnormal MRI findings are not necessarily epileptogenic, and even if they are it may be important to clarify the relation between anatomic and functional pathology in detail. Furthermore, if there is more than one lesion, those crucial to epileptogenicity must be determined. In a number of studies, epileptic activity

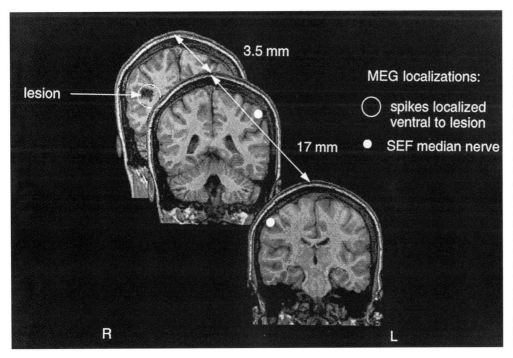

Fig. 29.2 Symptomatic parietal epilepsy: MSI focus localization (open circle, diameter representing mean dipole error of averaged spike activity) bordering ventrally on a lesion in the parietal lobe, projected onto the most anterior slice showing the lesion. SEF sources were found to be asymmetrical, with SEF ipsilateral to the lesion (white dot) being localized anterior to SEF on the unimpaired side (white dot). Distances are indicated by white double-headed arrows: the anteroposterior distance between the lesion and the contralateral SEF source is 3.5 mm; the distance between the planes of both SEF sources is 17 mm. (Modified from Stefan 1999 with permission from Lippincott, Williams and Wilkins.)

could be correctly localized in the vicinity of tumors, cysts, and other lesions.

On the other hand, sometimes there is no evidence preoperatively of morphologic pathology associated with epilepsy (Swartz *et al* 1989; Cascino *et al* 1992). Although with the availability of new powerful imaging systems, and more sophisticated software to identify discrete alterations, the number of patients with 'cryptogenic' etiology is decreasing, it is not yet possible to identify a structural abnormality to account for all epileptic foci. In these cases, the lack of morphologic clues renders the functional diagnostic methods more significant. MSI has been found to offer useful source locations of cryptogenic epileptic activity in accordance with other noninvasive results, thus facilitating the detailed planning of invasive interventions and the neurosurgical regimen.

In many patients with pharmacoresistant focal epilepsies, circumscribed clusters of localizations indicating centers of predominant focal epileptic activity were found (Stefan *et al* 1991). If MEG localizations in temporal lobe epilepsy showed more than one cluster in different regions, this indicated multifocal temporal lobe epilepsy.

Because MSI is noninvasive, it is not restricted to inpatients or to presurgical evaluation but is also applicable to projects screening outpatients as in postoperative follow-up. It may be particularly useful in cases where, after an operation, seizures have decreased, but not altogether ceased, and where the defect of the cranial vault and the cavity resulting after resection cause asymmetrical conductivities.

ICTAL RECORDING

As mentioned above, seizures very rarely occur during MEG recording sessions and, if they do, motor artifacts are likely to disturb the brain signals, as is known from EEG. Yet MEG data recorded during auras or seizure onset (Sutherling *et al* 1987; Stefan *et al* 1992, 1993a; Ebersole *et al* 1995; Seino *et al* 1995) may yield dipole localizations reflecting focal activity. Prolonged MEG recordings, split into repeated sessions and interspersed with breaks for the patient to stretch, might be a strategy to provide ictal data during spontaneous

seizures. Another way to obtain seizure-related MEG measurements is to take advantage of procedures that provoke the attacks. Sleep deprivation and withdrawal of antiepileptic drugs can be used for seizure precipitation.

The correlation of ictal and interictal localizations is one important issue that has to be assessed systematically in future research in different types of epilepsies.

MSI IN PREOPERATIVE EVALUATION OF PHARMACORESISTANT EPILEPSIES

Although enthusiastic hopes were aroused in the early years of MEG development that the 'elegant' new technique might be able to replace invasive EEG recordings, they have been less useful than anticipated. In spite of the specific limitations of the MSI technique, e.g. MEG being apt only to localize tangential dipoles, and the comparatively short recording periods that render spontaneous ictal recordings unlikely, the advantages of MSI are undeniable: its noninvasiveness, high spatial and temporal resolution, superior accuracy due to magnetic fields independence of conductivity, and its merging of functional and anatomic information suggest that MSI can play a role among the concert of diagnostic methods that contribute to finding epileptic foci. Yet, since publications on clinical applications of MSI have mostly reported small numbers of cases, the method still lacks statistical demonstration of clinical relevance backed up by large numbers of investigations. Studies comprising MEG as well as EEG data, recorded simultaneously (Ebersole *et al* 1993) and evaluated by means of source reconstruction programs, are of particular interest, enabling clinicians to take full advantage of the merits of both methods and to overcome their respective drawbacks. Indeed, numerous patients have already been investigated whose MSI localizations are being evaluated at present (for example, 250 cases were studied at the Erlangen Epilepsy Center). Another important issue that is being worked upon is the possibility of recording MEG ictal data under activation conditions (Kirchberger *et al* 1998).

KEY POINTS

The applications of MSI in epilepsies can be summarized as follows.

1. Delineation by means of evoked activity of functionally significant areas that should be spared in neurosurgery.

2. Localization of focal epileptic activity to guide invasive procedures and thus reduce invasive regimens.

3. Localization of focal epileptic activity to guide detailed planning of neurosurgical procedures, e.g. with neuronavigation, aimed at the removal of as little tissue as possible.

REFERENCES

Baumgartner C (1993) *Clinical Electrophysiology of the Somatosensory Cortex.* Wien: Springer-Verlag.

Baumgartner C, Barth DS, Levesque MF, Sutherling WW (1992) Detection of epileptiform discharges on magnetoencephalography in comparison to invasive measurements. In: Hoke M, Erne SM, Okada YC, Romani GL (eds) *Biomagnetism: Clinical Aspects*, pp 67–71. Amsterdam: Excerpta Medica.

Cascino GD, Jack JRJ, Parisi JE (1992) Magnetic resonance imaging in intractable frontal lobe epilepsy. Pathologic correlation and prognostic significance. *Epilepsy Research* 11:33–39.

Cheyne D, Kristeva R, Deecke (1991) Homuncular organization of human motor cortex as indicated by neuromagnetic recordings. *Neuroscience Letters* 122:17–20.

Deecke L, Kornhuber HH, Lang W, Lang M, Schreiber H (1985) Timing function of the frontal cortex in sequential motor and learning tasks. *Human Neurobiology* 4:143–154.

Ebersole JS, Squires K, Gamelin J, Lewine J, Scherg M (1993) Simultaneous MEG and EEG provide complementary dipole maps of temporal lobe spikes. *Epilepsia* 34:143.

Ebersole JS, Squires KC, Eliashiv SD, Smith JR (1995) Applications of magnetic source imaging in evaluation of candidates for epilepsy surgery. *Neuroimaging Clinics of North America* 5:267–288.

Eliashiv DS, Squires K, Fried I, Engel JJ (1998) Magnetic source imaging as a localization tool in patients with surgically remediable epilepsies. *Epilepsia* 39(6):80.

Fukao K, Watanabe Y, Kibota H *et al* (1998) The utility of MEG in the diagnosis of focalization related epilepsies. *Epilepsia* 37(5):61.

Gallen CC, Sobel DF, Iragui-Madoz V *et al* (1993) Use of MEG focal slow wave localizations to identify epileptic regions: comparisons with EEG monitoring. *Epilepsia* 34:84.

Ganslandt O, Steinmeier R, Kober H, Romstöck J, Strauss C, Fahlbusch R (1997) Magnetic source imaging combined with image guided frameless stereo surgery. *Neurosurgery* 41:621–628.

Hari R (1990) Magnetic evoked fields of the human brain: basic principles and applications. *Electroencephalography and Clinical Neurophysiology Suppl.* 41:3–12.

Hari R (1994) Magnetoencephalography as a tool of clinical neurophysiology. In: Niedermeyer E, Lopes da Silva F (eds) *Electroencephalography* 3, pp. 1035–1061. Baltimore: Williams and Wilkins.

Hari R, Ahonen A, Forss N *et al* (1993) Parietal epileptic mirror focus detected with a whole-head neuromagnetometer. *Neuroreport* 5:45–48.

Kettenmann B, Jousmaki V, Portin K, Salmelin R, Kobal G, Hari R (1996) Odourants activate the human superior temporal lobe. *Neuroscience Letters* 203:143–145.

Kirchberger K, Hummel C, Stefan H (1998) Postoperative multichannel magnetoencephalography in patients with recurrent seizures after epilepsy surgery. *Acta Neurologica Scandinavica* 98:1–7.

Knowlton RC, Laxer KD, Aminoff MJ, Roberts TPL, Wong STC, Rowley HA (1997) Magnetoencephalography in partial epilepsy:

clinical yield and localization accuracy. *Annals of Neurology* 42.622–631.

Morrell F, Whisler WW, Smith MC, Hoeppner TJ, Toledo-Morrell L, Pierre-Louis SJC (1995) Landau–Kleffner syndrome. Treatment with multiple subpial transection. *Brain* 118:1529–1546.

Nakasato N, Levesque MF, Barth DS, Baumgartner C, Rogers RL, Sutherling WW (1994) Comparisons of MEG, EEG, and ECoG source localization in neocortical partial epilepsy in humans. *Electroencephalography and Clinical Neurophysiology* 91:171–178.

Paetau R, Kajola M, Karhu J *et al* (1992) Magnetoencephalographic localization of epileptic cortex – impact on surgical treatment. *Annals of Neurology* 32:106–109.

Paetau R, Ahonen A, Salonen O, Sams M (1995) Auditory evoked magnetic fields to tones and pseudowords in healthy children and adults. *Journal of Clinical Neurophysiology* 12:177–185.

Papanicolaou AC, Breier JI, Gormley WB *et al* (1998) Comparison of language mapping using extra and intraoperative electrocortical stimulation and magnetoencephalography. *Epilepsia* 39(6):107.

Rose DF, Sato S, Smith PD *et al* (1987) Localization of magnetic interictal discharges in temporal lobe epilepsy. *Annals of Neurology* 22:348–354.

Seino M, Watanabe Y, Fukao K (1995) Interictal and ictal epileptic events observed by multichannel MEG. In: *Visualization of Information Processing in the Human Brain: Recent Advances in MEG and Functional MRI*, pp 35–38. Arcadia Ichigaya.

Smith JR, Gallen C, Orrison W *et al* (1994) Role of multichannel magnetoencephalography in the evaluation of ablative seizure surgery candidates. *Stereotactic and Functional Neurosurgery* 62:238–244.

Stefan H (1999) Plasticity in epilepsy: an outline of the problem. In Stefan H, Shovron S, Andermann F, Chauvel P (eds) *Plasticity in Epilepsy* (in press) Boston: Lippincott and Raven.

Stefan H, Hummel C (1999) Magnetoencephalography. In: Meinardi H (ed.) *Handbook of Neurology. The Epilepsies.* Amsterdam: Elsevier.

Stefan H, Bauer J, Neubauer U, Feistel H, Schulemann H, Huk W-J (1988) *Vergleich von Untersuchungsbefunden der präoperativen Epilepsiediagnostik unter Einbezug eines Mehrkanal-MEG. Deutsche EEG-Gesellschaft*, 33, Jahrestagung, Hamburg.

Stefan H, Schneider S, Abraham Fuchs K *et al* (1990) Magnetic source localization in focal epilepsy. Multichannel magnetoencephalography correlated with magnetic resonance brain imaging. *Brain* 113:1347–1359.

Stefan H, Schneider S, Abraham Fuchs K *et al* (1991) The neocortico to mesio-basal limbic propagation of focal epileptic activity during the spike-wave complex. *Electroencephalography and Clinical Neurophysiology* 79:1–10.

Stefan H, Schneider S, Feistel H *et al* (1992) Ictal and interictal activity in partial epilepsy recorded with multichannel magnetoelectroencephalography: correlation of electroencephalography/electrocorticography, magnetic resonance imaging, single photon emission computed tomography, and positron emission tomography findings. *Epilepsia* 33:874–887.

Stefan H, Abraham Fuchs K, Schneider S, Schuler P, Huk WJ (1993a)

Multichannel magneto-electroencephalography recordings of interictal and ictal activity. *Physiological Measurement* **14**(Suppl 4A):A109–111.

Stefan H, Hummel C, Schneider S *et al* (1993b) Use of mulitchannel MEG in focal epilepsies. In: *Proceedings of Biomagnetism,* Vienna, p 3.

Stefan H, Schuler P, Abraham Fuchs K *et al* (1994) Magnetic source localization and morphological changes in temporal lobe epilepsy: comparison of MEG/EEG, ECoG and volumetric MRI in presurgical evaluation of operated patients. *Acta Neurologica Scandinavica Supplementum* **152**:83–88.

Stefan H, Quesney LF, Feistel HK *et al* (1995) Presurgical evaluation in frontal lobe epilepsy. A multimethodological approach. *Advances in Neurology* **66**:213–220.

Sutherling WW, Crandall PH, Engel J, Jr, Darcey TM, Cahan LD, Barth DS (1987) The magnetic field of complex partial seizures agrees with intracranial localizations. *Annals of Neurology* **21**:548–558.

Sutherling WW, Crandall PH, Darcey TM, Becker DP, Levesque MF, Barth DS (1988) The magnetic and electric fields agree with intracranial localizations of somatosensory cortex. *Neurology* **38**:1705–1714.

Swartz B, Halgren E, Delgado-Escueta AV (1989) Neuroimaging in patients with seizures of probable frontal lobe origin. *Epilepsia* **30**(5):547–558.

30

Neuropsychologic deficits in temporal lobe epilepsy

SM OXBURY

Neuropsychologic function in people with epilepsy is influenced by many variables, including the age at seizure onset, frequency and type of seizures, duration of the habitual epilepsy, interictal EEG discharges, anticonvulsant medication and, of course, the nature and location of the underlying pathology. In focal epilepsy this last factor is the one of major interest, although it is still important to bear in mind the influence of the others. Much work has been devoted to the neuropsychologic status of people with intractable temporal lobe epilepsy (TLE), mainly because the condition may be amenable to surgical treatment; indeed, temporal lobe operations are performed more frequently than is any other surgery for epilepsy. This work has naturally concentrated on possible surgical candidates and hence on individuals with unilateral pathology and/or a predominantly unilateral EEG focus. There is relatively little literature on neuropsychologic deficits in those whose seizures arise from both temporal lobes, although every epilepsy center must be familiar with such patients. Furthermore, many neuropsychologic studies exclude individuals with an intelligence quotient (IQ) below 70 in order to avoid the confounding effects of more diffuse brain damage. Such selection may restrict our understanding of the neuropsychologic picture in the full range of people with TLE.

GENERAL INTELLIGENCE

A number of studies have shown that IQ, as a measure of general intellectual ability, is generally close to the normal range in adults with focal TLE, although the group mean may be shifted downwards by several points. Giordani et al (1985) studied 350 nonsurgical patients, comparing those with partial seizures and those with generalized seizures. The partial seizures were mostly complex partial and so, presumably, were mostly of temporal lobe origin, although this is not specifically stated. The mean WAIS (Wechsler Adult Intelligence Scale Full Scale IQ (FSIQ) was 88 in the partial seizure group, which was significantly higher than that of the generalized seizure group. More recently the Bozeman Epilepsy Consortium, a collaboration between eight epilepsy surgery centers (Strauss et al 1995), described a group of 1185 patients evaluated for possible surgical treatment, 92.6% of them with seizures originating in a temporal lobe. The distribution of IQ scores was negatively skewed, with the mean falling in the lower part of the average range. Patients with temporal lobe foci had a mean FSIQ of 88.8, which was significantly higher, though by only a few points, than that of the extratemporal group (mean FSIQ 85.6). However, defining intellectual impairment as IQ < 80, those with extratemporal disturbances were 1.35 times more likely to be intellectually impaired than those with temporal lobe disturbances. Similarly, Hermann et al (1995a) reported that group means for FSIQ were in the 85–90 range for a surgical series of 215 TLE patients restricted to those with IQ > 69 and excluding those with structural lesions other than mesial temporal sclerosis. The study by Selwa et al (1994) of 59 patients with refractory TLE found similar IQ means both in those treated medically and preoperatively in those treated surgically.

AGE AT SEIZURE ONSET

It is well established that, in general, the age at seizure onset influences IQ. An earlier age of onset is associated with a lower IQ (O'Leary et al 1983; Giordani et al 1985). This holds for the age of onset of habitual seizures in patients with TLE (Saykin et al 1989; Hermann et al 1995a; Strauss et al 1995). Saykin et al (1995) also found that a group of TLE patients who had an 'early risk factor' had lower IQ than TLE patients who had not been exposed to these risks. Early risk was defined as a CNS insult such as a febrile convulsion, encephalitis, or head trauma before the age of 6 years.

DURATION OF SEIZURE HISTORY

The duration of seizure history is another possible factor and is discussed further below. However, Selwa et al (1994) found no evidence of deterioration on reassessment after 1–8 years, in patients whose intractable TLE had been treated medically compared with healthy controls or with patients treated surgically, the majority of whom had become seizure-free.

LATERALITY

The side of the temporal lobe EEG focus, or of the relevant pathology, does not seem to have a consistent effect on general cognitive function (FSIQ), or specifically in the verbal (VIQ) or nonverbal (PIQ) domains.

1. FSIQ was found to be lower in those with left TLE (LTLE) by Strauss et al (1995) and in those undergoing surgery for left-sided pathology by Selwa et al (1994). On the other hand, McMillan et al (1987), Hermann et al (1995a), and Saykin et al (1995) did not find a significant laterality effect.
2. LTLE was associated with lower VIQ by Strauss et al (1995), but not by McMillan et al (1987), Saykin et al

(1995), or Hermann et al (1995a), and with both a lower VIQ and lower PIQ by Selwa et al (1994) in their presurgical patients.
3. No effects of right TLE (RTLE) on PIQ are reported in any of these studies.
4. Discrepancies between VIQ and PIQ, with PIQ higher in LTLE and VIQ higher in RTLE, have sometimes been reported but are a weak and variable finding. Hermann et al's (1995a) study of presurgical patients without structural lesions other than mesial temporal sclerosis on magnetic resonance imaging (MRI) concludes that 'there is no support for lateralising ability of WAIS-R VIQ/PIQ discrepancies.'

Hermann et al (1995a) performed further analyses of the WAIS-R scores in their presurgical groups, examining the 11 subtest scores separately in the groups with left- and right-sided pathology and also performing factor analyses. Laterality differences were found only for the Vocabulary and Similarities subtests, the group with left-sided pathology scoring lower than the group with right-sided pathology, although the Similarities difference ceased to be significant when age at onset was covaried (the group with LTLE having a younger age of onset than the group with RTLE). Factor analysis revealed that the three classic factors – Verbal-Comprehension (comprising Information, Vocabulary, Comprehension, and Similarities subtests), Perceptual-Organization (comprising Picture Completion, Picture Arrangement, Block Design, and Object Assembly subtests), and Freedom from Distraction (comprising Digit Span, Arithmetic, and Digit Symbol subtests) – emerged in this TLE population as in a normal population. Verbal-Comprehension was found to be significantly lower in LTLE than RTLE but again significance disappeared when age at onset was covaried.

NEUROPATHOLOGY

McMillan et al (1987) addressed the question of underlying neuropathology and cognitive function in their report of 40 patients who underwent en bloc temporal lobectomy in the New Maudsley Series. They were able to classify the patients' preexisting neuropathology by examining the resected temporal lobe specimens and to correlate it with the preoperative neuropsychologic function. A similar method was used in the 1980s in Los Angeles (Rausch and Babb 1987) and Oxford (Oxbury and Oxbury 1989) and has since been employed in many other centers.

In terms of general cognitive function or IQ, McMillan et al (1987) found that those with hippocampal sclerosis had lower VIQ and PIQ than a mixed group of other specific pathologies but there were no IQ effects dependent upon the side of the pathology. The studies of Rausch and Babb (1993) and Sass *et al* (1992a), which were concerned primarily with verbal memory and hippocampal neuron loss (see section Memory), reported no relationship between FSIQ or VIQ, respectively, and the degree of neuron loss in specific hippocampal zones. Indeed, one would not predict any particular correlation between neuronal density in a specific hippocampal zone and a general cognitive measure such as IQ.

Hermann *et al* (1997) have further examined the question of generalized cognitive impairment in patients with mesial temporal lobe epilepsy (MTLE). These authors recognize this as a distinct TLE syndrome, in which characteristic classical hippocampal sclerosis is a defining feature, early childhood febrile convulsions and subsequent relatively early onset of habitual epilepsy are common (Sagar and Oxbury 1987), and the response to surgery is usually good. They compared the preoperative neuropsychologic findings of two groups of patients defined by the subsequent neuropathologic examination of their excision specimens: those with classical hippocampal sclerosis fulfilling the criteria for the syndrome of MTLE and those without (non-MTLE). The syndrome of MTLE was associated with cognitive impairment in a considerable number of areas (the WAIS-R factors Verbal-Comprehension and Perceptual-Organization, other language and visuospatial functions, and academic achievement), while other cognitive domains were unimpaired (Freedom from Distraction, Executive Function). Material- and laterality-specific memory impairments were found, which are discussed below. The results were not unexpected as the MTLE group were younger than the others at the onset of their habitual epilepsy. The authors expressed their belief that these generalized neuropsychologic effects are not attributable to the consequences of hippocampal sclerosis *per se* but rather are associated with increasing duration of intractable seizure activity, longer exposure to antiepileptic medication, and other consequences of drug-resistant epilepsy. Their patients had on average 20 or more years of epilepsy, whereas the non-MTLE group had approximately half this duration. They raised the question as to whether the pattern of neuropsychologic findings would be evident in younger patients with a shorter seizure history, and suggested replication of the study with adolescents.

We have examined this question in our Oxford series (Oxbury *et al* 1998). We reviewed the preoperative neuropsychologic performance of 48 consecutive patients, aged 7–35 years, all of whom had suffered a prolonged convulsion before the age of 4 years and whose postoperative histopathology confirmed classical hippocampal sclerosis.

They were divided into two groups by a median split of their years of habitual epilepsy: those with up to 10 years of habitual epilepsy (mean 7.0 years) and those with more than 10 years (mean 16.5 years). A longer duration of habitual epilepsy was not associated with cognitive impairment as measured by IQ scores, verbal learning, or nonverbal memory, giving no support for the view of Hermann *et al* (1997). An earlier age of onset of habitual epilepsy was associated with a lower FSIQ, as expected, and also with lower scores on the Verbal-Comprehension factor. The effect of laterality was also examined. The groups with left-sided and right sided pathology each had 24 patients. They did not differ with respect to age at onset, age at assessment, seizures per year, or years of habitual epilepsy. Those with left-sided pathology were inferior to those with right-sided pathology in tests of verbal learning (an established finding, see below) and also in the Verbal-Comprehension score. To explain this latter finding we propose that the presence of a verbal learning deficit from early in life may lead to reduced acquisition of verbal semantic knowledge. This would be apparent in the Verbal-Comprehension subtests of the Wechsler scales. It might be particularly manifest in the Vocabulary and Information subtests, as was observed in this study.

LANGUAGE FUNCTION

CEREBRAL DOMINANCE

Cerebral language dominance is usually investigated in presurgical TLE patients by means of the intracarotid amobarbital test. Indeed, the survey by Snyder *et al* (1990) revealed that 80% of epilepsy surgery centers use this test routinely. So, there is much information relating to the cerebral language representation in these patients.

Typical left hemisphere language representation was found in approximately 90% of patients in both Loring *et al*'s (1990) study of 103 presurgical TLE patients and Strauss *et al*'s (1995) report of 1185 patients (the majority with TLE). Loring *et al* (1990) related this to handedness, showing left hemisphere language dominance in 90% of right-handers and 75% of those with left or mixed hand preferences. The remainder had right hemisphere language dominance or bilateral representation. Bilateral representation is inferred if there is significant language disturbance after both injections (Oxbury and Oxbury 1984). Bilateral representation does not necessarily imply equal representation in both hemispheres nor that the same language functions are represented in both. It may exist in various forms (Loring *et al* 1990; Snyder *et al* 1990).

Handedness

Both Loring *et al* (1990) and Strauss *et al* (1995) reported 10–12% left or mixed handedness in TLE patients, which is consistent with the normal population. It suggests that left-handedness is seldom acquired in TLE, confirming that the underlying pathology/dysfunction does not often interfere with the normal development of hand preference.

Development of language lateralization

The fact that the proportion of right-handed TLE patients who have left hemisphere language dominance (around 90%) is less than in the normal right-handed population (97% or more) suggests that TLE or an associated factor interferes with the normal development of language lateralization. The apparent shortfall in TLE patients may be at least partly because a significant number of them have bilateral representation, although 'pure' right hemisphere dominance is rare (Oxbury and Oxbury 1984; Loring *et al* 1990). We do not, of course, know how many normal people would make language errors after both a right and a left injection. However, if the finding in TLE patients is not an artifact, nor simply an uncharted 'normal' phenomenon, it implies that there has been some subtle effect on the development of language lateralization. Temporal lobe damage is present from early childhood in many TLE patients, for instance in those with hippocampal sclerosis or dysembryoplastic neuroepithelial tumors, and so an effect on the development of cerebral lateralization of function would not be surprising. Such an effect may not be limited to those with early damage on the left since bilateral representation is not significantly related to the laterality of seizure onset (Oxbury and Oxbury 1984; Powell *et al* 1987; Loring *et al* 1990). Furthermore, there are already suggestions that early risk factors might affect the organization of language *within* the left hemisphere (Stafiniak *et al* 1990; Saykin *et al* 1995). A comparison of the interhemispheric and intrahemispheric functional asymmetries in focal epilepsy patients and normal subjects may become possible with the use of functional MRI, which is already being piloted as a possible alternative to the intracarotid amobarbital test for the determination of cerebral dominance (Hertz-Pannier *et al* 1997).

LINGUISTIC DEFICIT

People with TLE do not usually have clinically obvious language disturbance or dysphasia but reports that they experience word-finding difficulty are not uncommon. The work of Mayeux *et al* (1980) is frequently cited. While investigating the relationship between memory and language impairment in people with TLE they compared non-surgical groups of patients with left temporal foci (LTLE), right temporal foci (RTLE), and generalized epilepsy on a number of verbal cognitive and memory measures. The groups differed only on the Boston Naming Test, where patients with LTLE were inferior to the other groups who scored within the normal range.

Several surgical centers have reported evaluation of language function in patients with LTLE and RTLE before surgery. The findings have not been entirely consistent. Hermann and Wyler (1988) and Hermann *et al* (1991), using the Multilingual Aphasia Examination, found that overall patients with LTLE were inferior to those with RTLE, although there was no significant difference on any individual subtest. A subsequent study (Hermann *et al* 1992) employing a greater number of subjects showed clearer differences between patients with LTLE and those with RTLE, subjects with LTLE being significantly inferior on visual naming, sentence repetition, the token test, reading comprehension, and aural comprehension; furthermore, subjects with RTLE were impaired on five of seven subtests.

Saykin *et al* (1995) reported patients with LTLE to be significantly inferior to those with RTLE on the Boston Naming Test but not on other language measures. Sass *et al* (1992a) also found presurgical LTLE patients inferior to RTLE patients on the Boston Naming Test, as did Davies *et al* (1994) in a group who were to have grid-directed surgery, although the difference did not emerge in those who were to have temporal lobe surgery without functional mapping (Davies *et al* 1995), despite this latter group of patients with LTLE being inferior to those with RTLE on other verbal measures (subtests of the WAIS-R).

Langfitt and Rausch (1996) found no preoperative differences between subjects with LTLE and those with RTLE on the sensitive full version of the Boston Naming Test (85 items), although *both* groups were significantly below the published norms. Ellis *et al* (1991) found that nonsurgical LTLE patients were inferior to RTLE patients on naming (Graded Naming Test; McKenna and Warrington 1983), reading (National Adult Reading Test; Nelson 1982), and a test of the comprehension of grammatical forms (Test for the Reception of Grammar; Bishop 1989). Both groups were inferior to normal controls in all tests.

Thus there are numerous suggestions that word-finding difficulty occurs among patients with LTLE, most frequently in visual naming tasks. There are also hints that LTLE patients may be mildly deficient in other areas of language function and that, furthermore, there may be some degree of deficit in RTLE patients. The few inconsistent findings may be due to factors such as sampling, differences in underlying pathology, size of samples, and the specific nature and sensitivity of the tests used.

Neuropathology and pathophysiology

Many patients have cell loss in their medial temporal lobe structures that usually would not be thought likely to be associated with naming disability. Nevertheless, functional mapping of the basal temporal areas has shown that there may be linguistic effects from electrical stimulation of the parahippocampal gyrus, which has been implicated in the mesial temporal epileptic process (Schäffler *et al* 1994).

Lateral cortical dysfunction is a more likely explanation for the language deficits. Such dysfunction could result from structural pathology, interictal discharges that might in turn cause transient cognitive impairment, or hypometabolism (or altered metabolism) that may be seen in areas considerably beyond the pathologic tissue or EEG focus (Arnold *et al* 1996). Indeed, Corcoran and Upton (1993) have shown that TLE patients with extrahippocampal pathology are inferior in word fluency tasks to those with MRI evidence of hippocampal sclerosis. All these factors may vary considerably between individuals, as may the exact extent and location of the language zones that would be vulnerable to their influence.

Another possibility is that some patients simply acquire less linguistic and verbal competence in a more general way. Most neuropsychologists who have experience of patients with severe classical hippocampal sclerosis in the dominant hemisphere will recognize the paucity of their linguistic competence, which may contrast sharply with their visuospatial ability. As described above, there are suggestions of lower VIQ factors, lower Vocabulary, and lower Information scores in this group, and their poor naming ability may partly reflect a less extensive lexicon or word store.

LOCATION OF CORTICAL LANGUAGE AREAS

It is well recognized that the precise location of the classical cortical language zones in the frontal lobe and the temporoparietal region, corresponding to Broca's and Wernicke's areas, may show considerable individual variability when mapped by stimulation studies prior to surgery for epilepsy (Ojemann *et al* 1989). Devinsky *et al* (1993) studied language localization in patients undergoing dominant temporal lobectomy. Those with naming deficits evoked by stimulation in the anterior part of the temporal lobe (4.5 cm from the temporal pole) had an earlier age of onset of their seizures than did those without such deficits. Surgery was tailored individually to spare these language

areas and there was no difference in postoperative linguistic outcome between those with, and those without, anterior language representation. The authors suggested that an early onset of dominant temporal lobe seizures leads to a more widespread or atypical distribution of the language areas in the cerebral cortex. Saykin *et al* (1995) reached a similar conclusion based on their observation of an acute decline in naming after anterior temporal lobectomy in those without early risk factors but not in those with early risks. They suggested that those with early risks involving the left temporal lobe may be protected from the disrupting acute effects of anterior temporal lobectomy because they have an atypically diffuse representation of their semantic stores or a more widespread distribution of pathways relevant to naming processes.

It is known that factors associated with left hemisphere dysfunction in early life may be associated with atypical laterality of hemispheric language representation. It is of particular interest that this may also apply to language localization within the left hemisphere in patients whose pathology and/or EEG focus is situated in the medial part of the temporal lobe.

MEMORY

The importance of medial temporal lobe structures in anterograde memory function has long been established. The case of H.M., who developed severe and lasting amnesia after bilateral removal of these structures (Scoville and Milner 1957), is well known. A similar memory disorder, accompanied by chronic focal epilepsy, can occur as a consequence of various bilateral temporal lobe pathologies such as herpes simplex virus encephalitis (Oxbury and MacCallum 1973). (The features of the severe amnesic syndrome are described in Chapter 60.)

The laterality- and material-specific deficits seen after unilateral temporal lobe surgery are also well established. Thus, verbal memory deficits are found after left dominant operations (Meyer and Yates 1955; Milner 1958; Frisk and Milner 1990) and nonverbal memory deficits after right nondominant operations (Kimura 1963; Milner 1965; Smith and Milner 1981). The verbal memory deficit is very consistent and reliable and has been found on a wide variety of tasks, both standardized memory tests, such as logical memory and paired associate learning from the Wechsler Memory Scale, and more experimental tasks. The nonverbal deficit is less reliably seen. The extent of hippocampal removal and the type of test paradigm are important factors related to these findings (Milner 1971; Jones-Gotman

1991). However, these postoperative findings do not tell us about the status of the unoperated or nonsurgical patient with TLE.

MIXED PATHOLOGY SERIES

Numerous studies have shown that patients with TLE have memory impairment compared with healthy controls and groups with other focal epilepsy. There have been many comparisons of patients with LTLE and those with RTLE on various measures of verbal and nonverbal memory, using groups of presurgical or nonsurgical patients, in the quest for laterality- and material-specific impairments. Many of the studies have been with mixed pathology groups or groups in which patients with structural lesions on MRI have been excluded but the presence or absence of hippocampal sclerosis has not been taken into account. The results have been inconsistent.

Verbal memory

Story recall tasks

Story recall tasks have shown patients with LTLE to be inferior to those with RTLE in the following studies: Delaney *et al* (1980) for delayed but not immediate story recall; Selwa *et al* (1994) for immediate but not delayed story recall; Moore and Baker (1996) for both immediate and delayed recall; and Prevey *et al* (1988) in the use of learning strategies and distortions of meaning, but not in immediate or delayed gist recall.

On the other hand, Mayeux *et al* (1980) and Saykin *et al* (1989) found no difference between LTLE and RTLE patients on immediate or delayed story recall, although those with early-onset epilepsy were clearly inferior to those with a later onset regardless of laterality. Breier *et al* (1996) found no difference between patients with LTLE and those with RTLE in delayed story recall.

Word list learning

Word list learning was found to be impaired in patients with LTLE compared with those with RTLE in the following studies: Hermann *et al* (1987) on several measures derived from the California Verbal Learning Test (CVLT); Helmstaedter *et al* (1995) on some measures from an equivalent German verbal learning test; Giovagnoli *et al* (1996) on multiple delayed trials on a verbal selective reminding test (VSRT); and Breier *et al* (1996) on the last trial only of a VSRT.

On the other hand, the study by Loring *et al* (1988) showed that LTLE and RTLE patients were not significantly different on a VSRT, although more patients with LTLE than those with RTLE tended to fall into the 'fail' category. A paired associate learning task (Wechsler Memory Scale) did not distinguish between patients with LTLE and those with RTLE in the study by Selwa *et al* (1994).

Other tests

A verbal distractor task based on the Brown–Peterson paradigm revealed that patients with LTLE were inferior to those with RTLE in the study by Giovagnoli and Avanzini (1996) but not in that by Mayeux *et al* (1980).

The Recognition Memory Test (Warrington 1984) for words did not distinguish between patients with LTLE and those with RTLE in the studies of Ellis *et al* (1991) and Hermann *et al* (1995b).

In many of these reports both LTLE and RTLE patients were inferior to normal controls and/or others with focal epilepsy. With the exception of the Recognition Memory Test, the patients in the LTLE group were almost never reported to be performing normally and those in the RTLE group only infrequently so.

Nonverbal memory

Only a few studies have reported patients with RTLE to be inferior to those with LTLE. They include Delaney *et al* (1980) who used a recurring figure memory task (Kimura 1963) and Ellis *et al* (1991) who used recognition of familiar faces. Helmstaedter *et al* (1991) used a learning task involving eight figures, each made up of five lines, presented over six trials. In this study patients with RTLE were inferior to those with LTLE and controls on five different measures: learning curve, first trial and last trial scores, total number correct, and tendency to make rotation errors. Patients with LTLE were also inferior to controls on three of the five measures.

Two *figural memory* tasks have been used frequently: the Visual Reproduction subtest of the Wechsler Memory Scale, comprising immediate and delayed recall and percent retained; and delayed recall of the Rey Osterrieth Complex Figure. Few significant differences have emerged between presurgical or nonsurgical groups of RTLE and LTLE patients. There have sometimes been postoperative differences but even this has been an inconsistent finding. Sass *et al* (1992b) found patients with RTLE to be inferior to those with LTLE on the Visual Reproduction subtest immediate recall. Conversely, no laterality differences were found by Mayeux *et al* (1980), Delaney *et al* (1980),

Loring *et al* (1988), Saykin *et al* (1989), Moore and Baker (1996), Breier *et al* (1996), or even by Barr *et al* (1997) reporting on 757 cases of unilateral TLE from the Bozeman Consortium of eight epilepsy centers.

There has been much discussion about the nature of these so-called nonverbal memory tasks and whether their failure to distinguish between RTLE and LTLE can be explained by the material being too easily verbalized and hence amenable to mediation by verbal memory systems (see below). Helmstaedter *et al* (1995) tackled this problem with another figural memory task, the Benton Visual Retention Test. There were no laterality differences on the conventional scores. However, reanalysis, after discarding the easily verbalizable figures and retaining only those items that contained too much information to lend themselves effectively to the verbal strategy, showed that patients with RTLE performed worse than those with LTLE who were inferior to controls.

HIPPOCAMPAL SCLEROSIS

Over the last 10 years neuropsychologic research in TLE has focused more on specific pathologies, particularly on patients with unilateral hippocampal sclerosis. In this discussion the term 'hippocampal sclerosis' is used, as far as possible, to refer to a severe depletion of hippocampal pyramidal neurons with gliosis, particularly in the CA1 and CA3–CA5 zones, and of the dentate granule cells. This corresponds to the state described as Ammon's horn sclerosis by Margerison and Corsellis (1966) and Sagar and Oxbury (1987), as 'classical' or 'total' Ammon's horn sclerosis by Bruton (1988), and as MTLE+ by Hermann *et al* (1997). In MRI terms this probably corresponds to hippocampal atrophy represented by a volume asymmetry at least two standard deviations beyond that of normal control values.

Hippocampal sclerosis is the most common single pathology underlying intractable TLE, and surgical outcome with respect to seizures is good. Can neuropsychologic assessment delineate the typical picture in those with right or left hippocampal sclerosis? Verbal memory has been studied in this context to a much greater extent than nonverbal memory because verbal memory impairment is more reliably seen and is clinically more relevant in that patients' self-reports more often suggest problems in this area.

The question has been addressed by investigating the relationship between preoperative memory performance and either the neuronal loss in the mesial temporal structures including the hippocampus, established by histopathologic examination of the excised specimen postoperatively, or various hippocampal measures seen on preoperative brain imaging. These methods have been reviewed by Baxendale (1995).

Verbal memory

The specific nature of the task must be taken into account when considering the relationship between verbal memory and the laterality of hippocampal sclerosis (Saling *et al* 1993). The tests most frequently used may be divided into two types: those requiring recall of semantically related verbal material, usually presented only once (story recall or logical memory); and those involving learning over several trials of word pairs or word lists that include unrelated material.

Story recall tasks

In studies that used preoperative story recall where the neuropathology was confirmed by examination of the subsequent excision specimens, the following findings have been reported.

1. Patients with left hippocampal sclerosis were inferior to those with right hippocampal sclerosis on delayed recall, but there were no differences on immediate recall (Miller *et al* 1993).
2. Patients with left hippocampal sclerosis and those with right hippocampal sclerosis did not differ on either immediate or delayed recall (McMillan *et al* 1987; Oxbury and Oxbury 1989; Saling *et al* 1993).
3. Patients with left hippocampal sclerosis and those with right hippocampal sclerosis performed worse than those with no, or only minor degrees of, hippocampal neuron loss (Oxbury and Oxbury 1989; Saling *et al* 1993); Hermann *et al* (1997) reported the same for patients with LTLE.
4. Recall was unrelated to the degree of sclerosis in either the group with left hippocampal sclerosis or that with right hippocampal sclerosis (Rausch and Babb 1993).

Some studies have examined the relationship using neuronal counts in specific hippocampal subfields. Sass *et al* (1992a) found no correlation between immediate and delayed recall and counts in hippocampal subfields, although in patients with left hippocampal sclerosis the percentage retained correlated with counts in both the CA3 and the hilar zones. Matkovic *et al* (1995a) found a correlation between delayed paragraph recall and counts in CA1 in patients with right hippocampal sclerosis.

In studies that used preoperative story recall where hippocampal sclerosis was assessed by MRI volumetrics, the following findings have been reported.

1. Kalviäinen *et al* (1997) found left hippocampal volume to be positively correlated with immediate and delayed story recall in newly diagnosed TLE patients.
2. Lencz *et al* (1992) found a correlation in patients with left hippocampal sclerosis only for the percentage retained score.
3. Trenerry *et al* (1993) found no correlation between the two measures in patients with either left or right hippocampal sclerosis.
4. Jones-Gotman (1996) found no differences between patients with left and those with right hippocampal sclerosis.

Verbal learning tasks

Verbal learning tasks have been more successful than story recall in characterizing left and right hippocampal sclerosis. These include a paired associate learning task (PALT) from the Wechsler Memory Scale, word list learning of the Rey Auditory Verbal Learning Test (RAVLT) type or CVLT type, and word list learning using a VSRT. On the whole, verbal learning appears to be more specifically associated with left dominant hippocampus than does story recall, which frequently fails to distinguish between left and right hippocampal sclerosis.

Using PALT, Rausch and Babb (1993), Saling *et al* (1993), Miller *et al* (1993), and Matkovic *et al* (1995a) have all reported differences between patients with left and those with right hippocampal sclerosis who had varying degrees of sclerosis; Sass *et al* (1990) found similar results using VSRT. Using CVLT, Arnold *et al* (1996) found LTLE patients, but not RTLE patients, to be impaired compared with normal controls. Also using CVLT, Hermann *et al* (1997) showed that those with severe left hippocampal sclerosis performed worse than those with only minor left-sided hippocampal neuron loss. Left, but not right, hippocampal neuron counts correlate with performance on verbal learning tasks. Thus, counts in the CA3 and hilar (CA4) zones correlate with VSRT (Sass *et al* 1990), and in CA4 with PALT (Matkovic *et al* 1995a).

Kalviäinen *et al* (1997) found that left hippocampal volume, measured on MRI, correlated with word list learning scores in newly diagnosed LTLE patients. Likewise, Kilpatrick *et al* (1997), but not Trenerry *et al* (1993) or Lencz *et al* (1992), found that left, but not right, hippocampal volume was positively correlated with several RAVLT measures. A word list learning task, but not PALT, distinguished between left and right hippocampal sclerosis, as determined by MRI, in the study of Jones-Gotman (1996).

Nonverbal memory

Figural memory tasks have frequently been used in patients with hippocampal sclerosis but, as with the mixed pathology groups, have not shown consistent differences between groups with right and those with left hippocampal sclerosis. Hermann *et al* (1997) found that patients with severe hippocampal sclerosis were impaired on the Visual Reproduction test, irrespective of the side of the pathology. Arnold *et al* (1996) found no differences between patients with right and those with left hippocampal sclerosis and controls on the Rey Osterrieth delayed recall. Jones-Gotman (1996) found no differences between patients with right and those with left hippocampal sclerosis on either Visual Reproduction or Rey Osterrieth recall, although she did find that patients with right hippocampal sclerosis were inferior to those with left hippocampal sclerosis in design learning (a task involving four trials to learn 13 designs or figures and additional testing after delays).

More specific correlations between performance on these figural tests and the degree of right hippocampal sclerosis have revealed only one positive result. Matkovic *et al* (1995b) reported significant correlations between neuronal counts and delayed recall of the Rey Osterrieth Figure for patients with RTLE (CA4) and those with LTLE (CA1 and CA4), and between the Benton Visual Retention Test and CA4 for patients with RTLE. Kilpatrick *et al* (1997) found no correlation between Rey Osterrieth recall, or Austin Maze learning, and the degree of right hippocampal smallness, compared with the left side, as measured on MRI. However, Rey Osterrieth delayed recall scores did correlate with the degree of left hippocampal smallness compared with the right side. Visual Reproduction scores did not correlate with hippocampal neuronal density in the study of Sass *et al* (1992b), nor did they correlate with MRI hippocampal volumes in the study of Trenerry *et al* (1993).

AMYGDALA SCLEROSIS

Hudson *et al* (1993) have described 16 patients with amygdala sclerosis demonstrated by histopathologic examination of their excision specimens; half had associated hippocampal sclerosis. Preoperative memory tests included Logical Memory, Visual Reproduction and PALT, Rey Osterrieth Figure recall, and the Warrington Recognition Memory Test (WRMT) for words and faces. Patients' performances were compared with those of 10 matched normal controls. Those with hippocampal sclerosis performed significantly worse on the WRMT for words and on Visual Reproduction than those without hippocampal sclerosis, who did not differ significantly from the normals. On PALT both those with, and those without, hippocampal sclerosis were inferior to normals, those without hippocampal sclerosis being intermediate between the other two groups. No information about the side of the pathology was given. The authors concluded that those with amygdala sclerosis alone had milder memory impairments than those with both amygdala and hippocampal sclerosis.

DUAL PATHOLOGY

Hippocampal sclerosis and cortical dysplasia

Baxendale (1997) examined recognition memory (WRMT for words and faces) in patients with unilateral hippocampal sclerosis and those with unilateral hippocampal sclerosis combined with cortical dysplasia. Those with hippocampal sclerosis alone were mildly impaired on both tasks with no laterality difference on either. Those with left dual pathology performed significantly worse on the word task than the other groups, whereas those with right dual pathology performed significantly better. The groups with right and left hippocampal sclerosis with dual pathology were both significantly impaired compared with normals on the faces task. Baxendale comments that although the Recognition Memory Test does not discriminate between left and right hippocampal sclerosis, it may provide a pointer to additional temporal lobe pathology such as cortical dysplasia.

Hippocampal sclerosis and other temporal lobe structural lesions

Sass et al (1995) examined the contribution of associated hippocampal neuronal loss to verbal memory impairment among TLE patients with structural lesions, mostly tumors and a few other pathologies such as vascular malformations and cortical dysplasia. Verbal memory was measured by the long-term retrieval score from VSRT and logical memory percentage retained, these having shown correlations with left hippocampal neuronal densities in previous studies (Sass et al 1990, 1992a). In patients with LTLE there were significant correlations between long-term retrieval and neuronal density in CA1, and between percentage retained and neuronal density in CA2, indicating that the pathologic status of the hippocampus is an important factor underlying memory performance in patients with structural temporal lobe lesions.

RHS AND NONVERBAL MEMORY: INCONSISTENT FINDINGS

There is relatively little evidence for an association between nonverbal memory impairment and right or nondominant

hippocampal sclerosis, or for the ability of nonverbal memory impairment to distinguish between right and left hippocampal sclerosis. Several explanations have been suggested for this.

The nature of the test material

Many figural memory stimuli are too easily verbalized. Thus those who might have difficulty remembering the figures can use verbal strategies to compensate; conversely those with verbal memory impairment might be at a disadvantage, further confounding the results. Other types of stimuli, particularly those with a greater spatial component, may be more relevant. Milner's (1965) visually guided maze learning task has consistently given results suggesting a strong hippocampal component in postoperative studies. The same is true of Smith and Milner's (1981) incidental spatial memory task. It is a pity that more effort has not been made to produce properly standardized tests for clinical use based on these findings.

The method of testing and the learning component of the task

Since the most consistent differences in verbal memory between patients with left and those with right hippocampal sclerosis have been found on verbal learning tasks, it is reasonable to attempt to devise similarly constructed tests of nonverbal memory. There has been some success with this approach. Both Jones-Gotman (1996) and Helmstaedter et al (1991) have used tasks that involve the learning of several unfamiliar figures over multiple trials. The Bonn group (Gleissner et al 1998) have recently reported that patients with right hippocampal sclerosis, but not RTLE patients without hippocampal sclerosis, show a preoperative deficit compared with normal controls on the Helmstaedter task, most clearly in a 'learning capacity' score. No comparison with LTLE patients was made.

The right hippocampus may be less specialized

The right hippocampus may be less specialized for visual and/or spatial learning than is the left for verbal learning. This may be so in normals. Patients with TLE based on early right hippocampal damage may have some cerebral reorganization such that the left hemisphere or other regions of the right hemisphere take over aspects of the nonverbal memory function of the right hippocampus. Such reorganization may be less possible in relation to verbal memory and learning capability of the left hippocampus following its early damage. In any case, memory function is not entirely lateralized, even in normals; rather there is a degree of specialization in each hemisphere.

EXECUTIVE FUNCTION

The performance of people with frontal lobe damage is impaired on so-called 'executive function' tasks (see Chapter 31). Several studies have reported that the performance of patients with TLE is also deficient on some of these tests.

The Wisconsin Card Sorting Test (WCST) tests mental flexibility and detects perseverative tendencies. It was originally shown to be sensitive to dorsolateral frontal lesions (Milner 1963). Reports that patients with TLE are impaired on the WCST include those of Hermann *et al* (1988), Corcoran and Upton (1993), Strauss *et al* (1993), Trenerry and Jack (1994), Hermann and Seidenberg (1995), and Horner *et al* (1996). Hermann *et al* (1988) found that impairment occurred more often in patients with RTLE than in those with LTLE. Similarly, Corcoran and Upton (1993), using the Modified WCST (Nelson 1976), found that patients with right hippocampal sclerosis performed worse than those with left hippocampal sclerosis. Strauss *et al* (1993), on the other hand, found a greater impairment in LTLE patients and in those with onset of seizures at a young age. Horner *et al* (1996) found no laterality difference. Corcoran and Upton (1993) found impairment to be more marked in patients with TLE due to hippocampal sclerosis than in those with TLE due to neocortical lesions or those with lesional frontal lobe epilepsy. The performance of these latter two groups did not differ. They proposed a role for the hippocampus in this task based on the concept of the hippocampus as a 'comparator,' whereby information about previous responses is used to guide behavior (Gray 1982). Subsequent work has provided little support for this hypothesis. Thus, Trenerry and Jack (1994), using MRI hippocampal volume measures, did not find any significant association between hippocampal sclerosis and preoperative WCST performance. Likewise, Hermann and Seidenberg (1995) found no significant difference between patients with, and those without, hippocampal sclerosis. Nor did they find any exacerbation of the impairment postoperatively, which the hippocampal hypothesis would have predicted for those who had removal of nonsclerotic hippocampus. Rather, the group with, and the group without, hippocampal sclerosis both tended to improve. Improvement was significantly more frequent in those who became seizure-free than in those who did not.

Their findings led Hermann and Seidenberg (1995) to reject the hippocampal explanation of executive deficits in TLE patients in favor of a 'nociferous cortex hypothesis,' which posits that discharges from epileptogenic medial temporal lobe structures adversely affect the extratemporal regions that mediate performance on executive tasks, thereby resulting in deficits. There is support for this view from studies of TLE using positron emission tomography (PET). These have shown hypometabolism in ipsilateral zones beyond the hippocampus and in bilateral frontal regions (Arnold *et al* 1996), and a relationship between prefrontal metabolism and performance on frontal lobe executive tests (Jokeit *et al* 1997).

Verbal fluency, the ability to rapidly produce words beginning with a specified letter or in a specified semantic category, has also been associated with frontal lobe function, particularly in the dominant hemisphere. Martin *et al* (1990) found deficits in a presurgical group of TLE patients, those with LTLE being inferior to those with RTLE who were also impaired compared with normal controls in both letter and semantic fluency tasks. Corcoran and Upton (1993) found that TLE patients with lateral temporal lobe pathology showed the same degree of impairment as those with frontal lobe epilepsy, while TLE patients with hippocampal sclerosis performed better. These findings support the view that both temporal and frontal regions participate in systems necessary for word fluency performance, as suggested by Parks *et al* (1988) in PET studies with normal subjects.

Thus, TLE patients may show deficits in at least two executive function tasks, WCST and word fluency, possibly due to distal effects of a discharging focus in one case and to the direct effects of temporal lobe damage in the other.

CHILDREN

Much has been written about cognitive function in children with epilepsy, although relatively few studies have focused specifically on TLE. In general, neuropsychologic function in children with epilepsy is influenced by the same factors as in adults (see above). To these, some would add secondary psychosocial factors, such as interruption of the learning process, due to frequent absences from school, and lowered self-esteem. One may also ask whether the nature and location of the pathology has different cognitive effects in children compared with adults, since early damage may modify the development of cerebral organization of function or be compensated by greater plasticity in the younger brain. In intractable TLE, however, this question may not be entirely relevant since many adults have early seizure onset and/or pathology that has been present from childhood. Indeed, many of them were children with epilepsy who grew up with unremitting seizures.

DEVELOPMENTAL LEVEL AND IQ

Overall, the developmental level and IQ in children with intractable TLE appears to vary from severe retardation to the normal range, with most falling in or near the average range. As with adult patients there is no consistent association between VIQ/PIQ differences and laterality of temporal lobe pathology.

Surgical series

Meyer *et al* (1986) described 50 children with a mean FSIQ of 91.6 when operated at 7–18 years of age. This is very similar to the median preoperative developmental quotient or FSIQ of 90 (range 33–112) in the 44 children reported by Adams *et al* (1990) who had surgery when aged 2–15 years. There were no significant differences according to laterality of TLE or type of pathology. PIQ tended to be higher than VIQ regardless of the side of pathology, particularly for those with hippocampal sclerosis.

Recently our group have reviewed 11 children aged 2–11 years with dysembryoplastic neuroepithelial tumors. The preoperative developmental quotients in the five preschool children (two average, two low, one severely delayed) indicated slower development than in the six older children, five of whom had average IQ. VIQ tended to be lower than PIQ, with individual discrepancies varying widely and unrelated to the laterality of the pathology (Knight *et al* 1998). Examination of a group of patients with severe hippocampal sclerosis aged 7–35 years has confirmed that age at onset is a significant factor in determining IQ level within this specific pathology group (Oxbury *et al* 1998).

VIQ and PIQ in nonsurgical studies

Fedio and Mirsky (1969) suggested that when there are large VIQ/PIQ discrepancies they are consistent with the side of EEG focus. In contrast, Camfield *et al* (1984), who studied 27 children with unilateral temporal lobe EEG foci, found no differences between patients with LTLE and those with RTLE with regard to FSIQ, VIQ, or PIQ. Similarly, Jambaqué *et al* (1993) reported that their RTLE and LTLE subgroups had average IQ and did not differ in VIQ/PIQ discrepancies. IQ was lower in those with

bilateral temporal lobe foci. All these studies excluded children who were cognitively retarded.

Gadian *et al* (1996) used magnetic resonance spectroscopy (MRS) to measure the extent of hippocampal sclerosis and related it to cognitive function in 22 children with intractable TLE. The group had a mean VIQ of 88 (range 51–118) and PIQ of 100 (56–142). VIQ was related to the MRS measure of pathology in the left temporal lobe and PIQ to the extent of pathology in the right temporal lobe, although less than 30% of the variance in IQ was attributable to this factor.

LANGUAGE

Published reports of the systematic evaluation of language function in children with TLE are sparse but there are indications that communication difficulties do exist. Caplan *et al* (1993) evaluated communication in children aged 5–16 years before and after temporal lobectomy. Preoperatively they were impaired, compared with normal children, in both a thought disorder (illogical thinking) and a discourse (cohesion) measure. The illogical thinking rating became normal after surgery, suggesting that the preoperative deficit may have been attributable to distal effects of the temporal lobe focus or pathology, possibly on the frontal lobes. Similarly, Kosciesza *et al* (1998) found that children aged 7–15 years with epilepsy and normal intelligence, including a subgroup with TLE, were impaired in syntactic and semantic elements of speech. Within the TLE group the deficit was more prominent in those patients with LTLE.

In children with early-onset severe TLE there is little evidence that language development in an overall sense is related to side of pathology. Thus, language development was not favored compared with other functions in the five children aged < 6 years with right temporal lobe dysembryoplastic neuroepithelial tumors mentioned above (Knight *et al* 1998).

MEMORY

There is some evidence of modality-specific memory impairment in children with TLE, although it is by no means invariable and usually LTLE and RTLE patients show deficits in both verbal and nonverbal memory.

Fedio and Mirsky (1969) found that children with LTLE were impaired on a delayed verbal memory task while those with RTLE were impaired on delayed nonverbal memory. Such a clear-cut result has not been replicated. Thus, Cohen (1992) reported that whereas children with LTLE scored significantly lower than normals on all his verbal memory tasks, they differed significantly from those with RTLE only on one (VSRT). Also, children with RTLE were inferior to normals on story recall. Children with RTLE and those with LTLE were impaired, compared with normals, on 2/5 visual or spatial subtests but did not differ from each other. Jambaqué *et al* (1993) found that children with LTLE were impaired compared with normals on all the verbal memory measures used, whereas those with RTLE differed from normals only on word list recall (a learning task); however, the authors did not compare the LTLE group with the RTLE group. Furthermore, children with RTLE and those with LTLE differed from normals on most of the visual or spatial tasks. A relative difference score (auditory/verbal minus visual/spatial) was negative in children with LTLE and positive in those with RTLE, indicating that overall verbal memory tended to be inferior to nonverbal memory in children with LTLE and vice versa in those with RTLE. Hershey *et al* (1998) also compared children with LTLE, those with RTLE, and normals on a variety of memory tasks, including a spatial short-term measure following the Brown–Peterson paradigm. Both groups with TLE were inferior to normals on most tasks, both verbal and spatial, but did not differ significantly from each other. Unusually, neither group with TLE differed from normal in the story recall task. In the study by Gadian *et al* (1996) of children with TLE, paired associate learning was associated with the left, but not the right, temporal lobe MRS measure.

Surgical groups

Meyer *et al* (1986) reported that the Wechsler Memory Scale Memory Quotient of their children was within the normal range (mean MQ 91.9). However, this is a composite score and no distinction was made between verbal and nonverbal measures or between children with LTLE and those with RTLE. Adams *et al* (1990) found no preoperative difference between the LTLE and RTLE groups on PALT, immediate and delayed story recall, or delayed Rey Osterrieth recall. Both groups scored below the average range on almost all measures, suggesting a general memory impairment.

KEY POINTS

1. The mean FSIQ of groups of patients with TLE falls in the lower part of the average range. IQ tends to be lower among those with early seizure onset and in those with hippocampal sclerosis, although the two factors are difficult to separate. People with left-sided hippocampal sclerosis seem to have reduced acquisition of verbal semantic knowledge.

2. LTLE patients may have word-finding difficulties and may be deficient in other areas of language function. There may also be some degree of language deficit in RTLE patients. Left hemisphere dysfunction early in life may be associated with atypical laterality of language dominance and with atypical localization of language function within the left hemisphere.

3. Intractable TLE is, in general, associated with poor memory irrespective of the underlying pathology or the side of the epileptogenic focus. This is particularly prominent for verbal memory in those with LTLE.

4. Left hippocampal sclerosis is consistently associated with impaired verbal learning. Recall of semantically related verbal material is usually impaired in patients with hippocampal sclerosis but without any clear difference between left and right hippocampal sclerosis.

5. There is, as yet, no evidence that the laterality of hippocampal sclerosis consistently affects performance on nonverbal memory tasks. A possible reason is that testing has mostly used techniques that do not sufficiently measure learning in the absence of verbal mediation. Never-theless, patients with right and those with left hippocampal sclerosis often show impairment on what are considered to be nonverbal memory tasks.

6. Bilateral medial temporal lobe damage can result in a severe anterograde memory deficit (severe amnesic syndrome).

7. Some TLE patients are impaired on some executive function tasks that are sensitive to frontal lobe damage.

8. Most children with TLE have IQ within or near the average range. They usually have an impairment of both verbal and nonverbal memory irrespective of the side of the temporal lobe pathology and/or the EEG focus.

REFERENCES

Adams CBT, Beardsworth ED, Oxbury SM, Oxbury JM, Fenwick PBC (1990) Temporal lobectomy in 44 children: outcome and neuropsychological follow-up. *Journal of Epilepsy* **3** (Suppl 1):157–168.

Arnold S, Schlaug G, Niemann H *et al* (1996) Topography of interictal glucose hypometabolism in unilateral mesiotemporal epilepsy. *Neurology* **46**:1422–1429.

Barr WB, Chelune GJ, Hermann BP *et al* (1997) The use of figural reproduction tests as measures of nonverbal memory in epilepsy surgery candidates. *Journal of the International Neuropsychology Society* **3**:435–443.

Baxendale SA (1995) The hippocampus: functional and structural correlations. *Seizure* **4**:105–117.

Baxendale SA (1997) The role of the hippocampus in recognition memory. *Neuropsychologia* **35**:591–598.

Bishop DVM (1989) *Test for the Reception of Grammar*, 2nd edn. Age and Cognitive Performance Research Centre, University of Manchester M13 9PL, UK.

Breier JI, Plenger PM, Wheless JW *et al* (1996) Memory tests distinguish between patients with focal temporal and extratemporal lobe epilepsy. *Epilepsia* **37**: 165–170.

Bruton CJ (1988) *The Neuropathology of Temporal Lobe Epilepsy*. Oxford: Oxford University Press.

Camfield PR, Gates R, Ronen G, Camfield C, Ferguson A, MacDonald GW (1984) Comparison of cognitive ability, personality profile, and school success in epileptic children with pure right versus left temporal lobe EEG foci. *Annals of Neurology* **15**:122–126.

Caplan R, Guthrie D, Shields WD, Peacock WJ, Vinters HV, Yudovin S (1993) Communication deficits in children undergoing temporal lobectomy. *Journal of the American Academy of Child and Adolescent Psychiatry* **32**:604–611.

Cohen M (1992) Auditory/verbal and visual/spatial memory in children with complex partial epilepsy of temporal lobe origin. *Brain and Cognition* **20**:315–326.

Corcoran R, Upton D (1993) A role for the hippocampus in card sorting. *Cortex* **29**:293–304.

Davies KG, Maxwell RE, Jennum P *et al* (1994) Language function following subdural grid-directed temporal lobectomy. *Acta Neurologica Scandinavica* **90**:201–206.

Davies KG, Maxwell RE, Beniak TE, Destafney E, Fiol ME (1995) Language function after temporal lobectomy without stimulation mapping of cortical function. *Epilepsia* **36**:130–136.

Delaney RC, Rosen AJ, Mattson RH, Novelly RA (1980) Memory function in focal epilepsy: a comparison of non-surgical unilateral temporal lobe and frontal samples. *Cortex* **16**:103–117.

Devinsky O, Perrine K, Llinas R, Luciano DJ, Dogali M (1993) Anterior temporal language areas in patients with early onset of temporal lobe epilepsy. *Annals of Neurology* **34**:727–732.

Ellis AW, Hillam JC, Cardno A, Kay J (1991) Processing of words and faces by patients with left and right temporal lobe epilepsy. *Behavioural Neurology* **4**:121–128.

Fedio P, Mirsky AF (1969) Selective intellectual deficits in children with temporal lobe or centrencephalic epilepsy. *Neuropsychologia* **7**:287–300.

Frisk V, Milner B (1990) The role of the left hippocampal region in the acquisition and retention of story content. *Neuropsychologia* **28**:349–359.

Gadian DG, Isaacs EB, Cross JH *et al* (1996) Lateralization of brain function in childhood revealed by magnetic resonance spectroscopy *Neurology* **46**:974–977.

Giordani B, Berent S, Sackellares, JC *et al* (1985) Intelligence test performance of patients with partial and generalized seizures. *Epilepsia*:**26**:37–42.

Giovagnoli AR, Avanzini G (1996) Forgetting rate and interference effects on a verbal distractor task in patients with temporal lobe epilepsy. *Journal of Clinical Neuropsychology* **18**:259–264.

Giovagnoli AR, Casazza M, Broggi G, Avanzini G (1996) Verbal learning and forgetting in patients with temporal lobe epilepsy. *European Journal of Neurology* **3**: 345–353.

Gleissner U, Helmstaedter C, Elger CE (1998) Right hippocampal contribution to visual memory: a presurgical and postsurgical study in patients with temporal lobe epilepsy. *Journal of Neurology, Neurosurgery and Psychiatry* **65**:665–669.

Gray JA (1982) *The Neuropsychology of Anxiety*. Oxford: Oxford University Press.

Helmstaedter C, Pohl C, Hufnagel A, Elger CE (1991) Visual learning deficits in non-resected patients with right temporal lobe epilepsy. *Cortex* **27**:547–555.

Helmstaedter C, Pohl C, Elger CE (1995) Relations between verbal and non-verbal memory performance: evidence of confounding effects particularly in patients with right temporal lobe epilepsy. *Cortex* **31**:354–355.

Hermann B, Seidenberg M (1995) Executive system dysfunction in temporal lobe epilepsy: effects of nociferous cortex versus hippocampal pathology. *Journal of Clinical and Experimental Neuropsychology* **17**:809–819.

Hermann BP, Wyler AR (1988) Effects of anterior temporal lobectomy on language function: a controlled study. *Annals of Neurology* **23**:585–588.

Hermann BP, Wyler AR, Richey ET, Rea JM (1987) Memory function and verbal learning ability in patients with complex partial seizures of temporal lobe origin. *Epilepsia* **28**:547–554.

Hermann BP, Wyler AR, Richey ET (1988) Wisconsin Card Sorting Test performance in patients with complex partial seizures of temporal lobe origin. *Journal of Clinical and Experimental Neuropsychology* **10**:467–476.

Hermann BP, Wyler AR, Somes G (1991) Language function following anterior temporal lobectomy. *Journal of Neurosurgery* **74**:560–566.

Hermann BP, Seidenberg M, Haltiner A, Wyler AR (1992) Adequacy of language function and verbal memory performance in unilateral temporal lobe epilepsy. *Cortex* **28**:423–433.

Hermann BP, Gold J, Pusakulich R *et al* (1995a) Wechsler Adult Intelligence Scale – Revised in the evaluation of anterior temporal lobectomy candidates. *Epilepsia* **36**:480–487.

Hermann BP, Connell B, Barr WB, Wyler AR (1995b) The utility of the Warrington Recognition Memory Test for temporal lobe epilepsy: pre- and postoperative results. *Journal of Epilepsy* **8**:139–145.

Hermann BP, Seidenberg M, Schoenfeld J, Davies K (1997) Neuropsychological characteristics of the syndrome of mesial temporal lobe epilepsy. *Archives of Neurology* **54**:369–376.

Hershey T, Craft S, Glauser TA, Hale S (1998) Short-term and long-term memory in early temporal lobe dysfunction. *Neuropsychology* **12**:52–64.

Hertz-Pannier L, Gaillard WD, Mott SH *et al* (1997) Noninvasive assessment of language dominance in children and adolescents with functional MRI: a preliminary study. *Neurology* **48**:1003–1012.

Horner MD, Flashman LA, Freides D, Epstein CM (1996) Temporal lobe epilepsy and performance on the Winconsin Card Sorting Test. *Journal of Clinical and Experimental Neuropsychology* **18**:310–313.

Hudson LP, Munoz DG, Miller L, McLachlan RS, Girvin JP, Blume T (1993) Amygdaloid sclerosis in temporal lobe epilepsy. *Annals of Neurology* **33**:622–631.

Jambaqué I, Dellatolas G, Dulac O, Ponsot G, Signoret J-L (1993) Verbal and visual memory impairment in children with epilepsy. *Neuropsychologia* **31**: 1321–1337.

Jokeit H, Seitz RJ, Markowitsch HJ, Neumann N, Witte OW, Ebner A (1997) Prefrontal asymmetric interictal glucose hypometabolism and cognitive impairment in patients with temporal lobe epilepsy. *Brain* **120**:2283–2294.

Jones-Gotman M (1991) Presurgical neuropsychological evaluation for localisation and lateralisation of seizure focus. In: Lüders H (ed) *Epilepsy Surgery*, pp 469–475. New York: Raven Press.

Jones-Gotman M (1996) Psychological evaluation for epilepsy surgery.

In: Shorvon S, Dreifuss F, Fish D, Thomas D (eds) *The Treatment of Epilepsy*, pp 621–630. Oxford: Blackwell Science.

Kalviäinen R, Partanen K, Aikiä M *et al* (1997) MRI-based hippocampal volumetry and T2 relaxometry: correlation to verbal memory performance in newly diagnosed epilepsy patients with left-sided temporal lobe focus. *Neurology* **48**:286–287.

Kilpatrick C, Murrie V, Cook M, Andrewes D, Desmond P, Hopper J (1997) Degree of left hippocampal atrophy correlates with severity of neuropsychological deficits. *Seizure* **6**:213–218.

Kimura D (1963) Right temporal lobe damage. *Archives of Neurology* **8**:264–271.

Knight ES, Oxbury JM, Oxbury SM, Middleton JA (1998) Cognitive development in children under 12 years of age following temporal lobe epilepsy surgery for dysembryoplastic neurepithelial tumour. *Epilepsia* **39**(suppl 6):172.

Kosciesza M, Stelmasiak Z, Kosciesza A (1998) Characteristics of language in children with epilepsy. *Epilepsia* **39** (Suppl 2):120–121.

Langfitt JT, Rausch R (1996) Word-finding deficits persist after left anteriotemporal lobectomy. *Archives of Neurology* **53**:73–76.

Lencz T, McCarthy G, Bronen RA (1992) Quantitative magnetic resonance imaging in temporal lobe epilepsy: relationship to neuropathology and neuropsychological function. *Annals of Neurology* **31**:629–637.

Loring DW, Lee GP, Martin RC, Meador KG (1988) Material specific learning in patients with complex partial seizures of temporal lobe origin: convergent validation of memory constructs. *Journal of Epilepsy* **1**:53–59.

Loring DW, Meador KJ, Lee GP *et al* (1990) Cerebral language lateralization: evidence from intracarotid amobarbital testing. *Neuropsychologia* **28**:831–838.

McKenna P, Warrington EK (1983) *The Graded Naming Test*. Windsor, UK: NFER Nelson.

McMillan TM, Powell GE, Janota I, Polkey CE (1987) Relationships between neuropathology and cognitive functioning in temporal lobectomy patients. *Journal of Neurology, Neurosurgery and Psychiatry* **50**:167–176.

Margerison JH, Corsellis JAN (1966) Epilepsy and the temporal lobes. A clinical, electroencephalographic and neuropathological study of the brain in epilepsy, with particular reference to the temporal lobes. *Brain* **89**:499–530.

Martin RC, Loring DW, Meador KJ, Gregory PL (1990) The effects of lateralized temporal lobe dysfunction on formal and semantic word fluency. *Neuropsychologia* **28**: 823–829.

Matkovic Z, Oxbury SM, Hiorns RW *et al* (1995a) Hippocampal neuronal density correlates with pre-operative verbal memory in patients with temporal lobe epilepsy. *Epilepsia* **36**(Suppl 3): S121.

Matkovic Z, Oxbury SM, Hiorns RW *et al* (1995b) Hippocampal neuronal density correlates with pre-operative non-verbal memory in patients with temporal lobe epilepsy. *Epilepsia* **36** (Suppl 3): S93.

Mayeux R, Brandt J, Rosen J, Benson F (1980) Interictal memory impairment in temporal lobe epilepsy. *Neurology* **30**:120–125.

Meyer FB, Marsh WR, Laws ER, Sharbrough FW (1986) Temporal lobectomy in children with epilepsy. *Journal of Neurosurgery* **64**:371–376.

Meyer V, Yates AJ (1955) Intellectual changes following temporal lobectomy for psychomotor epilepsy: preliminary communication. *Journal of Neurology, Neurosurgery and Psychiatry* **18**:44–52.

Miller LA, Munoz DG, Finmore M (1993) Hippocampal sclerosis and human memory. *Archives of Neurology* **50**:391–394.

Milner B (1958) Psychological defects produced by temporal lobe excision. *Proceedings of the Association for Research in Nervous and Mental Disease* **35**:244–257.

Milner B (1963) Effects of different brain lesions on card sorting. *Archives of Neurology* **9**:90–100.

Milner B (1965) Visually guided maze learning in man: effects of

bilateral hippocampal, bilateral frontal and unilateral cerebral lesions. *Neuropsychologia* **3**:317–338.

Milner B (1971) Interhemispheric differences in the localisation of psychological processes in man. *British Medical Bulletin* **27**:272–277.

Moore PM, Baker GA (1996) Validation of the Wechsler Memory Scale–Revised in a sample of people with intractable temporal lobe epilepsy. *Epilepsia* **37**:1215–1220.

Nelson HE (1976) A modified card sorting test sensitive to frontal lobe defects. *Cortex* **12**:313–324.

Nelson HE (1982) *National Adult Reading Test (NART)*, 2nd edn. Windsor, UK: NFER-Nelson.

Ojemann G, Ojemann J, Lettich E, Berger M (1989) Cortical language localization in left, dominant hemisphere. An electrical stimulation mapping investigation in 117 patients. *Journal of Neurosurgery* **71**:316–326.

O'Leary DS, Lovell MR, Sackellares JC *et al* (1983) Effects of age of onset of partial and generalized seizures on neuropsychological performance in children. *Journal of Nervous and Mental Disease* **171**:624–629.

Oxbury JM, MacCallum FO (1973) Herpes simplex virus encephalitis: clinical features and residual damage. *Postgraduate Medical Journal* **49**:387–389.

Oxbury JM, Oxbury SM (1989) Neuropsychology, memory and hippocampal pathology. In: Reynolds EH, Trimble MR (eds) *The Bridge between Neurology and Psychiatry*, pp 135–150. London: Churchill Livingstone.

Oxbury SM, Oxbury JM (1984) Intracarotid amytal test in the assessment of language dominance. *Advances in Neurology* **42**:115–123.

Oxbury SM, Campbell L, Baxendale SA, Oxbury JM (1998) Cognitive function in relation to duration of temporal lobe epilepsy due to Ammon's horn sclerosis. *Epilepsia* **39** (Suppl 2):120.

Parks RW, Lowenstien DA, Dodrill KL *et al* (1988) Cerebral metabolic effects of a verbal fluency test: a PET study. *Journal of Clinical and Experimental Neuropsychology* **10**: 565–575.

Powell GE, Polkey CE, Canavan AGM (1987) Lateralisation of memory functions in epileptic patients by use of the sodium amytal (Wada) technique. *Journal of Neurology, Neurosurgery and Psychiatry* **50**:665–672.

Prevey ML, Delaney RC, Mattson RH (1988) Gist recall in temporal lobe seizure patients. *Cortex* **24**:301–312.

Rausch R, Babb TL (1987) Evidence for memory specialisation within the mesial temporal lobe in man. In: Engel J, Ojemann G, Lüders H, Williamson P (eds) *Fundamental Mechanisms of Human Brain Function*, pp 103–109. New York: Raven Press.

Rausch R, Babb TL (1993) Hippocampal neuron loss and memory scores before and after temporal lobe surgery for epilepsy. *Archives of Neurology* **50**:812–817.

Sagar HJ, Oxbury JM (1987) Hippocampal neurone loss in temporal lobe epilepsy: correlation with early childhood convulsions. *Annals of Neurology* **22**:334–340.

Saling MM, Berkovic SF, O'Shea MF (1993) Lateralization of verbal memory and unilateral hippocampal sclerosis: evidence of task-specific effects. *Journal of Clinical and Experimental Neuropsychology* **15**:608–618.

Sass KJ, Spencer DD, Kim JH *et al* (1990) Verbal memory impairment correlates with hippocampal pyramidal cell density. *Neurology* **40**:1694–1697.

Sass KJ, Sass A, Westerveld M *et al* (1992a) Specificity in the correlation of verbal memory and hippocampal neuron loss: dissociation of memory, language and verbal intellectual ability. *Journal of Clinical and Experimental Neuropsychology* **14**:662–672.

Sass KJ, Sass A, Westerveld M *et al* (1992b) Russell's adaptation of the Wechsler Memory Scale as an index of hippocampal pathology. *Journal of Epilepsy* **5**:24–30.

Sass KJ, Buchanan CP, Kraemer S, Westerveld M, Kim JH, Spencer DD

(1995) Verbal memory impairment resulting from hippocampal neurone loss among epileptic patients with structural lesions. *Neurology* **45**:2154–2156.

Saykin AJ, Gur RC, Sussman NM, O'Connor MJ, Gur RE (1989) Memory deficits before and after temporal lobectomy: effects of laterality and age of onset. *Brain and Cognition* **9**:191–200.

Saykin AJ, Stafiniak P, Robinson LJ *et al* (1995) Language before and after temporal lobectomy: specificity of acute changes and relation to early risk factors. *Epilepsia* **36**:1071–1077.

Schäffler L, Lüders HO, Morris HH, Wyllie E (1994) Anatomic distribution of cortical language sites in the basal temporal language area in patients with left temporal lobe epilepsy. *Epilepsia* **35**:525–528.

Scoville W, Milner B (1957) Loss of recent memory after bilateral hippocampal lesions. *Journal of Neurology, Neurosurgery and Psychiatry* **20**:11–21.

Selwa LM, Berent S, Giordani B, Henry TR, Buchtel HA, Ross DA (1994) Serial cognitive testing in temporal lobe epilepsy: longitudinal changes with medical and surgical therapiest. *Epilepsia* **35**:743–749.

Smith ML, Milner B (1981) The role of the right hippocampus in the recall of spatial location. *Neuropsychologia* **19**:781–793.

Snyder PJ, Novelly RA, Harris LJ (1990) Mixed speech dominance in the intracarotid sodium amytal procedure: validity and criteria issues. *Journal of Clinical and Experimental Neuropsychology* **12**:629–643.

Stafiniak P, Saykin AJ, Sperling MR, *et al* (1990) Acute naming deficits following dominant temporal lobectomy. *Neurology* **40**:1509–1512.

Strauss E, Hunter M, Wada J (1993) Wisconsin Card Sorting performance: effects of age of onset of damage and laterality of dysfunction. *Journal of Clinical and Experimental Neuropsychology* **15**:896–902.

Strauss E, Loring D, Chelune G *et al* (1995) Predicting cognitive impairment in epilepsy: findings from the Bozeman Epilepsy Consortium. *Journal of Clinical and Experimental Neuropsychology* **17**:909–917.

Trenerry MR, Jack CR (1994) Wisconsin Card Sorting Test performance before and after temporal lobectomy. *Journal of Epilepsy* **7**:313–317.

Trenerry MR, Jack CR, Ivnik RJ *et al* (1993) MRI hippocampal volumes and memory function before and after temporal lobectomy. *Neurology* **43**:1800–1805.

Warrington EK (1984) *Recognition Memory Test*. Windsor, UK: NFER-Nelson.

31

Neuropsychologic deficits in frontal lobe epilepsy

RG MORRIS AND CM COWEY

Although neuropsychologic investigations of patients undergoing frontal lobe excisions span a period of over 50 years (see Milner 1995), there are relatively few data describing the neuropsychologic characteristics of patients with frontal lobe epilepsy (FLE) per se. Postoperative investigations are numerous, perhaps because of their theoretical importance, but patients not put forward for operations or those at the preoperative stage have not attracted the same attention, despite the diagnostic importance of defining their neuropsychologic status. This chapter reviews such studies as exist and comments on some of the theoretic and interpretive issues relating to this topic.

FRONTAL LOBE ANATOMY AND EARLY REPORTS ON COGNITIVE FUNCTION

FLE is the clinical manifestation of a range of brain abnormalities affecting the frontal lobes. These abnormalities can occupy disparate locations in what is a large region of the cortex with a highly distinct neuroanatomic organization (Milner 1988). The frontal cortex comprises approximately one-third of the cerebral cortex (Goldman-Rakic 1987).

Different methods of producing a geography of this area of the brain exist. Brodmann's (1909, 1925) framework of mapping of 13 distinct neuroanatomic regions is still the most widely used. The main areas comprise the premotor (area 6 and partially area 8), the prefrontal region (areas 9, 10, 45, 46) and the precentral or basiomesial region (areas 9, 10, 11, 12, 13, 24, 32), the latter including the motor cortex and the cingulate gyrus. Additional areas are the frontal eye field region (area 8), anterior to the premotor region, and Broca's area (partially area 44).

There have been considerable advances in understanding the cognitive role of the prefrontal cortex (see Chapter 59), the main areas of interest tending to be the dorsolateral region and the orbitofrontal region. These regions are implicated in a wide range of cognitive and behavioral functions. Examples of such functions are the organization and sequencing of cognition, the control of social behavior, and the processing of emotion. The clinical assessments outlined in the studies reviewed below have, in the main, concentrated on the cognitive function of the patient, focusing on intellectual, mnemonic, and executive abilities, examples of the latter being decision making and mental flexibility.

Early published reports of the cognitive function of patients with FLE are comparatively rare and tend to consider the postoperative outcome of those undergoing frontal lobectomies. Hebb (1939), in his study of four patients who underwent left frontal lobectomies, noted the Standford–Binet preoperative function in one of them. This patient had an intelligence quotient (IQ) of 124, placing her in the superior range, and, he commented, 'enough to guarantee a good physiological condition intracranially' (p 79). A subsequent report of two right frontal lobectomies had preoperative psychometric data for one patient, indicating an IQ of 92 (Hebb 1941). The famous patient K.M., studied by Hebb and Penfield (1940), who subsequently underwent a bilateral frontal lobectomy, had a preoperative Stanford–Binet IQ of 83. In each case, intellectual function remained stable or improved. Hebb and Penfield (1940) derived from these findings two main points: First, epileptogenic tissue had an interfering effect upon the function of neighboring brain areas; and secondly, the frontal lobes contributed less to intelligence than had hitherto been supposed.

NEUROPSYCHOLOGIC FUNCTION

In contrast to the limited nature of these early studies, four main centers have published group data, which comprise 'batteries' of psychometric tests:

1. Montreal Neurological Institute (Milner 1963, 1975)
2. VA Hospital Epilepsy Center and Seizure Clinic at the Yale-New Haven Hospital (Delaney *et al* 1980)
3. University Clinic of Bonn (Helmstaedter *et al* 1996; also reported initially as a pilot study by Kemper *et al* 1992, 1993)
4. National Society for Epilepsy, Chalfont St Peter, UK (Upton and Thompson 1996)

Additional data has been collected by Cowey and Green (1996) at the Institute of Neurology and later by Cowey *et al* in collaboration with the Maudsley Hospital, while based at the Institute of Psychiatry, London (CM Cowey *et al* unpublished data).

The paucity of studies permits a detailed review of each, which are presented below in chronologic order.

MONTREAL NEUROLOGICAL INSTITUTE (MNI)

Since 1950, most patients at the MNI receiving neurosurgical treatment for focal epilepsy have undergone a variety of preoperative neuropsychologic investigations. The data from selective cohorts of these patients have been reported by Milner (1963, 1964, 1975), in a comparative study of pre- and postoperative differences, as outlined below.

Intellectual function

Data on intellectual functioning has been collated (Milner 1975), describing 73 cases out of 955 patients seen since the early 1950s. These data showed that the IQ for those included was well within the normal range, with a full-scale Wechsler Adult Intelligence Scale (WAIS) score of 108 in patients who subsequently underwent left frontal lobectomies; and a score of 95 in those who underwent a right frontal lobectomy. The original observation by Hebb and Penfield (1940) of stable or improved postoperative functioning was tested, and discounted as partially an artifact of repeated testing. Milner (1975), however, also hypothesized that the presence of epileptogenic tissue was sufficient to disrupt the function of other cortical tissue.

Memory function

Data on memory function were collected from the same cohort. Memory was tested using delayed recall versions of the logical memory (prose recall) and paired associate tests from the Wechsler Memory Scale (WMS), producing a composite verbal memory score (Milner 1975). Preoperative scores in the FLE group indicated unimpaired function in groups with left- or right-sided damage. Memory function remained at approximately the same level postoperatively. These results contrasted with a left temporal lobe epilepsy group (TLE) which showed a lower performance, pre- and postoperatively.

Executive function

Executive functioning[1] has also been examined preoperatively (Milner 1963, 1964). Milner examined 71 patients who had undergone a unilateral operation and received both pre- and postoperative testing. These patients comprised 18 who subsequently had a dorsolateral-frontal operation (10 left and 8 right), and 53 with other cortical operations (33 who underwent temporal lobectomies, 8 with operations affecting the parietal lobe, and 12 with a mixture of operation sites, including, for example, the parietal, temporal, or occipital lobes). Of the 18 dorsolateral

---

[1] The term executive functioning came to be used in the 1980s to cover mental functions that are to do with the coordination or sequencing of cognition or behavior. It has since been widely used in this fashion and as such often replaces the concept of frontal lobe function, although the two are by no means synonymous.

patients, 7 had seizures due to penetrating head injuries, and 11 had seizures attributed to 'birth injury'.

Milner tested patients on the Wisconsin Card Sorting Test (WCST), selected as a sorting task over the Weigl test for its greater sensitivity. The WCST, now frequently used in clinical practice (Heaton 1981), had been modeled on testing techniques that had shown severe impairment in monkeys with frontal lobectomies (e.g. Brush *et al* 1961; Mishkin *et al* 1962), the theoretical impetus for use with these patients. The test involves sorting stimulus cards according to one of three categories (colour, shape, and number) and then switching the sorting rule (in this case, from colour to shape and then number, repeating this sequence again). In the full version used by Milner (see Heaton 1981), the sensitivity of the task is determined partially by the fact that the patient is not told the rule will change and that the stimulus cards may share more than one characteristic with the exemplar cards used for sorting. The test is known, *par excellence*, as a test of mental flexibility, sensitive to perseverative tendencies in patients.

Table 31.1 shows both the pre- and postoperative data of the patients. These results demonstrate a relative impairment of the preoperative dorsolateral group, which worsens following an operation. This pattern is seen both in terms of the number of categories achieved and the number of errors made by the patients, the latter achieving a statistically significant difference in the preoperative group when compared to controls. A breakdown of the errors is also given in Table 31.1, showing the number of perseverative errors, those that would have been correct on the immediately preceding stage of the test, or in the first stage, but as a continued response in terms of the patient's initial preference are erroneous. Again, the preoperative patients show a greater proportion of perseverative errors, compared to the control group, with the errors increasing postoperatively in the dorsolateral group. Notably, the reverse trend is seen for the nondorsolateral control patients, whose tendency to perseverate decreases following the reduction of epileptiform activity.

In summary, the data collected by Milner (1963, 1975) show the following pattern: intellectual functioning of preoperative FLE patients within the normal range, with unimpaired verbal memory, but significant impairment in executive function, namely on the WCST; performance on the WCST worsened postoperatively.

VA HOSPITAL EPILEPSY CENTER AND SEIZURE CLINIC AT THE YALE-NEW HAVEN HOSPITAL

Delaney *et al* (1980) examined patients at the above-mentioned center. They studied the memory function of 15 FLE patients (laterality of focus or damage not reported) and compared them to 30 TLE patients (15 left and 15 right) on tests of verbal and nonverbal memory. Verbal tests included prose recall (logical memory), from the WMS, tested immediately and after half an hour (scored following Russell 1975). The patients were also tested on lists of 10 words for subsequent recall, yes/no recognition, and cued recall using fragments of the words. Nonverbal tests included the WMS visual reproduction test with immediate and half-hour recall and a recurring figures test in which a series of abstract figures were presented and, after a certain number (20) had been shown, a selection of figures were re-presented, with the patient deciding whether or not they had been seen before.

A clear result was obtained, with the FLE patients unimpaired on all of the measures. The TLE patients showed impairment on the prose recall (both groups; the left more so for delayed recall); list learning (left only); visual reproduction (right only and with the delay); and the recurring figures test (right only). Notably, the performance profiles of the FLE group were very similar to the normal control group.

Table 31.1 Wisconsin Card Sorting Test performance of patients with frontal lobe epilepsy pre- and postoperatively (taken from Milner 1963, with permission). The comparison is between a dorsolateral-frontal group and respective control group (see text for details).

Patient group	Total categories achieved		Perseverative errors		Nonperseverative errors	
	Preoperative	Postoperative	Preoperative	Postoperative	Preoperative	Postoperative
Dorsolateral (*n* = 18)	3.3	1.4	39.5	51.5	15.4	21.7
Control (*n* = 53)	4.6	4.7	20.0	12.8	17.7	17.8

UNIVERSITY CLINIC OF BONN

Helmstaedter *et al* (1996) have focused their investigations on executive function and, because the study was more recent, were able to use more sophisticated diagnostic procedures, such as MRI.

They used a large battery of tests to examine the executive functioning of 23 patients with FLE and compared their ability to 38 patients with TLE. Extensive interictal and ictal video-EEG-electrocorticography (ECoG) monitoring and MRI findings in the FLE patients enabled an estimate of the primary epileptogenic zone to be made, as shown in Table 31.2. There were 17 FLE patients with right-sided zones, and 6 with left-sided zones. In contrast, 17 of the TLE patients had right-sided zones, and in 21 the primary epileptogenic zones were on the left. All patients were left-hemisphere dominant for language as investigated by the intracarotid sodium amobarbital (ISA) test.

The battery of tests employed (Fig. 31.1) are mainly concerned with attention or executive function, as described below:

Digit and Corsi block span

These are verbal and spatial counterparts of a test that measures immediate memory span. The patients have to recall increasing sequences of either digits or blocks in a serial order from immediate memory.

Letter cancellation

The patient 'cancels' target letters in a test of sustained selective attention and visuomotor speed.

The cI test

The first component involves counting squares out of a table with various other symbols, as fast as possible. This task measures visuoperceptual speed. The second component requires the patient to read two rows of As and Bs in an inverse fashion, for example, AABAB as BBABA. The aim of the task is to assess the effect of interference.

The stroop test

A modified version of this test was used which required the naming of either colored dots, words that do not refer to a color, or words that do refer to a color (for example, the word 'red' written in green ink).

Table 31.2 Localization of the primary epileptogenic zone in FLE patients by means of the EEG/ECoG monitoring and/or MRI findings. LFLE/RFLE = Left/right frontal lobe epilepsy (from Helmstaedter *et al* 1996, with permission).

Group	RFLE (n = 17)	LFLE (n = 6)
Central/premotor	4	2
Lateral	1	
Orbital	1	3
Polar	1	
Global	7	1
Bifrontal	4[a]	

[a] The classification of these patients into the RFLE group followed the right frontal localization of structural lesions.

Word fluency

This task was a variant of the controlled oral word association test, employing F, R, and K as the cue letters to assess initiation ability.

Five-point test

This test is a counterpart to verbal fluency, but is in the visual domain. The patient has to join the dots with firstly three, then four, and finally five lines to make different figures, with 1 min being allowed per level of difficulty.

Visual–verbal test

This task comprises two tests to assess concept formation and concept shift. It uses 42 cards with a four-letter string on each (A/B/C/D). Two triple sequences out of the four-letter presentations are similar with respect to color, form, structure, or position (ABC and BCD, for example). The patient has to name the two triples and the concept.

Maze test

A standard maze test of increasing difficulty designed to measure anticipation and planning ability.

Motor sequences

A set of motor coordination and sequencing tests based on Luria (1973), for example, complex bimanual alternating sequences.

Helmstaedter *et al* (1996) found, overall, that the FLE patients showed a poorer performance than the TLE group. In particular, consistent relative deficits were found on all the span measures, the cI (interference) test, the stroop measures, the five-point test, the visual–verbal test, the

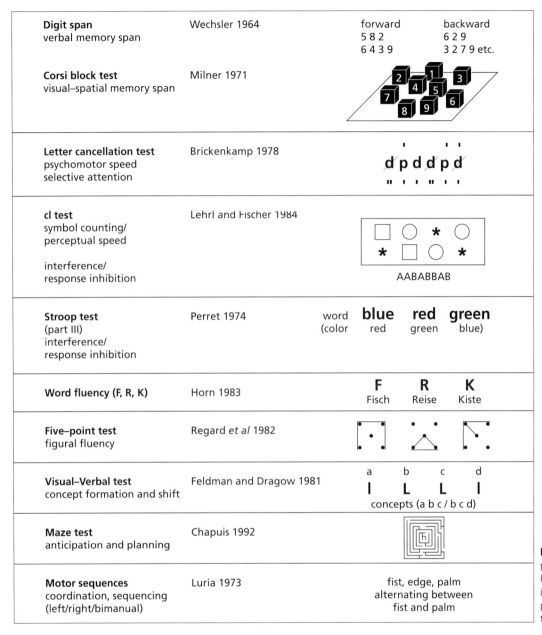

Digit span verbal memory span	Wechsler 1964	forward backward 5 8 2 6 2 9 6 4 3 9 3 2 7 9 etc.
Corsi block test visual–spatial memory span	Milner 1971	
Letter cancellation test psychomotor speed selective attention	Brickenkamp 1978	d p d d p d
cl test symbol counting/ perceptual speed interference/ response inhibition	Lehrl and Fischer 1984	AABABBAB
Stroop test (part III) interference/ response inhibition	Perret 1974	word **blue** **red** **green** (color red green blue)
Word fluency (F, R, K)	Horn 1983	**F** **R** **K** Fisch Reise Kiste
Five–point test figural fluency	Regard *et al* 1982	
Visual–Verbal test concept formation and shift	Feldman and Dragow 1981	a b c d I L L I concepts (a b c / b c d)
Maze test anticipation and planning	Chapuis 1992	
Motor sequences coordination, sequencing (left/right/bimanual)	Luria 1973	fist, edge, palm alternating between fist and palm

Fig. 31.1 Illustration of nine principal tests used by Helmstaedter *et al.* (1996) to investigate executive functions in patients with frontal lobe versus temporal lobe epilepsy

maze test and all of the motor sequencing tasks. Only letter cancellation and verbal fluency did not differentiate the patient groups.

A factor analysis of the results showed that rather than reflecting the degradation of one underlying 'central executive component', distinct patterns of impairment were present (Table 31.3). There were four factors:

1. psychomotor speed and attention
2. coordinating motor sequences
3. memory span
4. response inhibition

Factors (2) and (4) differentiated between the two groups, unlike factors (1) and (3) (note: individual tests contributing to these latter factors did discriminate the groups). This analysis highlights the discriminatory power of the motor impairments, which parallels Luria's (1980) observations of patients with frontal lobe pathology, and also what can be viewed broadly as the regulatory or monitoring aspects of executive function. This study did not produce differences between the left and right FLE patients, but this finding may reflect the low numbers in the former group, which may also explain the lack of verbal fluency impairment. Additionally, the authors suggested that widespread, bilateral and fast-propagating epileptic activity may also explain the lack of laterality effects.

To investigate how well the tests categorized patients, a cluster analysis was conducted to subgroup patients based

Table 31.3 Varimax rotated factor matrix resulting from factor analysis of all test parameters for the FLE and TLE patient data from Helmstaedter *et al* (1996) study. In addition, significant differences between the groups on individual measures are indicated.

Tests	Factors			
	1	2	3	4
Maze test (time)	−0.86			
Stroop (time)	−0.84[a]			
Five-point test (correct)	0.71			
Word fluency	0.61			
Letter cancellation	0.57			
Symbol counting (time)	−0.56[b]			
Motor sequencing (right)		0.89[a]		
Motor sequencing (bimanual alternating)		0.81[c]		
Motor sequencing (left)		0.76[a]		
Digits forward			0.80[a]	
Digits backward			0.78[b]	
Corsi backward			0.64[a]	
Corsi forward			(0.47)[a]	
Five-point test (errors)				−0.82[a]
Maze test (errors)				−0.74[c]
cI Interference (time)				−0.61[c]
Visual–verbal (correct)				0.60[a]

[a] $p < 0.01$; [b] $p < 0.05$; [c] $p < 0.001$. Significant differences represent those between FLE and TLE groups on the measures using a post hoc Tukey method.

on the factor scores. This produced three clusters, one principally reflecting motor coordination (mainly factor (2) above), a second, speed or attention (mainly factor (1)), and the third, response inhibition (mainly factor (4)). For the FLE group, group membership of these three clusters were 7, 9, and 7 patients, respectively. For the TLE group, the distribution of patients was 3, 35, and 0, respectively. An alternative way of expressing these results is that while the second cluster appeared in 79% of TLE patients, the first and third appeared in 82% of the FLE patients.

NATIONAL SOCIETY FOR EPILEPSY

A second major study of executive function was conducted recently by Upton and Thompson (1996). Following the same basic design as Helmstaedter *et al* (1996), they tested a larger sample of patients. Seventy-four patients with FLE (32 right and 42 left) and 57 with TLE (26 right and 31 left) were investigated. Upton and Thompson (1996) matched the IQ between the groups. All groups had a mean IQ of between 89 and 94. The etiology of FLE, as in the Helmstaedter *et al* (1996) study, was mixed. In the TLE group, however, over half of the patients had hippocampal sclerosis (n = 33). The battery included tests of executive and motor skills, as shown in Table 31.4.

As well as including the frequently used tests of executive function (the modified WCST, verbal fluency, stroop, trail making, cognitive estimates, and Porteus maze tests), Upton and Thompson (1996) introduced a 20-question task (Klouder and Cooper 1990), based on the parlor game

in which the patient had to guess which animal the experimenter had in mind, with the examiner responding either 'yes' or 'no' to the questions. They also had a cost estimation test where the patient had to estimate the cost of 10 common objects, where the accuracy and 'bizarreness' of the response is rated.

The executive task performance (Table 31.4) showed a mixed pattern of results. Some tasks demonstrated significant underperformance in the FLE group as compared to the TLE patients. Other tasks revealed hemisphere differences. Some tasks did not differentiate the groups. The tests that distinguished FLE patients were the stroop, trail making B, the 20-questions test, and the cost estimation test. Notably, Upton and Thompson (1996), in common with Helmstaedter *et al* (1996), found that the verbal fluency test failed to discriminate between the groups. This finding contrasts with the clear deficit that is frequently observed with left frontal excisions (e.g. Milner 1963). The modified WCST did show a right FLE versus left FLE difference in favor of the latter, but did not distinguish FLE from TLE overall. There were no group differences on perseverative errors. This result may have occurred due to the use of the modified form of the WCST with its known reduced sensitivity (Lezak 1995). Some of the tests, for example cognitive estimates and the Porteus maze, produced a right vs. left discrimination (combining the FLE and TLE patients), rather than frontal vs. temporal, which, as discussed below, may be a potentially useful diagnostic feature.

The only motor task which showed a relative FLE impairment was the motor sequencing test (Canavan *et al*

Table 31.4 Tests used by Upton and Thompson (1996) to compare right and left frontal lobe epilepsy (RFLE, LFLE) and right and left temporal lobe epilepsy (RTLE, LTLE) patients. The statistical outcome, comparing the four groups using Duncan's multiple range tests is given.

Test	Outcome	Reference
Executive		
Modified Wisconsin Card Sorting	RFLE more impaired than LFLE on category errors; no other group differences	Nelson 1976
Verbal fluency (S words and animals)	No group differences	
Stroop test	FLE groups more impaired than TLE, but no right–left lateralization effects	Dodrill 1978
Trail making	Frontal group more impaired than TLE on part B but no left–right lateralization effects	War Department 1944
Cognitive estimates test	Left hemisphere groups more impaired overall	Shallice and Evans 1978
Porteus maze test	Left hemisphere groups more impaired overall	Porteus 1965
Twenty questions	FLE groups more impaired than TLE, mainly due to LFLE impairment	Klouder and Cooper 1990
Cost estimation	FLE groups more impaired than TLE overall; right hemisphere groups more impaired	Smith and Milner 1984
Motor Skills		
Tapping	Right hemisphere group more impaired for both right and left hand tapping movements; relating to impairment in RTLE group	Wyke 1969
Bimanual hand movements	LFLE group more impaired than RFLE or LTLE	Laplane *et al* 1977
Motor sequences	FLE group more impaired that TLE overall	Canavan *et al* 1989
Gesture span	No significant differences between groups	Canavan *et al* 1989

1989). This task requires the subject to copy 10 three-item gestures, with the number of correct sequences being recorded. This test is similar to the motor sequencing task used by Helmstaedter *et al* (1996). A frontal lobe impairment was also reflected in the tendency for the left FLE group to be more impaired on the bimanual hand movement test than the right FLE or left TLE group. This task, which requires alternating fist and palm movements, also has sequencing or gestural components.

INSTITUTE OF PSYCHIATRY, INSTITUTE OF NEUROLOGY, AND THE MAUDSLEY HOSPITAL, LONDON

Cowey and colleagues (Cowey and Green 1996; CM Cowey, Goldstein, Polkey, and Morris, unpublished data) have conducted a series of experimentally orientated studies into executive functioning and memory. They investigated an additional feature of executive function, not addressed by the studies cited above. This feature is the ability to divide attention between simultaneous mental operations. In many 'real life' tasks, the patient has to carry out several mental activities in order to complete a task, either by rapidly switching between them or by keeping them in mind simultaneously.

In an initial study, Cowey and Green (1996) tested this ability in patients with FLE. They employed a task developed by AD Baddeley (personal communication, 1993). This task combined a memory span task with a concurrent spatial tracking task. The memory span task was the conventional digit span task, in which the patient has to recall lists of digits of increasing length in serial order until they are consistently failing. At the point of failure the patient's span can be determined. This span is then utilized in the dual task. The spatial tracking task involves the placing of crosses in boxes arranged in a maze-like fashion on a piece of paper and joined with arrows. In the dual task trials, the digit span test is given while the patient is completing the spatial tracking task (Baddeley *et al* 1997).

Cowey and Green (1996) compared the performance of 12 FLE patients (7 right and 5 left) and 12 TLE patients. The TLE group was matched with the FLE group for side of lesion, and all patients in the TLE group had hippocampal sclerosis. The results demonstrated that in healthy control subjects concurrent performance of tasks had a deleterious effect when compared to single task performance: the divided attention cost. This effect was clearly magnified in the FLE patients in comparison to the TLE patients and healthy controls. Indeed, the divided attention cost did not differ significantly between the TLE and

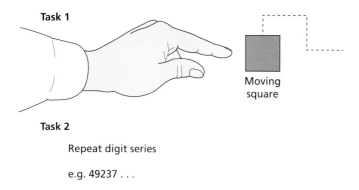

Task 1

Moving
square

Task 2

Repeat digit series

e.g. 49237 . . .

Fig. 31.2 Illustration of the divided attention test used by Cowey *et al* (unpublished data).

healthy control groups, suggesting unimpaired executive processes in the temporal lobe group.

Cowey, Goldstein, Polkey, and Morris (unpublished data) have since replicated this finding with a larger sample of patients, using computerized tasks (Fig. 31.2). The computerized tracking task involved the patient using their preferred index finger to track a moving 'square' on a touch-sensitive computer screen. The speed of the square, which moved in a random direction, altered until the patient maintained contact with the square for between 40 and 60% of the time. This method ensured that the difficulty of the task was titrated for each subject, as with digit span. This version of the task ensured that each component was matched for difficulty across groups. Nevertheless, the FLE patients continued to show a marked impairment when their attention was divided. Following Baddeley *et al* (1991), two additional levels of dual task performance were examined, namely tracking combined with tone detection (pressing a foot pedal when the computer emitted a tone) and articulatory suppression combined with tracking. Divided attention was found to be differently impaired in individuals with FLE. This finding of impaired divided attention in individuals with FLE contrasts with a subsequent experiment (CM Cowey *et al* unpublished data) in which a dual task experimental paradigm employing two memory tasks (a divided memory task), one visual and one verbal, does not differentially impair individuals with FLE.

The same study examined recognition and recall memory ability in individuals with FLE to explore Shallice's (1988) hypothesis that the supervisory attentional system, or its working memory equivalent, the central executive, is involved in recall memory. Tests of recall and recognition were equated by employing the Calev (1984) procedure and individuals with FLE, TLE, and healthy controls were examined.

The Calev procedure equates the difficulty of the recall and recognition tests. A measure was taken, therefore, of the difference in scores between recall and recognition and this variable was analyzed. The FLE group displayed the greatest disparity in scores and was significantly different to the healthy control group. The TLE group reached near-significant levels in its difference to the healthy control group and the FLE and TLE groups did not differ significantly. It was argued that the same impairment in these two patient groups arose from disparate underlying cognitive functions.

In order to explore this idea further, performance on recall and recognition tests was correlated with performance on the divided attention task outlined above. It was predicted that a positive relationship would exist between recall and the control of attentional tasks. It was also hypothesized that this relationship would differ from that between recognition and the control of attentional processes.

Correlation analyses supported the hypothesis that recall and recognition are qualitatively distinct memory processes. The results demonstrated a relationship between recall performance and central executive functioning. No such relationship was found between central executive functioning and recognition performance, which suggests that recognition memory does not rely to the same extent on the central executive.

Analysing the individual groups separately revealed that the relationship between recall and divided attention was demonstrated only for the frontal lobe group. A lack of correlation for the temporal lobe group supports the hypothesis that a recall deficit in this group is due to another mechanism. However, the lack of a demonstrated relationship between recall and divided attention in healthy controls challenges the relationship. No difference was found between left and right frontally damaged groups.

SUMMARY AND DISCUSSION

There is a paucity of studies examining neuropsychologic function in intractable FLE. However, existing studies can be employed to deduce general features.

1. There is evidence that intelligence is not grossly impaired in FLE. This finding is consistent with the general view concerning intellectual functioning and frontal lobe damage, which stems from Hebb's original findings (Hebb 1939, 1941; Hebb and Penfield 1940). The caveat to this conclusion is that epileptogenic tissue may, directly or otherwise, cause a general diminution of cognitive ability, as indicated by postoperative improvement despite large portions of the prefrontal cortex being removed.

2. There are impairments in executive functioning in FLE patients, although these may not be as pronounced as those associated with surgical lesions. These impairments are not seen in all patients or on all tasks when comparing groups of patients with FLE and appropriate controls. The major studies by Helmstaedter *et al* (1995) and Upton and Thompson (1996) show variations in patterns of impairment and it is difficult to discern common outcomes between the two studies. To some extent this may reflect the different approaches used by the two centers, but also a more fundamental property of executive function, namely the low correlations between executive tasks generally (Shallice and Burgess 1996). This outcome may be due to the neuroanatomic complexity of the brain systems that are implicated. It is possible that large batteries of frontal tests with aggregate scores, or at least those with subscales such as those that could be derived from the factors identified by Helmstaedter *et al* (1995), are needed to assess the executive dysfunction in these patients. The variable pattern suggests that it could be misleading to rely on single tests of executive function when assessing executive deficit.

3. In contrast to postoperative FLE patients, hemispheric differences are harder to detect in the preoperative group. Milner (1963, 1975) assessed patients who subsequently had unilateral operations, but did not discern differences in performance on tests of executive functioning or memory. This finding contrasts with the performance of patients with TLE. This pattern is similar in the other major studies detailed, with a few exceptions. Upton and Thompson (1996) tended to detect differences, sometimes specifically relating to FLE patients, or more generally showing hemispheric differences when including the TLE group (Table 31.4). The general pattern may be explained, in part, by the relatively small number of patients included in other studies, but may also reflect widespread, bilateral, and fast-propagating epileptic activity, as suggested by Helmstaedter *et al* (1995).

4. Memory is not impaired in the FLE patients to any gross extent (Milner 1975; Delaney *et al* 1980). Again, a caveat might apply when the memory task has a significant executive component, for example in the free recall test using the Calev procedure, in the study by Cowey, Goldstein, Polkey, and Morris (unpublished data), where FLE patients may perform worse due to a failure of efficient organization of the material. There is also the reported failure (not reviewed above) of difficulties on the delayed matching memory task, which

could be interpreted in terms of the executive demands (Swartz *et al* 1994).

5. Overall, the studies reviewed above demonstrate that the discrimination between FLE and TLE groups is not as striking as that which has been reported following neurosurgery. Both Helmstaedter *et al* (1995) and Upton and Thompson (1996) show considerable overlap between the two patient groups and inconsistent differences across tests of executive function. None of the major studies above presents a straightforward sensitivity and specificity of data profiles to discriminate between FLE and TLE patients. While the diagnostic utility of the tests in this context may be limited, their validity is not necessarily challenged. The numerous connections between the frontal and temporal regions suggest that they may form part of one functional system. It is possible, therefore, that the propagation of seizures originating in the mesiotemporal lobe via the prefrontal cortex would cause executive dysfunction, even though executive function has a prefrontal anatomic basis. Hermann *et al* (1988) suggest that the propagation of 'neural noise' anteriorly may make TLE patients show 'frontal-like' performance. Additionally, all executive tasks have nonexecutive features, making performance on them more vulnerable to deficits in, for example, language and perceptual functioning. Methods for improving discrimination should be considered; for example, while both FLE and TLE patients could be thought of as being prone to impairment on executive tasks, the FLE patients tend to be preserved on memory function of a 'nonexecutive' nature. Thus, FLE patients might be better discriminated by taking into account this additional information.

In conclusion, the studies reviewed above provide some indication of the expected deficits associated with FLE. Given that assessment of such patients is often routine practice (Jones-Gotman 1991), collating existing data or producing a systematic approach across centers should improve diagnostic procedures. In the past, this area may have been neglected by researchers, partly because the lack of demonstrable lesions makes FLE patients a less promising group for study. However, the advent of sophisticated neuroimaging techniques may encourage research in this field. The clinical implications of frontal lobe dysfunction are considerable, in terms of the pattern of behavioral dysfunction observed (Boone *et al* 1988). In this respect the refinement of diagnostic techniques, but also the ability to define and monitor cognitive and behavioral disturbance, will provide the impetus for future studies.

KEY POINTS

1. Relatively few data are available concerning the neuropsychologic status of FLE patients prior to brain surgery. The dorsolateral and orbitofrontal regions have, however, been implicated in a wide range of behavioral functions including sequencing of cognition, control of social behavior, and processing of emotions.

2. FLE patients show little if any impairment of general intelligence. Likewise, memory is not impaired to any gross extent.

3. Some, but not all, FLE patients are impaired on some tasks (including the WCST) which are considered to be tests of executive function. Likewise they are impaired, compared to healthy controls and TLE patients, in their ability to divide attention between simultaneous mental operations.

4. Consistent behavioral differences dependent upon the side of seizure origin have not been reported in FLE patients prior to brain surgery.

REFERENCES

Baddeley AD, Bressi S, Della Sala S, Logie R, Spinnler H (1991) The decline of working memory in Alzheimer's disease. *Brain* **114**:2521–2542.

Baddeley A, Della Sala S, Papagno C, Spinnler H (1997) Dual task performance in dysexecutive and nondysexecutive patients with a frontal lesion. *Neuropsychology* **11**:187–194.

Boone KB, Miller BB, Rosenberg L, Durazo, McIntyre H, Weil M (1988) Neuropsychological and behavioural disturbance in an adolescent with frontal seizures. *Neurology* **38**:583–586.

Brickenkamp R (1978) *d2–Aufmerksamkeits–belastungs-test*. Gottingen: Hogrefe.

Brodmann K (1909, 1925) *Vergleichende Lokalisations Lehre der Grosshirninde*. Leipzig: JA Barth.

Brush ES, Mishkin M, Rosvold HE (1961) Effects of object references and aversions on discrimination learning in monkeys with frontal lesions. *Journal of Comparative Physiology and Psychology* **54**:319–325.

Calev A (1984) Recall and recognition in chronic nondemented schizophrenics: use of matched tasks. *Journal of Abnormal Psychology* **93**:172–177.

Canavan AGM, Passingham RE, Marsden CD, Quinn N, Wyke M, Polkey CE (1989) Sequencing ability in Parkinsonians patients with frontal lobe lesions and patients who have undergone unilateral temporal lobectomies. *Neuropsychologia* **27**:787–798.

Chapuis F (1992) *Labyrinthtest*. Gottingen: Hogrefe.

Cowey CM, Green S (1996) The hippocampus: a 'working memory' structure? The effect of hippocampal sclerosis on working memory. *Memory* **4**(1):19–30.

Delaney DC, Rosen AJ, Mattson, Novelly RA (1980) Memory function in focal epilepsy: a comparison of nonsurgical, unilateral temporal lobe and frontal lobe samples. *Cortex* **16**:103–117.

Dodrill CB (1978) A neuropsychological test battery for epilepsy. *Epilepsia* **19**:611–623.

Feldman MJ, Dragow J (1981) *The Visual–Verbal Test (VVT)*. Los Angeles: Western Psychological Services.

Goldman-Rakic PS (1987) Circuitry of primate prefrontal cortex and regulation of behavior by representational memory. In: Plum F (ed.) *Handbook of Physiology. Section I: The Nervous System, Higher Functions of the Brain*, Vol V, pp 373–417. Bethesda, MD: American Physiological Society.

Heaton RK (1981) *Wisconsin Card Sorting Test Manual*. Odessa, FL: Psychology Assessment Resources.

Hebb DO (1939) Intelligence in man after large removal of cerebral tissue: report of four left frontal cases. *Journal of General Psychology* **21**:73–77.

Hebb DO (1941) Human intelligence after removal of cerebral tissue from the right frontal lobe. *Journal of General Psychology* **25**:257–264.

Hebb DO, Penfield W (1940) Human behavior after extensive bilateral removals from the frontal lobes. *Archives of Neurology and Psychiatry* **44**:421–438.

Helmstaedter C, Kemper B, Elger CE (1996) Neuropsychological aspects of frontal epilepsy. *Neuropsychologia* **34**:399–406.

Hermann BP, Wyler AR, Richey ET (1988) Wisconsin Card Sorting Test performance in patients with complex partial seizures of temporal origin. *Journal of Clinical and Experimental Neuropsychology* **10**:467–476.

Horn W (1983) *Leistungsprufsystem L-P-S*. Gottingen: Hogrefe.

Jones-Gotman M (1991) Localization of lesions by neuropsychological testing. *Epilepsia* **32**(Suppl 5):S41–S52.

Kemper B, Helmstaedter C, Elger CE (1992) Kognitive Profile von prachirurgischen Patienten mit Frontal und Temporallappenenepilepsie. In: Shcheffner D (ed) *Epilepsie 91*, pp 345–350. Reinbeck: Enihorn Presse Verlag.

Kemper B, Helmstaedter C, Elger CE (1993) Neuropsychological assessment in patients with frontal lobe epilepsy. *Epilepsia* **34**(Suppl 2):170.

Klouder GV, Cooper WE (1990) Information search following damage to the frontal lobes. *Psychology Reports* **67**:411–416.

Laplane D, Talairach J, Meininger V, Bancaud J & Bouchareine JM (1977) Motor consequences of ablation of motor area in man. *Journal of Neurological Science* **34**:29–39.

Lehrl S, Fischer B (1984) *CI-Test zur raschen objectivierung cerebraler insuffienzen*. Ebersberg: Vless-Test.

Lezak MD (1995) *Neuropsychological Assessment*, 3rd edn. New York: Oxford University Press.

Luria AR (1973) *The Working Brain*. London: Penguin Press.

Luria AR (1980) *Higher Cortical Functions in Man*, 2nd edn. New York: Basic Books.

Milner B (1963) The effects of different brain lesions on card sorting. *Archives of Neurology* **9**:90–100.

Milner B (1964) Some effects of frontal lobectomy in man. In: Warren JM, Akert K (eds) *The Frontal Granular Cortex and Behavior*. New York: McGraw-Hill.

Milner B (1971) Interhemispheric differences in the localization of psychological processes in man. *British Medical Bulletin* **27**:272–277.

Milner B (1975) Psychological aspects of focal epilepsy and its neurosurgical management. In: Purpura DP, Penry JK, Walter RD (eds) *Advances in Neurology, Vol 8, Neurosurgical Management of the Epilepsies*, pp 299–321. New York: Raven Press.

Milner B (1988) Patterns of neuropsychological deficit in frontal lobe epilepies. *Epilepsia* **29**:221.

Milner B (1995) Human frontal lobe function. In: Jasper HH, Riggio S, Goldman-Rakic PS (eds) *Epilepsy and the Functional Anatomy of the Frontal Lobe*, pp 67–82. New York: Raven Press.

Mishkin M, Prockop ES, Rosvold HE (1962) One trial object discrimination learning in monkeys with frontal lesions. *Journal of Comparative Physiology and Psychology* **55**:178–181.

Nelson HE (1976) A modified card sorting test sensitive to frontal lobe defects. *Cortex* **12**:313–324.

Perret E (1974) The left frontal lobe of man and the suppression of habitual responses in verbal categorical behavior. *Neuropsychologia* **12**:323–330.

Porteus SD (1965) *Porteus Maze Test. Fifty Years' Applications.* New York: Psychological Corporation.

Regard M, Strauss E, Knapp P (1982) Children's production on verbal and nonverbal fluency tasks. *Perceptions and Motor Skills* **55**:839–844.

Russell WR (1975) *Explaining the Brain.* London: Oxford University Press.

Shallice T (1988) *From Neuropsychology to Mental Structure.* Cambridge: Cambridge University Press.

Shallice T, Burgess P (1996) The domain of supervisory processes and temporal organization of behaviour. *Philosophical Transactions of the Royal Society* **B351**:1411–1413.

Shallice T, Evans ME (1978) The involvement of the frontal lobes in cognitive estimation. *Cortex* **14**:294–303.

Smith ML, Milner B (1984) Differential effects of frontal lobe lesions on cognitive estimation and spatial memory. *Neuropsychologia* **22**:6797–6805.

Swartz BE, Halgren E, Simkins F, Syndulko K (1994) Primary memory in patients with frontal and primary generalized epilepsy. *Journal of Epilepsy* **7**:232–241.

Upton D, Thompson PJ (1996) General neuropsychological characteristics of frontal lobe epilepsy. *Epilepsy Research* **23**:169–177.

War Department (1944) *Army Individual Test Battery, Manual of Directions and Scoring.* Washington DC: War Department, Adjunct General's Office.

Wechsler D (1964) Die Messung der Intelligenz Erwachsener. *Textband Zum Hamburg - Wechsler - Intelligenztest.* Bern: Hans Huber Verlag.

Wyke M (1969) Influence of direction on the rapidity of bilateral arm movements. *Neuropsychologia* **7**:189–194.

Ontogenetic specialization of hemispheric function

F VARGHA-KHADEM, E ISAACS, K WATKINS, AND M MISHKIN

INTRODUCTION

The division of labor between the two cerebral hemispheres has been recognized for over a century. In adults, the most impressive demonstration of this hemispheric specialization is the dramatic impairment in speech and language resulting from left hemisphere lesions that encroach on the perisylvian areas (Goodglass 1993; Willmes and Poeck 1993). Although some degree of improvement in function may occur after the onset of pathology in these cases, the impairment is typically chronic and, despite intensive efforts at rehabilitation, often remains severe enough to be referred to as an 'aphasia', rather than a 'dysphasia'. The complementary pattern of impairment, namely, a deficit in certain forms of visuospatial function, is produced in the adult by extensive right hemisphere lesions. Although in long-term follow-up these problems are less obvious than the linguistic disorder and tend to interfere less with everyday activities, they nonetheless seriously limit the capacity for cognitive and behavioral function generally and for nonverbal intelligence specifically. These complementary impairments resulting from extensive lesions of the left and right hemisphere of the mature brain have long provided what is perhaps our major source of information regarding hemispheric specialization of function.

In contrast to the vast literature on the cognitive and behavioral consequences of unilateral lesions in adults, there are relatively few studies addressing this issue in children. The dearth of such studies in children is at least partly due to the fact that cerebral lesions sustained during fetal development, infancy, or childhood are, fortunately, relatively rare. The low incidence rates, however, have commonly resulted in the collection of only small and heterogeneous study groups, allowing investigation of the effects of just one variable, usually hemispheric side of damage, even though cognitive outcome after injury is clearly the result of side of injury interacting with numerous other variables, including etiology of the lesion, site and size of damage, age at injury, time since injury, age and developmental status at assessment, presence or absence of epilepsy and, if present, type of epilepsy, etc. Furthermore, except for two recent investigations (Muter *et al* 1997; Bates *et al* 1999), the studies have been retrospective rather than longitudinal ones, and so have not taken into account the important changes in development and learning that are likely to occur after the onset of early lesions. Finally, few studies have examined the locus and extent of early injury in the detail made possible by modern noninvasive magnetic resonance imaging (MRI) techniques.

Despite these drawbacks in the existing literature, it is informative to review the studies on the consequences of early unilateral brain damage in order to trace the evolution of ideas concerning the ontogeny of hemispheric specialization. With that as the focus, we have excluded from this review other types of early damage that affect the development of specialized behavioral and cognitive abilities, in particular speech and language and other verbal functions, such as bilateral pathology (as in bilateral frontal opercular syndrome (Kuzniecky *et al* 1993), inherited forms of verbal dyspraxia (Vargha-Khadem *et al* 1998)) and developmental disorders that are associated with widespread and multifocal pathology (as in specific language impairment (Jernigan *et al* 1991), dyslexia (Paulesu *et al* 1996), William's syndrome (Bellugi *et al* 1988), and autism (Bachevalier 1994)).

THE EQUIPOTENTIALITY VIEW

Among the earliest studies on groups of children with unilateral hemispheric lesions are a series of reports in the 1960s by McFie (1961a; 1961b), Basser (1962), Alajouanine and Lhermitte (1965), and Lenneberg (1967). Although McFie (1961a) concluded that the pattern of intellectual outcome in children with unilateral damage sustained after 1 year of age approximated the pattern observed in adults, namely, deficits in verbal intelligence after left hemisphere damage and in nonverbal intelligence after right hemisphere damage, in fact he failed to obtain any significant differences between the two groups on either type of measure. Moreover, in long-term follow-up of a group of hemispherectomized children, McFie (1961b) found that, whereas verbal abilities were impaired more than nonverbal, this differential effect was independent of the side of the removal. Similarly, Basser (1962) failed to demonstrate hemisphere-dependent effects in speech and language function after hemispherectomy. Alajouanine and Lhermitte (1965) did report selective impairments in speech and written language following early-acquired lesions of the left hemisphere, but they concluded that in long-term follow-up the deficits had disappeared.

The results from these and other early group studies on the effects of early unilateral damage are concordant on two points: (a) compared to adults, children show an impressive degree of plasticity, such that by 1 or more years after injury, despite the chronicity of sensory and motor deficits, the majority of cases show normal or near normal levels of linguistic and intellectual ability; and (b) even in the presence of chronic behavioral and cognitive deficits, there is little evidence for differential hemispheric mediation of verbal and nonverbal functions.

Partly in an attempt to integrate the findings on preservation or recovery of function after early, focal, unilateral lesions, Lenneberg (1967) proposed the *equipotentiality* model, which states that the two cerebral hemispheres are equipotential at the start but gradually acquire specialization with increasing age and learning experience, particularly for speech and language. According to this view, increasing functional specialization with increasing age is accompanied by a gradual decline in neural plasticity, such that, by about the age of puberty, hemispheric specialization becomes 'crystalized', at which point it resembles the adult pattern. If unilateral brain injury occurs at any time during the prepubertal period, then an intact right hemisphere, say, can mediate the speech and language functions of the left hemisphere. The earlier the lesion, however, the more effective the compensatory takeover, and, consequently, the better the outcome.

This implication of the equipotentiality view, that specialized abilities like language should show different degrees of preservation depending on age at injury, has been difficult to test (for a detailed discussion of this issue, see Bates *et al* 1999). Although it is well documented that speech and language are rescued even after very extensive early lesions of the left hemisphere, the shape of the decline in this compensatory process as a function of increasing age at injury has been difficult to measure, mainly because groups of children with left and right hemispheric lesions sustained during each age level up to puberty have not been available for study. As a result, investigators have had to rely on case comparisons (e.g. Vargha-Khadem *et al* 1991) with all their attendant drawbacks. This issue is discussed further later in the chapter.

THE EARLY SPECIALIZATION VIEW

Lenneberg's model prevailed only until the mid-1970s, when a series of studies carried out on children with unilateral lesions (Woods and Teuber 1973; Hecaen 1976; Woods and Carey 1979; Woods 1980), including hemispherectomy (Kohn and Dennis 1974; Dennis and Kohn 1975; Dennis and Whitaker 1976, 1977), obtained evidence of material-specific impairments corresponding to the hemispheric side of insult. This wave of studies helped launch the *early specialization* view of the two cerebral hemispheres, a view that proved to be highly influential, remaining in force at least throughout the 1980s.

To appreciate why the early specialization view held sway for so long, it is necessary to examine developments that were taking place during this same period in disciplines allied to pediatric neuropsychology. For example, in the field of linguistics, Chomsky (1975, 1981) proposed the notion that language and grammar were *innate* properties and autonomous from other cognitive systems. This view of language fits well into Fodor's (1983) model of the modular organization of cognition and is consistent with the data on adult patients with focal brain injury and selective impairments in specific cognitive processes. In this model, a modular deficit is a selective impairment in one area of cognitive function that cannot be explained in terms of a more general loss of cognitive ability. The mapping of the innate module for language to an anatomic region in the brain was provided by the studies of Geschwind and Levitsky (1968), Wada *et al* (1975), and Witelson and Pallie (1973), whose post mortem examinations of the brains of both adults and newborns revealed an asymmetry favoring the left side in the length of the planum temporale within the sylvian fissure. The availability of techniques and paradigms to measure a wide range of psychophysiologic processes, such as long-latency evoked potentials (Molfese and Molfese 1980), heart rate deceleration (Glanville *et al* 1977), and nonnutritive sucking (Entus 1977; Bertoncini *et al* 1989), enabled researchers to investigate whether the anatomic asymmetries in normal infants led to differential responses to lateralized inputs of various types of stimuli. Most, though not all (e.g. Vargha-Khadem and Corballis 1979; Best *et al* 1982; Novak *et al* 1989; Molfese and Burger-Judisch 1991) of these types of studies concluded that hemispheric specialization of function could indeed be demonstrated even in the neonate, thus supporting the notion that the left and right cerebral hemispheres were innately organized to preferentially process verbal and nonverbal information, respectively.

It was against this background that the wave of neuropsychologic studies referred to earlier appeared. The main claim of these studies was that children with early left hemisphere disease or damage, despite the apparent recovery of their speech, continue to show subtle but selective impairments in both verbal intelligence and certain aspects of language. Thus, unlike early right hemidecortication, early left hemidecortication was found to cause deficits in comprehension of complex syntax, specifically of the word order in passive negative sentences (Dennis and Kohn 1975; Dennis and Whitaker 1976, 1977). Further, early acquired lesions on the left but not on the right were found to produce impairments not only in complex receptive grammar (Riva *et al* 1986), but also in expressive grammar (Aram *et al* 1986), lexical retrieval (Aram *et al* 1987), sentence repetition (Riva *et al* 1986), and verbal fluency (Aram *et al* 1990). Frank dysphasic symptoms were observed by Hecaen (1976) in long-term follow-up of a group of children with acquired left hemisphere lesions, although in this study comparative data were not provided for children with right hemisphere lesions. Even in cases with

congenital injury, impairments after left as compared with right hemisphere damage were observed in speech and language as well as in writing and spelling (Woods and Teuber 1973, 1978; Woods and Carey 1979). Finally, our own initial study on hemiplegic children with congenital or acquired hemispheric lesions (Vargha-Khadem *et al* 1985) revealed impairments in receptive language and in lexical retrieval after left as compared with right hemisphere damage, although these differential findings were no longer evident when patients with seizures were excluded from the analysis (Vargha-Khadem *et al* 1992).

During the period in which the early specialization view prevailed, the majority of studies reported in the literature concentrated on language functions, although there were a few reports in which visuospatial functions had been examined, either of small groups or of single cases in whom early neuropathology had led to hemispherectomy (Gott 1973; Kohn and Dennis 1974; Damasio *et al* 1975; Ogden 1989). The most pronounced evidence of hemisphere-dependent impairment was obtained by Kohn and Dennis (1974), who found that right hemispherectomized patients (*n* = 4) performed more poorly than left hemispherectomized patients (*n* = 4), but only on those aspects of visuospatial function, such as map-reading, that are late-maturing in the normal child. (It is worth noting, however, that a similar pattern of results, i.e. no impairment on simple visuospatial tasks but pronounced impairment on more demanding ones, was later reported by Ogden (1989) in two patients with infantile hemiplegia and seizures who underwent *left* hemispherectomy during adolescence.)

Although these neuropsychologic studies supporting the early specialization view suffered from many methodological shortcomings (for critical reviews, see Bishop 1983, 1988), their message reinforced the idea that had been forming simultaneously in the other disciplines that the hemispheric division of labor for processing verbal and nonverbal material begins as early as birth or shortly after.

THE ONTOGENETIC SPECIALIZATION VIEW

With the addition of several new investigations in the 1990s, there has by now been a sizable accumulation of reports on cognitive outcome in children with unilateral brain damage. For example, from 1977 to 1999, at least nine different studies have appeared wherein groups of children with left or right hemisphere lesions were directly compared on the well-standardized verbal and performance measures of the Wechsler Intelligence Scales (Table 32.1). Unfortunately, again largely because of small and heterogeneous groups in many of the studies, the findings continue to be divergent, and so a clear consensus has still not

Table 32.1 Summary of results for verbal and performance IQ in children with left vs. right hemisphere damage (adapted from Vargha-Khadem et al (1994) and Bates et al (1999)).

Study	n^a	Age at lesion onset	Time postlesion (years:months)^a	Seizure history (% incidence)^a	Verbal IQ^a	Performance IQ^a
Woods (1980)	L = 27 R = 23	Early = <1 year Late = >1 year	Le = 17:2 Re = 14:1 Ll = 8:6 Rl = 10:3	Le = 27 Re = 50 Ll = 19 Rl = 15	Le < normal Re < normal Ll < normal Rl = normal	Le < normal Re < normal Ll < normal Rl < normal
Riva and Cazzaniga (1986)	L = 22 R = 26	Early = <1 year Late = >1 year	Early = 8:5 Late = 4:2	None	Le < normal Re = normal Ll = normal Rl = normal	Le < normal Re < normal Ll = normal Rl < normal
Riva et al (1986)	L = 8 R = 8	Not divided by age of lesion onset	L = 6:8 R = 4:6	L = 37.5 R = 37.5	L < normal R = normal	L < normal R < normal
Nass et al (1989)	L = 15 R = 13	Pre/perinatal	L = 6:7 R = 8:5	Not indicated	L = normal R = normal	L < normal R < normal
Vargha-Khadem et al (1992)	L = 42 R = 40	Congenital/perinatal	L = 12:3 R = 11.5	Two seizure groups Two nonseizure groups	L + S < normal L – S < normal R + S < normal R – S = normal	L + S < normal L – S < normal R + S < normal R – S < normal
Ballantyne et al (1994)	L = 8 R = 9	Congenital/perinatal	L = 9:0 R = 11:2	L = 62.5 R = 55.5	L < normal R < normal L VIQ = PIQ R VIQ > PIQ	L < normal R < normal L VIQ = PIQ R VIQ > PIQ
Goodman and Yude (1996)	L = 51 R = 73	Congenital/perinatal	(range 6–10 years)	~40	L + R < normal L + R VIQ > PIQ	L + R < normal L + R PIQ < VIQ
Muter et al (1997)	L = 23 R = 15	Congenital/perinatal	L = 4:9 R = 4:9	L = 35 R = 27	L + S < normal L – S = normal R + S < normal R – S = normal	L + S < normal L – S < normal R + S < normal R – S < normal
Bates et al (1999)	L = 28 R = 15	Congenital/perinatal	L = 5:4 R = 5:5	L = 40.7 R = 46.7	L < normal R < normal L = R	L < normal R < normal L = R

^{a}L = Left hemisphere damage; R = right hemisphere damage; e = early lesion onset; l = late lesion onset; + S = with seizure history; – S = without seizure history.

emerged. It should be pointed out, however, that there is clear agreement between the findings in the two studies with the largest populations (Vargha-Khadem *et al* 1992 (*n* = 82); Goodman and Yude 1996 (*n* = 124), both of which report no significant differences between verbal and performance intelligence quotient (IQ) as a function of hemispheric side of damage.

The studies on speech and language after early unilateral damage are even more difficult to assess, because, in addition to containing small and heterogeneous samples, they have used different and often nonstandardized tests. In their review of numerous published and ongoing investigations spanning the period from 1961 to 1999, Bates *et al* (1999) concluded that a clear consensus had likewise not been reached regarding linguistic outcome. They acknowledged that delays in language production, particularly in expressive grammar, are more likely to occur in children with damage to the left hemisphere (Thal *et al* 1991; Kempler *et al* 1996; Reilly *et al* 1998), but these effects are neither robust nor stable. Furthermore, the most frequent reports regarding side-dependent effects were negative ones. Finally, an ongoing study by Vicari and colleagues on groups of children with left or right hemisphere lesions and normal controls matched for age, sex, and social class has so far concluded that 'there is absolutely no evidence for a difference between LH [left hemisphere] and RH [right hemisphere] children on any language measure' (quoted in Bates *et al* 1999).

Outcome studies of visuospatial ability after early unilateral cerebral damage are also difficult to evaluate. A leading group in this area (Stiles-Davis *et al* 1985; Stiles and Nass 1991; Stiles *et al* 1996, 1997) has obtained some evidence suggesting that the pattern of deficits in visuospatial processing in children with focal lesions resembles one that has been seen in adult patients with unilateral posterior lesions, namely, greater impairment in local processing after left-sided damage and in global processing after damage on the right. Like the linguistic impairments, however, the visuospatial deficits are neither robust nor consistently present on different measures. Furthermore, longitudinal follow-up revealed substantial recovery of function, such that by adolescence many of the patients had attained levels of performance that did not differ from those of normal controls (Stiles 1998; Stiles *et al* 1999).

In discussing the ontogeny of hemispheric specialization, and cognizant of the importance of developmental plasticity and its compatibility with the equipotentiality hypothesis, but cognizant also of the undeniable fact that in the absence of brain damage the majority of individuals go on to demonstrate hemispheric specialization in adulthood, Satz *et al* (1990) argued in favor of a middle ground between the extremes of equipotentiality and early specialization. This compromise position, which has been referred to as 'constrained plasticity' (Bates *et al* 1999), we shall call *ontogenetic specialization*. Unlike the equipotentiality position, the mediating view assumes that hemispheric specialization has an anatomic basis that is genetically determined, and further that, under normal circumstances, functional expression of this genetic disposition can begin to appear even very early in life. However, unlike the early specialization view, it also assumes that such functional expression is determined during development by the interaction between environmentally evoked neural activity and the special form of neural plasticity that appears to end during puberty (Lenneberg 1967). Accordingly, early brain damage may counteract the genetic disposition by affecting and modifying the activity/plasticity interaction.

The ontogenetic specialization view fits well with research on the normal development of linguistic functions. Studies of event-related potentials (ERPs) have shown that while even very young infants, just like adults, are electrophysiologically sensitive to a range of acoustic features that characterize speech as opposed to nonspeech sounds, such as temporal lag, voicing cue, etc., their ERP responses are not as clearly lateralized as they are in adults, suggesting that the two hemispheres may be more nearly equal in infancy than they are later in their ability to process these types of distinctions (Simos and Molfese 1997; Simos *et al* 1997). Similarly, Dehaene-Lambertz and Baillet (1998), studying phonologic processing with ERPs, found that infants, like adults, process phonemes categorically; but unlike adults, who show activation predominantly in the left temporal lobe (Naatanen *et al* 1997), infants show more bilaterally symmetrical processing, even though the voltages are higher on the left. A second study (Dehaene-Lambertz 1999) pursued this question of phoneme processing in infants by contrasting the effects of a phonemic change with a voice change or, separately, a change in timbre. Results again indicated higher voltages over the left hemisphere for the phonetic change, but, unlike in adults, there was no greater asymmetry for the phonetic than for the nonphonetic discrimination. When and how this asymmetry in response to both phonetic and nonphonetic stimuli eventually turns into left hemisphere specialization for linguistic processing selectively remains an open question. A possible answer suggested by connectionist theorists (Elman *et al* 1996), and one that is consistent with the position favored here, is that language experience itself propels the emerging specialization of the left hemisphere for this function (Elman *et al* 1996).

The ontogenetic specialization view also fits well with the increasing recognition that, in the aftermath of early brain injury, the ontogenetic trend toward hemispheric specialization is probably influenced by many variables that can counter this trend. Thus, one level of a variable, say a very small unilateral lesion, could well lead to a finding that accords with early specialization, while a level of the variable at the opposite extreme, in this case an extensive unilateral lesion, could result in a finding suggesting equipotentiality. The same could be true for widely divergent levels of many other variables. In attempting to resolve the discrepancies in the literature, numerous authors have touched on this issue, raising questions about the role of such factors as age at lesion onset (Goodman and Yude 1996; Vargha-Khadem *et al* 1997), lesion site as well as size (Banich *et al* 1990; Thal *et al* 1991; Isaacs *et al* 1996; Bates *et al* 1999), unsuspected contralateral pathology (Gadian *et al* 1996), presence of seizures (Vargha-Khadem *et al* 1992; Muter *et al* 1997), stage of development of the cognitive function under study (Marchman *et al* 1991; Thal *et al* 1991; Feldman *et al* 1992), age at testing (Feldman *et al* 1992; Dall'Oglio *et al* 1994), elapsed time since onset of the pathology (Levine *et al* 1987; Banich *et al* 1990; but see Bates *et al* 1999), and so on. However, none of these studies obtained definitive evidence regarding the role of such variables in tilting the results in favor of one or the other extreme theoretic position.

EFFECTS OF HEMIPLEGIA-CAUSING LESIONS ON INTELLIGENCE

The above review of previous research suggests that the ontogenetic specialization hypothesis probably provides the best fit to the available data. At the same time, this plausible notion, namely, that functional specialization of the hemispheres emerges and becomes consolidated only gradually during the course of normal development, and so can be overridden in cases of early unilateral injury, still lacks direct empirical support from brain-lesion studies. As already pointed out, all previous brain-injury studies, the authors' own included, were plagued by the presence of many uncontrolled and therefore potentially confounding variables. Because the total sample sizes were always relatively small, more homogeneous patient groups could not readily be formed, and so systematic investigation of these variables could not be undertaken. Among these variables, perhaps the most critical one for the issue under discussion is age at onset of injury. According to the ontogenetic specialization view, cognitive outcome after unilateral brain injury should vary depending on the age at which the damage occurred. Thus, congenital or very early-acquired

unilateral lesions should yield the same cognitive effects irrespective of lesion side, whereas comparable unilateral lesions sustained later in childhood, but before maturity, should begin to result in side-dependent deficits resembling those seen in brain-injured adults.

To test this prediction, we have here examined the IQ data obtained from the largest sample gathered to date of children who had suffered a single, nonprogressive, unilateral hemispheric insult resulting in a hemiplegia. The large sample size (nearly 200) allowed us to compare the effects of hemispheric side of damage on standardized measures of verbal and nonverbal intelligence as a function of age at injury, while controlling for the important variable of seizure history (see Vargha-Khadem *et al* 1992).

METHODS

Subjects

A total of 196 hemiplegic patients were divided into two groups according to hemispheric side of insult (left, $n = 106$; right, $n = 90$). The patients had all presented as children with neurologic problems to the neurology and/or neurosurgery departments of two pediatric hospitals, either for initial diagnosis or routine follow-up. The criterion for the selection of patients was the existence of a measurable degree of hemiparesis resulting from a unilateral brain lesion, sustained at some point during either gestational life or childhood. The unilateral nature of the injury was determined by neurologic examination and confirmed, when possible, by EEG (72 patients), and/or brain scans obtained with either CT or MR (90 patients). Patients with suspected bilateral involvement were excluded from the sample.

The patient groups with unilateral left or right hemisphere insult were each divided further into three age-at-injury groups, namely, a group with congenital injury ($n = 96$), one with early-acquired injury (i.e. 1 month to < 5 years; $n = 46$), and a third with late-acquired injury (i.e. 5–16 years; $n = 54$). The congenital group consisted of those who had sustained an injury prenatally, or, rarely, postnatally before the age of 1 month. In the latter cases, it was not possible to determine whether or not adverse prenatal conditions had predisposed the newborn infant to suffer from complications at or shortly after birth. The congenital origin of the brain injury was inferred from a normal course of pregnancy and the presence of either a unilateral deficit in motor coordination or a unilateral reduction in limb size documented by a physician within the first 6–9 months after birth, and/or an abnormally early demonstration of hand preference associated with disuse of the other hand during the same period of infancy. Because of the absence of a documented medical episode, it was inferred that the etiology of the cerebral insult was an ischemic event that had occurred at some stage during gestational development or shortly after birth. A section from the MR scan of a patient representative of the congenital group is shown in Fig. 32.1a.

The groups with early-acquired or late-acquired insult consisted of those children in whom a hemiplegia or hemiparesis became apparent after a single well-documented episode, nonprogressive in nature, and in whom previous neurologic development had been normal. The documented episode in these children, which occurred on average at the age of 7 years, was most frequently a cerebrovascular stroke. Other etiologies included tumor, trauma, cerebrovascular anomalies, Rasmussen encephalitis, infection, etc. Table 32.2 shows the main etiologic categories for both the early-acquired and late-acquired groups.

A section from the MR scan of a patient representative of these two groups is shown in Fig. 32.1b.

The six left and right hemisphere groups with congenital, early-acquired, or late-acquired injury were each further divided into two groups on the basis of the presence ($n = 52$) or absence ($n = 144$) of a history of clinical seizures of cerebral origin, excluding febrile convulsions or uncontrolled seizures. Patients with only febrile convulsions were included in the group without seizures. Patients with uncontrolled seizure disorders, i.e. those having convulsions on a daily basis and/or those who had suffered an episode of status epilepticus, were excluded from the sample. The great majority of the retained patients with a history of seizures had had their first seizure before the age of 4 years, and all were on anticonvulsant medication. In some cases, the medication resulted in complete seizure control, although others continued to have seizures, but with only a very few having them as frequently as once per week. Before psychologic testing, the adequacy of the blood levels for anticonvulsant agents was verified for the vast majority of the patients.

The 12 patient groups formed on the basis of the foregoing classification, and the numbers for each, are listed in Table 32.2. Table 32.3 shows each group's mean and standard deviation for age at insult, age at test, and elapsed time since insult.

Materials and procedures

All patients were given the age-appropriate Wechsler Intelligence Scales (WISC, WISC-R, WISC III, Wechsler-Bellevue, WAIS, WAIS-R) to provide measures of verbal, performance, and full-scale intelligence (VIQ, PIQ, FSIQ) (Wechsler 1955, 1976, 1981, 1990, 1992). The test was

Table 32.2 Etiologies of single-episode insult and their incidence.

Etiology	<5 years	No. of patients 5–16 years	Total
CVA[a]	27	32	59
HI[a]	5	5	10
AVM[a]	2	5	7
Tumor	2	4	6
Trauma	2	3	5
Other	1	3	4
RE[a]	0	3	3
Cyst	1	0	1
Total	40	55	95

[a]CVA = cerebrovascular accident; HI = hypoxia ischemia; AVM = arteriovenous malformation; RE = Rasmussen encephalitis.

Table 32.3 FSIQ scores and mean age at insult, age at test and elapsed time since insult.

Groups[a]	n	Mean age at injury (years: months (SD))	Mean age at test (years: months (SD))	Mean time to test (years: months (SD))	Mean FSIQ (SD)
LcNS	39	0 (0)	12:5 (3:7)	12:5 (3:7)	99.1 (16.0)
LcS	13	0 (0)	11:11 (2:8)	11:11 (2:8)	84.5 (13.3)
LeNS	19	2:5 (1:9)	8:10 (3:10)	6:5 (4:5)	88.7 (14.9)
LeS	6	2:8 (0.10)	12:4 (5:0)	9:7 (5:0)	89.5 (10.1)
LlNS	24	9:1 (2:8)	13:5 (4:5)	4:3 (4:0)	93.7 (18.4)
LlS	5	12:0 (3:5)	15:0 (4:4)	3:0 (2:3)	90.6 (20.8)
RcNS	28	0 (0)	11:6 (3:6)	11:6 (3:6)	98.6 (18.5)
RcS	16	0 (0)	11:7 (3:7)	11:7 (3:7)	89.2 (12.0)
ReNS	15	2:6 (1:7)	8:3 (4:5)	5:8 (4:5)	98.2 (13.0)
ReS	6	1:7 (1:5)	12:8 (3:10)	11:0 (4:0)	81.0 (5.8)
RlNS	19	9:6 (3:5)	12:6 (3:11)	3:0 (3:5)	96:9 (13.7)
RlS	6	9:0 (3:8)	12:3 (2:9)	3:3 (2:9)	89.8 (12.9)

[a] L = left hemisphere; R = right hemisphere; c = congenital injury; e = early-acquired injury; l = late-acquired injury; NS = nonseizure; S = seizure.

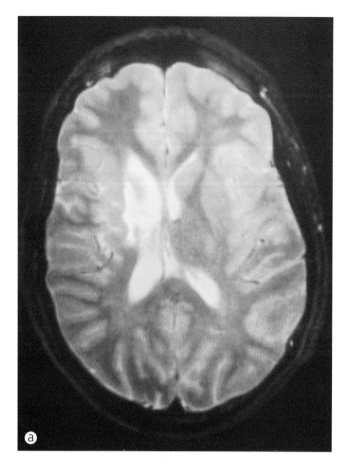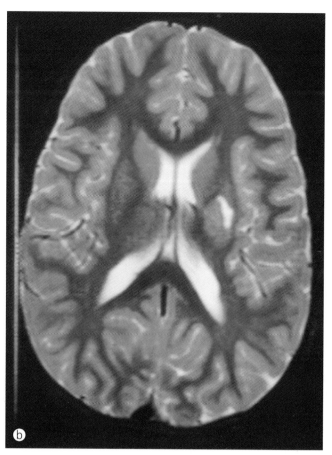

Fig. 32.1 Horizontal sections from MRI scans of two representative patients with strokes in the territory of the middle cerebral artery, each with lesion-severity ratings of 2 on a scale of 1–5 with 1 being most severe (Vargha-Khadem *et al* 1985 with permission from Oxford University Press). (a) Congenital lesion. (b) Acquired lesion.

administered in full to each child, individually, in a quiet room according to the instructions of the manual.

RESULTS

The FSIQ scores for each of the 12 groups are shown in Table 32.3, and those for VIQ and PIQ are shown in Table 32.4. The latter two scores were used as the dependent variables in an analysis of variance with repeated measures to determine the effects on verbal and nonverbal intelligence of the independent variables of hemispheric side of insult, age at insult, and presence or absence of seizures. Whenever appropriate, post hoc comparisons between groups were carried out using Student's two-tailed *t*-tests.

Effects of seizures on IQ

As indicated in Table 32.4, nearly all groups without seizures obtained mean VIQ and PIQ scores in the average range (90–109). In contrast, the groups with a history of seizures generally had lower scores on both

measures, with means often falling in the low average range (80–89) or even below. Across the entire group of 196 patients, this difference yielded the only significant main effect, indicating that patients with a history of seizures scored reliably lower than patients without seizures on both IQ measures (mean difference = –8.2 points, $P = 0.002$; Fig. 32.2). This strong impact of seizure history on IQ was totally independent of the effects of the other variables – side of injury and age at injury – in that there were no significant interactions with these other factors. Furthermore, it is interesting to note that these other variables did not independently exert any influence across the two types of IQ.

When the scores of the seizure and nonseizure groups were analyzed separately, the main effect of IQ type was found to be significant, but in the nonseizure group only. As shown in Fig. 32.2, regardless of hemispheric side of insult, the mean VIQ score of those without a history of seizures was slightly but significantly higher than their mean PIQ score (mean difference = 2.8 points, $P = 0.015$) suggesting that, in the absence of seizures, priority is assigned

Table 32.4 VIQ and PIQ scores following insult.

Groups[a]	n	VIQ (SD)	PIQ (SD)
LcNS	39	100.7 (17.1)	97.8 (15.6)
LcS	13	87.9 (12.9)	84.7 (12.4)
LeNS	19	90.8 (13.8)	89.0 (14.8)
LeS	6	90.7 (13.4)	89.8 (7.6)
LlNS	24	92.5 (20.4)	95.3 (16.6)
LlS	5	82.8 (25.0)	99.4 (15.8)
RcNS	28	100.5 (20.2)	96.5 (15.9)
RcS	16	90.1 (14.0)	90.2 (12.4)
ReNS	15	101.1 (10.6)	95.6 (16.6)
ReS	6	86.3 (11.0)	78.0 (12.1)
RlNS	19	100.5 (14.6)	93.7 (13.9)
RlS	6	92.0 (9.9)	89.3 (17.6)

[a] L = left hemisphere; R = right hemisphere; c = congenital injury; e = early-acquired injury; l = late-acquired injury; NS = nonseizure; S = seizure.

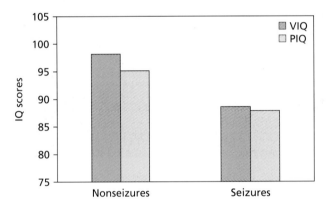

Fig. 32.2 Effects of seizures. Mean difference between the two groups is 8.2 IQ points, P = 0.002. Mean VIQ–PIQ difference in nonseizure group is 2.8 IQ points, P = 0.015.

to the preservation of verbal abilities. In the children with a history of seizures, however, this priority disappears.

Effects of hemispheric side of insult on IQ

Across the entire group of patients (i.e. both those with and those without a history of seizures), there was a significant interaction between hemispheric side of injury and IQ type (P = 0.025). Post hoc comparisons indicated that there were no significant differences between the left and right groups on either VIQ (mean difference = −3.1 points) or PIQ (mean difference = 0.7 points). Rather, the interaction resulted from the fact that, in the group with right hemisphere damage, VIQ was relatively better preserved than PIQ (mean difference = 4.2 points, P = 0.008; Fig. 32.3a). The same analysis performed on the scores of the seizure and nonseizure groups separately showed similar patterns, but ones which fell just short of significance (P = 0.071 and 0.055, respectively; Fig. 32.3b, c). None of the analyses

indicated a comparable sparing of PIQ after left hemisphere insult (mean difference = 0.4 points). As indicated below, the relative sparing of VIQ after right hemisphere damage was due mainly to the results obtained in the group with injuries that were acquired late in childhood.

Effects of age at insult on IQ

Across the entire group of patients, there was a significant three-way interaction between age at insult, hemispheric side of insult, and IQ type (P = 0.025; Fig. 32.4). Post hoc analyses indicated that this interaction was due mainly to the results obtained in the group with late-acquired injuries, as follows. First, the two-way interactions between side of injury and IQ type were analyzed for each of the three age-at-injury groups separately; only the interaction in the late-acquired group was significant (P = 0.008). Second, post hoc comparisons between VIQ and PIQ were run for each of the six side-of-injury by age-at-injury groups; again, the only difference that approached significance was the one for the right late-acquired group (mean difference = 5.9 points, P = 0.056). The comparison for the left late-acquired group also fell short of significance (mean difference = −5.2 points, P = 0.101).

The three-way interactions between age at injury, side of injury, and IQ type analyzed separately for the seizure and nonseizure groups again revealed patterns of results similar to the one obtained for the group as a whole, but these interactions were not significant.

DISCUSSION

Effects of seizures on IQ

The results of this large-scale study of hemiplegic children confirms an earlier finding with a smaller sample (Vargha-Khadem et al 1992), namely that seizures, even though their clinical manifestation is relatively well controlled by anticonvulsant medication, have a deleterious effect on intelligence. In the present study the seizure factor reduced both VIQ and PIQ by about 8 points in relation to patients without a history of seizures, and by about 12 points in relation to the hypothetic normal population means of 100. This deleterious effect was about the same regardless of which hemisphere was injured or when it was injured. In contrast, hemiplegia-causing lesions that did not result in seizures reduced VIQ and PIQ by only about 3 points in relation to the normal population means.

In the absence of the added burden of a history of seizures, there is a small but significant tendency for the preferential rescue of VIQ as compared with PIQ (mean

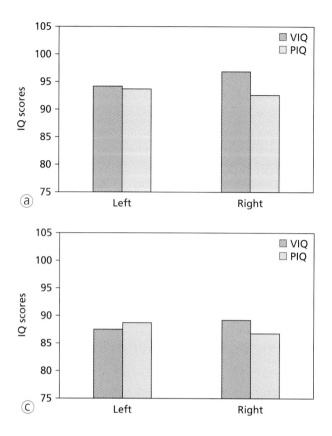

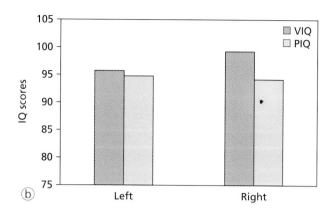

Fig. 32.3 Interaction between hemispheric side of injury and IQ type. (a) All patients ($n = 196$, $P = 0.025$); (b) nonseizure patients ($n = 144$, $P = 0.055$); (c) seizure patients ($n = 52$, $P = 0.073$).

scores of 98 and 95, respectively), with this effect also being independent of which hemisphere was injured and when it was injured. Thus, the net effect of an early hemiplegia-causing lesion that does not result in seizures is a slight but selective lowering of PIQ (see also Satz *et al* 1990). The cost paid by nonverbal functions for the sparing of verbal functions was labeled 'crowding' by Hans-Lukas Teuber and his colleagues (Woods and Teuber 1973; Milner 1974; Teuber 1975), but this phenomenon was assumed to be

hemisphere dependent, reflecting successful rescue of speech and language functions by a nondominant hemisphere (usually the right) after sufficiently early lesions of the dominant hemisphere. The results described above are consistent with previous reports from our group (Vargha-Khadem *et al* 1992; Muter *et al* 1997) and with those reported by Goodman and Yude (1996). They are also consistent with the notion that PIQ is 'crowded out' by the higher-priority VIQ. However, the effect in our hemiplegic cases without a history of seizures is only a small one and is clearly independent of whether the hemispheric damage is on the left or the right. Moreover, inasmuch as only a small minority of our patients with left hemisphere damage give any evidence of a shift of speech and language functions to the right (Isaacs *et al* 1996), our results imply, in addition, that the 'crowding' effect occurs regardless of whether or not there is postinjury reorganization of speech and language functions. Finally, in the patients with a history of seizures, the electrographic abnormality, the anticonvulsant medication, or both, apparently interfere sufficiently with the functions of undamaged tissue, whether in the intact portions of the damaged hemisphere or in the undamaged hemisphere, such that the priority which would otherwise be given to VIQ gives way to the more serious challenge of rescuing intellectual functions overall.

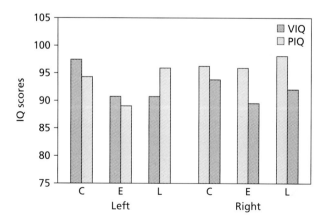

Fig. 32.4 Three-way interaction between age at injury, hemispheric side of injury, and IQ type. All patients ($n = 196$, $P = 0.025$). C = congenital lesion; E = early-acquired lesion; L = late-acquired lesion.

Effects of hemispheric side of injury on IQ

Unlike the results of large-scale investigations carried out on adults with unilateral cerebral lesions (Milner 1975; Warrington *et al* 1986), but like earlier findings on children with such lesions, as reported both in our own studies (Vargha-Khadem *et al* 1992, 1994; Muter *et al* 1997) and in many of the studies of others (e.g. Riva and Cazzaniga 1986; Riva *et al* 1986; Nass *et al* 1989; Goodman and Yude 1996; Bates *et al* 1999), there was no significant effect of side of lesions on either VIQ or PIQ. In the adult studies, left hemisphere lesions were found to result in a discrepancy of 7 to 9 points in favor of PIQ, and right hemisphere lesions in an even larger discrepancy of 12 points in favor of VIQ (Milner 1975; Warrington *et al* 1986). In the present study, on the other hand, there was no discrepancy in IQ type after left-sided injuries, and only a 4-point discrepancy in favor of VIQ after right-sided injuries. (The latter difference yielded the significant interaction between side of injury and IQ type.) Although both Milner and Warrington and her colleagues emphasized that the discrepancy scores they observed in their large adult samples (955 cases in Milner's study and 656 in the Warrington *et al* study) were quite variable, they nevertheless suggested that these discrepancies could be used as a first approximation in characterizing the specialized functions of the two cerebral hemispheres. This conclusion, however, is only applicable to the effects of unilateral lesions in adults, in whom hemispheric specialization has already been established before the injury. Clearly, the same conclusion cannot be applied to the effects of hemispheric lesions in children, presumably because hemispheric specialization of cognitive function emerges only gradually during development. One practical by-product of this difference in outcome after childhood vs. adult brain injury is that, whereas a large discrepancy between VIQ and PIQ scores can provide an important clue to the lateralization of a focal lesion in an adult, it cannot do so either in a child with a congenital brain injury or in one with a brain injury sustained before the age of about 5 years. The reason for suggesting this age as the tentative cut-off in the differential consequences of early vs. late hemispheric damage derives from the final results to be discussed.

Effects of age at injury on IQ

In addition to the interaction of side of injury with IQ type, there was also a three-way interaction involving age at injury. The analyses based on this interaction revealed that, whereas there was no influence of lesion side on IQ type in either the congenital or early-acquired groups, the group with lesions acquired at the age of 5 or later in childhood had a pattern of IQ scores that was at least qualitatively sim-

ilar to the one that has been reported in adults (see Fig. 32.4). In this age group only, there was a significant interaction between hemispheric side of injury and IQ type. Thus, in the patients with right hemisphere lesions, there was a VIQ–PIQ difference of 6 points, while in the patients with left hemisphere lesions, there was a PIQ–VIQ difference of 5 points. Although each of these discrepancy scores alone fell short of significance (i.e. only the interaction was reliable), and although each is roughly only half as large as that found after injuries acquired in adulthood (see above), the overall similarity in the pattern of results suggests that hemispheric specialization starts to become consolidated at about age 5 years, and then presumably becomes more firmly fixed gradually, i.e. less vulnerable to the effects of unilateral damage, throughout later childhood.

CONCLUSIONS

Our results suggest that hemispheric specialization of cognitive function, at least as indicated by a dissociation between verbal and performance IQ in children with unilateral, hemiplegia-causing brain injuries, begins to appear only at about age 5 years or later. Some cautions must of course be placed around this conclusion. First, the VIQ–PIQ discrepancies in the group with late-onset lesions were just at the borderline of detectability. It remains for future large-scale studies of children with unilateral lesions to determine whether more clear-cut or even earlier hemispheric dissociations might appear on particular linguistic and visuospatial tests that may tap more selective, and so perhaps earlier maturing, aspects of hemispheric function. Second, the exact age at which specialization in IQ appears is still uncertain. All that can be said at present is that, at some point between ages 5 and 16 years, functional development is sufficiently advanced and/or developmental neural plasticity is sufficiently attenuated that some degree of specialized hemispheric processing can be observed after unilateral injury sustained during this developmental period. Both of the above circumstances, i.e. advanced functional development and attenuated plasticity, are probably present when the injury occurs close to puberty. However, at least two very different scenarios can be imagined when the injury occurs in the early part of the period, closer to age 5 years, and further cognitive development over many childhood years must still take place in the presence of unilateral damage. Under these circumstances, one possibility is that the consolidation of hemispheric specialization has already been set in motion and the two hemispheres will continue undeflected on that course during further development, constrained only by the functional limitation of the damaged hemisphere. The other possibility is that environmental pressure combines with a still high degree of developmental plasticity to partially override the genetic disposition toward hemispheric specialization, just as it apparently does more fully when the injury occurs before age 5 years. Deciding between these and other alternatives will require a more fine-grained analysis of age at lesion onset than the one carried out here. With these caveats, however, it can be concluded that the results support at least the general notion of ontogenetic specialization, i.e. the gradual emergence and consolidation during development of hemispheric specialization for cognitive abilities.

When unilateral brain damage is incurred congenitally or even in early childhood before age 5 years, the anatomic disposition toward hemispheric specialization will be overridden by a fairly extensive, hemiplegia-causing lesion. In losing whatever cognitive advantage accrues to a clear division of labor between two normal hemispheres, the damaged brain may preserve the most effective performance possible of the cognitive functions that are under the greatest environmental demand. Perhaps the prime example of environmental demand on children is social communication through speech and language. If an early unilateral lesion of either hemisphere encroaches on this function's normal neural substrates, which are centered on the perisylvian region, the young child will need to recruit additional neuronal resources from one or both hemispheres depending on the site and extent of the damage. This recruitment, enabled by developmental neural plasticity, may ensure enough neuronal tissue to satisfy the demands of speech and language development. However, this type of reorganization can occur only at the cost of other cognitive systems, which may be 'crowded out' and become diffusely represented because the neuronal resources needed for their development have been siphoned off by the higher-priority function. The net effect of an early and extensive lesion of either hemisphere would thus be a nonspecialized pattern of hemispheric organization for intellectual functions, differing from the pattern in the normal adult not only in being nonlateralized, but also possibly lacking many of its *intra*hemispheric functional specializations.

ACKNOWLEDGEMENTS

We are indebted to the children and the children's families who participated in this study. We thank Alexandra Hogan for her help in collecting and analyzing the data on some of the patients with acquired stroke, and Fenella Kirkham for making these patients available to us. This study was supported in part by the Medical Research Council and the Wellcome Trust.

KEY POINTS

1. Hemispheric specialization for IQ measures is not evident in children who have sustained unilateral, hemiplegia-causing brain injuries before the age of 5 years.

2. Presumably, a genetic disposition toward hemispheric specialization is overridden in such cases by recruitment of the undamaged hemisphere to meet environmental demands (e.g. for social communication through language), and that such recruitment is possible only during early development, when neural plasticity is at its peak.

REFERENCES

Alajouanine T, Lhermitte F (1965) Acquired aphasia in children. *Brain* **88**:653–662.
Aram D, Ekelman B, Whitaker H (1986) Spoken syntax in children with acquired unilateral hemisphere lesions. *Brain and Language* **27**:75–100.
Aram D, Ekelman B, Whitaker H (1987) Lexical retrieval in left and right brain-lesioned children. *Brain and Language* **31**:61–89.
Aram D, Meyers S, Ekelman B (1990) Fluency of conversational speech in children with unilateral brain lesions. *Brain and Language* **38**:105–121.
Ballantyne AO, Scarvie KM, Trauner DA (1994) Verbal performance IQ patterns in children after perinatal stroke. *Developmental Neuropsychology* **10** (1): 39–50.
Bachevalier J (1994) Medial temporal lobe structures and autism: a review of clinical and experimental findings. *Neuropsychologia* **32**(6):627–648.
Banich M, Levine S, Kim H, Huttenlocher P (1990) The effects of developmental factors on IQ in hemiplegic children. *Neuropsychologia* **28**:35–47.
Basser L (1962) Hemiplegia of early onset and the faculty of speech with special reference to the effects of hemispherectomy. *Brain* **85**:427–460.

Bates E, Thal D, Trauner D *et al* (1997) From first words to grammar in children with focal brain injury. *Developmental Neuropsychology* **13**(3):447–476.

Bates E, Vicari S, Trauner D (1999) Neural mediation of language development: perspectives from lesion studies of infants and children. In: Tager-Flusberg H (ed) *Neurodevelopmental Disorders*, pp 533–581. Cambridge, MA: MIT Press.

Bellugi U, Marks S, Bihrle A, Sabo H (1988) Dissociation between language and cognitive functions in Williams syndrome. In: Bishop D, Mogford K *Language Development in Exceptional Circumstances*, pp 179–189. Edinburgh: Churchill Livingstone.

Bertoncini J, Morais J, Bijeljac-Babic R, McAdams S, Peretz Mehler J (1989) Dichotic perception and laterality in neonates. *Brain and Language* **37**:591–605.

Best C, Hoffman H, Glanville B (1982) Development of infant ear asymmetries for speech and music. *Perceptual Psychophysics* **31**:75–85.

Bishop D (1983) Linguistic impairment after left hemidecortication for infantile hemiplegia? A reappraisal. *Quarterly Journal of Experimental Psychology* **35**(A):199–207.

Bishop D (1988) Can the right hemisphere mediate language as well as the left? A critical review of recent research. *Cognitive Neuropsychology* **5**:353–367.

Chomsky N (1975) *Reflections on Language*. Pantheon.

Chomsky N (1981) *Lectures on Government and Binding*. Foris.

Dall'Oglio A, Bates E, Volterra V, Di Capua M, Pezzini G (1994) Early cognition, communication and language in children with focal brain injury. *Developmental Medicine and Child Neurology* **36**:1076–1098.

Damasio A, Lima A, Damasio H (1975) Nervous function after right hemispherectomy. *Neurology* **25**:89–93.

Dehaene-Lambertz G (1999) Cerebral specialization in speech and nonspeech stimuli in infants. *Journal of Cognitive Neuroscience* (in press).

Dehaene-Lambertz G, Baillet S (1998) A phonological representation in the infant brain. *NeuroReport* **9**:1885–1888.

Dennis M, Kohn B (1975) Comprehension of syntax in infantile hemiplegics after cerebral hemidecortication: left hemisphere superiority. *Brain and Language* **2**:472–482.

Dennis M, Whitaker H (1976) Language acquisition following hemidecortication: linguistic superiority of the left over the right hemisphere. *Brain and Language* **3**:404–433.

Dennis M, Whitaker H (1977) Hemispheric equipotentiality and language acquisition. In: Segalowitz S, Gruber F (eds) *Language Development and Neurological Theory*, pp 93–106. New York: Academic Press.

Elman E, Bates E, Johnson M, Karmiloff-Smith A, Parisi D, Plunkett K (1996) *Rethinking Innateness: a Connectionist Perspective on Development*. Cambridge, MA: MIT Press/Bradford Books.

Entus A (1977) Hemispheric asymmetry in processing of dichotically presented speech and nonspeech stimuli by infants. In: Segalowitz S, Gruber F (eds) *Language Development and Neurological Theory*, pp 63–73. New York: Academic Press.

Feldman H, Holland A, Kemp S, Janovsky J (1992) Language development after unilateral brain injury. *Brain and Language* **42**:89–102.

Fodor J (1983) *The Modularity of Mind*. Cambridge, MA: MIT Press.

Gadian D, Isaacs E, Cross J *et al* (1996) Lateralization of brain function in childhood revealed by magnetic resonance spectroscopy. *Neurology* **46**:974–977.

Geschwind N, Levitsky W (1968) Human brain: left–right asymmetries in temporal speech region. *Science* **161**:186–187.

Glanville B, Best C, Levenson R (1977) A cardiac measure of cerebral asymmetries in infant auditory perception. *Developmental Psychology* **13**:54–59.

Goodglass H (1993) *Understanding Aphasia*. San Diego: Academic Press.

Goodman R, Yude C (1996) IQ and its predictors in childhood hemiplegia. *Developmental Medicine and Child Neurology* **38**:881–890.

Gott P (1973) Cognitive abilities following right and left hemispherectomy. *Cortex* **9**:266–274.

Hecaen H (1976) Acquired aphasia in children and the ontogenesis of hemispheric specialization. *Brain and Language* **3**:114–134.

Isaacs E, Christie D, Vargha-Khadem F, Mishkin M (1996) Effects of hemispheric side of injury, age at injury, and presence of seizure disorder on functional ear and hand asymmetries in hemiplegic children. *Neuropsychologia* **34**(2):127–137.

Jernigan T, Hesselink J, Sowell E, Tallal P (1991) Cerebral structure on magnetic resonance imaging in language and learning-impaired children. *Archives of Neurology* **48**:539–545.

Kempler D, Van Lancker D, Marchman V, Bates E (1996) The effects of childhood vs. adult brain damage on literal and idiomatic language comprehension (abstract). *Brain and Language* **55**(1):167–169.

Kohn B, Dennis M (1974) Selective impairments of visuospatial abilities in infantile hemiplegics after right cerebral hemidecortication. *Neuropsychologia* **12**:505–512.

Kuzniecky R, Andermann F, Guerrini R (1993) Congenital bilateral perisylvian syndrome: study of 31 patients. The CBPS Multicenter Collaborative Study. *Lancet* **34**:608–612.

Lenneberg E (1967) *Biological Foundations of Language*. New York: John Wiley.

Levine S, Huttenlocher P, Banich M Duda E (1987) Factors affecting cognitive functioning in hemiplegic children. *Developmental Medicine and Child Neurology* **29**:27–35.

Marchman V, Miller R, Bates E (1991) Babble and first words in children with focal brain injury. *Applied Psycholinguistics* **12**:1–22.

McFie J (1961a) The effects of hemispherectomy on intellectual function in cases of infantile hemiplegia. *Journal of Neurology, Neurosurgery and Psychiatry* **24**:240–249.

McFie J (1961b) Intellectual impairment in children with localized postinfantile cerebral lesions. *Journal of Neurology, Neurosurgery and Psychiatry* **24**:361–365.

Milner B (1974) Sparing of language function after early unilateral brain damage. *Neurosciences Research Program Bulletin* **12**(2):213–217.

Milner B (1975) Psychological aspects of focal epilepsy and its neurosurgical management. In: Purpura D, Hendry J, Walter R (eds) *Advances in Neurology*, pp 299–321. New York: Raven Press.

Molfese D, Burger-Judisch L (1991) Dynamic temporal-spatial allocation of resources in the human brain: an alternative to the static view of hemisphere differences. In: Kitterle F (ed) *Cerebral Laterality: Theory and Research*, pp 71–102. Hillsdale, NJ: Lawrence Erlbaum Associates.

Molfese D, Molfese V (1980) Cortical responses of preterm infants to phonetic and nonphonetic speech stimuli. *Developmental Psychology* **16**:574–581.

Muter V, Taylor S, Vargha-Khadem F (1997) A longitudinal study of early intellectual development in hemiplegic children. *Neuropsychologia* **35**(3):289–298.

Naatanen R, Lehtokoski A, Lennes M *et al* (1997) Language-specific phoneme representations revealed by electric and magnetic brain responses. *Nature* **385**:432–434.

Nass R, Peterson H-C, Koch D (1989) Differential effects of congenital left and right brain injury on intelligence. *Brain and Cognition* **9**:258–266.

Novak G, Kurtzberg D, Kreuzer J, Vaughan H (1989) Cortical responses to speech sounds and their formants in normal infants: maturational sequence and spatiotemporal analysis. *Electroencephalography and Clinical Neurophysiology* **73**:295–305.

Ogden J (1989) Visuospatial and other 'right hemispheric' functions after long recovery periods in left hemispherectomized subjects. *Neuropsychologia* **27**:765–776.

Paulesu E, Frith U, Snowling M, Gallagher A, Morton J (1996) Is developmental dyslexia a disconnection syndrome? Evidence from PET scanning. *Brain* **119**:143–157.

Reilly J, Bates E, Marchman V (1998) Narrative discourse in children with early focal brain injury. *Brain and Language* 61(3):335–375.

Riva D, Cazzaniga L (1986) Late effects of unilateral brain lesions sustained before and after age one. *Neuropsychologia* 24:423–428.

Riva D, Cazzaniga L, Panaleoni C, Milani N, Fedrizzi E (1986) Acute hemiplegia in childhood: the neuropsychological prognosis. *Journal of Pediatric Neurosciences* 2:239–250.

Satz P, Strauss E, Whitaker H (1990) The ontogeny of hemispheric specialization: some old hypotheses revisited. *Brain and Language* 38:596–614.

Simos P, Molfese D (1997) Electrophysiological responses from a temporal order continuum in the newborn infant. *Neuropsychologia* 35(1):89–98.

Simos P, Molfese D, Brenden R (1997) Behavioral and electrophysiological indices of voicing-cue discrimination: laterality patterns and development. *Brain and Language* 57:122–150.

Stiles J (1998) The effects of early focal brain injury on lateralization of cognitive function. *Current Directions in Psychological Science* 7(1):21–26.

Stiles J, Nass R (1991) Spatial group ability in young children with congenital right or left hemisphere brain injury. *Brain and Cognition* 15:201–222.

Stiles J, Trauner D, Nass R (1996) Developmental change in spatial grouping activity among children with early focal brain injury: evidence from a modeling task. *Brain and Cognition* 31:46–62.

Stiles J, Trauner D, Engel M, Nass R (1997) The development of drawing in children with congenital focal brain injury: evidence for limited functional recovery. *Neuropsychologia* 35(3):299–312.

Stiles J, Bates EA, Thal D, Trauner D, Reilly J (1999) Linguistic, cognitive and affective development in children with pre- and perinatal focal brain injury: a 10-year overview from the San Diego Longitudinal Project. In Rovee-Collier C (ed) *Advances in Infancy Research,* pp 131–163. Norwood, NJ: Ablex.

Stiles-Davis J, Sugarman S, Nass R (1985) The development of spatial and class relations in four young children with right cerebral hemisphere damage: evidence for an early spatial-constructive deficit. *Brain and Cognition* 4:388–412.

Teuber H (1975) Recovery of function after brain injury in man. In Porter R, Fitzsimmons D (eds) *Outcome of Severe Damage to the Central Nervous System,* pp 159–190. Amsterdam: North Holland, Elsevier Excerpta Medica.

Thal D, Marchman V, Stiles J et al (1991) Early lexical development in children with focal brain injury. *Brain and Language* 40:491–527.

Vargha-Khadem F, Corballis M (1979) Cerebral asymmetry in infants. *Brain and Language* 8:1–9.

Vargha-Khadem F, O'Gorman AM, Waters GV (1985) Aphasin and handedness in relation to hemispheric side, age at injury and severity of cerebral lesion during childhood. *Brain* 108:677–696.

Vargha-Khadem F, Isaacs E, Papaleloudi H, Polkey C, Wilson J (1991) Development of language in six hemispherectomized patients. *Brain* 114:463–495.

Vargha-Khadem F, Isaacs E, Van der Wert S, Robb S, Wilson J (1992) Development of intelligence and memory in children with hemiplegic cerebral palsy: the deleterious consequences of early seizures. *Brain* 115:315–329.

Vargha-Khadem F, Isaacs E, Muter V (1994) A review of cognitive outcome after unilateral lesions sustained during childhood. *Journal of Child Neurology* 9(Suppl):2S67–2S73.

Vargha-Khadem F, Carr L, Isaacs E, Brett E, Adams C, Mishkin M (1997) Onset of speech after left hemispherectomy in a 9-year-old boy. *Brain* 120:159–182.

Vargha-Khadem F, Watkins K, Price C et al (1998) Neural basis of an inherited speech and language disorder. *Proceedings of the National Academy of Sciences* 95:12695–12700.

Wada J, Clark R, Hamm A (1975) Cerebral hemispheric asymmetry in humans. *Archives of Neurology* 32:239–246.

Warrington E, James M, Maciejewski C (1986) The WAIS as a lateralising and localising diagnostic instrument: a study of 656 patients with unilateral cerebral excisions. *Neuropsychologia* 24:223–239.

Wechsler D (1955) *Wechsler Adult Intelligence Scale.* New York: Psychological Corporation.

Wechsler D (1976) *Wechsler Intelligence Scale for Children* revised UK edn. Sidcup, Kent: Psychological Corporation, Harcourt Brace Jovanovich.

Wechsler D (1981) *Wechsler Adult Intelligence Scale* revised UK edn. Sidcup, Kent: Psychological Corporation, Harcourt Brace Jovanovich.

Wechsler D (1990) *Wechsler Preschool and Primary Scale of Intelligence.* Sidcup, Kent: Psychological Corporation, Harcourt Brace Jovanovich.

Wechsler D (1992) *Wechsler Intelligence Scale for Children,* 3rd edn, UK version. Sidcup, Kent: Psychological Corporation, Harcourt Brace Jovanovich.

Willmes K, Poeck K (1993) To what extent can aphasic syndromes be localized? *Brain* 116:1527–1540.

Witelson S, Pallie W (1973) Left hemisphere specialisation for language in the new-born: neuroanatomical evidence of asymmetry. *Brain* 88:653–662.

Woods B (1980) The restricted effects of right-hemisphere lesions after age one; Wechsler test data. *Neuropsychologia* 18:65–70.

Woods B, Carey S (1979) Language deficits after apparent clinical recovery from childhood aphasia. *Annals of Neurology* 6:405–409.

Woods B, Teuber H (1973) Early onset of complementary specialization of cerebral hemispheres in man. *Transcriptions of the American Association* 98:113–115.

Woods B, Teuber H (1978) Changing patterns of childhood aphasia. *Transcriptions of the American Neurological Association* 98:113–117.

Quality of life issues in intractable focal epilepsy

A JACOBY AND GA BAKER

Clinical definitions of 'intractability' in epilepsy focus on such factors as the duration of poorly controlled seizures, current seizure frequency and severity, and the need for polytherapy. In this book, for example, intractability is defined as 'a continuation of seizures beyond two years, despite treatment with three antiepileptics taken at optimal doses either individually or in combination.' A number of writers, however, have made the point that intractability should be assessed in relation to not only clinical but also psychosocial criteria (Janz 1989; Alving 1995). Any comprehensive evaluation of patients with intractable seizure disorders must therefore include consideration of the degree to which the seizures impact on daily functioning and quality of life (QoL). In this chapter, we examine available evidence about the impact of intractable epilepsy on patients' level of functioning and QoL, drawing attention where possible to any notable differences between individuals with focal epilepsy and those with other intractable epilepsies. We also consider methods for evaluating the impact of intractable epilepsy on QoL and potential treatment strategies by which this impact can be reduced.

DEFINING AND ASSESSING QUALITY OF LIFE IN INTRACTABLE EPILEPSY

Before examining the research evidence about the impact of intractable epilepsy on QoL, we briefly address the conceptual, definitional, and measurement issues upon which this evidence rests. It is not our intention to provide a comprehensive review of these issues, which we and other authors have dealt with in detail elsewhere (Avis and Smith 1994; Jacoby 1996; Spilker 1996; Hunt 1997). However, we do attempt to highlight some key points in the QoL assessment debate for the reader's consideration.

CONCEPTS AND DEFINITIONS

Though the term 'quality of life' entered the epilepsy literature only relatively recently, QoL studies in epilepsy are not new. Scambler (1993) points out that what he refers to as 'pre-formal studies' of QoL in epilepsy are, in fact, centuries old; and Meador (1993) cites examples of 'formal' studies dating back to the 1960s, which though not always comprehensive or systematic in their approach none the less addressed QoL issues. Since the beginning of the present decade, there has been increasing recognition (though undoubtedly also some skepticism) of the potential value of formal QoL assessments as measures of the outcome of epilepsy care. However, there is continuing debate in epilepsy, as elsewhere, about what to measure and how to measure it under the umbrella of 'quality of life' (Kendrick and Trimble 1994; Ruta *et al* 1994; Gilliam *et al* 1997a; Hunt 1997) and the need for this activity to be informed by theoretic models of QoL has been highlighted (Aaronson *et al* 1991; Hermann 1992; Baker *et al* 1993).

Among the reasons why the concept of QoL has proved so problematic are: (a) it is not a directly observable phenomenon; (b) it is multidimensional in nature, begging the question of whether it can be measured globally or only through delineation of its various components (and, if the latter, what those components are); (c) it involves both objective and subjective elements; and (d) the approach to its conceptualization rests largely on the academic discipline and perspective of the investigator (Rogerson 1995). Within the field of healthcare, a number of competing concepts have been proposed as informing the QoL debate (Schipper *et al* 1990) including the psychologic concept, the time trade-off concept, the community-centered concept, the reintegration concept, and the 'gap' principle. Unresolved difficulties about the conceptual basis for the measurement of QoL have meant, it has been argued (Hunt 1997), that efforts to do so have lacked coherence or consistency; and researchers have 'pressed into service' as QoL measures tools developed for rather different purposes. One manifestation of this lack of conceptual clarity is the interchangeable use in the literature of terms such as 'health status,' 'psychosocial functioning,' 'quality of life,' and 'health-related quality of life' (HRQoL), though the first two are, we would suggest, only surrogate measures of QoL. A number of writers (Brooks 1991; Guyatt *et al* 1993; Patrick and Erickson 1993) have expressed a clear preference for the term HRQoL over QoL, on the grounds that not all QoL dimensions are health or medical concerns. However, this preference has been challenged (Leplege 1997), since use of the term HRQoL implies that people can divide their QoL into its health and nonhealth components and 'fails to acknowledge the inter-connectedness of health status with other aspects of existence.' Largely because of its social meaning, epilepsy is, we would suggest, a condition where this interconnectedness is only too apparent. For this reason, we would support Hermann's (1992) proposition that in the HRQoL versus QoL debate in epilepsy, 'a broader vision may be appropriate and necessary.'

In our own research into QoL in patients with intractable epilepsy, we have opted to use as a theoretic framework the WHO definition of health (World Health Organization 1947) as 'a state of physical, mental and social well-being and not merely the absence of infirmity and disease'. The Liverpool QoL Battery (Baker *et al* 1993) thus comprises a series of validated scales and single items that focus on these three broad domains. The underlying assumption is that physical, social, and psychologic function are reduced to a greater or lesser degree by epilepsy and its treatment, although we acknowledge the caveat (Hunt 1997) that while reduced functional status may impact upon QoL, it is not necessarily synonymous with it. The representation of QoL by physical, social, and psychologic domains also formed the starting point for the development of the QoL inventory for epilepsy, QOLIE-89 (Devinsky *et al* 1995) and the Epilepsy Surgery Inventory, ESI-55 (Vickrey *et al* 1992). Other QoL researchers in the field of epilepsy have drawn upon the more recent WHO conceptualization of the consequence of disease at the level of impairment, disability, and handicap (Kendrick and Trimble 1994; O'Donoghue *et al* 1998).

MEASUREMENT

Rosenberg (1995) has argued that confronted with unresolved theoretic ambiguities with regard to QoL research in the healthcare setting, its practitioners have, by and large, opted to focus their efforts on pragmatic issues such as establishing the psychometric properties of their instruments. Without doubt, a considerable amount has been written both about the principles of validity, reliability, and responsiveness and about their representation in relation to specific QoL measures, both epilepsy related and others; thus we do not intend to revisit these topics in any detail here but refer readers to the standard texts (McDowell and Newell 1987; Streiner and Norman 1989; Jaeschke and Guyatt 1990). In summary, *validity* is concerned with whether or not an instrument measures what it purports to measure; *reliability* with its ability to produce the same results on repeated occasions under similar test conditions; and *responsiveness* with its ability to detect clinically significant within-patient changes over time. Information about the psychometric properties of the various epilepsy-specific QoL measures can be readily accessed in the literature; there is generally good evidence of their content and construct validity and of their reliability. Evidence of their responsiveness to change is so far generally sparse. This is an important gap, since prior knowledge of the responsiveness of potential instruments would, it has been argued (Deyo *et al* 1991), aid in the selection of measures, permit a more accurate estimation of required sample size, and assist in prioritizing outcomes to be assessed. This problem will, at least to some degree, be resolved as more studies are published in which data from the epilepsy QoL measures are reported.

One less well-addressed issue in QoL assessment concerns the interpretation of instrument scores. Once the impact of illness and its treatment has been quantified, researchers and clinicians then have to evaluate its significance (Fowler *et al* 1994); and there may be an important distinction between scale score differences that are statistically significant, those that have clinical significance, and those that are significant from the patient's own point of view. For this reason, guidelines have recently been proposed for the introduction of new QoL questionnaires in healthcare settings (Marquis 1998), which include specific interpretation strategies, derived from both statistical methods and external criteria. Establishing what constitutes a minimal important difference (defined as 'the smallest difference in score in the domain of interest which patients perceive as beneficial and which would mandate, in the absence of troublesome side-effects and excessive cost, a change in the patient's management'; Jaeschke *et al* 1989) is clearly an increasingly important topic on the QoL research agenda (Juniper *et al* 1994; Wagner and Vickrey 1995) though one as yet largely unaddressed for epilepsy.

Assuming the resolution of psychometric and interpretative problems, it has been suggested by Jaeschke and Guyatt (1990) that QoL measures can be applied in three broad healthcare contexts: to discriminate between individuals along a continuum of health, illness, or disability; to predict outcome or prognosis; and to evaluate within-person change over time. Within the epilepsy literature, we have identified studies employing QoL measures in both discriminative and evaluative contexts, and review them below. The recent development of several novel antiepileptic agents means that QoL assessments are now regarded as of particular importance in evaluating treatment outcome within the context of clinical trials.

METHODS FOR ASSESSMENT

Many of the preformal studies of QoL in epilepsy to which Scambler (1993) refers used qualitative research methods to explore the experiences and attitudes of people with epilepsy. Qualitative methods have traditionally formed an important part of the methodologic toolkit of social scientists, and their value in health and health services research has recently been given emphasis in the medical literature (Pope and Mays 1995). In the field of epilepsy, some important and highly illuminating qualitative studies of QoL issues include the one by Scambler (1989) and those by Schneider and Conrad (1983) and West (1979). However, the bulk of the work to investigate QoL in epilepsy has followed in the tradition of the clinical and biomedical sciences, using experimental quantitative methods. In this section we focus on these quantitative approaches, which can be subdivided into those involving the use of standardized QoL questionnaires and those which adopt an individualized patient focus.

Standardized approaches to QoL assessment in adults

To date, there have been three main approaches to developing standardized QoL assessments in epilepsy: (a) those involving a *de novo* QoL measure, such as the Washington Psychosocial Seizure Inventory (Dodrill *et al* 1980), the Social Effects Scale (Chaplin *et al* 1990), or the Subjective Handicap of Epilepsy Scale (O'Donoghue *et al* 1998); (b) those involving use of a single previously developed generic profile with customized additions, such as the Epilepsy Surgery Inventory (Vickrey *et al* 1992) or the Quality of Life in Epilepsy Inventory (Devinsky *et al* 1995); and (c) those that use a battery of scales addressing specific QoL domains, such as the Liverpool QoL Battery (Baker *et al* 1993).

Washington Psychosocial Seizure Inventory

The Washington Psychosocial Seizure Inventory (WPSI; Dodrill *et al* 1980) is one of the oldest and most widely used epilepsy-specific scales addressing QoL issues. It was designed to evaluate the psychosocial problems commonly seen in adults with seizure disorders and consists of 132 items across eight scales: family background, emotional adjustment, interpersonal adjustment, vocational adjustment, financial status, adjustment to seizures, medicines and medical management, and overall psychosocial functioning. WPSI has been criticized for its dichotomous response format, the fact that scale composition rests solely on statistical grounds, and the fact that because it is epilepsy specific it does not allow comparisons with other nonepilepsy populations (Vickrey *et al* 1992). Nevertheless it remains a much-used measure of psychosocial function. Recently, its authors, acknowledging the limitations of WPSI in relation to the concepts of QoL currently proposed in the literature, have developed a 36-item WPSI QoL scale (Dodrill and Batzel 1995) but as yet there is little information available about its psychometric properties.

Social Effects Scale

The Social Effects Scale (Chaplin *et al* 1990) was designed to investigate the social effects of their condition on adult patients with epilepsy of varying duration and severity. A large pool of statements about the impact of epilepsy was generated through in-depth interviews with patients; both patients and physicians were then asked to group the statements into distinct areas and other areas were generated from a search of the relevant literature. The most commonly used statement or statements in each of 21 areas thus generated were selected for inclusion in the final 42-item questionnaire. Among the areas covered are attitude towards epilepsy and seizures; fear of stigma; concern about personal and social relationships; lack of confidence to perform particular activities; problems with healthcare and medications; emotional problems and social isolation. The scale was developed for use in the UK National General Practice Study of Epilepsy (Chaplin *et al* 1992, 1995), where newly diagnosed patients are being followed prospectively to examine the perceived impact of their condition over time.

Subjective Handicap of Epilepsy Scale

The Subjective Handicap of Epilepsy Scale (O'Donoghue *et al* 1998) was developed to overcome some of the technical and conceptual difficulties in QoL measurement outlined above. Based on the WHO concept of handicap, it contains 32 items in six subscales: work and activities, social and personal, self-perception, physical, life satisfaction, and perceived life changes. From initial validation studies, the measure appears both reliable and valid and its authors recommend it as particularly suitable for longitudinal investigations into the effectiveness of interventions, such as epilepsy surgery, aimed at reducing the impact of chronic epilepsy.

Epilepsy Surgery Inventory

The Epilepsy Surgery Inventory (ESI-55; Vickrey *et al* 1992) is a composite measure based on the generic health status measure SF-36 (Ware and Sherborne 1992), supplemented by additional items that tap aspects of QoL seen as of particular relevance to epilepsy patients (five relating to cognitive function, eight to role limitations, four to health perceptions, and two to overall life quality). The final scale thus includes subscales to assess health perceptions, energy and fatigue, overall QoL, social function, emotional well-being, cognitive function, physical function, pain, and role limitations due to physical, emotional, and memory problems. Three composite scores (mental and physical health and cognitive role limitations) and an overall scale score can be derived by weighting and summing individual scale scores.

Quality of Life in Epilepsy Scales

The Quality of Life in Epilepsy (QOLIE) scales were developed by the QOLIE Development Group (Devinsky *et al*

1995). The SF-36 is also the basis of this series of scales referred to as QOLIE-89 (17 scales, 89 items), QOLIE-31 (seven scales, 31 items), and QOLIE-10 (10 items selected from the seven scales in the QOLIE-31). As for the ESI-55, an overall score and four composite scores (epilepsy-targeted, cognitive, mental health, and physical health) can be developed by weighting and summing individual scale scores on the QOLIE-89. These scales are intended for broad application in studies of people with epilepsy rather than the surgery-specific application developed by Vickrey and her colleagues. The domains covered by the two longer versions are shown in Table 33.1.

Health-related Quality of Life Model for Epilepsy

Rather than developing a single QoL scale to be applied across all studies of epilepsy, our own group has developed an epilepsy-specific QoL model (Baker *et al* 1993) that allows different combinations of domain-specific scales to be applied, depending on the particular research question under consideration (Table 33.2). Within the framework of the model, we have developed a series of QoL questionnaires specific to individuals with newly diagnosed seizures and epilepsy (Jacoby *et al* 1997; Baker *et al* 1998), patients with epilepsy in remission (Jacoby *et al* 1992), and patients with intractable epilepsy (Smith *et al* 1993; Espie *et al* 1997). Where we were able to identify relevant and psychometrically sound scales they were utilized; where we could not we developed them *de novo*. Though not all originally developed for epilepsy, all the scales in the model have

Table 33.1 Domains of the Quality of Life in Epilepsy (QOLIE-89) instrument. (From Cramer 1994 with permission.)

Health perceptions
Seizure worry[a]
Physical function
Role limitation
Physical
Emotional
Pain
Overall quality of life[a]
Emotional well-being[a]
Energy/fatigue[a]
Attention/concentration[a]
Memory
Language
Medication effects[a]
Social support
Social function[a]
Social isolation
Health discouragement
Sexual function
Overall health[a]

[a] The QOLIE-31 includes items taken from these scales.

Table 33.2 Liverpool Quality-of-Life Assessment Battery for epilepsy.

Scale	No. of items
Seizure Severity Scale (Baker *et al* 1991)	19
Nottingham Health Profile (Hunt *et al* 1981)	38
Hospital Anxiety and Depression Scale (Zigmond and Snaith 1983)	14
Affect Balance Scale (Bradburn 1969)	10
Self-esteem Scale (Rosenberg 1965)	10
Mastery Scale (Pearlin and Schooler 1978)	7
Stigma Scale (Jacoby 1994)	3
Life Fulfilment Scale (Baker *et al* 1994)	26
Impact of Epilepsy Scale (Jacoby *et al* 1993)	10
Adverse Drug Effects Profile (Baker *et al* 1995)	19

been validated in subjects with epilepsy of varying severity, from those with intractable epilepsy to those whose seizures are in remission. The most widely applied of the novel scales is the Seizure Severity Scale (Baker *et al* 1991), which has been used in a large number of clinical trials of novel antiepileptic drugs. Others include a measure of patient-perceived impact of epilepsy on daily functioning (Jacoby *et al* 1993), a measure of perceived stigma (Jacoby 1994), and an adverse drug effects profile (Baker *et al* 1995).

Recently, attempts have been made to compare the psychometric properties of these various standardized measures. Langfitt (1995) compared the reliability and validity of WPSI and ESI-55 and reported that WPSI had poorer face, content, and criterion validity, and so provides a less valid description of the impact of epilepsy on QoL than the ESI-55. Wagner *et al* (1995) evaluated the practicality and psychometric properties of a battery of generic and epilepsy-specific scales, including the SF-36 (Ware and Sherbourne 1992), the Impact of Epilepsy Scale (Jacoby *et al* 1993), the Liverpool Seizure Severity Scale (Baker *et al* 1991), a modified version of the Mastery Scale (Pearlin and Schooler 1978), and a novel two-item Epilepsy Distress Scale. They reported that data quality was high and that, with few exceptions, both the generic and epilepsy-specific measures satisfied standard psychometric criteria and were shown to be valid in relation to two clinical criteria, disease severity and symptoms. Further work is required to progress this debate, so that the task of selecting an appropriate QoL measure is simplified for the nonexpert.

Individualized QoL assessment

Some researchers have taken issue with the standardized approach to QoL assessment employed in the examples above, on the grounds that since it involves a process in which the researcher determines the core dimensions, domains and items, and the weightings attached to each, it inevitably fails to take account of the individual nature of QoL. They have therefore tried to develop a patient-elicited approach to QoL assessment. In the field of epilepsy, the main proponents of this approach is the group headed by Professor Trimble, who have used repertory grid technique to determine, within five core areas (physical, cognitive, social, emotional, economic) what specific aspects of functioning are important to individual patients (Kendrick and Trimble 1994). Within this framework, subjects then design their own QoL schedule, rating the degree to which each aspect they have identified is currently problematic. A problem recognized by the authors is that in its original form their patient-generated approach is complex and time-consuming to complete, and they are currently refining and simplifying the process.

Recently, attempts have been made by one group of researchers to combine the advantages of both standardized and individualized approaches by including within a standardized QoL assessment three to five 'individualized' activity items (Juniper *et al* 1996). Patients are asked at study baseline to identify activities that are important and undertaken frequently by them and limited by their condition. These activities are then retained as the focus of questioning for the individual during the course of the study. While simpler than the method developed by Trimble, this variant still depends on interviewer administration and so may be less than practicable in many research situations.

QoL measures for children

All the above examples relate to QoL assessment in adults with epilepsy and parallel work for children has been largely lacking, though interest in developing appropriate measures is gaining impetus in this condition as in others. The theoretic difficulties in assessing QoL in children are somewhat greater than in adults, largely because of the rapid physical, cognitive, and emotional changes that occur through childhood (Eiser 1993). Since it is unlikely that a single QoL assessment tool can take account of the different developmental phases, a more appropriate approach is to focus on the particular problems and stressors associated with each phase, and so develop a series of age-specific measures. Such an approach has been adopted elsewhere but has yet to be rigorously pursued for epilepsy. As mentioned earlier, the assumption has generally been made that children themselves cannot or should not be asked to report their QoL and, by and large, assessments have been based on proxy measures. However, research has highlighted serious limitations in using parents' reports of symptoms, impairments, and other general measures (Fink 1989) and suggests that even very young children can complete simple questionnaires, given some assistance (West 1995).

Recent developments in epilepsy include a generic measure with an add-on epilepsy-specific module (Bruil and Maes 1995) and a 65-item measure developed by the QOLIE Development Group for use in adolescents (Cramer *et al* in press). A generic health status measure for children, the Child Health Questionnaire (CHQ) (Landgraf *et al* 1996) has also recently been published. The CHQ Parent Form is available in three lengths (98, 50, and 28 items) and two modes of administration (self-completion and interview); the CHQ Child Form, designed for completion by children aged 10 and over, is currently available only in an 87-item version, but a short form is under development. The CHQ has been validated for a wide range of chronic childhood illnesses, including epilepsy.

USE OF ASSESSMENT IN CLINICAL SETTINGS

There have been a large number of studies, both qualitative and quantitative, that have described the QoL of adults (Schneider and Conrad 1983; Scambler 1989; Collings 1990a; Jacoby 1992) and children (West 1979; Hoare and Kerley 1991; Austin and Dunn 1993) with epilepsy. As noted earlier, however, QoL assessments have come to be seen as having a role beyond the merely descriptive, as measures of outcome in studies that seek to answer clinical questions about the management of epilepsy. Most commonly, this has been within the framework of clinical trials of alternative treatments, although those including a comprehensive QoL assessment are still relatively few in number. The proliferation of trials including QoL assessments indicates a much clearer recognition on the part of clinicians, the pharmaceutical industry, and the regulatory bodies of their relevance and importance. We would argue that this may be particularly the case in trials of patients with intractable epilepsy, where complete freedom from seizures is unlikely and even a marked reduction in seizure frequency is of little significance from the point of view of ability to function psychosocially.

Wagner and Vickrey (1995) have also made the case for including QoL assessments as a routine part of clinical practice: as a means of detecting functional limitations and psychologic distress; improving clinician–patient interaction; guiding management decisions, including in relation to nonclinical aspects of epilepsy; and informing resource use. We are aware of at least one attempt to do so in the UK, where a battery of QoL scales has been computerized. Patients complete the scales while waiting at the epilepsy

clinic and the results are then immediately available to them and their clinician for consideration during the ensuing consultation (McDonnell, personal communication).

REVIEW OF STUDIES ON THE IMPACT OF INTRACTABLE EPILEPSY ON QUALITY OF LIFE

The generally perceived wisdom in the epilepsy literature (Zielinski 1986; Trostle *et al* 1989) is that patients with intractable epilepsy are overrepresented, because their more regular attendance at hospital clinics renders them a more accessible research population than patients with seizures that are well controlled. While we accept this is the case, our MEDLINE search none the less identified relatively few comprehensive QoL studies specific to this group. If we return to the definition, given above, of medically intractable epilepsy as continuing seizures unresponsive to the range of drug therapies then, somewhat surprisingly to us, few studies have focused specifically on describing the QoL of individuals with intractable epilepsy. However, data are available from studies comparing QoL across epilepsy of varying severity and from studies that compare QoL of individuals with intractable epilepsy treated by surgery in a before-and-after design. Since the issue of QoL after surgery is addressed in chapter 49, we do not intend to review the latter in any detail here. In the analysis presented below, we focus largely on studies in adults with intractable epilepsy, but also present data from the relatively small number of studies in children that we have been able to locate.

STUDIES IN ADULTS

One of the earlier studies to systematically address QoL issues in patients with intractable epilepsy focused on 112 young adults admitted to a specialist assessment center (Thompson and Oxley 1988), the majority of whom had epilepsy of long duration and few of whom had experienced any substantial periods of remission. Three-quarters (73%) had complex partial seizures with, and a further 16% complex partial seizures without, secondary generalization; 89% had seizures at least weekly. The authors of the study used the Social Problems Questionnaire (SPQ) (Corney and Clare 1985) to assess subjects' satisfaction with current employment, financial matters, housing, social activities, and interpersonal relationships, in addition to which they collected information about educational and employment history. Almost half of the sample had received special schooling and their educational attainments were clearly skewed to lower-level qualifications; only 11% were in open employment at the time of their admission to the assessment center and of these, most were in unskilled jobs. Few of the sample were living independently at the time of assessment, the majority still being resident in the parental home; a few were married or cohabiting, 57% reporting that they had never had a stable relationship. Unsurprisingly, in the light of these figures, levels of dissatisfaction were high, 73% reporting themselves moderately or severely dissatisfied with their social life and activities, 71% with their work situation, 51% with their personal relationships, 37% with their financial situation, and 29% with their housing situation.

The authors of the study subsequently compared the responses of this group with those a second smaller group of 32 patients being considered for epilepsy surgery in whom duration of epilepsy and current seizure frequency was similar (Thompson and Oxley 1989). The surgical evaluation group were more likely to be working, more likely to be married or cohabiting, less likely to report financial problems, and much less likely to report problems in their social life than were the assessment center sample.

Smith *et al* (1991) also used the SPQ together with the Liverpool QoL Battery to examine the psychosocial consequences of intractable epilepsy in 100 patients with medically refractory partial seizures attending an epilepsy outpatient clinic; 33% of the patients were classified as being clinically anxious and 15% as clinically depressed, using a

well-validated measure, the Hospital Anxiety and Depression Scale (Zigmond and Snaith 1983). Their scores on the relevant measures indicated that 50% of the sample had poor self-esteem and 84% poor sense of control, the latter an unsurprising finding given that the mean seizure frequency per month was 22.9 for those with simple partial seizures and 28.7 for those with complex partial seizures. On a happiness scale (Bradburn 1969) one-third of these patients scored in the negative range, indicating that they did not perceive their lives as being particularly happy. None the less, compared with both groups of respondents in the survey by Thompson and Oxley this group reported markedly less dissatisfaction with their life (Table 33.3), emphasizing that even within the confines of the term 'intractable' there may be marked differences in the perceived impact of epilepsy on QoL.

To try to clarify further the degree to which intractable epilepsy impacts on QoL, Baker *et al* (1993) compared the psychologic profile and health status of patients in their study with that of a group at the opposite end of the epilepsy spectrum, namely patients whose epilepsy was now in remission and who were therefore eligible for withdrawal of antiepileptic medication. As expected, mean scores for self-esteem and sense of mastery were lower for those with intractable epilepsy than for those in remission; and for each of the six domains of a generic health status measure, the Nottingham Health Profile, a higher percentage of patients with intractable epilepsy had positive scores, indicating considerably greater dysfunction in these areas (Table 33.4).

Table 33.3 Reported dissatisfaction in different samples of patients with intractable epilepsy.

	Problem areas (%)					
	Work	Housing	Finance	Social	Marital	Family
Epilepsy outpatient clinic attenders (Smith *et al* 1991)	21	1	14	21	10	3
Assessment center sample (Thompson and Oxley 1989)	71	27	34	67	49	26
Surgical evaluation sample (Thompson and Oxley 1989)	34	6	22	22	28	16

Table 33.4 Comparison of quality-of-life scale scores for patients with intractable epilepsy and patients with epilepsy in remission.

Scale	Patients with intractable epilepsy	Patients with epilepsy in remission
Self-esteem (mean, 95% CI)	27.1 (25.9–28.3)	33.0 (32.6–33.4)
Mastery (mean, 95% CI)	18.1 (17.3–19.0)	21.7 (21.4–22.0)
Nottingham Health Profile (% positive scores)		
Energy	34	29
Pain	16	8
Emotional reaction	70	37
Sleep	41	28
Social isolation	51	15
Physical mobility	37	12

CI, confidence interval.

A similar comparison has been made by Chaplin *et al* (1995) who, using the Social Effects Scale (Chaplin *et al* 1990), explored psychosocial adjustment in matched samples of patients with chronic epilepsy and patients with a recent diagnosis of epilepsy. Though the chronic group do not fit strictly with our definition of intractability, they were individuals whose epilepsy was of at least 5 years' duration and who had had a minimum of 20 seizures. Of the 14 life areas addressed by the scale, there was only one where significant difficulties were reported by more than 50% of individuals with newly diagnosed epilepsy, that area being fear of seizures. In contrast, more than 50% of the individuals with chronic epilepsy reported significant difficulties in nine of the 14 areas: acceptance of the diagnosis, fear of seizures, fear of stigma in employment, lack of confidence about the future, adverse effects of epilepsy on social life and leisure, change in outlook, increased social isolation, and lack of energy. The authors concluded that 'a potent factor affecting psychosocial adjustment is chronicity.'

Data about the impact of intractable epilepsy on QoL can also be gleaned from community-based studies that include in their samples patients across the range of epilepsy severity. In our own community study (Jacoby *et al* 1996a), we compared QoL in adult patients seizure-free in the last year (51% of all subjects), those experiencing fewer than one seizure per month (25% of all subjects), and those experiencing at least one seizure per month. Since only 14% of this latter group had ever had a 2-year remission, we think that they may reasonably be regarded as a group with medically intractable epilepsy. There was a clear relationship between seizure activity and psychologic well-being, with the percentages classified as clinically anxious and depressed increasing from 13% and 4%, respectively, in those currently seizure-free to 44% and 21% in those with frequent seizures. Of subjects with frequent seizures 62% reported feeling stigmatized by their epilepsy compared with only 25% of those who were seizure-free. Current seizure activity also clearly influenced subjects' perceptions about the impact of their condition on their daily functioning. Mean scores on the Impact of Epilepsy Scale (Jacoby *et al* 1993) increased from 12.9 (95% confidence interval 12.34–13.42) for individuals who were seizure-free to 19.3 (95% confidence interval 18.36–20.18) for those with frequent seizures, and there were marked differences in their responses to the individual items within the Impact of Epilepsy Scale (Table 33.5). While none of the seizure-free group felt it to be the case, more than half of the group reporting frequent seizures felt their condition significantly affected their social activities, overall health, feelings about themselves, and plans for the future. Fewer

subjects with frequent seizures were married and more reported that they had never been married.

As part of our analysis, we examined the employment status of this community sample in some detail and found that employment status varied with reported seizure frequency in the expected direction for both men and women of working age (Jacoby *et al* 1998). The percentages of men in full- or part-time employment fell from 66% among those who were seizure-free to only 21%, while in women the equivalent figures were 50% and 24%. The percentages of men and women registered as permanently sick increased from 16% and 7%, respectively, in those who were seizure-free to 53% and 27%, respectively, in those with frequent seizures.

We also examined the physical impact of epilepsy in this sample and found that, among those whose seizures were active, individuals with frequent seizures were significantly more likely than those whose seizures were infrequent to report seizure-related injuries, particularly burns, scalds, and dental injuries (Buck *et al* 1997). Thus, it appeared that across all the major domains, physical, psychologic, social, and employment, QoL was significantly poorer in people with intractable epilepsy than the rest.

Although intended as a psychometric exercise to compare validity and reliability of three QoL measures, the study by Langfitt (1995) provides some useful descriptive data on QoL in intractable epilepsy. Langfitt studied three groups of patients: the first, patients with complex partial seizures with secondary generalization (*n* = 18), and the second, patients with complex partial seizures only (*n* = 22), were both admitted to the Comprehensive Epilepsy Program at Rochester, Minnesota; the third group (*n* = 31) had previously undergone anterior temporal lobectomy and were now seizure-free. The three groups were largely similar in relation to demographic and clinical characteristics. As might be expected, the more severe the epilepsy,

Table 33.5 Perceived impact of epilepsy reported by patients (%) vs. seizure activity in the previous year.

	Seizure activity		
	None (n = 322)	<1 per month (n = 163)	>1 per month (n = 160)
Relationship with family members	13	28	37
Social activities	18	37	55
Ability to work	18	31	45
Overall health	21	46	60
Relationship with friends	11	24	41
Feelings of self	25	45	55
Plans for the future	24	33	56
Standard of living	16	35	49

the poorer the reported QoL on all three measures examined (Table 33.6), although the differences were somewhat less apparent on the one (WPSI) than on the other two measures. Since the third group were patients rendered seizure-free by surgery, the data provide some indication as to which areas and to what extent QoL can, potentially, be improved by this means for patients with intractable seizures, a point addressed in considerably greater detail in Chapter 64.

There are a number of other studies in adults with epilepsy that, although not examining QoL issues comprehensively, none the less shed some further light on this matter since they have focused on specific QoL domains. In particular, such studies have addressed the issues of psychopathology in

epilepsy, the impact on employment and, to a lesser degree, the impact on interpersonal relations.

Psychopathology

The question of the psychopathology associated with epilepsy has been widely researched, though again it is difficult to locate studies that directly compare rates of psychopathology in patients with intractable epilepsy and others. For example, Edeh *et al* (1990) compared psychiatric morbidity in 26 attenders at epilepsy outpatient clinics and 62 patients with epilepsy registered in UK general practices and not attending any hospital clinic and reported much higher proportions in the former

Table 33.6 Quality of life of people with intractable epilepsy compared with those rendered seizure-free by surgery.

	Group 1: intractable CPS + SG	Group 2: intractable CPS only	Group 3: seizure-free after surgery	P value
WPSI[a]				
Family background	3.67	2.04	2.71	NS
Emotional adjustment	17.10	8.50	9.30	<0.01
Adjustment to seizures	8.67	5.18	3.29	<0.01
Interpersonal adjustment	8.60	5.09	5.42	NS
Vocational adjustment	6.78	4.73	4.32	NS
Financial status	2.22	2.32	2.13	NS
Medical management	2.56	1.78	0.94	<0.01
Overall functioning	26.55	16.59	15.74	<0.05
ESI-55[b]				
Physical function	79.35	83.41	95.97	<0.05
Physical role limitations	44.44	74.55	87.58	<0.01
Pain	60.69	78.52	84.76	<0.05
Emotional well-being	58.44	72.55	75.87	<0.05
Cognitive function	48.07	72.48	74.62	<0.01
Emotional role limitations	54.44	85.91	87.10	<0.01
Memory problems	68.24	84.71	84.14	NS
General health perceptions	53.40	66.52	82.70	<0.01
Energy/fatigue	43.61	59.77	68.71	<0.05
Overall quality of life	61.81	70.23	76.53	NS
Social function	59.58	73.75	88.55	<0.01
SIP[c]				
Ambulation	5.09	1.08	0.34	NS
Mobility	11.54	8.36	0.78	<0.01
Body care	7.81	3.19	0.87	<0.01
Social interaction	14.76	9.09	6.21	NS
Communication	13.69	8.51	5.94	NS
Alertness behavior	41.91	13.35	11.19	<0.01
Emotional behavior	25.60	14.92	8.25	<0.01
Sleep and rest	31.03	21.10	6.49	<0.01
Eating	5.34	5.11	2.16	NS
Work	49.76	28.59	21.05	<0.05
Home management	13.82	9.41	1.34	<0.05
Recreation	17.80	16.33	2.88	<0.05

CPS, complex partial seizures; NS, not significant; SG, secondary generalization.
[a]Washington Psychosocial Seizure Inventory (Dodrill *et al* 1980): Lower means indicate better functioning.
[b]Epilepsy Surgery Inventory (Vickrey *et al* 1992): range 0–100; higher means indicate better functioning.
[c]Sickness Impact Profile (Bergner *et al* 1976): range 0–100; lower means indicate better functioning.

group than the latter of anxiety neurosis (26.9% compared with 9.7%) and depressive neurosis (26.9% compared with 19.4%). In their paper, these authors make a clearly articulated assumption that clinic attenders 'constitute a hard core of drug-resistant patients characterised by poor seizure control [and] polypharmacy,' yet examination of the reported characteristics of their subjects reveals that 23% of clinical attenders were seizure-free (compared with 35% of nonattenders) and that the mean number of antiepileptic drugs prescribed to the two groups was not markedly different. However, there was an excess of patients with focal seizures among the clinic attenders.

Collings (1990a) examined psychologic well-being in a group of people with epilepsy recruited through the UK epilepsy support groups. Although no information is given about the severity of epilepsy, we can make some judgment about this based on the information that half of the study sample were taking two antiepileptic drugs and a further 13% were taking three at the time of completing the questionnaire. Compared with a control group matched for age, gender, and geographic location, respondents with epilepsy had lower self-esteem, lower life satisfaction, more health, interpersonal and money worries, and more negative affect. On an overall well-being scale, which also included items relating to physical symptoms and social difficulties, lower well-being was found to be significantly associated with, among other factors, high seizure frequency, though not with seizure type or number of antiepileptic medications.

Several authors have pointed out that, with regard to psychopathology, clinical variables such as the level of seizure activity have, in fact, only limited explanatory power *per se* (Robertson and Trimble 1983; Hermann and Whitmann 1986; Robertson *et al* 1987; Gehlert 1994). Other nonclinical factors, such as the coping strategies patients evolve and their ability to adjust to epilepsy at whatever level of severity it manifests, may be more important predictors. For example, Mittan (1986) places the fear of having seizures high on the list of factors contributing to psychopathology, reporting extremely high levels of depression arising from the 'unpredictable terror' of seizures causing death or brain damage; it is clear from the work by Chaplin *et al* (1995) that this unpredictable terror is not confined to people with chronic or intractable epilepsy. Likewise, Goldstein *et al* (1990) reported that while poor seizure control was associated with higher rates of emotional and behavioral difficulties, fear of seizures was also significantly and independently related to psychologic functioning in adults with epilepsy.

Employment

According to Mittan (1986) fear of seizures not only influences psychopathology in people with epilepsy but also acts as a barrier to them obtaining and maintaining employment. In his study, where respondents were all patients whose epilepsy could reasonably be described as intractable, the workplace was seen as an extremely hazardous environment. Fears that work conditions would trigger seizures limited the kinds of employment subjects were willing to consider, and fears that work stress would precipitate seizures was one of the commonest reasons for quitting employment. Fear of seizures is, of course, only one of many reasons why epilepsy increases the risk of both under-employment and unemployment. There are also many formal and informal societal barriers to employability (Thompson and Oxley 1993). However, there is ample evidence that people with epilepsy are at risk and that intractability of their seizures, together with the disabling effects of antiepileptic medication, constitute major threats (Espir and Floyd 1986; Hauser and Hesdorffer 1990). Most of the studies we identified have only reported differences in employment rates between individuals whose seizures are successfully controlled and those whose seizures are continuing (Rodin et al 1972; Elwes *et al* 1991; Collings 1992), but two studies also examined the effects of seizure type. Emlen and Ryan (1985) found that for all seizure types the more frequent the seizures, the higher the percentage of unemployed; however, unemployment was highest (50%) for individuals experiencing at least one tonic–clonic seizure per year and lowest (13%) for those experiencing fewer than five 'minor' seizures per year. Scambler and Hopkins (1980) reported that of the subjects unemployed in their community study 32% were having generalized seizures and 43% partial seizures at least once monthly compared with 2% and 7%, respectively, among those who were in employment.

Social activities and relationships

As for the other domains of functioning that we have covered, much of what we can conclude about this topic must be extrapolated from available data, which in the main focus on chronicity rather than intractability of epilepsy. The broad message from the various studies, some involving samples recruited from epilepsy support groups (Collings 1990a,b) and tertiary epilepsy clinics (Dansky *et al* 1980) and population-based patient cohorts (Jalava and Sillanpaa 1997), is that people with epilepsy are less likely to marry and have children than people without epilepsy. However, this message can be refined by data which demonstrate that whereas epilepsy with onset in childhood may reduce the likelihood of marrying (Dansky *et al* 1980), early remission of childhood epilepsy may increase the likelihood (Lindsay *et al* 1979) and rates of marriage are little different in those with epilepsy uncomplicated by other related problems than in people without epilepsy (Britten *et al* 1986).

The reasons why people with epilepsy are less likely to marry have been the focus of considerable speculation. It has been suggested that such people restrict their social encounters out of fear of having seizures in public and the resultant stigma potential and threat to their personal safety (Mittan 1986); that the need for regular living habits to minimize the threat of seizures and the statutory restrictions on holding a driving licence reduces leisure activities and, in turn, the opportunities for making social relationships (Thompson and Oxley 1988); and that those whose epilepsy develops in childhood may be overprotected by other family members to the degree that they remain, in adulthood, immature and socially inept so that their interpersonal relationships are problematic (Scambler 1989). Whatever the causes, the data suggest that the problems are likely to be more acute for people whose epilepsy is chronic and intractable than for those whose condition is mild.

STUDIES IN CHILDREN

As for adults, there is an increasing literature on the QoL of children following epilepsy surgery (Yang *et al* 1996; Gilliam *et al* 1997b; Rougier *et al* 1997) to which we make only passing reference here, the broad message being that successful surgery is accompanied by marked improvements across a number of QoL domains. As for adults also, we face the problem of identifying studies specifically concerned with intractable epilepsy. One author who has written widely on the topic is Hoare (Hoare 1984; Hoare and Kerley 1991; Hoare and Russell 1995), who examined psychosocial adjustment in children with chronic and difficult-to-control epilepsy. Subjects were children aged 5–15 years attending a tertiary pediatric epilepsy clinic. Hoare and Kerley (1991) used three measures of psychosocial adjustment: the Rutter Behavioural Checklist (parent and teacher questionnaires) (Rutter *et al* 1970), the Piers–Harris Self-esteem Questionnaire (Piers 1984), and the Self-administered Dependency Questionnaire (Berg 1974). Psychologic morbidity of siblings and parents was also assessed, using the Rutter questionnaires for the siblings and the General Health Questionnaire (Tarnopolosky *et al* 1979) for the parents. The authors report high rates of behavioral disturbance, neurotic disorder being the most common diagnostic category, with no significant difference

in the rate of disturbance between boys and girls (53 and 49%, respectively). Interestingly, given the generally held view that self-esteem is impaired in people with epilepsy, total and subscale scores on the Piers–Harris scale were no different for the study children than the general population, nor were their scores on the dependency measure. However, those children who were psychiatrically disturbed were also shown to have poorer self-esteem. Hoare and Kerley examined the contribution of four sets of variables (demographic and family, clinical, maternal attitude, and child characteristics) to psychosocial adjustment and reported that among the clinical variables psychiatric disturbance was predicted by high seizure frequency, partial or focal EEG abnormalities, and combination drug treatment. Hoare (1984) also compared the rate of psychiatric disturbance in children with newly diagnosed and chronic epilepsy and concluded that in both groups those with focal EEG abnormalities and/or complex partial seizures were particularly vulnerable to psychiatric disturbance.

Austin *et al* (1996) compared QoL in adolescents with varying severity of epilepsy and asthma. A severity classification was determined by summing scores, which for epilepsy was related to seizure type, seizure frequency, and number of antiepileptic drugs, and for asthma to frequency of attacks, medication side-effects, hospitalization and emergency room visits, and school absences. Based on this classification, the condition was inactive in half of the epilepsy sample and one-fifth of the asthma sample, but was classified as 'high severity' in roughly one-quarter of both samples. The authors explored 19 dimensions across three broad QoL domains, psychologic, social, and school. Overall, QoL was poorer for the adolescents with epilepsy than those with asthma. There were significant differences on 13 of the 19 QoL dimensions and across all three QoL domains. Illness severity was also clearly important. Adolescents with active epilepsy fared worse than the other three groups on 10 of the 19 dimensions; in general, adolescents with active epilepsy fared worst and those with inactive asthma fared best. Adolescents with high-severity epilepsy, who can reasonably be thought of as having intractable epilepsy, had more internalizing problems, poorer peer relations, lower activity scores, more social problems, and higher attention problems than the other adolescents with epilepsy. The authors suggest that the poorer QoL in adolescents with epilepsy may be because of the social stigma attached to it, which means that it is more difficult to adjust to than asthma; may be related to associated neurologic dysfunction, which persists even after seizures remit; and may also be the product of impaired cognitive performance associated with antiepileptic medication. With regard to this last, there is ample evidence of the effects of antiepileptic drugs, and in particular of polytherapy, both on cognitive and emotional development (Thompson 1995) and so, potentially, on overall QoL.

Our own community study of epilepsy also showed differences in QoL between children with continuing seizures and those without (Jacoby *et al* unpublished data). We identified 93 children with active epilepsy through UK general practitioner medical records, one-third of whom were reported to have been seizure-free in the previous year and two-fifths of whom had seizures at least monthly. QoL was assessed using the Rutter Behavioural Checklist (Rutter *et al* 1970) and child versions of the Liverpool Seizure Severity Scale (Baker *et al* 1991), and the Impact of Epilepsy Scale (Jacoby *et al* 1993). Seizure frequency was the strongest predictor both of Rutter scale scores and scores on the Impact of Epilepsy Scale (Table 33.7), followed by age of onset and duration of epilepsy. Seizure frequency was also associated with the likelihood of receiving either special schooling or remedial help those with frequent seizures being almost twice as likely to be doing so than children with infrequent or inactive seizures.

Carlton-Ford *et al* (1995) also investigated social and psychologic adjustment in a study involving 32 children with active epilepsy (defined as seizures in the previous year) and 86 with a history of seizures drawn from the 1988 US National Health Interview Survey. Initially, the same pattern emerged as for our own and Austin's analyses. Compared with both controls and children with a history of epilepsy, those in whom the condition was active did significantly worse in relation to the numbers of days lost from school and were perceived (by the parent) as having poor general health, life-threatening illness, concomitant illnesses, and clumsiness. However, a rather different picture emerged when the authors used multivariate techniques to examine the influence of active and inactive epilepsy on home and school behavior problems, depressed mood, and impulsiveness. They found that once family process variables and concomitant illnesses were accounted for, the effect of epilepsy, whether active or not, on home and school behavior was nonsignificant; however, both groups of children with epilepsy were at increased risk of depression and impulsiveness compared with controls and the magnitude of the risk was similar. The authors interpret the lack of difference between children with active epilepsy and those with inactive epilepsy as demonstrating that poor social and psychologic adjustment is not a product of the condition *per se* but of self-fulfilling prophecies stemming from parental attitudes to epilepsy. Other studies of psychopathology (Pazzaglia and Frank-Pazzaglia 1976) and psychosocial adjustment in children and adolescents (Kokkonen *et al* 1997) also appear to confirm the relative unimportance of the clinical features of the epilepsy, including epilepsy duration, seizure frequency, and seizure type, and reinforce the comments by Schachter (1993) that clinical and psychosocial judgments of intractability are not necessarily one and the same.

One point to note in these studies of childhood epilepsy is that samples generally exclude children at the extreme worst end of the epilepsy severity spectrum, those with the so-called 'malignant epilepsies' (Renier 1995), which are frequently accompanied by significant learning disabilities and multiple handicaps. The problems of assessing QoL in such children are complex and have yet to be robustly addressed.

QUALITY OF LIFE AS A MEASURE OF TREATMENT OUTCOME

The studies referenced in the review above are descriptive ones in which QoL measures were used to discriminate between groups of people with epilepsy of varying type and severity. As we noted earlier, QoL measures are now increasingly used as measures of the outcome of treatment,

Table 33.7 Perceived impact of epilepsy on daily functioning of children reported by parent.

| | Seizure frequency | |
	Seizure-free in last 12 months (n = 26)	One or more seizures in last month (n = 36)
Relationship with parent responder	15	25
Relationship with responder's spouse/partner	12	17
Relationship with siblings	12	28
Relationship with other children	12	31
Hobbies and interests	12	31
Schooling	23	50
Overall health	4	39
Feelings about self	19	31
Plans for the future	24	50

both pharmacologic and surgical. One of the first published studies of treatment outcome that systematically assessed QoL was our own on the use of lamotrigine as add-on therapy in patients with intractable epilepsy (Smith *et al* 1993). This provided evidence that lamotrigine not only decreased seizure frequency and severity but also improved psychologic well-being. Similar findings have recently been reported for lamotrigine in children and adolescents with a severe and intractable form of epilepsy, Lennox–Gastaut syndrome (Jacoby *et al* 1996b). Dodrill *et al* (1993) have also used a QoL measure, the WPSI, to evaluate the effects of another novel antiepileptic drug, vigabatrin, as add-on therapy in patients with difficult-to-control focal epilepsy and found it to have no significant impact, either positive or negative, upon QoL. Though the use of QoL outcomes is relatively recent, we are aware of several studies currently ongoing in the field of epilepsy into which they have been incorporated and we think it likely that their inclusion will become routine given the emphasis on the importance now accorded to patient-based assessments.

REDUCING THE IMPACT OF INTRACTABLE EPILEPSY ON QUALITY OF LIFE

Despite limitations in the available data and problems of definition such as those discussed above, it is clear that intractable epilepsy is frequently associated with reduced QoL across all its domains. Recent research from our own group and others demonstrates that these QoL costs are mirrored by the large financial costs associated with intractable epilepsy (Murray *et al* 1996; Jacoby *et al* 1998). In this last section, we briefly mention the various nonsurgical approaches for reducing the impact.

A considerable amount has been written about the management of intractable epilepsy by pharmacologic and psychologic means. With regard to the use of pharmacologic agents, suffice it to say that though they can bring huge QoL benefits they are not without costs, particularly with regard to their potential impact on cognitive function (Mattson *et al* 1985; Trimble 1988; Aldenkamp 1995) and so, in turn, on daily functioning and QoL. Schachter (1993) points out that while only a relatively small percentage of patients with intractable seizures can expect to achieve any significant level of control through the use of polytherapy, the addition of a single antiepileptic drug to existing therapy may result in a marked increase of unwanted side-effects. The hope is that with the advent of new drugs with better-defined mechanisms of action, it will

be possible to identify 'combination regimens with synergistic properties' (Chadwick 1994) that will maximize seizure control while maintaining QoL.

Psychologic approaches can be divided into two broad categories: (a) those aimed at reducing seizure frequency; and (b) those that target the psychologic adjustment of the individual with epilepsy, which as we have shown may be less than optimal. A variety of relaxation strategies have been advanced in the management of seizures, including progressive muscle relaxation techniques and cognitive and behavioral approaches (Tan and Bruni 1986; Goldstein 1990). Though there has been little formal investigation of the efficacy of such approaches, there is none the less some evidence of their effectiveness in patients with otherwise intractable seizures (Betts 1997). The role of the clinical psychologist also extends to helping people with epilepsy to accept their diagnosis and to self-manage their condition effectively. People with epilepsy who are better informed about their condition perceive themselves as being in better control and subsequently have significantly better psychologic profiles than those who are less informed (Hills and Baker 1992). Cognitive behavioral techniques may be useful for modifying the underlying core beliefs people have about their condition, which are at the root of their psychologic impairments. Interestingly, the use of such techniques in one study (Tan and Bruni 1986) did result in an increase in patients' ratings of their well-being, although they did not significantly reduce seizure frequency.

Lastly, we support those who argue the case for an epilepsy specialist nurse as another key member of the multidisciplinary team. The concept of the nurse specialist has been slow to find favor in the UK (Appleton and Sweeney 1995), although in one UK pediatric epilepsy clinic its incorporation into the multidisciplinary team has, in the view of its protagonists, facilitated closer liaison with schools, community health personnel, and the voluntary groups for people with epilepsy, and so ensured the more comprehensive management of children under its care.

CONCLUSIONS

Epilepsy is a 'lived-with illness' (Conrad 1987) that is not generally life-threatening but where the affected person, whether child or adult, has to learn to cope with the consequences for their QoL. The broad message is that these consequences are generally more marked for those with more severe epilepsy, although the relationship is not perfectly linear. Despite the difficulties of definition in relation both to the notion of epilepsy intractability and the concept of QoL, many studies linking the two show that as the severity of the epilepsy increases so QoL diminishes. Against this general rule of thumb, it is important to remember that not all people with poorly controlled epilepsy report a poor QoL and that not all those with inactive epilepsy report a good one. This finding simply reinforces the very individual nature of QoL, the fact that health or the lack of it constitutes only one QoL domain among many, and the need to recognize the social as well as the clinical nature of the condition. If the QoL problems of people with intractable epilepsy are to be minimized, attending to the medical management of their condition, though critically important, is insufficient. Care must also be taken to determine their rehabilitation needs and their needs for counseling and support. Additionally, continuing efforts must be made to educate those without epilepsy in order to increase their understanding of this complex condition.

KEY POINTS

1. Intractability in epilepsy rests on QoL as well as clinical criteria.
2. QoL assessments are valuable across a range of healthcare contexts.
3. QoL measures are being used increasingly as measures of the outcome of treatment and healthcare provision for epilepsy.
4. Though the concept of QoL is problematic, QoL assessments should be informed by robust theoretic models.
5. QoL assessments should also satisfy standard psychometric criteria.
6. QoL assessments in epilepsy have employed both standardized and individualized approaches. There are advantages and disadvantages of each approach.
7. QoL assessments in children with epilepsy are less well advanced than for adults, because the theoretic difficulties are more marked.
8. Though the relationship is not perfectly linear, the broad conclusion from QoL research is that QoL is reduced in people with intractable epilepsy.
9. However, even within the confines of 'intractable epilepsy', there are marked differences in QoL.
10. Medical management of epilepsy alone is insufficient; attention must also be given to needs for rehabilitation, counseling, and support to improve QoL.

REFERENCES

Aaronson NK, Meyerowitz BE, Bard B, *et al* (1991) Quality of life research in oncology: past achievements and future priorities. *Cancer* 67:839–843.

Aldenkamp AP (1995) Cognitive side effects of antiepileptic drugs. In: Aldenkamp AP, Reiner WO, Suurmeijer TPBM (eds) *Epilepsy in Children and Adolescents*, pp 161–182. Boca Raton, FL: CRC Press.

Alving J (1995) What is intractable epilepsy? In: Johannessen SI, Gram L, Sillanpaa M, Tomson T (eds) *Intractable Epilepsy*, pp 1–12. Stroud: Wrightson Biomedical Publishing.

Appleton RE, Sweeney A (1995) The management of epilepsy in children: the role of the clinical nurse specialist. *Seizure* 4:287–291.

Austin JK, Dunn DW (1993) Children with newly diagnosed epilepsy: impact on quality of life. In: Baker GA, Jacoby A (eds) *Quality of Life and Quality of Care in Epilepsy: Update 1993*, pp 14–26. London: Royal Society of Medicine.

Austin JK, Huster GA, Dunn DW, Risinger MW (1996) Adolescents with active or inactive epilepsy or asthma: a comparison of quality of life. *Epilepsia* 37:1228–1237.

Avis NE, Smith KW (1994) Conceptual and methodological issues in selecting and developing quality of life measures. In: Fitzpatrick R (ed) *Advances in Medical Sociology*, pp 255–280. London: JAI Press.

Baker GA, Smith DF, Dewey M, Morrow J, Crawford PM, Chadwick DW (1991) The development of a seizure severity scale as an outcome measure in epilepsy. *Epilepsy Research* 8:245–251.

Baker GA, Smith DF, Dewey M, Jacoby A, Chadwick DW (1993) The initial development of a health-related quality of life model as an outcome measure in epilepsy. *Epilepsy Research* 16:65–81.

Baker GA, Jacoby A, Smith DF, Dewey ME, Chadwick DW (1994) Development of a novel scale to assess life fulfilment as part of the further refinement of a quality-of-life model for epilepsy. *Epilepsia* 35:591–596.

Baker GA, Jacoby A, Francis P, Chadwick DW (1995) The Liverpool adverse drug events profile. *Epilepsia* 36(suppl 3):S59.

Baker G, Jacoby A, Abetz L *et al* (1998) Evaluating the severity of newly diagnosed epilepsy patients using a quality-of-life instrument (abstract). *Epilepsia* 39:63.

Berg I (1974) A self administered dependency questionnaire (SADQ) for use with the mothers of school children. *British Journal of Psychiatry* 124:1–9.

Bergner M, Bobbitt RA, Pollard WE (1976) The sickness impact profile: validation of a health status measure. *Medical Care* 14:57–67.

Betts T (1997) Can anything be done if medical treatment fails? (abstract). *Epilepsia* 38:107.

Bradburn NM (1969) *The Structure of Psychological Well-being.* Chicago: Aldine.

Britten N, Morgan K, Fenwick PBC, Britten H (1986) Epilepsy and handicap from birth to age thirty-six. *Developmental Medicine and Child Neurology* 28:719–728.

Brooks RG (1991) *Health Status and Quality of Life Measurement: Issues and Developments.* Lund, Sweden: Institute for Health Economics.

Bruil J, Maes S (1995) Assessing quality of life among children with a chronic illness: the development of a questionnaire (poster). Presented at First Dutch Conference on Psychology and Health.

Buck D, Baker GA, Jacoby A, Smith DF, Chadwick D (1997) Patients' experiences of injury as a result of epilepsy. *Epilepsia* 9:87–93.

Carlton-Ford S, Miller R, Brown M, Nealeigh N, Jennings P (1995) Epilepsy and children's social and psychological adjustment. *Journal of Health and Social Behavior* 36:285–301.

Chadwick D (1994) Standard approach to antiepileptic drug treatment in the United Kingdom. *Epilepsia* 35(suppl 4):S3–S10.

Chaplin JE, Yepez R, Shorvon S, Floyd M (1990) A quantitative approach to measuring the social effects of epilepsy. *Neuroepidemiology* 9:151–158.

Chaplin JE, Yepez Lasso R, Shorvon SD, Floyd M (1992) National general practice study of epilepsy: the social and psychological effects of a recent diagnosis of epilepsy. *British Medical Journal* 304:1416–1418.

Chaplin JE, Shorvon SD, Floyd M, Yepez Lasso R (1995) Psychosocial factors in chronicity of epilepsy. *Journal of Neurology, Neurosurgery and Psychiatry* 58:112–113.

Collings J (1990a) Psychosocial well-being and epilepsy: an empirical study. *Epilepsia* 31:418–426.

Collings JA (1990b) Correlates of wellbeing in a New Zealand epilepsy sample. *New Zealand Medical Journal* 103:301–303.

Collings J (1992) *Epilepsy and the Experience of Employment. A Report of a National Survey by the British Epilepsy Association*. Leeds: British Epilepsy Association.

Conrad P (1987) The experience of illness: recent and new directions. In: Roth JA, Conrad P (eds) *Research in the Sociology of Health Care*, Vol 6. Greenwich, CT: JAI Press.

Corney RH, Clare AW (1985) The construction, development and testing of a self-report questionnaire to identify social problems. *Psychological Medicine* 15:637–649.

Cramer JA (1994) Quality of life for people with epilepsy. *Neurologic Clinics* 12:1–13.

Cramer *et al* (in press). *Epilepsia*

Dansky LV, Andermann E, Andermann F (1980) Marriage and fertility in epileptic patients. *Epilepsia* 21:261–271.

Devinsky O, Vickrey BG, Cramer J *et al* (1995) Development of the quality of life in epilepsy inventory. *Epilepsia* 36:1089–1104.

Deyo RA, Diehr P, Patrick DL (1991) Reproducibility and responsiveness of health status measures. Statistics and strategies for evaluation. *Controlled Clinical Trials* 12:142S–158S.

Dodrill CB, Batzel LW (1995) The Washington psychosocial seizure inventory: new developments in the light of the quality of life concept (abstract). *Epilepsia* 36:S220.

Dodrill CB, Batzel LW, Queisser HR, Temkin NR (1980) An objective method for the assessment of psychological and social problems among epileptics. *Epilepsia* 21:123–135.

Dodrill CB, Arnett JL, Sommerville KW, Sussman NM (1993) Evaluation of the effects of vigabatrin on cognitive abilities and quality of life in epilepsy. *Neurology* 43:2501–2507.

Edeh J, Toone BK, Corney RH (1990) Epilepsy, psychiatric morbidity and social dysfunction in general practice: comparison between hospital clinic patients and clinic nonattenders. *Neuropsychiatry, Neuropsychology, and Behavioural Neurology* 3:180–192.

Eiser C (1993) *Growing Up with a Chronic Disease: The Impact on Children and Their Families*. London: Jessica Kingsley.

Elwes RDC, Marshall J, Beattie A, Newman PK (1991) Epilepsy and employment: a community based survey in an area of high unemployment. *Journal of Neurology, Neurosurgery and Psychiatry* 54:200–203.

Emlen AC, Ryan R (1985) Personal communication to R. Masland. In: Porter RJ, Morselli PL (eds) *The Epilepsies*, p 361. London: Butterworth.

Espie CA, Kerr M, Paul A *et al* (1997) Learning disability and epilepsy. 2. A review of available outcome measures and position statement on development priorities. *Seizure* 6:337–350.

Espir M, Floyd M (1986) Epilepsy and recruitment. In: Edwards F, Espir M, Oxley J (eds) *Epilepsy and Employment: A Medical Symposium on Current Problems and Best Practices*, pp 39–45. London: Royal Society of Medicine.

Fink R (1989) Issues and problems in measuring children's health status in community health research. *Social Science and Medicine* 29:715–719.

Fowler FJ, Cleary PD, Magaziner J, Patrick DL, Benjamin KL (1994) Methodological issues in measuring patient-reported outcomes: the agenda of the work group on outcomes assessment. *Medical Care* 32:JS65–JS76.

Gehlert S (1994) Perceptions of control in adults with epilepsy. *Epilepsia* 35:81–88.

Gilliam F, Kuzniecky R, Faught E, Black L, Carpenter G, Schrodt R (1997a) Patient-validated content of epilepsy-specific quality of life measurement. *Epilepsia* 38:233–236.

Gilliam F, Wyllie E, Kashden J *et al* (1997b) Epilepsy surgery outcome: comprehensive assessment in children. *Neurology* 48:1368–1374.

Goldstein J, Seidenberg M, Peterson R (1990) Fear of seizures and behavioural functioning in adults with epilepsy. *Journal of Epilepsy* 3:101–106.

Goldstein LH (1990) Behavioural and cognitive-behavioural treatments for epilepsy: a progress review. *British Journal of Clinical Psychology* 29:257–269.

Guyatt G, Feeny DH, Patrick DL (1993) Measuring health-related quality of life. *Annals of Internal Medicine* 118:622–629.

Hauser WA, Hesdorffer DC (1990) Employment. In: Hauser WA, Hesdorffer DC (eds) *Epilepsy: Frequency, Causes and Consequences*, pp 273–296. Maryland: Epilepsy Foundation of America.

Hermann BP (1992) Quality of life in epilepsy. *Journal of Epilepsy* 5:153–165.

Hermann BP, Whitmann S (1986) Psychopathology in epilepsy: a multi-etiological model. In: Whitman S, Hermann BP (eds) *Psychopathology in Epilepsy: Social Dimensions*, pp 5–37. Oxford: Oxford University Press.

Hills MD, Baker PG (1992) Relationships among epilepsy, social stigma, self-esteem and social support. *Journal of Epilepsy* 5:231–238.

Hoare P (1984) The development of psychiatric disorder among schoolchildren with epilepsy. *Developmental Medicine and Child Neurology* 26:3–13.

Hoare P, Kerley S (1991) Psychosocial adjustment of children with chronic epilepsy and their families. *Developmental Medicine and Child Neurology* 33:201–215.

Hoare P, Russell M (1995) The quality of life of children with chronic epilepsy and their families: preliminary findings with a new assessment measure. *Developmental Medicine and Child Neurology* 37:689–696.

Hunt SM (1997) The problem of quality of life. *Quality of Life Research* 6:205–212.

Hunt S, McKenna SP, McEwan J, Williams J, Papp E (1981) The Nottingham Health Profile: subjective health status and medical consultations. *Social Science and Medicine* 15A:221–229.

Jacoby A (1992) Epilepsy and the quality of everyday life: findings from a study of people with well-controlled epilepsy. *Social Science and Medicine* 43:657–666.

Jacoby A (1994) Felt versus enacted stigma: a concept revisited. *Social Science and Medicine* 38:269–274.

Jacoby A (1996) Assessing quality of life in patients with epilepsy. *Pharmaco Economics* 9:399–416.

Jacoby A, Johnson AL, Chadwick DW (1992) Psychosocial outcomes of antiepileptic drug discontinuation. *Epilepsia* 33:1123–1131.

Jacoby A, Baker GA, Smith DF, Dewey M, Chadwick DW (1993) Measuring the impact of epilepsy: the development of a novel scale. *Epilepsy Research* 16:83–88.

Jacoby A, Baker GA, Steen N, Chadwick DW (1996a) The clinical course of epilepsy and its psychosocial correlates: findings from a UK community study. *Epilepsia* 37:148–161.

Jacoby A, Baker G, Bryant-Comstock L, Phillips S, Bamford C (1996b) Lamotrigine add-on therapy is associated with improvement in mood in patients with severe epilepsy. *Epilepsia* **37** (suppl 5):S202.

Jacoby A, Buck D, Chadwick DW (1997) Impact of newly diagnosed seizures and epilepsy: findings from a prospective study. *Epilepsia* **38**(suppl 3):S104.

Jacoby A, Buck D, Baker G, McNamee P, Graham-Jones S, Chadwick D (1998) Uptake and costs of care for epilepsy: findings from a UK regional study. *Epilepsia* **39**:776–786.

Jaeschke R, Guyatt G (1990) How to develop and validate a new quality of life instrument. In: Spilker B (ed) *Quality of Life Assessments in Clinical Trials*. New York: Raven Press.

Jaeschke R, Singer J, Guyatt G (1989) Measurements of health status: ascertaining the minimally important difference. *Controlled Clinical Trials* **10**:407–415.

Jalava M, Sillanpaa M (1997) Reproductive activity and offspring health of young adults with childhood-onset epilepsy: a controlled study. *Epilepsia* **38**:532–540.

Janz D (1989) How does one assess the severity of epilepsy? In: Trimble MR (ed) *Chronic Epilepsy: its Prognosis and Management*, pp 21–36 Chichester: John Wiley & Sons.

Juniper EF, Guyatt GH, Willan A, Griffith LE (1994) Determining a minimal important change in a disease-specific quality of life questionnaire. *Journal of Clinical Epidemiology* **47**:81–87.

Juniper EF, Guyatt GH, Jaeschke R (1996) How to develop and validate a new health-related quality of life instrument. In: Spilker B (ed) *Quality of Life and Pharmacoeconomics in Clinical Trials*, pp 49–55. Philadelphia: Lippincott-Raven.

Kendrick AM, Trimble MR (1994) Repertory grid in the assessment of quality of life in patients with epilepsy: the quality of life assessment schedule. In: Trimble M, Dodson W (eds) *Epilepsy and Quality of Life*, pp 151–163. New York: Raven Press.

Kokkonen J, Kokkonen E-R, Saukkonen A-L, Pennanen P (1997) Psychosocial outcome of young adults with epilepsy in childhood. *Journal of Neurology, Neurosurgery and Psychiatry* **62**:265–268.

Landgraf JM, Abetz L, Ware JE (1996) *The Child Health Questionnaire Users' Manual*. Boston: Health Institute, New England Medical Center.

Langfitt JT (1995) Comparison of the psychometric characteristics of three quality of life measures in intractable epilepsy. *Quality of Life Research* **4**:101–114.

Leplege A (1997) The problem of quality of life in medicine. *Journal of the American Medical Association* **278**:47–50.

Lindsay J, Ounsted C, Richards P (1979) Long-term outcome in children with temporal lobe seizures. II. Marriage, parenthood and sexual indifference. *Developmental Medicine and Child Neurology* **21**:433–440.

McDowell I, Newell C (1987) *Measuring Health: A Guide to Rating Scales and Questionnaires*. Oxford: Oxford University Press.

Marquis P (1998) Strategies for interpreting quality of life questionnaires. *Quality of Life Newsletter* March 3–4.

Mattson RH, Cramer JA, Collins JF *et al* (1985) Comparison of carbamazepine, phenobarbital, phenytoin and primidone in partial and secondarily generalised tonic–clonic seizures. *New England Journal of Medicine* **313**:145–151.

Meador KJ (1993) Research use of the new Quality-of-life in Epilepsy Inventory. *Epilepsia* **34**(suppl 4):S34–S38.

Mittan RJ (1986) Fear of seizures. In: Whitman S, Hermann B (eds) *Psychopathology in Epilepsy: Social Dimensions*, pp 90–121. Oxford: Oxford University Press.

Murray MI, Halpern MT, Leppik IE (1996) Cost of refractory epilepsy in adults in the USA. *Epilepsy Research* **23**:139–148.

O'Donoghue MF, Duncan JS, Sander JWAS (1998) The subjective handicap of epilepsy: a new approach to measuring treatment outcome. *Brain* **121**:100–127.

Patrick DL, Erickson P (1993) Assessing health-related quality of life for

clinical decision-making. In: Walker SR, Rosser RM (eds) *Quality of Life Assessment: Key Issues in the 1990s*, pp 11–63. Lancaster: Kluwer Academic Publishers.

Pazzaglia P, Frank-Pazzaglia L (1976) Record in grade school of pupils with epilepsy: an epidemiological study. *Epilepsia* **17**:361–366.

Pearlin L, Schooler C (1978) The structure of coping. *Journal of Health and Social Behavior* **19**:2–21.

Piers E (1984) *Piers–Harris Children's Self-concept Scale: Revised Manual*. Los Angeles: Western Psychological Services.

Pope C, Mays N (1995) Reaching the parts other methods cannot reach: an introduction to qualitative methods in health and health services research. *British Medical Journal* **311**:42–45.

Renier WO (1995) The malignant epilepsies of childhood and adolescence. In: Aldenkamp AP, Dreiffus FE, Renier WO, Suurmeijer TPBM (eds) *Epilepsy in Children and Adolescents*, pp 43–58. Boca Raton, FL: CRC Press.

Robertson MM, Trimble MR (1983) Depressive illness in patients with epilepsy: a review. *Epilepsia* **24**(suppl 2):S109–S116.

Robertson MM, Trimble MR, Townsend HRA (1987) Phenomenology of depression in epilepsy. *Epilepsia* **28**:364–372.

Rodin E, Rennick P, Denerll R, Lin Y (1972) Vocational and educational problems of epileptic patients. *Epilepsia* **13**:149–160.

Rogerson RJ (1995) Environmental and health-related quality of life: conceptual and methodological similarities. *Social Science and Medicine* **41**:1373–1382.

Rosenberg M (1965) *Society and the Adolescent Self-image*. Princeton: Princeton University Press.

Rosenberg R (1995) Health-related quality of life between naturalism and hermeneutics. *Social Science and Medicine* **41**:1411–1415.

Rougier A, Claverie B, Pedespan JM, Marchal C, Loiseau P (1997) Callosotomy for intractable epilepsy: overall outcome. *Journal of Neurosurgical Sciences* **41**:51–57.

Ruta DA, Garratt AM, Leng M, Russell IT, MacDonald LM (1994) A new approach to the measurement of quality of life. *Medical Care* **32**:1109–1123.

Rutter M, Graham P, Yule W (1970) *A Neuropsychiatric Study in Childhood*. Clinics in Developmental Medicine nos 35/36. London: Spastics International and Heinemann Medical.

Scambler G (1989) *Epilepsy*. London: Tavistock.

Scambler G (1993) Epilepsy and quality of life research. *Journal of the Royal Society of Medicine* **86**:449–450.

Scambler G, Hopkins A (1980) Social class, epileptic activity and disadvantage at work. *Journal of Epidemiology and Community Health* **34**:129–133.

Schachter SC (1993) Advances in the assessment of refractory epilepsy. *Epilepsia* **34** (suppl 5):S24–S30.

Schipper H, Clinch J, Powell V (1990) Definitions and conceptual issues. In: Spilker B (ed) *Quality of Life Assessments in Clinical Trials*, pp 11–24. New York: Raven Press.

Schneider JW, Conrad P (1983) *Having Epilepsy: The Experience and Control of Illness*. Philadelphia: Temple University Press.

Smith DF, Baker GA, Dewey M, Jacoby A, Chadwick DW (1991) Seizure frequency, patient perceived seizure severity and the psychosocial consequences of intractable epilepsy. *Epilepsy Research* **9**:231–241.

Smith DF, Baker GA, Davies G, Dewey M, Chadwick DW (1993) Outcomes of add-on treatment with lamotrigine in partial epilepsy. *Epilepsia* **34**:312–322.

Spilker B (1996) *Quality of Life and Pharmacoenomics in Clinical Trials*, 2nd edn. Philadelphia: Lippincott-Raven.

Streiner DL, Norman GR (1989) *Health Measurement Scales: A Practical Guide to their Development and Use*. Oxford: Oxford Medical Publications.

Tan SY, Bruni J (1986) Cognitive-behaviour therapy with adult patients with epilepsy: a controlled outcome study. *Epilepsia* **27**:225–233.

Tarnopolosky A, Hand D, MacLean E, Roberts H, Wiggins RD (1979) Validity and use of a screening questionnaire (GHQ) in the community. *British Journal Psychiatry* **134**:508–515.

Thompson PJ (1995) The impact of epilepsy on behaviour and emotional development. In: Aldenkamp AP, Reiner WO, Suurmeijer TPBM (eds), *Epilepsy in Children and Adolescents*, pp 239–250. Boca Raton, FL: CRC Press.

Thompson PJ, Oxley J (1988) Socioeconomic accompaniments of severe epilepsy. *Epilepsia* **29**(suppl 1):S9–S18.

Thompson PJ, Oxley J (1989) Social difficulties and severe epilepsy: survey results and recommendations. In: Trimble MR (ed) *Chronic Epilepsy: Its Prognosis and Management*, pp 113–131. Chichester: John Wiley & Sons.

Thompson P, Oxley J (1993) Social aspects of epilepsy. In: Laidlaw J, Richens A, Chadwick DW (eds) *A Textbook of Epilepsy*, 4th edn., pp 661–704. Edinburgh: Churchill Livingstone.

Trimble MR (1988) Anticonvulsant drugs: mood and cognitive function. In: Trimble MR, Reynolds EH (eds) *Epilepsy: Behaviour and Cognitive Function*, pp 135–143. Chichester: John Wiley and Sons.

Trostle JA, Hauser WA, Sharbrough FW (1989) Psychological and social adjustment to epilepsy in Rochester, Minnesota. *Neurology* **39**:633–637.

Vickrey BG, Hays RD, Graber J, Rausch R, Engel J, Brook RH (1992) A health-related quality of life instrument for patients evaluated for epilepsy surgery. *Medical Care* **30**:299–319.

Wagner AK, Vickrey BG (1995) The routine use of health-related quality of life measures in the care of patients with epilepsy: rationale and research agenda. *Quality of Life Research* **4**:169–177.

Wagner AK, Keller SD, Kosinski M *et al* (1995) Advances in methods for assessing the impact of epilepsy and antiepileptic drug therapy on patients' health-related quality of life. *Quality of Life Research* **4**:115–134.

Ware JE, Sherbourne CD (1992) The MOS 36-item Short-Form Health Survey (SF-36). I. Conceptual framework and item selection. *Medical Care* **30**:473–483.

West A (1995) Methodological issues in the assessment of quality of life in childhood asthma: what educational research has to offer. In: Christie M, French D (eds) *Assessment of Quality of Life in Childhood Asthma*, pp 121–130. Chur, Switzerland: Harwood Academic Publishers.

West P (1979) *Investigation into the social construction and consequences of the label 'epilepsy'*, PhD thesis, University of Bristol.

World Health Organization (1947) The constitution of the World Health Organisation. *Bulletin of the World Health Organization* **1**:29.

Yang T-F, Wong T-T, Kwan S-Y, Chang K-P, Lee Y-C, Hsu T-C (1996) Quality of life and life satisfaction in families after a child has undergone corpus callosotomy. *Epilepsia* **37**:76–80.

Zielinski JJ (1986) Selected psychiatric and psychosocial aspects of epilepsy as seen by an epidemiologist. In: Whitman S, Hermann BP (eds) *Psychopathology in Epilepsy: Social Dimensions*, pp 38–68. New York: Oxford University Press.

Zigmond AS, Snaith RP (1983) The hospital anxiety and depression scale. *Acta Psychiatrica Scandinavica* **67**:361–370.

Quality of life with reference to children and adolescents

33b

P DEAN AND S LANNON

The 1990s saw an increasing awareness of the importance of quality of life (QoL) issues for people with epilepsy. QoL remains a difficult concept to define since it is such a subjective phenomenon. It is influenced by the person's age at seizure onset, how the patient and family adjust to the diagnosis, and the support available to them. Intractable partial epilepsy affects QoL in multiple areas, such as physical and psychologic well-being, level of independence, education, employment, leisure activities, and other social aspects of life. Some very good instruments have been developed to objectively measure the concept and develop effective interventions. However, there are some limitations to these tools.

INTRODUCTION

Recognition of the importance of quality of life (QoL) in patients with epilepsy began in 1990 when members of the International League Against Epilepsy (ILAE) and the International Bureau for Epilepsy (IBE) presented a consensus opinion on behalf of the World Health Organization (WHO). Entitled *Initiative of Support to People with Epilepsy* (Bertolote 1994), the document focused global attention on personal aspects regarding the care of people

with epilepsy, especially in developing countries, and fostered a Global Campaign Against Epilepsy that began in 1997. Provision of medical care and services for all people with epilepsy, and increasing public awareness regarding its treatment, are fundamental to the WHO initiative (Epigraph 1998).

The importance of improving QoL was further emphasized in a special, day-long symposium dedicated exclusively to QoL at the 22nd International Epilepsy Congress. With more widespread awareness of QoL, through the collaboration of the WHO with ILAE and IBE, epilepsy is finally being understood in the full context of the individual's life.

This chapter addresses factors known to influence QoL in individuals with intractable partial seizures. Tools to assess QoL and their contribution and limitations are presented. Finally, interventions to improve QoL are reviewed.

DEFINITION OF QUALITY OF LIFE

QoL, also defined as well-being, life satisfaction, or happiness, is difficult to define satisfactorily (Hartshorn and Byers 1992). The term is highly subjective as it involves individual perceptions within cultural, societal, and family contexts. Personal values, goals, expectations, experiences, and standards are factored into the overall equation (Orley

1994). Age, gender, state of health, self-image, emotional support, independence, and feelings of control over events also play prominent roles. Ultimately the person living with epilepsy must define QoL for himself or herself (Santilli *et al* 1994).

QoL also affects family dynamics in a significant way whenever one member is diagnosed. Hunt and McKenna (1995) convey this point succinctly by stating: 'the ripples caused by the experience of epilepsy extend far beyond the human boundaries of the individual patient'. Thus, full assessment must include the primary supporters and interventions must be developed from a family-centered perspective. Even from a global perspective, QoL is influenced by variables beyond family control including socioeconomic status, access to medical care, and inherent coping skills of family members (Burckhardt 1987).

FACTORS INFLUENCING QOL IN INTRACTABLE FOCAL EPILEPSY

AGE AT SEIZURE ONSET

The influence of age at seizure onset on QoL is complex. Jacoby *et al* (1996) report that the impact of early seizure onset is largely negative. Many patients with childhood-onset epilepsy, with or without neurologic deficits, display impaired social adjustment and diminished competence in adulthood (Jalava *et al* 1997); by contrast, depression is more frequent if seizures begin in adolescence (Upton and Thompson 1992). However, early seizure onset may also foster positive adjustment and good coping strategies with respect to education, employment, and social independence.

In contrast, adult seizure onset produces different issues often revolving around loss of independence (driving, employment). With adequate coping skills, individuals with adult-onset seizures may be better able to transfer that previous experience to their new situation. Elderly persons are particularly devastated by the diagnosis of epilepsy, particularly if it compromises retirement or feeds into preconceived negative stereotypes regarding the diagnosis (Lannon 1993). Luhdorf (1986) found that a significant number of single, elderly people became homebound or institutionalized once seizures became medically resistant.

ADJUSTMENT

A diagnosis of epilepsy may establish a chain of events that significantly and permanently alters lifestyle. Initially, the lifestyle changes of the individual and their family constitute a form of loss that must be grieved, analyzed, internalized in terms of personal meaning, and ultimately resolved. Self-esteem, dignity, expectations, family roles, and perceptions of self-control must be utilized to achieve successful reintegration (Burckhardt 1987). Successful resolution is critical to achieving positive life quality, and requires coping skills that must be sustained for many years.

The chronicity and unpredictability of seizures influence the adjustment process and patients with chronic seizures need to establish healthy lifestyles, adhere to medication compliance, and maintain medical follow-up. Previous experiences with health care and illness often influence perceptions of a chronic medical condition (Aguilar 1997). The value attached to health status negatively or positively influences modification in lifestyle in relation to epilepsy and its treatment (Lannon 1997). The unpredictability and fear of seizures in public, and the perception of loss of control, has a greater impact on QoL than the actual seizures themselves (Collings 1995).

Ethnic, cultural, and religious factors may contribute to acceptance by family and community, and influence interaction with health care providers (Dean 1996). Ancient perceptions of epilepsy as a disease related to demon possession, mysticism, a curse from God, and madness still persist in many parts of the world and are not limited to developing countries (Lebrun 1992; McLin and de Boer 1995). Media representations of people with epilepsy as being tragic, helpless, aggressive, or out of control strongly influence public perceptions and may cause rejection or social isolation (Coyle and Brown 1997).

SUPPORT

Acceptance of the diagnosis of epilepsy by family and friends is essential to healthy QoL (Upton 1993). QoL also improves with access to ordinary life pursuits including education, employment, relationships, social interactions, and leisure activities. This may be facilitated by raising public awareness about epilepsy, debunking existing myths, correcting misconceptions, and rescinding restrictive legislation.

SPECIFIC EFFECTS OF INTRACTABLE PARTIAL SEIZURES ON QOL

PHYSICAL HEALTH

Sixty-one percent of patients with epilepsy report some form of adverse drug effect (Roper Poll 1992). Depression, behavior changes, difficulty concentrating, drowsiness, and lethargy are the symptoms most frequently reported. Barbiturates are especially likely to impair cognition, but all drugs, to a greater or lesser degree, affect higher cortical processing, especially when administered in high doses or as polytherapy (Buchanan 1992; Devinsky 1995). Physical problems such as hirsutism, acne, gingival hyperplasia, hair loss, and weight gain negatively influence self-esteem, particularly in adolescence. Potential teratogenicity, gastrointestinal, liver, and hematological effects also negatively influence lifestyle.

Some individuals with intractable partial seizures take toxic doses or multiple drug regimens which increase adverse drug effects (Wagner *et al* 1996). While the new antiepileptic drugs (AEDs) are designed to obviate these problems, not all patients have access to these drugs, or investigational agents and clinical drug trials. Discouraged by persistent seizures and/or intolerable side-effects, it is not surprising that in the 1992 Roper Poll 14% of patients reported intentionally missing drug doses.

The potential for injury and seizure-related death may further compromise QoL (Baker *et al* 1997b; McLachlan *et al* 1997). Lacerations, fractures, contusions, scalds, and dental/mouth trauma (Buck *et al* 1997) increase the use of medical, hospital, and emergency services (Donker *et al* 1997). Severe and uncontrolled seizures cause a two- to threefold risk of sudden unexplained death in epilepsy (SUDEP) above the general population (Brown 1992; Nashef and Shorvon 1997).

PSYCHOLOGIC HEALTH

Loss of control is probably the single most important fear in individuals with seizures, and perceived helplessness can affect all aspects of the person's life (Gehlert 1994). As one patient eloquently stated, 'having epilepsy is like standing on a trap door which someone else controls. You never know from one moment to the next when the bottom is going to fall out of your world.' The sense of helplessness in witnessing a seizure is equally stressful for the family (Thompson and Upton 1992).

Depression is common in individuals with epilepsy and is typical of patients who are medically uncontrolled (Hermann *et al* 1996). In one study, 21% of people with intractable seizures experienced depressive symptomatology compared to 4% of individuals who were well controlled (Baker *et al* 1997a). Inability to drive, earn income, or raise children are additional concerns (Pollock 1987).

Anxiety due to fear of recurrent seizures, lowered expectations, feelings of rejection and embarrassment, and an overall sense of hopelessness may lead to an external locus of control. Learned helplessness associated with negative events is closely related to the person's degree of seizure control (Gehlert 1994), with severe and frequent seizures requiring further monitoring to prevent a crisis (Braden 1990). Negative experiences thus tend to promote a system that reinforces feelings of helplessness and depression. Family members may also foster learned helplessness through overprotection, which inhibits the maturational process (Murray and Haynes 1996).

LEVEL OF INDEPENDENCE

The ability to drive, find gainful employment, have access to education, and an opportunity to live independently greatly affect QoL for people with epilepsy. However, since the first reported seizure-related motor vehicle accident in 1906, there have been prohibitions against driving for individuals suffering from epilepsy (Fisher *et al* 1994). Countries, states, and provinces within countries have different regulations regarding epilepsy and driving (Fisher *et al* 1996). Loss of driving privilege is particularly significant in areas where public transportation is limited. The ability to drive is pivotal for employment, education, and choice of residence.

The Joint Commission on Drivers' Licensing of the ILAE and IBE recommended that blanket prohibitions against driving be amended to allow for individual differences (Fisher *et al* 1994). These prohibitions not only fail to recognize the vast differences in seizure severity, type, and frequency but do not recognize that many people with epilepsy drive safely. In a study of 1089 patients with epilepsy, road accidents were few and generally minor (Beaussart *et al* 1997), possibly due to restrictions on obtaining the initial driving license.

The Commission also concluded that individual situations should be evaluated individually. Thus, someone who is deemed medically unfit to drive should be given a legitimate reason for this classification such as daytime seizures with loss of consciousness. Unfortunately, even when individuals with epilepsy obtain a driving license, they are often assigned to a high-risk pool for automobile insurance and may not be able to afford necessary coverage (Krumholz 1994). An epilepsy diagnosis also prohibits certain forms of commercial driving, particularly public transport.

EMPLOYMENT

The existence of frequent seizures with their physical and psychologic sequelae, the need to rely on medications which can have cognitive effects, and the fear of employers about the person's reliability and performance restricts many people with epilepsy from gainful employment (Fisher *et al* 1996). Underemployment, which is working at a job below one's training or potential, is also a common experience for people with epilepsy. Poor self-image, lack of social skills, and lack of good work habits are self-limiting characteristics which impede job search and placement (Jacoby 1995; Lipsey 1996). In the Republic of Ireland, 61% unemployment was observed in young people with epilepsy compared to UK and USA rates of 25–42% (Carroll 1992).

In the USA, the Americans with Disabilities Act (ADA) has eliminated certain stigmas attached to hiring people with epilepsy. The ADA states that each person who has the qualifications for a position must be given an equal opportunity to prove their ability to do the job (Troxell 1997).

EDUCATION

Early-onset and symptomatic seizures correlate with poor school performance and lower intelligence quotient (IQ) scores (Dodson 1993; Fisher *et al* 1996). Cognitive effects of AEDs, school absence, frequent medical appointments, and diminished expectations all negatively affect school performance (Thompson and Oxley 1988). As the academic and social advantages of school attendance enhance the chances for future independence, every effort should be made to encourage placement in an ordinary school environment.

LIVING SITUATIONS

In one study, 59% of adults lived at home and remained fully dependent on their families for support (Thompson and Oxley 1988). In countries like the UK, supported living accommodations enable some young people to be autonomous and leave home; an understanding and supportive roommate is another feasible alternative.

LEISURE ACTIVITIES

The benefits of physical exercise include decreased levels of depression (Roth *et al* 1994), increased social interaction opportunities and even a slight decrease in seizure activity (Eriksen *et al* 1994). Unfortunately, access to leisure activities is often restricted for fear of seizures. Adults with epilepsy are likely to be less physically fit and select more passive activities, typically preferring television or radio compared to age-matched controls (Steinhoff *et al* 1996). Fear of embarrassment of having a seizure during more strenuous activity in public, like playing a sport, was a frequent reason for this choice.

SOCIAL

Seizure patients have fewer friends and lower marriage rates. Thompson and Oxley (1988) found that 68% of patients at the Chalfont Center reported having 'no personal friends'. People with epilepsy describe 'loneliness' at a rate six times higher than matched controls (Jalava *et al* 1997). Many women fear they will not be able to have healthy children and avoid relationships leading to marriage. Both men and women doubt their parenting skills.

QOL ISSUES IN CHILDHOOD

Although the concept of QoL is universal and applies to all ages, it has been extremely difficult to define the effects of epilepsy in childhood (Dodson 1994). Children have a limited knowledge of cause–effect relationships (Sanger *et al* 1993) and different age groups may perceive these issues quite differently.

In a study of children with well-controlled epilepsy utilizing a modified Quality of Life in Epilepsy scale (QoLIE-89) concerns about their epilepsy varied depending on the age group of the child (Wildrick *et al* 1996).

Austin *et al* (1994) compared children with epilepsy and asthma and showed that children with epilepsy have greater compromise in psychologic, social, and educational areas, even for conditions beginning at a later age with fewer episodes. These results suggest that epilepsy is specifically responsible for deteriorated QoL in children in the psychologic, social, and educational domain.

The risk of injury and death from seizures is less clear in children than for adults but is still a significant issue in the pediatric population. While there are no studies that look at injuries from seizures specifically in children, children with seizures commonly injure themselves. Children with epilepsy are also 3 to 7.5 times more likely to experience a submersion incident (Pearn *et al* 1978; Orlowski *et al* 1982; Kemp and Sibert 1993). Death as a result of seizures is also not rare in childhood. Harvey *et al* (1993) found an increased risk of death during childhood in children with epilepsy, with SUDEP accounting for 12% of these deaths.

Studies show that children have a great deal of concern in regard to their seizures. Some of their greatest concerns center on how they will be perceived by their friends (Austin 1993; Wildrick *et al* 1996). Personal dissatisfaction and feelings of being different from or not as good as others are common in children with epilepsy (Austin 1993). Loss of control undermines a sense of competence, and fear of injuries often leads to exclusion from social activities or prohibition from sports. Limitation of recreational activity further jeopardizes a sense of competence. While adults express depression and anxiety more directly, pediatric patients may present with symptoms such as disruptive behavior or irritability, which may not be readily identified (Ettinger *et al* 1998).

Academic achievement is poorer in children with epilepsy in comparison to children with asthma (Austin *et al* 1998). Even children with controlled seizures and a normal IQ may have trouble concentrating in school and finishing assignments because of medication side-effects. Children are also afraid of being teased by other students if a seizure occurs and may feel singled out as different if they need to take medications during school time (Thompson 1995).

QOL ASSESSMENT

Quality of Life in Epilepsy (QoLIE) questionnaires were developed in the USA in the 1990s. The validity of the QoLIE was initially piloted at epilepsy centers throughout the USA (Devinsky *et al* 1995). Two longer versions, QoLIE-31 and QoLIE-89, provide formal testing, while the QoLIE-10 is a screening tool for outpatient evaluation (Cramer *et al* 1996). The QoLIE-10 can be administered to patients with limited reading skills. An adolescent QoLIE has also been developed.

The Epilepsy Self-Efficacy Scale (Dilorio *et al* 1992) measures behavior in relation to competence in self-management domains. It assesses perceptions of control ranging from medication compliance to social situations.

QoL inventories should be appropriate for the patient groups to which they are applied (Gilliam *et al* 1997). Most current versions have limited use for patients in developing countries and future assessment tools should be ethnically and culturally sensitive. Illiterate people with epilepsy require different testing paradigms.

Assessment also requires access to resources and a support team trained in vocational and rehabilitation techniques. The Epilepsy Foundation, British Epilepsy Association, and National Society for Epilepsy are excellent resources.

OTHER MEANS OF ASSESSMENT
Structured and semistructured interview
This has an open-ended format to encourage elaboration on issues of special concern.

Neuropsychologic evaluation

This examines specific information regarding cognition and emotional stability.

Family APGAR

This is a simple five-item questionnaire assessing family functioning. It measures adaptation, partnership, growth, affection, and resolve. The Family APGAR, evaluates individual family responses including internal strength, support, and needs. Formal tools to assess children are not yet available (Smilkstein 1979).

Child Behavior Checklist, the Child Attitude Toward Illness Scale (CATIS) and the Child's Version of the Family APGAR

These measure several QoL variables in children. The CATIS measures the children's attitudes toward epilepsy. The APGAR assesses interaction with family members. All are reliable and valid (Austin 1993).

Child Health Questionnaire (CHQ)

This gives a profile of 14 health concepts and measures physical and psychosocial functioning in children of 5 years or older. Concepts assessed include general health, physical functioning, limitation in schoolwork, and activities with friends due to physical problems, self-esteem, and family cohesion (Landgraf *et al* 1996).

INTERVENTIONS

While physicians and nurses provide primary educational support, allied specialists address specific patient needs. A survey at a specialized epilepsy assessment and treatment unit in the UK (Upton *et al* 1996) revealed that 90% of patients believed their physical and social situation improved as a result of attendance. Epilepsy specialist nurses provide patient, family, and community education, observe responses to drug changes and monitor stable patients (Ridsdale *et al* 1997; Russell 1997).

In the USA, the TAPS (Training and Placement Success) service of the Epilepsy Foundation has sites in 16 states where trained staff help individuals with epilepsy to develop interviewing and job-searching skills. TAPS also provides education for potential employers and explains the provisions of the Americans with Disabilities Act to people with epilepsy seeking employment. Further practical interventions include departments of vocational rehabilitation available throughout the USA and supported work schemes in other countries.

SUMMARY

Quality of life for people with epilepsy is contingent upon a constellation of both internal and external factors. Seizure control, access to adequate medical care, and the ability of the family to adjust to the diagnosis are important. Public understanding, acceptance, and support of the person are critical. Professional organizations, support associations, and initiatives like the WHO Global Campaign offer hope that, as we face the new century, people with epilepsy worldwide will be accepted as productive, valued citizens.

KEY POINTS

1. Quality of life is highly subjective and is best defined by the individual.
2. The ability of the person and family to adjust to the diagnosis of epilepsy is of more importance than the age of onset.
3. Social perception and cultural beliefs about epilepsy affect how the person is accepted within his/her community.
4. Adverse effects of antiepileptic drugs may decrease the perception of quality of life.
5. Inability to drive, underemployment, restrictions in education settings, and social isolation negatively affect psychosocial well-being.
6. Depression is a common coexisting problem in people with epilepsy.
7. Quality of life assessment questionnaires can be helpful in screening for major issues requiring intervention.
8. Interventions to improve quality of life include patient/family education about epilepsy, support groups, employment assistance, and community education programs to enhance public understanding of epilepsy.

REFERENCES

Aguilar N (1997) Counseling the patient with chronic illness: strategies for the health care provider. *Journal of the American Academy of Nurse Practitioners* 9:171–175.

Austin JK (1993) Concerns and fears of children with seizures. *Clinical Nursing Practice in Epilepsy* 1:1–10.

Austin JK, Smith MS, Risinger MW, McNelis AM (1994) Childhood epilepsy and asthma: comparison of quality of life. *Epilepsia* 35(3):608–615.

Austin JK, Huberty TJ, Huster GA, Dunn DW (1998) Academic achievement in children with epilepsy or asthma. *Developmental Medicine and Child Neurology* 40(4):248–255.

Baker GA, Jacoby A, Buck D *et al* (1997a) Quality of life of people with epilepsy: a European study. *Epilepsia* 38:353–362.

Baker GA, Nashef L, van Hout BA (1997b) Current issues in the management of epilepsy: the impact of frequent seizures on cost of illness, quality of life and mortality. *Epilepsia* 38(Suppl 1): S1–S8.

Beaussart M, Beaussart-Defaye J, Lamiaux JM *et al* (1997) Epileptic drivers – a study of 1089 patients. *Medicine and Law* 16:295–306.

Bertolote JM (1994) Epilepsy as a public health problem. *Tropical and Geographical Medicine* 46(3):28–30.

Braden CJ (1990) A test of the self-help model: learned response to chronic illness experience. *Nursing Research* 39:42–47.

Brown S (1992) Sudden death and epilepsy. *Seizure* 1:71–73.

Buchanan N (1992) The occurrence, management and outcome of antiepileptic drug side-effects in 767 patients. *Seizure* 1:89–98.

Buck D, Baker GA, Jacoby A *et al* (1997) Patients' experiences of injury as a result of epilepsy. *Epilepsia* 38:439–444.

Burckhardt CS (1987) Coping strategies of the chronically ill. *Nursing Clinics of North America* 22:543–551.

Carroll D (1992) Employment among young people with epilepsy. *Seizure* 1:127–131.

Collings JA (1995) Life fulfillment in an epilepsy sample from the United States. *Social Science and Medicine* 40(11): 1579–1584.

Coyle HP, Brown S (1997) Epilepsy, the law and the media. *Medicine and Law* 16:323–337.

Cramer JA, Perrine K, Devinsky O *et al* (1996) A brief questionnaire to screen for quality of life in epilepsy: the QOLIE-10. *Epilepsia* 37:577–582.

Dean P (1996) Cultural issues and epilepsy. In: Santilli N (ed) *Managing Seizure Disorders: A Handbook for Health Care Professionals*, pp 229–237. Philadelphia: Lippincott-Raven.

Devinsky O (1995) Cognitive and behavioral effects of antiepileptic drugs. *Epilepsia* 36 (Suppl 2):S46–S65.

Devinsky O, Vickery BC, Cramer J *et al* (1995) Development of the quality of life in epilepsy inventory. *Epilepsia* 36:1089–1104.

Dilorio C, Faherty B, Manteuffel B (1992) The development and testing of an instrument to measure self-efficacy in individuals with epilepsy. *Journal of Neuroscience Nursing* 24:9–13.

Dodson WE (1993) Epilepsy and IQ. In: Dodson WE, Pellock JM (eds) *Pediatric Epilepsy: Diagnosis and Therapy*, pp 373–385. New York: Demos.

Dodson WE (1994) Quality of life measurements in children with epilepsy. In: *Epilepsy and Quality of Life*, pp 217–226. New York: Raven Press.

Donker GA, Foets M, Spreeuwenberg P (1997) Epilepsy patients: health status and medical consumption. *Journal of Neurology* 244:365–370.

Epigraph (1998) Global Campaign Against Epilepsy launched. *Newsletter of the International League Against Epilepsy*, Issue 2.

Eriksen HR, Ellertson B, Gronningsaeter H *et al* (1994) Physical exercise in women with intractable epilepsy. *Epilepsia* 35:1256–1264.

Ettinger AB, Weisbrot DM, Nolan EE *et al* (1998) Symptoms of depression and anxiety in pediatric epilepsy patients. *Epilepsia* 39(6):595–599.

Fisher RS, Parsonage M, Beaussart M *et al* (1994) Epilepsy and driving: an international perspective. *Epilepsia* 35:675–684.

Fisher RS, Parks-Trusz SL, Lehman C (1996) Social issues in epilepsy. In: Shorvon S, Dreifuss FE, Fish D, Thomas D (eds) *The Treatment of Epilepsy*, pp 357–369. Oxford: Blackwell Science.

Gehlert S (1994) Perceptions of control in adults with epilepsy. *Epilepsia* 35:81–88.

Gilliam F, Kuzniecky R, Faught E *et al* (1997) Patient-validated content of epilepsy-specific quality-of-life measurement. *Epilepsia* 38:233–236.

Hartshorn JC, Byers VL (1992) Impact of epilepsy on quality of life. *Journal of Neuroscience Nursing* 24:24–29.

Harvey AS, Nolan T, Carlin JB (1993) Community-based study of mortality in children with epilepsy. *Epilepsia* 34(4):597–603.

Hermann BP, Trenerry MR, Colligan RC *et al* (1996) Learned helplessness, attributional style, and depression in epilepsy. *Epilepsia* 37:680–686.

Hunt SM, McKenna SP (1995) The measurement of quality of life of people with epilepsy. In: Hopkins A, Shorvon S, Cascino G (eds) *Epilepsy*, 2nd edn, pp 581–591. London: Chapman & Hall.

Jacoby A (1995) Impact of epilepsy on employment status: findings from a UK study of people with well-controlled epilepsy. *Epilepsy Research* 21:125–132.

Jacoby A, Baker GA, Steen N *et al* (1996) The clinical course of epilepsy and its psychosocial correlates: findings from a UK community study. *Epilepsia* 37:148–161.

Jalava M, Sillanpää M, Camfield C, Camfield C (1997) Social adjustment and competence 35 years after onset of childhood epilepsy: a prospective controlled study. *Epilepsia* 38(6):708–715.

Kemp AM, Sibert JR (1993) Epilepsy in Children and the Risk of *Drowning*. University of Health of Wales College of Medicine.

Krumholz A (1994) Driving and epilepsy: a historical perspective and review of current regulations. *Epilepsia* 35:666–674.

Landgraf J, Abetz L, Ware J (1996) *The Child Health Questionnaire (CHQ): A User's Manual*. Health Institute.

Lannon SL (1993) Epilepsy in the elderly. *Journal of Neuroscience Nursing* 25:273–282.

Lannon SL (1997) Using a health promotion model to enhance medication compliance. *Journal of Neuroscience Nursing* 9:170–178.

Lebrun Y (1992) The language of epilepsy. *Seizure* 1:207–212.

Lipsey DC (1996) Impact of epilepsy on employability. In: Santilli N (ed.) *Managing Seizure Disorders: A Handbook for Health Care Professionals*, pp 199–210. Philadelphia: Lippincott-Raven.

Luhdorf K, Jensen LK, Plesner AM (1986) Epilepsy in the elderly: incidence, social function and disability. *Epilepsia* 27:135–141.

McLachlan RS, Rose KJ, Derry PA *et al* (1997) Health-related quality of life and seizure control in temporal lobe epilepsy. *Annals of Neurology* 41:482–489.

McLin WM, de Boer HM (1995) Public perceptions about epilepsy. *Epilepsia* 36:957–959.

Murray JA, Haynes MP (1996) The benevolent overreaction: nursing assessment and intervention in families coping with seizure disorder. *Journal of Neuroscience Nursing* 28:252–258.

Nashef L, Shorvon SD (1997) Mortality in epilepsy. *Epilepsia* 38:1059–1061.

Orley J (1994) The World Health Organization (WHO) quality of life project. In: Trimble MR, Dodson WE (eds) *Epilepsy and Quality of Life*, pp 99–108. New York: Raven Press.

Orlowski J, Rothner AD, Lueders H (1982) Submersion accidents in children with epilepsy. *American Journal of Disease of Childhood* 136:777–780.

Pearn J, Bart R, Yamaoka R (1978) Drowning risks to epileptic children: a study from Hawaii. *British Medical Journal* 2:1284–1285.

Pollock SE (1987) Adaptation to chronic illness. *Nursing Clinics of North America* 22(3):631-644.

Ridsdale L, Robins D, Cryer C *et al* (1997) Feasibility and effects of nurse-run clinics for patients with epilepsy in general practice: randomized controlled trial. *British Medical Journal* 314 (7074) 120–122.

Roper Poll (1992) *Living with epilepsy: report of a Roper poll of patients on quality of life*. Storrs, CT: Roper Organization.

Roth DL, Goode KT, Williams VL *et al* (1994) Physical exercise, stressful life experience and depression in adults with epilepsy. *Epilepsia* 35(6) 1248–1255.

Russell A (1997) How nurses can support people with epilepsy. *Nursing Times* 93(27): 50–51.

Sanger MS, Perrin EC, Sandler HM (1993) Development in children's causal theories of their seizure disorders. *Developmental and Behavioral Pediatrics* 14(2):88–93.

Santilli N, Kessler BL, Schmidt WT (1994) Quality of life in epilepsy: perspectives of patients. In: Trimble MR, Dodson WE (eds) *Epilepsy and Quality of Life*, pp 1–18. New York: Raven Press.

Smilkstein G (1979) The family APGAR: a proposal for a family function test and its use by physicians. *Journal of Family Practice* 6:1231–1239.

Steinhoff BJ, Neususs K, Thegeder H *et al* (1996) Leisure time activity and physical fitness in patients with epilepsy. *Epilepsia* 37:1221–1227.

Thompson PJ (1995) Managing the patient and their family. In: Duncan JS, Shorvon SD, Fish DR (eds) *Clinical Epilepsy* , pp 283–298. New York: Churchill Livingston.

Thompson PJ, Oxley J (1988) Socioeconomic accompaniments of severe epilepsy. *Epilepsia* 29 (Suppl 1):S9–S18.

Thompson PJ, Upton D (1992) The impact of chronic epilepsy on the family. *Seizure* 1:43–48.

Troxell J (1997) Epilepsy and employment: the Americans with Disabilities Act and its protections against employment discrimination. *Medicine and Law* 16:375–384.

Upton D (1993) Social support and emotional adjustment in people with chronic epilepsy. *Journal of Epilepsy* 6:105–111.

Upton D, Thompson PJ (1992) Effectiveness of coping strategies employed by people with chronic epilepsy. *Journal of Epilepsy* 5:119–127.

Upton D, Thompson PJ, Duncan JS (1996) Patient satisfaction with specialized epilepsy assessment and treatment. *Seizure* 5:195–198.

Wagner AK, Bungay KM, Kosinski M *et al* (1996) The health status of adults with epilepsy compared with that of people without chronic conditions. *Phamacotherapy* 16:1–9.

Wildrick D, Parker-Fisher S, Morales A (1996) Quality of life in children with well-controlled epilepsy. *Journal of Neuroscience Nursing* 28(3):192–198.

Psychiatric comorbidity

MV LAMBERT AND AS DAVID

'The good physician is concerned not only with turbulent brain waves but with disturbed emotions and with social injustice, for the epileptic is not just a nerve–muscle preparation; he is a person ...' (Lennox and Markham 1953; cited in Standage and Fenton 1975).

EPIDEMIOLOGY

The incidence and prevalence of psychiatric disorders in people with epilepsy (PWE) is not known. Most studies have been criticized for being retrospective, for using non-representative hospital samples and inadequate or absent controls, and for not clearly identifying the seizure and syndrome type. Interpretation and comparison are further complicated by differing methods of determining psychiatric cases, ranging from self-report questionnaires to structured clinical interviews using operational criteria.

There are few large prevalence studies; most have been of patients with medically intractable partial epilepsy being evaluated for epilepsy surgery. The findings of the major studies are summarized in Table 34.1 along with those of community studies. Cockerell *et al* (1996) performed a prospective study of PWE developing an 'acute psychological disorder' of sufficient severity to warrant specialist attention, during a 1-year period, using the British Neurological Surveillance Unit reporting scheme (Cockerell *et al* 1995); 64 cases were reported giving a *minimum* estimate of the annual rate of new cases of psychiatric disorder of 0.1%. The main reported diagnoses were delirium (27%), schizophreniform (31%), affective (30%), and delusional disorder (5%). The majority (81%) occurred in patients with localization-related epilepsy (Cockerell *et al* 1996).

Jalava and Sillanpää (1996) assessed psychiatric morbidity in 94 patients with childhood-onset epilepsy after a mean follow-up period of 35 years. Of these patients 19% had psychiatric comorbidity compared with 5% of controls and 65% had a psychosomatic comorbidity compared with 57% of controls, regardless of whether they were still receiving anticonvulsant medication. Patients received psychotropic drugs 8.6 times more frequently than controls. Thus, it would appear that epilepsy *per se*, rather than medication, was associated with psychiatric comorbidity.

Table 34.1 Epidemiologic studies of psychiatric comorbidity in people with epilepsy.

Reference	Population	Number	Findings
Gibbs (1951)	Anterior temporal lobe focus	163	49% psychiatric disorder (32% personality disorder; 17% psychosis)
	Midtemporal lobe focus	37	13% psychiatric disorder (all personality disorder)
	Occipital focus	30	12% psychiatric disorder (10% personality disorder; 2% psychosis)
	Frontal focus	19	5% psychiatric disorder (all personality disorder)
	Parietal Focus	26	0% psychiatric disorder
Pond and Bidwell (1959/60)	GP survey, all ages all seizure types	245	29% psychologic difficulties 7% psychiatric hospital admissions
	TLE	39	51% psychologic difficulties
Gudmundsson (1966)	PWE in Iceland, all seizure types	987	52% nonpsychotic psychiatric disorder 7% history of/current psychosis
Rutter et al (1970)	All 5–14 year olds, Isle of Wight	11 865	Psychiatric disorder in: 6.6% 'well' children 11.6% nonneurologic physical disorder 28.6% uncomplicated epilepsy 37.5% CNS lesion without epilepsy 58.3% CNS lesion with epilepsy
Mignone et al (1970)	Hospital sample of PWE	151	30.3% psychiatric disorder
Currie et al (1971)	Hospital sample of TLE	666	44% abnormal MSE (19% anxious; 11% depressed; 7% aggressive; 6% obsessive)
Taylor (1972)	Medically intractable epilepsy	100	87% any psychiatric disorder 48% 'psychopathy' 30% neurosis (17% depressed; 7% anxious 4%; obsessional)
Standage and Fenton (1975)	Hospital sample of PWE	27	22% past psychiatric history 60% depression 75% depressed mood 50% anxiety
Roy (1979)	Hospital sample of PWE	42	54.7% depressed (65% CPS; 42% other seizures)
Jensen and Larsen (1979)	Medically intractable CPS	74	52.7% history of psychiatric illness
Pritchard et al (1980)	Hospital sample of TLE, 15–30 years	56	36% psychopathology
Kogeorgos et al (1982)	Hospital sample of PWE	66	45.5% psychiatric cases
Mendez et al (1986)	Community study of PWE	175	55% depression
Brown et al (1986)	Hospital sample of PWE	28	26.7% subjectively depressed 31.1% objectively depressed 22.2% subjectively anxious 11.1% objectively anxious
Edeh and Toone (1987)	PWE > 16 years	88	47.7% psychiatric cases 21.6% depressive neurosis 14.8% anxiety neurosis

Table 34.1 (Cont.)

Reference	Population	Number	Findings
Edeh et al (1990)	PWE	88	47.7% psychiatric cases
	Community sample	62	40.3% psychiatric cases (9.7% anxiety neurosis; 19.4% depressive neurosis)
	Hospital sample	26	65.4% psychiatric cases (26.9% depressive neurosis; 26.9% anxiety neurosis;
Victoroff et al (1990)	Medically intractable epilepsy	47	62% history of depression 38% currently depressed
Gureje (1991)	Hospital sample of PWE, Nigeria	204	37.3% psychiatric cases 53% neurosis 29% psychosis 7% personality disorder
Manchanda et al (1992)	Medically intractable epilepsy	71	45% psychiatric cases
Fiordelli et al (1993)	Cryptogenic epilepsy (only 28% TLE; excluded documented brain lesions)	100 (only 90 with seizures in previous 2 years)	19% psychiatric cases
Victoroff (1994)	Medically intractable CP	60	Lifetime prevalence (DSMIIIR) of: 88.3% any psychiatric disorder 70% axis I diagnosis 58.3% depression 31.7% anxiety 10% psychosis 5% bipolar disorder 18.3% axis II diagnosis (personality disorder)
Robertson et al (1994)	Hospital sample of PWE	18	27% depressed
Blumer et al (1995)	PWE undergoing EEG monitoring	75	56% psychiatric disorder requiring treatment
Manchanda et al (1996)	Medically intractable epilepsy	300 (231 with TLE)	DSMIIIR: 47.3% psychiatric case 29.3% axis I diagnosis 10.7% anxiety 3% mood disorder 4.3% SLPE 18% axis II diagnosis
Jacoby et al (1996)	Community sample All PWE	696	25% anxious 9% depressed
	Seizure-free	350	13% anxious 4% depressed
	Frequent seizures (>1month)	168	44% anxious 21% depressed
Baker et al (1996)	Community sample of PWE (as in Jacoby et al 1996)	696	Perceived seizure severity predicted anxiety and depression
Ring et al (1998)	Medically intractable epilepsy	60	52% psychiatric disorder 21% depression 18% anxiety
Blumer et al (1998)	Medically intractable TLE	44	57% interictal dysphoric disorder
	Medically intractable FLE	6	67% interictal dysphoric disorder

CPS, complex partial seizure; DSMIII R, *Diagnostic and Statistical Manual*, 3rd edn revised; FLE, frontal lobe epilepsy; MSE, Mental State Examination; PWE, people with epilepsy; SLPE, schizophrenia-like psychosis of epilepsy; TLE, temporal lobe epilepsy.

Table 34.2 Psychiatric disorders associated with epilepsy.

Seizure related
Prodromal
Periictal (aura, ictus)
Postictal
Paraictal (associated with increased seizures/clusters)
Forced normalization (associated with cessation of seizures)

Interictal
Affective disorders
    Depressive reaction/feelings
    Depressive illness
    Interictal dysphoric disorder
    Bipolar disorder and hypomania
Anxiety disorders
    Generalized anxiety disorder
    Panic disorder
Neurotic/somatoform disorder
    Obsessional compulsive disorder
    Nonepileptic attack disorder
Psychosis
    Brief interictal psychosis
    Chronic interictal psychosis (schizophrenia-like psychosis of epilepsy)
Personality disorder
    Religiosity
    Hypergraphia
    Viscosity
    Sexual dysfunction
Disorders of impulse control
    Anger/irritability
    Drug/alcohol abuse

Table 34.3 Etiology of psychiatric disorder in people with epilepsy.

Etiology of epilepsy/underlying pathology
    Brain damage associated with head injury, cerebrovascular accident, space-occupying lesion
    Underlying condition responsible for epilepsy and psychiatric disorder (e.g. multiple sclerosis, porphyria)
    Genetic/environmental factors contributing to development of the psychiatric disorder
Epilepsy factors
    Age of onset of epilepsy
    Duration of epilepsy
    Seizure type
    Number of different seizure types
    Localization of focus (LRE vs. PGE; TLE vs. extra-TLE)
    Lateralization of focus
    Seizure frequency
    Seizure severity
    Secondary generalization of seizure
Iatrogenic
    Type of AED
    Number of AED
    Serum level of AED
    Secondary effects of AED, e.g. hormonal, serum folate deficiency
Psychosocial
    Stigma
    Discrimination
    Locus of control
    Fear of seizures
    Attributional style
    Adjustment to epilepsy
    Parental overprotection
    Social support
    Socioeconomic status

AED, antiepileptic drug; LRE, localization-related epilepsy; PGE, primary generalized epilepsy; TLE, temporal lobe epilepsy.

There have been few studies assessing psychiatric disorder in patients with both learning disability and epilepsy. Lund (1985) found that among those with learning disability the addition of epilepsy increased the prevalence of psychiatric illness (including behavioral disorder and autism) and doubled the rate, if seizures had occured in the previous year. Surprisingly, the two other major studies in this group (Deb and Hunter 1991; Pary 1993) did not find an increase of psychiatric disorder in patients with or without epilepsy. This may reflect the difficulty of diagnosing psychiatric comorbidity in patients with learning disability, especially if it is severe.

In summary, about 30–50% of PWE appear to suffer at some time from a psychiatric disorder, usually anxiety or depression. Psychiatric disorders can occur perictally or interictally, or may be unrelated in time to seizure occurrence. However, differentiation may be difficult in patients with frequent seizures. The major psychiatric disorders associated with epilepsy are shown in Table 34.2 and the major etiologic factors in Table 34.3 (Hermann and Whitmann 1992; Murray *et al* 1994). The importance of recognizing psychiatric disorder in PWE is not only to enable treatment to be considered but also to identify those at risk of suicide.

Temporal lobe epilepsy (TLE) may be associated with more psychiatric comorbidity than the other focal epilep-

sies, with the lowest rates occurring in patients with parietal lobe foci (Gibbs 1951). Early studies comparing patients cared for solely by their general practitioner, with those managed by hospital specialists, revealed that psychologic disturbance was a more important factor in determining referral than severity of epilepsy (Pond and Bidwell 1959/60). However, more recent work has reported that patients attending hospital clinics tend to have an earlier age of onset of epilepsy and less well-controlled complex partial seizures (CPS) (Edeh *et al* 1990). Generally, the rate of psychiatric disorder increases with seizure frequency (Jacoby *et al* 1996) and is higher in those attending hospital clinics (Edeh *et al* 1990).

DELIBERATE SELF-HARM AND SUICIDE

The reported incidence of suicide and deliberate self-harm is thought to be at least four to five times that of the general population (Barraclough 1981; Harris and Barraclough 1997), while those with TLE have an increased risk by a factor of up to 25 (Barraclough 1981; Harris and Barraclough 1997). Robertson (1998) reviewed 17 studies detailing causes of death in PWE and found the average incidence of suicide to be nine to ten times that of the general population (13.2% compared with 1.4%). Two reports have also shown a 5–7% increase in self-poisoning in PWE (Mackay 1979; Hawton *et al* 1980). Suicide has been reported in patients with severe epilepsy, epilepsy with other disabilities, and those seen in specialist clinics (Robertson 1998) but may also follow an improvement in seizure control (Blumer and Benson 1982). Risk factors for completed suicide have been found to include previous history of deliberate self-harm, family history of suicide, stressful life events, poor morale and stigma, along with psychiatric disorders such as alcohol and drug abuse, depression, psychosis, and personality disorder (Harris and Barraclough 1997; Robertson 1998).

PREICTAL, ICTAL, AND POSTICTAL DEPRESSION

PREICTAL DEPRESSION

Prodromal moods of depression or irritability occur hours to days before a seizure and are often relieved by the convulsion (Devinsky and Bear 1991). Blanchet and Frommer (1986) found that patients tended to report more depression on the days immediately preceding their seizures than on interictal days, along with improvement of mood after convulsions. A more recent study evaluated 148 adult PWE of whom 128 had partial seizures (Hughes *et al* 1993). One-third of those with partial seizures reported premonitory symptoms (usually preceding secondarily generalized seizures) compared with none of those with primary generalized epilepsy. Half of the symptoms were 'emotional' in nature, usually irritability, depression, fear, elation, or anger, and lasted between 10 minutes and 3 days.

The mechanism for the development of prodromal mood changes is not known. The same biologic processes may cause both the change in affect and the seizure, or the dysphoric mood itself may precipitate the seizure.

ICTAL DEPRESSION

Williams (1956) observed depression occurring as part of an aura, or simple partial seizure, in approximately 1% of a series of 2000 PWE, although fear occurred more

frequently. Ictal depression appears to be more common in patients with TLE (Williams 1956), in whom rates of more than 10% have been reported (Weil 1959; Devinsky *et al* 1991). No association with laterality of seizure focus has been found (Williams 1956; Weil 1959; Devinsky *et al* 1991).

Classically, ictal depression is of sudden onset and occurs out of context, not being related to environmental stimuli. The severity ranges from mild feelings of sadness to profound hopelessness and despair (Devinsky and Bear 1991). Lim *et al* (1986) described a patient with nonconvulsive status epilepticus presenting as a case of psychotic depression, and both deliberate self-harm and suicide have been reported during ictal depression (Mendez and Doss 1992; Betts 1993). Complex (formed) hallucinations may accompany the depressive feelings (Williams 1956). Several workers have found ictal depression to be of prolonged duration, often persisting into the postictal period, which may represent underlying subclinical seizure activity (Williams 1956; Weil 1959).

POSTICTAL DEPRESSION

Blumer (1992) described three cases who developed depression lasting hours to days immediately following seizures. However, these patients also experienced episodes of interictal depression and Blumer commented that it was rare to find a patient who suffered postictal depression alone. Devinsky *et al* (1994) also noted depressed affect following CPS originating in right temporal lobe structures in patients with medically intractable epilepsy; more prominent changes were seen with bilateral limbic dysfunction. However, these findings do not appear to be consistent with those of an earlier single case report of a patient who developed postictal depression after left-sided CPS and hypomania after right-sided seizures (Hurwitz *et al* 1985).

TREATMENT OF PREICTAL AND PERIICTAL DEPRESSION

Although prodromal and periictal depression does not usually require treatment *per se*, improvement in seizure frequency should reduce the occurrence of these forms of depression. Depressive preictal and periictal feelings may be regarded by some patients as an 'early warning system.' They may have time to alert people that they need help and the warning may enable them to move to a place of safety. Medication such as fast-acting benzodiazepines may abort or prevent the development of the attack, as may behavioral methods (Gillham 1990; Betts *et al* 1995; Goldstein 1997).

INTERICTAL DEPRESSION

EPIDEMIOLOGY

Interictal depression is thought to be much more common than periictal depression; however, the prevalence is not known. Mendez *et al* (1986) found that four times as many PWE had been hospitalized for depression compared with a control group with similar socioeconomic and disability levels. Hospital studies have found a history of depression or depressive symptoms in up to two-thirds of patients with medically intractable epilepsy (Standage and Fenton 1975; Roy 1979; Victoroff *et al* 1990), whereas community studies have only demonstrated affective disorder in one-quarter (Edeh and Toone 1985).

ETIOLOGY

Most authors have found no correlation between depression and epilepsy variables such as age of onset (Roy 1979; Robertson *et al* 1987, 1994; Altshuler *et al* 1990; Mendez *et al* 1993), duration of epilepsy (Roy 1979; Altschuler *et al* 1990; Indaco *et al* 1992; Robertson *et al* 1994), the presence of an intracranial lesion, or seizure frequency (Mendez *et al* 1986). However, CPS (Currie *et al* 1971; Roy 1979; Dikmen *et al* 1983; Mendez *et al* 1986; Robertson *et al* 1987; Indaco *et al* 1992) and TLE, especially of left-sided origin, have been associated with depression (Dongier 1959/60; Rodin *et al* 1976a; Brown *et al* 1986; Robertson 1997), whilst the severity of the depression has been found to correlate with the duration of the epilepsy (Robertson *et al* 1987). More recent studies have found frequent seizures to be associated with increased anxiety, depression, and stigma (Baker *et al* 1995) and the number of seizure types to be correlated with greater risk of psychiatric disorder (Fiordelli *et al* 1993). However, other studies have found no association between seizure type and psychiatric comorbidity (Trimble and Perez 1980; Kogeorgos *et al* 1982). Some authors (Robertson *et al* 1987), but not all (Mendez *et al* 1986; Indaco *et al* 1992), have found a significant family history of psychiatric disorder, suggesting a genetic predisposition to the development of depression. Several studies have reported a decrease in seizure frequency prior to the onset of the depressive illness (Dongier 1959/60; Flor-Henry 1969; Betts 1974; Standage and Fenton 1975) and depression has been reported *de novo* following epilepsy surgery.

Psychosocial factors are thought to play a major role in the development of depression in PWE. Hermann (1979) proposed that the exposure to unpredictable, uncontrol-

lable, aversive events (seizures) may produce depression. This idea has been developed into the concept of locus of control, and preoperative depression has been correlated with an external locus of control (a perception of events not being attributable to the patient's own efforts but rather to the effects of fate) (Hermann and Wyler 1989). More recently, a pessimistic attributional style (attributing global difficulties to epilepsy) has been associated with the development of depression in PWE (Hermann *et al* 1996). Hermann and Whitman (1989) showed that increased stressful life events, poor adjustment to seizures, and financial stress were predictive of increased depression. However, other workers have found no relationship between depression and psychosocial factors such as socioeconomic status (Indaco *et al* 1992), education (Altschuler *et al* 1990; Indaco *et al* 1992), and employment status (Altschuler *et al* 1990).

DIAGNOSIS

Making the correct diagnosis is an essential prerequisite to treating depression in PWE. Betts (1981) has differentiated between a depressive *reaction* (reactive depression) and a depressive *illness* (endogenous depression). Depressive feelings usually respond to circumstance and tend to be understandable as a reaction to being given the diagnosis of epilepsy. The main features of depressive illness are low mood, loss of interest and enjoyment, and reduced energy. In addition, reduced concentration, attention, and self-esteem or self-confidence, ideas of guilt and unworthiness, pessimistic views of the future, ideas or acts of self-harm, disturbed sleep, and diminished appetite may be present (World Health Organization 1992). However, making the diagnosis can be difficult and Betts (1981) has stressed that drug intoxication (especially with phenytoin) can resemble depression.

PHENOMENOLOGY

Patients with epilepsy and depression tend to have significantly fewer 'neurotic' traits, such as anxiety, guilt, rumination, hopelessness, low self-esteem, and somatization, and more 'psychotic' symptoms, such as paranoia, delusions, and persecutory auditory hallucinations. Between episodes of major depression, PWE tend to be dysthymic with irritability and humorlessness (Mendez *et al* 1986). Betts (1981) also reports that depression in PWE tends to be endogenous in nature, with a sudden onset and fluctuating markedly until it suddenly ends.

Blumer *et al* (1995) described the interictal dysphoric disorder, which was noted in 44% of patients with medically intractable epilepsy. The syndrome comprises eight symptoms, including depressive moods, insomnia, euphoria, intermittent paroxysmal irritability, anxiety, and phobic fears. Patients with several of the symptoms may be at increased risk of suicidal behavior (Blumer *et al* 1995).

PSYCHOLOGIC TREATMENT

Depressive reactions should be treated with supportive therapy provided by trained therapists, social workers, or epilepsy nurse specialists. Betts (1981) has stressed that these reactions should not be treated medically unless prolonged, and therefore atypical, as such episodes may become protracted if treated with antidepressants or tranquillizers. More severe reactions may require specialized psychotherapy such as cognitive behavioral therapy (Davis *et al* 1984). Psychotherapy can also be used to improve coping skills and this has been shown to improve mild depressive illness and anxiety as well as reducing seizure frequency (Gillham 1990).

Patient support groups introduce patients to fellow sufferers, who can provide emotional support and have been found to modify depression and dysthymia in PWE (Becú *et al* 1993).

ADJUSTMENT OF ANTIEPILEPTIC DRUGS

Polytherapy has been shown to be associated with depression in PWE (Fiordelli *et al* 1993; Mendez *et al* 1993a); Shorvon and Reynolds (1979) reported an improvement in alertness, concentration, drive, mood, and sociability on reducing to monotherapy.

Certain anticonvulsants have been found to be psychotropic, whereas others have been associated with behavioral changes and depression. Phenobarbital has been associated with depression in adults (Rodin *et al* 1976b; Robertson *et al* 1987; Smith and Collins 1987; Dodrill 1991) and children and adolescents (Brent *et al* 1987). Positive behavioral changes have been associated with carbamazepine, including decreased anxiety and depression, and valproic acid, including improved mood and increased happiness (Dodrill 1991). Phenytoin has been said to produce positive and negative effects approximately equally often (Dodrill 1991).

Fewer studies have been performed with the newer anticonvulsants. Vigabatrin seems to be particularly associated with depression, which develops in up to 10% of patients (Sander and Duncan 1996), typically within a few weeks of the drug being introduced or following dose increments. A past history of psychiatric disturbance may be a major risk factor (Ring *et al* 1993). Lamotrigine has been shown to be at least as effective in producing seizure freedom as carbamazepine while being better tolerated (Reunanen *et al* 1996) and improvements in well-being and increased 'happiness' have been demonstrated (Smith *et al* 1993; Betts 1994).

ANTIDEPRESSANT TREATMENTS

Approximately 60–70% of acute major depressive episodes respond to antidepressant treatment (Klerman 1990) and *early* intervention has been shown to reduce the duration of the episodes by almost 50% (Kupfer *et al* 1989). Antidepressant therapy should be continued for at least 4 months following complete remission of symptoms in order to reduce the chance of a relapse (Prien and Kupfer 1986).

Choice of antidepressant

Choice of drug depends on efficacy, interactions with concomitant medication, and the side-effect profile, in particular epileptogenic potential. These factors have been reviewed recently (Lambert and Robertson 1999). It is widely believed that the newer antidepressants do not significantly differ with respect to efficacy compared with the tricyclic antidepressants (Kasper *et al* 1992; Series 1992; Swinkels and de Jonghe 1995). There has only been one double-blind placebo-controlled study of antidepressants in PWE (Robertson and Trimble 1985), which showed that after 12 weeks nomifensine was superior to amitriptyline.

Most antidepressants are either metabolized by, or inhibit to varying degrees, one or more of the cytochrome P450 isoenzymes located in the liver (Nemeroff *et al* 1996). Clinically relevant interactions for PWE mainly involve the concomitant use of antidepressants with phenytoin and carbamazepine. Most published studies consist of single case reports. In clinical practice fluoxetine or fluvoxamine could produce toxic anticonvulsant levels, whereas sertraline, paroxetine, and citalopram should have little effect (Gailer and Edwards 1996; Jeppesen *et al* 1996; Nemeroff *et al* 1996). The anticonvulsants phenobarbital, primidone, phenytoin and, carbamazepine are potent inducers of liver enzymes (Brodie 1992), which can result in reduced plasma levels of antidepressants metabolized by the same isoenzymes and thus reduced efficacy. Clinically significant interactions have been reported with tricyclic antidepressants (Spina *et al* 1996) and paroxetine (Boyer and Blumhardt 1992).

The incidence of seizures occurring with therapeutic doses of antidepressants varies from 0.1 to 4% (Rosenstein *et al* 1993), which is not much higher than the annual incidence of first seizures in the general population. Some authors have suggested that various risk factors may predispose to the

Table 34.4 Factors associated with increased risk of antidepressant-induced seizures.

Patient related
  History of previous seizures
  Family history of a seizure disorder
  Abnormal pretreatment EEG
  Brain damage, head injury
  Dementia
  Learning disability
  History of electroconvulsive treatment
  Alcohol/substance abuse/withdrawal
  Reduced renal/hepatic drug elimination capacity
Drug related
  High dose/plasma level of antidepressant or metabolites
  Overdose of antidepressant
  Rapid dose escalation
  Concurrent use of drugs that lower seizure threshold
  Concurrent use of drugs that inhibit metabolism of antidepressant

precipitation of drug-induced seizures and may be either patient or drug related (Table 34.4) (Wroblewski *et al* 1990; Preskorn and Fast 1992; Skowron and Stimmel 1992; Rosenstein *et al* 1993). Seizures may be more likely to occur during the first week of antidepressant treatment or after an increase in the dose, especially following rapid dose escalation (Rosenstein *et al* 1993).

There have been reports of seizures with the use of selective serotoninergic reuptake inhibitors. These have mainly been single case studies, however, and the seizure often occurs when the drug is administered with, or shortly after, another drug known to lower the seizure threshold or in patients at risk of seizures (see Lambert and Robertson 1999 for review).

In summary, the older antidepressants especially the tricyclics appear to lower seizure threshold, especially in vulnerable individuals. There is less evidence for such an effect with the newer antidepressants, especially moclobemide and citalopram, which are the only drugs not to state epilepsy as a reason for 'special precaution' in their data sheet. Antidepressants should be introduced at a low dose and gradually increased to therapeutic levels, and continued for at least 4 months after complete clinical recovery. Other medication known to reduce the seizure threshold should be avoided. Patients and anticonvulsant levels should be carefully monitored; if seizures develop, the patient should be changed to an antidepressant with lower risk. A patient with severe, uncontrolled epilepsy or who develops an exacerbation in their seizures may be best managed as an inpatient.

ELECTROCONVULSIVE THERAPY

Electroconvulsive therapy (ECT) is not contraindicated in PWE and may be life-saving in patients with severe or psychotic depression not responding to antidepressants (Betts 1981). Although there have been reports of spontaneous seizures occurring in patients following ECT (Devinsky and Duchowny 1983; Grogan *et al* 1995), major studies have found the incidence of spontaneous seizures to be lower than that of epilepsy in the general population (Blumenthal 1955; Blackwood *et al* 1980). The efficacy of ECT may be reduced if antiepileptic drugs decrease the intensity of the induced seizures (Krystal and Weiner 1993). Hence, Weiner and Coffey (1993) recommend that, with the exception of patients at high risk of status epilepticus or with recent generalized tonic–clonic seizures, antiepileptic drugs should be omitted on the morning prior to each ECT treatment.

HYPOMANIA AND BIPOLAR AFFECTIVE DISORDER

Maniacal episodes were described in 4.8% of Dongier's series of PWE (Dongier 1959/60) and Williams (1956) reported periictal elation in 3 of 2000 patients. Since then, reports of mania and hypomania have mainly described single cases or have been studies involving small numbers of patients (Wolf 1982; Joseph 1986; Barczak *et al* 1988; Byrne 1988; Gillig *et al* 1988; Humphries and Dickinson 1988; Morphew 1988; Shukla *et al* 1988; Taylor 1991; Betts 1993; Lyketsos *et al* 1993; Sanders and Mathews 1994), often with nondominant TLE (Barczak *et al* 1988; Byrne 1988; Gillig *et al* 1988; Humphries and Dickinson 1988; Betts 1993; Sanders and Mathews 1994). This may be explained by cases of mania being classified as 'schizo-affective psychosis' and thus included in the epilepsy and psychosis literature. Alternatively, the use of antiepileptic drugs such as carbamazepine and valproic acid, which are known to be effective in the treatment of bipolar affective disorder (Post *et al* 1985; Balfour and Bryson 1994), may reduce the occurrence of hypomania in these patients. Hypomania has been described occurring *de novo* after temporal lobe surgery (Kanemoto 1995).

PHENOMENOLOGY AND DIAGNOSIS

To diagnose mania, the following should be present and of sufficient severity to disrupt work and social activities for at least 1 week.

1. Mood is elevated out of keeping with the individual's circumstances (alternatively, irritability or suspiciousness may be the predominant mood state) and is

accompanied by increased energy, resulting in overactivity, pressure of speech, and decreased need for sleep.
2. Normal social inhibitions are lost and there is increased self-esteem; grandiose ideas, reduced attention, and marked distractibility.

A more severe form may occur, with psychotic symptoms such as delusions (usually grandiose or persecutory) along with hallucinations (World Health Organization 1992).

Hypomania is defined as a lesser degree of mania, persisting for several days but not to the extent that severe disruption of work or social rejection is experienced (World Health Organization 1992).

TREATMENT

Lithium is the traditional treatment of bipolar affective disorder. However, controversy remains as to its proconvulsant properties despite small open studies of PWE treated without adverse effect (Shukla *et al* 1988; Lyketsos *et al* 1993). Several studies have reported seizures in patients treated with lithium at both toxic serum levels (Schou *et al* 1968; Wharton 1969; Spring 1979) and therapeutic serum levels (Wharton 1969; Baldessarini and Stephens 1970; Demers *et al* 1970; Jus *et al* 1973; Moore 1981; Julius and Brenner 1987). EEG changes have also been reported in patients (Spring 1979; Rosen and Stevens 1983; Julius and Brenner 1987) and normal volunteers (Thau *et al* 1988). A recent paper by Bell *et al* (1993) included preexisting EEG abnormalities as a risk factor for the development of neurotoxicity at therapeutic lithium levels.

Carbamazepine is efficacious as an antidepressant in patients without epilepsy and is prophylactic in the control of manic-depressive illness (Post *et al* 1985), as are valproic acid (Balfour and Bryson 1994), lamotrigine (Calabrese *et al* 1996; Walden *et al* 1996), and gabapentin (Ryback *et al* 1997; Schaffer and Schaffer 1997). Thus, these drugs should be used for the treatment of epilepsy in patients with coexistent bipolar disorder and additional therapy with lithium may then be avoided.

ANXIETY DISORDERS

Ictal fear and anxiety have been described (Williams 1956) and can complicate management, as such experiences may be mistaken for anxiety or panic attacks (Young *et al* 1995; Lee *et al* 1997). Conversely, anxiety attacks may be misdiagnosed as seizures, especially in people with temporal lobe epileptiform EEG activity or a history of epilepsy (Hirsch *et al* 1990; Genton *et al* 1995). Guidelines have been determined to help differentiate these conditions (Young *et al* 1995; Lee *et al* 1997). Ictal anxiety or fear is usually stereotyped, with a rapid onset and shorter duration than panic attacks. Anxiety occurring as part of a simple partial seizure may evolve into a typical CPS with disturbance of consciousness, during which aphasia may occur, and may be followed by fatigue, confusion, and memory disturbance.

The most commonly encountered anxiety disorders experienced interictally in PWE are generalized anxiety disorder and phobic and panic disorders. Anxiety can also coexist with a depressive disorder and is particularly common in patients with late-onset epilepsy (Robertson *et al* 1987). Treatment of the underlying depression should also alleviate the anxiety.

Anxiety can be a reaction to acquiring the label of epilepsy and the accompanying social and family problems (Betts 1981). A self-reinforcing situation may occur, in which the patient is fearful of leaving the house in case they have a seizure, becomes anxious, hyperventilates, and thus increases the likelihood of convulsions. This in turn increases anxiety levels and a phobic anxiety state may ensue (Betts 1981).

Treatment of anxiety in PWE consists of relaxation training, biofeedback, counseling, behavioral and cognitive therapy and, if necessary, formal psychotherapy. Minor tranquilizers should be avoided, as most are also anticonvulsants and thus are particularly difficult to withdraw in PWE.

OBSESSIONAL COMPULSIVE DISORDER

There have been several single case reports, and also small studies, demonstrating an association between epilepsy and obsessional compulsive disorder (OCD), in both adults (Jenike 1984; Kroll and Drummond 1993; Bystritsky and Strausser 1996; Koopowitz and Berk 1997) and children (Kettl and Marks 1986; Levin and Duchowny 1991; Caplan *et al* 1992). Some studies have also found patients with OCD to have an abnormal EEG, predominantly temporal sharp wave activity (Jenike 1984). However, a review of 50 Irish patients with OCD (Lucey *et al* 1994) only revealed one with concomitant epilepsy. One case report described a patient who appeared to have an inverse relationship between seizures and OCD, in that he suffered more severely from compulsive cutting behavior when his seizures were well controlled but had no such behavior on the days when he experienced seizures (Bystritsky and Strausser 1996).

Although Schmitz *et al* (1997) did not find any association between obsessionality, measured using the Leyton obsessionality inventory, and laterality of seizure focus, patients with right-sided foci exhibited a positive correlation between higher obsessionality scores and cerebral hyperperfusion in the ipsilateral temporal and bilateral frontal regions, as measured by single-photon emission computed tomography (SPECT) using hexamethylpropylenamine oxime (HMPAO).

PHENOMENOLOGY AND DIAGNOSIS

The disorder is characterized by recurrent obsessional thoughts or compulsive acts, which should be present on most days for at least 2 weeks. Obsessional thoughts are ideas, images, or impulses that enter the individual's mind repeatedly in a stereotyped form. They are perceived as distressing and the sufferer often tries, unsuccessfully, to resist them. Compulsive acts are stereotyped behaviors that the individual repeats despite being aware of the futility of the ritual. Mounting anxiety, usually experienced while the subject attempts to resist the act, is relieved by performing the ritual (World Health Organization 1992).

TREATMENT

Behavioral and pharmacologic therapies (Perse 1988) are effective in the treatment of OCD; psychosurgery has been used for some very severe cases (Levin and Duchowny 1991). Serotoninergic drugs such as fluoxetine (Jenike *et al* 1989) are most commonly prescribed. However, several case studies have demonstrated the proconvulsant properties of fluoxetine, especially in PWE (Lambert and Robertson 1999), and carbamazepine has been shown to be an effective, safer alternative for these patients (Jenike and Brotman 1984; Caplan *et al* 1992; Kroll and Drummond 1993; Koopowitz and Berk 1997).

NONEPILEPTIC ATTACK DISORDER

Nonepileptic seizures (NES) have been defined as 'paroxysmal events that alter or appear to alter neurologic function to produce motor signs or sensory, autonomic, or psychic symptoms that at least superficially resemble those occurring during epileptic seizures' (Vossler 1995). The terminology of nonepileptic attack disorder (NEAD) is contentious, with many different pseudonyms existing for the attacks themselves including nonepileptic seizures

(NES), nonepileptic seizure events (NESLEs), pseudoseizures, and psychogenic seizures. In this chapter, the disorder will be referred to as NEAD and the attacks as NES.

NES can be of psychologic (emotional or psychiatric) or physiologic (medical) origin. Psychiatric causes of NES include panic, somatization, conversion, and dissociative disorder, along with malingering and factitious disorder. Medical causes include migraine and disorders of sleep and the cardiovascular and cerebrovascular systems. The discussion of NEAD in this chapter focuses on the etiology, clinical features, diagnosis, and management of nonepileptic conversion or dissociative disorders.

The clinical significance of a diagnosis of NEAD includes providing appropriate treatment rather than ever-increasing polypharmacy and the avoidance of such medical complications as respiratory arrest, septicemia, and pneumonia when emergency interventions are instigated for 'pseudostatus' (Lesser 1996). Also, some patients with apparently medically unresponsive seizures and temporal spikes on the interictal EEG may be needlessly investigated for epilepsy surgery until EEG monitoring reveals fully treated epileptic seizures but medically intractable nonepileptic seizures (Henry and Drury 1997).

EPIDEMIOLOGY

NES have been reported in 22–24% patients undergoing video-EEG monitoring for medically refractory seizures (Blumer *et al* 1995; Vossler 1995). They may coexist with real epileptic seizures in 4–58% (Gates and Erdahl 1993; Holmes *et al* 1993; Ramsay *et al* 1993; Vossler 1995), further complicating diagnosis and treatment.

DIAGNOSIS

The differentiation between epileptic and nonepileptic seizures may be difficult even for experienced observers (King *et al* 1982). Diagnosis entails careful history-taking from both the patient and observers and certain special investigations.

DEMOGRAPHIC CHARACTERISTICS

NEAD has been reported in patients of all ages. The average age of onset, however, is 14–30 years (Kuyk *et al* 1997). It appears to be much more common in women, who account for three-quarters of cases (Lesser 1996). There is usually a model on which the NES is based, often a witnessed attack of epilepsy; hence NES often occur in healthcare workers.

PHENOMENOLOGY

The clinical features of NES may help to differentiate them from real seizures. The most diagnostically helpful of these features are listed in Table 34.5 (Luther *et al* 1982; Gates *et al* 1985; Meierkord *et al* 1991; Leis *et al* 1992; Saygi *et al* 1992; Bergen and Ristanovic 1993; Fenwick and Aspinal 1993; Binnie 1994; Kuyk *et al* 1995; Peguero *et al* 1995; Benbadis *et al* 1996; Devinsky *et al* 1996; Lesser 1996).

ETIOLOGY

NES usually serve a function. They may be an expression of emotional needs or they may help the patient to cope with emotional difficulties. The attacks may provide 'secondary gain' such as increased attention, avoidance of activities, and decreased pressure to succeed academically or socially. The details and circumstances of the first NES may reveal clues as to the underlying etiology. NES have also been reported to occur *de novo* following epilepsy surgery (Krahn *et al* 1995; Parra *et al* 1998).

Previous childhood sexual and/or physical abuse has been associated with the development of NES by many workers (Shen *et al* 1990; Alper *et al* 1993; Bowman 1993; Arnold and Privitera 1996; Bowman and Markand 1996; Aldenkamp and Mulder 1997; Harden 1997). Betts and Bowden (1992a) describe the 'swoon' type of NES as an automatic reaction to intrusion into consciousness of unpleasant memories/flashbacks of childhood sexual abuse (dissociation) and 'abreactive' attacks as a symbolic replay of the abuse experience (conversion reaction).

PSYCHIATRIC COMORBIDITY

The following have been reported to coexist in patients with NEAD:

1. anxiety disorders, especially panic disorder with or without agoraphobia and posttraumatic stress disorder (Betts and Bowden 1992a; Snyder *et al* 1994; Bowman and Markand 1996);
2. mood disorders, mainly major depression (Snyder *et al* 1994; Bowman and Markand 1996);
3. somatization disorder (Eisendrath and Valan 1994; Snyder *et al* 1994; Bowman and Markand 1996; Aldenkamp and Mulder 1997);
4. personality disorder (Pakalnis *et al* 1991; Eisendrath and Valan 1994; Bowman and Markand 1996; Aldenkamp and Mulder 1997).

Aldenkamp and Mulder (1997) have developed a model for the development of NEAD. The patients tend to have an underlying personality disorder along with a tendency to somatize when stressed. The development of seizures rather than other somatic symptoms reflects a prior knowledge of epilepsy.

INVESTIGATIONS

Prolactin

Trimble (1978) demonstrated a rise in serum prolactin within 20 min of a spontaneous generalized seizure, contrasting with no change following NES. Others have also found that most patients with generalized seizures (Abbott *et al* 1980; Aminoff *et al* 1984; Rao *et al* 1989) and 43–100% of those with CPS (Pritchard *et al* 1983; Trimble *et al* 1984; Wyllie *et al* 1984; Sperling *et al* 1986; Rao *et al* 1989) have rises in serum prolactin. However, elevations may not follow frontal lobe seizures (Kuyk *et al* 1997) and only follow up to 10% of simple partial seizures (Trimble *et al* 1984; Wyllie *et al* 1984). A serum prolactin level threshold of $700\,\mu U\,ml^{-1}$ has been reported to differentiate between NES and 80% of tonic–clonic seizures and 39% of CPS (Bauer *et al* 1992). Tharyan *et al* (1988) found that elevation of the level to three times baseline should differentiate epileptic from nonepileptic seizures. The baseline level should be taken several hours following the episode, as prolactin may remain elevated for up to 1 hour (Abbott *et al* 1980; Aminoff *et al* 1984). However, prolactin levels may be misleading in patients with coexistent psychiatric disorders, as levels can be elevated by most neuroleptics and by stress (Kuyk *et al* 1997).

Electroencephalography

EEG studies need to be interpreted with caution as 50% of single waking interictal EEGs in PWE are normal. Sleep recordings help to increase the diagnostic yield, although even repeated awake and sleep recordings fail to reveal epileptiform discharges interictally in 8% of patients (Binnie 1993). EEG recordings during convulsive epileptic attacks should show epileptiform activity. These recordings may be obscured by muscle artifacts but the postictal record usually reveals slowing (Binnie 1994). Movement artifacts during NES may even resemble epileptiform activity (Burnstine *et al* 1991). The EEG may be normal during simple partial seizures, especially with visceral or psychic symptoms (Binnie 1994). The EEG of patients with frontal lobe CPS may also be normal and ictal frontal slowing may be mistaken for an artifact. Frontal lobe seizures are often nocturnal and the attack can be assumed to be epileptic if the seizure onset precedes EEG evidence of waking (Binnie 1994; Bazil and

Table 34.5 Clinical features of nonepileptic seizures (NES). (Modified from Devinsky and Thacker 1995.)

Characteristic	Nonepileptic seizure	Comment
Precipitant	Emotion/stress or environmental factors	Similar factors may also precipitate ES
Onset	Often gradual over minutes Rarely occurs when alone May arise from 'pseudosleep'	ES may be preceded by prodrome/SPS ES may arise from sleep
Symptoms at onset	Vocalizations, palpitations, malaise, choking, numbness, peripheral sensory disturbances, pain and olfactory, gustatory or visual hallucinations	Similar symptoms may occur during prodrome or SPS
Duration	May be prolonged (>5 min); mean 134 s, range 20–805 s	GTCS usually lasts < 4 min; mean 70 s, range 50–92 s GTCS lasting > 5 min usually accompanied by cyanosis and decreased oxygen saturation
Clinical features of seizure	Ranges from unresponsiveness with no motor manifestation to movements including thrashing, flailing, struggling, side-to-side rocking of head, back arching with forward pelvic thrusting If subject is placed on one side, the eyes will be directed towards the floor. If patient is turned, the eye deviation is reversed ('geotropic eye movement') Avoidance reactions to noxious/painful stimuli (e.g. hand being dropped onto face) Clinical features may fluctuate from one seizure to next.	Bizarre movements including hand clapping, pedaling, and pelvic thrusting may occur during frontal lobe seizures. However frontal lobe seizures are usually brief (< 1 min) and nocturnal. Patient tends to assume prone position and tonic abduction of upper limbs may occur Avoidance reactions may occur during SPS ES are usually stereotyped. In patients with ES and NES, both events may be stereotyped and distinguishable
Motor activity	Intermittent, arrhythmic out-of-phase jerking	In GTCS, jerking is rhythmic and in phase, with alternating brisk contraction and relaxation. Usually slows before stopping
Consciousness	May be preserved, with ability to talk during bilateral motor activity Amnesia is common during NES, but subsequent recall may occur during hypnosis	Speech may occur during CPS. ES from supplementary motor area may produce bilateral motor activity with preserved consciousness and speech
Reflexes	Usually normal May resist attempt to open eyes	Dilated pupils, reduced corneal reflexes, and extensor plantars may occur during NES
Injury	Occurs in up to 40% Most injuries consist of bruising Fractures and other serious injuries may occur in NES	Biting of hands, lips, or *tip* of tongue may occur in NES. In ES usually biting of *side* of tongue 'Carpet burns' on elbows and face are common in NES. 'Heat'-induced burns (from hot water, falling into fires, etc.) more common in ES
Incontinence	Urinary incontinence occurs in up to 44% Bowel incontinence is rare in NES	Combination of incontinence, injury, and tongue-biting during NES, associated with deliberate self-harm and suicide
Postictal features	Lack of headache, drowsiness, or confusion Crying common	Recovery may be rapid after frontal lobe seizures
Response to medication	Frequent seizures despite therapeutic AED levels	AED toxicity may exacerbate seizures or cause behavioral symptoms suggestive of NES

AED, antiepileptic drug; CPS, complex partial seizure; ES, epileptic seizure; GTCS, generalized tonic–clonic seizure; SPS, simple partial seizure.

Walczak 1997). It should also be noted that generalized epileptiform discharges can occur during antiepileptic drug (especially barbiturate) withdrawal, regardless of whether the patient has epilepsy. A normal EEG with preserved alpha rhythm during a typical attack manifest by apparent loss of consciousness is virtually diagnostic of NEAD (Lesser 1996; Kuyk *et al* 1997).

EEG monitoring plus video recording is often performed to help confirm the diagnosis. It is essential that the recorded seizure is the same as the patient's habitual seizure, and so a close family member should either be an observer during the monitoring or, failing that, should review the recorded seizure.

Provocative tests

Activation procedures (hyperventilation, sleep deprivation, and medication withdrawal) are routinely used in most epilepsy centers for the provocation of real epileptic seizures. Nevertheless, the provocation of NES remains the most controversial area of the management of patients with NEAD. This has recently been discussed (Devinsky and Fisher 1996; Devinsky 1998).

Generally, suggestion is used along with physical 'placebo' procedures, such as intravenous saline (Cohen and Suter 1982; Drake 1985; Wyllie *et al* 1990; Bauer *et al* 1993; Bazil *et al* 1994; Walczak *et al* 1994; Slater *et al* 1995; Bhatia *et al* 1997); alternatively a stressful psychiatric interview may be tried (Cohen *et al* 1992). Various studies have reported that NES can be provoked in 77–91% of patients thought to have NEAD (Lancman *et al* 1994a; Walczak *et al* 1994; Slater *et al* 1995) and many workers have found them to be a useful screening method that may reduce the length of video-EEG monitoring, an important factor in units with limited resources (Bhatia *et al* 1997).

Concern has been expressed by several authors (Drake 1985; Bazil *et al* 1994) that provoked seizures may not be typical of the patient's habitual NES or that NES may be mimicked by, or provoked in, PWE resulting in a false-positive diagnosis of NEAD. Walczak *et al* (1994) provoked typical seizures in two patients with epilepsy (10%), one of whom had reflex epilepsy, and nonepileptic events in three patients with epilepsy (15%). They also found the provocation procedure to be stressful for many patients, resulting in increased heart rate and blood pressure that may have contributed to the development of genuine seizures. However, the most widely expressed criticism of these methods relates to ethical issues. Some workers prefer not to use a provocative or suggestive techniques as they feel that it tends to interfere with the formation of a trusting relationship and may alienate the patient from the treatment or care team

thereby compromising therapy (Fenwick and Aspinal 1993; Gates 1998; McConnell and Duncan 1998).

Functional neuroimaging

Varma *et al* (1996) found that HMPAO SPECT scans were normal in 7 of 10 NEAD patients yet showed the typical hypoperfusion in 8 of 10 patients with localization-related epilepsy. One patient with NEAD showed hypoperfusion indistinguishable from that seen in PWE. De León *et al* (1997) performed ictal SPECT in patients with suspected NEAD and reported that hyperperfusion did not occur during NES. Thus, the presence of a normal interictal and ictal SPECT scan would support a diagnosis of NEAD.

Neuropsychologic tests

Pakalnis *et al* (1991) found Minnesota Multiphasic Personality Inventory (MMPI) scale elevations indicative of psychopathology in 15 of 16 patients with a history of nonepileptic status. Using the MMPI-2, Derry and McLachlan (1996) found a classification accuracy of 92% for NES and 94% for PWE and demonstrated that it could help identify PWE who also has NES.

TREATMENT

The majority of workers believe that the most important aspect of management after correct diagnosis of NEAD is the nonjudgmental presentation of the diagnosis (Shen *et al* 1990; Buchanan and Snars 1993; Lesser 1996; Aboukasm *et al* 1998; Devinsky 1998). Treatment should usually be provided by a multidisciplinary team. Fenwick and Aspinal (1993) describe giving patients the 'good news' that they do not have epilepsy but have 'emotional attacks,' at a time when they have begun to accept that there may be emotional precipitants of their attacks. These authors stress the importance of ensuring that the patient does not feel rejected by the team and emphasize the possibility of treatment and recovery. McDade and Brown (1992) and Betts and Bowden (1992b) advocate the use of 'operant conditioning,' attempting to prevent 'rewarding' of seizure activity by ignoring it, while nonseizure activity is positively reinforced by verbal praise and encouragement. Fenwick and Aspinal (1993) describe a behavioral program addressing antecedents, behavior during the attack, and the consequences, along with the use of relaxation as a counter measure. Finally both the patient and his or her family should be encouraged to readjust to a life without seizures (Fenwick and Aspinal 1993). Other therapeutic interventions include anxiety management, abreaction, hypnosis, counseling, formal psychotherapy, and pharmacotherapy usually with major tranquillizers (Betts and Bowden 1992b; Lesser 1996; Aboukasm *et al* 1998; Devinsky 1998). Patients with a history of childhood sexual abuse need specific therapy directed at disclosure and ventilation of the abuse experience (Betts and Bowden 1992a). Coexistent psychiatric disorders should be treated appropriately.

PROGNOSIS

Buchanan and Snars (1993) followed up a series of patients with NEAD (some with coexistent epilepsy). Three-quarters of the patients derived 'significant benefit' from management, consisting of confrontation with the diagnosis in half, formal psychotherapy in almost one-third, and supportive therapy or ongoing support in the remainder. Antiepileptic drugs were stopped in 32% and reduced in 14%. The patient, family, and treating physician considered that 48% made a complete recovery and 28% improved; only 16% were unaffected by management. Conversion symptoms developed in 6%, although NES stopped or improved. Betts and Bowden (1992b) reported that 63% of patients no longer had NES on discharge from their unit, but on follow-up only 31% were free from attacks. Many had restarted their anticonvulsant medication, often following pressure from the family.

Good prognostic factors include the recent onset of seizures (Lempert and Schmidt 1991), a short interval between any stressor and the diagnosis of NEAD (Lempert and Schmidt 1991; Betts and Bowden 1992b), a normal psychiatric evaluation (Lempert and Schmidt 1991), female sex (Meierkord *et al* 1991), living an independent life (Meierkord *et al* 1991), and the lack of coexistent epilepsy (Meierkord *et al* 1991). Bad prognostic factors include low IQ (McDade and Brown 1992), a history of violent behavior (McDade and Brown 1992), a prolonged history of NEAD (Wyllie *et al* 1991; Buchanan and Snars 1993), and personality disorder (Pakalnis *et al* 1991). Patients with both NEAD and epilepsy may be particularly difficult to treat because when the real seizures are under control the nonepileptic seizures may increase, thus maintaining the same number of 'events.' These patients need to be helped to recognize the different types of attack so that both can be monitored and treated appropriately.

PERI-ICTAL AND POSTICTAL PSYCHOSES

Psychosis can be temporally related to the seizure (periictal) or occur interictally when the episode may be either brief or chronic.

PERIICTAL PSYCHOSIS

Psychotic symptoms may occur as part of the seizure and can be prolonged in cases of nonconvulsive status epilepticus, where concurrent EEG studies may be required to make the diagnosis. A wide range of experiential phenomena may occur, including affective, behavioral, and perceptual experiences, often accompanied by automatisms. Consciousness is usually impaired but not in cases of simple partial status; insight tends to be maintained but amnesia usually follows. There is debate as to the mechanism of ictal psychosis – whether the seizure discharge activates a behavioral mechanism originating from part of the limbic system (positive effect) or whether behaviors are released by the inactivation of structures that normally suppress them (negative effect) (Sachdev 1998).

The most common and well-investigated periictal psychosis is that occurring postictally. It is thought to account for one-quarter of the cases of psychosis in PWE (Dongier 1959/60).

POSTICTAL PSYCHOSIS

Logsdail and Toone (1988) developed operational criteria for the diagnosis of postictal psychosis (PIP) that have become widely accepted.

1. Onset of confusion or psychosis within 1 week of the return of apparently normal mental function.
2. Duration of 1 day to 3 months.
3. Mental state characterized by:

   (a) clouding of consciousness, disorientation, or delirium;
   (b) delusions, hallucinations, in clear consciousness;
   (c) a mixture of (a) and (b).

4. No evidence of factors that may have contributed to the abnormal mental state:

   (a) anticonvulsant toxicity;
   (b) previous history of interictal psychosis;
   (c) EEG evidence of status epilepticus;
   (d) recent history of head injury or alcohol or drug intoxication.

The incidence and prevalence of PIP are not known. However, rates of up to 18% have been reported in patients with medically intractable focal epilepsy (Umbricht *et al* 1995; Kanner *et al* 1996).

Various risk factors have been identified for the development of PIP:

1. bilateral cerebral dysfunction (Logsdail and Toone 1988; So *et al* 1990; Savard *et al* 1991; Devinsky *et al* 1995; Umbricht *et al* 1995);
2. ictal fear (Savard *et al* 1991; Kanemoto *et al* 1996);
3. clusters of seizures (Logsdail and Toone 1988; So *et al* 1990; Mendez and Grau 1991; Savard *et al* 1991; Lancman *et al* 1994b; Devinsky *et al* 1995; Umbricht *et al* 1995; Kanemoto *et al* 1996; Kanner *et al* 1996);
4. absence of history of febrile convulsions (Umbricht *et al* 1995) or mesial temporal sclerosis (Roberts *et al* 1990);
5. preexisting personality disorder (Logsdail and Toone 1988; Savard *et al* 1991).

Although one of the patients in Logsdail and Toone's (1988) series had a family history of excess alcohol consumption, other studies have not found a positive family psychiatric history in patients with PIP (So *et al* 1990; Mendez and Grau 1991; Savard *et al* 1991). PIP has also been reported following convulsions induced by ECT (Zwil and Pomerantz 1997).

Clinical features and phenomenology

PIP mostly develops in patients with CPS (often with secondary generalization). However, it has also been described in patients with primary generalized epilepsy (Logsdail and Toone 1988; Devinsky *et al* 1995). There tends to be a delay between the onset of habitual seizures and the development of PIP ranging from 1 month to 56 years (Devinsky *et al* 1995), with a mean ranging from 13.1 years (Kanner *et al* 1996) to 21.7 years (Devinsky *et al* 1995).

Most authors have described a 'lucid interval,' which can last for up to 72 hours, between the restoration of an apparently 'normal mental state' following the seizure and the beginning of the psychosis (Logsdail and Toone 1988; So *et al* 1990; Mendez and Grau 1991; Savard *et al* 1991; Lancman *et al* 1994b; Devinsky *et al* 1995; Kanemoto *et al* 1996; Kanner *et al* 1996). PIP itself is often preceded by a period of confusion (Logsdail and Toone 1988; Mendez and Grau 1991).

The phenomenology of PIP appears to vary widely both within and between series. Logsdail and Toone (1988) found that only one patient had primary delu-

sions and thought disorder, nine had an abnormal mood, and six had paranoid delusions. Visual, auditory, or somatic hallucinations were reported in six, six, and two cases, respectively. Savard *et al* (1991) reported that seven of nine patients developed a paranoid delusional syndrome with prominent persecutory delusions; six patients had further generalized seizures while psychotic and five of these experienced a deterioration in psychotic symptoms. Lancman *et al* (1994b) described paranoid delusions, mysticism, and religious preoccupations along with auditory and visual hallucinations. These authors noted that in most cases the patients could recall what had happened during the psychotic episodes. Devinsky *et al* (1995) reported fluctuating combinations of delirium, persecutory delusions, hallucinations, and affective changes. Kanner *et al* (1996) reported that most patients exhibited an abnormal affect, depressed in 90%, alternating with hypomania in 70%; 70% were irritable and 20% had suicidal ideation. Delusions were experienced by 90% (paranoid, grandiose, somatic, and religious) and hallucinations by 40% (mainly auditory). All patients were orientated in time, place, and person. Kanemoto *et al* (1996) described sexual indiscretions, sudden unprovoked aggressive behavior, and religious and grandiose delusions in patients with PIP.

In some studies, an EEG was performed when the patient was psychotic. In some cases the abnormalities were exacerbated (Logsdail and Toone 1988; So *et al* 1990; Mendez and Grau 1991), while in others there was an improvement (Logsdail and Toone 1988) or only a minimal diffuse background slowing (Lancman *et al* 1994b).

The duration of PIP ranged from 1 to 90 days (Logsdail and Toone 1988), with a mean varying from approximately 3 days (Devinsky *et al* 1995; Kanner *et al* 1996) to 14.3 days (Logsdail and Toone 1988). There have been few long-term follow-up studies but PIP seems to recur, often in a stereotyped way (Logsdail and Toone 1988; Savard *et al* 1991; Lancman *et al* 1994b), and some patients go on to develop a chronic interictal psychosis (Logsdail and Toone 1988; Kanner *et al* 1996).

Management and treatment

Logsdail and Toone (1988) reported that over half of their patients needed to be treated with major tranquilizers and one with lithium. However, Lancman *et al* (1994b) did not demonstrate any benefits from either neuroleptics or psychotherapy and noted that most patients returned to their premorbid state within 1 week regardless of intervention. Some patients responded well to mild sedation with benzodiazepines or choral hydrate, given in a supportive environment.

The clinical significance of PIP in patients with intractable focal epilepsy is that it tends to follow a cluster of seizures often provoked by a reduction of medication during video-EEG monitoring as part of presurgical assessment. Savard *et al* (1991) suggested that patients with risk factors for PIP, including an interictal psychotic profile on the MMPI, should have a more cautious and gradual reduction of medication. Kanner *et al* (1996) treated one patient with a previous history of PIP prophylactically with neuroleptics, prior to depth electrode recording, and no psychosis occurred despite a cluster of seizures.

INTERICTAL PSYCHOSIS

ACUTE

Brief psychotic episodes are characterized by paranoid delusions and auditory hallucinations. They tend to last days to weeks and are more common when seizures are infrequent or fully controlled. Such episodes have been reported to alternate with periods of increased seizure activity and may be terminated by a seizure. Premonitory symptoms such as anxiety and insomnia have been reported; Wolf (1991) suggested that anxiolytic treatment may prevent the development of the psychosis. Landolt (1958) noted that the EEG normalized during such episodes of psychosis, generating the term 'forced' or 'paradoxical normalization' accompanying the 'alternative psychosis.'

These episodes of psychosis are considered to be rare, only occurring in 3 of 697 patients with epilepsy in one series (Schmitz and Wolf 1995). However, they have been reported as occurring more commonly when seizures have been treated with ethosuximide (Wolf 1991) or vigabatrin (Sander and Duncan 1996).

CHRONIC: SCHIZOPHRENIA-LIKE PSYCHOSIS OF EPILEPSY

In 1963, Slater *et al* described the 'schizophrenia-like psychoses of epilepsy' in 69 patients who had a combination of epilepsy (mostly TLE) and schizophrenia-like states; 11 had a chronic psychosis that had been preceded by recurrent confusional states of short duration, 46 had a psychosis suggestive of paranoid schizophrenia, and 12 had hebephrenic schizophrenia. There was no family history of psychiatric illness and the premorbid personality was normal. The mean age of onset of the psychosis was 29.8 years and it

occurred after the epilepsy had been present for a mean of 14.1 years. In some cases the psychotic symptoms appeared when the fit frequency was falling. Most patients had delusions without any change in level of consciousness, mystical delusions being common. Since then many studies have looked at chronic psychosis and rates of up to 9.25% have been reported in PWE (Mendez *et al* 1993b). Overall, schizophrenia-like psychosis is thought to occur 6–12 times more often in PWE than in the general population (Sachdev 1998).

The mechanism for the development of chronic psychosis in PWE is not known. One theory is that the psychosis may be a direct consequence of the epileptic discharge either directly or through the development of neurophysiologic (such as kindling) or neurochemical changes. The other major theory is that both the psychosis and the epilepsy have a shared etiology (Sachdev 1998).

Clinical features and phenomenology

The clinical picture is usually that of a paranoid psychosis and most studies have found it difficult to differentiate between the schizophrenia-like psychosis of epilepsy and schizophrenia, although in the former there tends to be

Table 34.6 Risk factors for the development of chronic interictal psychosis

Age of onset:	before/around puberty (10–14 years before onset of psychosis)
Seizures	lack of history of febrile convulsions
	multiple types
	CPS>PGE
	history of status epilepticus
	medically intractable
Epilepsy syndrome:	localization-related, especially temporal lobe epilepsy
Seizure frequency:	diminished (especially after temporal lobectomy)
Sex bias:	female > male
Neurology	sinistrality
Premorbid personality:	normal
Family psychiatric history	none
EEG	mesiobasal focus
	left > right or bilateral
Functional neuroimaging (SPECT)	left temporal hypoperfusion perhaps independent of seizure focus
Pathology:	ganglioglioma/hamartoma

CPS, complex partial seizure; PGE, primary generalized epilepsy; SPECT, single-photon emission computed tomography.

better preservation of affect with a relative lack of negative symptoms. Risk factors for the development of schizophrenia-like psychosis of epilepsy are shown in Table 34.6 (Slater *et al* 1963; Flor-Henry 1969; Taylor 1975; Perez and Trimble 1980; Marshall *et al* 1993; Umbricht *et al* 1995; Mellers *et al* 1998; Sachdev 1998; Trimble and Schmitz 1998).

Treatment

Generally, management of acute psychosis necessitates treatment with neuroleptic drugs in a calm environment, preferably a ward experienced in managing such neuropsychiatric patients. Trimble (1995) has suggested that the neuroleptics of choice for patients whose psychosis is clearly related to a fall in seizure frequency (such as cases of 'alternative' psychosis) may be those that lower the seizure threshold (such as chlorpromazine).

All neuroleptic medication reduces the seizure threshold to some degree, with rates of seizures ranging from 0.5 to 1.2% (Whitworth and Fleischhacker 1995). Patients most likely to suffer an exacerbation of their epilepsy are those with cerebral damage and the increase in seizures tends to occur early in treatment or following a dose increment, especially if the escalation was rapid.

Choice of neuroleptic depends on many factors. These have recently been reviewed and summarized (McConnell and Duncan 1998). Clozapine, chlorpromazine, and loxapine should be avoided in PWE because these drugs seem to be the most epileptogenic. Of the conventional neuroleptics, haloperidol appears to be relatively safe. If long-term treatment is required, sulpiride and risperidone have little effect on seizure threshold and have fewer extrapyramidal side-effects. Although depot neuroleptics improve compliance, they are more difficult to titrate slowly and if adverse effects do occur they will last longer. Thus, oral doses are preferable in PWE. When possible, only one neuroleptic drug should be given, starting at the lowest possible dose and gradually increasing while monitoring seizure frequency.

PERSONALITY CHANGES

Interictal behavioral changes have been documented for centuries, although most PWE have normal personality and thus the concept of the 'epileptic personality' has been disbanded. Nevertheless, many authors agree that some PWE do have personality changes.

Waxman and Geschwind (1975) described the interictal behavior syndrome of TLE, consisting of religiosity, hypergraphia, viscosity or stickiness, circumstantiality, meticulousness, and attention to detail. Bear and Fedio (1977) reported that patients with TLE appeared to differ from normal controls and patients with other neurologic diseases on certain personality traits recorded using their inventory. They also noted that patients with right TLE exhibited more emotional traits and tended to deny their negative behavior, whereas those with a left-sided focus displayed more ideational traits and tended to be more self-critical. However, the study has been criticized for assessing small numbers of patients: 15 with right temporal foci, 12 with left temporal foci, and no patients with other forms of epilepsy. The authors did not control for the presence or absence of psychiatric disorder nor did they specify anticonvulsant medication. Since then, there has been controversy regarding replication of these findings. Mungas (1982) found that the Bear–Fedio Inventory did not differentiate patients with TLE from other neurologic groups but merely reflected the presence or absence of concomitant psychiatric illness. Dodrill and Batzel reviewed the literature in 1986 and reported that PWE show more behavioral problems than normal controls and differ from patients with nonneurologic medical problems in that they show more 'psychotic-like' symptoms. Rodin and Schmaltz (1984) concluded that the Bear-Fedio Inventory is a general measure of emotional maladjustment but provides no support for a specific TLE syndrome. It seems that the number of seizure types, and the presence of 'cephalic' auras (dizziness, pressure, heaviness) especially when not followed by secondary generalization and hence amnesia (Mendez *et al* 1993c), are more predictive of behavioral abnormalities than the presence or absence of TLE (Rodin *et al* 1976a; Hermann *et al* 1982; Dodrill 1984). Hermann *et al* (1980) found that onset of TLE during adolescence was associated with more maladjustment in the MMPI. Naugle and Rogers (1992) reported differences between male patients with intractable seizures and medical, psychiatric, and normal controls using the MMPI and the California Psychological Inventory, but concluded that these differences merely represented logical, adaptive responses to their epilepsy.

Certain personality traits, including increased concern with philosophic, moral, or religious issues, hypergraphia (often associated with circumstantiality and viscosity), hyposexuality, and irritability, have been assessed in more detail in PWE and some authors refer to these traits as the Geschwind syndrome (Geschwind 1979; Benson 1991).

RELIGIOSITY

Sudden religious conversions have been reported in PWE, closely related to the first seizure or an increase (or more rarely a decrease) in seizure frequency (Dewhurst and Beard 1970). However, other studies have failed to demonstrate a relationship between religiosity and either seizure type or lateralization of TLE (Tucker *et al* 1987).

HYPERGRAPHIA

Waxman and Geschwind (1975) were the first to document the occurrence of hypergraphia (a tendency to excessive and compulsive writing) in patients with TLE. They reported meticulous and detailed writing, often concerned with moral, ethical, or religious issues. Since then, it has been observed in 8% of PWE (Hermann *et al* 1988) and has been associated with previous psychiatric episodes, emotional maladjustment, CT abnormalities, and focal epilepsy, especially TLE (Okamura *et al* 1993), along with affective disturbance, especially hypomania, and nondominant foci (Sanders and Mathews 1994).

VISCOSITY

This refers to the tendency to talk repetitively and circumstantially about a restricted range of topics. It appears to be more common in patients with TLE, especially with left or bilateral seizure foci, and is also correlated with duration of epilepsy and left-handedness (Rao *et al* 1992). It is widely believed that viscosity may result from impaired linguistic skills (Mayeux *et al* 1980; Rao *et al* 1992).

SEXUAL DISORDERS

Despite sexual dysfunction being described in PWE since the nineteenth century (Blumer 1985), there is still debate as to the etiology of the dysfunction and even the extent to which epilepsy increases the risk of sexual disorder (Jensen *et al* 1990).

Self-mutilation (Taylor 1969), transvestism (Davies and Morgenstein 1960), sadomasochism (Taylor 1969), exhibitionism (Hooshmand and Brawley 1969; Taylor 1969), and fetishism (Hill *et al* 1957) have been reported in PWE, especially those with TLE, and may resolve when the attacks cease with medical or surgical treatment (Toone 1986). The most common sexual dysfunction experienced by PWE is the interictal disorder of hyposexuality, which Toone (1986) defined as 'a global reduction in sexual interest, awareness and activity.' The prevalence varies from study to study, with rates ranging from 22% (Murialdo *et al* 1995) to 67% (Taylor 1969), although some workers have found less dysfunction (Jensen *et al* 1990; Duncan *et al* 1997).

Toone *et al* (1989) compared the sexual functioning of adult male epileptics attending their general practitioners with controls. They found that 56% of patients with epilepsy had experienced previous sexual intercourse compared with 98% of controls, with only 43% having sexual activity in the last month compared with 91% of controls.

Fewer studies have focused on sexual dysfunction in women. Ndegwa *et al* (1986) found that women with epilepsy, all of whom had a regular heterosexual partner, had less frequent sexual activity, more vaginismus, and generally less interest in sex than controls. Bergen *et al* (1992) found that 34% of 50 female outpatients attending a tertiary referral centre were hyposexual.

The sexual dysfunction in both sexes seems to have a neurophysiologic component (Morrell *et al* 1994). Men with epilepsy have an increased rate of erectile dysfunction, as much as 57% in one study (Toone *et al* 1989) compared with 9% in the general population (Frank *et al* 1978). It can occur in isolation (Hierons and Saunders 1966; Saunders and Rawson 1970) or in conjunction with hyposexuality (Gastaut and Collomb 1954; Blumer and Walker 1967; Shukla *et al* 1979). Nocturnal penile tumescence testing has shown that the erectile dysfunction is probably physiologic in origin (Guldner and Morrell 1996).

There are many theories regarding the etiology of sexual dysfunction, in particular hyposexuality, in PWE. It is probably multifactorial in origin, involving neurologic, endocrine, psychiatric, cognitive, and psychosocial factors (Morrell 1998). Many workers have found that PWE do not complain of their hyposexuality, especially if their seizures began before puberty (Blumer and Walker 1967; Taylor 1969; Shukla *et al* 1979). Physicians and other healthcare workers should discuss sexuality when interviewing PWE, as sexual dysfunction, whether of physiologic or psychologic cause, may be treatable (Schover and Jensen 1988).

DISORDERS OF IMPULSE CONTROL

IRRITABILITY AND AGGRESSION

Various studies have investigated whether epilepsy is more common in violent and aggressive people. Riley and Niedermeyer (1978) reviewed the EEG of more than 200 patients who had been referred for problems with aggression or outbursts of anger; less than 7% had an abnormal

EEG and in none were the abnormalities epileptiform. The prevalence of epilepsy among prisoners has been found to be up to four times that of the general population (Gunn 1977; Whitman *et al* 1984). Several reasons for this have been suggested: there may have been differential sentencing for PWE; people with disordered brain function are more liable to imprisonment; prisoners are often from socioeconomic groups III and IV, in whom there is also an increased prevalence of epilepsy; antisocial behavior may result in posttraumatic epilepsy; and finally there may be a true increase in criminal activity in PWE secondary to reduced self-esteem and social stigma (Gunn 1977; Fenwick 1986). An increased rate of epilepsy has not been observed in those convicted of violent crimes compared with those committing nonviolent offences (Gunn and Bonn 1971).

ICTAL VIOLENCE

Ictal violence has been classified by Treiman (1991), although its frequency is unclear and remains controversial. Misconceptions about such aggressive outbursts further stigmatize PWE. Ictal aggression usually consists of spontaneous nondirected stereotyped behavior. However, there are a few reports of cases in which violent crimes and arson have been thought to be committed during an ictal or postictal confusional state or automatism (Fenwick 1984; Byrne and Walsh 1989; Carpenter and King 1989; Borum and Appelbaum 1996). Automatism has been defined as:

> 'an involuntary piece of behaviour over which an individual has no control. The behaviour itself is usually inappropriate to the circumstances, and may be out of character for the individual. It can be complex, coordinated, and apparently purposeful and directed, though lacking in judgement. Afterwards, the individual may have no recollection, or only partial and confused memory, for his actions,' (Fenwick 1990).

Ictal violence is generally considered to be uncommon. Treiman (1986) has reviewed violent crimes in which epilepsy was used as a defence: in 26 of 60 cases, the crime was premeditated; in 36 of 57, the episode was provoked by anger; and in only 12 of 50 was there any evidence of amnesia. An international panel of epileptologists reviewed video-EEG studies of suspected aggressive behavior during seizures and concluded that directed ictal aggression was extremely rare (Delgado-Escueta *et al* 1981). However, it is now widely acknowledged that the form taken by an epileptic seizure depends not only on the spread of discharge through the brain but also on the thought content of the patient at the time of the attack. Thus, patients having a fit in the clinical setting of a recording laboratory would not be expected to show ictal aggression (Fenwick 1986).

INTERICTAL VIOLENCE

Paroxysmal interictal irritability has been reported in 30% of PWE compared with 2% of neurologic or normal controls (Devinsky *et al* 1991). There have also been reports of aggressive interictal behavior (Devinsky and Bear 1984). The most likely explanations for this association are (a) that there are shared risk factors for epilepsy and aggression, including exposure to violence as a child, male sex, low socioeconomic status, cognitive impairment, and neurologic lesions (Stevens and Hermann 1981; Herzberg and Fenwick 1988; Mendez *et al* 1993d), or (b) that the violence is associated with other psychopathology such as psychosis (Mendez *et al* 1993d).

EPISODIC DYSCONTROL

This term has been used to describe patients who manifest paroxysmal outbursts of violent behavior with little or no provocation. There is doubt as to whether it should be regarded as a separate entity or categorized as a form of personality disorder, such as 'intermittent explosive disorder.' Lucas (1994) has suggested that such behavior may be considered as one extreme of a continuum including normality.

Bach-y-Rita *et al* (1971) described 130 patients with 'explosive violent behaviour'; 25 of them had a history of childhood febrile convulsions or adult seizures (seven with TLE) and a further 30 reported seizure-like episodes consisting of loss of contact with the environment. A variety of 'soft' neurologic signs, such as general awkwardness in gesture and gait, mixed cerebral dominance, left–right disorientation, clumsiness, and dyslexia, that are suggestive of neurodevelopmental disorders are often reported in such patients (Maletzky 1973).

Some workers have questioned whether episodic dyscontrol is a form of complex seizure originating from the temporal lobes, as there are several shared characteristics including violent family background, low socioeconomic status, and underlying brain damage. Prodromal altered mood states, anticipatory fear, hyperacusis, and derealization, along with inaccessibility during the episode, subsequent amnesia, drowsiness, and remorse, have been reported (Fenton 1986; Sugarman 1992). However, the violent outbursts are often provoked and EEG abnormalities have not been consistently observed. Drake *et al* (1992) found nonspecific diffuse or focal EEG slowing in only 7 of 23 patients, the rest having normal records. Fenton (1986) observed that the slowing of the EEG, which tended to occur over the posterior temporal lobes, was attenuated by sleep and augmented by overbreathing. In contrast, the EEG changes in TLE, which tended to be maximal over the anterior temporal lobes, were augmented by sleep and not affected by overbreathing. Further evidence for the association between dyscontrol and epilepsy has been the improvement in outbursts following treatment with anticonvulsant medication (Maletsky 1973; Gardner and Cowdry 1986; Munroe 1989; Giakas *et al* 1990; Lewin and Sumners 1992; Sugarman 1992; Ryback and Ryback 1995). Treiman (1986) concluded that although he believed the syndrome existed, it was not epileptic in nature but arose from damage to frontal lobe structures, resulting in impairment of the normal inhibitory mechanisms that usually govern social and interactive behavior.

The issue of whether episodic dyscontrol does exist and whether it is a form of epilepsy thus remains unresolved. It has important legal implications, however, because if such violent behavior was considered epileptic it could be used as an example of an insane automatism in legal defences.

DRUG AND ALCOHOL ABUSE

Alcohol can complicate the management of epilepsy. Alcohol abuse can produce poor seizure control by several mechanisms, including a stimulant effect of the drug, a withdrawal effect associated with decreasing blood alcohol levels, enhancement of antiepileptic drug metabolism through hepatic enzyme induction, alteration in absorption of antiepileptic drugs, and noncompliance with medication (Hauser *et al* 1988). Although there have been no recent studies, there appears to be no evidence that PWE drink alcohol to excess. Lennox (1941) showed that more PWE had never used alcohol and less drank a 'large' amount compared with controls. A double-blind study performed by Höppener *et al* (1983) compared the effects of vodka added to orangeade over a 16-week period. There was no significant change in seizure frequency, epileptiform activity on the EEG, or antiepileptic drug levels and the authors concluded that social drinking had little adverse effect in PWE. Most epileptologists agree that a moderate alcohol intake is acceptable (Betts 1993).

Illicit drug abuse has also been found to be a risk factor for seizure exacerbation, especially in women (Earnest 1993; Stimmel and Dopheide 1996). High-dose cocaine appears to pose the highest risk, followed by opioids and, to a lesser extent, amphetamines, phencyclidine, and LSD (Earnest 1993; Stimmel and Dopheide 1996).

Alcohol and drug abuse are associated with increased rates of depression, deliberate self-harm, and suicide, which should be considered when assessing PWE with psychiatric comorbidity.

KEY POINTS

1. Psychiatric disorder and suicide are common in PWE and are thought to be in the region of four times that in the 'normal' population. Patients with medically intractable epilepsy, especially of temporal lobe origin, appear to be most at risk and the risk increases with the frequency of the seizures.

2. Interictal depression has been reported in up to two-thirds of PWE assessed in hospital studies. Etiologic factors include (a) biologic (TLE, especially of left-sided origin), (b) iatrogenic (polytherapy, treatment with barbiturates or vigabatrin), and (c) psychosocial (stressful life events, poor adjustment to seizures, and financial difficulties).

3. Patient support groups and psychotherapy should be sufficient to treat depressive *reactions*, whereas antidepressants are usually necessary to treat depressive *illness*. Older antidepressants, especially the tricyclics, have been reported to be epileptogenic, particularly in high-risk groups; this risk appears to be lower with newer drugs such as moclobemide and citalopram. Antidepressants should be started at low doses, gradually increased to therapeutic levels, and continued for at least 4 months after complete clinical recovery.

4. NES have been reported in over 20% of patients undergoing video-EEG investigation of medically refractory seizures. They may be interspersed with true epileptic seizures. Their recognition is very important to enable *appropriate* treatment rather than unnecessary and toxic polypharmacy.

5. PIP, which may last weeks, has been reported in up to 18% of patients with medically intractable focal epilepsy. There tends to be a 'lucid interval' between the seizure and the onset of the psychosis. PIP tends to follow a cluster of seizures such as may be precipitated by antiepileptic drug dose reduction during presurgical video-EEG monitoring.

6. Chronic interictal psychosis has been documented in up to 9.25% of PWE and tends to occur several years after the onset of the seizures. Risk factors include female sex, sinistrality, early onset of seizures, and medically intractable CPS especially of temporal lobe origin. Immediate management may necessitate treatment with haloperidol, and long-term neuroleptic

REFERENCES

Abbott RJ, Browning M, Davidson DLW (1980) Serum prolactin and cortisol concentrations after grand-mal seizures. *Journal of Neurology, Neurosurgery and Psychiatry* **43**:163–167.

Aboukasm A, Mahr G, Gahry BR, Thomas A, Barkley GL (1998) Retrospective analysis of the effects of psychotherapeutic interventions on outcomes of psychogenic nonepileptic seizures. *Epilepsia* **39**:470–473.

Aldenkamp AP, Mulder OG (1997) Behavioural mechanisms involved in pseudoepileptic seizures: a comparison between patients with epileptic seizures and patients with pseudoepileptic seizures. *Seizure* **6**:275–282.

Alper K, Devinsky O, Perrine K, Vazquez B, Luciano D (1993) Nonepileptic seizures and childhood sexual and physical abuse. *Neurology* **43**:1950–1953.

Altshuler LL, Devinsky O, Post RM, Theodore W (1990) Depression, anxiety, and temporal lobe epilepsy. Laterality of focus and symptoms. *Archives of Neurology* **47**:284–288.

Aminoff MJ, Simon RP, Wiedemann E (1984) The hormonal responses to generalised tonic–clonic seizures. *Brain* **107**:569–578.

Arnold LM, Privitera MD (1996) Psychopathology and trauma in epileptic and psychogenic seizure patients. *Psychosomatics* **37**:438–443.

Bach-y-Rita G, Lion JR, Climent CE, Ervin FR (1971) Episodic dyscontrol: a study of 130 violent patients. *American Journal of Psychiatry* **127**:1473–1478.

Baker GA, Nashef L, van Hout BA (1995) Current issues in the management of epilepsy: the impact of frequent seizures on cost of illness, quality of life and mortality. *Epilepsia* **38** (Suppl 1):S1–S8.

Baker GA, Jacoby A, Chadwick DW (1996) The associations of psychopathology in epilepsy: a community study. *Epilepsy Research* **25**:29–39.

Baldessarini RJ, Stephens JH (1970) Lithium carbonate for affective disorders. *Archives of General Psychiatry* **22**:72–77.

Balfour JA, Bryson HM (1994) Valproic acid. A review of its pharmacology and therapeutic potential in indications other than epilepsy. *CNS Drugs* **2**:144–173.

Barczak P, Edmunds E, Bets T (1988) Hypomania following complex partial seizures: a report of three cases. *British Journal of Psychiatry* **152**:137–139.

Barraclough B (1981) Suicide and epilepsy. In: Reynolds FH, Trimble MR (eds) *Epilepsy and Psychiatry*, pp 72–76. Edinburgh: Churchill Livingstone.

Bauer J, Stefan H, Schrell U *et al* (1992) Serum prolactin concentrations and epilepsy. A study which compares healthy subjects with a group of patients in presurgical evaluation and circadian variations with those related to seizures. *European Archives of Psychiatry and Clinical Neuroscience* **241**:365–371.

Bauer J, Elger CE, Hefner G, Güldenberg V (1993) Psychogenic seizures provoked by suggestion: an analysis of ictal characteristics in 100 patients documented by video-telemetry. *Epilepsia* **34** (Suppl 2):147.

Bazil CW, Walczak TS (1997) Effects of sleep and sleep stage on epileptic and nonepileptic seizures. *Epilepsia* **38**:56–62.

Bazil CW, Kothari M, Luciano D *et al* (1994) Provocation of non-epileptic seizures by suggestion in the general population. *Epilepsia* **35**:768–770.

Bear DM, Fedio P (1977) Quantitative analysis of interictal behavior in temporal lobe epilepsy. *Archives of Neurology* **34**:454–467.

Becú M, Becú N, Manzur G, Kochen S (1993) Self-help epilepsy groups: an evaluation of effect on depression and schizophrenia. *Epilepsia* **34**:841–845.

Bell AJ, Cole A, Eccleston D, Ferrier IN (1993) Lithium neurotoxicity at normal therapeutic levels. *British Journal of Psychiatry* **162**:689–692.

Benbadis SR, Lancman ME, King LM, Swanson SJ (1996) Preictal pseudosleep: a new finding in psychogenic seizures. *Neurology* **47**:63–67.

Benson DF (1991) The Geschwind syndrome. In: Smith DB, Treiman DM, Trimble MR (eds) *Neurobehavioral Problems in Epilepsy*, pp 411–421. New York: Raven Press.

Bergen D, Ristanovic R (1993) Weeping as a common element of pseudoseizures. *Archives of Neurology* **50**:1059–1060.

Bergen D, Daugherty S, Eckenfels E (1992) Reduction of sexual activities in females taking antiepileptic drugs. *Psychopathology* **25**:1–4.

Betts TA (1974) A follow-up study of a cohort of patients with epilepsy admitted to psychiatric care in an English city. In: Harris P, Mawdsley C (eds) *Epilepsy: Proceedings of the Hans Berger Centenary Symposium*, pp 326–338. Edinburgh: Churchill Livingstone.

Betts TA (1981) Depression, anxiety and epilepsy. In: Reynolds EH, Trimble MR (eds) *Epilepsy and Psychiatry*. Edinburgh: Churchill Livingstone.

Betts TA (1993) Neuropsychiatry. In: Laidlaw J, Richens A, Chadwick D (eds) *A Textbook of Epilepsy*, pp 397–457. Edinburgh: Churchill Livingstone.

Betts T (1994) Lamotrigine in the context of non-pharmacological therapies for epilepsy. *Reviews of Contemporary Pharmacotherapy* **5**:141–146.

Betts T, Bowden S (1992a) Diagnosis, management and prognosis of a group of 128 patients with non-epileptic attack disorder. Part II. Previous childhood sexual abuse in the aetiology of these disorders. *Seizure* **1**:27–32.

Betts T, Bowden S (1992b) Diagnosis, management and prognosis of a group of 128 patients with non-epileptic attack disorder. Part I. *Seizure* **1**:19–26.

Betts T, Fox C, MacCallum R (1995) Using olfactory stimuli to abort or prevent seizures: countermeasures or cue-controlled arousal manipulation? Is there something special about smell? *Epilepsia* **36** (Suppl 3):S25.

Bhatia M, Sinha PK, Jain S, Padma MV, Maheshwari MC (1997) Usefulness of short-term video EEG recording with saline induction in psedoseizures. *Acta Neurologica Scandinavica* **95**:363–366.

Binnie CD (1993) Electroencephalography. In: Laidlaw J, Richens A,

Chadwick D (eds) *A Textbook of Epilepsy*, pp 277–348. Edinburgh: Churchill Livingstone.

Binnie CD (1994) Non-epileptic attack disorder. *Postgraduate Medical Journal* **70**:1–4.

Blackwood DHR, Cull RE, Freeman CPL *et al* (1980) A study of the incidence of epilepsy following ECT. *Journal of Neurology, Neurosurgery and Psychiatry* **43**:1098–1102.

Blanchet P, Frommer GP (1986) Mood change preceding epileptic seizures. *Journal of Nervous and Mental Disease* **174**:471–476.

Blumenthal IJ (1955) Spontaneous seizures and related electroencephalographic findings following shock therapy. *Journal of Nervous and Mental Disorders* **122**:581–588.

Blumer D (1985) The psychiatric dimension of epilepsy: historical perspective and current significance. In: Blumer D (ed) *Psychiatric Aspects of Epilepsy*, pp 1–65. Washington, DC: American Psychiatric Press.

Blumer D (1992) Postictal depression: significance for the neurobehavioral disorder of epilepsy. *Journal of Epilepsy* **5**:214–219.

Blumer D, Benson DF (1982) Psychiatric manifestations of epilepsy. In: Blumer D, Benson DF (eds) *Psychiatric Aspects of Neurological Disease*, Vol II, pp 25–48. New York: Grune and Stratton.

Blumer D, Walker A (1967) Sexual behavior in temporal lobe epilepsy. *Archives of Neurology* **16**:31–43.

Blumer D, Montouris G, Hermann B (1995) Psychiatric morbidity in seizure patients on a neurodiagnostic monitoring unit. *Journal of Neuropsychiatry and Clinical Neurosciences* **7**:445–456.

Blumer D, Wakhlu S, Davies K, Hermann B (1998) Psychiatric outcome of temporal lobectomy for epilepsy: incidence and treatment of psychiatric complications. *Epilepsia* **39**:478–486.

Borum R, Appelbaum KL (1996) Epilepsy, aggression and criminal responsibility. *Psychiatric Services* **47**:762–763.

Bowman ES (1993) Etiology and clinical course of pseudoseizures: relationship to trauma, depression and dissociation. *Psychosomatics* **34**:333–342.

Bowman ES, Markand ON (1996) Psychodynamic and psychiatric diagnoses of pseudoseizure subjects. *American Journal of Psychiatry* **153**:57–63.

Boyer WF, Blumhardt CL (1992) The safety profile of paroxetine. *Journal of Clinical Psychiatry* **53** (Suppl 2):61–66.

Brent DA, Crumrine PK, Varma RR *et al* (1987) Phenobarbital treatment and major depressive disorder in children with epilepsy. *Pediatrics* **80**:909–917.

Brodie MJ (1992) Drug interactions in epilepsy. *Epilepsia* **33** (Suppl 1):S13–S22.

Brown SW, McGowan MEL, Reynolds EH (1986) The influence of seizure type and medication on psychiatric symptoms in epileptic patients. *British Journal of Psychiatry* **148**:300–304.

Buchanan N, Snars J (1993) Pseudoseizures (non epileptic attack disorder): clinical management and outcome in 50 patients. *Seizure* **2**:141–146.

Burnstine TH, Lesser RP, Cole AJ (1991) Pseudepileptiform EEG patterns during pseudoseizures. *Journal of Epilepsy* **4**:165–171.

Byrne A (1988) Hypomania following increased epileptic activity (letter). *British Journal of Psychiatry* **153**:573–574.

Byrne A, Walsh JB (1989) The epileptic arsonist (letter). *British Journal of Psychiatry* **155**:268.

Bystritsky A, Strausser BP (1996) Treatment of obsessive–compulsive disorder with naltrexone (letter). *Journal of Clinical Psychiatry* **57**:423–424.

Calabrese JR, Fatemi SH, Woyshville MJ (1996) Antidepressant effects of lamotrigine in rapid cycling bipolar disorder. *American Journal of Psychiatry* **153**:1236.

Caplan R, Comair Y, Shewmon DA, Jackson L, Chugani HT, Peacock WJ (1992) Intractable seizures, compulsions and coprolalia: a pediatric case study. *Journal of Neuropsychiatry and Clinical Neuroscience* **4**:315–319.

Carpenter PK, King AL (1989) Epilepsy and arson. *British Journal of Psychiatry* **154**:554–556.

Cockerell OC, Catchpole M, Sander JWAS, Shorvon SD (1995) The British Neurological Surveillance Unit: a nation-wide scheme for the ascertainment of rare neurological disorders. *Neuroepidemiology* **14**:182–187.

Cockerell OC, Moriarty J, Trimble M, Sander JWAS, Shorvon SD (1996) Acute psychological disorders in patients with epilepsy: a nation-wide study. *Epilepsy Research* **25**:119–131.

Cohen LM, Howard GF, Bongar B (1992) Provocation of psuedoseizures by psychiatric interview during EEG and video monitoring. *International Journal of Psychiatry in Medicine* **22**:131–140.

Cohen RJ, Suter C (1982) Hysterical seizures: suggestion as a provocative EEG test. *Annals of Neurology* **11**:391–395.

Currie S, Heathfield W, Henson R, Scott D (1971) Clinical course and prognosis of temporal lobe epilepsy: a survey of 666 patients. *Brain* **94**:173–190.

Davies B, Morgenstern FS (1960) A case of cysticercosis, temporal lobe epilepsy and transvestism. *Journal of Neurology, Neurosurgery and Psychiatry* **23**:247–249.

Davis GR, Armstrong HE, Donovan DM, Temkin NR (1984) Cognitive-behavioural treatment of depressed affect amongst epileptics: preliminary findings. *Journal of Clinical Psychology* **4**:930–935.

Deb S, Hunter D (1991) Psychopathology of people with mental handicap and epilepsy. II. Psychiatric illness. *British Journal of Psychiatry* **159**:826–830.

De León OA, Blend MY, Jobe TH, Pontón M, Gaviria M (1997) Application of ictal SPECT for differentiating epileptic from nonepileptic seizures. *Journal of Neuropsychiatry and Clinical Neurosciences* **9**:99–101.

Delgado-Escueta A, Mattson R, King L (1981) The nature of aggression during epileptic seizures. *New England Journal of Medicine* **305**:711–716.

Demers R, Lukesh R, Prichard J (1970) Convulsion during lithium therapy (letter). *Lancet* **ii**:315–316.

Derry PA, McLachlan RS (1996) The MMPI-2 as an adjunct to the diagnosis of pseudoseizures. *Seizure* **5**:35–40.

Devinsky O (1998) Nonepileptic psychogenic seizures: quagmires of pathophysiology, diagnosis, and treatment. *Epilepsia* **39**:458–462.

Devinsky O, Bear D (1984) Varieties of aggressive behaviour in temporal lobe epilepsy. *American Journal of Psychiatry* **141**:651–656.

Devinsky O, Bear DM (1991) Varieties of depression in epilepsy. *Neuropsychiatry, Neuropsychology and Behavioral Neurology* **4**:49–61.

Devinsky O, Duchowny MS (1983) Seizures after convulsive therapy: a retrospective case survey. *Neurology* **33**:921–925.

Devinsky O, Fisher R (1996) Ethical use of placebos and provocative testing in diagnosing nonepileptic seizures. *Neurology* **47**:866–870.

Devinsky O, Thacker K (1995) Nonepileptic seizures. *Neurologic Clinics* **13**:299–319.

Devinsky O, Feldmann E, Bromfield E, Emoto S, Raubertis R (1991) Structured interview for simple partial seizures: clinical phenomenology and diagnosis. *Journal of Epilepsy* **4**:107–116.

Devinsky O, Kelley K, Yacubian EMT *et al* (1994) Postictal behavior. A clinical and subdural electroencephalographic study. *Archives of Neurology* **51**:254–259.

Devinsky O, Abramson H, Alper K *et al* (1995) Postictal psychosis: a case control series of 20 patients and 150 controls. *Epilepsy Research* **20**:247–253.

Devinsky O, Sanchez-Villasenor F, Vazquez B, Kothari M, Alper K, Luciano D (1996) Clinical profile of patients with epileptic and nonepileptic seizures. *Neurology* **46**:1530–1533.

Dewhurst K, Beard AW (1970) Sudden religious conversions in temporal lobe epilepsy. *British Journal of Psychiatry* **117**:497–507.

Dikmen S, Hermann BP, Witensky AJ, Rainwater G (1983) Validity of the Minnesota Multiphasic Personality Inventory (MMPI) to psychopathology in patients with epilepsy. *Journal of Nervous and Mental Disease* **171**:114–122.

Dodrill CB (1984) Number of seizure types in relation to emotional and psychosocial adjustment in epilepsy. In: Porter RJ, Ward Jr AA, Mattson RH, Dam M (eds) *Advances in Epileptology: XVth Epilepsy International Symposium*, pp 541–544. New York: Raven Press.

Dodrill CB (1991) Behavioral effects of antiepileptic drugs. *Advances in Neurology* **55**:213–224.

Dodrill CB, Batzel LM (1986) Interictal behavioral features of patients with epilepsy. *Epilepsia* **27**(Suppl 2):S64–76.

Dongier S (1959/60) Statistical study of clinical and electroencephalographic manifestations of 536 psychotic episodes occurring in 516 epileptics between clinical seizures. *Epilepsia* **1**:117–142.

Drake ME (1985) Saline activation of pseudoepileptic seizures: clinical, EEG and neuropsychiatric observations. *Clinical Electroencephalography* **16**:171–176.

Drake ME, Hietter SA, Pakalnis A (1992) EEG and evoked potentials in episodic-dyscontrol syndrome. *Neuropsychobiology* **26**:125–128.

Duncan S, Blacklaw J, Beastall GH, Brodie MJ (1997) Sexual function in women with epilepsy. *Epilepsia* **38**:1974–1081.

Earnest MP (1993) Neurologic complications of drug and alcohol abuse. Seizures. *Neurologic Clinics* **1**:563–575.

Edeh J, Toone BK (1985) Antiepileptic therapy, folate deficiency and psychiatric morbidity: a general practice survey. *Epilepsia* **26**:434–440.

Edeh J, Toone B (1987) Relationship between interictal psychopathology and the type of epilepsy. Results of a survey in general practice. *British Journal of Psychiatry* **151**:95–101.

Edeh J, Toone BK, Corney RH (1990) Epilepsy, psychiatric morbidity, and social dysfunction in general practice. Comparison between hospital clinic patients and clinic nonattenders. *Neuropsychiatry, Neuropsychology and Behavioral Neurology* **3**:180–192.

Eisendrath SJ, Valan MN (1994) Psychiatric predictors of pseudoepileptic seizures in patients with refractory seizures. *Journal of Neuropsychiatry and Clinical Neurosciences* **6**:257–260.

Fenton GW (1986) The EEG, epilepsy and psychiatry. In: Trimble MR, Reynolds EH (eds) *What is Epilepsy?* pp 139–160. Edinburgh: Churchill Livingstone.

Fenwick P (1984) Epilepsy and the law. *British Medical Journal* **288**:1938–1939.

Fenwick P (1986) Aggression and epilepsy. In: Trimble MR, Bolwig TG (eds) *Aspects of Epilepsy and Psychiatry*, pp 31–60. Chichester: John Wiley and Sons.

Fenwick P (1990) Automatism, medicine and the law. *Psychological Medicine* Suppl 17.

Fenwick P, Aspinal A (1993) Non-epileptic seizures: treatment. In: Gran L, Johannesson SI, Ostermann PO, Sillanpää M (eds) *Pseudo-epileptic Seizures*, pp 123–132. Petersfield: Wrightson Biomedical Publishing.

Fiordelli E, Beghi E, Bogliun G, Crespi V (1993) Epilepsy and psychiatric disturbance. A cross-sectional study. *British Journal of Psychiatry* **163**:446–450.

Flor-Henry P (1969) Psychosis and temporal lobe epilepsy: a controlled investigation. *Epilepsia* **10**:363–395.

Frank E, Anderson C, Rubinstein D (1978) Frequency of sexual dysfunction in normal couples. *New England Journal of Medicine* **299**:111–115.

Gailer JL, Edwards SM (1996) SSRIs and anticonvulsants. *Australian Journal of Hospital Pharmacy* **26**:587–588.

Gardner DL, Cowdry RW (1986) Positive effects of carbamazepine on behavioral dyscontrol in borderline personality disorder. *American Journal of Psychiatry* **143**:519–522.

Gastaut H, Collomb H (1954) Etude du comportement sexuel chez les épileptiques psychomotors. *Annales Medico-Psychologiques* **112**:657–696.

Gates JR (1998) Diagnosis and treatment of nonepileptic seizures. In:

McConnell HW, Snyder PJ (eds) *Psychiatric Comorbidity in Epilepsy. Basic Mechanisms, Diagnosis, and Treatment*, pp 187–204. Washington, DC: American Psychiatric Press.

Gates JR, Erdahl P (1993) Classification of non-epileptic events. In: Rowan AJ, Gates JR (eds) *Non-epileptic Seizures*, pp 21–30. Boston: Butterworth-Heinemann.

Gates JR, Ramani V, Whalen S, Loeweson R (1985) Ictal characteristics of pseudoseizures. *Archives of Neurology* **42**:1183–1187.

Genton P, Bartolomei F, Guerrini R (1995) Panic attacks mistaken for relapse of epilepsy. *Epilepsia* **36**:48–51.

Geschwind N (1979) Behavioural changes in temporal lobe epilepsy. *Psychological Medicine* **9**:217–219.

Giakas WJ, Seibyl JP, Mazure CM (1990) Valproate in the treatment of temper outbursts (letter). *Journal of Clinical Psychiatry* **51**:525.

Gibbs FA (1951) Ictal and non-ictal psychiatric disorders in temporal lobe epilepsy. *Journal of Nervous and Mental Disease* **113**:522–528.

Gillham RA (1990) Refractory epilepsy: an evaluation of psychological methods in outpatient management. *Epilepsia* **31**:427–432.

Gillig P, Sackellares J, Greenberg H (1988) Right hemisphere partial complex seizures: mania, hallucinations, and speech disturbances during ictal events. *Epilepsia* **29**:26–29.

Goldstein LH (1997) Effectiveness of psychological interventions for people with poorly controlled epilepsy. *Journal of Neurology, Neurosurgey and Psychiatry* **63**:137–143.

Grogan R, Wagner DR, Sullivan T *et al* (1995) Generalised nonconvulsive status epilepticus after electroconvulsive therapy. *Convulsive Therapy* **11**:51–56.

Gudmundsson G (1966) Epilepsy in Iceland: a clinical and epidemiological investigation. *Acta Neurologica Scandinavica* **43**(Suppl 25):64–90.

Guldner GT, Morrell MJ (1996) Nocturnal penile tumescence and rigidity evaluation in men with epilepsy. *Epilepsia* **37**:1211–1214.

Gunn J (1977) *Epileptics in Prison*. London: Academic Press.

Gunn J, Bonn J (1971) Criminality and violence in epileptic prisoners. *British Journal of Psychiatry* **118**:337–343.

Gureje O (1991) Interictal psychopathology in epilepsy. Prevalence and pattern in a Nigerian clinic. *British Journal of Psychiatry* **158**:700–705.

Harden CL (1997) Pseudoseizures and dissociative disorders: a common mechanism involving traumatic experiences. *Seizure* **6**:151–155.

Harris EC, Barraclough B (1997) Suicide as an outcome for mental disorders. A meta-analysis. *British Journal of Psychiatry* **170**:205–228.

Hauser WA, Ng SKC, Brust JCM (1988) Alcohol, seizures, and epilepsy. *Epilepsia* **29** (Suppl 2):S66–S78.

Hawton K, Fagg J, Marsack P (1980) Association between epilepsy and attempted suicide. *Journal of Neurology, Neurosurgery and Psychiatry* **43**:168–170.

Henry TR, Drury I (1997) Non-epileptic seizures in temporal lobectomy candidates with medically refractory seizures. *Neurology* **48**:1374–1382.

Hermann BP (1979) Psychopathology in epilepsy and learned helplessness. *Medical Hypotheses* **5**:723–729.

Hermann BP, Whitman S (1989) Psychosocial predictors of interictal depression. *Journal of Epilepsy* **2**:231–237.

Hermann B, Whitman S (1992) Psychopathology in epilepsy. The role of psychology in altering paradigms of research, treatment, and prevention. *American Psychologist* **47**:1134–1138.

Hermann BP, Wyler AR (1989) Depression, locus of control, and the effects of epilepsy surgery. *Epilepsia* **30**:332–338.

Hermann BP, Schwartz MS, Karnes WE, Vahdat P (1980) Psychopathology in epilepsy: relationship of seizure type to age of onset. *Epilepsia* **21**:15–23.

Hermann BP, Dikmen S, Wilensky AJ (1982) Increased psychopathology associated with multiple seizure types: fact or artifact? *Epilepsia* **23**:587–596.

Hermann BP, Whitman S, Wyler AR, Richey ET, Dell J (1988) The neurological, psychosocial and demographic correlates of hypergraphia in patients with epilepsy. *Journal of Neurology, Neurosurgery and Psychiatry* **51**:203–208.

Hermann BP, Trenerry MR, Colligan RC (1996) Learned helplessness, attributional style and depression in epilepsy. *Epilepsia* **37**:680–686.

Herzberg JL, Fenwick PBC (1988) The aetiology of aggression in temporal-lobe epilepsy. *British Journal of Psychiatry* **153**:50–55.

Hierons R, Saunders M (1966) Impotence in patients with temporal lobe lesions. *Lancet* **ii**:761–764.

Hill D, Pond DA, Mitchell W, Falconer MA (1957) Personality changes following temporal lobectomy for epilepsy. *Journal of Mental Science* **103**:18–27.

Hirsch E, Peretti S, Boulay C, Sellal F, Maton B (1990) Panic attacks misdiagnosed as partial epileptic seizures. *Epilepsia* **31**:636.

Holmes MD, Wilkus RJ, Dodrill CB, Batzell LB, Wilensky AJ, Ojemann LM (1993) Coexistence of epilepsy in patients with nonepileptic seizures. *Epilepsia* **34** (Suppl 2):13.

Hooshmand H, Brawley BW (1969) Temporal lobe seizures and exhibitionism. *Neurology* **19**:1119–1124.

Höppener RJ, Juger A, van der Ligt PJM (1983) Epilepsy and alcohol: the influence of social alcohol intake on seizures and treatment in epilepsy. *Epilepsia* **26**:459.

Hughes J, Devinsky O, Feldmann E, Bromfield E (1993) Premonitory symptoms in epilepsy. *Seizure* **2**:201–203.

Humphries SR, Dickinson PS (1988) Hypomania following complex partial seizures (letter). *British Journal of Psychiatry* **152**:571–572.

Hurwitz TA, Wada JA, Kosaka BD, Strauss EH (1985) Cerebral organization of affect suggested by temporal lobe seizures. *Neurology* **35**:1335–1337.

Indaco A, Carrieri PB, Nappi C *et al* (1992) Interictal depression in epilepsy. *Epilepsy Research* **12**:45–50.

Jacoby A, Baker GA, Steen N, Potts P, Chadwick DW (1996) The clinical course of epilepsy and its psychosocial correlates: findings from a UK community study. *Epilepsia* **37**:148–161.

Jalava M, Sillanpää M (1996) Concurrent illnesses in adults with childhood-onset epilepsy: a population-based 35-year follow-up study. *Epilepsia* **37**:1155–1163.

Jenike MA (1984) Obsessive compulsive disorder: a question of a neurologic lesion. *Comprehensive Psychiatry* **25**:298–304.

Jenike MA, Brotman AW (1984) The EEG in obsessive–compulsive disorder. *Journal of Clinical Psychiatry* **45**:122–124.

Jenike MA, Buttolph L, Baer L, Ricciardi J, Holland A (1989) Open trial of fluoxetine in obsessive–compulsive disorder. *American Journal of Psychiatry* **146**:909–911.

Jensen I, Larsen JK (1979) Mental aspects of temporal lobe epilepsy. *Journal of Neurology, Neurosurgery and Psychiatry* **42**:256–265.

Jensen P, Jensen SB, Sørensen PS (1990) Sexual dysfunction in male and female patients with epilepsy: A study of 86 outpatients. *Archives of Sexual Behaviour* **19**:1–14.

Jeppesen U, Gram LF, Vistisen K, Loft S, Poulson HE, Brøsen K (1996) Dose-dependent inhibition of CYP1A2, CYP2C19 and CYP2D6 by citalopram, fluoxetine, fluvoxamine and paroxetine. *European Journal of Clinical Pharmacology* **51**:73–78.

Joseph AB (1986) A hypergraphic syndrome of automatic writing, affective disorder and temporal lobe epilepsy in two patients. *Journal of Clinical Psychiatry* **47**:255–257.

Julius SC, Brenner RP (1987) Myoclonic seizures with lithium. *Biological Psychiatry* **22**:1184–1190.

Jus A, Villeneuve A, Gauthier J *et al* (1973) Influence of lithium carbonate on patients with temporal lobe epilepsy. *Canadian Journal of Psychiatry* **18**:77–78.

Kanemoto K (1995) Hypomania after temporal lobectomy: a sequela to the increased excitability of the residual temporal lobe? (letter). *Journal of Neurology, Neurosurgery and Psychiatry* **59**:448–449.

Kanemoto K, Kawasaki J, Kawai I (1996) Postictal psychosis: a comparison with acute interictal and chronic psychoses. *Epilepsia* **37**:551–556.

Kanner AM, Stagno S, Kotagal P, Morris HH (1996) Postictal psychiatric events during prolonged video-electroencephalographic monitoring studies. *Archives of Neurology* **53**:258–263.

Kasper S, Fuger J, Möller HJ (1992) Comparative efficacy of antidepressants. *Drugs* **43**:11–22.

Kettl PA, Marks IM (1986) Neurological factors in obsessive compulsive disorder. Two cases and a review of the literature. *British Journal of Psychiatry* **149**:315–319.

King DW, Gallagher BB, Murvin AJ *et al* (1982) Pseudoseizures: diagnostic evaluation. *Neurology* **32**:18–32.

Klerman GL (1990) Treatment of recurrent unipolar major depressive disorder: commentary on the Pittsburg Study. *Archives of General Psychiatry* **47**:1158–1161.

Kogeorgos J, Fonagy P, Scott DF (1982) Psychiatric symptom patterns of chronic epileptics attending a neurological clinic: a controlled investigation. *British Journal of Psychiatry* **140**:236–243.

Koopowitz LF, Berk M (1997) Response of obsessive compulsive disorder to carbamazepine in two patients with co-morbid epilepsy. *Annals of Clinical Psychiatry* **9**:171–173.

Krahn LE, Rummans TA, Sharborough FW, Jowsey SG, Cascino GD (1995) Pseudoseizures after epilepsy surgery. *Psychosomatics* **36**:487–493.

Krystal AD, Weiner RD (1993) ECT seizure adequacy. *Convulsive Therapy* **10**:153–164.

Kroll L, Drummond LM (1993) Temporal lobe epilepsy and obsessive–compulsive symptoms. *Journal of Nervous and Mental Disorders* **181**:457–478.

Kupfer DJ, Frank E, Perel JM (1989) The advantage of early treatment intervention in recurrent depression. *Archives of General Psychiatry* **46**:771–775.

Kuyk J, Dunki Jacobs L, Spinhoven Ph, Van Dyck R (1995) Diagnosis of pseudoepileptic and epileptic seizures. *Epilepsia* **36** (Suppl 3): S173.

Kuyk J, Leijten F, Meinardi H, Spinhoven Ph, Van Dyck R (1997) The diagnosis of psychogenic non-epileptic seizures: a review. *Seizure* **6**:243–253.

Lambert MV, Robertson MM (1999) Depression in epilepsy: etiology, phenomenology and treatment. *Epilepsia* **40** (Suppl 10): S21–S46.

Lancman ME, Asconape JJ, Craven WJ, Howard G, Penry JK (1994a) Predictive value of induction of psychogenic seizures by suggestion. *Annals of Neurology* **35**:359–361.

Lancman ME, Craven WJ, Asconape JJ, Penry JK (1994b) Clinical management of recurrent postictal psychosis. *Journal of Epilepsy* **7**:47–51.

Landolt H (1958) Serial electroencephalographic investigations during psychotic episodes in epileptic patients and during schizophrenic attacks. In: deHass L (ed) *Lectures on Epilepsy*, pp 91–133. London: Elsevier.

Lee DO, Helmers SL, Steingard RJ, DeMaso DR (1997) Case study: seizure disorder presenting as panic disorder with agoraphobia. *Journal of the American Academy of Child and Adolescent Psychiatry* **36**:1295–1298.

Leis AA, Ross MA, Summers AK (1992) Psychogenic seizures: ictal characteristics and diagnostic pitfalls. *Neurology* **42**:95–99.

Lempert T, Schmidt D (1991) Natural history and outcome of psychogenic seizures: a clinical study in 50 patients. *Journal of Neurology* **237**:35–38.

Lennox WG (1941) Alcohol and epilepsy. *Quarterly Journal of Studies on Alcohol* **2**:1–11.

Lennox WG, Markham CH (1953) The socio-psychological treatment of epilepsy. *Journal of the American Medical Association* **152**:1690–1694.

Lesser RP (1996) Psychogenic seizures. *Neurology* **46**:1499–1507.

Levin B, Duchowny M (1991) Childhood obsessive–compulsive disorder and cingulate epilepsy. *Biological Psychiatry* **30**:1049–1055.

Lewin J, Sumners D (1992) Successful treatment of episodic dyscontrol with carbamazepine. *British Journal of Psychiatry* **161**:261–262.

Lim J, Yagnik P, Schraeder P, Wheeler S (1986) Ictal catatonia as a manifestation of nonconvulsive status epilepticus. *Journal of Neurology, Neurosurgery and Psychiatry* **49**:833–836.

Logsdail SJ, Toone BK (1988) Post-ictal psychosis. A clinical and phenomenological description. *British Journal of Psychiatry* **152**:246–252.

Lucas P (1994) Episodic dyscontrol: a look back at anger. *Journal of Forensic Psychiatry* **5**:371–407.

Lucey JV, Butcher G, Clare AW, Dinan TG (1994) The clinical characteristics of patients with obsessive compulsive disorder: a descriptive study of an Irish sample. *Irish Journal of Psychological Medicine* **11**:11–14.

Lund J (1985) Epilepsy and psychiatric disorder in the mentally retarded adult. *Acta Psychiatrica Scandinavica* **72**:557–562.

Luther JS, McNamara JO, Carwile S, Miller P, Hope V (1982) Pseudoepileptic seizures: methods and video analysis to aid diagnosis. *Annals of Neurology* **12**:458–462.

Lyketsos CG, Stoline AM, Longstreet P *et al* (1993) Mania in temporal lobe epilepsy. *Neuropsychiatry, Neuropsychology and Behavioral Neurology* **6**:19–25.

McConnell HW, Duncan D (1998) Treatment of psychiatric comorbidity in epilepsy. In: McConnell HW, Snyder PJ (eds) *Psychiatric Comorbidity in Epilepsy. Basic Mechanisms, Diagnosis, and Treatment*, pp 245–362. Washington, DC: American Psychiatric Press.

McDade G, Brown SW (1992) Non-epileptic seizures: management and predictive factors of outcome. *Seizure* **1**:7–10.

Mackay A (1979) Self poisoning: A complication of epilepsy. *British Journal of Psychiatry* **34**:277–282.

Maletzky BM (1973) The episodic dyscontrol syndrome. *Diseases of the Nervous System* **34**:178–185.

Manchanda R, Schaefer B, McLachlan RS, Blume WT (1992) Interictal psychiatric morbidity and focus of epilepsy in treatment-refractory patients admitted to an epilepsy unit. *American Journal of Psychiatry* **149**:1096–1098.

Manchanda R, Schaefer B, McLachlan RS *et al* (1996) Psychiatric disorders in candidates for surgery for epilepsy. *Journal of Neurology, Neurosurgery and Psychiatry* **61**:82–89.

Marshall EJ, Syed GMS, Fenwick PBC, Lishman WA (1993) A pilot study of schizophrenia-like psychosis in epilepsy using single-photon emission computerized tomography. *British Journal of Psychiatry* **163**:32–36.

Mayeux R, Brandt J, Rosen J, Benson DF (1980) Interictal memory and language impairment in temporal lobe epilepsy. *Neurology* **30**:120–125.

Meierkord H, Will B, Fish D, Shorvon S (1991) The clinical features and prognosis of pseudoseizures diagnosed using video-EEG telemetry. *Neurology* **41**:1643–1646.

Mellers JDC, Adachi N, Takei N, Cluckie A, Toone BK, Lishman WA (1998) SPET study of verbal fluency in schizophrenia and epilepsy. *British Journal of Psychiatry* **173**:69–74.

Mendez MF, Doss RC (1992) Ictal and psychiatric aspects of suicide in epileptic patients. *International Journal of Psychiatry in Medicine* **22**:231–237.

Mendez MF, Grau R (1991) The postictal psychosis of epilepsy: investigation in two patients. *International Journal of Psychiatry in Medicine* **21**:85–92.

Mendez MF, Cummings JL, Benson DF (1986) Depression in epilepsy. Significance and phenomenology. *Archives of Neurology* **43**:766–770.

Mendez MF, Doss RC, Taylor JL, Salguero P (1993a) Depression in epilepsy. Relationship to seizures and anticonvulsant therapy. *Journal of Nervous and Mental Disorder* **181**:444–447.

Mendez MF, Grau R, Doss RC, Taylor JL (1993b) Schizophrenia in epilepsy: seizure and psychosis variables. *Neurology* **43**:1073–1077.

Mendez MF, Doss RC, Taylor JL, Arguello R (1993c) Relationship of seizure variables to personality disorders in epilepsy. *Journal of Neuropsychiatry and Clinical Neurosciences* **5**:283–286.

Mendez MF, Doss RC, Taylor JL (1993d) Interictal violence in epilepsy. Relationship to behaviour and seizure variables. *Journal of Nervous and Mental Disorder* **181**:566–569.

Mignone RJ, Donnelly EF, Sadowsky D (1970) Psychological and neurological comparisons of psychomotor and non-psychomotor epileptic patients. *Epilepsia* **11**:345–359.

Moore DP (1981) A case of petit mal epilepsy aggravated by lithium. *American Journal of Psychiatry* **138**:690–691.

Morphew JA (1988) Hypomania following complex partial seizures (letter). *British Journal of Psychiatry* **152**:572.

Morrell MJ (1998) Sexuality in epilepsy. In: Engel J Jr., Pedley TA (eds) *Epilepsy – A Comprehensive Textbook*, pp 2021–2026. Philadelphia: Lippincott-Raven.

Morrell MJ, Sperling MR, Stecker M, Dichter MA (1994) Sexual dysfunction in partial epilepsy: a deficit in physiologic sexual arousal. *Neurology* **44**:243–247.

Mungas D (1982) Interictal behavior abnormality in temporal lobe epilepsy. *Archives of General Psychiatry* **39**:108–111.

Munroe RR (1989) Dyscontrol syndrome: long term follow-up. *Comprehensive Psychiatry* **30**:489–497.

Murialdo G, Galimberti CA, Fonzi S *et al* (1995) Sex hormones and pituitary function in male epileptic patients with altered or normal sexuality. *Epilepsia* **36**:360–365.

Murray RE, Abou-Khalil B, Griner L (1994) Evidence for familial association of psychiatric disorders and epilepsy. *Biological Psychiatry* **36**:428–429.

Naugle RI, Rogers DA (1992) Personality inventory responses of males with medically intractable seizures. *Journal of Personality Assessment* **59**:500–514.

Ndegwa D, Rust J, Golombok S, Fenwick P (1986) Sexual problems in epileptic women. *Sexual and Marital Therapy* **1**:175–177.

Nemeroff CB, De Vane CL, Pollock BG (1996) Newer antidepressants and the cytochrome P450 system. *American Journal of Psychiatry* **153**:311–320.

Okamura T, Fukai M, Yamadori A *et al* (1993) A clinical study of hypergraphia in epilepsy. *Journal of Neurology, Neurosurgery and Psychiatry* **56**:556–559.

Pakalnis A, Drake ME, Phillips B (1991) Neuropsychiatric aspects of psychogenic status epilepticus. *Neurology* **41**:1104–1106.

Parra J, Iriarte J, Kanner AM, Bergen DC (1998) *De novo* psychogenic nonepileptic seizures after epilepsy surgery. *Epilepsia* **39**:474–477.

Pary R (1993) Mental retardation, mental illness, and seizure diagnosis. *American Journal of Mental Retardation* **98**:S58–S62.

Peguero E, Abou-Khalil B, Fakhoury T, Mathews G (1995) Self-injury and incontinence in psychogenic seizures. *Epilepsia* **36**:586–591.

Perez MM, Trimble MR (1980) Epileptic psychosis: psychopathological comparison with process schizophrenia. *British Journal of Psychiatry* **137**:245–249.

Perse T (1988) Obsessive-compulsive disorder: a treatment review. *Journal of Clinical Psychiatry* **49**:48–55.

Pond DA, Bidwell BH (1959/60) A survey of epilepsy in fourteen general practices. 2. Social and psychological aspects. *Epilepsia* **1**:285–299.

Post RM, Uhde TW, Joffe RT *et al* (1985) Anticonvulsant drugs in psychiatric illness: new treatment alternatives and theoretical implications. In: Trimble MR (ed) *The Psychopharmacology of Epilepsy*, pp 95–105. Chichester: Wiley.

Preskorn SH, Fast GA (1992) Tricyclic antidepressant-induced seizures and plasma drug concentration. *Journal of Clinical Psychiatry* **53**:160–162.

Prien RF, Kupfer DJ (1986) Continuation drug therapy for major depressive episodes: how long should it be maintained? *American Journal of Psychiatry* **143**:18–23.

Pritchard PB III, Lombroso CT, McIntyre M (1980) Psychological complications of temporal lobe epilepsy. *Neurology* **30**:227–232.

Pritchard PB III, Wannamaker BB, Sagel J, Nair R, De Villier C (1983) Endocrine function following complex partial seizures. *Annals of Neurology* **14**:27–32.

Ramsay RE, Cohen A, Brown MC (1993) Coexisting epilepsy and non-epileptic seizures. In: Rowan AJ, Gates JR (eds) *Non-epileptic Seizures*, pp 47–54. Boston: Butterworth-Heinemann.

Rao ML, Stefan H, Bauer J (1989) Epileptic but not psychogenic seizures are accompanied by simultaneous elevation of serum pituitary hormones and cortisol levels. *Neuroendocrinology* **49**:33–39.

Rao SM, Devinsky O, Grafman J et al (1992) Viscosity and social cohension in temporal lobe epilepsy. *Journal of Neurology, Neurosurgery and Psychiatry* **55**:149–152.

Reunanen M, Dam M, Yuen A (1996) A randomised open multicentre comparative trial of lamotrigine and carbamazepine as monotherapy in patients with newly diagnosed or recurrent epilepsy. *Epilepsy Research* **23**:149–155.

Riley T, Niedermeyer E (1978) Rage attacks and episodic violent behaviour. Electroencephalographic findings and general consideration. *Journal of Clinical Electroencephalography* **9**:113–139.

Ring HA, Crellin R, Kirker S, Reynolds EH (1993) Vigabatrin and depression. *Journal of Neurology, Neurosurgery and Psychiatry* **56**:925–928.

Ring HA, Moriatry J, Trimble MR (1998) A prospective study of the early postsurgical psychiatric associations of epilepsy surgery. *Journal of Neurology, Neurosurgery and Psychiatry* **64**:601–604.

Roberts GW, Done DJ, Crow TJ (1990) A 'mock-up' of schizophrenia: temporal lobe epilepsy and schizophrenia-like psychosis. *Biological Psychiatry* **28**:127–143.

Robertson MM (1997) Depression in neurological disorders. In: Robertson MM, Katona CLE (eds) *Depression and Physical Illness*, pp 305–340. Chichester: John Wiley and Sons.

Robertson MM (1998) Suicide, parasuicide, and epilepsy. In: Engel J Jr, Pedley TA (eds) *Epilepsy: A Comprehensive Textbook*, pp 2141–2151. Philadelphia: Lippincott-Raven.

Robertson MM, Trimble MR (1985) The treatment of depression in patients with epilepsy. *Journal of Affective Disorders* **9**:127–136.

Robertson MM, Trimble MR, Townsend HRA (1987) Phenomenology of depression in epilepsy. *Epilepsia* **28**:364–372.

Robertson MM, Channon S, Baker J (1994) Depressive symptomatology in a general hospital sample of outpatients with temporal lobe epilepsy: a controlled study. *Epilepsia* **35**:771–777.

Rodin E, Schmaltz S (1984) The Bear–Fedio personality inventory and temporal lobe epilepsy. *Neurology* **34**:591–596.

Rodin EA, Katz M, Lennox K (1976a) Differences between patients with temporal lobe seizures and those with other forms of epileptic attacks. *Epilepsia* **17**:313–320.

Rodin EA, Rim CS, Kitano H et al (1976b) A comparison of the effectiveness of primidone versus carbamazepine in epileptic outpatients. *Journal of Nervous and Mental Disorder* **163**:41–46.

Rosen RB, Stevens R (1983) Action myoclonus in lithium toxicity. *Annals of Neurology* **13**:221–222.

Rosenstein DL, Nelson JC, Jacobs SC (1993) Seizures associated with antidepressants: a review. *Journal of Clinical Psychiatry* **54**:289–299.

Roy A (1979) Some determinants of affective symptoms in epileptics. *Canadian Journal of Psychiatry* **24**:554–556.

Rutter M, Graham P, Yule W (1970) *A Neuropsychiatric Study in Childhood*. Clinics in Developmental Medicine nos 35/36. London: Heinemann/Spastics International Medical Publications.

Ryback R, Ryback L (1995) Gabapentin for behavioral dyscontrol (letter). *American Journal of Psychiatry* **152**:1399.

Ryback RS, Brodsky L, Munasilfi F (1997) Gabapentin in bipolar

disorder. *Journal of Neuropsychiatry and Clinical Neuroscience* **9**:301.

Sachdev P (1998) Schizophrenia-like psychosis and epilepsy: the status of the association. *American Journal of Psychiatry* **155**:325–336.

Sander JWAS, Duncan JS (1996) Vigabatrin. In: Shorvon S, Dreifuss F, Fish D, Thomas D (eds) *The Treatment of Epilepsy*, pp 491–499. Oxford: Blackwell Science.

Sanders RD, Mathews TA (1994) Hypergraphia and secondary mania in temporal lobe epilepsy. Case reports and literature review. *Neuropsychiatry, Neuropsychology and Behavioral Neurology* **7**:114–117.

Saunders M, Rawson M (1970) Sexuality in male epileptics. *Journal of Neurology* **10**:577–583.

Savard G, Andermann F, Olivier A, Rémillard GM (1991) Postictal psychosis after partial complex seizures: a multiple case study. *Epilepsia* **32**:225–231.

Saygi S, Katz A, Marks DA, Spencer SS (1992) Frontal lobe partial seizures and psychogenic seizures: comparison of clinical and ictal characteristics. *Neurology* **42**:1274–1277.

Schaffer CB, Schaffer LC (1997) Gabapentin in the treatment of bipolar disorder. *American Journal of Psychiatry* **154**:291–292.

Schmitz B, Wolf P (1995) Psychosis in epilepsy: frequency and risk factors. *Journal of Epilepsy* **8**:295–305.

Schmitz EB, Moriarty J, Costa DC, Ring HA, Ell PJ, Trimble MR (1997) Psychiatric profiles and patterns of cerebral blood flow in focal epilepsy: interactions between depression, obsessionality, and perfusion related to the laterality of the epilepsy. *Journal of Neurology, Neurosurgery and Psychiatry* **62**:458–463.

Schou M, Amdisen A, Trap-Jensen J (1968) Lithium poisoning. *American Journal of Psychiatry* **125**:520–527.

Schover LR, Jensen SB (1988) Physiological factors and sexual problems in chronic illness. In: Schover LR, Jensen SB (eds) *Sexuality and Chronic Illness: A Comprehensive Approach*, pp 78–105. New York: Guildford Press

Series HG (1992) Drug treatment of depression in medically ill patients. *Journal of Psychosomatic Research* **36**:1–16.

Shen W, Bowman ES, Markand ON (1990) Presenting the diagnosis of pseudoseizures. *Neurology* **40**:756–759.

Shorvon S, Reynolds EH (1979) Reduction in polypharmacy for epilepsy. *British Medical Journal* **2**:1023–1025.

Shukla GD, Sirvastava OM, Katiyar BC (1979) Sexual disturbances in temporal lobe epilepsy: a controlled study. *British Journal of Psychiatry* **134**:288–292.

Shukla S, Mukherjee S, Decina P (1988) Lithium in the treatment of bipolar disorders associated with epilepsy: an open study. *Journal of Clinical Psychopharmacology* **8**:201–204.

Skowron DM, Stimmel GL (1992) Antidepressants and the risk of seizures. *Pharmacotherapy* **12**:18–22.

Slater E, Beard AW, Glithero E (1963) The schizophrenia-like psychoses of epilepsy. *British Journal of Psychiatry* **109**:95–150.

Slater JD, Brown MC, Jacobs W, Ramsey RE (1995) Induction of pseudoseizures with intravenous saline placebo. *Epilepsia* **36**:580–585.

Smith DB, Collins JB (1987) Behavioral effects of carbamazepine, phenobarbital, phenytoin and primidone. *Epilepsia* **28**:598.

Smith D, Baker G, Davies G, Dewey M, Chadwick DW (1993) Outcomes of add-on treatment with lamotrigine in partial epilepsy. *Epilepsia* **34**:312–322.

Snyder SL, Rosenbaum DH, Rowan DH, Strain JJ (1994) SCID diagnosis of panic disorder in psychogenic seizure patients. *Journal of Neuropsychiatry and Clinical Neurosciences* **6**:261–266.

So NK, Savard G, Andermann F et al (1990) Acute postictal psychosis: a stereo EEG study. *Epilepsia* **31**:188–193.

Sperling MR, Pritchard PB III, Engel J Jr, Daniel C, Sagel J (1986)

Prolactin in partial epilepsy: an indicator of limbic seizures. *Annals of Neurology* **20**:716–722.

Spina E, Pisani F, Perucca E (1996) Clinically significant pharmacokinetic drug interactions with carbamazepine. An update. *Clinical Pharmacokinetics* **31**:198–214.

Spring GK (1979) EEG observations in confirming neurotoxicity (letter). *American Journal of Psychiatry* **136**:1099–1100.

Standage KF, Fenton GW (1975) Psychiatric symptom profiles of patients with epilepsy: a controlled investigation. *Psychological Medicine* **5**:152–160.

Stevens JR, Hermann BP (1981) Temporal lobe epilepsy, psychopathology, and violence: the state of the evidence. *Neurology* **31**:1127–1132.

Stimmel GL, Dopheide JA (1996) Psychotropic drug-induced reductions in seizure threshold. Incidences and consequences. *CNS Drugs* **5**:37–50.

Sugarman P (1992) Carbamazepine and episodic dyscontrol (letter). *British Journal of Psychiatry* **161**:721.

Swinkels JA, de Jonghe F (1995) Safety of antidepressants. *International Clinical Psychopharmacology* **9** (Suppl 4):19–25.

Taylor DC (1969) Sexual behaviour and temporal lobe epilepsy. *Archives of Neurology* **21**:510–516.

Taylor DC (1972) Mental state and temporal lobe epilepsy: a correlative account of 100 patients treated surgically. *Epilepsia* **13**:727–765.

Taylor DC (1975) Factors influencing the occurrence of schizophrenia-like psychosis in patients with temporal lobe epilepsy. *Psychological Medicine* **5**:249–254.

Taylor DC (1991) Epilepsy and organic mania. *Biological Psychiatry* **2**:202–203.

Tharyan P, Kuruvilla K, Prabhakar S (1988) Serum prolactin changes in epilepsy and hysteria. *Indian Journal of Psychiatry* **30**:145–152.

Thau K, Rappelsberger P, Lovrek A, Petsche H, Simhandl Ch, Topitz A (1988) Effect of lithium on the EEG of healthy males and females. *Neuropsychobiology* **20**:158–163.

Toone BK (1986) Sexual disorders in epilepsy. In: Pedley TA, Meldrum BS (eds) *Recent Advances in Epilepsy*, Vol 3, pp 233–259. Edinburgh: Churchill Livingstone.

Toone BK, Edeh J, Nanjee MN, Wheeler M (1989) Hyposexuality and epilepsy: a community survey of hormonal and behavioural changes in male epileptics. *Psychological Medicine* **19**:937–943.

Treiman DM (1986) Epilepsy and violence: medical and legal issues. *Epilepsia* **27**: (Suppl 2):S77–S104.

Treiman D (1991) Psychobiology of ictal aggression. *Advances in Neurology* **55**:341–356.

Trimble MR (1978) Serum prolactin in epilepsy and hysteria. *British Medical Journal* **ii**:1682.

Trimble MR (1995) Long-term treatment of dysfunctional behaviour in epilepsy. *Baillière's Clinical Psychiatry* **1**:667–682.

Trimble M, Perez M (1980) The phenomenology of the chronic psychoses of epilepsy. *Advances in Biology and Psychiatry* **8**:98–105.

Trimble MR, Schmitz B (1998) The psychoses of epilepsy. A neurobiological perspective. In: McConnell HW, Snyder PJ (eds) *Psychiatric Comorbidity in Epilepsy. Basic Mechanisms, Diagnosis, and Treatment*, pp 169–186. Washington, DC: American Psychiatric Press.

Trimble MR, Dana-Haeri J, Oxley J, Baylis PH (1984) Some neuroendocrine consequences of seizures. In: Porter RJ, Ward Jr AA, Mattson RH, Dam M (eds) *Advances in Epileptology: XVth Epilepsy International Symposium*, pp 201–208. New York: Raven Press.

Tucker DM, Novelly RA, Walker PJ (1987) Hyperreligiosity in temporal lobe epilepsy: redefining the relationship. *Journal of Nervous and Mental Disorder* **175**:181–184.

Umbricht D, Degreef G, Barr WB *et al* (1995) Postical and chronic psychoses in patients with temporal lobe epilepsy. *American Journal of Psychiatry* **152**:224–231.

Varma AR, Moriaty J, Costa DC *et al* (1996) HMPAO SPECT in non-epileptic seizures: preliminary results. *Acta Neurologica Scandinavica* **94**:88–92.

Victoroff J (1994) DSMIIIR psychiatric diagnoses in candidates for epilepsy surgery: lifetime prevalence. *Neuropsychiatry, Neuropsychology and Behavioral Neurology* **7**:87–97.

Victoroff JI, Benson DF, Engel J Jr *et al* (1990) Interictal depression in patients with medically intractable complex partial seizures: electroencephalography and cerebral metabolic correlates. *Annals of Neurology* **28**:221.

Vossler DG (1995) Nonepileptic seizures of physiologic origin. *Journal of Epilepsy* **8**:1–10.

Walczak TS, Williams DT, Berten W (1994) Utility and reliability of placebo infusion in the evaluation of patients with seizures. *Neurology* **44**:394–399.

Walden J, Hesslinger B, van-Calker D, Berger M (1996) Addition of lamotrigine to valproate may enhance efficacy in the treatment of bipolar affective disorder. *Pharmacopsychiatry* **29**:193–195.

Waxman SG, Geschwind N (1975) The interictal behaviour syndrome of temporal lobe epilepsy. *Archives of General Psychiatry* **32**:1580–1586.

Weil AA (1959) Ictal emotions occurring in temporal lobe dysfunction. *Archives of Neurology* **1**:87–97.

Weiner RD, Coffey CE (1993) Electroconvulsive therapy in the medical and neurologic patient. In: Stoudemire A Fogel BS (eds) *Psychiatric Care of the Medical Patient*, pp 207–224. New York: Oxford University Press.

Wharton RN (1969) Grand mal seizures with lithium treatment. *American Journal of Psychiatry* **125**:152.

Whitman S, Coleman TE, Patmon C, Desai BT, Cohen R, King LN (1984) Epilepsy in prison: elevated prevalence and no relationship to violence. *Neurology* **141**:651–656.

Whitworth AB, Fleischhacker WW (1995) Adverse effects of neuroleptic drugs. *International Clinical Psychopharmacology* **9** (Suppl 5):21–27.

Williams D (1956) The structure of emotions reflected in epileptic experiences. *Brain* **79**:29–67.

Wolf P (1982) Manic episodes in epilepsy. In: Akimoto H, Kazamatsuri H, Seino M, Ward AA (eds) *Advances in Epileptology: 13th Epilepsy International Symposium*, pp 237–240. New York: Raven Press.

Wolf P (1991) Acute behavioral symptomatology at disappearance of epileptiform EEG abnormality: paradoxical or 'forced' normalization. *Advances in Neurology* **55**:127–142.

World Health Organization (1992) *ICD-10 Classification of Mental and Behavioural Disorders: Clinical Descriptions and Diagnostic Guidelines*. Geneva: WHO.

Wroblewski BA, McColgan K, Smith K *et al* (1990) The incidence of seizures during tricyclic antidepressant drug treatment in a brain-injured population. *Journal of Clinical Psychopharmacology* **10**:124–128.

Wyllie E, Lüders H, MacMillan JP, Gupta M (1984) Serum prolactin levels after epileptic seizures. *Neurology* **34**:1601–1604.

Wyllie E, Friedman D, Rothner AD *et al* (1990) Psychogenic seizures in children and adolescents: outcome after diagnosis by ictal video and electroencephalographic recording. *Pediatrics* **85**:480–485.

Wyllie E, Friedman D, Luders H *et al* (1991) Outcome of psychogenic seizures in children and adolescents compared with adults. *Neurology* **41**:742–744.

Young GB, Chandarana PC, Blume WT, McLachlan RS, Munoz DG, Girvin JP (1995) Mesial temporal lobe seizures presenting as anxiety disorders. *Journal of Neuropsychiatry and Clinical Neurosciences* **7**:352–357.

Zwil AS, Pomerantz A (1997) Transient postictal psychosis associated with a course of ECT. Case report. *Convulsive Therapy* **13**:32–36.

Medical management

Drug treatment: adults

JM OXBURY

Between 20 and 40% of people with epilepsy continue to have seizures despite 'optimum' medication. In the British National General Practice Study of Epilepsy (BNGPSE), 20% of those with a partial seizure disorder, newly diagnosed during 1984–1987, did not achieve a 3-year remission within 9 years of the index seizure (Cockerell *et al* 1995, 1997).

The prevalence of focal seizure disorders manifest by at least one seizure per month is considered to be around 0.78/1000 population overall. The age-adjusted figure for men (0.93) is significantly higher than for women (0.64), and the age-related prevalence peaks at age 30–40 years (see Chapter 3). Hauser and Hesdorffer (1996) considered that despite optimal antiepileptic drug (AED) treatment, 5–10% of all incidence cases of epilepsy ultimately develop a truly intractable disease of sufficient severity to merit consideration of surgery. Merging this figure with the BNGPSE data would lead to the suggestion that between one-quarter and one-half of those who do not enter 3-year remission will continue to have epilepsy that is of such a severity. Data derived from a UK study mentioned by Aicardi and Shorvon (1998) indicate that around 40% of people experiencing seizures while on AED may be having more than 12 per year.

Intractability has been defined in various ways but none has been universally adopted (Aicardi and Shorvon 1998). The large majority of those with partial seizures who entered a 3-year remission in the BNGPSE did so within 2 years of the index seizure (Cockerell *et al* 1995, 1997). In line with that finding, the editors of this book decided to take an operational definition of medical intractability as *a continuation of seizures beyond two years despite treatment with three of phenobarbital, phenytoin, carbamazepine, sodium valproate, or lamotrigine taken at 'optimal' doses either individually or in combination.* These have all been regarded as 'first-line' AED licensed in the UK for monotherapy. This definition of intractability is similar to that suggested by Gilman *et al* (1994) for the evaluation of children prior to epilepsy surgery. It is also in line with the view of Schmidt and Gram (1995) that diagnostic reevaluation should be undertaken after three AEDs, given either sequentially or in combination, have failed to achieve adequate control of the epilepsy. The proportion of patients classed as medically intractable would be slightly lower if the definition required a continuation of seizures for longer than 2 years. The number of patients who will spontaneously enter remission after 2 years is, however, relatively small and the disadvantages of continuing seizures are usually great. So, especially if the seizures are frequent, there is good reason to consider that the epilepsy may be medically intractable and to undertake detailed assessment no later than the third year after diagnosis and the initiation of medication.

THE ASSESSMENT OF APPARENT MEDICAL INTRACTABILITY

The first step that should be taken in the face of apparent medically intractable focal (partial) epilepsy is to check that the diagnosis is correct and that *appropriate* medication has been taken regularly at 'optimal' doses.

DIAGNOSIS

Is it epilepsy?

The diagnosis should be reviewed firstly to confirm that the patient's episodic symptoms are truly epileptic and that the seizures are focal rather than primary generalized, and secondly, to try to establish the cause or underlying pathology. The history of the presumed epilepsy should be re-examined particularly with respect to:

1. The precise semeiology of the habitual episodic symptoms (the presumed seizures). The symptoms should be stereotyped and conform to a recognized pattern for focal seizures. If there are doubts the possibility of an alternative diagnosis should be considered.
2. The age of onset of the habitual epilepsy and whether there was any significant previous history – especially early childhood complicated convulsions, as might suggest a liability to hippocampal sclerosis, or any cerebral condition including brain injury. Such data may give a clue to the cause or pathology underlying the epilepsy.
3. A family history of epilepsy.
4. Any associated neurologic condition or the presence of abnormal neurologic signs on examination.
5. The drug history (see below).
6. The previous investigations including EEG and neuroimaging (CT and magnetic resonance imaging (MRI)). MRI may need to be repeated using protocols suitable for the investigation of intractable epilepsy (see Chapter 24) and/or for assessing the state of the hippocampi (see Chapter 44). Routine MRI often fails to detect hippocampal atrophy, particularly when it is undertaken in a unit that does not specialize in the management of difficult to control epilepsy. Routine EEG may need to be repeated to exclude the presence of abnormalities suggestive of a primary generalized seizure disorder and prolonged

monitoring, with ambulatory cassette or video-telemetry, may be undertaken particularly if the episodic symptoms are frequent.

Nonepileptic conditions that may mimic epileptic seizures in adults are listed in Table 35.1. (See also Andermann 1993.) Particular attention should be given to the possibility that either the nonepileptic attack disorder or one of the various causes of syncope may underlie the apparently intractable epileptic symptoms. Lambert and David describe the features of the nonepileptic attack disorder in Chapter 34. Suffice it to say here that nonepileptic seizures have been reported in up to 25% patients undergoing video-EEG monitoring for the investigation of medically refractory seizures and that they may coexist with real epileptic seizures in up to 55% of cases.

Are the seizures focal (partial) rather than primary generalized?

Some primary generalized seizures, especially absence seizures and myoclonic jerks, may be exacerbated by carbamazepine and to some extent by phenytoin. Consequently it is important to establish correctly the seizure type(s) before defining a drug treatment regimen. This is best done by a combination of the clinical history and EEG. It must be remembered that some patients may have both primary generalized and focal seizures.

Table 35.1 Nonepileptic conditions that may mimic medically refractory focal epilepsy in adults.

Nonepileptic attack disorder
Syncope
   Cardiogenic syncope (Stokes–Adams attacks and other cardiac arhythmias, aortic stenosis, mitral valve prolapse, hypertrophic cardiac myopathy) ± secondary anoxic seizures
   Cough syncope
   Micturition syncope
Cataplexy
Parasomnias
   Night terrors
   Sleep walking
Dyscontrol syndrome
Idiopathic drop attacks
Paroxysmal dystonia, hemifacial spasm, dyskinesias
Multiple sclerosis tonic spasms
Metabolic
   Hypoglycemia
   Hypocalcemia
   Hypomagnesemia

Can the epilepsy syndrome be defined?

A very small number of adults with intractable focal epilepsy have the condition on the basis of an idiopathic localization-related epilepsy syndrome. The very large majority has it on the background of a symptomatic localization-related syndrome (see Chapter 2). A definite pathologic diagnosis should be achievable in at least 80% of this latter group. The more common forms of pathology are listed in Table 35.2. The diagnosis is usually based on data acquired from a detailed clinical history, as is described above, and from high-resolution brain imaging (see also Chapter 2). The importance of making a correct diagnosis of the epilepsy syndrome is that a more accurate prognosis can then be given and realistic treatment options, including possible surgery, can be defined.

SEIZURE-PRECIPITATING FACTORS

These should be carefully assessed. There is much individual variation but it is sometimes possible to recognize circumstances that increase the chances of a person suffering a seizure. Such circumstances include irregular antiepileptic medication with missed doses (see below), unaccustomedly high alcohol intake especially if followed by sleep deprivation, stress and other psychologic factors, and the taking of other medication that lowers the seizure threshold. Some women have the impression that their seizures are exacer-

bated in relation to a particular phase of their menstrual cycle but the keeping of a strict diary only rarely confirms this impression.

Many patients ignore advice to abstain from alcohol completely at all times. Consequently, it may be more practical to advise that intake should never exceed 2 units day^{-1}. Late nights, especially if accompanied by high alcohol intake, followed by early rising next morning can be a powerful stimulation to a seizure in people with focal seizure disorders, just as they can be for those with juvenile myoclonic epilepsy. Stress and other psychologic states may also increase the liability to seizures. The seizure frequency of people who are prone to such states may be reduced by psychologic techniques (see Chapter 38).

A number of therapeutic agents may precipitate or exacerbate seizures in some of those who take them. The drugs that may be important in relation to the apparent inability of medication to control focal epilepsy include tricyclic and other antidepressants, lithium, neuroleptics, baclofen, theophylline, and the higher-dose estrogen oral contraceptives (Brust 1999a). Drug abuse, especially with heroin, amphetamine, and cocaine, may also precipitate seizures (Brust 1999b).

DRUG HISTORY

A very careful history of AED use must be obtained. It is not always easy! By the author's definition the patient will have taken three of phenobarbital, phenytoin, carbamazepine, sodium valproate, and lamotrigine at 'optimal' doses either alone or in combination. An optimal dose is the maximum that can be tolerated, and/or the dose that gives the lowest seizure frequency, without any significant unwanted effect. It is not necessarily dependent upon any particular blood level. It may be achieved by increasing the dose until unwanted effects develop and then reducing the dose to the last level that was free from such effects. The aim is to determine which drug if any has been the most effective by ascertaining the seizure frequency during a period of stable dose on each. The patient's view of the relative severity of unwanted effects from each drug should also be recorded.

Compliance

This must be assessed. It will not necessarily be the same for all drugs. By *noncompliance* is meant that the patient does not take the medication regularly according to the regimen that has been agreed with the physician and that the latter believes to be operative. It is thought that around 25–50% of patients are noncompliant in this sense.

Table 35.2 Common causes of chronic intractable focal epilepsy in adults.

Cerebral vascular disease
  Cerebral infarction/hemorrhage
  Arteriovenous malformations
  Cavernous angioma
  Late effect of aneurysmal subarachnoid hemorrhage
Brain tumor
  Oligodendroglioma and low-grade astrocytoma
  Dysembryoplastic neuroepithelioma, ganglioglioma, hamartoma
  (these usually, but not invariably, have their habitual epilepsy
  commencing in childhood)
Brain trauma
Mesial temporal sclerosis (epilepsy usually commences in childhood or adolescence)
CNS infection
  Cysticercosis and tuberculoma (in some geographic areas)
  Late effects of subdural empyema and cerebral abscess, viral
  encephalitis (especially arborviruses, cytomegalovirus, herpes
  simplex, HIV, Japanese B, measles) and bacterial meningitis
  including tuberculous
Cerebral developmental disorders
  Cortical dysplasia
  Neuronal migration defects
Chronic alcoholism

Serial measurement of the blood AED concentrations is probably the most reliable generally available method for checking on compliance. On the whole, the best compliance is achieved with a drug that the patient perceives as well tolerated taken on a simple dose regimen once, or at most twice, per day at convenient times. Compliance falls when the number of doses rises above two per day (Cramer *et al* 1995).

DRUG REGIMENS FOR MEDICALLY INTRACTABLE FOCAL EPILEPSY

MONOTHERAPY

From the data quoted above it is clear that around 70% of those with newly diagnosed focal seizures enter remission relatively quickly. They are usually treated with only one of carbamazepine (CBZ), sodium valproate (SVP), lamotrigine (LAM), phenytoin (DPH), phenobarbital (PB), or primidone (PRIM). These six are licensed in the UK for monotherapy for epilepsy.

The advantages of monotherapy, if seizures can be controlled thereby, include lower toxicity and the avoidance of AED interactions. Furthermore, monotherapy gives the best opportunity to select the drug that is least likely to give any unwanted effects that might be especially disadvantageous for the individual patient (e.g. weight gain in an already overweight person, or a higher risk of teratogenicity in a woman contemplating pregnancy).

Control of complex partial seizures in newly diagnosed epilepsy

Heller *et al* (1995) did not find any significant difference in efficacy between PB, DPH, CBZ, and SVP for the control of newly diagnosed complex partial seizures. Likewise, Brodie *et al* (1995) found the efficacy of CBZ and LAM to be the same. Mattson *et al* (1985), however, found that CBZ achieved significantly better control than either PB or PRIM, and better control than DPH although the latter difference did not achieve statistical significance.

CBZ achieved better control of complex partial seizures than did SVP in the study of Mattson *et al* (1992) from the Veterans Affairs (VA) medical centers. The efficacy of the two drugs did not, however, differ significantly in the study of Richens *et al* (1994). These latter authors attributed the difference between their results and those from the VA centers to three aspects of study design. First, the patient

groups probably differed. More than 90% of the patients in the VA study were male, their mean age was >45 years, and around 30% had trauma-related epilepsy. The patients in the Richens *et al* (1994) study were younger, their mean age being only 33–34 years, and there was no stated predominance of a particular pathology. Second, more than half of those in the VA study had taken AEDs previously, whereas those in the Richens *et al* (1994) study were all newly diagnosed and previously untreated. Third, the VA study had a higher drop-out rate.

Another possible explanation of the difference between the findings of the two studies is that the epilepsy of the VA patients was more difficult to control and that CBZ is more efficacious than SVP for 'difficult to control' complex partial seizures. It is not easy to make a direct comparison between the two studies. Nevertheless, around 50% of patients in the Richens *et al* (1994) study seem to have remained seizure-free during the first year after starting treatment with either CBZ or SVP compared to only 30–34% in the VA study. This is consistent with the view that the latter group contained a higher proportion of patients with intractable epilepsy. A similar explanation might underlie the difference between the finding of Mattson *et al* (1985) that CBZ is more efficacious than PB, and that of Heller *et al* (1995) that the two do not differ significantly.

Control of secondarily generalized seizures in newly diagnosed epilepsy

PB, DPH, CBZ, SVP, and LAM appear to be of essentially the same efficacy (Mattson *et al* 1985; 1992; Brodie *et al* 1995; Heller *et al* 1995).

Toxicity and patient acceptability

Drug treatment failure, that is withdrawal of the drug because of unacceptable seizure frequency and/or untoward side-effects, occurred more often with PB and PRIM than with CBZ or DPH in the study of Mattson *et al* (1985). Similarly, in the Heller *et al* (1995) study the number withdrawn from the PB group (22%) was higher than for the DPH (3%), CBZ (11%), and SVP (5%) groups. In this latter study, the initial daily dose of each drug was low (PB 60 mg, DPH 200 mg, CBZ 400 mg, SVP 400 mg). The doses were increased to achieve plasma levels in the top half of the optimal range (PB 20–40 μg ml^{-1}, DPH 10–20 μg ml^{-1}, CBZ 4–11 μg ml^{-1}, SVP 50–100 μg ml^{-1}) only if seizures recurred despite good compliance. The unwanted symptoms leading to the withdrawal of PB are mostly drowsiness or lethargy and cognitive effects such as poor memory or concentration, depression, and loss of libido.

CBZ was withdrawn because of unacceptable side-effects more often than was SVP in both the study of Mattson *et al* (1992) and that of Richens *et al* (1994). In both, rash occurred significantly more often with CBZ and large weight gain and tremor occurred significantly more often with SVP. Withdrawal of CBZ because of rash usually occurred during the first 3 months of treatment. In the Brodie *et al* (1995) study, 49% of the CBZ group had withdrawn by the forty-eighth week, usually because of an adverse event, compared to only 35% of the LAM group (*P* < 0.02) even though the incidence of rash did not differ between the groups.

These rather sparse data suggest that PB and PRIM are the least acceptable of the six drugs because of their unwanted effects, and that SVP and LAM may be more acceptable than CBZ. The position of DPH is not clear. Overtly it seems as acceptable as CBZ and SVP but it may lead to less good compliance (Heller *et al* 1995). Although DPH, CBZ, SVP, and LAM seem equally efficacious for newly diagnosed focal seizures, it is not known whether they are equally efficacious for seemingly intractable focal seizures. Indeed, even though monotherapy is the treatment mode that has been recommended for intractable focal seizures (Aicardi and Shorvon 1998), few data concerning the differential effectiveness of the various AED for this form of epilepsy are available. There is simply the hint from the VA studies that CBZ may be better than DPH or SVP. Furthermore, there are other factors in AED selection that are important.

Alternative monotherapy

Schmidt and Gram (1995) suggest that up to 35% of newly diagnosed patients with focal seizures who do not respond adequately to one of CBZ or DPH taken as monotherapy may achieve complete seizure control with the second taken as monotherapy. Alternative monotherapy may also significantly reduce the seizure frequency of patients with intractable epilepsy. The converse must, however, be equally recognized. Thus, a change in medication may be followed by a deterioration of the seizure control rather than by the hoped-for improvement. A very careful drug history should be taken during the evaluation of a patient with intractable epilepsy. The purpose is to try to ascertain the drug, or drug combination, that has previously achieved the best seizure control without unacceptable side-effects, and also whether the previously tried drugs have been taken at optimal doses.

POLYTHERAPY

Only a small number of those whose seizures are not fully controlled by monotherapy achieve better control from a drug combination. Eighty-two patients whose seizures were not adequately controlled by monotherapy in the Mattson *et al* (1985) study were subsequently treated with a two-drug combination. The seizure frequency of 39% was reduced, at the expense of increased adverse effects, but only 11% became seizure-free.

The data presented by Schmidt and Gram (1995) indicate that 15% of patients who had failed to respond adequately to each of CBZ and DPH taken as monotherapy did so when the two were taken together. Presented in a different way, 67% of their patients were fully controlled by either CBZ or DPH taken as monotherapy and 5% by the two in combination, but 28% remained uncontrolled by these drugs taken either singly or in combination. With DPH and CBZ the adverse effect rate approximately doubles when the two are taken together compared to when either is taken alone. Thus, the antiepileptic effects of CBZ and DPH (pharmacodynamic interaction) are additive but the usefulness of this is limited because the neurotoxic effects are also additive. In contrast, with CBZ and SVP the pharmacodynamic effects are additive but the neurotoxic effects are infra-additive (Levy and Bourgeois 1998). This drug combination can be clinically useful.

Add-on of 'new' AED

A systematic review (Marson *et al* 1996) of published and unpublished randomized controlled trials of various new AEDs used as add-on treatment for intractable focal epilepsy suggested that:

1. There is a 50% reduction in the frequency of partial seizures of all types in 41% of patients given topiramate (TOP) compared to 10% for those given placebo, with a plateau for the therapeutic effect at 600 mg day^{-1}. The equivalent figures for the other five drugs considered are shown in Table 35.3.

Table 35.3 Seizure reduction with new AED. (After Marson *et al* 1996.)

Drug	% 50% responders	% Placebo 50% responders
Topiramate	41	10
Vigabatrin	40	14
Tiagabine	21	6
Zonisamide	25	11
Gabapentin	20	9
Lamotrigine	20	9

The studies with gabapentin (doses up to 1800 mg day^{-1}) and tiagabine (doses up to 56 mg day^{-1}) did not give any suggestion of a plateau effect. The authors stated that they did not have conclusive evidence of a difference in efficacy between the drugs, but they noted that TOP appeared to be the most effective and to be twice as effective as gabapentin, which seemed the least effective.

2. Gabapentin and lamotrigine appeared to be the best tolerated and patients were no more likely to withdraw from them than from placebo. Zonisamide appeared to be the worst tolerated.

As yet, in late 1999, no one of these drugs is licensed for monotherapy in the UK.

CONCLUSIONS

Ideas concerning the efficacy of the older drugs (PB, PRIM, DPH, CBZ, SVP) depend largely upon trials conducted with newly diagnosed patients or patients who have previously been inadequately treated. In contrast, ideas about the new AED depend upon trials where they are added to preexisting and necessarily variable drug regimens of patients with severe intractable focal seizure disorders. Only LAM spans the two groups. Paradoxically it appears the equal of the older drugs when used as monotherapy for newly diagnosed patients, but one of the least effective of the new drugs when used as add-on to treat patients with chronic intractable disorders. There are no large-scale trials comparing the new and the old beyond that of LAM vs. CBZ (Brodie *et al* 1995).

Some tentative conclusions may be drawn.

1. PB and PRIM should no longer be considered as first-line drugs because there is no evidence that they have greater efficacy than CBZ, SVP, DPH, or LAM and their adverse effects make them less acceptable to patients.
2. DPH, CBZ, SVP, and LAM seem equally efficacious for newly diagnosed patients, but few data are available for patients with intractable seizures beyond a hint that CBZ may give better control than SVP and DPH.
3. CBZ is rejected by patients more often than are SVP or LAM. Overtly DPH seems as acceptable as CBZ and SVP, at least in the short term, but it may lead to less good compliance. Furthermore, the long-term taking of DPH can lead to unwanted effects (see below and Chapter 40), as can the long-term taking of SVP (especially unacceptable weight gain constituting a health hazard). These effects could lead to DPH and SVP

losing their status as a first-line drugs for the treatment of intractable focal epilepsy.

4. Provided that CBZ can be tolerated, and that there is no particular contraindication to SVP (see below), each of CBZ, LAM, and SVP, and possibly also DPH, should be tried as monotherapy at the maximum tolerable doses before a decision is taken to give an extended trial of polytherapy.
5. For polytherapy, two of CBZ, SVP, LAM, and possibly DPH might be combined, such as, for instance, CBZ + SVP. Alternatively, one of the four might be combined with TOP or vigabatrin (VIG), these being the most powerful of the new add-on drugs. Possibly tiagabine (TIA) should also be considered especially as it is as yet little tried and VIG may pass out of favor because of its unwanted effects especially on vision (see below).
6. As with monotherapy, great care must be taken over possible toxic effects of polytherapy, and the precise combination that is chosen must depend upon the side-effect constraints of the individual patient.

SOME INDIVIDUAL ANTIEPILEPTIC DRUGS

For the reasons given above, currently most patients with medically intractable focal epilepsy will be best served by treatment with one of CBZ, LAM, SVP, and DPH, or with two of the four in combination, or with one of the four combined with TOP or VIG or possibly TIA. Brief profiles of these seven are given below. These descriptions have drawn heavily on the manufacturers' summaries of product characteristics or data sheets, given in the *1998–1999 Association of British Pharmaceutical Industries Compendium of Data Sheets and Summaries of Product Characteristics*, for: Epanutin (phenytoin) – Parke-Davis; Tegretol and Tegretol Retard (carbamazepine) – Novartis; Epilim (sodium valproate) – Sanofi Winthrop; Lamictal (lamotrigine) – Wellcome UK; Topamax (topiramate) – Janssen-Cilag Ltd; Sabril (vigabatrin) – Hoechst Marion Roussel Ltd. Information has also been taken from the *Summary of Product Characteristics* for Gabitril (tiagabine) – Sanofi Winthrop, which is too recent for the *1998–1999 Compendium*.

Neither PB nor PRIM are included because their side-effect profiles are such that they are no longer first-line drugs for long-term administration to patients with intractable focal epilepsy, although the occasional patient may require PB if unable to tolerate the other AEDs. Also, PB is a first-line drug for the management of convulsive status epilepticus (see below).

PHENYTOIN

DPH was introduced to clinical practice as an AED in 1938 (Merritt and Putnam 1938). Along with PB, it was the mainstay of AED treatment until well after the introduction of CBZ and SVP during the 1970s. Indeed, it was only during the 1990s that its popularity markedly declined, probably because of its recognized potential to cause irreversible unwanted effects after long-term use, and because its non-linear kinetics and complex interactions can make it difficult to use, particularly in combination with other drugs.

The comparative study of Heller *et al* (1995) showed that its efficacy in the treatment of newly diagnosed focal seizure disorders is the equal of PB, CBZ, and SVP, and only 3% of patients in the DPH-treated group of that study were withdrawn because of serious unwanted effects. There was, however, a suggestion of worse compliance with DPH than with CBZ or SVP, possibly because of subtle DPH-induced side-effects. The unwanted consequences of long-term treatment would not have been expected in a short-term (3-year) study. These latter include cosmetic effects (gum hypertrophy and gingivitis, hirsutism, acne, and coarsening of the features) and cerebellar atrophy.

Preparations

Capsules/tablets, infatabs, suspension, injectable.

Dose

For adults the oral maintenance dose should be sufficient to give blood concentrations in the range of 10–20 mg L^{-1} (40–80 μmol L^{-1}). This is usually achieved with 200–500 mg day^{-1}. It can be taken on once/day or twice/day regimens. The stable maintenance dose should be reached by increments over 3–4 weeks with dose changes being made no more frequently than once/7–10 days. Doses may need to be lower in the elderly and in those with liver damage.

Contraindications

Hypersensitivity to hydantoins; porphyria.

Interactions

1. Drugs raising blood DPH levels include: amiodarone, antifungals, chloramphenicol, chlordiazepoxide, diazepam, dicoumarol, disulfiram, H_2-antagonists, isoniazid, methylphenidate, omeprazole, estrogens, phenothiazines, phenylbutazone, salicylates, succinimides, sulfonamides, tolbutamide, trazodone, viloxazine; acute alcohol intake.

2. Drugs lowering blood DPH levels include: carbamazepine, folic acid, reserpine, sucralfate, VIG; chronic alcoholism.
3. Drugs having unpredictable effects on blood DPH levels: PB, SVP, antineoplastics.
4. DPH may impair the action of: antifungals, antineoplastics, oral contraceptives and estrogens, clozapine, warfarin, corticosteroids, digitoxin, rifampicin, dicoumarol, frusemide, theophylline.

Oral contraception

For the 'combined' pill a preparation containing at least 50 μg estrogen should be used. Breakthrough bleeding indicates that contraception cannot be assured (O'Brien and Gilmore-White 1993). The dose of the progestogen-only preparation should also be increased.

Pregnancy

There is an increased risk of fetal malformations, especially cleft lip or palate and cardiac anomalies, and there is risk of the fetal hydantoin syndrome (prenatal growth deficiency, microencephaly, mental deficiency). There have been isolated reports of malignancies, including neuroblastoma, in children whose mothers took DPH during pregnancy.

The lowest antiepileptic dose should be used preferably as monotherapy, folic acid supplements should be taken starting at least 3 months before conception, and antenatal screening (α-fetoprotein estimation and high-resolution ultrasound examination of the fetus) should be offered.

Plasma DPH levels should be monitored.

Vitamin K as a prophylactic against bleeding disorders in the newborn should be administered to the mother during the last 4 weeks of pregnancy and to the baby at birth.

Breast-feeding is not recommended by Parke-Davis (see *Data Sheet for Epanutin 1998–1999*).

Common dose-dependent side-effects

These include ataxia/nystagmus/vertigo, slurred speech, drowsiness, and encephalopathy (confusion, delirium) at high blood levels.

Serious unwanted effects

CNS

Dose-related ataxia/nystagmus, dyskinesias, irreversible cerebellar dysfunction and atrophy (which may present acutely), peripheral neuropathy.

Gastrointestinal

Toxic hepatitis and liver damage.

Bone

Osteomalacia, hypocalcemia, and rickets due to impaired vitamin D metabolism.

Skin

Allergic rash, other severe dermatitides, Stevens–Johnson syndrome, gum hypertrophy, hirsutism, acne, coarsening of features.

Blood

Bone marrow aplasia, megaloblastic anemia.

Immune system

Lupus erythematosus, lymphadenopathy ± features of serum sickness, immunoglobulin abnormalities.

Sex

Impotence and decreased libido.

CARBAMAZEPINE

Many authorities consider that CBZ is the AED of first choice for the control of focal seizures. Its efficacy in newly diagnosed focal seizure disorders, both complex partial and secondarily generalized, is at least equal to that of PB, DPH, SVP (Mattson *et al* 1985; 1992; Richens *et al* 1994; Heller *et al* 1995), and LAM (Brodie *et al* 1995). It does, however, have some disadvantages. Thus:

1. Around 10% of patients develop a hypersensitivity rash during the early weeks of treatment and this often results in withdrawal of the drug (Mattson *et al* 1992; Richens *et al* 1994; Brodie *et al* 1995; Heller *et al* 1995). Otherwise it has a good side-effect profile.
2. It is an enzyme-inducer that may reduce the therapeutic effectiveness of a number of other medications, including the contraceptive pill and other AEDs. From the clinical viewpoint these interactions are at least as complex as those of DPH.
3. It depresses cardiac atrioventricular conduction and thus may occasionally precipitate clinical features of cardiac arrhythmia. This can be a problem particularly in the elderly.
4. Absence seizures may be exacerbated.

Preparations

Tablets, retard tablets (to reduce peak plasma levels), chewtabs, liquid, suppositories.

Dose

The maintenance oral dose for adults is usually in the range of 800–1200 mg day^{-1} taken in two or three divided doses, irrespective of whether it is the standard or the retard preparation. The maintenance should be achieved via gradually increasing doses, over several weeks, from an initial 100 mg twice per day. Some patients have unwanted effects on 800 mg day^{-1} and will only tolerate lower doses. Others tolerate up to 2000 mg day^{-1}. Some patients require a higher dose when changing from the standard to the retard preparation. The dose should be increased by 25% when changing from an oral preparation to suppositories, except that the daily dose with suppositories is limited to 1000 mg. Optimum blood levels are 4–12 mg L^{-1} (20–50 μmol L^{-1}).

Contraindications

Previous sensitivity to CBZ or structurally related drugs (e.g. tricyclic antidepressants); treatment with monoamine oxidase inhibitors during the previous 2 weeks; cardiac atrioventricular conduction defects; previous bone marrow depression; porphyria.

Interactions

1. Drugs raising blood CBZ levels include: erythromycin, isoniazid, verapamil, diltiazem, dextropropoxyphene, viloxazine, fluoxetine, cimetidine, acetazolamide, danazol.
2. Drugs lowering blood CBZ levels include: PB, DPH, primidone, theophylline.
3. Complex interactions may occur with:

   (a) isoniazid – its hepatotoxicity may be increased
   (b) lithium – enhanced neurotoxicity despite lithium plasma concentrations within the therapeutic range
   (c) haloperidol/thioridazine/metoclopramide – increased neurologic side-effects
   (d) diuretics – leading to symptomatic hyponatremia
   (e) nondepolarizing muscle relaxants – unexpectedly rapid recovery from neuromuscular blockade
   (f) isotretinoin – unpredictable alteration of CBZ bioavailability.

4. CBZ may decrease the effectiveness of: contraceptive

pill, various AEDs (clobazam, clonazepam, etho-suximide, primidone, SVP, DPH), corticosteroids, alprazolam, cyclosporin, digoxin, doxycycline, felodipine, haloperidol, imipramine, methadone, theophylline, warfarin.

Oral contraception

For the 'combined' pill a preparation containing at least 50 μg estrogen should be used. Breakthrough bleeding indicates that contraception cannot be assured (O'Brien and Gilmore-White 1993). The dose of the progestogen-only preparation should also be increased.

Pregnancy

The risk of fetal malformations, including spina bifida, may be increased.

The lowest antiepileptic dose should be used preferably as monotherapy, folic acid supplements should be taken starting at least 3 months before conception, and antenatal screening (α-fetoprotein estimation and high-resolution ultrasound examination of the fetus) should be offered.

Plasma CBZ levels should be monitored.

Vitamin K as a prophylactic against bleeding disorders in the newborn should be administered to the mother during the last 4 weeks of pregnancy and to the baby at birth.

CBZ in breast milk is not considered a hazard to the baby.

Common dose-dependent side-effects

These include blurred vision, drowsiness or fatigue, dizziness or ataxia, nausea or vomiting, and headache.

Serious unwanted effects

Skin

Allergic skin reactions, Stevens–Johnson syndrome, various other dermatitides, hirsutism, hair loss, systemic lupus erythematosus-like syndrome.

Hematological

Aplastic anemia, agranulocytosis, thrombocytopenia, pure red cell aplasia, megaloblastic anemia, folic acid deficiency, acute intermittent porphyria.

CNS

Headache, abnormal involuntary movements, activation of psychosis, aggression, depression, loss of appetite.

Immune system

Multiorgan hypersensitivity disorder, aseptic meningitis with myoclonus and peripheral eosinophilia.

Cardiac

Arrhythmias, aggravation of coronary artery disease.

Endocrine

Hyponatremia and water retention leading to symptoms of water intoxication, gynecomastia, galactorrhea, impaired male fertility and abnormal spermatogenesis, hyperlipidemia.

Bone

Osteomalacia.

Liver

Jaundice.

Recommended monitoring

1. Blood counts – asymptomatic leukopenia occurs in around 10% of patients. CBZ needs be withdrawn only if the leukopenia is progressive, severe, or symptomatic.
2. Liver function tests – mild elevation of γ-glutamyl transferase and alkaline phosphatase is not an indication for withdrawing CBZ.

SODIUM VALPROATE

SVP is highly efficacious, and possibly the most efficacious, AED for managing primary generalized seizure disorders. It is not clear, however, whether it is the equal of CBZ for difficult to control complex partial seizures as has been mentioned above.

A major advantage of SVP is that it is only mildly enzyme-inducing and consequently has fewer drug interactions than CBZ. In particular it does not interfere with use of the oral contraceptive. There are, however, some important interactions with other drugs (see below).

Its disadvantages include a greater tendency than CBZ to cause unacceptable weight gain (Richens *et al* 1994) which can be to the extent of constituting a health hazard, a possibly greater tendency to cause maldevelopment (Anonymous 1994) and perhaps a tendency to cause abnormalities of insulin metabolism leading to hyperandrogenism and polycystic ovaries (Isojarvi *et al* 1996).

Preparations

Enteric coated tablets, crushable tablets, controlled-release tablets (to reduce peak plasma levels and give more even concentrations throughout the day), syrup, and an intravenous preparation.

Dose

Adults usually require a maintenance dose of 1000–2000 mg day^{-1}, in two or three divided doses, irrespective of whether the standard or the controlled-release form is taken. This range can be entered within 2–3 weeks of initiating treatment at lower doses.

Contraindications

Hypersensitivity to SVP; active liver disease and possibly a family history of severe drug-related liver dysfunction; porphyria.

Interactions

The effects of neuroleptics, monoamine oxidase inhibitors, and other antidepressants may be potentiated. The metabolism of LAM is inhibited and the dose of this drug should be reduced when combined with SVP. There may be interactions with: aspirin, warfarin, DPH, CBZ, PB.

Oral contraception

This is not affected by SVP.

Pregnancy

The risk of fetal malformations (including neural tube defects, facial dysmorphia, and multiple malformations) is increased. The incidence of neural tube defects in the babies of mothers taking SVP during the first trimester of pregnancy has been estimated as around 1–2%, and it is not certain that this is reduced by folic acid.

The lowest antiepileptic dose should be used in divided doses and preferably as monotherapy; the recommendation is that folic acid supplements should be taken starting at least 3 months before conception, and antenatal screening

(α-fetoprotein estimation and high-resolution ultrasound examination of the fetus) should be offered.

The concentration of SVP in breast milk is low and not considered a hazard to the baby.

Common dose-dependent side-effects

These include ataxia, tremor (occasionally permanent rather than dose dependent), sedation, lethargy, or stupor, or hallucinations.

Severe unwanted effects

Hematologic

Prolonged bleeding time and thrombocytopenia, reduced fibrinogen, red cell hypoplasia, leukopenia, pancytopenia.

CNS

Increased alertness, hyperactivity, aggression, hearing loss.

Skin

Hair loss, hair curliness, rashes, systemic lupus erythematosus-like syndrome.

Endocrine

Unacceptable weight gain, possibly related to altered insulin metabolism, polycystic ovaries.

Liver

Fatal liver failure.

Metabolic

Hyperammonemia (especially in association with ornithine transcarbamylase deficiency).

Pancreas

Fatal pancreatitis.

Recommended monitoring

Liver function tests during the first 6 months of treatment. Raised enzymes during the early stages of treatment are common. Monitoring (including prothrombin time) should be continued until they return to normal and treatment with aspirin should be avoided during that time. Blood clotting if spontaneous bruising occurs or surgery is intended.

LAMOTRIGINE

The results of the trial conducted by Brodie *et al* (1995) suggested that LAM is as effective as CBZ for the control of newly diagnosed partial seizures and more acceptable to the patients. It is not, however, known whether it exerts as good control as CBZ for intractable focal epilepsy. Furthermore, the meta-analysis of Marson *et al* (1996) suggested that LAM does not have particular potency when it is used as an add-on drug for refractory epilepsy.

A disadvantage of LAM is that the dose must be built up only very slowly to keep the risk of developing a rash to a minimum and so several weeks may elapse before therapeutically effective levels are achieved.

Preparations

Tablets, dispersible tablets.

Dose

For adult monotherapy: 25 mg day^{-1} for 2 weeks followed by 50 mg day^{-1} for 2 weeks, thereafter increasing by 50–100 mg every 1–2 weeks to a maintenance dose usually of 100–200 mg day^{-1} in one or two divided daily doses. Some patients may need doses up to 500 mg day^{-1}.

For add-on to SVP: 25 mg on alternate days for 2 weeks followed by 25 mg day^{-1} for 2 weeks, thereafter increasing by a maximum 25–50 mg day^{-1} every 1–2 weeks to a maintenance dose of 100–200 mg day^{-1}.

For add-on to enzyme-inducing drugs without SVP: 50 mg day^{-1} for 2 weeks followed by 100 mg day^{-1} for 2 weeks in two divided doses, thereafter increasing by a maximum of 100 mg day^{-1} every 1–2 weeks to a maintenance dose usually of 200–400 mg day^{-1}.

Contraindications

Hypersensitivity to lamotrigine; significantly impaired liver function.

Interactions

LAM does not effect the pharmacokinetics of other AEDs. Enzyme-inducers such as CBZ and DPH reduce the half-life of LAM to around 14 hours. SVP increases the half-life to around 70 hours.

Oral contraception

No effect.

Pregnancy

Insufficient data available, no teratogenic effects in animal studies.

Common dose-dependent side-effects

These include tiredness or drowsiness, headache, nausea or vomiting, dizziness, and insomnia.

Severe unwanted effects

Skin

Rash is usually maculopapular, appearing within 8 weeks of starting treatment. It can be severe including Stevens–Johnson syndrome or as part of a hypersensitivity syndrome with multiorgan failure. The risk of rash is <1/100 if the dose increase is slow, as recommended especially in the presence of SVP.

CNS

Tremor.

Blood

Leukopenia, thrombocytopenia.

Recommended monitoring

None.

TOPIRAMATE

TOP was the add-on drug with the most powerful seizure reduction effect in the meta-analysis of Marson *et al* (1996).

Many patients lose weight when taking TOP. This rarely constitutes a clinical problem and it is welcomed by many patients who have started treatment with a weight well above the ideal.

Preparations

Tablets.

Dose

The maximum recommended daily dose for adults is 800 mg taken in two divided doses. In the author's experience, the best chance of avoiding rejection by the patient because of unwanted effects is achieved by starting at 25 mg day^{-1} and increasing the daily dose by no more than 25 mg day^{-1} every 2 weeks.

Contraindications

Sensitivity to topiramate; history, or family history, of renal tract stone formation or concomitant medication that may increase the risk of stone.

Interactions

TOP may increase the plasma concentration of DPH. The plasma concentration of TOP may be reduced by DPH and by CBZ. There may be an interaction with digoxin.

Oral contraception

For the 'combined' pill, a preparation containing at least 50 µg estrogen should be used. Breakthrough bleeding indicates that contraception cannot be assured (O'Brien and Gilmore-White 1993).

Pregnancy

No information. Breast-feeding is not advised.

Common dose-dependent side-effects

These include fatigue or somnolence, impaired concentration, confusion or abnormal thinking, nausea or dizziness, limb paraesthesiae, taste perversion, paucity of speech, slowness, and amnesia.

Severe unwanted effects

These include increased risk of renal tract stone – most cases resolve by passage of the stone and the patient continues on the medication (Shorvon 1996).

Recommended monitoring

None

VIGABATRIN

Preparations

Tablets, sachets containing powder.

Dose

For adults an initial dose of 1000 mg day^{-1} in two divided doses increasing by 500 mg day^{-1} each week to a maximum daily maintenance dose of 2000–4000 mg day^{-1}.

Contraindications

Hypersensitivity to VIG; pregnancy; history of psychosis; defective visual fields.

Interactions

Blood DPH level may fall by around 20%.

Oral contraception

No effect.

Pregnancy

Insufficient information; breast-feeding not advised.

Common dose-dependent side-effects

These include drowsiness or fatigue, nervousness or irritability, headache, ataxia or tremor, impaired concentration or poor memory, and confusion or paresthesiae.

Severe unwanted effects

Psychiatric

Depression, psychosis (Ferrie *et al* 1996), hypomania.

Vision

Visual field constriction affecting peripheral vision (Krauss *et al* 1998) – the incidence of this unwanted effect is as yet unknown.

Weight

Weight gain.

Recommended monitoring

Close observation for adverse effects on neurologic function. Regular visual field measurements for early detection of visual field constriction.

TIAGABINE

There is as yet very little experience of the use of this drug.

Preparations

Tablets.

Dose

The recommendation is that the initial dose for adults already taking enzyme-inducing AEDs should be 10 mg day^{-1} in two divided doses during the first week followed by increments of 5–10 mg day^{-1} at weekly intervals to a maintenance dose of 30–45 mg day^{-1}.

For those not taking enzyme-inducing AEDs, the maintenance dose should be 15–30 mg day^{-1}.

For those with mild or moderate hepatic dysfunction, the maintenance dose should be 10–20 mg day^{-1}.

Contraindications

Severe hepatic dysfunction; history of serious behavioral problems.

Interactions

Enzyme-inducing AEDs enhance the metabolism of TIA and may reduce its plasma concentration by a factor of 1.5–3.0.

TIA reduces the plasma concentration of SVP by around 10%.

Oral contraception

No effect.

Pregnancy

Insufficient information. Breast-feeding is not advised.

Common dose-dependent side-effects

These include tiredness, dizziness, nervousness, concentration difficulties, diarrhea, tremor, depression and emotional lability.

Severe unwanted effects

None known as yet.

Recommended monitoring

Hematologic for leukopenia.

THE TREATMENT OF STATUS EPILEPTICUS

Status epilepticus has an incidence of around 5 cases per 10 000 population per year, of which approximately 50% are convulsive. Other forms that may occur in adults as a consequence of partial seizure disorders are complex partial status and epilepsia partialis continua.

Convulsive status has been defined as a convulsion continuing unabated for more than 30 min, or separate convulsions that are recurrent over a period of more than 30 min without recovery of consciousness between them. A convulsion of any duration may, however, cause irreparable damage and should be terminated as soon as possible. The commonest causes of status epilepticus in already established epilepsy are AED withdrawal, intercurrent illness, and progression of the underlying pathology. The risk of death directly attributable to the convulsive seizure has been estimated as 1–2%.

Complex partial status has been defined as a prolonged epileptic confusional state, with variable clinical symptoms due to frequently recurring epileptic discharges that may continue for days. Treatment is with intravenous benzodiazepine, or DPH, or PB.

Epilepsia partialis continua is defined as simple partial motor seizures with repetitive regular or irregular clonic jerks, of cortical origin, on a part of one side of the body without loss of consciousness. It may progress to generalized convulsive status. It can be extremely difficult to control with medication, and treatment (including surgical) should be directed at the underlying pathology.

TREATMENT OF CONVULSIVE STATUS EPILEPTICUS

This can be considered under the headings of general measures, immediate medication, second-stage medication, and third-stage management.

General measures

1. Secure the airway + give oxygen ± intubate and control respiration.

2. Examine the patient and attempt to establish the cause of the status. Failure to treat the prime cause may lead to failure to control the status.
3. Set up an intravenous line for the administration of fluids and drugs.
4. Initiate clinical monitoring and set up continuous ECG + oximetry.
5. Send blood for gases, full blood count, glucose, urea and electrolytes, liver function indices, and calcium.
6. Ensure that routine AED doses are maintained for those already on medication. Failure to do so may lead to failure to control the status.
7. Ensure that the patient has *epileptic* status since non-epileptic status is probably the more common condition.

Immediate medication for adults

This is usually with a benzodiazepine provided there is no history of benzodiazepine sensitivity, no acute pulmonary insufficiency, and no respiratory depression.

1. Intravenous *diazepam* 10–20 mg (0.15–0.25 mg kg^{-1} body weight) should be administered at a rate of <2–5 mg min^{-1} because of the risk of sudden apnea with faster injection (Valium Roche ampules contain diazepam 10 mg in 2 ml). Facilities for resuscitation should always be available when administering a benzodiazepine intravenously. The dose should not be repeated more than twice, or to a total dose >40 mg, because of the risks of respiratory depression and hypotension. Second-stage medication should be instituted if control is not achieved within a maximum of three doses or diazepam 40 mg.
2. Rectal *diazepam* 5–10 mg which can be repeated after 5–10 min is an alternative for situations where intravenous administration is not possible.
   or
3. Intravenous *clonazepam*, initially 1 mg, diluted as instructed, slowly over 30–60 s to keep the risk of apnea to a minimum. (Rivotril ampules contain clonazepam 1 mg in 1 ml solvent and are accompanied by an ampule containing 1 ml water for injection; the two should be mixed, giving clonazepam 1 mg in 2 ml, immediately prior to administration.) Clonazepam has a longer duration of action than diazepam. Up to 4 mg may be administered in the first hour.

   Intravenous maintenance therapy may then continue by a titrated infusion according to the following regimen:

   (a) Use clonazepam 3 mg (three ampoules) in 300 ml sodium chloride and dextrose solution (0.45% NaCl and 2.5% dextrose); this must be used within 12 hours of mixing.
   (b) Administer hourly:

       (i) 50 ml if there has been a seizure, during the previous hour.
       (ii) 10 ml less than previous dose if there has been no fit in the previous hour.

   Thus, the dose progressively falls if the convulsions have been aborted, but if they continue intermittently the total daily dose does not exceed clonazepam 12 mg (in addition to any loading dose).
   or
4. Intravenous *lorazepam* 0.07 mg kg^{-1} body weight to a maximum of 4 mg which can be repeated once after 20 min (Shorvon 1997). Ampules (Ativan Injection) contain lorazepam 4 mg in 1 ml. The contents should be diluted 1:1 with water for injection and should not be mixed with other drugs.

Second-stage medication for adults

One of these should be instituted without delay if there is any suggestion that the convulsion(s) will not be halted by the initial benzodiazepine or controlled by a continuing clonazepam infusion.

1. Intravenous *phenobarbital*. This is the drug of choice (Shorvon 1997) because it has excellent prolonged antiepileptic properties of rapid onset, most patients will not have been taking it as a routine AED, and it may have a cerebral protective action. The disadvantages are that it may cause respiratory depression and hypotension. Acute intermittent porphyria is a contraindication to its use.
   The dose is 10 mg kg^{-1} body weight to a maximum 1000 mg administered at a rate of 100 mg min^{-1}, followed by 1–4 mg kg^{-1} body weight per day given intravenously, intramuscularly, or orally. Suboptimal doses may be ineffective.
   Ampules (Gardenal Sodium) contain phenobarbital 200 mg in 1 ml. This must be diluted with water for injection to a concentration not >20 mg ml^{-1} immediately before administration.
2. Intravenous *phenytoin*. This is a first-choice drug for patients not using it as a maintenance AED, because it has excellent prolonged antiepileptic properties and causes relatively little respiratory depression. The disadvantages are that administration must be slow, and effective blood levels are not achieved until 20–30 min after the infusion commences. It is contraindicated for patients with sinus bradycardia, sinoatrial block,

second- and third-degree atrioventricular block, and Stokes–Adams syndrome.

The dose is 15–18 mg/kg^{-1} body weight, or approximately 1000 mg for an average-sized person. This must be administered slowly, not exceeding 50 mg min^{-1} (<30 mg min^{-1} in the elderly) because of the risk of potentially fatal cardiac arrhythmia. Suboptimal doses may be ineffective.

Ampules contain phenytoin (Epanutin Ready Mixed Parenteral) 250 mg in 5 ml, which should be diluted in normal saline to a concentration no greater than 10 mg ml^{-1}. Check that there is no precipitate. The infusion should be completed within 1 hour of mixing and carried out with continuous ECG and blood pressure monitoring.

3. Intravenous *fosphenytoin sodium* (Pro-Epanutin Parke-Davis). This is rapidly and completely converted to phenytoin *in vivo*. It is said to have the following advantages over DPH:

   (a) Fosphenytoin can be infused at three times the speed.
   (b) Fosphenytoin is significantly better tolerated at infusion sites.

   (c) Fosphenytoin can be administered intramuscularly with a rapid and predictable absorbtion *but this route should not be used for the treatment of status epilepticus* because therapeutic concentrations of phenytoin are not achieved as rapidly as with intravenous administration.

It is possible that intravenous fosphenytoin will replace intravenous phenytoin as a treatment for status epilepticus.

Third-stage management

This should be instituted, in an attempt to reduce permanent brain damage, if the convulsion has continued unabated for longer than 60 min. It can, however, be delayed if the seizures have become intermittent even though consciousness has not been regained, especially if there is a facility for EEG monitoring. Third-stage management consists of intubation, if that has not already been undertaken, along with the institution of intermittent positive pressure respiration and the administration of *thiopental* or *propofol* with EEG monitoring and under anesthetist control.

KEY POINTS

1. For the purposes of this book medical intractability has been defined operationally as a continuation of seizures beyond two years despite treatment with three of phenobarbital, phenytoin, carbamazepine, sodium valproate, or lamotrigine taken at 'optimal' doses either individually or in combination. Around 20% of people who develop focal epilepsy do not enter long-term remission within 10 years. The prevalence of focal epilepsy manifest by at least 12 seizures/year is considered to be around 0.75/1000 population.

2. The assessment of apparent medical intractability must consider the diagnosis of epilepsy, the seizure syndrome, and any underlying cerebral pathology, seizure precipitating factors, the anti-epileptic drug history, and compliance.

3. Only a small number of those whose seizures are not fully controlled by monotherapy achieve better control from a drug combination. The advantages of monotherapy include lower toxicity than with polytherapy and the avoidance of drug interactions. Carbamazepine, sodium valproate, lamotrigine, phenytoin, phenobarbital, and primidone are licensed in the UK for use as monotherapy for epilepsy.

4. In monotherapy comparisons these six drugs seem to be equally efficacious for the control of secondarily generalised seizures. Carbamazepine may achieve marginally better control of complex partial seizures than barbiturates, phenytoin, or valproate but no difference between carbamazepine and lamotrigine has been demonstrated.

5. Patient acceptability of a drug is determined by a combination of its efficacy and its unwanted effects. For monotherapy, lamotrigine probably achieves the highest acceptability amongst newly diagnosed patients, and barbiturates the least, but this might not be so amongst those with medically intractable seizures.

6. For those patients who may gain better control from a drug combination than from monotherapy, the drugs should be chosen to achieve additive pharmacodynamic effects but sub- or infra-additive neurotoxic effects. Carbamazepine with sodium valproate is an example of such a combination.

7. Of the drugs that do not have a UK monotherapy licence for partial seizure disorders, topiramate and vigabatrin seem the mostly likely to

KEY POINTS

bring about a 50% reduction in seizure frequency when added to a pre-existing drug regimen. They may also be the most likely to create unwanted effects.

8. The choice of a drug should take into account factors such as the probability of permanent unwanted effects arising, i.e. cerebellar atrophy with phenytoin and visual

failure with vigabatrin, and also whether the patient is likely to become pregnant.

REFERENCES

Aicardi J, Shorvon SD (1998) Intractable epilepsy. In: Engel J Jr, Pedley TA (eds) *Epilepsy: A Comprehensive Textbook*, pp 1325–1331. Philadelphia: Lippincott-Raven.

Andermann F (1993) Nonepileptic paroxysmal neurologic events. In: Rowan AJ, Gates JR (eds) *Nonepileptic Seizures*, pp 111–121. Boston: Butterworth-Heinemann.

Anonymous (1994) Epilepsy and pregnancy. *Drug and Therapeutics Bulletin* **32**:49–51.

Brodie MJ, Richens A, Yuen AWC (1995) Double-blind comparison of lamotrigine and carbamazepine in newly diagnosed epilepsy. *Lancet* **345**:476–479.

Brust JCM (1999a) Sezures and commonly prescribed drugs. In: Kotaga P, Luders HO (eds) *The Epilepsies: Etiologies and Prevention*, pp 427–436. San Diego: Academic Press.

Brust JCM (1999b) Seizures, ethanol, and recreationally abused drugs. In: Kotagal P, Luders HO (eds) *The Epilepsies: Etiologies and Prevention*, pp 449–455. San Diego: Academic Press.

Cockerell OC, Johnson AL, Sander JWAS, Hart YM, Shorvon SD (1995) Remission of epilepsy: results from the National General Practice Study of Epilepsy. *Lancet* **346**:140–144.

Cockerell OC, Johnson AL, Sander JWAS, Shorvon SD (1997) Prognosis of epilepsy: a review and further analysis of the first 9 years of the British National General Practice Study of Epilepsy, a prospective population-based study. *Epilepsia* **38**:31–46.

Cramer J, Vachlon L, Desforges C, Sussman NM (1995) Dose frequency and dose interval compliance with multiple antiepileptic medications during a controlled clinical trial. *Epilepsia* **36**:1111–1117.

Ferrie CD, Robinson RO, Panayiotopoulos CP (1996) Psychotic and severe behavior reactions with vigabatrin: a review. *Acta Neurologica Scandinavica* **93**:1–8.

Gilman JT, Duchowny M, Jayakar P, Resnick TH (1994) Medical intractability in children evaluated for epilepsy surgery. *Neurology* **44**:1341–1343.

Hauser WA, Hesdorffer DC (1996) The natural history of seizures. In: Wyllie E (ed) *The Treatment of Epilepsy: Principles and Practice*, pp 173–178. Baltimore: Williams and Wilkins.

Heller AJ, Chesterman P, Elwes RDC *et al* (1995) Phenobarbitone, phenytoin, carbamazepine, or sodium valproate for newly diagnosed adult epilepsy: a randomized comparative monotherapy trial. *Journal of Neurology, Neurosurgery and Psychiatry* **58**:44–50.

Isojarvi JIT, Laatikainen TJ, Knip M, Pakarinen AJ, Juntunen KTS, Myllyla VV (1996) Obesity and endocrine disorders in women taking valproate for epilepsy. *Annals of Neurology* **39**:579–584.

Krauss GL, Johnson MA, Miller NR (1998) Vigabatrin-associated retinal cone system dysfunction: electroretinogram and ophthalmologic findings. *Neurology* **50**:614–618.

Levy RH, Bourgeois FD (1998) Drug–drug interactions. In: Engel J Jr, Pedley TA (eds) *Epilepsy: A Comprehensive Textbook*, Vol 2, pp 1175–1179. Philadelphia: Lippincott-Raven.

Marson AG, Kadir ZA, Chadwick DW (1996) New antiepileptic drugs: a systematic review of their efficacy and tolerability. *British Medical Journal* **313**:1169–1174.

Mattson RH, Cramer JA, Collins JF *et al* (1985) Comparison of carbamazepine, phenobarbital, phenytoin, and primidone in partial and secondarily generalized seizures. *New England Journal of Medicine* **313**:145–151.

Mattson RH, Cramer JA, Collins JF; The Department of Veterans Affairs Epilepsy Cooperative Study No. 264 Group (1992) A comparison of valproate with carbamazepine for the treatment of complex partial seizures and secondarily generalized tonic–clonic seizures in adults. *New England Journal of Medicine* **327**:765–771.

Merritt HH, Putnam TJ (1938) A new series of anticonvulsant drugs tested by experiments on animals. *Archives of Neurology and Psychiatry* **39**:1003–1015.

O'Brien MD, Gilmore-White S (1993) Epilepsy and pregnancy. *British Medical Journal* **307**:492–495.

Richens A, Davidson DLW, Cartlidge NEF, Easter DJ (1994) A multicenter comparative trial of sodium valproate and carbamazepine in adult-onset epilepsy. *Journal of Neurology, Neurosurgery and Psychiatry* **57**:682–687.

Schmidt D, Gram L (1995) Monotherapy versus polytherapy in epilepsy: a reappraisal. *CNS Drugs* **3**:194–208.

Shorvon SD (1996) Safety of topiramate: adverse events and relationship to dosing. *Epilepsia* **37**(Suppl 2):S18–S22.

Shorvon S (1997) Tonic–clonic status epilepticus. In: Hughes RAC (ed) *Neurological Emergencies*, pp 123–150. London: BMJ Publishing.

Drug treatment: children

JT GILMAN

Children with medically refractory seizures are a distinct biologic subgroup of all epileptic children for whom repeated attempts to control seizures are unlikely to be successful. The burden of recurrent epileptic seizures exposes these children to increased risks of adverse drug effects, psychosocial morbidity and, in rare circumstances, death. The specific risk factors predictive of medical intractability can often be identified early in the course of the disorder, allowing clinicians to treat seizures aggressively while remaining objective regarding future outcomes. The nature of epileptic disorders found in children often differs from that in adults. For example, epilepsies in childhood are more likely to be developmentally or genetically based than those found in adults. In addition to differences in the epileptic disorders, there are biotransformation and drug disposition differences in children that necessitate special dosage considerations.

The pharmacotherapy of children with intractable focal epilepsy must account for a number of specific treatment issues that may not be applicable in the adult population. Treatment choices should be based on an equal comparison of efficacy and tolerability of individual antiepileptic drugs (AEDs). The spectrum of toxicity is often different in younger patients compared with adults. Adverse effects that are acceptable in adults may be cause for discontinuation of therapy in children. Intellectual, cognitive, and behavioral toxicity are particularly unacceptable and, if unavoidable, may justly lead to the label of intractability. Maintaining sustained effective AED serum concentrations in children

also requires specific attention. Accelerated gastrointestinal transit times, interactions with milk and infant formulas, and rapid drug elimination may present special management problems. Children may be mistaken as medically intractable if treatment is not individualized with these differences in mind. This chapter focuses on issues related to the treatment of intractable focal epilepsy in children and special management problems in the effective administration of AEDs.

DEVELOPMENTAL PHARMACOLOGY

EFFECTS OF CEREBRAL MATURATION

Evidence from experimental animal data suggests that differences exist between the mature and immature brain that may potentially influence antiepileptic efficacy, especially in newborns. It is known that the immature brain has increased susceptibility to both focal and generalized seizures, the etiology of which is probably multifaceted (Gottlieb et al 1977; Zouhar et al 1989; Mares and Trojan 1991; Velisek et al 1992). Excessive postsynaptic potentials increase excitability in the immature brain, while developmentally low concentrations of γ-aminobutyric acid (GABA) and GABA receptors diminish inhibitory processes (Coyle and Enna 1976; Swann and

Brady 1984; Michelson and Lothman 1989). This provides a fertile environment for the propagation of seizures in susceptible individuals. Additionally, the immaturity of the substantia nigra alters seizure expression and increases excessive electrical activity, presumably promoting intractability (Xu *et al* 1992; Moshe and Garant 1996). These features help to explain the changing seizure semeiology when epilepsy is developed early in life and furthermore may ultimately explain some of the epilepsy syndromes and seizure types that occur predominantly in young children.

Developmental differences in seizure susceptibility suggest the possibility of concurrent alterations in AED response. Moshe (1993) has proposed both qualitative and quantitative age-dependent differences. Qualitative differences are illustrated by the proconvulsant effects of baclofen in early life compared with an anticonvulsant action in older animals (Veliskova *et al* 1996). Developmental differences in GABA receptors suggest possible quantitative changes for antiepileptic agents targeted at the GABA receptor (e.g. phenobarbital). For example, higher serum phenobarbital concentrations are necessary to control seizures in most newborns. Efficacy rates can be increased from 32–39% (Painter *et al* 1978; Lockman *et al* 1979) to 77–85% (Gal *et al* 1982; Gilman *et al* 1989) by using higher serum concentrations than typically utilized in adults.

Drug concentration at receptor sites also affects drug efficacy in a quantitative fashion. The entry of drugs into the brain and cerebrospinal fluid depends on a number of properties, including blood–brain barrier permeability; active transport across the choroid plexus, cerebral capillaries, neuronal membranes, and glial cells; and extracellular fluid volume. Human brain specimens collected during neurosurgery or after neonatal death reveal that brain tissue uptake of therapeutic agents follows developmental trends. For example, brain/plasma ratios of phenobarbital increase with age from newborns to adults (Sherwin *et al* 1973; Houghton *et al* 1975; Painter *et al* 1981; Onishi *et al* 1984).

The clinical relevance of many developmental differences is still not completely understood. However, these pathophysiologic differences may explain the difficulty in controlling some neonatal seizures. Much has been learned about the hazards of extrapolating pediatric pharmacotherapy from adult data. For example, valproate-induced hepatotoxicity in children was entirely unforeseen based on adult safety data. As more data are collected from testing the newer AEDs in children, perhaps pharmacotherapy in the context of cerebral ontogenesis will become better defined.

DEVELOPMENTAL PHARMACOKINETICS

Changing drug disposition throughout the lifespan is associated with continual maturation and is particularly rapid in neonates and infants. Pharmacokinetic parameters obtained in early infancy are typically valid for only a very brief time due to rapid developmental changes (Gilman and Gal 1992). Figure 36.1 illustrates age-related drug disposition in relation to body size. These changes can have dramatic effects on AED serum concentrations and potential seizure control. Knowledge of maturational effects on drug disposition improves the ability to identify and solve problems with childhood AED therapy (Gilman 1990, 1994).

Absorption

Extravascular drug absorption depends on several important patient variables, including pH-dependent diffusion, gastric contents, gastric emptying time, and gastrointestinal motility (Radde 1985a). Although variable, these physiologic processes are clearly age dependent. Gastric pH displays a biphasic pattern postnatally, with the highest acid concentration between 1 and 10 days after birth and the lowest between 10 and 30 days after birth. The lower limit of adult values are achieved by approximately 3 months of age (Agunod *et al* 1969). Gastrointestinal absorption of enterally administered AEDs may be variable during this time and leads to poor seizure control.

The rate of gastric emptying is probably the most important single determinant of drug absorption. Gastric emptying rate is affected by gestational age, postnatal age, and type of feeding. Adult values are reached by the age of 6–8 months (Grand *et al* 1976). Gastric emptying is prolonged in the neonate (relative to adult standards), and peristaltic activity is irregular. Early data suggest that enteral phenytoin may be poorly absorbed in newborns (Painter *et al* 1978). Unfortunately, phenytoin absorption

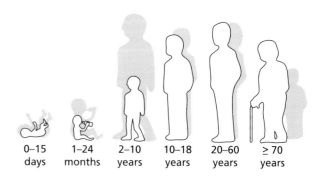

| 0–15 days | 1–24 months | 2–10 years | 10–18 years | 20–60 years | ≥ 70 years |

Fig. 36.1 Effect of age on drug disposition relative to adult standards. (Adapted from Gilman 1994.)

characteristics are complicated by its chemical and pharmacokinetic properties. Later studies have shown that low neonatal serum phenytoin concentrations can likewise be related to rapid metabolism (Whelan *et al* 1983; Leff *et al* 1986). In infants and children, gastric emptying time is shortened and splanchnic blood flow is higher, leading to faster drug absorption and, consequently, higher peak drug concentrations. Faster absorption rates have been reported for phenobarbital, carbamazepine, valproic acid, ethosuximide, and diazepam (Morselli 1983). When medications are absorbed more quickly, the variation in peak-to-trough serum drug concentration is larger and can lead to more adverse effects, less effective seizure control, or both.

Intestinal transit time and absorptive surface area are also diminished in young children (Grand *et al* 1976). Shorter transit time reduces the duration of drug contact with absorptive surfaces and decreases absorption. Products that have a long absorption phase (e.g. Tegretol 200 mg tablets), extended-release products, or products requiring larger absorptive surfaces (e.g. cyclosporin) may be incompletely absorbed in children (Gilman *et al* 1988). These differences are probably responsible for some of the variations in intrapatient serum concentrations observed in pediatric patients. Maturational changes in medication absorption also have important implications for serum drug concentrations. Product forms that are more easily absorbed (liquids, suspension, chewable/crushed tablets, etc.) should be used when low serum AED concentrations are attributable to poor oral absorption. AEDs are frequently abandoned as failures when high daily doses fail to achieve serum concentrations sufficient for seizure control. Poor gastrointestinal drug absorption should always be considered in the differential for low serum drug concentrations.

Acute diarrhea and other intestinal disorders are frequent in children and may intermittently affect drug absorption (Nelson *et al* 1972). Impaired drug absorption may also occur when medications are coadministered with formula or milk products. In older infants and children, most agents are absorbed into the systemic circulation at a rate and extent similar to that observed in adults (Heimann 1980).

Drug distribution

Drug distribution is influenced by such age-dependent factors as body compartment size and protein binding. The greatest disparity between fat and water compartments occurs during the first year of life (Friis-Hansen 1971). Alterations in drug distribution are seen with agents that are highly water or lipid soluble. These changes become important as they affect serum drug concentrations, particularly those obtained following a bolus or loading dose. Because AEDs have a slightly larger volume of distribution in newborns, serum concentrations may be lower than expected. Developmental differences in body compartments after the first year of life are insufficient to impact drug disposition (Kearns and Reed 1989).

Protein-binding changes have clinical significance usually only for agents with plasma protein binding of at least 90% (e.g. phenytoin and valproate). Agents with lower binding characteristics require large changes in protein binding to elicit clinical effects (Radde 1985b). The unbound (free) fraction of a drug is a pharmacokinetic variable that can change in various situations, including age, disease states, and concomitant therapy. Changes in protein binding either enhance or reduce tissue diffusion and have pharmacologic and therapeutic implications.

Physiologic factors that alter drug protein binding in newborns are covered extensively elsewhere (Radde 1985b). In general, however, protein binding in neonates is lower than that in older patient populations. This difference increases free drug fraction, tissue diffusion, and may alter effective serum concentration. Total proteins and plasma globulin concentrations are also decreased in infancy, with approximate adult values reached by 1 year of age. Developmental characteristics of α_1-acid glycoprotein, a major protein for drug binding, are still unclear in early childhood. It appears that drug protein binding may be altered in newborns and early infancy but should be similar to adult values by age 1 year (Radde 1985b).

Phenobarbital increases α_1-acid glycoprotein production and protein binding of some basic drugs (Brinkschulte and Breyer-Pfaff 1982). Other enzyme-inducing AEDs (carbamazepine, phenytoin, and primidone) also increase α_1-acid glycoprotein when administered as monotherapy (Tiula and Neuvomen 1982; Riva *et al* 1985). However, lower concentrations of α_1-acid glycoprotein have been reported in epileptic patients on polytherapy (Bruguerolle *et al* 1984). Similar to adults, protein-binding abnormalities also occur with certain illnesses (renal disease, carcinomas, diabetes, inflammatory disease, etc.), malnutrition, burns, and trauma (Zini *et al* 1990). Protein-binding displacements can sometimes create difficulties in AED management. Problems are more likely to be encountered when using combination therapy. Determination of the free (unbound) drug concentration in serum can also be met with technical difficulties. Drug can dissociate from protein *in vitro* if ultrafiltration of the specimen is not performed shortly after it is drawn (Albani *et al* 1983). This results in erroneously elevated free drug concentrations. If specimens are sent to a reference laboratory, ultrafiltration should be performed prior to shipping. In general, however, routine sampling of 'free' drug concentrations of AEDs is not necessary unless a problem is suspected.

Biotransformation, metabolism, and excretion

Most important drug biotransformations occur in the liver, although they can occur in almost any body tissue and at various subcellular sites within the tissues. An example of this is the transformation of fosphenytoin to phenytoin, which can occur almost anywhere in the body. This biotransformation reaction appears to be unaffected by age, as pharmacokinetic studies suggest complete conversion even in premature neonates (Morton et al 1997). These biotransformation reactions are typically classified into phase I and phase II reactions. Phase I reactions involve microsomal enzymes and include oxidation, reduction, and hydrolysis biotransformations. These pathways are thought to mature rapidly, reaching rates that are similar to, or in excess of, adult values by 6 months of age. It is interesting to note that agents which undergo biotransformation via phase I pathways frequently display faster elimination rates in children. AEDs with initial or primary biotransformation through phase I pathways include carbamazepine, phenobarbital, phenytoin, and primidone. Phase II reactions involve extramolecular changes that may be catalyzed by microsomal, mitochondrial, and/or cytoplasmic enzymes. These pathways include acetylation, glucuronidation, and conjugation and are thought to mature by 3 months of age (Kearns and Reed 1989). AEDs that undergo biotransformation via phase II pathways include valproic acid and lamotrigine.

During the first year of life, the metabolism of most AEDs is transformed from a state of reduced capacity to a level that exceeds adult values. Increased metabolic capacity is found in both phase I and phase II pathways. Changes in the ratio of liver to total body size occurs during periods of growth, with dramatic consequences for drug metabolism (Bach et al 1981). It is important to realize that when children are in a hypermetabolic phase where drug elimination is rapid, high AED doses are necessary to maintain effective serum concentrations (Gilman 1990, 1991). Frequently, agents are abandoned as failures after the perceived maximum dose has been tried. It is also worthwhile remembering that the manufacturer's recommended maximum daily dosages are based on adult elimination rates. Some children require almost twice the recommended dosage, particularly if agents are coadministered with enzyme inducers. In children, serum AED concentrations should be used as the dosage guide instead of the total $mg\,kg^{-1}day^{-1}$ dose administered (Gilman 1990, 1991).

Increased drug clearance in children is particularly prominent and troublesome with carbamazepine (Battino et al 1980), phenytoin (Bach et al 1981), and valproic acid (Hall et al 1985). Distinct correlations with drug clearance and age are well documented with these agents. Clearance rates decrease with increasing age in children older than 4 years. The need to administer high phenytoin doses is particularly bothersome because of its capacity-limited metabolism and risk for toxicity even with small dosage changes. However, the requirements necessary to maintain adequate serum concentrations in early infancy may be as high as $25\,mg\,kg^{-1}$ daily (Whelan et al 1983).

Another consequence of rapid metabolic capacity is the production of metabolites in quantities sufficient to elicit adverse or unwanted effects. Children typically have higher concentrations of the active metabolite of carbamazepine (carbamazepine 10,11-epoxide) compared with adults and a higher conversion of primidone to phenobarbital (Pynnonen et al 1977). This faster transformation from parent drug to metabolite exceeds the capacity to eliminate the metabolite, permitting metabolite accumulation. Other adverse effects that may be related to increased metabolite formation include valproic acid-induced hepatotoxicity, hypersensitivity reactions with carbamazepine, phenytoin, phenobarbital, and primidone, and cutaneous reactions with lamotrigine.

As children approach puberty, AED biotransformation begins to slow toward adult values. The reduction in drug clearance may increase serum concentrations and result in toxicity. However, the change in body size during this time usually compensates for the slower clearance by permitting the child to outgrow the dose (Pippenger 1983).

Renal function also displays age-dependent maturity. Glomerular filtration rate approaches adult values by approximately 3–5 months of age. Tubular secretory and reabsorptive capacity matures at a slower rate, with adult values attained at approximately 7 months of age (Kearns and Reed 1989). The role of renal elimination may become more important with some of the newer agents (gabapentin and vigabatrin).

ASSESSMENT OF DRUG-RESISTANT EPILEPSY

DEFINITION

Pharmacoresistant or medically intractable epilepsy are synonymous terms to describe epileptic individuals who have not achieved desirable seizure control. It is difficult to ascribe a universal definition of these terms because many different situations can render intractability. Treatment failure may relate to intolerance of adverse drug effects or simply the inability to suppress seizure activity despite maximally tolerated drug doses. Clinicians are often pressed for a definitive definition since most patients are required to demonstrate pharmacologic intractability prior to consideration for epilepsy surgery. The term 'intractability' has also been used to describe the duration patients have remained uncontrolled. A minimum period of 2 years is generally considered reasonable, although some patients may exhibit such frequent seizures that a 2-year wait prior to surgical intervention would be regarded as unethical. In our own investigations, it appears that ultimate seizure control is unlikely if therapy has been unsuccessful with at least three first-line agents as high-dose monotherapy and at least one combination trial (Gilman *et al* 1994). While a 'cookbook' definition and time period may be helpful, each case requires individual assessment.

THERAPY EVALUATION

Efficacy assessments

The diagnosis of pharmacoresistant epilepsy can be made easier with an accurate medication history that documents serum AED concentrations, seizure frequency, and adverse effects. When assessing pharmacoresistance, it is often helpful to have a standardized medication list to ensure a good therapeutic trial of each agent. A methodical examination of the child's treatment history can often uncover pseudorefractory epilepsy. Up to 10% of patients derive significant benefit by correcting treatment flaws if a major agent has been inadvertently overlooked or serum concentrations have not been adequate. The likelihood of achieving freedom from seizures with pharmacotherapy is greatly diminished if there is documented failure to three or more agents in different mechanistic categories (Gilman *et al* 1994).

Maximizing serum concentrations without adverse effects is a difficult task in children. Their rapid metabolism and potentially poor oral absorption, and the lack of suitable product formulations constitute treatment problems that are not easily overcome. In the assessment of children with uncontrolled seizures, it may be helpful to obtain serum concentrations before both the evening and morning doses as morning troughs may be very low in young children. If it is determined that the inability to sustain sufficient serum concentrations has compromised therapy, clinicians should refer to the section on treatment strategies later in this chapter for methods aimed at resolving these problems.

In any therapy assessment, compliance should be evaluated. Similar to adults, compliance is problematic in children with chronic illnesses. Noncompliance is listed as a primary etiology for low or widely fluctuating serum concentrations. Noncompliance rates are 30–40% in pediatric patients and increase proportionately with the number of medications the child is required to take (Gilman 1990; Cramer 1995). The preferred method of compliance assessment is pharmacokinetic analysis of multiple specimens obtained within the same dosing interval. If this is unavailable, then serial monitoring of steady-state AED serum concentrations, several days to a week apart, can be used as a tool. These specimens should not vary by more than 10% if drawn at approximately the same time of day on the same dosage schedule. Pill counts and prescription refill rates have also been used as a measure of compliance.

Adverse drug effects

The occurrence of adverse drug reactions is felt to be the single most important determinant in successful AED therapy. Most of the noncompliance and inability to retain patients on AEDs relates to the extent of drug-related side-effects (Mattson *et al* 1985). Since adverse drug events and uncontrolled seizures both erode quality of life, it is often difficult to separate their relative contributions for any given patient. Quality of life has become as important as seizure frequency in making a diagnosis of intractable epilepsy. As a result, patients with controlled seizures may also be medically intractable if they experience a poor quality of life related to unavoidable adverse drug effects. The most prominent adverse effects leading to AED withdrawal in children are behavioral changes (irritability, sleeplessness, hyperactivity, aggressiveness) and declining cognitive function (Herranz *et al* 1988). Often, these behaviors are attributed to parenting issues, underlying neurologic disorders, and/or periictal events and are not recognized as adverse drug effects. There are notable changes in behavior and alertness when children are withdrawn from AEDs for epilepsy surgery evaluation. Figure

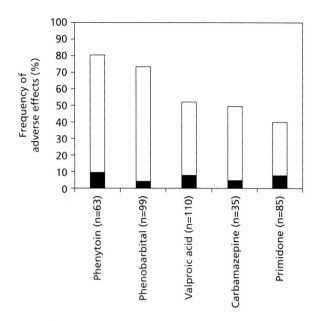

Fig. 36.2 Frequency of adverse effects of monotherapy with antiepileptic agents in 392 pediatric outpatients. Hatched area indicates the percentage of children withdrawn from therapy; total bar height represents the overall frequency of adverse effects with each agent. (Adapted from Herranz *et al* 1988.)

36.2 illustrates the frequency of adverse drug effects with some of the older AEDs.

Parents are likely to request a therapy change even in the face of good seizure control if a decline in school performance is perceived. For most AEDs, cognitive changes are probably subtle and only discernible with neuropsychologic testing (Meador *et al* 1990). The most demonstrative cognitive changes are associated with phenobarbital therapy. Farwell *et al* (1990) studied the effect of phenobarbital on the intelligence of 217 young children with febrile seizures. This study demonstrated a mean drop in IQ of 8.4 points ($P = 0.005$) in the phenobarbital-treated children (over a 2-year period) compared with the placebo group. Although there were some methodologic limitations, other reports of cognitive problems with phenobarbital seem to substantiate this report (Bourgeois *et al* 1983; Vining *et al* 1987).

The other AEDs have varying effects on cognition. Phenytoin is usually associated with some cognitive impairments, although these effects are less evident with valproate and minimal with carbamazepine (Aman *et al* 1987, 1990; Gallassi *et al* 1988). Neuropsychologic functioning has not been formally investigated with the more recently released AEDs, except for vigabatrin. Multiple studies have shown that vigabatrin has no detrimental effects on cognitive function and some suggest improved cognitive effects (Monaco 1996; Provinciali *et al* 1996; Monaco *et al* 1997).

Allergic hypersensitivity reactions can be unfortunate adverse events, particularly if the child is well controlled. The most notable group of AEDs that share this reaction are the aromatic compounds (carbamazepine, phenytoin, phenobarbital, primidone). Among these agents, phenytoin has been reported to cause the highest incidence of rash requiring hospitalization for 5 days or more (Snodgrass 1997). Hypersensitivity reactions can range from a simple skin rash to Stevens–Johnson syndrome, toxic epidermal necrolysis and, rarely, death. A postulated mechanism includes the accumulation of arene oxide metabolites, a phenomenon that may be more prevalent in children with a rapid metabolism. Cross-reactivity between these agents is high ($\geq 70\%$) but can be tested *in vitro*. If this reaction occurs, it is likely that other agents in this group will elicit a similar reaction (Schlienger and Shear 1998). It should be noted that the benzodiazepines should be used for seizure management in the acute stage of the reaction. Sodium valproate is generally a safe agent in hypersensitive children but should be avoided until the rash clears because it may further delay the elimination of arene oxide metabolites (Griebel 1998). Hypersensitivity poses a real treatment dilemma in susceptible children because its occurrence eliminates treatment with some of the most effective AEDs.

Lamotrigine-induced cutaneous eruptions do not seem to be related to the production of arene oxide. The incidence of this reaction is much higher in children, particularly if they are comedicated with valproate. Often this rash can be avoided with a very slow dosage titration when therapy is initiated. If the rash is mild, children may respond without hypersensitivity to a rechallenge at a lower dose and slower titration. However, if the reaction is more severe, a rash is likely to reemerge with a rechallenge (Besag *et al* 1995; Dooley *et al* 1996).

Valproic acid is a drug of choice in many childhood syndromes and generalized epilepsies, and an alternate agent for focal epilepsies. Other agents seem to be considerably less effective in some of these disorders. Treatment can become problematic when serious adverse reactions such as hepatotoxicity or pancreatitis limit therapy. Alterations in liver function tests are expected with valproate treatment, although once it becomes clear that these changes are higher than expected, therapy should be discontinued (Dreifuss *et al* 1987). Likewise, pancreatitis is a well-documented adverse effect of valproate; therapy should be immediately discontinued and patients should not be rechallenged (Wyllie *et al* 1984). Other adverse effects that are not life-threatening but which may affect compliance include weight gain, alopecia, and hyperactivity.

Drug interactions

Drug interactions can complicate therapy and render assessments more difficult. Understanding the occurrence and basis for drug interactions can provide valuable information in determining if therapy can be improved. Interactions occur on one of three levels: biotransformation, pharmacokinetics, and pharmacodynamics. The most dramatic interactions occur when biotransformation pathways are affected. Biotransformation reactions create three distinct mechanisms that influence a drug's pharmacologic effect.

1. Conversion of an inactive precursor or prodrug to a pharmacologically active compound, an example being the conversion of fosphenytoin to phenytoin.
2. Extension of pharmacologic effect through the transformation of the active parent compound to an active metabolite, an example of which is the biotransformation of diazepam to its active metabolites and oxcarbazepine to the active 10-monohydroxy derivative.
3. Inactivation of the active parent compound to an inactive metabolite, such as that seen with phenytoin.

Agents are considered accomplices if they either inhibit or induce biotransformation pathways and substrates if their serum concentrations are affected by accomplice isoenzyme alterations (Virani et al 1997; Gilman 2000). Many of the AEDs can act as either accomplices or substrates. The enzyme-inducing agents (carbamazepine, phenobarbital, phenytoin) are inducer accomplices and increase the metabolism of agents that undergo biotransformation through those pathways, which in the case of carbamazepine can be itself (autoinducer). On the other hand, many of these agents themselves undergo biotransformation and are susceptible to substrate interactions. Carbamazepine acts as a substrate when coadministered with the macrolide antibiotics (erythromycin, clarithromycin), and in this situation serum carbamazepine concentrations can increase twofold (Wong et al 1983; Tatum and Gonzalez 1994).

Pharmacokinetic interactions tend to be less dramatic than those interfering with biotransformation pathways. Interference with gastrointestinal absorption can complicate phenytoin therapy, especially in young infants. The interaction between phenytoin and enteral feedings has been recognized for over a decade (Bauer 1982; Krueger et al 1987). Since phenytoin's elimination half-life is concentration dependent, when absorption is impeded with enteral or infant feedings the maintenance of adequate serum concentrations becomes difficult. If serum phenytoin concentrations fail to rise after several attempts at optimizing absorption, it is probably better to seek treatment with an alternate AED.

Although there has been considerable investigation regarding the role of protein binding and AED therapy, protein-binding displacement interactions usually do not lead to serious adverse effects. Only agents with ≥ 90% protein binding can be displaced enough to create a clinical concern. Among the AEDs, this applies only to valproic acid and phenytoin. When these two agents are administered in tandem, unbound phenytoin concentrations are higher than expected and effective total concentrations are lower. It is usually not necessary to monitor unbound concentrations as long as the treating physician realizes that lower total phenytoin concentrations are still therapeutic. In most instances, when unbound concentrations begin to rise, clinical toxicity manifests and signals that a dosage reduction is in order. When adding agents from other therapeutic categories to a phenytoin regimen, it is prudent to check the protein-binding affinity of the added agent. High-dose salicylates are known displacing agents from protein-binding sites. The displacement of valproic acid usually is not problematic since its protein binding is saturable (Zaccara et al 1988); among the AEDs, this applies only to valproic acid and phenytoin.

Pharmacodynamic interactions are harder to predict than those dependent upon pharmacokinetic or biotransformation mechanisms. This reaction is evidenced by the production of a synergism or antagonism between two agents that leads to unexpected adverse or therapeutic effects. The interaction is more than additive, is unrelated to a change in serum concentrations, and presumably occurs at the receptor site. An example of this is the enhanced cerebellar dysfunction observed when lamotrigine is added to existing carbamazepine therapy. Neither carbamazepine nor carbamazepine 10,11-epoxide serum concentrations change significantly under controlled conditions (Maly et al 1997). These symptoms usually resolve when carbamazepine dosages are lowered.

When determining if a patient is pharmacologically intractable it is important to determine if drug interactions are responsible for either the lack of response due to compromised serum concentrations or intolerable adverse effects. If this is the case, therapy may be improved by implementing changes that would eliminate or compensate for the adverse interaction. A more extensive discussion of AED interactions appears in Gilman (2000).

TREATMENT STRATEGIES

Treatment success largely depends on seizure type and the underlying neurologic disorder. Seizure control for partial seizures is generally achieved in 72% of children (Scarpa and Carassini 1982), while less than 40% with complex partial seizures attain seizure remission (Resnick 1990). Data from adults suggest that carbamazepine and phenytoin are comparable first-line treatments for partial and secondarily generalized tonic–clonic seizures. Phenobarbital offers intermediate success, primidone the lowest, primarily because of drug intolerance (Mattson *et al* 1985). Valproic acid is equivalent to carbamazepine for secondarily generalized seizures but is less beneficial for complex partial seizures (Mattson *et al* 1992). Despite the comparable efficacy of carbamazepine and phenytoin (Ramsay *et al* 1983), carbamazepine is the preferred agent for chronic therapy in children because of the potential cosmetic and cognitive side-effects of phenytoin. If carbamazepine is ineffective, other agents, including the newer AEDs, should be substituted. The adverse effects of the second-line agents should be carefully weighed against the expected benefit of treatment.

Table 36.1 lists the AEDs of choice for use in pediatric seizure disorders. It should be noted that these selections differ somewhat from adult recommendations. Historically, AED selection for childhood seizures relied on comparative adult efficacy studies. Over the past decade, it has become clear that adverse drug effects often emerge as a major determinant in the ultimate choice of chronic therapy in children. Treatment must therefore strike a reasonable balance between efficacy and toxicity. Table 36.1 reflects these considerations and consequently many agents considered as first choice in adults are used as second or even third choices in children.

Once a therapeutic agent has been selected, maintaining effective serum concentrations can be pivotal in successful treatment. Pediatric dosing strategies must be tailored to individual metabolisms. Low serum AED concentrations in children are frequently attributed to their rapid metabolism. However, the differential should also include poor or erratic oral absorption and noncompliance. This assessment is best accomplished with three serial serum concentrations obtained within the same dosing interval. In order for enough time to elapse between specimens, it may be necessary to delay the next dose. The first specimen should be obtained two or more hours after the dose is administered. Rapid drug elimination is evidenced by large differences in the peak and trough serial specimens. Poor or erratic absorption typically has smaller variations, with low peak concentrations and a serum concentration–time curve that is frequently more flattened.

Younger children commonly have subtherapeutic morning trough concentrations due to the 12-hour span between doses. This frequently results in low early morning serum concentrations and potentially compromised seizure

Table 36.1 Therapeutic recommendations for childhood epilepsy.

Disorder	Drugs of first choice	Drugs of second choice	Drugs of third choice	Adjunctive agents
Epileptic disorders				
Primary generalized tonic–clonic seizures	Carbamazepine, valproic acid	Lamotrigine, oxcarbazepine	Felbamate, phenobarbital, phenytoin, primidone, topiramate	Benzodiazepines, ethotoin
Partial seizures[a] (simple and complex)	Carbamazepine	Gabapentin, lamotrigine, oxcarbazepine, vigabatrin	Phenobarbital, phenytoin primidone, tiagabine, topiramate, valproic acid	Ethotoin
Atypical absence, atonic, myoclonic seizures	Valproic acid	Benzodiazepines, lamatrigine	Felbamate, phenobarbital, primidone	
Childhood syndromes				
Juvenile myoclonic epilepsy	Valproic acid	Benzodiazepines, lamotrigine	Acetazolamide	Corticosteroid
Lennox–Gastaut syndrome	Valproic acid	Benzodiazepines, felbarnate, lamotrigine, topiramate, vigabatrin	Carbamazepine, oxcarbazepine, phenytoin	Corticosteroids
Typical absence seizures	Ethosuximide	Lamotrigine, valproic acid	Benzodiazepines	
West syndrome (infantile spasms)	Vigabatrin[b]	Corticosteroids, valproic acid	Benzodiazepines	

[a] Partial seizures with and without secondary generalization.
[b] In countries where available.

protection. Waking a child for nighttime medication is generally not recommended. Frequently a higher bedtime dose or alternate product formulation resolves this problem. Oral solid formulations (carbamazepine tablets, Depakote Sprinkles) or sustained-release products (Carbatrol, Tegretol XR) have a slower absorption rate and avoid low morning troughs (Gilman 1990).

Large variations in serum peak-to-trough AED concentrations are common in children. This creates a greater risk for breakthrough seizures, adverse effects, and intractability. In children 1–10 years of age most AEDs should be administered thrice daily due to their shorter half-lives. Even with frequent dosage administration, swings in peak-to-trough serum concentrations may be unacceptably large, especially in younger children. Solid oral dosage forms (compared with liquids) overcome this problem by providing a longer absorption phase that reduces peak and increases trough concentrations. Crushed tablets are generally preferable to liquids in younger children with a rapid metabolism (Gilman 1990; Gilman and Duchowny 1994). Carbamazepine sustained-release formulations provide minimal changes in serum concentrations in older children but may require thrice-daily dosing schedules in some children.

Stabilizing serum concentrations in some children may not be attainable. In these situations, the child is best served by changing drugs. Conversely, therapy may simply be ineffective despite maximal serum concentrations. Older treatments such as methsuximide (Tennison *et al* 1991), amantadine (Shields *et al* 1985), allopurinol (Tada *et al* 1991), bromide therapy (Woody 1990), and ketogenic diet (Kinsman *et al* 1992; Craig *et al* 1997) have met with varying success in children with intractable epilepsy. In most cases, patients respond better to simplified regimens using as few AEDs as possible (Schmidt 1983). Many of the newer agents have the advantage of lacking dependency on serum concentrations for efficacy and have fewer toxicities than older remedies reserved for intractable epilepsy.

ROLE OF NEW AND INVESTIGATIONAL AGENTS

WHEN TO USE THESE AGENTS

There is a continual need for the development of more selective and less toxic AEDs, especially for children. The research, development, and marketing thrust of the newer agents is focused on quality of life as much as efficacy issues. The use of most investigational AEDs significantly benefits 20–25% of children with intractable epilepsy. However, freedom from seizures is achieved in probably less than 5%. The availability of investigational agents is essential in providing hope for these children's families, especially when other options have been exhausted. The added benefit is the generation of valuable pediatric data under controlled conditions, which enhances our knowledge of pediatric use prior to marketing.

The newer AEDs are creating a niche in the selection scheme for childhood seizure disorders. It remains to be determined, however, whether these agents will significantly affect the long-term care and outcome of refractory childhood epilepsies. Some of these agents offer significant advantages over older treatments, particularly in the area of adverse effects. It seems clear that while the newer agents may not be first-line treatment choices at this point, they should probably be considered earlier rather than later if first-line agents fail. Suggestions of where these new agents may benefit children have been incorporated into Table 36.1.

AVAILABLE PEDIATRIC DATA

The pediatric initiative has resulted in well-organized, double-blind, placebo-controlled, multicenter studies for most of the new and investigational agents that have provided valuable pediatric data. Ongoing investigations are underway with topiramate, tiagabine, vigabatrin, lamotrigine, oxcarbazepine, and remacemide.

Among the newer agents the most pediatric experience has been gained with vigabatrin, although much has been in uncontrolled, open-label investigations. There have been no double-blind vigabatrin studies in children with partial seizures published to date. A meta-analysis of five large open-label pediatric studies indicated that 43% of the treated children experienced at least a 50% reduction in seizures (Ferrie and Robinson 1995). Of particular interest is the efficacy of vigabatrin in the treatment of infantile spasms, especially if coexisting with tuberous sclerosis. Children with tuberous sclerosis and infantile spasms respond well to vigabatrin therapy, with a remission rate of up to 96% (Chiron *et al* 1991, 1997; Aicardi *et al* 1996). In children with other etiologies, the response rate appears to be comparable to that with adrenocorticotropic hormone (ACTH) (Aicardi *et al* 1996). Response is also reportedly good in children with tuberous sclerosis and other seizure types (Curalto 1994). Behavioral side-effects (hyperactivity, psychosis), excessive sedation, and change in muscle tone in infants are commonly reported problems (Gram *et al* 1992). Of more concern, however, are the reports of irreversible visual field loss which in some cases may progress to complete blindness (Krauss *et al* 1988). This serious adverse effect will undoubtedly limit the use of vigabatin to only the most intractable patients.

Lamotrigine has been well studied in the pediatric population. It possesses a wide clinical spectrum, effective in both partial and generalized epilepsies. Currently, much of the pediatric data is still unpublished, although lamotrigine has been investigated in randomized trials for intractable childhood partial seizures (Graf *et al* 1997), Lennox–Gastaut syndrome (Motte *et al* 1997), absence epilepsy and a pediatric single-dose pharmacokinetic trial (Chen *et al* 1997). In Lennox–Gastaut syndrome, 33% of the patients experienced at least a 50% reduction in seizure frequency (Motte *et al* 1997). Open-label studies in children indicate that approximately 34% with intractable epilepsies demonstrate at least a 50% seizure reduction (Wallace 1994; Besag *et al* 1995, 1997). Although uncontrolled, some open-label studies suggest that the rate of seizure freedom achieved in intractable children can be as high as 10–18% (Battino *et al* 1993; Uvebrant and Bauziene 1994). It has also been suggested that lamotrigine is beneficial in combination with valproate in the treatment of infantile spasms (Veggiotti *et al* 1994). The major disadvantage has been the higher incidence of cutaneous reactions in children and the necessity of initiating therapy slowly to avoid this hypersensitivity. If the dosage is titrated carefully, it appears that the rash rate is probably no higher than that seen with carbamazepine (Besag *et al* 1995). However, families are often reluctant to wait a month to reach effective doses. Short-term benzodiazepine usage may be necessary for controlling seizures during titration.

Gabapentin was studied early in clinical testing for the treatment of drug-naive childhood absence epilepsy but was temporarily withdrawn from development. The pediatric study was not completed when clinical testing resumed. However, data analysis of children randomized suggested that gabapentin has little effect against absence epilepsy at doses up to 20 mg kg^{-1} daily (Trudeau *et al* 1996). There have been no large pediatric, randomized, placebo-controlled trials published to date. Gabapentin has been used in refractory partial seizures, with 34% of treated children exhibiting at least a 50% reduction in seizure frequency (Khurana *et al* 1996). Oral gabapentin relies on an active transport system for gastrointestinal absorption, creating a dose-dependent bioavailability and lower extent of absorption (60%). Plasma drug concentrations are not directly proportional to the dose administered and absorption rates decline further (about 35%) as daily doses are increased over 4 g (McLean 1994). Smaller more frequent doses may yield improved absorption and efficacy rate. Gabapentin has become known as an agent with minimal adverse effects, although excessive sedation can occur if dosage escalation is too rapid. Severe behavioral

problems have been reported in children with developmental delay or attention deficit hyperactivity disorder (Wolf *et al* 1995; Lee *et al* 1996; Tallian *et al* 1996).

Topiramate demonstrates a broad spectrum of anticonvulsant activity in both cryptogenic and symptomatic partial and generalized epilepsies. Large multicenter pediatric trials have been conducted in refractory partial seizures, primary generalized tonic–clonic seizures, and Lennox–Gastaut syndrome. Data analysis for some of these trials is ongoing. In children with refractory partial seizures topiramate was shown to be superior to placebo, with 39% experiencing at least a 50% decline in seizure frequency (Elterman *et al* 1999). Open-label studies mirror the effectiveness of topiramate in children (Glauser 1997a). Preliminary reports in children with Lennox–Gastaut syndrome are also encouraging, with the best results observed in tonic–atonic, atypical absence, and generalized tonic–clonic seizures (Glauser 1997b). Topiramate has also been reported as possibly effective in cryptogenic infantile spasms (Yeung *et al* 1997). Adverse effects reported include emotional lability, fatigue, and difficulty with concentration, attention, and memory (Elterman *et al* 1999). Because of the potential cognitive effects, topiramate will probably be reserved for the more intractable childhood epilepsies.

Oxcarbazepine appears to mirror the efficacy of carbamazepine but with less dosage- and nondosage-related toxicity. Oxcarbazepine may be used successfully in up to 70% of children who have experienced carbamazepine hypersensitivity (Gram 1994). In an open-label study of young children (< 7 years of age) with intractable focal epilepsy, 27% (12 of 44) became seizure-free and an additional 36% exhibited at least a 50% decline in seizure frequency. Hyponatremia may occur in up to 15% of treated children (Gaily *et al* 1997). Clinical efficacy studies are currently in progress for the active metabolite of oxcarbazepine (10-monohydroxy derivative) as a new injectable antiepileptic agent. With these advantages, oxcarbazepine may virtually replace carbamazepine in countries where it is available.

There are insufficient pediatric data on tiagabine to draw any conclusions regarding its effectiveness in children. Two large multicenter trials are currently underway in children with refractory partial seizures. Two small pilot studies have provided some information. Boellner and colleagues studied 25 children with refractory complex partial seizures and examined both single-dose pharmacokinetics and long-term follow-up safety (Boellner *et al* 1996; Gustavson *et al* 1997). Tiagabine was initiated at doses of 0.1 mg kg^{-1} daily and titrated to effect or toxicity. Of the 25 children 16 were converted to monotherapy and were seizure-free for at least 2 months (mean dose 0.31 mg kg^{-1} daily). A single-blind, multicenter trial has also been completed in 47 children with various types of medically intractable seizures and

Table 36.2 Dosing guidelines for the new antiepileptic drugs.

	Initial dose		Usual maintenance dose[a]	
	mg kg^{-1} daily	Interval	mg kg^{-1} daily	Interval
Felbamate	15	t.i.d.	45	t.i.d. to q.i.d.
Gabapentin	15	t.i.d.	30–60	t.i.d. to q.i.d.
Lamotrigine[b]				
Monotherapy	0.5	q.d. to b.i.d.	2–10	q.d. to b.i.d.
With enzyme-inducing antiepileptic drugs	2.0	b.i.d. to t.i.d.	5–15	b.i.d. to t.i.d
With valproate	0.2	q.d.	1–5	q.d.
Oxcarbazepine	20	b.i.d.	50–90	b.i.d. to t.i.d.
Topiramate	1.0	q.d.	6–10	b.i.d.
Tiagabine	0.1	q.d.	0.3–1.5	t.i.d. to q.i.d
Vigabatrin	40	b.i.d.	60–80	b.i.d.
			100–150[c]	

[a] Dosage can be doubled at 2-week intervals with lamotrigine and topiramate.
[b] Only increase dosage every 2 weeks due to potential of rash.
[c] Doses required to treat infantile spasms are frequently higher than those used for partial seizures.

syndromes (Uldall *et al* 1995). Of these children, seven were still in dose titration at the time of the report, 20 withdrew due to lack of efficacy, while 20 completed the trial with 17 going into long-term extension. Children with partial seizures derived the most benefit at doses between 0.37 and 1.25 mg kg^{-1} daily. Tiagabine did not appear beneficial in children with generalized epilepsies.

DOSAGES AND MONITORING PARAMETERS

Tentative dosing guidelines for the newer agents are listed in Table 36.2. As more pediatric experience is gained, these guidelines are likely to change. Although lamotrigine is normally recommended for twice-daily dosing, because of the faster elimination rate in children a thrice-daily schedule may improve response in children with seizures that are more difficult to control (Yuen and Rafter 1992; Gilman 1995; Chen *et al* 1997). Likewise, mean topiramate clearance is 44–45% higher in children compared with adults (Rosenfeld *et al* 1995; Glauser 1997b). Three times daily dosage with this agent in children may reduce some of the adverse effects

related to high peak concentrations. Tiagabine clearance in children has also been reported as higher in comparison with adult data (Gustavson *et al* 1997). It is unclear at this time if this difference is clinically significant.

SUMMARY

The medical management of intractable focal childhood seizures differs from adults in several important respects. Although similar medications are used, the choice of agents is often based on considerations of adverse effects as much as potential efficacy. The metabolic differences of children compared with adults also present unique management challenges, since children, especially infants and younger children, metabolize drugs more rapidly than adults and may even produce different metabolites. Failure to appreciate these issues could result in unacceptable adverse effects, medication noncompliance, seizure relapses, and intractable epilepsy.

KEY POINTS

1. Children with intractable focal epilepsy are a distinct biologic subgroup.
2. Children pose biotransformation and drug disposition differences which complicated pharmacotherapy.
3. Spectrum of drug toxicity and adverse drug effects is often different in younger patients.
4. Attention to these nuances is critical in the sucessful treatment of epileptic children.

REFERENCES

Aicardi J, Mumford JP, Duman C, Wood S (1996) Vigabatrin as initial therapy for infantile spasms: a European retrospective survey. Sabril IS investigator and peer review groups. *Epilepsia* **37**:638–642.

Agunod M, Yonaguchi N, Lopez R *et al* (1969) Correlative study of hydrochloric acid, pepsin and intrinsic factor secretion in newborns and infants. *American Journal of Digestive Diseases* **14**:400–414.

Albani F, Riva R, Procaaccianti G, Baruzzi A, Perucca E (1983) Free fraction of valproic acid: *in vitro* time-dependent increase and correlation with free fatty acid concentration in human plasma and serum. *Epilepsia* **24**:65–73.

Aman MG, Werry JS, Paxton JW, Turbott SH (1987) Effect of sodium valproate on psychomotor performance in children as a function of dose, fluctuations in concentration, and diagnosis. *Epilepsia* **28**:115–124.

Aman MG, Werry JS, Paxton JW, Turbott SH, Stewart AW (1990) Effects of carbamazepine on psychomotor performance in children as a function of drug concentration, seizure type and time of medication. *Epilepsia* **31**:51–60.

Bach B, Hansen JM, Kampmann JP *et al* (1981) Disposition of antipyrine and phenytoin correlated with age and liver volume in man. *Clinical Pharmacokinetics* **6**:389–396.

Battino D, Bossi L, Croci D *et al* (1980) Carbamazepine plasma levels in children and adults: influence of age, dose and associated therapy. *Therapeutic Drug Monitoring* **2**:315–322.

Battino D, Buti D, Croci D *et al* (1993) Lamotrigine in resistant childhood epilepsy. *Neuropediatrics* **24**:332–336.

Bauer LA (1982) Interference of oral phenytoin absorption by continuous nasogastric feedings. *Neurology* **32**:570–572.

Besag FMC, Wallace SJ, Dulac O *et al* (1995) Lamotrigine for the treatment of epilepsy in childhood. *Journal of Pediatrics* **127**:991–997.

Besag FM, Dulac O, Alving J, Mullens EL (1997) Long-term safety and efficacy of lamotrigine (Lamictal) in pediatric patients with epilepsy. *Seizure* **6**:51–56.

Boellner S, McCarthy J, Mercante D, Sommerville K (1996) Pilot study of tiagabine in children with partial seizures. *Epilepsia* **37**:92.

Bourgeois BFD, Prensky AL, Palkes HS, Talent BK, Bush SG (1983) Intelligence in epilepsy: a prospective study in children. *Annals of Neurology* **14**:438–444.

Brinkschulte M, Breyer-Pfaff V (1982) Increased binding of desmethyl-imipramine in plasma of phenobarbital-treated rats. *Biochemical Pharmacology* **31**:1749–1754.

Bruguerolle B, Jadot G, Bussiere H (1984) Together, phenobarbital and carbamazepine lower alpha₁-acid glycoprotein concentration in plasma of epileptic patients. *Clinical Chemistry* **30**:590.

Chen C, Sorie AM, Casale EJ *et al* (1997) Single-dose pharmacokinetics and safety of lamotrigine in children with epilepsy. *Epilepsia* **38** (Suppl 8):192.

Chiron C, Dulac O Beaumont D *et al* (1991) Therapeutic trial of vigabatrin in refractory infantile spasms. *Journal of Child Neurology* **6** (Suppl 2):53–59.

Chiron C, Dumas C, Jambaque I *et al* (1997) Randomized trial comparing vigabatrin and hydrocortisone in infantile spasms due to tuberous sclerosis. *Epilepsy Research* **26**:389–395.

Coyle JT, Enna SJ (1976) Neurochemical aspects of the ontogenesis of GABAergic neurons in the rat brain. *Brain Research* **111**:119–133.

Craig N, Gurbani SG, Miller L, Baram TZ (1997) Ketogenic diet: evaluation of its efficacy in children with intractable epilepsy. *Epilepsia* **38** (Suppl 8):197.

Cramer JA (1995) Optimizing long-term patient compliance. *Neurology* **45** (Suppl 1):S25–S28.

Curalto P (1994) Vigabatrin for refractory partial seizures in children with tuberous sclerosis. *Neuropediatrics* **25**:55.

Dooley J, Camfield P, Gordon K, Camfield C, Wirrell E, Smith E (1996) Lamotrigine-induced rash in children. *Neurology* **46**:240–242.

Dreifuss FE, Santilli N, Langer DH, Sweeney KP, Moline KA, Menander KB (1987) Valproic acid hepatic fatalities: a retrospective review. *Neurology* **37**:379–385.

Elterman RK, Glauser T, Wyllie E, Reife R, Wu SC, Pledger G (1999) A double-blind, placebo-controlled trial of topiramate for the treatment of partial onset seizures in children. YP study group. *Neurology* **56**:1338–1344.

Farwell JR, Lee YJ, Hirtz DG, Sulzbacher SI Ellenberg JH, Nelson KB (1990) Phenobarbital for febrile seizures: effects on intelligence and on seizure recurrence. *New England Journal of Medicine* **322**:364–369.

Ferrie CD, Robinson RO (1995) The clinical efficacy of vigabatrin in children. *Reviews of Contemporary Pharmacotheraeutics* **6**:469–476.

Friis-Hansen B (1971) Body composition during growth: *in vivo* measurements and biochemical data correlated to differential anatomical growth. *Pediatrics* **47**: (Suppl):264–274.

Gaily E, Granstrom ML, Liukkonen E (1997) Oxcarbazepine in the treatment of early childhood epilepsy. *Journal of Child Neurology* **12**:496–498.

Gal P, Toback J, Boer HR *et al* (1982) Efficacy of phenobarbital monotherapy in treatment of neonatal seizures in relationship to blood levels. *Neurology* **32**:1401–1404.

Gallassi R, Morreale A, Lorusso S, Procaccianti G, Lugaresi E, Baruzzi A (1988) Carbamazepine and phenytoin: comparison of cognitive effects in epileptic patients during monotherapy and withdrawal. *Archives of Neurology* **45**:892–894.

Gilman JT (1990) Intractable childhood epilepsy: issues in pharmacotherapy. *Journal of Epilepsy* **3**: (Suppl):21–24.

Gilman JT (1991) Carbamazepine dosing for pediatric seizure disorders: the highs and lows. *The Annals of Pharmacotherapy* **25**:1109–1112.

Gilman JT (1994) Developmental principles of antiepileptic drug therapy. *Journal of Child Neurology* **9** (Suppl):S20–S25.

Gilman JT (1995) Lamotrigine: an antiepileptic agent for the treatment of partial seizures. *The Annals of Pharmacotherapy* **29**:144–151.

Gilman JT (2000) Perspectives on AED interactions. In Pellock JM, Dodson WE, Bourgeois B (eds) *Pediatric Epilepsy Diagnosis and Therapy*, 2nd edn in press. New York: Demos.

Gilman JT, Duchowny M (1994) Childhood epilepsy: current therapeutic recommendations. *CNS Drugs* **1**:180–192.

Gilman JT, Gal P (1992) Pharmacokinetic and pharmacodynamic data collection in children and neonates. *Clinical Pharmacokineics* **23**:1–9.

Gilman JT, Duchowny MS, Resnick TJ, Hershorin ER (1988) Carbamazepine malabsorption: a case report. *Pediatrics* **82**:518–519.

Gilman JT, Gal P, Duchowny MS *et al* (1989) Rapid sequential phenobarbital treatment of neonatal seizures. *Pediatrics* **83**:674–678.

Gilman JT, Duchowny M, Jayakar P, Resnick TJ (1994) Medical intractability in children evaluated for epilepsy surgery. *Neurology* **44**:1341–1343.

Glauser TA (1997a) Topiramate. *Seminers in Pediatric Neurology* **4**:34–42.

Glauser TA (1997b) Preliminary observations on topiramate in pediatric epilepsies. *Epilepsia* **38** (Suppl 1):S37–S41.

Gottlieb A, Keydor I, Epstein HT (1977) Rodent brain growth stages. An analytical review. *Biology of the Neonate* **32**:166–167.

Graf WD, Pellock JM, Duchowny M, Womble G, Manasco P (1997) Lamictal is effective for add-on treatment of partial seziures in children and adolescents. *Epilepsia* **38** (Suppl 8):193.

Gram L (1994) Clinical experience with oxcarbazepine. *Epilepsia* **35** (Suppl 3):S21–S22.

Gram L, Sabers A, Dulac O (1992) Treatment of pediatric epilepsies with gamma-vinyl GABA (Vigabatrin). *Epilepsia* **33** (Suppl 5):S26–S29.

Grand RJ, Watkins JB, Torti FM (1976) Development of the human gastrointestinal tract: a review. *Gastroenterology* **70**:400–414.

Griebel ML (1998) Acute management of hypersensitivity reactions and seizures. *Epilepsia* **39** (Suppl 7):S17–S21.

Gustavson LE, Boellner SW, Granneman GR *et al* (1997) A single-dose study to define tiagabine pharmacokinetics in pediatric patients with complex partial seizures. *Neurology* **48**:1032–1037.

Hall K, Otten N, Johnston B *et al* (1985) A multivariable analysis of factors governing the steady-state pharmacokinetics of valproic acid in 52 young epileptics. *Journal of Clinical Pharmacology* **25**:261–268.

Heimann G (1980) Enteral absorption and bioavailability in relation to age. *European Journal of Clinical Pharmacology* **18**:43–50.

Herranz JL, Armijo JA, Arteaga R (1988) Clinical side effects of phenobarbital, primidone, phenytoin, carbamazepine and valproate during monotherapy in children. *Epilepsia* **29**:794–804.

Houghton GW, Richens A, Toseland PA *et al* (1975) Brain concentrations of phenytoin, phenobarbitone and primidone in epileptic patients. *European Journal of Clinical Pharmacology* **9**:73–78.

Kearns GL, Reed MD (1989) Clinical pharmacokinetics in infants and children: a reappraisal. *Clinical Pharmacokinetics* **17** (Suppl 1):29–67.

Khurana DS, Riviello J, Helmers S *et al* (1996) Efficacy of gabapentin therapy in children with refractory partial seizures. *Journal of Pediatrics* **128**:829–833.

Kinsman SL, Vining EPG, Quaskey SA, Mellits D, Freeman JM (1992) Efficacy of the ketogenic diet for intractable seizure disorders: review of 58 cases. *Epilepsia* **33**:1132–1136.

Krauss SL, Johnson MA, Miller NR (1988) Vigabatrin-associated retinal cone system dysfunction. *Neurology* **50**: 614–618.

Krueger KA, Garnett WR, Comstock TJ *et al* (1987) Effect of two administration schedules of an enteral nutrient formula on phenytoin bioavailability. *Epilepsia* **28**:706–712.

Lee DO, Steingard RJ, Cesena M, Helmers SJ, Riviello JJ, Mikati MA (1996) Behavioral side effects of gabapentin in children. *Epilepsia* **37**:87–90.

Leff RD, Fischer LJ, Roberts RJ (1986) Phenytoin metabolism in infants following intravenous and oral administration. *Developmental Pharmacology and Therapeutics* **9**:217–223.

Lockman LA, Driel R, Zaske D *et al* (1979) Phenobarbital dosage for control of neonatal seizures. *Neurology* **29**:1445–1449.

McLean MJ (1994) Clinical pharmacokinetics of gabapentin. *Neurology* **44** (Suppl 5):S17–S22.

Maly MM, Gidal BE, Rutecki P, Shaw R, Collins DM, Pitterle ME (1997) Effect of lamotrigine on carbamazepine epoxide/carbamazepine serum-concentration ratios. *Epilepsia* **38** (Suppl 8):101.

Mares P, Trojan S (1991) Ontogenetic development of isonicotine-hydrazide-induced seizures in rats. *Brain and Development* **13**:121–125.

Mattson RH, Cramer JA, Collins JF *et al* (1985) Comparison of carbamazepine, phenobarbital, phenytoin and primidone in partial and secondarily generalized tonic–clonic seizures. *New England Journal of Medicine* **313**:145–151.

Mattson RH, Cramer JA, Collins JF *et al* (1992) A comparison of valproate with carbamazepine for the treatment of complex partial seizures and secondarily generalized tonic–clonic seizures in adults. *New England Journal of Medicine* **327**:765–771.

Meador KJ, Loring DW, Huh K, Gallagher BB, King DW (1990) Comparative cognitive effects of anticonvulsants. *Neurology* **40**:391–394.

Michelson HB, Lothman EW (1989) An *in vivo* electrophysiologic study of the ontogeny of excitatory and inhibitory processes in rat hippocampus. *Developmental Brain Research* **46**:113–122.

Monaco F (1996) Cognitive effects of vigabatrin: a review. *Neurology* **47** (Suppl 1):S6–S11.

Monaco F, Torta R, Cicolin A *et al* (1997) Lack of association between vigabatrin and impaired cognition. *Journal of International Medical Research* **25**:296–301.

Morselli PL (1983) Development of physiological variables important for drug kinetics. In: Morselli PL, Pippenger CE, Penry JK (eds) *Antiepileptic Drug Therapy in Pediatrics*, pp 1–12. New York: Raven Press.

Morton LD, Pellock JM, Maria BL *et al* (1997) Fosphenytoin safety and pharmacokinetics in children. *Epilepsia* **38** (Suppl 8):194.

Moshe SL (1993) Seizures in the developing brain. *Neurology* **43** (Suppl 5):S3–S7.

Moshe SL, Garant DS (1996) Substantia nigra GABA receptors can mediate anticonvulsant or proconvulsant effects. *Epilepsy Research* (Suppl 12):247–256.

Motte J, Trevathan E, Arvidsson JFV *et al* (1997) Lamotrigine for generalized seizures associated with the Lennox–Gastaut syndrome. *New England Journal of Medicine* **337**:1807–1812.

Nelson JD, Shelton S, Kusmiesz HT, Haltalin KC (1972) Absorption of ampicillin and nalidixic acid by infants and children with acute shigellosis. *Clinical Pharmacology and Therapeutics* **13**:879–886.

Onishi S, Yoshihi O, Nishimura Y *et al* (1984) Distribution of phenobarbital in serum, brain and other organs from pediatric patients. *Developmental Pharmacology and Therapeutics* **7**:153–159.

Painter MJ, Pippenger C, MacDonald H, Pitlick W (1978) Phenobarbital and diphenylhydantoin levels in neonates with seizures. *Journal of Pediatrics* **92**:315–319.

Painter MJ, Pippenger CE, Wasterlein C *et al* (1981) Phenobarbital and phenytoin in neonatal seizures: metabolism and tissue distribution. *Neurology* **31**:1107–1112.

Pippenger EC (1983) Maturation of biotransformation rates. In: Morseli PL, Pippenger CE, Penry JK (eds) *Antiepileptic Drug Therapy In Pediatrics*, pp 333–338. New York: Raven Press.

Provinciali L, Bartolini M, Mari F, Del-Pesce M, Ceravol MG (1996) Influence of vigabatrin on cognitive performances and behaviour in patients with drug-resistant epilepsy. *Acta Neurologica Scandinavica* **94**:12–18.

Pynnonen S, Sillanpaa M, Frey H, Lisalo E (1977) Carbamazepine and its 10,11-epoxide in children and adults with epilepsy. *European Journal of Clinical Pharmacology* **11**:129–133.

Radde IC (1985a) Mechanisms of drug absorption and their development. In: MacLeod SM, Radde ID (eds) *Textbook of Pediatric Clinical Pharmacology*, pp 17–31. Littleton, MA: PSG Publishing.

Radde IC (1985b) Drugs and protein binding. In: MacLeod SM, Radde IC (eds) *Textbook of Pediatric Clinical Pharmacology*, pp 32–43. Littleton, MA: PSG Publishing

Ramsay ER, Wilder BJ, Berger JR, Bruni J (1983) A double-blind study comparing carbamazepine with phenytoin as initial seizure therapy in adults. *Neurology* **33**:904–910.

Resnick TJ (1990) Criteria for surgical evaluation in children with uncontrolled seizures. *Journal of Epilepsy* **3** (Suppl):35–40.

Riva R, Contin M, Albani F, Baruzzi A (1985) High alpha$_1$-acid glycoprotein concentrations in serum of epileptic children being treated with carbamazepine. *Clinical Chemistry* **31**:151.

Rosenfeld WE, Doose DR, Walker SA, Schaefer P, Reife RA (1995) The steady-state pharmacokinetics of topiramate as adjunctive therapy in pediatric subjects with epilepsy. *Epilepsia* **36** (Suppl 2):158.

Scarpa P, Carassini B (1982) Partial epilepsy in childhood. Clinical and EEG study of 261 cases. *Epilepsia* **23**:333–341.

Schlienger RG, Shear NH (1998) Anticonvulsant hypersensitivity syndrome. *Epilepsia* **39** (Suppl 7):S3–S7.

Schmidt D (1983) Reduction of two-drug therapy in intractable epilepsy. *Epilepsia* **24**:368–376.

Sherwin AL, Eisen AA, Sokolowski CD (1973) Anticonvulsant drugs in human epileptogenic brain. *Archives of Neurology* **29**:73–77.

Shields WD, Lake JL, Chugani HT (1985) Amantadine in the treatment of refractory epilepsy in childhood: an open trial in 10 patients. *Neurology* **35**:579–581.

Snodgrass R (1997) Anticonvulsants and rashes in children. *Epilepsia* **38** (Suppl 8):193.

Swann JW, Brady RJ (1984) Penicillin-induced epileptogenesis in immature rats' CA3 hippocampal pyramidal cells. *Developmental Brain Research* **12**:243–254.

Tada H, Morooka K, Arimoto K, Matsuo T (1991) Clinical effects of allopurinol on intractable epilepsy. *Epilepsia* **32**:279–283.

Tallian KB, Nahata MC, Lo W, Tsao CY (1996) Gabapentin associated with aggressive behavior in pediatric patients with seizures. *Epilepsia* **37**:501–502.

Tatum WO, Gonzalez MA (1994) Carbamazepine toxicity in an epileptic induced by clarithromycin. *Hospital Pharmacy* **29**:45–46.

Tennison MB, Greenwood RS, Miles MV (1991) Methsuximide for intractable childhood seizures. *Pediatrics* **87**:186–189.

Tiula E, Neuvomen PJ (1982) Antiepileptic drugs and alpha$_1$-acid glycoprotein. *New England Journal of Medicine* **307**:1148.

Trudeau V, Myers S, LaMoreaus L *et al* (1996) Gabapentin in naive childhood absence epilepsy: results from two double-blind, placebo-controlled, multicentre studies. *Journal of Child Neurology* **11**:470–475.

Uldall P, Bulteau C, Pedersen SA, Dulac O, Meinild H, Lassen LC (1995) Single-blind study of safety, tolerability and preliminary efficacy of tiagabine as adjunctive treatment of children with epilepsy. *Epilepsia* **36**:S147.

Uvebrant P, Bauziene R (1994) Intractable epilepsy in children. The efficacy of lamotrigine treatment, including non-seizure-related benefits. *Neuropediatrics* **25**:284–289.

Veggiotti P, Cieuta C, Rey E, Dulac O (1994) Lamotrigine in infantile spasms. *Lancet* **344**:1375–1376.

Velisek L, Kubova H, Pohl M *et al* (1992) Pentylenetetrazol-induced seizures in rats: an ontogenetic study. *Naunyn Schmiedebergs Archives of Pharmacology* **346**:588–591.

Veliskova J, Velisek L, Moshe SL (1996) Age-specific effects of baclofen on pentylenetetrazol-induced seizures in developing rats. *Epilepsia* **37**:718–722.

Vining EPG, Mellits ED, Dorsen MM *et al* (1987) Psychologic and behavioral effects of antiepileptic drugs in children: a double-blind comparison between phenobarbital and valproic acid. *Pediatrics* **80**:165–174.

Virani A, Mailis A, Shapiro LE, Shear NH (1997) Drug interactions in human neuropathic pain pharmacotherapy. *Pain* **73**:3–13.

Wallace SJ (1994) Lamotrigine: a clinical overview. *Seizure* **3** (Suppl A):47–51.

Whelan HT, Hendeles L, Haberkern CM, Neims AH (1983) High intravenous phenytoin dosage requirement in a newborn infant. *Neurology* **33**:106–108.

Wolf SM, Shinnar S, Kang H *et al* (1995) Gabapentin toxicity in children manifesting as behavioral changes. *Epilepsia* **36**:1203–1205.

Wong YY, Ludden TM, Bell RD (1983) Effect of erythromycin on carbamazepine kinetics. *Clinical Pharmacology and Therapeutics* **33**:460–464.

Woody RC (1990) Bromide therapy for pediatric seizure disorder intractable to other antiepileptic drugs. *Journal of Child Neurology* **5**:65–67.

Wyllie E, Wyllie R, Cruse RP, Erenberg G, Rothner D (1984) Pancreatitis associated with valproic acid therapy. *American Journal of Diseases of Children* **138**:912–914.

Xu SG, Garant DS, Sperber EF *et al* (1992) The proconvulsant effect of nigral infusion of THIP on flurothyl-induced seizures in rat pups. *Developmental Brain Research* **68**:275–277.

Yeung S, Murdoch-Eaton D, Ferrie CD, Livingston JH (1997) Topiramate for drug-resistant epilepsies in children. *European Journal of Paediatric Neurology* **1**:A81.

Yuen AWC, Rafter JEW (1992) Lamotrigine (Lamictal) as add-on therapy in pediatric patients with treatment-resistant epilepsy. An overview. *Epilepsia* **33** (Suppl 3):82–83.

Zaccara G, Messori A, Moroni F (1988) Clinical pharmacokinetics of valproic acid: 1988. *Clinical Pharmacokinetics* **15**:367–389.

Zini R, Riant P, Barre J, Tillement JP (1990) Disease-induced variations in plasma protein levels. Implications for drug dosage regimen, part I. *Clinical Pharmacokinetics* **19**:147–159.

Zouhar A, Mares P, Liskova-Bernaskova K *et al* (1989) Motor and electrocorticographic epileptic activity induced by bicuculline in developing rats. *Epilepsia* **30**:501–510.

Development of new antiepileptic drugs

GDS WRIGHT

Around 80% of patients with epilepsy are controlled on one drug with relative ease (Shorvon and Reynolds 1982). A few more gain control with different drug combinations. Nevertheless, in absolute terms, there are many thousands of individuals with uncontrolled epilepsy in the UK alone. Epilepsy surgery is the treatment of choice for some. For most, hope lies in the discovery of more effective drugs. A second, but no less important, reason for seeking new drugs is that existing ones all fall short of the ideal. New drugs are needed to gain greater efficacy, greater tolerability, and greater ease of administration.

THE IDEAL ANTIEPILEPTIC DRUG

The ideal antiepileptic drug (AED) is yet to be discovered. The attributes sought in such a drug are 100% efficacy in all seizure types and complete tolerability; a wide therapeutic index or range, i.e. a large difference between the smallest effective dose and the dose at which toxicity occurs; and a sufficiently long half-life to enable once or twice daily dosage. The drug should be easy to take and available in a number of different formulations including a parenteral form. It should not interact with other drugs; thus, it should have low (or no) protein binding and no human metabolism. It should be antiepileptogenic as well as anticonvulsant. It should not be teratogenic. It should be cost-effective. The heterogeneity of the epilepsies and their underlying mechanisms impose further constraints on finding the ideal drug. It seems unlikely that any one drug will be found that can act 'cleanly' in multiple ways at multiple sites. Nevertheless, new drugs are designed with these principles in mind to try to find the ideal drug and to make up for the specific deficiencies of currently available products.

The cost of drug development is another barrier. As new drugs have to show their value in patients unresponsive to, or intolerant of, existing AEDs, it is clear that each successful new drug will reduce the field for future drugs. Eventually it will become economically nonviable to develop new AEDs in the current way since they will not produce a sufficient return on investment.

In the past, AEDs have been discovered by serendipity (Mattson 1996). A development has been to create similar molecules to those known to have antiepileptic effects and to try them in animal models, seeking similar or greater efficacy and fewer side-effects. The current trend is to design a drug to have an action at a particular site to counter the effects of epileptogenic activity in a specific way (Patsalos and Sander 1994). This requires knowledge of the underlying mechanisms responsible for the epileptogenic activity. Computer modeling is increasingly used. It is a much quicker way to eliminate compounds unlikely to show the desired effects since their properties can be predicted without actually making them. Combinatorial chemistry and mass screening of chemical databases has increased the number of compounds that can be made and screened each year (Taylor and Marks 1998). Bioinformatics is tackling the analysis of the vast quantities of data generated by molecular biology (Kingsbury 1997).

UNDERLYING MECHANISMS OF THE EPILEPSIES

The epilepsies are a heterogeneous group of disorders etiologically, electrically, and clinically. Action specifically at a final common path, if such exists, might produce a universally effective drug. In its absence, drugs with different mechanisms and actions are effective in different seizure types. Complementary combinations of these are necessary until the ideal single drug arrives.

Understanding what is known about neuronal membranes, synapses, neurotransmitters, the basic mechanisms of normal and abnormal neuronal behavior, and the mechanisms involved in focal and generalized seizures is necessary to understand where chemical intervention might have an anticonvulsant effect. Knowledge of cellular pathophysiology has come from the study of acute focal 'epileptic' discharges in brain slice preparations. These are created *in vitro*, or are maintained *in vitro* having been taken from brains of animal epilepsy models. These models allow an understanding of the human epilepsies and all are important in the study and development of AEDs. The basic mechanisms have been reviewed by a number of authors (Jefferys and Roberts 1987; Richens 1991; Heinemann *et al* 1996; Johnston 1996; Dichter 1997). A summary is given below.

DEPOLARIZATION

The neuronal membrane has a resting negative potential of approximately 80 mV. If this is reduced, depolarization occurs and an action potential results when a particular threshold below the resting potential is reached. Following the action potential, there is a brief period of hyperpolarization before the normal resting membrane potential returns.

EXCITATION

The depolarizing effect leading to an action potential is called the excitatory postsynaptic potential (EPSP), which is the result of excitatory neurotransmitter release from synapses. Not all EPSPs result in an action potential as they may be too small to reach the threshold value. However, small EPSPs may summate collectively to produce depolarization leading to an action potential; some EPSPs may be sufficient in their own right to generate an action potential.

INHIBITION

Some synaptic contacts may be inhibitory and activation of these leads to brief hyperpolarization, the so-called inhibitory postsynaptic potential (IPSP) that makes an action potential less likely to occur. Neurons typically have a mixture of inhibitory and excitatory contacts and the eventual firing of the cell depends upon the balance between these two influences. These processes are involved in normal and abnormal neuronal function and play an important part in the genesis and manipulation of seizure activity. However, epilepsy is not simply an excess of excitation over inhibition but involves many other processes only some of which are currently understood. Furthermore, a straightforward increase in discharge frequency is not epilepsy. Other factors are necessary to synchronize the neuronal discharges to generate seizures.

EXCITATORY AND INHIBITORY NEUROTRANSMITTERS

These cause excitatory and inhibitory postsynaptic potentials. The same neurotransmitter may have different actions at different sites. Many neurotransmitters have been identified: glutamate and aspartate are excitatory neurotransmitters; γ-aminobutyric acid (GABA) has been identified as an important inhibitory neurotransmitter.

Excitatory neurotransmission

Several glutamate receptors have been identified and are named after their preferential agonists. The N-methyl-D-aspartate (NMDA) receptor and the γ-amino-3-hydroxy-5-methyl-4-isoxazolepropionic acid (AMPA) receptor appear most closely associated with epileptogenic activity (Rogawski 1998). The NMDA receptor has been most closely studied. This receptor is also important in the process of ischemic damage and much current research is attempting to modulate its activity in this pathologic condition.

NMDA receptor

After release from presynaptic nerve terminals the neurotransmitter binds to a specific postsynaptic recognition site on the receptor. At the NMDA receptor, in addition to a glutamate site there is an adjacent recognition site at which glycine facilitates glutamate transmission, a process known as upregulation. When both sites are activated, Na^+ and Ca^{2+} ions move into the cell and K^+ ions pass out of the cell, leading to an action potential if the threshold depolarization is reached. However, the ion channel can be blocked by Mg^{2+} ions in a voltage-dependent gate. If depolarization occurs, Mg^{2+} ions move out of the channel and allow current flow from glutamate action. This voltage-dependent channel blockade is believed to be involved in burst firing in epileptogenic activity. Other processes and molecules can affect the ion channel, for example it is blocked by activation of the phencyclidine-binding site. Some drugs influence this but only in response to glutamate release and are therefore 'use-dependent.'

Competitive agonists block the NMDA site and prevent excitatory transmission. By virtue of their action some have psychomimetic effects and are proving intolerable in humans.

Inhibitory neurotransmission

Two forms of CNS synaptic inhibitory mechanism are known: presynaptic and postsynaptic inhibition. In the former, an inhibitory nerve terminal makes contact with an excitatory nerve terminal, inhibiting release of its neurotransmitter. In the latter, the inhibitory nerve terminal synapses directly with the neuron. Nonsynaptic inhibition also occurs.

When the inhibitory neurotransmitter GABA is released at a synapse and binds with the postsynaptic membrane, an ion channel opens that allows chloride ions to pass into the neuron, producing hyperpolarization and reduced cellular excitability. Blocking of the GABA receptor may produce convulsive activity.

Analogous to the glycine site in excitatory neurotransmission, modulation with other compounds can occur at sites on the inhibitory postsynaptic membrane. One is the benzodiazapine-binding site, although the naturally endogenous ligands have not been identified. Inhibition can therefore be influenced by increasing GABA synthesis, reducing GABA breakdown and release, decreasing GABA reuptake, use of GABA agonists, co-site activity, and a direct effect on chloride channels causing them to open. Phenobarbital acts partly in this way.

In nonsynaptic inhibition, there is reduced membrane excitability. Phenytoin, carbamazepine, and lamotrigine limit sustained high-frequency firing of the type associated with epileptic seizure activity. This reduces ion conduction in voltage-gated sodium channels.

SEIZURE GENERATION

Changes in ion flux may lead to burst discharges in individual neurons but this alone does not constitute epileptic activity. The discharges of many neurons must be synchronized to generate epileptic phenomena. Different mechanisms occur in focal and generalized epilepsies.

Focal seizures and interictal discharges arise from cortical areas that are excessively excitable. Interictal discharges occur when a group of pyramidal neurons synchronously depolarize and fire a burst of action potentials. The depolarizing shift in the neurons is followed by a large, prolonged hyperpolarization. Neurons are alternately excited then inhibited (Dichter 1997). The depolarizing shift appears to be generated by a combination of synaptic currents, mediated by the excitatory neurotransmitters glutamate and aspartate, and by voltage-dependent depolarizing currents, especially calcium currents. Hyperpolarization is also produced by a combination of events, including voltage-dependent potassium currents, calcium-dependent potassium currents and possibly chloride currents in membranes, and synaptic currents mediated by GABA A and B receptors.

Seizures may develop from interictal discharges or independent of them (Dichter 1997). A sequence of events can be observed in animal models. The hyperpolarization becomes progressively smaller with each interictal discharge and then disappears. Eventually the neuron becomes tonically depolarized and fires repetitively along with surrounding neurons, creating seizure activity. Once a small group of neurons begins to fire hypersynchronously, seizure development in areas not primarily epileptogenic is a likely consequence. When inhibitory synapses are repeatedly activated they tend to become less efficient (Dichter 1988; Diesz and Prince 1989). The converse appears to be true for excitatory synapses (Zucker 1989). Therefore, an unstable state is reached in certain circumstances of sustained repetitive activity. The local discharge loses its inhibitory control; it involves nearby neurons and may spread further (Dichter and Spencer 1969). Synaptic and nonsynaptic mechanisms are at work. Nonsynaptic mechanisms include electrotonic junctions (electric synapses), ephaptic interaction through electric field effects, and fluctuations in extracellular ion concentrations. Each of these mechanisms might be a target for intervention and a reason for AED development.

Table 37.1 Summary of animal models of epilepsy.

Generalized tonic–clonic seizures	Neocortical partial seizures	Complex partial seizures
Maximal electroshock	Application of topical convulsant, e.g. penicillin or tetanus toxoid	Focal stimulation
Systemic injection of convulsant drugs	Focal afterdischarges	Kindling
Photic-induced epilepsy in photosensitive baboons	Freeze focus	Kainic acid
Genetically prone rodent models		Tetanus toxoid
		Brain slices *in vitro* with physical and chemical stimulation

Sources: Jefferys and Roberts (1987), Kupferburg (1993) and White *et al* (1998).

ANIMAL MODELS OF SEIZURES

A number of animal models are used to evaluate potential AEDs (Table 37.1). Only those particularly pertinent to focal epilepsy are discussed in this section.

MAXIMAL ELECTROSHOCK

Meritt and Putnam (1938) pioneered the use of the maximal electroshock (MES) model, which predicts anticonvulsant activity against tonic–clonic seizures and set the scene for screening potential AEDs. In the MES model, a seizure is induced in mice by applying a supramaximal current via corneal electrodes. If the test substance abolishes hindleg tonic extension during the seizure, this is interpreted as preventing seizure spread. In general, MES identifies drugs of use in complex partial and secondarily generalized seizures by identifying compounds that block sustained, rapid, repetitive firing in isolated neurons dependent on prolonging inactivation of voltage-dependent sodium channels (Meldrum 1997).

SYSTEMIC INJECTION OF CONVULSANT DRUGS

Pentylenetetrazol-induced seizures, described by Goodman *et al* (1946), are used as a model of absence and tonic–clonic seizures depending on the dose used (Jefferys and Roberts 1987). A previously determined convulsive dose of pentylenetetrazol is injected at the time of peak effect of the test substance. The absence of clonic activity for 5 s or more during the 30 min following the injection suggests that the drug elevates seizure threshold. In general, this test tends to identify benzodiazepine-like compounds that potentiate the action of GABA A receptors (Meldrum 1997). Other convulsant drugs include bicuculline, picrotoxin, and strychnine.

KINDLING

Kindling models of epilepsy have been used as predictors of drug effects in partial epilepsies (McNamara *et al* 1980; McNamara 1989). Kindling is the phenomenon whereby repeated subclinical stimuli progressively lead to potentially permanent reduction in seizure threshold and spontaneous epileptogenic activity, with increased liability to seizures. The stimuli can be focal or systemic and electrical or chemical (Jefferys and Roberts 1987). The underlying pathophysiology is not completely understood.

MECHANISM OF ACTION OF DRUGS

Most studies have been carried out on drugs with actions on neuronal membranes and synapses. Other mechanisms of action that a drug with antiepileptic properties might possess include induction of metabolic, hormonal, and ionic changes, alteration of trophic changes following nerve damage, or alteration in genetic expression of proteins involved in synaptic transmission (Waterhouse and Delorenzo 1996). Any proposed mechanism of action should be consistent with a known alteration of neuronal function occurring during seizure activity. An ideal drug would have this mode of action without significant effects on the CNS in the interictal state.

Table 37.2 summarizes the mechanisms of action that are best understood and form the focus of most attention. Other mechanisms include potassium channel modulation, excitatory amino acid receptor regulation, regulation of second messenger effects in neurons, inhibition of carbonic anhydrase, and alteration of genetic expression (Waterhouse and Delorenzo 1996). The known modes of action of various AEDs are shown in Table 37.3.

Table 37.2 The mechanisms of action of antiepileptic drugs that are best understood.

Sodium channel	Calcium channel	GABA receptor/chloride ion complex
Use-dependent block	T-channel blockers L-channel blockers N-channel blockers Receptor regulated	GABA receptor Chloride channel regulation GABA reuptake inhibition GABA transaminase inhibition

GABA, γ- aminobutyric acid.

Table 37.3 Currently understood modes of action of antiepileptic drugs in use or soon to become available.

	Sodium channel	GABA receptor	T-type calcium channel	NMDA receptor
Barbiturates	+	+	–	
Primidone	+	–	?	
Phenytoin	++	–	–	–
Ethosuximide	–	–	++	
Carbamazepine	++	–	–	–
Valproic acid	++	?/+	?/+	–
Benzodiazepines	+	++	–	–
Vigabatrin	?	+	?	?
Lamotrigine	++	–/?	–/?	?
Gabapentin	+/?	–	–	–
Felbamate	+/?	+/?	?	+/?
Oxcarbazepine	+/?	?	?	?
Topiramate				
Tiagabine		+		

GABA, γ-aminobutyric acid; NMDA, N-methyl-D-aspartate.
Sources: MacDonald and Kelly (1994); Leach and Brodie (1995); Waterhouse and Delorenzo (1996).

DRUG DEVELOPMENT

The development of a new drug can be divided into a number of phases: research, preexploratory development, exploratory development, full development, registration, and launch.

In the research phase, a candidate drug is identified using a number of methods ranging from computer modeling to *in vitro* and *in vivo* studies. Implicit in this phase is the ability to manufacture the drug on a laboratory scale. The patent is applied for during preexploratory development and it is here that the commercial 'clock' starts ticking. The longer a drug takes to develop, the less time remains in the life of the patent when it is launched. In this phase, basic pharmacologic and biochemical screening takes place, as well as analytic characterization of the active substance. Dose range finding, toxicology, and preliminary genotoxicity tests are carried out, along with preliminary studies of metabolism.

In exploratory development there is small-scale synthesis of the active substance. Specific analytic methods must be developed to determine the active substance, its metabolites, degradation products, and impurities. Methods of drug synthesis are considered. There are studies of the formulations that may be possible, for example a parenteral form. Different formulations are prepared for clinical and toxicologic evaluation. The radiolabeled version is prepared for pharmacokinetic studies and there is development of analytic methods for stability testing. At the same time the animal safety studies are in progress. There is assessment of acute toxicity, with single administration in two animal species, and subacute toxicity, with repeated medium-term administration in two species. There are reproductive toxicity studies, further genotoxicity studies, detailed pharmacologic studies (main effects, side-effects, duration of effects), and pharmacokinetic studies examining drug absorption, distribution, metabolism, and excretion. When these are complete, phase I clinical studies in healthy volunteers start. Full development then follows, with double-blind studies in patients in phase II and III trials which, if successful, lead to registration and launch.

SCREENING OF ANTIEPILEPTIC DRUGS IN ANIMAL MODELS

New drugs undergo stringent tests in animals before testing in humans begins. The initial evaluation of an AED involves a number of stages. In the 1970s, the National Institute of Neurologic and Communicative Disorders and Stroke sponsored a screening program for potential AEDs that has played a major role in facilitating the development of new drugs (Waterhouse and Delorenzo 1996). It is summarized below and is similar to that followed generally (Swinyard 1989; White *et al* 1995, 1998).

The first stage is *detection of anticonvulsant effect.* The test drug is injected intraperitoneally into mice at varying doses. The MES and subcutaneous pentylenetetrazol epilepsy models are used to detect anticonvulsant activity and minimal neural toxicity is sought using the rotorod test. In this test a mouse is placed on a rod of 2.5 cm diameter rotating at a rate of 6 r.p.m. A normal mouse can maintain its balance for long periods of time. Neurologic deficit is indicated by inability to maintain equilibrium for 1 min in each of three trials. The various tests are carried out 30 min and 4 hours after drug administration.

Compounds active in mice are tested in rats, the drug being given orally. The same seizure models are used and minimal neurotoxicity is assessed using the positional sense test, gait and stance test, or the muscle tone test. Compounds found to be inactive in mice using the intraperitoneal route are administered subcutaneously to mice using the threshold tonic extension test and the effect measured at 15 min, 30 min, 1, 2, and 4 hours.

The next stage is *anticonvulsant quantification.* A drug shown to have antiepileptic activity is given to mice intraperitoneally. The time of peak effect is noted using the MES, pentylenetetrazol, and rotorod tests. Likewise, the median effective dose is calculated. The same measures are then made in rats.

The third stage is *anticonvulsant differentiation.* The drug is administered intraperitoneally in mice and the median effective dose is measured in the bicuculline and picrotoxin models and in audiogenic seizure-susceptible animals. It is then given orally to rats with EEGs altered by γ-hydroxybutyrate, a spike-and-wave model of absence. The drug is also tested in kindling models.

The fourth stage is assessment of *proconvulsant potential.* The active compound is administered to mice intraperitoneally. A timed intravenous infusion of pentylenetetrazol is then given. This test measures the minimal seizure threshold of each animal that has received the median effective dose of the drug.

Subchronic studies are then carried out. The drug is administered to rats orally in order to assess *in vivo* tolerance and any lasting effect of subchronic dosing on MES and pentylenetetrazol seizures. The effect of subchronic dosing on liver enzymes and drug-metabolizing enzymes is also assessed.

In the sixth stage, *mechanism of action studies* are carried out *in vitro* using imaging techniques and patch clamp analysis of chloride, potassium, calcium, and sodium currents. Anticonvulsant properties and toxicity are further evaluated in another species. Finally, *lethal dose tests* are carried out and prolonged administration is tested. At this stage receptor binding assays, pharmacodynamic studies, and comparison of the new compound with commonly used AEDs are also carried out.

Preclinical evaluation is vital; however, promising drugs from studies in animal models may not show the same success in humans since both beneficial and unwanted effects may be species-specific.

CLINICAL TRIALS

Clinical trials have evolved over the last 30–40 years. Previously, it was accepted that a drug would have a clinical effect if an effect could be shown in animals (Dam *et al* 1995). Since then there has been progressive development of clinical trial methodology and biostatistics (Gram and Schmidt 1993; French 1998). Clinical testing begins once the animal studies are completed. The trials are designed to give an accurate profile of the drug for registration purposes. Currently, two large prospective double-blind trials are required.

Since trials are designed for registration the late-phase clinical trials are unlikely to truly reflect clinical practice. There are also a number of other imperfections (Walker and Sander 1996; Chadwick 1997). Initially, AEDs are tested as add-on therapy in patients with intractable epilepsy. Therefore, the test is really of drug combinations rather than of any separate effect of the new compound. In addition, the value and safety of a new drug as monotherapy cannot be elucidated by add-on studies. The patients in these trials usually have partial seizures, with or without secondary generalization, as this reflects the drug-resistant group. Clinical trials for registration tend to look at seizure frequency rather than other equally important aspects, such as seizure severity and quality of life. Alternative endpoints have been discussed by Cramer (1998), Mizrahi (1998), and Nabulsi and Karrar (1998).

Registration trials are not necessarily carried out on populations representative of those that may need to use the drug, for example there are restrictions on the inclusion of women of childbearing age. Finally, trials for registration usually compare a new compound with well-established older compounds and the comparative value of different new drugs is hard to ascertain unless they are examined in the same clinical trial.

In the UK since 1990, an AED has had to demonstrate efficacy in a particular seizure type or epilepsy syndrome before it can be licensed for use in that condition. Previously, efficacy in whatever seizure types were tested enabled the drug to be licensed for epilepsy in general. Consequently, the task of developing a new AED is now rather cumbersome, time-consuming, and costly.

Clinical trials, which have been reviewed by Dam *et al* (1995), are conventionally divided into four phases.

PHASE I STUDIES

A well-tolerated dose range and the highest tolerated dose is defined in healthy volunteers. Information on pharmacodynamic and pharmacokinetic properties is obtained. Firstly, variable single-dose studies are carried out in placebo-controlled double-blind trials. Careful safety monitoring and basic pharmacokinetic parameters, including elimination half-life, protein binding, and excretion, should be established. It is particularly important to determine the effect of dose on half-life and clearance.

Multiple dose studies are then carried out, once again using a double-blind placebo-controlled trial design. The dosing intervals are based on the half-life data from the single-dose studies. Several different dosing levels should be examined. The behavior of the drug in particular subpopulations, such as the elderly and those with hepatic or renal impairment, is examined.

Finally, preliminary evaluation of the drug takes place in patients with epilepsy. The ideal form of trial is once again a double-blind design with placebo. This is the first stage at which the physician is able to assess the drug clinically in order to gain a preliminary idea of its efficacy and its potential interactions with other AEDs.

PHASE II STUDIES

The new drug is tested in a controlled randomized trial in patients with epilepsy. The safety and tolerability profile is carefully monitored and the dose range established as far as possible. It must be borne in mind that it is really the effect of the drug in combination which is being assessed. The trials may be crossover or parallel in design.

PHASE III STUDIES

The efficacy and tolerability of the safety profile are studied in larger groups of patients and over longer periods of time. Randomized, double-blind, placebo-controlled trials with crossover and parallel design are used. Occasionally the new drug is compared with an active comparator.

PHASE IV STUDIES

The postmarketing performance of the drug is evaluated. More trials occur with an active comparator. Also, different seizure types and epilepsy syndromes are studied with a view to license extension.

AVAILABLE ANTIEPILEPTIC DRUGS

Table 37.4 shows the year of general release in the UK of some of the better-known AEDs. Others have had a period of popularity before being withdrawn because of insufficient efficacy or unacceptable side-effects (Table 37.5).

Table 37.4 Year of introduction of better-known antiepileptic drugs.

	Year of introduction
Bromide	1853
Phenobarbital	1912
Phenytoin	1938
Primidone	1952
Ethosuximide	1960
Carbamazepine	1963
Clonazepam	1974
Sodium valproate	1974
Clobazam	1982
Vigabatrin	1989
Lamotrigine	1991
Gabapentin	1993
Topiramate	1995

Table 37.5 Drugs that have been marketed and then withdrawn in the UK.

Beclamide
Benzchlorpropamide
Mephenytoin
Metharbital
Methylphenobarbital
Mesuximide
Paramethadione
Phenacemide
Phensuximide
Phenthenylate
Sulthiam
Trimethadione

ANTIEPILEPTIC DRUGS THAT MAY BECOME AVAILABLE

A number of new compounds are undergoing phase III clinical trials or have not yet been released in the UK, including eterobarb, levetiracetam, losigamone, ralitoline, remacemide, stiripentol, taltrimide, tiagabine, and zonisamide. Their properties have been reviewed by a number of authors (Patsalos and Sander 1994; Leach and Brodie 1995; Leppik and Gil-Nagel 1995; Stables *et al* 1995; Walker and Sander 1996; Blum 1998). Many more are in the early phases of clinical trials. A recent survey suggests that there are at least eight in phase II trials and a further eight at the phase I stage, with many more in the earlier stages of development. Only the drugs in phase III clinical trials are summarized here.

ETEROBARB

Eterobarb is a phenobarbital derivative. It is rapidly converted to phenobarbital and *N*-monomethoxymethylphenobarbital (Rapport and Kupferberg 1973). Its mode of action is the same as phenobarbital. It has a short half-life of 3–4 hours compared with phenobarbital (5 days). In animal studies, it has been shown to have the same potency as phenobarbital but produces less sedation (Wolter 1991).

Eterobarb has been compared with phenobarbital in open-label and double-blind studies, which suggest that higher levels of phenobarbital can be tolerated in patients on eterobarb; a significant number of patients experience better seizure control on eterobarb; and eterobarb has a side-effect profile similar to phenobarbital but is better tolerated. Interestingly, there was some resolution of hyperactivity in children when eterobarb was substituted for phenobarbital (Smith 1977).

LEVETIRACETAM

Levetiracetam is an ethyl analog of piracetam and is one of the class of 'nootropic' drugs (Gouliaev and Senning 1994). The mode of action is unclear and may be via a variety of systems, including the cholinergic, dopaminergic, and glutaminergic. This class of drugs modulates AMPA glutamate receptors *in vitro* (Copani *et al* 1992). Levetiracetam is rapidly absorbed following oral administration. It is renally excreted and has an elimination half-life of 5–8 hours (Edelbroeck *et al* 1993). There is clear evidence from experiments with amygdala kindled seizures of its potential in partial seizures. Furthermore, there is

evidence that it might have an antiepileptogenic as well as an anticonvulsant effect (Gower *et al* 1992; Loscher and Honack 1993). It is currently in phase II and III studies and appears to be both effective and well tolerated. Side-effects include drowsiness, unsteadiness, and mood change (De Deyn *et al* 1992).

REMACEMIDE

Remacemide is a novel water-soluble anticonvulsant and is a racemic mixture of two enantiomers. It has a number of active metabolites and could be viewed as a prodrug. The desglycine metabolite, FPL 12495, shows greater anticonvulsant activity. The other metabolites have varying degrees of anticonvulsant activity. Remacemide itself has a half-life of 4 hours but the desglycine metabolite has an apparent elimination half-life of 12–24 hours (Muir and Palmer 1991). It is effective in the MES model and hippocampal kindling-induced seizures but not in pentylenetetrazol-induced seizures. It inhibits convulsions in mice subject to audiogenic seizures, and inhibits seizures induced by NMDA (Garske *et al* 1991). It has weak affinities with glycine-sensitive and noncompetitive ion channel subsites of the NMDA receptor complex (Garske *et al* 1991). In cell culture, remacemide hydrochloride prevents sustained repetitive firing through action on voltage-sensitive sodium channels.

It is currently undergoing phase III clinical trials. Results so far indicate efficacy in complex partial and secondarily generalized seizures (Crawford *et al* 1992). Side-effects include gastrointestinal upsets and dizziness.

STIRIPENTOL

Stiripentol is structurally unrelated to other AEDs. It increases brain GABA but the mode of action is unknown. Its pharmacokinetics are complicated: it has a multiphasic elimination curve (Levy *et al* 1983), is extensively bound to plasma, extensively metabolized in the liver, and demonstrates nonlinear pharmacokinetics (Levy *et al* 1984). It is effective in a wide range of animal seizure models including electrically and chemically induced seizures, absence seizures in a genetic rat model, and focal seizures in an alumina-gel monkey model. Studies in relatively small numbers of patients have shown efficacy in refractory complex partial seizures and atypical absence seizures (Vincent 1991). Side-effects are dose related and include anorexia, nausea, vomiting, and lethargy. Trials using the drug as add-on medication have proved difficult.

TIAGABINE

Tiagabine is a nipecotic acid derivative. It raises extracellular GABA concentrations by specific inhibition of GABA uptake by nerve terminals and glial cells (Fink-Jensen *et al* 1992), which enhances GABAergic neurotransmission; the action is reversible. It is quickly absorbed by the oral route but this is affected by food. Peak concentration occurs in 1 hour. It is 95% bound to plasma proteins and is extensively metabolized by the liver. It has a half-life of 7 hours in healthy volunteers, although this is halved in comedicated patients. It is effective in a variety of chemically induced seizure models and some genetic models of epilepsy, including light-induced myoclonic seizures in photosensitive baboons and sound-induced seizures in DBA/Z mice (Pierce *et al* 1991).

In clinical trials it has proved effective in the management of partial seizures and is now licensed in the UK. Side-effects are dose dependent and primarily CNS related, and include sedation, headache, poor concentration, dizziness, and tremor. There is some concern that, like vigabatrin, it may become associated with visual field defects although there is no evidence of this currently.

ZONISAMIDE

Zonisamide is a 1,2-benzisoxole derivative. The mechanism of action is unclear but may be at voltage-gated sodium channels and T-type calcium channels. It is rapidly and well absorbed. It has a half-life of 60 hours, which is reduced to 28 hours in patients taking enzyme-inducing drugs (Ojermann *et al* 1986). It is effective in the MES model and pentylenetetrazol-induced seizures and suppresses kindled seizures. These suggest a wide spectrum of activity, with the exception of absence seizures. However, in clinical trials efficacy has been demonstrated here too (Yagi and Seino 1992). It has a license in Japan where it was developed. However, a high incidence of renal stones in a study in the USA halted further work there and in Europe until recently (Leppik *et al* 1993). Other side-effects include anorexia, ataxia, and mental slowing.

COST OF NEW DRUG DEVELOPMENT

Approximately 12 years pass from the time of the discovery of a new chemical entity (NCE) to the procurement of a license and the drug becoming generally available. Currently, the patent lasts for 20 years from the time of registration. Thus the different trial phases take up many commercially important years. Of 4000 NCEs synthesized only about five reach the stage of testing in humans. Of these only one will achieve registration and of these only about one in three recaptures the development costs, which are now in the order of several billion pounds and increasing.

THE FUTURE

Some improvement in the overall profile of new AEDs is likely during the next 10 years but a major breakthrough and the emergence of a panacea is unlikely. Greater understanding of the genetics of epilepsy and increased ability to affect gene expression will lead to improved control of certain conditions. However, increasing cost consciousness in healthcare will be a major factor limiting the development of new AEDs.

KEY POINTS

1. The ideal antiepileptic drug (AED) would have 100% efficacy in all seizure types, complete tolerability, a wide therapeutic index, and a sufficiently long half-life to enable once or twice daily dosage, and it would be easy to take and available in a number of different formulations, including parenteral. It would not interact with other drugs nor be teratogenic. New drugs are designed with these principles in mind, but it seems unlikely that one will be found that can act cleanly in multiple ways at multiple sites.

2. A current trend is to aim for a drug to have an action at a particular site to counter epileptogenic activity in a specific way. This requires knowledge of the mechanism underlying the genesis of seizures.

3. The possible substrates of drug actions that have received most attention are ion (sodium, calcium, potassium, chloride) channel modulation, GABA receptors, and NMDA receptors.

4. Clinical trials, carried out after animal studies have been

---

KEY POINTS

completed, are designed for registration purposes. Initially drugs are tested as add-on therapy for patients with intractable epilepsy. Thus, drug combinations are under trial rather than any separate effect of the new compound.

5. Trials usually examine seizure frequency ignoring important aspects,

such as seizure severity and quality of life. Thus, they may not reflect the realities of how the drug may be used in clinical practice.

6. After initial add-on trials, a new drug is usually compared with a well-established older drug, or a number of these, in monotherapy trials.

7. In the UK a drug must be shown to be efficacious in a particular seizure type or epilepsy syndrome before it can be licensed for use in that condition.

8. The whole process of developing a new AED is very costly.

REFERENCES

Anhut H, Satzinger G, von Hoedenberg A (1991) Ralitoline. *Epilepsy Research* Suppl 3: 141–145.

Blum DE (1998) New drugs for persons with epilepsy. *Advances in Neurology* 76:57–88.

Cesa-Bianchi MG, Macia M, Mutani R (1967) Experimental epilepsy induced by cobalt powder in lower brainstem and thalamic structures. *Electroencephalography and Clinical Neurophysiology* 22:526–536.

Chadwick DW (1997) Monotherapy clinical trials of new antiepileptic drugs: design, indications, and controversies. *Epilepsia* 38(Suppl 9):S16–S20.

Chadwick DW, Marson T, Kadir Z (1996) Clinical administration of new antiepileptic drugs: an overview of safety and efficacy. *Epilepsia* 37(Suppl 6):S17–S22.

Chapman AG (1995) Excitatory neurotransmission and antiepileptic drug development: a status report. In: Pedley TA, Meldrum BS (eds) *Recent Advances in Epilepsy*, Vol 6, pp 1–22. Edinburgh: Churchill Livingstone.

Copani A, Genazzini AA, Aleppo G *et al* (1992) Nootropic drugs positively modulate α-amino-3-hydroxy-5-methyl-4-isoxazole-propionic acid-sensitive glutamate receptors in neuronal cultures. *Journal of Neurochemistry* 58:1199–1204.

Cramer J (1998) Alternate endpoints for seizure measurement. *Advances in Neurology* 76:189–194.

Crawford P, Richens A, Mower G *et al* (1992) A double-blind placebo-controlled cross-over study of remacemide hydrochloride as adjunctive therapy in patients with refractory epilepsy. *Seizure* 1 (Suppl A):P7/13.

Dam M, Gram L, Mumford JP (1995) Design of clinical trials of new antiepileptic drugs. In: Levy RH, Mattson RH, Meldrun BS (eds) *Antiepileptic Drugs*, 4th edn, pp 00–00. New York: Raven Press.

De Deyn PP, Bielen E, Sazena V *et al* (1992) Assessment of the safety of orally administered usb L059 as add-on therapy in patients treated with antiepileptice drugs. *Seizure* (Suppl A):7–15.

Dichter MA (1997) Basic mechanisms of epilepsy: targets for therapeutic intervention. *Epilepsia* 38 (Suppl 9):S2–S6.

Dichter M (1998) Modulation of inhibition and the transition to seizures. In: Dichter M (ed) *Mechanisms of Epileptogenesis: The Transition to Seizure*, pp 169–181. New York: Plenum Press.

Dichter MA (1998) Mechanism of action of new antiepileptic drugs. *Advances in Neurology* 76:1–10.

Dichter M, Spencer W (1969) Penicillin induced interictal discharges from cat hippocampus. II. Mechanisms underlying origin and restriction. *Journal of Neurophysiology* 32:663–687.

Diesz RA, Prince DA (1989) Frequency-dependent depression of inhibition in guinea-pig neocortex *in vitro* by GABA_B receptor feedback on GABA release. *Journal of Physiology* 412:513–541.

Edelbroeck PM, de Wilde-Ockeleon JM, Kasteleijn-Nolst Trendite DGA *et al* (1993) Evaluation of the pharmacokinetics and neuropsychometric parameters in chronic comedicated epileptic patients of three increasing dosages of a novel, antiepileptic drug ucb L059:250-mg capsules per each dose for one week followed by two weeks of placebo. *Epilepsia* 34 (Suppl 2):7.

Fink-Jensen A, Suzdak PD, Swedberg MDB *et al* (1992) The γ-aminobutyric acid (GABA) uptake inhibitor, tiagabine, increases extracellular brain levels of GABA in awake rats. *European Journal of Pharmacology* 220:197–201.

Fisher W, Bodewei R, Satzinger G (1992) Anticonvulsant and sodium channel blocking effects of ralitoline in different screening models. *Naunyn Schmiedebergs Archives of Pharmacology* 346:442–452.

French JA (1998) The art of antiepileptic trial design. *Advances in Neurology* 76:113–123.

Garske GE, Palmer GC, Napier JJ *et al* (1991) Pre-clinical profile of the anticonvulsant remacemide and its enantiomers in the rat *Epilepsy Research* 9:161–174.

Gloor P (1984) Electrophysiology of generalised epilepsy. In: Schwartzkroin PA, Wheal H (eds) *Electrophysiology of Epilepsy*, pp 107–136. London: Academic Press.

Goodman L, Toman J, Swinyard E (1946) The anticonvulsant properties of Tridione: laboratory and clinical investigations. *American Journal of Medicine* 1:213.

Gouliaev AH, Senning A (1994) Piracetam and other structurally related nootropics. *Brain Research Reviews* 19:180–222.

Gower AJ, Noyer M, Verloes R *et al* (1992) ucb L059, a novel anticonvulsant: pharmacological profile in animals. *European Journal of Pharmacology* 222:193–203.

Gram L (1996) Pharmacokinetics of new antiepileptic drugs. *Epilepsia* 37 (Suppl 6):S12–S16.

Gram L, Schmidt D (1993) Innovative designs of controlled clinical trials in epilepsy. *Epilepsia* 34 (Suppl 7):S1–S6.

Guerrero-Figuero R, Barros A, de Balbian Verster F, Health RG (1963) Experimental 'petit mal' in kittens. *Archives of Neurology* 9:297–306.

Hayashi T (1953) A physiological study of epileptic seizures following cortical stimulation in animals and its application to human clinics. *Japanese Journal of Physiology* 3:46–64.

Heinemann U, Draguhn A, Meierkord H (1996) The pathophysiology of seizure generation. In: Shorvon S, Dreifuss F, Fish D, Thomas D (eds) *The Treatment of Epilepsy*, pp 3–19. Oxford: Blackwell Science.

Jefferys JGR, Roberts R (1987) The biology of epilepsy. In: Hopkins A (ed) *Epilepsy*, pp 19–81. London: Chapman and Hall Medical.

Johnston MV (1996) Developmental aspects of epileptogenesis. *Epilepsia* 37 (Suppl 1):S2–S9.

Kingsbury DT (1997) Bioinformatics in drug discovery. *Drug Development Research* 41:129–141.

Kreindler A, Zuckermann E, Steriade M, Chimian D (1958) Electroclinical features of the convulsive fit induced experimentally through stimulation of the brainstem. *Journal of Neurophysiology* 21:525–536.

Kupferberg HJ (1993) Animal models for identifying new anticonvulsant drugs. In: Wyllie E (ed) *The Treatment of Epilepsy: Principles and Practice*, pp 743–751. Philadelphia: Lea and Febiger.

Leach JP, Brodie MJ (1995) New antiepileptic drugs: an explosion of activity. *Seizure* 4:5–17.

Leach JP, Brodie MJ (1998) Tiagabine. *Lancet* 351:203–207.

Leppik IE, Gil-Nagel A (1995) New antiepileptic drugs. In: Pedley TA, Meldrum BS (eds) *Recent Advances in Epilepsy*, Vol 6, pp 117–138. Edinburgh: Churchill Livingstone.

Leppik IE, Willmore LJ, Homan RW et al (1993) Efficacy and safety of zonisamide: results of a multicenter study. *Epilepsy Research* 14:145–173.

Levy RH, Lin HS, Blehaut HM, Tor JA (1983) Pharmacokinetics of stiripentol in normal man: evidence of nonlinearity. *Journal of Clinical Pharmacology* 23:523–533.

Levy RH, Loiseau P, Guyot M et al (1984) Stiripentol kinetics in epilepsy: nonlinearity and interactions. *Clinical Pharmacology and Therapeutics* 36:661–669.

Loscher W, Honack D (1993) Profile of ucb-L059, a novel anticonvulsant drug in models of partial and generalised epilepsy in mice and rats. *European Journal of Pharmacology* 232:147–158.

Loskota WJ, Lomax P, Rich ST (1974) The gerbil as a model for the study of the epilepsies. *Epilepsia* 15:109–119.

MacDonald RL, Kelly KM (1994) Mechanisms of action of new anticonvulsant drugs. In: Trimble MR (ed) *New Anticonvulsants: Advances in the Treatment of Epilepsy*, pp 35–50. New York: John Wiley & Sons.

MacDonald RL, Meldrum BS (1995) Principles of antiepileptic drug action. In: *Antiepileptic Drugs*, 4th edn, pp 61–77. New York: Raven Press.

McNamara JO (1989) Development of new pharmacological agents for epilepsy: lessons from the kindling model. *Epilepsia* 30:S513–S518.

McNamara JO, Byrne MC, Dasheiff RM, Fitz JG (1980) The kindling model of epilepsy: a review. *Progress in Neurobiology* 15:139–159.

Marson AG, Kadir ZA, Hutton JL, Chadwick DW (1997) The new antiepileptic drugs: a systemic review of their efficacy and tolerability. *Epilepsia* 38:859–880.

Mattson RH (1996) Introduction and symposium overview. *Epilepsia* 37 (Suppl 6):S1–S3.

Meldrum BS (1995) Neurotransmission in epilepsy. *Epilepsia* 36 (Suppl 1):S30–S35.

Meldrum BS (1996) Update on the action of antiepileptic drugs. *Epilepsia* 37 (Suppl 6):S4–S11.

Meldrum BS (1997) Identification and preclinical testing of novel antiepileptic compounds. *Epilepsia* 38 (Suppl 9):S7–S15.

Merritt HH, Putnam TJ (1938) Sodium diphenylhydantoinate in treatment of convulsive disorders. *Journal of the American Medical Association* 111:1068–1073.

Mizrahi EM (1998) Alternate endpoint: EEG assessment of antiepileptic drug efficacy and toxicity. *Advances in Neurology* 76:209–222.

Muir KT, Palmer GC (1991) Remacemide. *Epilepsy Research* Suppl 3:147–152.

Nabulsi A, Karrar HA (1998) Alternate endpoints: studies in quality of life and health economics of epilepsy. *Advances in Neurology* 76:195–208.

Naquert R, Meldrum BS (1972) Photogenic seizures in baboon. In: Purpura DP et al (eds) *Experimental Models of Epilepsy*, pp 373–406. New York: Raven Press.

Noebels JL (1984) Single gene control of excitability in central neurones. In: Schwartzkroin PA, Wheal H (eds) *Electrophysiology of Epilepsy*, pp 201–218. London: Academic Press.

Ojermann LM, Shastri RA, Wilensky AJ, Friel PN, Levy RH (1986) Comparative pharmacokinetics of zonisamide (CL-912) in epileptic patients on carbamazepine or phenytoin monotherapy. *Therapeutic Drug Monitoring* 8:293–296.

Patsalos PN, Sander JWAS (1994) Newer antiepileptic drugs. Towards an improved risk–benefit ratio. *Drug Safety* 11:37–67.

Penfield W, Jasper H (1954) *Epilepsy and Functional Anatomy of the Human Brain*. Boston: Little, Brown.

Pierce MW, Suzdak PD, Gustavson LE, Mengel HB, McKelvy JF, Mant T (1991) Tiagabine. *Epilepsy Research* Suppl 3:157–160.

Pollen DA (1964) Intracellular studies of cortical neurones during thalamic induced wave and spike. *Electroencephalography and Clinical Neurophysiology* 17:398–404.

Rapport R, Kupferberg H (1973) Metabolism of dimethoxy-methylphenobarbital in mice. Relationship between brain phenobarbital levels and anticonvulsant activity. *Journal of Medicinal Chemistry* 16:559–602.

Richens A (1991) The basis of the treatment of epilepsy: neuropharmacology. In: Dam M (ed) *A Practical Approach to Epilepsy*, pp 75–85. Oxford: Pergamon Press.

Rogawski MA (1998) Mechanism-specific pathways for new antiepileptic drug discovery. *Advances in Neurology* 76:11–28.

Seyfried TN, Glaser GH (1985) A review of mouse mutants as genetic models of epilepsy. *Epilepsia* 26:143–150.

Shorvon S, Reynolds EH (1982) Early prognosis of epilepsy. *British Medical Journal* 285:1699–1701.

Smith D (1977) A clinical evaluation of eterobarb in epileptic children. In: Meinardi H, Rowan AJ (eds) *Advances in Epileptology*, pp 318–321. Amsterdam: Swetz and Zeitlinger.

Stables JP, Bialer M, Johannessen SI et al (1995) Progress report on new antiepileptic drugs. A summary of the second Eilat conference. *Epilepsy Research* 22:235–246.

Stefani A, Spadoni F, Benardi G (1997) Voltage-activated calcium channels: targets of antiepileptic drug therapy?

Stein U, Klessing K, Chattergee S (1991) Losigamone. *Epilepsy Research* Suppl 3:129–133.

Swinyard EA, Woodhead JH, White HS, Franklin MR (1989) General principles: experimental selection, quantification and evaluation of anticonvulsants. In: Levy R, Meldrum B, Penry JK, Dreifuss FE (eds) *Antiepileptic Drugs*, 3rd edn, pp 85–102. New York: Raven Press.

Taylor CP, Marks JL (1998) Pharmaceutical industry screening for new antiepileptic drugs. *Advances in Neurology* 76:41–47.

Tukel K, Jasper H (1952) The electroencephalogram in parasagittal lesions. *Electroencephalography and Clinical Neurophysiology* 4:481–494.

Vergnes M, Marescaux C, Micheletti G et al (1982) Spontaneous paroxysmal electroclinical patterns in rat: a model of generalised non-convulsive epilepsy. *Neuroscience Letters* 33:97–101.

Vincent JC (1991) Stiripentol. *Epilepsy Research* Suppl 3:153–166.

Walker MC, Sander JWAS (1996) Antiepileptic drugs in clinical trials. In: Shorvon S, Dreifuss F, Fish D, Thomas D (eds) *The Treatment of Epilepsy*, pp 509–515. Oxford: Blackwell Science.

Waterhouse E, Delorenzo RJ (1996) Mechanisms of action of antiepileptic drugs: an overview. In: Shorvon S, Dreifuss F, Fish D, Thomas D (eds) *The Treatment of Epilepsy*, pp 123–137. Oxford: Blackwell Science.

White SH (1997) Clinical significance of animal seizure models and mechanism of action studies of potential antiepileptic drugs. *Epilepsia* 38(Suppl 1):S9–S17.

White SH, Woodhead JH, Franklin MR Swinyard EA, Wolf HH (1995) Experimental selection, quantification and evaluation of antiepileptic drugs. In: Levy RH, Mattson RH, Meldrun BS (eds) *Antiepileptic Drugs*, 4th edn, pp 99–110. New York: Raven Press.

White SH, Wolf HH, Woodhead JH, Kupfberg H (1998) The National Institutes of Health Anticonvulsant Drug Development Program: screening for efficacy. *Advances in Neurology* **76**:29–39.

Wolter KD (1991) Eterobarb. *Epilepsy Research* Suppl 3:99–102.

Yagi K, Seino M (1992) Methodological requirements for clinical trials in refractory epilepsies: our experience with zonisamide. *Progress in Neuropsychopharmacology and Biological Psychiatry* **16**:79–85.

Zucker R (1989) Short-term synaptic plasticity. *Annual Review of Neuroscience* 13–32.

Psychologic methods

LH GOLDSTEIN

Most individuals with epilepsy, around 70%, have their seizures successfully controlled pharmacologically. However, some may need to explore other methods of management, and knowledge is growing about psychologic approaches to seizure control. This chapter reviews psychologic techniques for improving seizure control and their potential for more widespread application.

People with epilepsy may experience a range of psychologic problems, including anxiety, depression, and low self-esteem (Baker 1997). Effective psychologic treatments for such disorders have been applied in other patient populations. Evidence is reviewed to demonstrate their applicability to individuals with poorly controlled epilepsy.

PSYCHOLOGIC PRECIPITANTS OF SEIZURES

Behavioral interventions for seizures were described in the last century (Dahl 1992), although systematic evaluations of psychologic treatments of epilepsy are relatively recent. However, theoretic models explaining how psychologic factors can affect seizure occurrence are relatively limited. The assumption that the cause of seizures resides in 'the interaction of the person with epilepsy and the environment'

(Dahl 1992, p 30) underpins the available models. Engel (1989) recognized this possible interaction by dividing potential causes of epilepsy into nonspecific predisposing factors producing individual differences in predisposition to seizures, specific epileptogenic disturbances responsible for chronic epilepsy in susceptible individuals, and precipitating factors, which can be internal or external to the person and which can provoke seizures acutely in people with chronic epilepsy (Dahl 1992, p 30). Antebi and Bird (1992) suggested that both psychologic and physiologic factors can temporarily alter seizure thresholds, thereby influencing seizure occurrence. Facilitation of seizures occurs when stimuli, including psychologic states, make it more likely that seizures will develop (Antebi and Bird 1992). Evocation of seizures involves a stimulus almost certainly leading to a seizure within seconds. Antebi and Bird generally viewed seizure triggers as falling on a continuum between evocation and facilitation.

A much-discussed model of seizure genesis (Fenwick and Brown 1989; Goldstein 1990, 1997a,b; Dahl 1992) has been developed from Lockard and Ward's (1980) experimental research with monkeys. Two groups of neurons were considered important in seizure development. Damaged neurons at the center of an epileptic focus, called group 1 neurons, fire continuously in an abnormal, paroxysmal manner, acting as a 'pacemaker' for epileptic discharges. Surrounding these are group 2 neurons that, being partially deafferented, either fire normally (thereby limiting the spread of a seizure) or paroxysmally (thereby producing a focal seizure); if they then recruit normal neurons into seizure activity, the seizure generalizes. Fenwick and Brown (1989) suggested that group 2 neuronal activity may be influenced by environmental factors and behavior, and on this basis seizure activity may come under environmental or behavioral control. Dahl (1992) developed this model, postulating that while an initial seizure may not have been influenced by learning, some degree of learning or conditioning would always subsequently be involved in the elicitation or inhibition of a seizure. Thus, if conditioning factors can produce seizures, they should be of potential use in seizure reduction.

Other models have considered the specific role of anxiety and stress in seizure genesis (Fried 1993; Mostofsky 1993; Joëls *et al* 1997). Mostofsky (1993) suggested that anxiety might affect levels of corticosteroids, cerebral blood flow, or acidosis or alkalosis. Research has begun to consider the levels of corticosteroids in the hippocampus during acute episodes of stress, emphasizing the changed balance between mineralocorticoid and neurohormones. Joëls *et al* (1997) noted that calcium currents in the CA1 field of the hippocampus and thus seizure threshold, vary with corticosteroid levels, providing a possible mechanism whereby stress can potentiate seizure occurrence. Repeated exposure to stress might therefore provide the physiochemical setting for seizure precipitation and might also involve a learned association between stressful situations and seizure genesis, along the general lines suggested by Dahl (1992).

Hyperventilation, which often accompanies anxiety, has also been linked with seizure occurrence. Carbon dioxide loss, consequent upon hyperventilation, exhibits an almost linear relationship to EEG frequency decrease and the onset of seizures (see Fried 1993). Training in diaphragmatic breathing used to alter breathing patterns in hyperventilating individuals, when accompanied by biofeedback of percentage end-tidal carbon dioxide levels, resulted in EEG normalization and seizure frequency reduction. Since the development of hyperventilation may follow an environmental stressor, this too would be consistent with Dahl's (1992) concept that the 'cause' of seizures lies in the dynamic interaction between the person's brain and their environment.

SELF-REPORT OF SEIZURE TRIGGERS

Seizure onset

A number of studies have addressed the ability of people with epilepsy and their carers to identify settings in which

seizures are more or less likely to occur. From these, a broad consensus has emerged (Table 38.1).

Situations with a high risk for seizures appear to be characterized predominantly by stress and anxiety. Tiredness is another commonly identified seizure risk, possibly reflecting variations in neurohormonal responses to stress within the circadian rhythm (see Myslobodsky 1993). The studies by Dahl (1992) and Løyning *et al* (1993) also suggest that rapid changes in arousal may precipitate seizures.

An individual's subjective appraisal of the consistency of triggers may confound assessment of an environment–seizure contingency. However, Spector's (1997) sample of 100 adults with poorly controlled seizures reported considerable consistency between the presence of certain settings and seizure occurrence when presented with a list of 11 possible seizure precipitants.

Some people with epilepsy report being able to induce seizures at will. The percentage of patients reporting this varies between studies (15%, Spector 1997; 8.9%, Cull *et al* 1996; 3%, Antebi and Bird 1993; 69%, Dahl 1992; 22.6%,

Table 38.1 Common seizure precipitants. (Adapted from Spector 1997.)

Reference	Most common seizure precipitants
Finkler *et al* (1990)	
76 adult outpatients with epilepsy and psychiatric diagnosis	Anxiety (69%), mood (60%), tired (44%)
36 adult outpatients with epilepsy without psychiatric diagnosis	Tired (52%), anxiety (37%), mood (37%)
Dahl (1992)	
160 patients	Drowsiness (84%), after physical activity (83%), negative stress (78%)
Hayden *et al* (1992)	
475 adults and children with epilepsy	Stress (41%), fatigue (19%), lack of sleep (14%)
Antebi and Bird (1993)	
100 adults from neurology (50) and neuropsychiatry outpatient clinics, low IQ levels	Anxiety (66%), depression (44%), menstruation (44%)
Løyning *et al* (1993)	
48 patients (aged 13–60) and 16 parents of patients with epilepsy	Stress (42%), arousal change (26%)
Hart and Shorvon (1995)	
1628 adults and children (46% seizure-free in previous year)	Stress (28%), tired (11%), menstruation (7%)
Cull *et al* (1996)	
79 young people (aged 14–22) with severe epilepsy (IQ 40–103)	Stress (38.5%), visual stimuli (20.8%)
Spector (1997)	
86 adults attending neurology or neuropsychiatry clinics, at least average IQ	Tension/anxiety (53%), menstruation (35.3%), tiredness/rundown (30%)

Finkler *et al* 1990). It may seem perverse that anyone should deliberately seek to induce seizures. Nevertheless, Dahl (1992) has indicated that seizure behavior can have positive consequences, for example enabling the person to avoid demands made of them. Continuing epilepsy can also have economic advantages. In addition, for some individuals seizures may be perceived as pleasurable, and seizure occurrence may maintain the status quo in family dynamics. Clearly any of these factors need to be considered when formulating a psychologic treatment plan.

Seizure inhibition

In addition to individuals' attempts to induce seizures, patients' ability to abort seizures has been documented (Pritchard *et al* 1985; Dahl 1992; Fenwick 1994; Betts *et al* 1995a; Spector 1997). Such techniques may postpone, abort, or shorten an ongoing seizure (Dahl 1992). Such self-control techniques do not necessarily always work (e.g. Betts *et al* 1995a) and it is unclear why patients persist with such techniques when this is the case.

In summary, when considering reports on patients' identification of seizure precipitants, their recognition of low-risk situations for seizures, and their tendency to abort or to induce seizures, it is apparent that such factors are specific to the individual. Thus, in order to assess which psychologic methods might be used to reduce seizure frequency, individual-based assessments must consider likely seizure precipitants in addition to seizure-maintaining factors in the person's life (Goldstein 1997a). Since seizure precipitants and attempts at self-control vary between individuals, patients may respond differently if a uniform treatment package is administered. Surprisingly, this has not been discussed in many published treatment studies and it is addressed alongside the treatment methods documented below.

PSYCHOLOGIC TECHNIQUES USED TO REDUCE SEIZURE OCCURRENCE

The literature on psychologic methods of seizure control has many weaknesses (see Mostofsky and Balaschak 1977; Krafft and Poling 1982; Goldstein 1990). Many published studies are weak because of various factors, including poor study design, small sample sizes, inadequate descriptions of treatments, insufficient follow-up of patients, and the inclusion of patients with multiple seizure types. Furthermore, explicit indications that treatments have incorporated features specific to the onset of the individual's seizures are frequently absent. None the less, systematic reviews do support the effectiveness of various forms of psychologic treatment in reducing the frequency of seizure occurrence (Powell 1981; Goldstein 1990, 1997a,b; Fenwick 1994).

OPERANT AND CLASSICAL CONDITIONING

Dahl (1992), discussing conditioning factors in epilepsy, considers that a seizure is not, at least initially, a learned behavior but is, in learning theory terms, an unconditioned response 'caused' by underlying pathology. Once a seizure occurs, however, it becomes susceptible to conditioning factors (Powell 1981). This chapter cannot fully describe models of classical and operant conditioning, but both can contribute valuably to the understanding of patterns of seizure occurrence.

Powell (1981) reviewed studies that were based on either operant or classical conditioning as seizure-reduction techniques and which employed methods that took account of the patients' seizure behavior. For example, Cautela and Flannery (1973) gave positive reinforcement (attention, talking to a 22-year-old man with learning disabilities, social praise, candy) for seizure-free time, but not if a seizure occurred. Zlutnick *et al* (1975) used individual-specific interruptions of early seizure behavior, with all five of their subjects showing an initial response to treatment and three gaining longer-term benefit. Ince (1976) used systematic desensitization to treat a 12-year-old boy who was unhappy at school because of others' reactions to his seizures. Hierarchies of emotionally relevant and stressful scenes were constructed and applied once the boy had learned relaxation techniques. This resulted in markedly reduced seizure occurrence.

Dahl (1992) discussed the use of EEG biofeedback as an operant technique for seizure control. This work assumes that patients can discriminate early seizure signals and then generate an 'anticonvulsant' EEG rhythm. Reviews of such work (Powell 1981; Dahl 1992; Fenwick 1994; Sterman 1996; Thompson and Baxendale 1996) have demonstrated the possible use of several EEG rhythms (sensorimotor rhythms, slow cortical potentials) in training seizure control. Results have been generally positive in outcome (Thompson and Baxendale 1996), although training can be very intensive (Rockstroh *et al* 1993). While age may determine a patient's ability to learn to produce a particular EEG pattern (Rockstroh *et al* 1993), studies have assumed that the EEG rhythm under investigation will be anticonvulsant for all individuals in the particular study without demonstrating this for each person.

Further use of classical conditioning to treat seizures has been reviewed by Powell (1981) and Dahl (1992). Seminal work here is that of Effron (1956, 1957) and Forster (1969, 1977). Effron (1956) described the pairing of an unpleasant odor with early seizure signals to interrupt and abort seizures. Subsequently, the smell of jasmine, previously effective in interrupting a seizure, was paired with the presentation of a silver bracelet. After 8 days of conditioning, seeing the bracelet elicited the recollection of the smell of jasmine and seizures were aborted when the patient stared at the bracelet at seizure onset (Effron 1957).

Forster treated seizures elicited by specific evoking stimuli. Using conditioning techniques of successive approximation and habituation he demonstrated that patients' sensitivity to trigger stimuli could be modified. He also demonstrated that seizure thresholds could be modified (Forster *et al* 1964). In addition seizures could be prevented by requiring the person to perform a distracting behavior when a seizure trigger was presented (Forster *et al* 1969).

In summary, a range of operant and classical conditioning techniques have been effective in reducing seizure occurrence. This is consistent with the view that seizures can be influenced by both conditioning processes. Dahl (1992) proposed that early seizure occurrence may be more susceptible to classical conditioning where seizures (unconditioned responses) are paired with environmental, conditioned stimuli, which leads the person to expect seizures to occur in certain situations. Via operant learning, the consequences of that seizure will come to be associated with its occurrence, which may, if pleasant for the person, lead to increased seizure frequency until the consequence of having seizures is modified. This complex model emphasizes the need for a comprehensive assessment of seizure occurrence patterns in the individual being treated. This has not always been undertaken in published studies.

RELAXATION

Given that anger, stress, and tension have frequently been identified as situations that aggravate the risk of seizures, and since anxiety is frequently reported by people with epilepsy, it is appropriate that attempts have been made to use relaxation training to reduce seizure frequency.

Three studies (Rousseau *et al* 1985; Whitman *et al* 1990; Puskarich *et al* 1992) employed progressive muscular relaxation with adults with mixed seizure types, although training schedules varied between studies. Only Puskarich *et al* (1992) used an independent control group, and the sample sizes were small in all three studies. In none were patients encouraged to employ relaxation in likely seizure situations, although they had to practice it at least twice daily.

Common to all three studies is the finding that most subjects experienced fewer seizures following relaxation training, e.g. seizure decrease ranged from 38 to 100% in Rousseau *et al*'s (1985) study. However in each study some subjects obtained no benefit from relaxation training, occasionally showing increased seizure frequency or showing improvement during sham training. Positive results may relate to the tendency for tension, anxiety or stress to be common seizure precipitants. The authors did not investigate whether the individuals for whom relaxation training was ineffective in reducing seizures would identify different seizure precipitants from those who did respond, although individual differences in treatment response may have resulted from inappropriate matching of treatments to the patients' seizure triggers. Miller (1994a) has also expressed similar concerns about the blanket use of relaxation training.

Relaxation was used in a more patient-specific way by Dahl *et al* (1987). Subjects were trained in relaxation and to identify high-risk seizure situations and early signs of seizure onset. They also learned to recognize physical symptoms or situations that were relatively incompatible with seizure occurrence. Subjects then combined awareness of these safe symptoms or situations with a relaxed state, and subsequently applied this relaxed state to the high-risk situations in fantasy, role play and, finally, real-life situations. Those receiving this treatment ($n = 5$) showed greater reduction in mean seizure frequency (66%) than subjects in attention ($n = 5$; 68% increase) and waiting list ($n = 6$; 2% reduction) control groups. Dahl *et al* (1987) speculated that relaxation facilitated better coping with seizures by reducing negative emotional states. They also queried whether relaxation, in an alert state, inhibits epileptic activity or serves to distract the person from the seizure triggers. If relaxation serves the latter function, then it may be only one of a range of suitable coping behaviors.

COUNTERMEASURES

Where a rapid change in arousal level is an identifiable seizure precipitant, then a specific behavior designed to counteract the arousal change may prevent a seizure from developing, if applied at the person's first awareness of its impending occurrence. Such behaviors, termed 'countermeasures' (Dahl *et al* 1988), may involve physical and/or mental activity. Countermeasures represent many of the techniques people use to limit their seizures (Pritchard *et al* 1985; Fenwick 1994; Betts *et al* 1995a), although these techniques are not always effective (Betts *et al* 1995a).

Dahl *et al* (1988) evaluated the use of countermeasures by three children with intractable epilepsy (mixed seizure types). Countermeasures ('a change in the arousal level relevant to and contingent on early seizure cues, situation, and arousal level') were devised for each child so that they were discrete, could be performed rapidly, controlled arousal or attention, and entailed probable seizure incompatibility (Dahl *et al* 1988, p 176). These produced a significant decrease in seizure behavior for all three children. Applications of cue-controlled relaxation or arousal (Brown and Fenwick 1989), or of individual patient-selected pairings of aromatherapy oils and autohypnotic suggestions of relaxation or arousal (Betts *et al* 1995b), have further demonstrated the potential effectiveness of countermeasures in seizure reduction involving patient-specific treatments.

MULTICOMPONENT TREATMENTS

The environmental triggers for a person's seizures can be complex (Dahl 1992). It is understandable therefore that a number of studies have incorporated multiple techniques into training self-control of seizures. Implicit in these studies is that techniques are modified or applied in a manner particular to the individual concerned, although specific details of such modifications are generally absent.

For example, Dahl *et al* (1985) divided 18 children into three treatment groups. The behavior modification group learned to discriminate early seizure signals and then to apply relaxation in high-risk situations. Parents and teachers were taught to respond to the children's seizures in a neutral way and were also encouraged to be less overprotective towards the children. The superior effectiveness of this treatment package, compared with an attention control or traditional epilepsy management approach, was demonstrated at the end of training and at 1-year and 8-year follow-ups (Dahl *et al* 1985, 1992).

Gillham (1990) compared different treatment approaches in two groups of adult outpatients with inadequate seizure control (mixed seizure types) and psychologic disorder. She compared one treatment based on teaching seizure prediction and control with another based on alleviating patients' particular psychologic distress. Each treatment involved three sessions of patient contact once a stable baseline of seizure frequency had been obtained. A third group of patients without psychologic disorder received one treatment following baseline. Although the interventions differed in content, Gillham (1990) viewed them as being broadly educational and designed to develop patients' coping skills. All three groups of patients showed improved seizure control; for patients receiving two treatments, seizure control improved after each. Reduction in seizures of at least 50% was found for 48.5% of patients. Intervention directed at psychologic problems also resulted in improved psychologic status. However, Gillham did not

discuss interindividual variability in treatment response with a view to matching specific seizure treatments to patients.

Andrews and Schonfeld (1992) reviewed which patients derived benefit from their 'taking control' approach to seizure treatment (Reiter *et al* 1987). This multicomponent treatment contained elements that were applied to all patients (EEG alpha activity biofeedback, relaxation training), in addition to individually tailored features such as training seizure trigger recognition or avoidance and dealing with emotional difficulties. Of 83 adults undergoing treatment between 1980 and 1985, 83% had achieved good seizure control (which was not defined) by the end of the program. Good treatment outcome is not surprising since the treatment package was designed for highly motivated individuals and contained multiple interventions that were specific in their application to the patient.

Cognitive-behavior therapy, widely used to treat anxiety and depression in people without epilepsy (Beck *et al* 1979), has been useful in reducing seizures where mood changes constitute a seizure prodrome (Brown and Fenwick 1989). Given the high prevalence of anxiety and depression in patients with epilepsy, and that anxiety and depression may serve to trigger seizures, Tan and Bruni (1986) attempted to teach seizure reduction to a group of patients of mixed seizure type using cognitive-behavior methods. Little support was found for the effectiveness of eight 2-hour sessions of cognitive-behavior therapy applied on a group basis in reducing seizure frequency. However, there was an overall improvement in therapists' ratings of patients' well-being. Tan and Bruni (1986) subsequently suggested that eight sessions were insufficient and that individual treatment may be more effective than group-based sessions. In addition, an active coping skills-based treatment may only have been suitable for individuals already demonstrating a predisposition to employ active coping skills. It is also possible that the strict treatment protocol permitted insufficient flexibility for patients' specific problems to be dealt with in a group setting.

Oosterhuis (1994) applied a 'psychoeducational approach' to seizure reduction to five adults with stress-induced seizures. Treatment included discussion of seizures and seizure behavior, provision of epilepsy-related information, application of self-management of epilepsy techniques adapted from behavior therapy, and self-monitoring of seizures. The treatment, conducted across eight 2-hour group sessions, produced an average reduction in seizures of 51%. However, there was considerable variation in seizure frequency prior to treatment and in percentage reduction following treatment.

Williams *et al* (1979) evaluated patients with stress-exacerbated seizures, both epileptic and nonepileptic, receiving at least two sessions with a psychiatrist. Treatment was individually designed, with family assessments included in the evaluation of the role of psychologic causes of the seizure disorder. Patients with partial seizures did better than those with generalized seizures and at the end of treatment (ranging from 2 to 70 sessions) over half of the 37 patients were either seizure-free or had improved seizure control.

In summary, various therapeutic approaches have been applied to adults and children with poorly controlled seizures in order to reduce seizure occurrence; these have incorporated single-case and group studies. Group studies have used individually applied and group format interventions. Generally, research has yielded positive outcomes with respect to seizure reduction, although variability in response to treatment has occurred within group studies. Little attempt has been made to account for this variability and it remains unclear whether poor treatment outcome relates to seizure features or to poor matching of treatment to patient.

INTERVENTIONS FOR PSYCHOLOGIC DISTURBANCE ASSOCIATED WITH EPILEPSY

Individuals with poorly controlled seizures are at increased risk for a range of psychiatric and psychologic problems (Fiordelli *et al* 1993; Cockerell *et al* 1996; Perini *et al* 1996; Baker 1997). Baker *et al* (1996), in a large cross-sectional community study, demonstrated that 25% of patients with epilepsy reported depression and 39% symptoms of anxiety. Epilepsy-associated stigma was reported by 38%. Seizure frequency significantly predicted anxiety and depression scores, as well as the degree of perceived stigma and the impact of epilepsy on the subjects' lives. For patients experiencing seizures in the year preceding the study, the perceived seizure severity (rather than frequency) predicted anxiety, depression, and the impact on life scores. Hospital-based studies (Smith *et al* 1991) have also demonstrated the importance of seizure severity in predicting anxiety, self-esteem, and perceived locus of control.

In individuals with epilepsy, anxiety may stem from fears that seizures may be fatal, as well as from other people's reactions to witnessing seizures (Baker 1997). The latter may be addressed by showing patients videos of their seizures, in a controlled setting (Sanders *et al* 1995). Depression may result from biochemical changes or may constitute a reaction to living with a stigmatizing illness. 'Endogenous' and 'reactive' depression may coexist in a

person with epilepsy (Betts 1992), and a range of symptoms may be experienced (Baker 1997). Low self-esteem may result from being overprotected, failing to achieve desired goals, and perceived stigma.

Thus many of the psychologic problems found in people with epilepsy resemble those present in other populations.

COGNITIVE-BEHAVIOR APPROACHES

Cognitive-behavior therapy, focusing on changing patients' thought patterns and behavior, has successfully reduced anxiety and depression in individuals without epilepsy and has also been used effectively in people with seizures. Thompson and Baxendale (1996) cite work by Upton and Thompson that evaluated this treatment in adults with poorly controlled epilepsy who had been identified as having poor coping strategies. Of 85 subjects, 25 formed a waiting list control group, while 50 were given a specifically written self-help manual. Although this group showed improved emotional and social adjustment, an additional 10 patients who also received individual sessions demonstrated even greater improvement.

Cognitive-behavior therapy was also effective in treating seizure phobia in a 26-year-old female with a 9-year history of complex partial and tonic–clonic seizures (as well as troubling auras) that developed following the evacuation of a left-sided occipitoparietal hematoma (Newsom-Davis *et al* 1998). Her deep fear of the seizures was disproportionate to the actual threat they posed to her safety. Although much of her anxiety related to their unpleasant nature, her greatest fear was that she would die during a seizure. She coped with her seizures by self-medicating with clonazepam, and avoided situations where having a seizure might be dangerous. Cognitive-behavior therapy was initiated as an inpatient once she had discontinued clonazepam. The program included education about epilepsy, anxiety, and phobias, systematic desensitization using graded exposure to increasingly anxiety-inducing situations, encouragement to identify and challenge maladaptive thoughts about her seizures and herself, and enhancement of her self-esteem. After 10 treatment sessions, her anxiety had decreased markedly, as had her measure of depression. Improvement persisted at follow-up and was accompanied by increased social and occupational activities and improved self-esteem. This case demonstrated the value of cognitive-behavior techniques in tackling the anxiety and hopelessness that the patient experienced, which were more restricting than the seizures themselves.

Cognitive-behavior and psychodynamic techniques reduced panic symptoms in a 32-year-old man whose symptoms were being attributed to his complex partial seizures

(Reisner 1990). Hyperventilation, seen in panic attacks, was treated using behavioral relaxation training in a profoundly learning-disabled 6-year-old boy who also experienced seizures (Kiesel *et al* 1989). Episodes of hyperventilation were reduced and hyperventilation-related seizure occurrence fell by more than 50%.

COUNSELING

Counseling has begun to be offered in a relatively systematic way to adults with epilepsy. Usiskin (1993) provided counseling for 83 adults attending a specialist center. Although treatment outcome was not formally evaluated and the number of counseling sessions varied (51 patients had between two and six sessions), most patients were satisfied with the outcome of counseling.

GROUP THERAPY

A small number of studies have documented the use of group therapy for patients with poorly controlled seizures.

Lessman and Mollick (1978) assumed that patients' psychologic reactions to their seizures, their ability to cope with them, family dynamics, and epilepsy-related stigma would determine how people cope with their illness. They described their work with small groups of six to eight patients who met with two therapists for 10–15 weekly 90-min sessions. Although the impact of the group was not formally evaluated, the authors indicated that their patients generally felt less lonely and alienated, and had increased self-esteem. Not all participants derived equal benefit from the treatment.

Appolone and Gibson (1980) described three short-term groups for adults with epilepsy all under 35 years of age. The groups met weekly for 12 sessions and focused on changing their main view of themselves as being epileptic and on changing the patients' sick role to a more appropriate and assertive role. The group meeting schedule included education about epilepsy and involvement of family members. Again this study failed to incorporate objective evaluation of treatment outcome, although the authors reported that all group members had made at least some progress by the end of the group sessions.

Mathers (1992) ran a psychodynamically oriented, closed, fixed-length group (10 sessions) for eight females with poorly controlled seizures. There was no formal evaluation of the group members' psychologic state after therapy and six of them reported increased seizure frequency during the lifetime of the group, possibly due to stressful issues being confronted during treatment. Mathers concluded that the greatest benefit to her

patients was being in a group with other people with the same illness.

Thus, despite the absence of formal evaluation, studies have reported beneficial effects for some patients undergoing group therapy. However, key elements in the therapeutic process cannot be identified due to the absence of properly controlled systematic evaluations of group work.

INDIVIDUAL PSYCHODYNAMIC PSYCHOTHERAPY

While poorly controlled and not permitting systematic evaluation of treatment outcome, psychodynamic psychotherapy has been applied to individuals with inadequately controlled seizures (see Taube and Calman 1992; Miller 1994a,b). The complex issues addressed within such treatment include the meaning of seizures for the patient, denial of the disorder, guilt about having epilepsy, unconscious emotional conflicts, dependency–autonomy conflicts, the impact of epilepsy on the person's development, and the formation of an 'integrated form of self' (see Taube and Calman 1992; Miller 1994a,b). Gandolfi and Martinelli (1990) and Taube and Calman (1992) stress that it is important for patients' families to collaborate with treatment in order for it to be successful.

A number of single-case studies, dealing with both adults and children, suggest the possible effectiveness of psychodynamic treatments for people with epilepsy. Problems tackled have included anxiety, aggression, and sleep disorder (Tancredi and Guerrini 1992), lack of self-esteem (Grasso *et al* 1992), weak and insecure sense of self due to epilepsy-provoked anxiety (Muratori *et al* 1992), and poor family and school relationships (Paladin *et al* 1989), as well as feelings of worthlessness, hopelessness, depression, and inability to establish lasting heterosexual relationships (Dorwart 1984). In addition, psychotherapy to reduce anxiety has complemented medical treatment of reflex epilepsy (Espadaler-Medina *et al* 1992). The systematic evaluation of these different approaches remains a pressing need.

In summary, the diverse psychologic difficulties faced by people with epilepsy appear, from the poorly controlled studies available, to be amenable to a range of psychotherapeutic interventions. Although most objective evaluation has been undertaken for cognitive-behavior approaches, psychodynamic psychotherapy, individual and group based, seems to offer patients potential benefit, although patient selection for particular treatments may require further consideration (Mathers 1992).

OUTSTANDING ISSUES

Two areas where psychologic interventions may help people with epilepsy have been considered, namely reducing seizure occurrence and dealing with psychologic problems accompanying epilepsy. It seems that psychologic treatments for seizure reduction may improve psychologic status and vice versa. The distinction between the two approaches is less clear in clinical practice than would appear from research reports, although some studies have been mindful of both areas of intervention (Rousseau *et al* 1985; Tan and Bruni 1986; Gillham 1990; Mathers 1992).

Research into psychologic treatments to reduce seizure frequency continues to pose methodologic difficulties. These include difficulty in matching treatments to seizure types and patients, and differences between studies in treatment outcome measures and variable follow-up periods (Goldstein 1990; Dahl 1992). In addition, some studies have used an identical treatment for all their patients (Rousseau *et al* 1985; Whitman *et al* 1990; Puskarich *et al* 1992), while other studies have applied similar treatments to all patients although adapting them to suit individual patients' needs (Dahl *et al* 1987; Reiter *et al* 1987; Gillham 1990). This, together with frequently poor descriptions of treatments used, makes outcome comparisons difficult. A further problem in evaluation arises from the observations that some individuals develop their own strategies for seizure inhibition and, occasionally, precipitation. Dahl (1992) confirms that it is unknown how these self-developed strategies interact with treatment approaches designed to reduce seizure occurrence.

A crucial issue for clinicians is the matching of treatments to seizure types for specific patients. Goldstein (1997b) suggested that for focal seizures with clear well-defined auras approaches such as cue-controlled arousal or relaxation or the use of other countermeasures may be effective in promoting seizure avoidance or abortion. Cognitive-behavior interventions may be helpful for seizures with a prodrome characterized by a mood change, as may also be the case when anxiety and interpersonal difficulties seem to be significant seizure precipitants.

Dahl (1992) attempted to identify who might benefit from psychologic interventions for their seizures. Although considering children with epilepsy, many of her recommendations apply to adults, as she believes that almost everyone can influence their seizure occurrence to some degree. With increasing length of seizure history, there is a greater chance that operant learning will have influenced seizure occurrence patterns. Dahl proposed that seizure control techniques for children might be most effective if applied before the child has learned to use seizure occurrence as a means of controlling factors such as people in its environment. She also suggested that if seizure control techniques were taught soon after seizure onset, psychosocial problems experienced by people with epilepsy might be avoided to some extent (see also Goldstein and Cull 1997).

It is conceivable that different approaches to seizure reduction might conflict with each other. Dahl (1992) and Reiter *et al* (1987) have discussed whether psychologic treatments are most effective for decreasing seizure frequency when combined with a level of antiepileptic medication that does not leave the person too sedated to be able to identify auras and seizure precipitants. Other conflicts may arise, for example between psychologic and neurosurgical interventions. As discussed elsewhere (Goldstein 1997b; Goldstein and Cull 1997) psychologic interventions place the onus for change in seizure patterns upon the patient, whereas the success of neurosurgical interventions will be seen to depend upon the neurosurgeon's skill rather than the patient's behavior. It is important therefore that decisions about which treatment path to adopt are made on an interdisciplinary basis so that patients are not advised to follow two apparently contradictory courses of investigation and treatment.

As in other areas of adult mental health, benzodiazepines (often used as antiepileptic drugs) may need to be withdrawn prior to the treatment of anxiety (Newsom-Davis *et al* 1998). Medication should not contribute unnecessarily to patients' cognitive difficulties, such that patients cannot remember suggestions made during therapy. As it is, neuropsychologic impairments may require adaptation of cognitive-behavior techniques to facilitate their use (see Newsom-Davis *et al* 1998).

Finally, when considering psychologic aspects of seizure control, more refined models linking organic (neurophysiologic, neurohormonal, metabolic) and psychologic factors are required to assist the design of optimal treatment methods. Greater understanding of the role of seizure-related neurotransmitter effects on psychologic states is also important when deciding how best to treat psychologic disturbance.

CONCLUSIONS

Psychologic interventions have much to benefit people with epilepsy and should be considered routinely for such patients (see Wallace *et al* 1997). Patients themselves recognize the value of having access to psychologists (Jain *et al*

1993; Goldstein *et al* 1997) and the development of interventions along the lines already discussed will ensure that people with epilepsy will derive optimal benefit from such approaches.

KEY POINTS

1. Psychologic factors that may more commonly precipitate seizures acutely in people with epilepsy include stress, possibly acting through the effects of corticosteroids on hippocampal neurons, hyperventilation consequent upon anxiety, and tiredness.
2. Each individual's likely seizure precipitants, and any seizure-maintaining factors, should be assessed before deciding which psychologic method might be most effective for reducing their seizure frequency.
3. Operant and classical conditioning techniques, relaxation training, biofeedback, and countermeasures, used either individually or in various combinations, may be effective in reducing seizure frequency in some cases. A 50% reduction in seizure frequency in around 50% of patients has been reported in at least one study.
4. Cognitive-behavior therapy may improve emotional and social adjustment.
5. A multidisciplinary team should advise on how to integrate psychologic methods of treatment with medication regimens and possible surgery for medically intractable epilepsy.

REFERENCES

Andrews D, Schonfeld WH (1992) Predictive factors for controlling seizures using a behavioural approach. *Seizure* 1:111–116.
Antebi D, Bird J (1992) The facilitation and evocation of seizures. *British Journal of Psychiatry* 160:154–164.
Antebi D, Bird J (1993) The facilitation and evocation of seizures: a questionnaire study of awareness and control. *British Journal of Psychiatry* 162:759–764.
Appolone C, Gibson P (1980) Group work with young adult epilepsy patients. *Social Work in Health Care* 6:23–32.
Baker GA (1997) Psychological responses to epilepsy. Their development, prognosis and treatment. In: Cull C, Goldstein LH (eds) *The Clinical Psychologist's Handbook of Epilepsy. Assessment and Management*, pp 96–112. London: Routledge.
Baker GA, Jacoby A, Chadwick DW (1996) The associations of psychopathology in epilepsy: a community study. *Epilepsy Research* 25:29–39.
Beck AT, Rush J, Shaw B, Emery G (1979) *Cognitive Therapy of Depression*. New York: Wiley.
Betts TA (1992) Epilepsy and stress. Time for proper studies of the association. *British Medical Journal* 305:378–379.
Betts T, Fox C, MacCallum R (1995a) Assessment of countermeasures used by people to attempt to control their own seizures. *Epilepsia* 36 (Suppl 3): S130.
Betts T, Fox C, MacCallum R (1995b) An olfactory countermeasures treatment for epileptic seizures using a conditioned arousal response to specific aromatherapy oils. *Epilepsia* 36 (Suppl 3): S130–S131.
Brown SW, Fenwick PBC (1989) Evoked and psychogenic epileptic seizures. II. Inhibition. *Acta Neurologica Scandinavica* 80:541–547.
Cautela JR, Flannery RB (1973) Seizures: controlling the uncontrollable. *Journal of Rehabilitation* 39:34–36.
Cockerell OC, Moriarty J, Trimble M *et al* (1996) Acute psychological disorder in patients with epilepsy: a nationwide study. *Epilepsy Research* 25:119–131.
Cull CA, Fowler M, Brown SW (1996) Perceived self-control of seizures in young people with epilepsy. *Seizure* 5:131–138.

Dahl J (1992) *Epilepsy. A Behavior Medicine Approach to Assessment and Treatment in Children*. Seattle: Hogrefe & Huber.
Dahl J, Mellin L, Brorson L-O, Schollin J (1985) Effects of a broad-spectrum behavior modification treatment program on children with refractory epileptic seizures. *Epilepsia* 26:303–309.
Dahl J, Mellin L, Lund L (1987) Effects of a contingent relaxation treatment program on adults with refractory epileptic seizures. *Epilepsia* 28:125–131.
Dahl J, Mellin L, Leissner P (1988) Effects of a behavioral intervention on epileptic seizure behavior and paroxysmal activity: a systematic replication of three cases of children with intractable epilepsy. *Epilepsia* 29:172–183.
Dahl J, Brorson L-O, Melin L (1992) Effects of a broad-spectrum behavioral medicine treatment program on children with refractory epileptic seizures: an 8-year follow-up. *Epilepsia* 33:98–102.
Dorwart RA (1984) Psychotherapy and temporal lobe epilepsy. *American Journal of Psychotherapy* 38:286–294.
Effron R (1956) Effect of olfactory stimuli in uncinate fits. *Brain* 79:267–281.
Effron R (1957) The conditioned inhibition of uncinate fits. *Brain* 80:251–261.
Engel J (1989) *Seizures and Epilepsy*. Philadelphia: Davis.
Espadaler-Medina JM, Espadaler-Gamissans JM, Seoane JL (1992) Reflex epilepsy. *Clinical Neurology and Neurosurgery* 94 (Suppl): S70–S72.
Fenwick PBC (1994) The behavioral treatment of epilepsy generation and inhibition of seizures. *Neurologic Clinics* 12:175–202.
Fenwick PBC, Brown SW (1989) Evoked and psychogenic epileptic seizures. I. Precipitation. *Acta Neurologica Scandinavica* 80:535–540.
Finkler J, Lozar N, Fenwick P (1990) Der Zusammenhang Zwischen spezifischen Situationen emotionalen Zuständen und Anfallschäufigkeit: Vergleich einer psychiatrischen mit einer nichtpsychitriaschen population von epilepsie patienten. In: Scheffner D (ed) *Epilepsie 90*, pp 114–121. Berlin: Einhorn Presse.
Fiordelli E, Beghi E, Boglium G, Crespi V (1993) Epilepsy and

psychiatric disturbance. A cross-sectional study. *British Journal of Psychiatry* **163**:446–450.

Forster FM (1969) Conditional reflexes and sensory-evoked epilepsy: the nature of the therapeutic process. *Conditional Reflex* **4**:103–114.

Forster FM (1977) *Reflex Epilepsy, Behavior Therapy and Conditional Reflexes.* Springfield, Illinois: Charles C Thomas.

Forster F, Ptacek L, Peterson W *et al* (1964) Stroboscopic-induced seizure discharges: modification by extinction techniques. *Archives of Neurology* **11**:603–608.

Forster F, Paulsen W, Baughman F (1969) Clinical therapeutic conditioning in reading epilepsy. *Neurology* **19**:717–723.

Fried R (1993) Breathing training for the self-regulation of alveolar CO_2 in the behavioral control of idiopathic epileptic seizures. In: Mostofsky DI, Løyning Y (eds) *The Neurobehavioral Treatment of Epilepsy*, pp 19–66. Hillsdale, New Jersey: Lawrence Erlbaum Associates.

Gandolfi M, Martinelli F (1990) The child in family therapy: a systematic revision of the Sceno Test. *Terapia Familiare* **34**:17–30.

Gillham RA (1990) Refractory epilepsy: an evaluation of psychological methods in outpatient management. *Epilepsia* **31**:427–432.

Goldstein LH (1990) Behavioural and cognitive-behavioural treatments for epilepsy: a progress review. *British Journal of Clinical Psychology* **29**:257–269.

Goldstein LH (1997a) Psychological control of seizures. In: Cull C, Goldstein LH (eds) *The Clinical Psychologist's Handbook of Epilepsy. Assessment and Management*, pp 113–129. London: Routledge.

Goldstein LH (1997b) Effectiveness of psychological interventions for people with poorly controlled epilepsy. *Journal of Neurology, Neurosurgery and Psychiatry* **63**:137–142.

Goldstein LH, Cull C (1997) The way forward. In: Cull C, Goldstein LH (eds) *The Clinical Psychologist's Handbook of Epilepsy. Assessment and Management*, pp 203–212. London: Routledge.

Goldstein LH, Minchin L, Stubbs P, Fenwick PBC (1997) Are what people know about their epilepsy and what they want from an epilepsy service related? *Seizure* **6**:435–442.

Grasso G, Bailo P, Crivelli E (1992) Mental development integration in dynamic psychotherapy of an adolescent with partial seizures. *Giornale di Neuropsichiatria dell'Eta Evolutiva* **12**:271–290.

Hart YM, Shorvon SD (1995) The nature of epilepsy in the general population. I. Characteristics of patients receiving medication for epilepsy. *Epilepsy Research* **21**:43–49.

Hayden M, Penna C, Buchanan N (1992) Epilepsy: patient perceptions of their condition. *Seizure* **1**:191–197.

Ince LP (1976) The use of relaxation training and a conditioned stimulus in the elimination of epileptic seizures in a child: a case study. *Journal of Behavior Therapy and Experimental Psychiatry* **17**:39–42.

Jain P, Patterson NH, Morrow JI (1993) What people with epilepsy want from a hospital clinic. *Seizure* **2**:75–78.

Joëls M, Karst H, Wadman WJ, deKloet ER (1997) Steroids, calcium and epilepsy. *Epilepsia* **38** (Suppl 3):552.

Kiesel KB, Lutzker JR, Campbell RV (1989) Behavioural relaxation training to reduce hyperventilation and seizures in a profoundly retarded epileptic child. *Journal of the Multihandicapped Person* **2**:179–190.

Krafft KM, Poling AD (1982) Behavioral treatments of epilepsy: methodological characteristics and problems of published studies. *Applied Research in Mental Retardation* **3**:151–162.

Lessman SE, Mollick LR (1978) Group treatment of epileptics. *Health and Social Work* **3**:105–121.

Lockard JS, Ward AS (1980) *Epilepsy: A Window to Brain Mechanisms.* New York: Raven Press.

Løyning Y, Bjørnaes H, Larsson PG *et al* (1993) Influence of psychosocial factors on seizure occurrence. In: Mostofsky DI,

Løyning Y (eds) *The Neurobehavioural Treatment of Epilepsy*, pp 253–283. Hillsdale, New Jersey: Lawrence Erlbaum Associates.

Mathers CBB (1992) Group therapy in the management of epilepsy. *British Journal of Medical Psychology* **65**:279–287.

Miller L (1994a) Psychotherapy of epilepsy: seizure control and psychosocial adjustment. *The Journal of Cognitive Rehabilitation* **12**:14–30.

Miller L (1994b) The epilepsy patient: personality psychodynamics, and psychotherapy. *Psychotherapy* **31**:735–743.

Mostofsky DI (1993) Behavior modification and therapy in the management of epileptic disorders. In: Mostofsky DI, Løyning Y (eds) *The Neurobehavioral Treatment of Epilepsy*, pp 67–81. Hillsdale, New Jersey: Lawrence Erlbaum Associates.

Mostofsky DI, Balaschak BA (1977) Psychobiological control of seizures. *Psychological Bulletin* **84**:723–750.

Muratori F, Masi G, Passani G, Patarnello MG (1992) Memory experience and rationalisation defences: a case of an adolescent with partial epilepsy. *Giornale di Neuropsichiatria dell'Eta Evolutiva* **12**:245–259.

Myslobodsky MS (1993) Neuroactive steroids and epilepsy. In: Mostofsky DI, Løyning Y (eds) *The Neurobehavioural Treatment of Epilepsy*, pp 159–195. Hillsdale, New Jersey: Lawrence Erlbaum Associates.

Newsom-Davis I, Goldstein LH, Fitzpatrick D (1998) Fear of seizures: an investigation and treatment. *Seizure* **7**:101–106.

Oosterhuis A (1994) A psycho-educational approach to epilepsy. *Seizure* **3**:23–24.

Paladin F, Cantele P, Pinkus L, Mattarollo L (1989) ESES: multidisciplinary approach to a case of focal cortical dysplasia. *Archivo di Psicologia Neurologia e Psichiatria* **50**:613–627.

Perini GI, Tosin C, Carraro C *et al* (1996) Interictal mood and personality disorders in temporal lobe epilepsy and juvenile myoclonic epilepsy. *Journal of Neurology, Neurosurgery and Psychiatry* **61**:601–605.

Powell GE (1981) *Brain Function Therapy.* Aldershot, Hampshire: Gower.

Pritchard PB, Holmstrom VL, Giacinto J (1985) Self-abatement of complex partial seizures. *Annals of Neurology* **18**:265–267.

Puskarich CA, Whitman S, Dell J *et al* (1992) Controlled examination of effects of progressive relaxation training on seizure reduction. *Epilepsia* **33**: 674–680.

Reisner AD (1990) A case of rapid reduction of panic symptoms: an eclectic approach. *Phobia Practice and Research Journal* **3**:87–93.

Reiter J, Andrews D, Janis C (1987) *Taking Control of Your Epilepsy. A Workbook for Patients and Professionals.* Santa Rosa: BASICS Publishing

Rockstroh B, Elbert T, Birbaumer N *et al* (1993) Cortical self-regulation in patients with epilepsies. *Epilepsy Research* **14**:63–72.

Rousseau A, Hermann BP, Whitman S (1985) Effects of progressive relaxation on epilepsy: analysis of a series of cases. *Psychological Reports* **57**:1203–1212.

Sanders PT, Bare MA, Lesser RP (1995) It is not harmful for patients with epilepsy to view their own seizures. *Epilepsia* **36**:1138–1141.

Smith DF, Baker GA, Dewey M *et al* (1991) Seizure frequency, patient-perceived seizure severity and the psychological consequences of intractable epilepsy. *Epilepsy Research* **9**:231–241.

Spector S (1997) *Self-control of seizures in adults with epilepsy.* PhD thesis, University of London.

Sterman MB (1996) Physiological origins and functional correlates of EEG rhythmic activities: implications for self-regulation. *Biofeedback* **21**:3–33.

Tan S-Y, Bruni J (1986) Cognitive-behaviour therapy with adult patients with epilepsy: a controlled outcome study. *Epilepsia* **27**:225–233.

Tancredi R, Guerrini R (1992) Aggressiveness and libido in early psychotherapeutic work of a child with partial epilepsy. *Giornale di Neuropsichiatria dell'Eta Evolutiva* **12**:261–269.

Taube SL, Calman NH (1992) The psychotherapy of patients with complex partial seizures. *American Journal of Orthopsychiatry* **62**:35–43

Thompson PJ, Baxendale SA (1996) Non-pharmacological treatment of epilepsy. In: Shorvon S, Dreifuss F, Fish D, Thomas D (eds) *The Treatment of Epilepsy*, pp 345–356. Oxford: Blackwell Science.

Usiskin S (1993) The role of counselling in an out-patient clinic: a three-year study. *Seizure* **2**:111–114.

Wallace H, Shorvon SD, Hopkins A, O'Donoghue M (1997) *Adults with Poorly Controlled Epilepsy*. London: Royal College of Physicians.

Whitman S, Dell J, Legion V *et al* (1990) Progressive relaxation for seizure reduction. *Journal of Epilepsy* **3**:17–22.

Williams DT, Gold AP, Shrout P *et al* (1979) The impact of psychiatric intervention on patients with uncontrolled seizures. *Journal of Nervous and Mental Disease* **167**:626–631.

Zlutnick SI, Mayville WT, Moffat S (1975) Modification of seizure disorders: the interruption of behaviour chains. *Journal of Applied Behavior Analysis* **8**:1–12.

Dietary measures

DR NORDLI JR AND DC DE VIVO

INTRODUCTION

The ketogenic diet is an effective and safe medical treatment for epilepsy. It is a high-fat, low-carbohydrate and protein regimen that has been used for more than 70 years on thousands of patients. It must be judiciously applied and carefully monitored, but it may show impressive results in correctly selected patients.

The proper way to identify patients for the ketogenic diet is not, however, entirely clear. Traditionally, the diet has been prescribed for children with symptomatic or cryptogenic generalized epilepsies that are refractory to antiepileptic medications. These patients may suffer from a variety of seizures, particularly of the myoclonic variety. In this group, the diet may perform very well, but modern experience with other patients outside this spectrum is limited. It is probably more important to consider the epilepsy syndrome, etiology, or both, rather than seizure type, in determining candidacy for the diet. This chapter reviews information regarding the long-chain triglyceride (LCT) ketogenic diet and will focus on its role in the treatment of patients with partial epilepsies.

HISTORICAL HIGHLIGHTS

There are biblical references to the salutary effects of starvation upon seizure control, but the earliest scientific reports emerged in the 1920s. Geyelin (1921) at the Presbyterian Hospital, New York, carefully studied the beneficial effects of starvation upon seizures. Shortly thereafter, Wilder (1921) proposed a high-fat diet to mimic the effects of starvation. Since this high-fat diet increased the production of ketone bodies, the regimen became known as a 'keto' or ketogenic diet. It was known that ketone bodies could be found in the urine of patients with diabetes and that they were produced when fatty acids were oxidized. This led to the notion that ketone bodies were potentially toxic metabolites of fatty acid degradation, and that the anticonvulsant effect was due to a sedative property, similar to the mechanisms of action of the available anticonvulsants of that era: bromides and phenobarbital.

Later, a different function of ketone bodies was suspected when, in the 1950s, it was discovered that a separate pathway synthesized the ketone bodies, acetoacetate and 3-hydroxybutyrate. Krebs (1961) suggested that ketone bodies were fuels for respiration. In 1967, Owen *et al* proved that ketone bodies were the major fuel for brain metabolism during starvation. Appleton and De Vivo (1974) developed an animal model and showed that the utilization of ketone bodies during starvation alters brain metabolites and increases cerebral energy reserves. Hasselbach *et al* (1994) showed that the human brain adapts to the changes in energy supply as early as 3 days following the initiation of starvation. Huttenlocher (1976) showed that the level of ketosis correlated with efficacy. Livingston *et al* (1977) reported extensive (41-year) experience with the diet in the treatment of myoclonic seizures of childhood. They stated that it completely controlled seizures in 54% of their patients, and markedly improved control in another 26%. Therefore, only 20% of patients did not respond.

SCIENTIFIC BASIS OF THE DIET

Scientific studies of the ketogenic diet have revealed important biochemical and metabolic observations. Appleton and De Vivo (1974) developed an animal model to permit study of the effect of the ketogenic diet on cerebral metabolism. Adult male albino rats were placed on either a high-fat diet containing (by weight) 38% corn oil, 38% lard, 11% vitamin-free casein, 6.8% glucose, 4% United States Pharmacopeia (USP) salt mixture, and 2.2% vitamin diet fortification mixture; or a high-carbohydrate diet containing (by weight) 50% glucose, 28.8% vitamin-free casein, 7.5% corn oil, 7.5% lard, 4% USP salt mixture, and 2.2% vitamin diet fortification mixture. Parallel studies were conducted to evaluate electroconvulsive shock responses and biochemical alterations. These studies revealed that the mean voltage necessary to produce a minimal convulsion remained constant for 12 days before the high-fat diet was started and for about 10 days after beginning the feedings (69.75 ± 1.88 V). About 10–12 days after starting the high-fat diet, the intensity of the convulsive response to the established voltage decreased, necessitating an increase in voltage to reestablish a minimal convulsive response. Approximately 20 days after beginning the high-fat diet, a new convulsive threshold was achieved (81.25 ± 2.39 V) ($P < 0.01$). When the high-fat diet was replaced by the high-carbohydrate diet, a rapid change in response to the voltage was observed. Within 48 hours the animal exhibited a maximal convulsion to the electrical stimulus which had previously produced only a minimal convulsion, and the mean voltage to produce a minimal convulsion returned to a value similar to prestudy (70.75 ± 1.37 V).

Blood concentrations of β-hydroxybutyrate, acetoacetate, chloride, esterified fatty acids, triglycerides, cholesterol, and total lipids increased in the rats fed on the high-fat diet. Brain levels of β-hydroxybutyrate and sodium were significantly increased in the fat-fed rats.

Subsequently, De Vivo *et al* (1978) reported the change in cerebral metabolites in chronically ketotic rats, and found no changes in brain water content, electrolytes, or pH. As expected, fat-fed rats had significantly lower blood glucose concentrations and higher blood β-hydroxybutyrate and acetoacetate concentrations. More importantly, the brain concentrations of adenosine triphosphate (ATP), glycogen, glucose 6-phosphate, pyruvate, lactate, β-hydroxybutyrate, citrate, α-ketoglutarate, and alanine were higher and the brain concentrations of fructose 1,6-diphosphate, aspartate, adenosine diphosphate (ADP), creatine, cyclic nucleotides, acid-insoluble coenzyme A (CoA), and total CoA were lower in the fat-fed group. Cerebral energy reserves were significantly higher in the fat-fed rats (26.4 ± 0.6) compared to controls (23.6 ± 0.2) ($P < 0.005$). Many of these changes in metabolites could be explained by the higher energy state of the brain cells in the fat-fed group, specifically by the ratio of ATP to ADP. In addition, the normal oxaloacetate, elevated α-ketoglutarate, and decreased succinyl-CoA imply maximal tricarboxylic acid (TCA) cycle activity – quite contrary to the metabolite profile seen with anesthetic-sedative agents. Nakazawa *et al* (1983) also noted that chronic ketosis increased the brain ATP content. Elevated α-ketoglutarate raises the possibility of increased flux through the γ-aminobutyric acid (GABA) shunt. Al-Mudallal *et al* (1996) recently showed that in adult male rats fed a high-fat ketogenic diet, neither cerebral pH nor total cerebral GABA levels were altered in the ketotic rats when compared with controls. However, Erecinska *et al* (1996) demonstrated that ketone bodies increase the synaptosomal content of GABA. Finally, it is worth speculating about possible GABA mimetic effects of ketosis given the chemical structural similarities of GABA, β-hydroxybutyrate, and acetoacetate.

These observations suggest that the ketogenic diet favorably influences cerebral energetics and that increased cerebral energy reserves and increased GABA shunt activity may be important factors bestowing an increased resistance to seizures in ketotic brain tissue (Nordli and De Vivo 1997).

ADMINISTRATION OF THE DIET

IMPLEMENTATION

Patients should be hospitalized for the initiation of the ketogenic diet. Close observation is important because children with certain underlying inborn errors of metabolism, particularly ones that interfere with utilization of ketone bodies, could quickly decompensate (De Vivo *et al* 1977). Hospitalization also provides the opportunity for family members to be instructed on the maintenance of the diet.

The first step is to promote ketosis by a fast. This can be done by fasting the patient after dinner (6 p.m.) on the evening of admission and continuing the fast until breakfast at 8 a.m. on the third day (38 hours). This allows metabolic adaptation to the state of ketosis, and an opportunity to screen the child for any severe hypoglycemic predisposition. It is typical to see a transient hypoglycemia during the first few days, which does not require any treatment unless the child demonstrates symptoms. Treatment of asymptomatic hypoglycemia delays the metabolic adaptation of the child to the state of chronic ketosis. During the fast, the patient is offered water, sugar-free beverages, and unsweetened gelatin.

When the urine reveals medium to large ketones, the diet is begun. The LCT diet consists of three or four parts fat to one part nonfat (carbohydrate and protein) calculated on the basis of weight. It is computed to provide 75–100 kilocalories per kg body weight and 1–2 g dietary protein per kg body weight per day. Caloric requirements are adjusted to minimize weight gain and to maximize ketonemia. If a 3:1 (fat-to-nonfat) ratio is insufficient to produce the required ketosis, then a ratio of 4:1 is used.

Conventional ketogenic diet or long-chain triglyceride diet

Prior to initiating the conventional ketogenic or LCT diet, a dietary prescription is made. Calculation of this prescription is straightforward. For example, if a 10 kg child is to be started on a 3:1 diet, one begins by estimating the calorie requirements of the child:

$$10\,\text{kg} \times 100\text{ kilocalories day}^{-1} = 1000\text{ kilocalories day}^{-1}$$

Alternatively, consulting a table of recommended daily allowances (RDA) may derive this figure. In either case, it may require adjustment based upon the child's individual metabolic needs.

The 3:1 ratio of the diet stipulates that 4 g of food must contain 3 g of fat and 1 g of nonfat. The nonfat consists of both carbohydrate and protein. One gram of fat has the calorie equivalent of 9 calories, whereas 1 g of protein or carbohydrate has the calorie equivalent of approximately 4 calories. Four grams of food (arbitrarily referred to as 1 unit here) on a 3:1 diet is then equal to 31 calories:

1 g fat = 9 calories $\times$ 3 = 27 calories
1 g protein and carbohydrate = 4 calories $\times$ 1 = 4 calories
Total calories = 27 + 4 = 31 calories per unit

To calculate the daily fat intake, one first divides the daily requirements of calories by this figure of 31 calories unit^{-1}, which generates the number of units required for the day:

1000 calories day^{-1} 31 calories^{-1} unit^{-1} = 32.25 units day^{-1}

Next, multiplying by 27 calories of fat per unit provides the daily fat requirement:

32.26 units day^{-1} $\times$ 27 calories of fat per unit = 871 calories of fat per day

which is equivalent to 96 g.

The protein requirement is 10 kg $\times$ 2 g kg^{-1} or 20 g day^{-1} (80 calories). Alternatively, one may consult the RDA table to determine the protein requirement.

So far, the combination of 871 calories of fat and 80 calories of protein leaves only 49 calories (1000 − 951) not accounted for in the daily allowance. The carbohydrate intake is then calculated to supply the necessary remaining calories (49 calories), which here is approximately 12 g.

The diet prescription for this 10 kg patient on a 3:1 LCT diet is then:

Fat: 96 g day^{-1} or 32 g per meal
Protein: 20 g day^{-1} or 6.6 g per meal
Carbohydrate: 12 g day^{-1} or 4 g per meal

Although the calculation of the calorie requirements is straightforward, the generation of the actual food prescription requires more time and effort. The approach may vary from institution to institution. In the authors' institution, the nutrition support team does this, and in order to provide a successful regimen, the constituents are customized to fit the individual's preferences and special needs. In so doing, the various elements of the diet may be 'juggled' to conform to the nutritional requirements. A food substitution approach may be used, analogous to that used for diabetic diets. This approach is simple to implement and increases the flexibility of the diet (Carroll and Koenigsberger 1998).

MAINTENANCE OF THERAPY

After initiation of the diet, the patient remains in the hospital for another 2–3 days. This time is utilized to carefully instruct the parents, or caretakers, on the techniques of providing the diet, weighing the food, providing food substitutions and monitoring ketosis. Patients on the ketogenic diet are often supplemented with calcium, iron, folate, and multivitamins including vitamin D to provide the RDA requirements. Protein requirements are carefully monitored and increased on an individual basis to allow for weight gain and growth.

After discharge from the hospital, the child is initially seen on a monthly basis by the nutrition support team or registered dietitian. At each visit the child's height, weight, and head circumference are charted. Electrolytes, liver function tests, serum lipids and proteins, and a complete blood count (CBC) are periodically checked. On average, the calorie and nutritional needs are readjusted monthly for infants and every 6–12 months for children.

TERMINATION OF THE KETOGENIC DIET

The ketogenic diet should be stopped gradually. A sudden stop of the diet or sudden administration of glucose may aggravate seizures and precipitate status epilepticus (Nordli et al 1992). Livingston (1972) advocates maintaining the diet at a ratio 4:1 for 2 years and, if successful, weaning down to a 3:1 diet for 6 months, followed by 6 months of a 2:1 diet. At this point a regular diet is given. The authors have not utilized such a rigorous protocol.

ADVERSE EVENTS

The ketogenic diet may be lethal in certain circumstances where cerebral energy metabolism is deranged. An example of this is pyruvate carboxylase deficiency, where patients may present early in life with refractory myoclonic seizures (De Vivo et al 1977). Mitochondria disorders or diseases that involve the respiratory chain, such as myoclonic epilepsy with ragged-red fibers (MERRF); mitochondrial encephalopathy, lactic acidosis, and strokelike episodes (MELAS); and cytochrome oxidase deficiency, would also probably be contraindications for use of the ketogenic diet, because of the increased stress on respiratory chain and TCA cycle function. Patients with fatty acid oxidation problems would also be adversely affected by the ketogenic diet, but such patients do not, as a rule, present with seizures.

COMPLICATIONS

Patients on the ketogenic diet exhibit a significantly reduced quantity of bone mass, which improves in response to vitamin D supplementation (5000 IU day^{-1}) (Hahn et al 1979). Renal calculi may develop but are rarely seen. Lipemia retinalis developed in two of Livingston's (1972) patients. Bilateral optic neuropathy has been reported in two children who were treated with a 4:1 'classic' ketogenic diet. These patients were not originally given vitamin B supplements. After administration of vitamin B supplements, vision was restored in both patients. Thinning of hair and, rarely, alopecia may occur. Cardiovascular complications have not been seen in those adults examined (Livingston 1972). In a recent prospective study, Ballaban-Gil et al (1998) reported serious adverse events in 5 of 52 children: severe hypoproteinemia (two patients), lipemia and hemolytic anemia (one patient), renal tubular acidosis (one patient), and marked increases in liver function tests (two patients). Four of these patients were comedicated with valproate.

POTENTIAL ADVERSE DRUG INTERACTIONS

Carbonic anhydrase inhibitors such as acetazolamide and topiramate should be avoided, particularly in the early stages of treatment with the ketogenic diet. Valproate is an inhibitor of fatty acid oxidation and a mitigator of hepatic ketogenesis. In addition, the authors have encountered marked elevation of liver transaminases in two patients during coadministration of valproate and the diet, as have Ballaban-Gil et al (1998). When possible, therefore, the authors avoid use of this agent.

Carnitine supplementation is complex. It is often used to supplement the diet of patients with various metabolic derangements whose defects allow a build-up of undesirable intermediates. It is also not uncommon in patients who need the ketogenic diet that a metabolic disorder of this sort is either suspected or confirmed (another reason to avoid valproate if possible). Carnitine supplementation may be desirable for these patients; however, high doses of carnitine may interfere with ketogenesis. These factors must be weighed up in each patient, and the decision to use the supplementation should be individualized. This topic has recently been thoroughly reviewed (De Vivo et al 1998).

CLINICAL INDICATIONS FOR USE (TABLE 39.1)

Primary therapy

The ketogenic diet is first-line therapy for the treatment of seizures in association with glucose transporter protein deficiency and pyruvate dehydrogenase deficiency (De Vivo et al 1991; Wexler et al 1997). In both cases, the diet effectively treats seizures while providing essential fuel for brain metabolic activity. In this manner, the diet is not only an anticonvulsant treatment but it also treats the other nonepileptic manifestations of these diseases.

Table 39.1 Indications for treatment with the ketogenic diet.

Primary therapy
   Glucose transporter protein deficiency
   Pyruvate dehydrogenase deficiency

Secondary treatment
   Generalized epilepsies refractory to multiple antiepileptic medications
   Other generalized myoclonic epilepsies, after failure of valproate

Other possible indications
   Partial epilepsies

These disorders illustrate an important and fundamental point regarding the efficacy of the ketogenic diet. Both may present with partial seizures in early life, and then later show evolution to a more generalized, clinical, interictal EEG, and ictal EEG pattern. The authors have noted these specific changes in patients with the glucose transporter protein deficiency. Specifically, 10 of 16 patients had interictal EEG abnormalities. In eight of ten there were interictal epileptiform discharges; four of these patients had generalized spike-wave discharges and four had focal spikes. In three of four patients with focal spikes, the abnormality was in the temporal lobe. The authors realized that these EEG findings and the clinical presentations were age specific: children presenting in infancy had partial seizures characterized by behavioral arrest and focal interictal epileptiform discharges. The older children had a mixture of generalized convulsions with other generalized seizures (absence, drop attacks, myoclonus) and presented with generalized spike-wave discharges on EEG.

This clearly indicates that patients with a form of generalized symptomatic epilepsy complicating a specific disease state (2.3.2 according to the International League Against Epilepsy classification scheme) may exhibit exclusively partial seizures at a certain stage of neurologic development. As is discussed later, some authors have concluded that the diet may be least effective against partial seizures (Prasad *et al* 1996). The importance of this fact, as it relates to the use of the ketogenic diet, is that the diet may not be considered in these patients if the focus of attention is directed towards the partial nature of the seizure and not towards the epilepsy syndrome, or etiology of the disorder. In these circumstances, the broader epilepsy syndrome and etiology are more important than the seizure diagnosis.

Secondary treatment

Based upon extensive clinical data, the ketogenic diet has clearly been shown to be effective in the treatment of patients with symptomatic or cryptogenic forms of general-

ized epilepsy. Prasad *et al* (1996) have compiled a summary of the efficacy data. It is clear from this compilation that the diet may be particularly helpful when the symptomatic epilepsy manifests with myoclonic and related seizures. For these reasons, the ketogenic diet may be considered as an alternate treatment, usually after the failure of valproate, for generalized epilepsies, particularly those with myoclonic seizures. The particular type of ketogenic diet used may not be critically important, although there may be some differences in efficacy. In 63 studies of 55 patients conducted by Schwartz *et al* (1989), a total of 51 studies (81%) showed a greater than 50% reduction in seizure frequency regardless of the type of diet used. Others, however, have found that the medium-chain triglyceride (MCT) diet is slightly less efficacious with 44% of patients achieving greater than 50% reduction in the number of seizures (Sills *et al* 1986). A corn oil ketogenic diet was found to be equally beneficial when compared with the MCT diet (Woody *et al* 1988). Regardless of the type of diet used, seizure control may be inconsistently accompanied by electroencephalographic improvement (Janaki *et al* 1976). In addition to improved seizure control, the diet may have a calming effect on behavior, which contrasts with the effect of some antiepileptic drugs.

Appropriate epilepsy syndromes to consider early treatment with the ketogenic diet include early myoclonic epilepsy (EME), early infantile epileptic encephalopathy (EIEE), and myoclonic-absence epilepsy. Given the effectiveness of the diet in the treatment of myoclonic epilepsies, it could also be considered as *first line* treatment for patients with those very severe epileptogenic encephalopathies that are notoriously difficult to control with medications, namely Lennox–Gastaut syndrome, myoclonic-astatic epilepsy, and severe infantile myoclonic epilepsy. However, in the authors' experience, most parents prefer the convenience of a medication, and it is unusual to try the ketogenic diet before at least one or two antiepileptic drugs have failed. The ketogenic diet can be beneficial in infants with West syndrome who are refractory to corticosteroids and other medications (Nordli *et al* 1995). Based upon Keith's (1963) data and the authors' own experience, the ketogenic diet may also be useful in the treatment of children with refractory-absence epilepsy without myoclonus.

FURTHER POSSIBLE INDICATIONS

Partial epilepsies

It is very difficult to precisely determine the efficacy of the diet in the treatment of partial seizure disorders. Livingston (Livingston 1972; Livingston *et al* 1977) stated that the diet was not effective in treating patients with partial seizures. Keith (1963) did not classify his patients in a manner that allows one to determine the effectiveness in partial seizures. In current use, the diet is usually prescribed for children with other forms of refractory epilepsy.

In a recent scientific study of the efficacy of the diet in kindled animals, the diet was shown to have at least transient anticonvulsant properties. Hori *et al* (1997) studied 32 male Sprague–Dawley rats, 20 of which were kindled and underwent behavioral testing, and 12 others underwent behavioral testing alone. Rats were kindled from P56–60 and then randomized (10 in each group) to either treatment with a ketogenic diet or regular rat chow. After-discharge threshold and seizure thresholds were tested at 1, 2, 4, and 5 weeks. Behavioral testing using both a water maze test and an open field test was done on week 3. During the period of administration of the ketogenic diet there were statistically significant elevations of β-hydroxybutyrate. Both the after-discharge thresholds and seizure thresholds were raised for the first 2 weeks of the diet; however, this effect disappeared by weeks 4 and 5. There were no differences in behavioral performances between the ketogenic-diet rats and controls. This scientific observation bolsters the consideration of its use in children with refractory partial epilepsy.

In contrast, Livingston *et al* (1977) found the diet ineffective in controlling either true 'petit mal' or temporal lobe epilepsy.

Kinsman *et al* (1992) reported on the efficacy of the diet in 58 children, all of whom had severe neurologic handicaps, including 84% with mental retardation. The authors showed that 39 children had improved seizure control, and seizure type was not of predictive value in determining success with the diet, either in terms of frequency of seizures or length of time on the diet.

Schwartz *et al* (1989) studied the treatment of 55 children with the ketogenic diet. Nine of these children appeared to have partial seizures as their main seizure type. Overall, 81% of patients showed a greater than 50% reduction in seizures. Although the number of children in each group was small, seizure type did not seem to predict response to the treatment.

Taken together, these scientific and clinical observations support the use of the ketogenic diet in patients with localization-related epilepsy, but there are no compelling clinical data to favor its use over newer medications or potentially curative surgery. Therefore, children with refractory partial seizures should be evaluated to determine if they are candidates for focal respective surgery. If they are, then surgery need not be delayed to institute a trial of the ketogenic diet, in the authors' opinion. On the other hand, if drugs have failed and the patient

is deemed to be a poor surgical candidate, then the diet should be tried. A more definitive statement would require data comparing efficacy of the diet in patients with localization-related epilepsy to those with generalized forms of epilepsy. It would seem inappropriate to treat children with otherwise benign seizure disorders, such as febrile seizures, benign rolandic epilepsy, benign occipital epilepsy, and benign familial neonatal convulsions with the ketogenic diet.

CONCLUSIONS

It is remarkable that 70 years and scores of drugs later, the ketogenic diet still retains a role in the modern treatment of children with refractory epilepsy. The diet has repeatedly been shown to be effective for children with refractory generalized cryptogenic or symptomatic epilepsies, but it is of unclear efficacy with refractory localization-related epilepsy. Comments have been made that the diet is less effective in this group, but the numbers of patients treated with isolated focal epileptogenic lesions is small and this markedly limits the power of these observations. Data exist to suggest that it may be of benefit to patients exhibiting partial seizures.

Even with our new pharmacologic armamentarium, there remain patients whose epilepsy is resistant to the effects of antiepileptic medications. Indeed, once several antiepileptic drugs with multiple different mechanisms of action have failed, it is unlikely that another will demonstrate good efficacy. In a sense, these patients may be declaring that they are not candidates for drugs and that they require alternate forms of treatment such as the ketogenic diet or surgery. Yet it is still difficult to determine who these patients are at the onset and the only reliable way to determine the refractory nature of their epilepsy is by trying treatment with various antiepileptic drugs. In children with refractory focal epilepsy, scientific and clinical observations support the use of the ketogenic diet, but there are no compelling clinical data to favor its use over newer medications or potentially curative surgery. Therefore, children with refractory partial seizures should be evaluated to determine if they are candidates for focal resective surgery. If they are, then surgery need not be delayed to institute a trial of the ketogenic diet, in the authors' opinion. On the other hand, if drugs have failed and the patient is deemed to be a poor surgical candidate, then the diet should be tried. Improvements in the classification of epilepsy, animal models, clinical studies, and deeper insights into the basic pathogenesis of refractory epilepsy will most likely provide useful information in this regard.

KEY POINTS

1. The standard ketogenic diet consists of three to four parts of fat to one part non-fat (carbohydrate and protein), calculated on the basis of weight, computed to provide 75–100 kcal/kg of body weight and 1–2 g dietary protein each day. This diet appears to influence cerebral energetics, so that in some cases increased energy reserves and increased GABA shunt activity lead to an increased resistance to seizures.

2. The diet is a first-line therapy for seizures associated with glucose transporter protein deficiency and pyruvate dehydrogenase deficiency. Both conditions may present with partial seizures in early life. It may also be considered a first-line treatment for Lennox–Gastaut syndrome, myoclonic-astatic epilepsy and severe infantile myoclonic epilepsy, these being severe epileptogenic encephalopathies that are notoriously difficult to control with medication.

3. The diet is an alternative treatment for generalized epilepsies manifest by myoclonic seizures that have failed to respond to valproate. It should also be considered for patients with partial seizures who have failed to respond to antiepileptic drugs and are deemed poor surgical candidates.

4. Patients should be hospitalized for initiation of the ketogenic diet. Children with certain inborn errors of metabolism, especially those that interfere with the utilization of ketone bodies, could quickly decompensate.

5. The diet may be lethal in certain conditions, such as pyruvate carboxylase deficiency, where cerebral energy metabolism is deranged. It should probably be avoided in patients with mitochondrial disorders and in those with disorders of fatty acid oxidation. It should also be avoided in patients taking valporate, topiramate, and acetazolamide.

6. The diet is often supplemented with calcium, iron, folate, and multivitamins including vitamin D.

7. Sudden termination of the diet, or the sudden administration of glucose, may aggravate seizures and precipitate status epilepticus.

8. Reported complications of the diet include a reduced bone density, renal calculi, optic atrophy, hair loss, hypoproteinemia, lipemia and hemolytic anemia, and renal tublar acidosis.

REFERENCES

Al-Mudallal AS, LaManna JC, Lust WD, Harik SI (1996) Diet-induced ketosis does not cause cerebral acidosis. *Epilepsia* **37**(3):258–261.

Appleton DB, De Vivo DC (1974) An animal model for the ketogenic diet. *Epilepsia* **15**(2):211–227.

Ballaban-Gil K, Callahan C, O'Dell C, Pappo M, Moshé S, Shinnar S (1998) Complications of the ketogenic diet. *Epilepsia* **39**:744–748.

Carroll J, Koenigsberger D (1998) The ketogenic diet: a practical guide for caregivers. *Journal of the American Dietetic Association* **98**(3):316–321.

De Vivo DC, Haymond MW, Leckie MP, Bussmann YL, McDougal DB, Pagliara AS (1977) The clinical and biochemical implications of pyruvate carboxylase deficiency. *Clinical Endocrinology and Metabolism* **45**(6):1281–1296.

De Vivo DC, Leckie MP, Ferrendelli JS, McDougal DB (1978) Chronic ketosis and cerebral metabolism. *Annals of Neurology* **3**:331–337.

De Vivo DC, Trifiletti RR, Jacobson RI, Ronen GM, Behmand RA, Harik SI (1991) Defective glucose transport across the blood–brain barrier as a cause of persistent hypolycorrhachia, seizures, and developmental delay. *New England Journal of Medicine* **325**:713–721.

De Vivo DC, Bohan TP, Coulter DL *et al* (1998) L-Carnitine supplementation in childhood epilepsy: current perspectives. *Epilepsia* (in press)

Erecinska M, Nelson D, Daikhin Y, Yudkoff M (1996) Regulation of GABA level in rat brain synaptosomes: fluxes through enzymes of the GABA shunt and effects of glutamate, calcium, and ketone bodies. *Journal of Neurochemistry* **67**(6):2325–2334.

Geyelin HR (1921) Fasting as a method for treating epilepsy. *Medical Record* **99**:1037–1039.

Hahn TJ, Halstead LR, De Vivo DC (1979) Disordered mineral metabolism produced by ketogenic diet therapy. *Calcified Tissue International* **28**(1):17–22.

Hasselbach SG, Knudsen GM, Jakobsen J, Hageman LP, Holm S, Paulson OB (1994) Brain metabolism during short-term starvation in humans. *Journal of Cerebral Blood Flow and Metabolism* **14**(1):125–131.

Hori A, Tandon P, Holmes GL, Stafstrom C (1997) Ketogenic diet: effects on expression of kindled seizures and behavior in adult rats. *Epilepsia* **38**:750–758.

Huttenlocher PR (1976) Ketonemia and seizures: metabolic and anticonvulsant effects of two ketogenic diets in childhood epilepsy. *Pediatric Research* **10**(5):536–540.

Janaki S, Rashid MK, Gulati MS, Jayaram SR, Baruah JK, Saxena VK (1976) A clinical electroencephalographic correlation of seizures on a ketogenic diet. *Indian Journal of Medical Research* **64**(7):1057–1063.

Keith HM (1963) *Convulsive Disorders in Children: with Reference to Treatment with Ketogenic Diet*. Boston: Little Brown.

Kinsman SL, Vining EPG, Quaskey SA, Mellits D, Freeman JM (1992) Efficacy of the ketogenic diet for intractable seizure disorders: review of 58 cases. *Epilepsia* **33**:1132–1136.

Krebs HA (1961) The physiological role of the ketone bodies. *Biochemical Journal* **80**:225–233.

Livingston S (1972) *Comprehensive Management of Epilepsy in Infancy, Childhood and Adolescence.* Springfield, IL: Charles C Thomas.

Livingston S, Pauli LL, Pruce I (1977) Ketogenic diet in the treatment of childhood epilepsy. *Developmental Medicine and Child Neurology* **19**:833–834.

Nakazawa M, Kodama S, Matsuo T (1983) Effects of ketogenic diet on electroconvulsive threshold and brain contents of adenosine nucleotides. *Brain Development* **5**(4):375–380.

Nordli DR, De Vivo DC (1997) The ketogenic diet revisited: back to the future. *Epilepsia* **38**:743–749.

Nordli DR, Koenigsberger D, Schroeder J, De Vivo DC (1992) Ketogenic diets. In: Resor S, Kutt H (eds) *The Medical Treatment of Epilepsy*, pp 455–472. New York: Marcel Dekker.

Nordli DR, Koenigsberger D, Carroll J, De Vivo DC (1995) Successful treatment of infants with the ketogenic diet (Abstract). *Annals of Neurology* **38**:523.

Owen OE, Morgan AP, Kemp HG, Sullivan JM, Herrera MG, Cahill GF (1967) Brain metabolism during fasting. *Journal of Clinical Investigation* **46**:1589–1595.

Prasad AN, Stafstrom CE, Holmes GL (1996) Alternative epilepsy therapies: the ketogenic diet, immunoglobulins, and steroids. *Epilepsia* **37**:S81–S95.

Schwartz RH, Eaton J, Bower BD, Aynsley-Green A (1989) Ketogenic diets in the treatment of epilepsy: short-term clinical effects. *Developmental Medicine and Child Neurology* **31**(2):145–151.

Sills MA, Forsythe WI, Haidukewych D, MacDonald A, Robinson M (1986) The medium-chain triglyceride diet and intractable epilepsy. *Archives of Disease in Childhood* **61**:1168–1172.

Wexler ID, Hemalatha SG, McConnell J *et al* (1997) Outcome of pyruvate dehydrogenase deficiency treated with ketogenic diets. Studies in patients with identical mutations. *Neurology* **49**:1655–1661.

Wilder RM (1921) Effects of ketonuria on the course of epilepsy. *Mayo Clinic Bulletin* **2**:307–314.

Woody RC, Brodie M, Hampton DK, Fiser RH Jr (1988) Corn oil ketogenic diet for children with intractable seizures. *Journal of Child Neurology* **3**(1):21–24.

Adverse events during long-term medical treatment: adults

40

PM CRAWFORD AND JM OXBURY

Intractable epilepsy reduces the quality of life. People afflicted with the condition have a higher incidence of psychiatric morbidity and they are at greater risk of death than are the 'normal population'. These aspects are the subjects of other chapters and are mentioned here only briefly. In the main this chapter is given firstly to injuries arising in people with intractable epilepsy, and secondly to some long-term unwanted consequences of medication.

Chronic intractable epilepsy imposes considerable psychosocial disadvantage. There are reduced employment opportunities for various reasons, including difficulty traveling to the workplace and because of the increased physical risks especially as perceived by employers. Intractable epilepsy creates difficulties for independent living and it imposes financial disadvantage (Trostle, 1998). It creates low self-esteem, lack of confidence, and a fear of the seizures themselves. These quality-of-life issues are fully described in Chapter 33.

Psychiatric disorder and suicide are thought to occur four times more often in people with intractable epilepsy than in the normal population (see Chapter 34). Interictal depression is particularly common and chronic interictal psychosis has been documented in up to 9%, most often several years after the onset of the seizures. The chances of marriage and stable relationships are reduced. Hyposexuality is particularly common in men with temporal lobe epilepsy that has commenced before puberty and has been treated with enzyme-inducing drugs, such as phenobarbital, phenytoin, and carbamazepine. A tendency to depression may be accentuated by treatment with various antiepileptic drugs, including phenobarbital, phenytoin, vigabatrin, topiramate, and tiagabine, and vigabatrin may precipitate psychosis (see below).

Increased mortality is due to a number of factors including the underlying pathology if it is progressive, accidents (see below) including especially drowning, suicide (see Chapter 34), status epilepticus, and sudden unexpected death in epilepsy (SUDEP) (see Chapter 4). SUDEP appears to be mostly seizure related. It is more common among those with severe intractable symptomatic and focal epilepsy, especially if they are prone to generalized convulsions and if they are noncompliant with medication or if their medication is withdrawn too rapidly. The best preventative measure is better seizure control.

INJURIES

Injuries are common during seizures, particularly tonic–clonic seizures. Most studies of injuries during seizures relate to patients attending specialist epilepsy clinics or under institutional care. Most are not community based and the seizure disorder is usually not classified. Injuries vary in severity from cuts and bruises, to burns, head injuries and other serious injuries that very rarely prove fatal. Sonnen et al (1984) in a 3–7 months follow-up study of 604 patients (371 outpatients) reported one 'accident' per 500 seizures but the term 'accident' was not further defined. Interestingly, patients with epilepsy appear not to be more prone to sport- or play-related injuries (Aisenson 1948; Berman 1984).

A study from Norway of 62 institutionalized patients with epilepsy and multiple handicaps, 81% of them with localization-related epilepsy, found that the risk of seizure-related injury was 1.2% for partial seizures. During the assessment period, 6889 seizures were recorded of which 2805 were complex partial. Tonic–clonic seizures were frequent (1984) but the majority (1489) occurred in one patient. Ten patients were seizure-free but two patients had 2581 seizures between them (37.4% of the total seizure numbers). The mean number of seizures per patient was 111. Simple partial seizures did not result in injuries. A higher injury rate occurred in tonic–clonic seizures accompanied by falls (2.9%). Thirty-nine percent of seizures were accompanied by falls. Overall 20 patients (32%) had 80% of the seizure-related injuries, all in conjunction with seizures accompanied by a fall – approximately 67 seizures per injury (seizure-related injury rate = 1.5%). Of the seizure-related injuries, 61 (76%) were localized to the head and face and most were to soft tissues (74%). In this study, six injuries were considered serious – five fractures and one subdural hematoma in a 91-year-old woman who fell during a complex partial seizure; she died during the operation to remove the hematoma (Nakken and Lossius 1993).

Some patients with refractory epilepsy experience intellectual deterioration. It has been proposed that the etiology in some cases is secondary to repeated head trauma, as in boxers' encephalopathy (Thompson and Sander 1987). Seizure-related injuries are conditioned not only by the seizure type but also by the place and circumstances of the seizure. For example, 17% of all seizure-related injuries occur in the bathroom (Nakken and Lossius 1993). A Swedish study reported that more than 60% of seizure-related injuries occurred at home (Lund and Hellstrom 1989).

BURNS

In a study from Colorado, 25 of 244 patients attending an epilepsy clinic reported burns secondary to seizures. Twelve needed hospitalization (Spitz et al 1994). Most burns occurred after seizures in the home and there were avoidable factors. Five patients had burns while showering with water that was too hot. Three burnt themselves on unprotected room heaters and 10 burnt themselves while cooking. Burns secondary to epileptic seizures are a very frequent complication of epilepsy in the Third World. This was reported in 24% of people with epilepsy in a prevalence study from rural Tanzania (Rwiza et al 1993).

FRACTURES

An increased incidence of fractures in people with epilepsy results not only from an increased incidence of falls but also from possible antiepileptic drug-induced osteomalacia and/or osteoporosis secondary to inactivity. A UK study analyzed 185 000 seizures among an institutional population with epilepsy to calculate the incidence of the five commonest fractures. Only 25% of the fractures occurred during a seizure. When age and sex were matched against a 'normal' population, there was a fivefold increase in femoral neck fractures, a 10-fold increase in intertrochanteric and ankle fractures, and a fourfold increase in fractures of the proximal humerus. Overall, there was a fourfold increase in the risk for all fractures and a threefold increase in the risk of fractures not related to seizures. There was no evidence that the first fracture occurred at a younger age than in the general population (Desai et al 1996).

HEAD INJURY

In a study of head injuries in New York, 1.7% were found to be secondary to epileptic seizures. The patients with epilepsy tended to have a higher mortality than the other head injury patients (Hauser et al 1984). In the UK study of institutionalized patients observed for a year, there were 766 significant head injuries, 1.2% of which required sutures. In this study, one patient sustained a fractured skull, another had an extradural hematoma, and a third had subdural hematoma. This was out of a total of 12 626 falls (Russell-Jones and Shorvon 1989). It is estimated that the risk of a skull fracture or subdural or extradural hematoma is 1:9311 seizures or 1:4208 seizures associated with falls.

DROWNING

Other accidents include drowning. A study of 306 children under the age of 15 who drowned or nearly drowned suggested that a child with epilepsy is 7.5 times more likely to drown or nearly drown than other children (Kemp and Sibert 1993).

UNWANTED CONSEQUENCES DURING LONG-TERM MEDICATION

Nonspecific side-effects of antiepileptic drugs (AEDs) are very common. A recent British Epilepsy Association survey is based on the answers to a questionnaire from 4449 people with epilepsy, of whom 44% were experiencing seizures at least once every 3 months, more than half of them at least once per week. The details are given in the British Epilepsy Association (1996) publication. *The Treatment of Epilepsy – A Patient's Viewpoint.* Overall, 81% of the total sample experienced tiredness, 74% difficulty concentrating, 69% loss of memory, and 59% feelings of confusion. Other unwanted effects experienced by at least 50% were: funny moods (58%), headaches (54%), sluggishness (54%), weight gain (51%), and feelings of aggression (50%). Half of the sample was on treatment with carbamazepine (CBZ), 31% with sodium valproate (SVP), 29% with phenytoin (DPH), and 11% with lamotrigine (LAM). Only 6% were taking phenobarbital (PB). Around 40% were on polytherapy. Although 97% stated that they would not be willing to accept less seizure control for fewer side-effects, nevertheless 28% would not have been prepared to tolerate yet more side-effects for total seizure control.

SPECIFIC ANTIEPILEPTIC DRUGS

Unwanted consequences of AEDs arising during long-term treatment are particularly associated with PB and DPH but may also be seen with CBZ, SVP, and vigabatrin (VIG). Drugs such as LAM, topiramate, and tiagabine have been in use for periods too short to determine whether they will manifest unwanted effects in the long term.

Phenobarbital

PB is a cheap and effective drug for the control of focal seizures but it has fallen out of favor in Western industrialized societies because it generates unacceptable side-effects in around 25% of those who take it (Heller *et al* 1995). Unwanted effects of long-term treatment with PB include:

1. Cognitive disturbances of various sorts. These are the most usual reason for its rejection. They include sedation, slowing of thought processes, irritability and

aggression especially in children and adolescents, and psychiatric depression.
2. Decreased libido (Mattson *et al* 1985).
3. Physical dependence.
4. Osteomalacia and megaloblastic anemia as for DPH (see below) and probably most often when PB and DPH are taken in combination.
5. Dupuytren's contracture and thickening of the heel pad and other connective tissue disorders (Mattson and Cramer 1989).
6. A tendency to precipitate convulsions when attempts are made to withdraw the drug even very slowly.

Phenytoin

Reynolds (1989) has reviewed the unwanted consequences of long-term DPH treatment. They include:

1. Gingival hyperplasia that develops in up to 50% within 1 year of starting the medication, especially when there is high dose and poor dental hygiene. It usually resolves after the DPH is withdrawn. It is possible that DPH may also lead to coarsening of the features associated with calverial thickening, hirsutism and acne, all contributing to a poor cosmetic effect, especially when it is combined with PB.
2. Ataxia and cerebellar atrophy that are usually irreversible after withdrawal of the drug. Ney *et al* (1994) reported that cerebellar atrophy, as measured by magnetic resonance imaging (MRI), was significantly more pronounced in patients with partial seizures taking DPH long term than in healthy sex- and age-matched volunteers or in · patients simply complaining of headache or dizziness. The condition usually develops insidiously after several years of treatment, but it can present acutely and irreversibly after treatment at toxic doses for only brief periods (Masur *et al* 1989, 1990).
3. Overt encephalopathy, manifest by deteriorating mental function and memory impairment, and sometimes accompanied by dyskinesia, may develop insidiously without ataxia or nystagmus (Reynolds 1989). There may be failure to recognize that the condition is due to DPH toxicity for some considerable while. The blood DPH level is usually elevated at toxic levels and the encephalopathy is reversible once the blood level is restored to the nontoxic range.
4. Peripheral neuropathy, as manifest by reduced or absent lower limb tendon reflexes and mild electrophysiologic abnormalities, usually without symptoms, may develop in up to 20% patients taking DPH long term, especially when the blood DPH levels have

tended to be high, and/or when there has been folic acid deficiency and/or when there has been polytherapy including PB.

5. Megaloblastic anemia, due to folic acid deficiency, occurs in a small number. Nonanemic macrocytosis is considerably more common.

6. Osteomalacia and rickets. Minor abnormalities of the blood calcium (lowered) and alkaline phosphatase (increased) levels are considerably more common than clinically apparent metabolic bone disease.

Carbamazepine

Patients who reject CBZ usually do so during the first few months of treatment as a consequence of rash or sometimes sedation, dizziness, diplopia, or headache (Richens *et al* 1994; Heller *et al* 1995). Unwanted effects that may occur during long-term medication include:

1. Weight gain in up to 10% (Mattson 1998).
2. Hyponatremia and water retention that is usually asymptomatic but can lead to peripheral edema and occasionally to encephalopathic symptoms (Mattson *et al* 1992).
3. Heart rhythm disorders including Stokes–Adams attacks and aggravation of the sick sinus syndrome.
4. A hypersensitivity syndrome involving multiple organs may develop after several months of treatment. The condition may resemble systemic lupus erythematosus and there may be involvement of the liver, kidneys, lungs, and heart (Gram and Jensen 1989; Salzman *et al* 1997).
5. Bone marrow suppression leading to aplastic anemia is rare, at around 1:287 000 cases treated (Pellock and Willmore 1991), and routine blood count monitoring is not generally recommended.

Sodium valproate

Unacceptable weight gain is the most frequent serious unwanted consequence of long-term treatment with SVP. It was reported in 12% of the SVP group in the Richens *et al* (1994) study, usually after at least 3 months on treatment. It was reported in 20% of the SVP group at 12 months after the initiation of treatment in the Veterans Affairs (VA) study (Mattson *et al* 1992). More than half of them gained more than 5.5 kg.

Other serious unwanted effects that have been attributed to SVP include:

1. Polycystic ovaries associated with hyperandrogenism and hyperinsulinemia (Isojarvi *et al* 1996).

2. Fatal hepatotoxicity, which is most often seen in young children with developmental delay and coincident metabolic disorders on polytherapy. It is very rare, at around 1:470 000 treated, in adults on monotherapy rising to 1:50 000 in those on polytherapy (Bryant and Dreifuss 1996). A number of rare specific biochemical defects may be associated with a tendency to SVP hepatotoxicity (Pellock and Willmore 1991).
3. A tendency to bleed secondary to thrombocytopenia and inhibition of platelet aggregation should be recognized if surgery is planned.
4. Acute pancreatitis that may be fatal.

Vigabatrin

Serious unwanted effects include weight gain, that occurs in around 8% treated (Ben-Menachem and French 1998), behavior disturbances including psychosis that mostly occur during the early weeks after the initiation of treatment, and visual failure.

1. Psychosis is mostly seen during the early weeks of treatment and the probability of its occurring increases with increasing dose. It emerges during long-term treatment in only around 1% of cases (Ferrie *et al* 1996).
2. Visual field constriction that is severe, symptomatic, and persistent has been reported in patients receiving VIG (Eke *et al* 1997). The incidence is uncertain but it has been said that the overall prevalence in asymptomatic patients may be around 28% (Sankar and Wasterlain 1999). It seems that the onset may be from 1 month to several years after the initiation of treatment (Committee on Safety of Medicines 1998). The defect appears to arise from retinal cone dysfunction (Krauss *et al* 1998). Sankar and Wasterlain (1999) suggest that the retinal toxicity may be exacerbated by SVP.

UNWANTED COGNITIVE EFFECTS OF ANTIEPILEPTIC DRUGS

A meta-analysis of studies on the cognitive effects of AED carried during the period 1970–1994 (Vermeulen and Aldenkamp 1995) led to the following conclusions:

1. There are very few monotherapy studies that satisfy basic criteria of method, design, and analysis using control group data for comparison and employing appropriate forms of repeated measures. Consequently the effects of medication on cognition are difficult to assess.
2. There are probably only small differences between the cognitive effects of PB, DPH, CBZ, and SVP administered at therapeutic doses.

3. Nevertheless even small differences may be of clinical importance when the drugs are being taken long term.

Inevitably, with changes over time there is the very difficult matter of trying to separate the components attributable to medication from those due to the ongoing seizure disorder itself (Jokiet and Ebner 1999).

A general consensus seems to be (Dodrill 1998) that:

1. For the established AEDs (PB, DPH, CBZ, SVP),

   (a) all are likely to have a mild general adverse effect on cognitive performance;

   (b) PB has the most prominent detrimental effect but it is difficult to demonstrate differences between the others (benzodiazepines are also clearly detrimental).

2. None of the newer AEDs has been completely evaluated when used as monotherapy and they need to be kept under close scrutiny.

There is also general agreement that the chances of cognitive impairment are much increased by polytherapy.

DISTURBANCES RELEVANT TO REPRODUCTION

There is an increased prevalence of hyposexuality and decreased potency with decreased sperm counts and abnormal sperm morphology or motility in males, especially if they have developed their epilepsy before puberty and taken AEDs ever since. This may be at least partly secondary to long-term AED-taking (Herzog 1998). DPH, CBZ, and PB in particular appear to lower testosterone levels leading to testicular malfunction. Females may have an increased prevalence of menstrual abnormalities, anovular cycles, and decreased fertility. Again, this may be at least partly due to medication. As has been mentioned above, it has been suggested that SVP may be a factor contributing to decreased fertility with the polycystic ovary syndrome.

Contraception

There may be oral contraceptive failure as a consequence of the coincident taking of enzyme-inducing AEDs (PB, DPH, CBZ) and topiramate. Failure of implanted contraceptives has also been recorded. For the 'combined' pill, a preparation containing at least 50 µg estrogen should be used. Breakthrough bleeding indicates that contraception cannot be assured (O'Brien and Gilmore-White 1993).

Teratogenicity

The risk of a woman who is taking an AED giving birth to a child with a malformation is around two times higher than for pregnant women in general (Independent reviewer 1994). The following points are pertinent:

1. Abnormalities occur with PB, DPH (see Table 40.1), CBZ, and SVP (see Table 40.2) (D'Souza *et al* 1990; Lindhout and Omtzigt 1994; Steegers-Theunissen *et al* 1994; Clayton-Smith and Donnai 1995). The risk from PB monotherapy may be relatively low. Likewise, the risk from CBZ monotherapy may be low apart from for spina bifida (see below). The risks with LAM, if any, are not yet established. The manufacturer's data sheet for Lamictal (see Association of British Pharmaceutical Industries 1998) states that the reproductive toxicology studies in animals at doses in excess of the human therapeutic dose showed no teratogenic effects. The position of the more recently introduced AEDs is not known.

2. All women should take daily doses of folic acid 4–5 mg during the 3 months before conception and for at least the first 12 weeks of the pregnancy although the value of this to counteract AED-induced teratogenicity is not established.

3. At least those women taking CBZ or SVP should be offered α-fetoprotein measurement and high-resolution ultrasound examination of the fetus during the second trimester of the pregnancy, because both drugs

Table 40.1 Fetal malformations associated with phenytoin treatment of the mother during pregnancy (increased risk).

Cleft lip and palate
Cardiac defects
Cranial anomalies
   Facial dysmorphism
Limb anomalies
   Hypoplasia and irregular ossification
   of the distal phalanges
Hypospadias
Intestinal atresia

Table 40.2 Fetal malformations associated with sodium valproate treatment of the mother during pregnancy (increased risk).

Neural tube defects
   Spina bifida
   Microcephaly
Cranial anomalies
   Facial dysmorphism
Limb anomalies

increase the risk of spina bifida. Data from cohort studies presented by Rosa (1991) indicated that the general risk of a woman producing a spina bifida baby is 1:1500. This compares with risks of 1:68 for a woman taking SVP, 1:109 for a woman taking CBZ, and 1:748 for women taking other AEDs.

4. The best possible seizure control should be maintained. It is probably best if this is with the regimen that gave the best control prior to conception. In principle, however, the ideal is monotherapy with the lowest effective dose. The seizure frequency increases in pregnancy in around 33% of mothers, possibly in association with decreased plasma concentrations of AED. Voluntary noncompliance may be a significant factor. There is an increased risk to the fetus from maternal convulsions during pregnancy and labor.

5. Mothers taking SVP should divide the total daily dose into at least three portions so that relatively small amounts are taken on each occasion.

There have been suggestions that AED-induced teratogenicity may also be manifest by neurologic *dysfunction* that does not show itself until infancy or childhood rather than simply by overt structural abnormality (Koch *et al* 1996).

Hemorrhagic disease of the newborn

This condition is due to a deficiency of vitamin K-dependent clotting factors in the neonate. It is manifest by internal bleeding during the first 24 hours of life. It has been reported in the babies of mothers who have been taking barbiturate, benzodiazepine, DPH, CBZ, and ethosuximide (Yerby and Collins 1998). The condition is mostly prevented if the mother ingests vitamin K during the last month of the pregnancy. The risk without such prophylaxis is said to be around 10%. The recommendation is that women should take vitamin K_1 (20 mg day^{-1} orally) during the last month of their pregnancy and that the infant should receive vitamin K_1 (1 mg intramuscularly) at birth (Duncan 1996). Fresh frozen plasma should be administered to the infant intravenously if there is bleeding or if the concentration of two or more of factors II, VII, IX, or X fall to <25% normal.

KEY POINTS

1. The risk of a seizure-related injury is around 1% for partial seizures and 3% for tonic–clonic seizures accompanied by a fall. Most injuries (around 75%) are to the head and face, especially the soft tissues, and most occur in the home.

2. People with intractable epilepsy have an increased risk of fracture both seizure and nonseizure related. The risk of skull fracture, subdural or extradural hematoma is around 1:4200 seizures with a fall.

3. The child with epilepsy has a sevenfold increased risk of drowning.

4. Unwanted consequences of long-term antiepileptic medication include, depending on which drug is being taken, cognitive disturbances, depression and psychosis, decreased libido and fertility, serious weight gain, cerebellar atrophy, visual failure, osteomalacia and rickets, and megaloblastic anemia. Aplastic anemia and fatal liver failure are rare.

5. Monotherapy at nontoxic doses with antiepileptic drugs other than phenobarbital and benzodiazepines should not cause major cognitive impairment.

6. Antiepileptic drugs increase the risk of fetal malformation and hemorrhagic disease of the newborn baby.

7. Folic acid should be taken prior to conception and during the early part of the pregnancy. Antiepileptic drug treatment during pregnancy should preferably be with monotherapy at the lowest dose able to control the epilepsy. The mother should take oral vitamin K during the month prior to delivery and vitamin K should be administered to the baby intramuscularly shortly after birth.

8. Mothers taking sodium valproate or carbamazepine should be offered blood α-fetoprotein level measurement and high-resolution ultrasound examination of the fetus during the second trimester of the pregnancy, because both drugs increase the risk of spina bifida.

REFERENCES

Aisenson MR (1948) Accident injuries in epileptic children. *Pediatrics* 2:85–88.

Association of British Pharmaceutical Industries (1998) *Compendium of Data Sheets and Summaries of Product Characteristics, 1998–1999.* London: Datapharm Publications Ltd.

Ben-Menachem E, French J (1998) Vigabatrin. In: Engel J Jr, Pedley TA (eds) *Epilepsy: A Comprehensive Textbook*, Vol 2, pp 1609–1618. Philadelphia: Lippincott-Raven.

Berman W (1984) Sports and the child with epilepsy. *Pediatrics* 74:320–321.

British Epilepsy Association 1996. *The Treatment of Epilepsy: A Patient's Viewpoint.* London: British Epilepsy Association Publishers.

Bryant AE, Dreifuss FE (1996) Valproic acid hepatic fatalities. III. US experience since 1986. *Neurology* 46:465–469.

Clayton-Smith J, Donnai D (1995) Fetal valproate syndrome. *Journal of Medical Genetics* 32:724–727.

Committee on Safety of Medicines (1998) Vigabatrin (Sabril) and visual fields. *Current Problems in Pharmacovigilance* 24:1.

Desai KB, Ribbans WJ, Taylor GJ (1996) Incidence of five common fracture types in an institutional epileptic population. *Injury* 27:758–759.

Dodrill CB (1998) Effects of seizures and various AEDs on cognition. In: *Cognitive Organisation of the Brain: Considerations Relative to Epilepsy Populations.* Symposium at American Epilepsy Society meeting, San Diego, December.

D'Souza SW, Robertson IG, Donnai D, Mawer G (1990) Fetal phenytoin exposure, hypoplastic nails, and jitteriness. *Archives of Diseases in Childhood* 65:320–324.

Duncan JS (1996) Reproductive aspects of epilepsy treatment. In: Shorvon S, Dreifuss F, Fish D, Thomas D (eds) *The Treatment of Epilepsy*, pp 318–323. Oxford: Blackwell Science.

Eke T, Talbot JF, Lawden MC (1997) Severe persistent visual field constriction associated with vigabatrin. *British Medical Journal* 314:180–181.

Ferrie CD, Robinson RO, Panayiotopoulos CP (1996) Psychotic and severe behavior reactions with vigabatrin: a review. *Acta Neurologica Scandinavica* 93:1–8.

Gram L, Jensen PK (1989) Carbamazepine toxicity. In: Levy R, Mattson R, Meldrum B, Penry JK, Dreifuss FE (eds) *Antiepileptic Drugs*, 3rd edn, pp 555–565. New York: Raven Press.

Hauser W, Tabaddor K, Factor P, Finer C (1984) Seizures and head injury in an urban community. *Neurology* 34:746–751.

Heller AJ, Chesterman P, Elwes RDC *et al* (1995) Phenobarbitone, phenytoin, carbamazepine, or sodium valproate for newly diagnosed adult epilepsy: a randomized comparative monotherapy trial. *Journal of Neurology, Neurosurgery and Psychiatry* 58:44–50.

Herzog AG (1998) Disorders of reproduction and fertility. In: Engel J Jr, Pedley TA (eds) *Epilepsy: A Comprehensive Textbook*, Vol 2, pp 2013–2019. Philadelphia: Lippincott-Raven.

Independent reviewer (1994) Epilepsy and pregnancy. *Drug and Therapeutics Bulletin* 32:49–51.

Isojarvi JIT, Laatikainen TJ, Knip M, Pakarinen AJ, Juntunen KTS, Myllyla VV (1996) Obesity and endocrine disorders in women taking valproate for epilepsy. *Annals of Neurology* 39:579–584.

Jokiet H, Ebner A (1999) Long-term effects of refractory temporal lobe epilepsy on cognitive abilities: a cross-sectional study. *Journal of Neurology, Neurosurgery and Psychiatry* 67:44–50.

Kemp AM, Sibert JR (1993) Epilepsy in children and the risk of drowning. *Archives of Disease in Childhood* 68:684–685.

Koch S, Jager-Roman E, Losche G, Nau H, Rating D, Helge H (1996) Antiepileptic drug treatment in pregnancy: drug side-effects in the neonate and neurological outcome. *Acta Paediatrica* 84:739–746.

Krauss GL, Johnson MA, Miller NR (1998) Vigabatrin-associated retinal cone system dysfunction: electroretinogram and ophthalmologic findings. *Neurology* 50:614–618.

Lindhout D, Omtzigt JGC (1994) Teratogenic effects of antiepileptic drugs: implications for the management of epilepsy in women of childbearing age. *Epilepsia* 35(Suppl 4):S19–S28.

Lund L, Hellstrom (1989) 2000 allvarliga skador varje ar. *Svenska Epilepsia* 2:30–31.

Masur H, Elger CE, Ludolph AC, Galanski M (1989) Cerebellar atrophy following acute intoxication with phenytoin. *Neurology* 39:432–433.

Masur H, Fahrendorf G, Oberwittler C, Reuther G (1990) Cerebellar atrophy following acute intoxication with phenytoin. *Neurology* 40:1800.

Mattson RH (1998) Carbamazepine. In: Engel J Jr, Pedley TA (eds) *Epilepsy: A Comprehensive Textbook*, Vol. 2, pp 1491–1502. Philadelphia: Lippincott-Raven.

Mattson RH, Cramer JA (1989) Phenobarbital toxicity. In: Levy R, Mattson R, Meldrum B, Penry JK, Dreifuss FE (eds) *Antiepileptic Drugs*, 3rd edn, pp 341–355. New York: Raven Press.

Mattson RH, Cramer JA, Collins JF *et al* (1985) Comparison of carbamazepine, phenobarbital, phenytoin, and primidone in partial and secondarily generalized seizures. *New England Journal of Medicine* 313:145–151.

Mattson RH, Cramer JA, Collins JF; The Department of Veterans Affairs Epilepsy Cooperative Study No. 264 Group (1992) A comparison of valproate with carbamazepine for the treatment of complex partial seizures and secondarily generalized tonic–clonic seizures in adults. *New England Journal of Medicine* 327:765–771.

Nakken KO, Lossius R (1993) Seizure-related injuries in multihandicapped patients with therapy-resistant epilepsy. *Epilepsia* 34:836–840.

Ney GC, Lantos G, Barr WB, Schaul N (1994) Cerebellar atrophy in patients with long-term phenytoin exposure and epilepsy. *Archives of Neurology* 51:767–771.

O'Brien MD, Gilmore-White S (1993) Epilepsy and pregnancy. *British Medical Journal* 307:492–495.

Pellock JM, Willmore LJ (1991) A rational guide to blood monitoring in patients receiving antiepileptic drugs. *Neurology* 41:961–964.

Reynolds EH (1989) Phenytoin toxicity. In: Levy R, Mattson R, Meldrum B, Penry JK, Dreifuss FE (eds) *Antiepileptic Drugs*, 3rd edn, pp 241–255. New York: Raven Press.

Richens A, Davidson DLW, Cartlidge NEF, Easter DJ (1994) A multicenter comparative trial of sodium valproate and carbamazepine in adult-onset epilepsy. *Journal of Neurology, Neurosurgery and Psychiatry* 57:682–687.

Rosa FW (1991) Spina bifida in infants of women treated with carbamazepine during pregnancy. *New England Journal of Medicine* 324:674–677.

Russell-Jones DL, Shorvon SD (1989) The frequency and consequences of head injury in epileptic seizures. *Journal of Neurology, Neurosurgery and Psychiatry* 52:659–662.

Rwiza HT, Mteza I, Matuja WBP (1993) The clinical and social characteristics of epileptic patients in Ulanga district, Tanzania. *Journal of Epilepsy* 6:162–169.

Salzman MB, Valderrama E, Sood SK (1997) Carbamazepine and fatal eosinophilic myocarditis. *New England Journal of Medicine* 336:878–879.

Sankar R, Wasterlain CG (1999) Is the devil we know the lesser of two evils? Vigabatrin and visual fields. *Neurology* 52:1537–1538.

Sonnen A, van Eil A, Erhens A *et al* (1984) Is epilepsy a dangerous condition? Breda, Holland. Monograph Dr. Hans Berger clinic.

Spitz MC, Towbin JA, Shantz D, Adler LE (1994) Risk factors for burns as a consequence of seizures in persons with epilepsy. *Epilepsia* 35:764–767.

Steegers-Theunissen RPM, Renier WO, Borm GF *et al* (1994) Factors influencing the risk of abnormal pregnancy outcome in epileptic women: a multicenter prospective study. *Epilepsy Research* **18**:261–269.

Thompson P, Sander J (1987) Intellectual deterioration in severe epilepsy. In: Wolf P, Dam M, Jenz D, Dreifuss F, *et al* (eds) *Advances in Epileptology,* p 34, XVIth Epilepsy International Symposium. New York: Raven Press.

Trostle JA (1998) Social aspects: stigma, beliefs, and measurement. In:

Engel J Jr, Pedley TA (eds) *Epilepsy: A Comprehensive Textbook*, Vol 2, pp 2183–2189. Philadelphia: Lippincott-Raven.

Vermeulen J, Aldenkamp AP (1995) Cognitive side-effects of chronic antiepileptic drug treatment: a review of 25 years of research. *Epilepsy Research* **22**:65–95.

Yerby MS, Collins SD (1998) Teratogenicity of antiepileptic drugs. In: Engel J Jr, Pedley TA (eds) *Epilepsy: A Comprehensive Textbook*, Vol 2, 1195–1203. Philadelphia: Lippincott-Raven.

Outcome after long-term medical treatment: children

41

M DUCHOWNY

While the long-term prognosis of many childhood epilepsies is generally known, localization-related disorders, with the exception of idiopathic syndromes, are much less well understood. Several factors add to the complexities of prognostic certainty. The diversity of symptoms associated with activation of specific brain regions has made the classification of partial seizures extremely challenging. Second, it is not always possible to differentiate primary from secondary generalized seizures, despite off-line analysis of seizure semeiology through video-EEG monitoring. Finally, and perhaps most importantly, as deterioration in many cases of partial seizures may be subtle and gradual, the clear delineation of long-term prognosis requires carefully designed long-term analysis.

It is becoming increasingly clear that the consequences of medically uncontrolled symptomatic and cryptogenic partial seizures in childhood may be considerable, and ultimately interfere with the ability to lead a normal life. The negative impact results from disturbances in a variety of domains that are reviewed in this chapter.

MATURATIONAL CONSIDERATIONS

IMMATURE CORTEX: SUSCEPTIBILITY VERSUS STABILITY TO INSULT

The vulnerability of immature cortex to epileptic seizures is a topic of considerable controversy (Camfield 1997; Wasterlain 1997). While it is often stated that the CNS in infants and children is more prone to insult by noxious events such as epileptogenic discharging than in adults, experimental and clinical data bearing on this issue are often conflicting and open to challenge.

Experimental studies in young animals suggest that neuroprotection rather than susceptibility is common in developing neural tissue (Holmes 1997). Experimentally induced seizures in young postnatal animals produce fewer histologic or behavioral abnormalities. Rat pups with kainic acid-induced seizures exhibit more restricted changes in the hippocampus and fewer deficits in learning and behavior if kainic acid is administered earlier in the postnatal period. Unilateral injections of glutamate into the CA1 hippocampal subfield generate less cell loss earlier in postnatal development (Liu *et al* 1996). It is currently unknown whether this pathophysiologic 'sparing' results from intrinsic neuro-protection or cellular plasticity with recovery of function.

Alternatively, electrographic discharges can produce sustained biochemical and neurobehavioral alterations. Kainic acid exposure increases binding sites in the fascia dentata and CA3 regions of the hippocampus (Represa and Ben Ari 1997), while even brief seizure episodes induce mossy fiber sprouting, synaptic reorganization, long-lasting alterations in gene expression, and potentiated neural excitability (Sutula et al 1989; Ben Ari and Represa 1990). Similar changes have been found in anterior temporal lobectomy specimens (Sutula et al 1988; Houser 1990), emphasizing that regulatory disturbances of neural excitation and abnormal cellular architecture are features of human epilepsy as well.

Other factors in childhood predispose to limbic dysfunction and cellular change. Prolonged early febrile seizures in some patients predispose to hippocampal sclerosis (HS) and temporal lobe epilepsy (Davidson and Falconer 1975; Sagar and Oxbury 1987; Verity et al 1993). Timing appears critical as febrile attacks in older individuals are rarely injurious (Kotagal et al 1987). Bacterial meningitis and viral encephalitis before the age of 4 years are linked to later HS (Ounsted et al 1985; Marks et al 1992).

While HS is the predominant pathology in adults with chronic temporal lobe epilepsy, it is more prevalent in early life than formerly believed. Of 53 children (mean age 10 years) with temporal lobe seizures undergoing detailed MRI evaluations, 30 demonstrated either HS or abnormal signal in the absence of a mass lesion (Grattan Smith et al 1993). HS was subsequently confirmed in 11 of 13 patients treated surgically. Similar results are reported by others (Kuks et al 1993). While further studies of HS in childhood are likely to yield additional insights, the available information suggests that hippocampal damage can occur early and the antecedents of temporal lobe epilepsy may be present in early life.

PREDICTORS OF MEDICAL INTRACTABILITY

The diagnosis of intractable partial epilepsy in children relies on clinical experience. Two practical issues are particularly subjective – choosing the 'best' antiepileptic drug (AED), and the perceptions of individual well-being and quality of life by physician and family. Surgical therapy is an option for seizures deemed to interfere with daily function at home and at school. Physicians rarely perceive issues similarly.

High serum AED concentrations and the judicious application of polytherapy are the cornerstone of rational drug treatment. Parents are sensitive to adverse effects and may resist potentially useful AEDs. Diagnosing of medical 'intractability' is rarely straightforward and requires a close relationship with patient and family.

Several factors predict medical intractability (Chevrie and Aicardi 1979). Frequent seizures (daily or weekly), clustering (Aicardi 1988), and early seizure onset (particularly infancy) favor seizure persistence (Lindsay et al 1980) while infantile hemiconvulsive status epilepticus is linked to later temporal lobe epilepsy (Gastaut et al 1959; Cendes et al 1993; Harvey et al 1995). Motor convulsions in nonconvulsive disorders worsen the prognosis in proportion to the overall number of convulsive episodes (Ousted and Lindsay 1981). Children with brain damage are more prone to persistent seizures (Aicardi 1990; Huttenlocher and Hapke 1990), especially in the most severely damaged (Trevathan et al 1988).

Gilman et al (1994) reevaluated the diagnosis of medical intractability in 21 children with significant treatment omissions referred for epilepsy surgery. Omissions consisted primarily of nonutilization of first or second-line AEDs and a lack of high serum levels. Correction did not benefit 19 children (90%) while two improved on high-dose AED monotherapy. This suggests that although medically refractory patients occasionally respond to further therapeutic manipulation, definitive remission is unusual.

SEIZURE OUTCOME

PARTIAL SEIZURES IN INFANTS

Only a small proportion of afebrile localization-related seizures in infancy are benign. A high proportion will remain treatment resistant, and produce significant morbidity and mortality. Poor prognosis is well known for West syndrome, with localization-related features, but applies equally to other seizure types as well. All are associated with epilepsy, mental handicap and, in some cases, neurologic deterioration and death. The onset of epilepsy in infancy is thus itself a significant risk factor for later intractability at any later time.

Studies of partial seizures in the infant are influenced by technical considerations. Clinical seizure patterns often do not conform to guidelines set out in the International Classification (Nordli et al 1997). Assessing the level of consciousness is also difficult, and many authors have abandoned efforts to differentiate simple from complex partial seizure subtypes. Video-EEG has been extremely useful for subtle features, but the interpretation of clinical seizure manifestations in the infant remains challenging.

Partial seizures display a strong tendency to access motor pathways in immature cortex. Propagation is typically rapid, suggesting that seizures involve motor or premotor cortex; brief loss of awareness is thus easily overlooked, and is an important diagnostic pitfall. A small proportion of severely brain damaged infants manifest migratory ictal motor phenomena in conjunction with a multifocal EEG (Coppola *et al* 1995).

Seizure persistence

Infants with partial seizures are prone to recurrent seizures in later life. Chevrie and Aicardi (1979) found that 68% of infants with recurrent afebrile partial seizures and without acquired brain insult were still symptomatic 5 years after initial presentation. Seizure persistence was more likely in patients with abnormal neurologic and cognitive status. By comparison, only 52% of patients with infantile spasms were experiencing seizures at 5-year follow-up. Partial seizure recurrence was highly correlated to the presence of cryptogenic or symptomatic etiologies.

Similarly poor seizure outcomes have been noted by other investigators (Matsumoto *et al* 1983; Cavazzuti *et al* 1984). Czochanska *et al* 1994 performed a long-term prospective analysis of 133 patients diagnosed with epilepsy in the first year of life. Of the 118 patients still alive at age 3 years, 52 (44%) had active epilepsy. There was no difference in outcome between children with West syndrome and other seizure types. More ominously, deterioration in mental development occurred significantly more often in children with active epilepsy.

Kramer *et al* (1997) reported the outcome of seizures in the first year of life in patients classified according to criteria established by the Commission on Classification and Terminology of the International League Against Epilepsy (1989). While 19 of 38 patients (50%) were still experiencing seizures at follow-up, 71% had partial seizures and 25% had generalized convulsions. The cohort represented 27.6% of all patients with seizure onset before the age of 16 years.

Cognitive status

The poor prognosis for mental development in patients with West syndrome is well recognized, but the neurocognitive prognosis for recurrent partial seizures in infants is equally unfavorable. From an initial cohort of 437 infants, Chevrie and Aicardi (1978) followed 313 patients for 1 year or more and found the outlook for mental status and neurologic handicap to be similar for cases of West syndrome and partial seizures. Both groups were more likely to experience seizure onset before age 6 months, to have negative

family histories, and to show a higher incidence of developmental brain anomalies associated with cryptogenic and symptomatic etiologies. These features confirm that partial epileptic seizures presenting in the first year of life are the expression of severe, prenatally acquired brain damage, and their poor prognosis is not surprising.

Although cognitive deterioration may partially be medication related, patients responding promptly to drug therapy have a more favorable prognosis with respect to seizures and mental status (Kramer *et al* 1997).

PARTIAL SEIZURES IN CHILDREN AND ADOLESCENTS

In contrast to the outcome for infants, the prognosis of partial epilepsy in older pediatric patients is less certain. Much of this variation is explained by differences in etiology, with more favorable prognoses in idiopathic disorders. Earlier studies typically lumped together patients now recognized to have idiopathic partial epilepsies (e.g. syndromes of benign epilepsy with centrotemporal spikes and benign occipital epilepsy) with cryptogenic and symptomatic cases.

Chao *et al* (1962) reported on 156 children with complex partial seizures, the majority of whom had EEG evidence of temporal lobe involvement. Seizure control was achieved in 45%, although no long-term follow-up data were given. Currie *et al* (1971) reported a large cohort of 666 patients with temporal lobe seizures including 171 children; 32% obtained adequate seizure control. Kotagal *et al* (1987) reported a 5-year follow-up of 29 carefully studied children with clinical and EEG criteria of complex partial seizures. Only 12 patients were seizure-free, 8 of whom had surgical therapy. There were no spontaneous remissions without AED treatment, and only one patient discontinued medication after surgery. This outcome was obtained at a referral center, and despite community-based studies of temporal lobe seizures in childhood (Harvey *et al* 1997), there are few community-based investigations of long-term seizure prognosis.

Ounsted and Lindsay (1981) followed a subgroup of 100 children with temporal lobe seizures from an unselected population of 1000 children with all types of epilepsy. The study began in 1948 with the inception of the UK National Health Service and was followed until 1977. As adults, roughly one-third became seizure-free, one-third had seizures but supported themselves socially and economically, and one-third had seizures and led fully dependent lives.

Does early and aggressive AED therapy alter long-term seizure prognosis? Advocates of early aggressive drug treatment point to experimental paradigms such as kindling to suggest that seizures lower threshold. However, clinical studies of long-term seizure prognosis do not provide convincing support (Shinnar and Berg 1996). The number of pretreatment seizures (<10) in children does not reduce the likelihood of remission once treatment is started (Camfield *et al* 1996), and data from the British National General Practice Study of Epilepsy (Cockerell *et al* 1995), suggests that pretreatment seizures do not affect the prognosis of newly diagnosed epilepsy. Population-based studies of the incidence and prevalence of epilepsy in developing countries, where treatment is often lacking, reveal high spontaneous remission rates for epilepsy, especially within the first two decades (Osuntokun *et al* 1987).

While there is little conclusive clinical evidence of seizures facilitating seizures, they may contribute to the development of HS (Kalviainen *et al* 1998). HS was found in 57% of an unselected group of children with video-EEG-confirmed temporal lobe epilepsy (Grattan Smith *et al* 1993), almost half of whom were under the age of 10 years (Harvey *et al* 1995); magnetic resonance imaging (MRI) of unaffected individuals from families with febrile seizures and temporal lobe epilepsy reveal significantly reduced left hippocampal volumes (Fernandez *et al* 1998). This observation suggests that a developmental malformation of the hippocampus may predispose to febrile convulsions. Isolated reports of serial MRI studies after prolonged convulsions confirm that HS can develop over time after nervous system insult. It is therefore possible that in early postnatal life, genetically predisposed individuals are at risk for developing seizures and hippocampal damage.

NEUROBEHAVIORAL OUTCOME

COGNITION

As early as 1961, Chaudhry and Pond documented intellectual and social deterioration in selected epileptic children. The majority had partial epilepsy with secondary generalized seizures; the authors noted a correlation with increased seizure frequency, medical resistance, and the occurrence of both focal and generalized EEG abnormalities. The degree of seizure control is a critical variable, as seizure recurrence is highly correlated with diminished intellectual ability compared to patients whose seizures are controlled or in remission (Farwell *et al* 1985; Rodin *et al* 1986).

Recurrent temporal lobe seizure activity shows a predilection for memory impairment (Loiseau *et al* 1983). The left temporal lobe is specialized for learning and retention of

verbal information while the right temporal lobe processes visuospatial and nonverbal material. Children with left temporal lobe epilepsy are prone to verbal memory impairment, while children with right temporal lobe epilepsy exhibit performance difficulty and disordered visual memory (Fedio and Martin 1983). Children with persistent focal spike discharges also manifest lower reading levels and diminished reading accuracy compared to nonepileptic matched controls (Stores and Hart 1976). A laterality effect for focal interictal spiking has also been shown whereby localized recurrent discharges interrupt hemispheric-specific cognitive tasks (Rivas *et al* 1993). While absence of a laterality effect for cognitive impairment was reported in one study of children with temporal lobe seizures (Camfield *et al* 1984), this series included a high proportion of normal children with well-controlled disorders.

In detailed neuropsychologic studies of memory impairment in 60 children with epilepsy (two-thirds with partial seizures), and 60 normal controls (Jambaque *et al* 1993), memory scales were consistently lower in the epilepsy group, and showed more impairment in partial compared to generalized epilepsy. Furthermore, children with left and right temporal lobe epilepsy demonstrated significant memory deficits related to hemispheric specialization. Seizure frequency, age at seizure onset, and AEDs could not account for the observed memory impairment.

These observations suggest that in some children, recurrent partial seizures are associated with long-term cognitive impairments, and that memory is particularly vulnerable. Cognitive deterioration is more likely to occur with higher rates of seizure recurrence, but may be absent or so subtle as to escape detection when seizures are well controlled. It therefore seems likely that cognitive impairment is a feature of a select group of children with chronic partial epilepsy, with severity falling along a continuum based on the degree of interictal spiking and seizure frequency.

PSYCHOLOGIC STATUS

The first description of behavioral disturbance in children with epilepsy by Charles Bradley (1951) enumerated five traits that clustered in affected children including – 'erratic variability in mood', 'hypermotility', irritability, short attention span, and selective difficulty in math. While they may be typical of children with brain damage (the last trait is arguable), studies have tended to confirm these observations while suggesting that children with partial seizure disorders were particularly vulnerable (Pond and Bidwell 1954; Grunberg and Pond 1957; Nuffield 1961).

The special contribution of the temporal lobe to behavioral problems in childhood epilepsy was also noted fairly early (Lennox 1951; Bray 1962). Outbursts of catastrophic rage were seen in 36 of the 100 children in the temporal lobe cohort of Ounsted and Lindsay (Ounsted *et al* 1966; Ounsted 1969). Hyperactivity was also common with or without aggression. There was no relationship to the frequency of complex partial seizures or grand mal attacks. Boys were more prone to physical rage than girls while aggression in girls was largely limited to severely retarded patients (Ounsted and Lindsay 1981).

Affective disturbances of mood and anxiety are common. Standardized checklists reveal increased rates of self-reported symptoms of anxiety and depression among children with epilepsy (Ettinger *et al* 1998). As these findings are consistent with the higher rate of depression in adults with epilepsy, it is likely that many young children with epilepsy go unrecognized and contribute to the higher incidence of depression in adults with epilepsy (Robertson and Trimble 1983).

When does psychiatric disability first develop? Although recurrent seizures and epileptic discharges produced widespread disturbance, the evolution of neuropsychologic dysfunction is poorly understood. In a comparison of newly diagnosed and chronic epileptic children, Hoare (1984a) found similar rates of psychiatric disturbance. Both groups were significantly more disturbed than children with chronic illness outside the CNS and healthy children in the population. Children with focal EEG abnormalities and complex partial seizures were especially vulnerable, and severity was related to seizure frequency. The high frequency of psychiatric disturbance in newly diagnosed children with epilepsy points to a common underlying biologic mechanism.

The relative strength of family relationships also influences behavior. Family stress negatively correlates with childhood behavior, while extended family support improves behavioral symptoms (Austin 1996). At the same time, raising a child with seizures is more emotionally stressful than raising a child with other chronic handicaps (Rutter *et al* 1970). Treatment of psychiatric disability should therefore aim to reduce symptoms of anxiety and stress in the parents.

DRUG EFFECTS

Recognition of the potential adverse and long-term consequences of AEDs on behavior and cognition led to the Committee on Drugs of the American Academy of Pediatrics to recommend factoring neurobehavioral consequences into the initial treatment decisions. Hyperactivity, attentional deficit, depression, and irritability are most common, especially with long-term administration of barbiturates. In practice, it is often difficult to identify the specific contribution of drug effects, as they must be distinguished from the effects of seizures and underlying brain damage. A clear understanding requires careful testing on and off drug therapy, controlling for the amount of seizure activity.

In an open, parallel-design study of the neuropsychologic effects of four AEDs using the Child Behavior Checklist (Miles *et al* 1988), hyperactivity and aggression were observed with phenobarbital and primidone, whereas patients switched to carbamazepine showed improved behavior. A reduction in AEDs improves certain cognitive domains (Durwen *et al* 1989). After medication reduction patients with left temporal lobe epilepsy exhibit improved verbal memory performance. By contrast, patients with right temporal lobe epilepsy showed a trend towards improved nonverbal memory function.

There is little information about long-term stability of cognitive status factoring the effect of AEDs. This issue is critical, as maturational factors in the developing nervous system may determine different responses to drug treatment at different periods of brain growth. In a prospective study of 72 noninstitutionalized children with normal mean intelligence quotient (IQ) scores, Bourgeois *et al* (1983) found that compared to sibling pairs, children with seizures demonstrate stability in cognition with a subset showing persistent decreases of 10 IQ points or more. Drug toxicity, particularly to phenobarbital, was a better predictor of diminished IQ than seizure control. Children showing a decline in IQ had seizure onset at a younger age.

SOCIAL AND REHABILITATIVE STATUS

The negative impact of medically uncontrolled childhood epilepsy was initially demonstrated in the long-term prospective study of 100 children with temporal lobe epilepsy at the Park Hospital for Children, Oxford, UK (Lindsay *et al* 1984). If seizures did not remit by adolescence, behavioral and cognitive deterioration were virtually assured, and often prevented patients from functioning as independent adults. Psychosocial morbidity was the most important determinant of outcome; if schooling was compromised, less than 5% functioned normally (Lindsay *et al* 1979a). Females were more likely to marry and have children (Lindsay *et al* 1979b). While individuals with chronic epilepsy have lower overall levels of schooling and lower socioeconomic status (Camfield *et al* 1993; Jalava *et al* 1997), the ability to be economically productive adults also correlates with good marital and work adjustment (Wilson *et al* 1959).

Community-based studies confirm early seizure remission as a predictor of psychosocial functioning (Jacoby *et al* 1996). Earlier age at seizure onset is associated with a reduced likelihood of marriage for both males and females. Interestingly, an older age of seizure onset is more likely to produce feelings of depression and stigmatization. While seemingly counterintuitive, the lower incidence of these symptoms with earlier seizure onset may reflect superior adaptive mechanisms.

Children with epilepsy are more likely to be inappropriately dependent and to manifest greater psychiatric disturbance compared to diabetic children or children in the general population (Hoare 1984a). Higher rates of psychiatric morbidity are found in mothers and siblings of children with chronic epilepsy (Hoare 1984b). In contrast, the psychologic health of mothers of newly diagnosed children

with epilepsy does not differ from controls. It has been suggested that social assistance should be offered to children and their families in the early stages of treatment (Mulder and Suurmeijer 1977).

While reasons for the poor long-term social and rehabilitative status of children with epilepsy are complex, continuing epilepsy, especially seizures that are severe and/or frequent, is likely to precipitate social and vocational problems for the patient and family members (Ward and Bower 1978). Apart from seizures, additional factors act as coprecipitants, including educational disadvantage, social isolation and, possibly, sexual dysfunction. The reaction of the family to the child's epilepsy also exerts a strong influence, either directly through feedback to the child, or indirectly through deficient parental coping mechanisms, as, for example, competence in seeking community resources. Anxiety among relatives and ignorance and prejudice in the general population may compound these problems.

KEY POINTS

1. The outcome after long-term medical treatment of partial seizures in childhood is extremely variable.

2. In infants, partial seizures may occur in the context of benign syndromes with favorable prognoses, or result from brain damage and carry a poor prognosis for seizure remission and mental status.

3. Maturational factors strongly influence seizure expression but evidence that immature cortex is specifically vulnerable is often conflicting.

4. In older children and adolescents, chronic partial seizures are associated with increasing neurobehavioral deterioration and social isolation.

5. Risk factors for medical intractability can often be identified at the outset, and the importance of properly diagnosing and fully controlling partial seizures cannot be overemphasized.

REFERENCES

Aicardi J (1988) Clinical approach to the management of intractable epilepsy. *Developmental Medicine and Child Neurology* **30**:429–440.

Aicardi J (1990) Epilepsy in brain-injured children. *Developmental Medicine and Child Neurology* **32**:191–202.

Austin JK (1996) A model of family adaptation to new-onset childhood epilepsy. *Journal of Neuroscience Nursing* **28**:82–92.

Ben Ari Y, Represa A (1990) Brief seizure episodes induce long-term potentiation and mossy fiber sprouting in the hippocampus. *Trends in Neurological Science* **13**:312–318.

Bourgeois BF, Prensky AL, Palkes HS, Talent BK, Busch SG (1983) Intelligence in epilepsy: a prospective study in children. *Annals of Neurology* **14**:438–444.

Bradley C (1951) Behavior disturbances in epileptic children. *Journal of the American Medical Association* **146**:436–491.

Bray F (1962) Temporal lobe syndrome in children: a longitudinal review. *Pediatrics* **29**:339–346.

Camfield PR (1997) Recurrent seizures in the developing brain are not harmful. *Epilepsia* **38**:735–737.

Camfield PR, Gates R, Ronen G, Camfield C, Ferguson A, MacDonald GW (1984) Comparison of cognitive ability, personality profile, and school success in epileptic children with pure right versus left temporal lobe EEG foci. *Annals of Neurology* **15**:122–126.

Camfield C, Camfield P, Smith B, Gordon K, Dooley J (1993) Biologic factors as predictors of social outcome of epilepsy in intellectually normal children: a population-based study. *Journal of Pediatrics* **122**:869–873.

Camfield C, Camfield P, Gordon K, Dooley J (1996) Does the number of seizures before treatment influence ease of control or remission of childhood epilepsy? *Neurology* **464**:41–44.

Cavazzuti GB, Ferrari F, Lalla M (1984) Follow-up study of 482 cases with convulsive disorders in the first year of life. *Developmental Medicine and Child Neurology* **26**:425–437.

Cendes F, Andermann F, Dubeau F *et al* (1993) Early childhood prolonged febrile convulsions, atrophy and sclerosis of mesial structures, and temporal lobe epilepsy: an MRI volumetric study. *Neurology* **43**:1083–1087.

Chao D, Sexton JA, Pardo SS (1962) Temporal lobe epilepsy in children. *Journal of Pediatrics* **60**:686–693.

Chaudhry MR, Pond DA (1961) Mental deterioration in epileptic children. *Journal of Neurology, Neurosurgery and Psychiatry* **24**:213.

Chevrie JJ, Aicardi J (1978) Convulsive disorders in the first year of life: neurological and mental outcome and mortality. *Epilepsia* **19**:67–74.

Chevrie JJ, Aicardi J (1979) Convulsive disorders in the first year of life: persistence of epileptic seizures. *Epilepsia* **20**:643–649.

Cockerell OC, Johnson AL, Sander JW, Hart YM, Shorvon SD (1995) Remission of epilepsy: results from the National General Practice Study of Epilepsy [see comments]. *Lancet* **346**:140–144.

Commission on Classification and Terminology of the International League Against Epilepsy (1989) Proposal for revized classification of epilepsies and epileptic syndromes. *Epilepsia* **30**:389–399.

Coppola G, Plouin P, Chiron C, Robain O, Dulac O (1995) Migrating partial seizures in infancy: a malignant disorder with developmental arrest. *Epilepsia* **36**:1017–1024.

Currie S, Heathfield KWG, Henson RA (1971) Clinical course and prognosis of temporal lobe epilepsy: a survey of 666 patients. *Brain* **94**:173–190.

Czochariska J, Langner-Tyszka B, Losiowski Z, Schmidt-Sidor B (1994) Children who develop epilepsy in the first year of life: a prospective study. *Developmental Medicine and Child Neurology* **36**:344–350.

Davidson S, Falconer MA (1975) Outcome of surgery in 40 children with temporal lobe epilepsy. *Lancet* i:1260–1263.

Durwen HF, Elger CE, Helmstaedter C, Penin H (1989) Circumscribed improvement of cognitive performance in temporal lobe epilepsy patients with intractable seizures following reduction of anticonvulsant medication. *Journal of Epilepsy* **2**:147–153.

Ettinger AB, Weisbrot DM, Nolan EE *et al* (1998) Symptoms of depression and anxiety in pediatric epilepsy patients. *Epilepsia* **39**:595–599.

Farwell JR, Dodrill CB, Batzel LW (1985) Neuropsychological abilities of children with epilepsy. *Epilepsia* **26**:395–400.

Fedio P, Martin A (1983) Ideative–emotive behavioral characteristics of patients following left or right temporal lobectomy. *Epilepsia* **24**:S117–S130.

Fernandez G, Effenberger O, Vinz B *et al* (1998) Hippocampal malformation as a cause of familial febrile convulsions and subsequent hippocampal sclerosis. *Neurology* **50**:909–917.

Gastaut H, Poirier F, Payan H, Salamon G, Toga M, Vigouroux M (1959) HHE syndrome, hemiconvulsions, hemiplegia, epilepsy. *Epilepsia* **1**:418–447.

Gilman JT, Duchowny M, Jayakar P, Resnick TJ (1994) Medical intractability in children evaluated for epilepsy surgery. *Neurology* **44**:1341–1343.

Grattan Smith JD, Harvey AS, Desmond PM, Chow CW (1993) Hippocampal sclerosis in children with intractable temporal lobe epilepsy: detection with MR imaging. *American Journal of Roentgenology* **161**:1045–1048.

Grunberg F, Pond DA (1957) Conduct disorders in epileptic children. *Journal of Neurology, Neurosurgery and Psychiatry* **20**:65.

Harvey AS, Grattan Smith JD, Desmond PM, Chow CW, Berkovic SF (1995) Febrile seizures and hippocampal sclerosis: frequent and related findings in intractable temporal lobe epilepsy of childhood. *Pediatric Neurology* **12**:201–206.

Harvey AS, Berkovic SF, Wrennall JA, Hopkins IJ (1997) Temporal lobe epilepsy in childhood: clinical, EEG, and neuroimaging findings and syndrome classification in a cohort with new-onset seizures. *Neurology* **49**:960–968.

Hoare P (1984a) Does illness foster dependency? A study of epileptic and diabetic children. *Developmental Medicine and Child Neurology* **26**:20–24.

Hoare P (1984b) Psychiatric disturbance in the families of epileptic children. *Developmental Medicine and Child Neurology* **26**:14–19.

Holmes GL (1997) Epilepsy in the developing brain: lessons from the laboratory and clinic. *Epilepsia* **38**:12–30.

Houser CR (1990) Granule cell dispersion in the dentate gyrus of humans with temporal lobe epilepsy. *Brain Research* **535**:195–204.

Huttenlocher PR, Hapke RJ (1990) A follow-up study of intractable seizures in childhood [see comments]. *Annals of Neurology* **28**:699–705.

Jacoby A, Baker GA, Steen N, Potts P, Chadwick D (1996) The clinical course of epilepsy and its psychosocial correlates: findings from a UK community study. *Epilepsia* **37**:148–161.

Jalava M, Sillanpaa M, Camfield C, Camfield P (1997) Social adjustment and competence 35 years after onset of childhood epilepsy: a prospective controlled study. *Epilepsia* **38**:708–715.

Jambaque I, Dellatolas G, Dulac O, Ponsot G, Signoret JL (1993) Verbal and visual memory impairment in children with epilepsy. *Neuropsychologia* **31**:1321–1337.

Kalviainen R, Salmenpera T, Partanen K, Vainio P, Riekkinen PJ Sr, Pitkanen A (1998) Recurrent seizures may cause hippocampal damage in temporal lobe epilepsy. *Neurology* **50**:1377–1382.

Kotagal P, Rothner AD, Erenberg G, Cruse RP, Wyllie E (1987) Complex partial seizures of childhood onset. A five-year follow-up study. *Archives of Neurology* **44**:1177–1180.

Kramer U, Phatal A, Neufeld MY, Leitner Y, Harel S (1997) Outcome of seizures in the first year of life. *European Journal of Pediatric Neurology* **5**(6):165–171.

Kuks JB, Cook MJ, Fish DR, Stevens JM, Shorvon SD (1993) Hippocampal sclerosis in epilepsy and childhood febrile seizures [see comments]. *Lancet* **342**:1391–1394.

Lennox WG (1951) *Epilepsy and Related Disorders.* Boston: Little Brown.

Lindsay J, Ounsted C, Richards P (1979a) Long-term outcome in children with temporal lobe seizures. I: Social outcome and childhood factors. *Developmental Medicine and Child Neurology* **21**:285–98.

Lindsay J, Ounsted C, Richards P (1979b) Long-term outcome in children with temporal lobe seizures. II: Marriage, parenthood and sexual indifference. *Developmental Medicine and Child Neurology* **21**:433–440.

Lindsay J, Ounsted C, Richards P (1980) Long-term outcome in children with temporal lobe seizures. IV: Genetic factors, febrile convulsions and the remission of seizures. *Developmental Medicine and Child Neurology* **22**:429–439.

Lindsay J, Ounsted C, Richards P (1984) Long-term outcome in children with temporal lobe seizures. V: Indications and contraindications for neurosurgery. *Developmental Medicine and Child Neurology* **26**:25–32.

Liu Z, Stafstrom CE, Sarkisian M *et al* (1996) Age-dependent effects of glutamate toxicity in the hippocampus. *Brain Research and Development* **97**:178–184.

Loiseau P, Strube E, Brouset D, Battellochi S, Gomeni C, Morselli PL (1983) Learning impairment in epileptic patients. *Epilepsia* **24**:183–192.

Marks DA, Kim J, Spencer DD, Spencer SS (1992) Characteristics of intractable seizures following meningitis and encephalitis. *Neurology* **42**:1513–1518.

Matsumoto A, Watanabe K, Sugiura M, Negoro T, Takaesu E, Iwase K (1983) Etiologic factors and long-term prognosis of convulsive disorders in the first year of life. *Neuropediatrics* **14**:231–234.

Miles VM, Tennison MB, Greenwood RS (1988) Assessment of antiepileptic drug effects on child behavior using the child behavior checklist. *Journal of Epilepsy* **1**:209–213.

Mulder HC, Suurmeijer TPBM (1977) Families with a child with epilepsy: a sociological contribution. *Journal of Biosocial Science* **9**:13–24.

Nordli DRJ, Bazil CW, Scheuer ML, Pedley TA (1997) Recognition and classification of seizures in infants. *Epilepsia* **38**:553–560.

Nuffield EJA (1961) Neurophysiology and behavior disorders in epileptic children. *Journal of Mental Science* **107**:438–458.

Osuntokun BO, Adeuja AOG, Nottidge VA (1987) Prevalence of the epilepsies in Nigerian Africans: a community-based study. *Epilepsia* **28**:272–279.

Ounsted C (1969) Aggression and epilepsy rage in children with temporal lobe epilepsy. *Journal of Psychosomatics Research* **13**:237–242.

Ounsted C, Lindsay J (1981) The long-term outcome of temporal lobe epilepsy in childhood. In: Reynolds EH, Trimble MR (ed.) *Epilepsy and Psychiatry*, pp 185–215. Edinburgh: Churchill Livingstone.

Ounsted C, Lindsay J, Norman R (1966) *Biological Factors in Temporal Lobe Epilepsy. Clinics in Developmental Medicine No 22.* London: Spastics International Medical Publications with Heinemann Medical; Philadelphia: Lippincott.

Ounsted C, Glaser GH, Lindsay J, Richards P (1985) Focal epilepsy with mesial temporal sclerosis after acute meningitis. *Archives of Neurology* **42**:1058–1060.

Pond DA, Bidwell B (1954) Management of behavior disorders in epileptic children. *British Medical Journal* 1520–1523.

Represa A, Ben Ari Y (1997) Molecular and cellular cascades in seizure-induced neosynapse formation. *Advances in Neurology* **72**:25–34.

Rivas D, Pataleoni C, Milani N, Giorgi C (1993) Hemispheric specialization in children with unilateral epileptic focus, with and without computed tomography-demonstrated lesion. *Epilepsia* **34**:69–73.

Robertson MM, Trimble MR (1983) Depressive illness in patients with epilepsy: a review. *Epilepsia* **22**:515–524.

Rodin EA, Schmaltz S, Twitty G (1986) Intellectual functions of patients with childhood-onset epilepsy. *Developmental Medicine and Child Neurology* **28**:25–33.

Rutter M, Graham P, Yule W (1970) *A Neuropsychiatric Study in Childhood. Clinics in Developmental Medicine.* London: Spastics International Medical Publications and Heinemann.

Sagar HJ, Oxbury JM (1987) Hippocampal neuron loss in temporal lobe epilepsy: correlation with early childhood convulsions. *Annals of Neurology* **22**:334–340.

Shinnar S, Berg AT (1996) Does antiepileptic drug therapy prevent the development of 'chronic' epilepsy? *Epilepsia* **37**:701–708.

Stores G, Hart J (1976) Reading skills of children with generalized or focal epilepsy attending ordinary school. *Developmental Medicine and Child Neurology* **18**:705–716.

Sutula T, Xiao-Xian H, Cavazos J, Scott G (1988) Synaptic reorganization in the hippocampus induced by abnormal functional activity. *Science* **239**:1147–1150.

Sutula T, Cascino G, Cavazos J et al (1989) Mossy fiber synaptic reorganization in the epileptic human temporal lobe. *Annals of Neurology* **26**:321–330.

Trevathan E, Yeargin-Allsop M, Murphy CC, Ding G (1988) Epilepsy among children with mental retardation. *Annals of Neurology* **24**:321.

Verity M, Ross EM, Golding J (1993) Outcome of childhood status epilepticus and lengthy febrile convulsions: findings of national cohort study. *British Medical Journal* **307**:225–228.

Ward F, Bower BD (1978) A study of certain social aspects of epilepsy in childhood. *Developmental Medicine and Child Neurology* **20**:S39.

Wasterlain CG (1997) Recurrent seizures in the developing brain are harmful. *Epilepsia* **38**:728–734.

Wilson WP, Stewart LF, Parker JB (1959) A study of the socioeconomic effects of epilepsy. *Epilepsia* **1**:300.

Surgical treatment

Syndromes amenable to surgery 42

JM OXBURY

The pioneers of modern epilepsy surgery were well aware of the need to remove pathology if relief from the seizures was to be obtained (Penfield and Jasper 1954; Falconer 1971). The introduction of the en-bloc method of temporal lobectomy by Falconer (1953) provided the opportunity for detailed histopathologic analysis of the excision specimen (Bruton 1988). This in turn led to better understanding of the clinicopathologic correlations and hence easier preoperative diagnosis of the underlying pathology.

The advent of MRI has enabled a proper exploration of the relationship between the nature of the pathology underlying the epilepsy, the feasibility of surgery, and postoperative seizure outcome. As a consequence it is becoming recognized that there are certain pathologic conditions that commonly present with intractable focal epilepsy and carry a particularly good prognosis for successful postoperative outcome. Thus, it is beginning to be possible to predict the outcome of proposed surgery with greater reliability because both the nature of the pathology and its precise location can be determined preoperatively with considerable accuracy. Indeed, it has been suggested that high-quality MRI should be the first step in the evaluation for epilepsy surgery and that, if it does not reveal pathology, the patient should be carefully counseled before proceeding to complex neurophysiologic or other investigations (Scott et al 1999). This is because the probability of successful excisional surgery is low when the MRI is negative.

This chapter is concerned with the conditions that commonly present with intractable focal epilepsy amenable to successful treatment by surgical resection of the underlying pathology (Table 42.1). All have been described in detail elsewhere in this book, some of them over a number of chapters. The purpose here is simply to summarize the salient features for those who require a distillate of what can be appropriately treated surgically. The chapter is best read in conjunction with Chapter 57. Conditions possibly amenable to functional neurosurgical techniques, such as the Landau–Kleffner syndrome treated by multiple subpial transection or frequent drop attacks treated by callosotomy, are noted in Table 42.1, but no consideration is given to them in the text. Neville describes the former in

Chapter 22. See also Polkey in Chapters 54 and 55. Finally, no consideration is given to the evaluation of patients in whom no pathology can be detected preoperatively and in whom the decision to operate must be based primarily on complex neurophysiologic data.

The large majority of patients undergoing successful epilepsy surgery, whether children or adolescents or adults, have mesial temporal sclerosis/hippocampal sclerosis, a low-grade glioma or a benign tumor such as a dysembryoplastic neuroepithelioma, or a cavernous angioma as the basis of their epilepsy. Another considerable number of those treated at some centers have their epilepsy on a background of focal cortical dysplasia, but the success rate with that pathology is less good even with complex preoperative investigation protocols, including intracranial EEG monitoring.

The common substrata among children undergoing hemispherectomy are pre- or perinatal cerebral infarction or hemorrhage, Rasmussen encephalitis, Sturge–Weber syndrome, the hemiconvulsions–hemiplegia–epilepsy (HHE) syndrome, and a malformation of cortical development (MCD). The latter needs to be extensive but, as far as can be ascertained, confined to one hemisphere if it is to merit consideration of hemispherectomy. A large area of cortical dysplasia with already established hemiplegia, and also hemimegalencephaly, are examples.

There are in addition reports of relatively small numbers of patients who have undergone epilepsy surgery for a wide range of other pathologic conditions with varying degrees of success. These include traumatic scar, old abscess cavity, arteriovenous malformation, and tuberous sclerosis. These conditions have all been described in other chapters and will not be described further here.

MESIAL TEMPORAL SCLEROSIS/HIPPOCAMPAL SCLEROSIS

This condition gives rise to the mesial temporal lobe epilepsy syndrome. It is the commonest condition amenable to successful surgical treatment. Wieser, Aguzzi, Hajek, and Goos give a full description in Chapter 11. Salient features are:

- The seizures usually commence in childhood or adolescence, at a median age of 5–8 years.
- The typical pattern consists of partial seizures, particularly an epigastric-rising sensation associated with psychic phenomena such as fear, and complex partial seizures, especially oroalimentary and gestural automatisms, sometimes with secondary generalization.
- A history of a prolonged convulsion in early childhood, or some other cerebral insult, prior to the onset of the habitual epilepsy is common, as is a family history of febrile convulsions.
- MRI shows hippocampal smallness and increased T2 signal that may be unilateral, bilateral but asymmetric, or symmetrically bilateral (see Chapter 44). If smallness is bilateral the possibility of surgery should be approached with great caution.
- The characteristic EEG findings are
  Interictal blunt sharp waves predominating at the basal anterior electrodes on scalp EEG.
  A generalized attenuation of background rhythms and disappearance of interictal spikes at seizure onset.
  Fairly regular theta-rhythms of about $5 \, s^{-1}$ ictally with a crescendo-like increase of amplitude and slowing of the discharge rhythms.
- Characteristically there is ipsilateral temporal lobe hyperperfusion on ictal SPECT (see Duncan in Chapter 26) and ipsilateral temporal lobe hypometabolism on interictal FDG-PET.
- Neuropsychologic assessment reveals variable degrees of memory and learning deficit (see Chapter 30).

Unilateral resection of the atrophic medial temporal lobe structures from those with predominantly unilateral hippocampal sclerosis renders 80% seizure-free, or virtually so, without producing additional clinically relevant deficits.

Table 42.1 Conditions considered amenable to successful epilepsy surgery when they are causing intractable epilepsy. (Other conditions (e.g. tuberous sclerosis) may also be amenable occasionally but are not usually so.)

1. *Focal pathology amenable to restricted excisions (usually unilobar)*
   - Hippocampal sclerosis/mesial temporal sclerosis
   - Malformations of cortical development
   - Benign/low-grade tumors
     Dysembryoplastic neuroepithelioma/hamartoma
     Ganglioglioma
     Low-grade glioma
   - Cavernous angioma
   - Other, e.g. abscess cavity, trauma scar
2. *Conditions that may require more extensive, multilobar excisions or hemispherectomy*
   - Cortical dysplasia including hemimegalencephaly and other disorders of cerebral development including Sturge–Weber syndrome
   - Pre- and perinatal vascular lesions
   - Hemiconvulsions–hemiplegia–epilepsy syndrome
   - Rasmussen syndrome
3. *Conditions amenable to disconnection surgery (including callosotomy and subpial transection)*
   - Landau–Kleffner
   - Frequent drop attacks

DUAL PATHOLOGY

Hippocampal sclerosis may accompany other cerebral pathology, particularly malformations of cortical development including dysembryoplastic neuroepithelial tumor, especially when there is a history of a prolonged convulsion in early childhood (Cendes *et al* 1995).

MALFORMATIONS OF CORTICAL DEVELOPMENT

Sisodiya, Squier, and Anslow describe the classification, clinical features, and management of MCD in detail in Chapter 10. Only a very brief summary will be given here. Focal cortical dysplasia, polymicrogyria, and heterotopia are the most common.

Raymond *et al* (1995) noted that around 80% of the seizure disorders attributable to MCD, excluding dysembryoplastic neuroepithelioma, are localization-related rather than generalized and that up to 15% of patients had a history of status epilepticus. Nevertheless, there are relatively few instances of surgical treatment leading to a complete cessation of these seizures. Such success has been reported mostly for focal cortical dysplasia and occasionally for polymicrogyria, schizencephaly, lissencephaly, focal nodular heterotopia, and hemimegalencephaly. Routine MRI may fail to detect these conditions in around 50% of cases. CT misses a higher proportion.

FOCAL CORTICAL DYSPLASIA

This term was introduced to describe focal areas of macroscopically evident loss of cortical lamination with associated abnormal giant cells and heterotopic (see below) white-matter neurons. It is clear, however, that microscopic areas of abnormality may exist beyond the macroscopic areas. Larger areas of dysplasia may be detected on high-resolution MRI but not necessarily smaller areas, thus making the extent of the pathology difficult to define by clinical methods. The epilepsy usually presents before 16 years of age (Raymond *et al* 1995). The presentation can be as epilepsia partialis continua, without any MRI abnormality, resistant to medication, and necessitating surgical treatment, but this is rare.

POLYMICROGYRIA

This is the second commonest variety of MCD. It is associated with ischemic, traumatic, and infectious etiologies and only arises before the 28th week of gestation. The cortex may appear to have small, irregular, closely packed gyri and may appear on MRI to be thicker than normal. Polymicrogyria may be found in small areas bordering a porencephalic cyst or it may be more extensive. The constant histologic feature is fusion of the pial surfaces of adjacent gyri. The presentation can be with epilepsy and/or developmental delay and/or abnormal neurologic signs such as hemiplegia.

HETEROTOPIA

These are clusters of immature irregularly orientated neurons situated in white matter. *Focal nodular heterotopia* may be single or multiple. *Bilateral periventricular nodular heterotopia* are often contiguous, lining the walls of the lateral ventricles and bulging into the lumen so that they are clearly seen on MRI. Epilepsy usually begins during adolescence or in early adult life. Affected females are usually otherwise normal. Epilepsy tends to begin at a younger age in males and may be associated with other features including developmental delay (see Chapter 10 for further details). *Band heterotopia* consists of a band of irregularly arranged neurons separated from the cortex by a layer of white matter. It appears on MRI as 'double cortex.' Epilepsy does not necessarily begin at a particularly young age and may be associated with normal intellect.

LISSENCEPHALY

This is a condition in which a major part of one cerebral hemisphere, or both, lacks gyri. In type I lissencephaly the neuronal content of the cortex is poor, there is no laminar pattern, and the white–gray border is indistinct. In type II lissencephaly there seems to have been an overmigration of neurons such that they are found in the leptomeninges. Epilepsy usually begins during the first few months of life and is accompanied by severe developmental delay and motor system abnormalities.

SCHIZENCEPHALY

This consists of a complete cleft through the cerebral hemisphere from the ventricle to the surface. The cleft is usually lined with dysplastic cortex. It is unclear whether it is a primary defect or a response to injury during early development. The epilepsy usually begins in early childhood; there is usually developmental delay and there may be hemiparesis.

HEMIMEGALENCEPHALY

In this rare condition there is macroscopic enlargement of the whole or most of one cerebral hemisphere. The gyri are coarse, the cortex is thickened and shows a wide variety of dysplastic abnormalities, the white matter may be gliotic with cystic areas and calcification, and the ventricle is dilated. The opposite hemisphere may contain dysplastic areas. Seizures usually commence during the neonatal period; there is developmental delay with other abnormal neurologic signs, and there may be other somatic features (see Chapter 10).

BENIGN AND LOW-GRADE TUMORS

In my experience, dysembryoplastic neuroepithelioma and ganglioglioma are the commonest forms of tumor in patients aged less than 20 years presenting with intractable epilepsy as surgical candidates. Low-grade glioma is the commonest variety in those aged 20 years and over.

DYSEMBRYOPLASTIC NEUROEPITHELIAL TUMOR

These tumours, originally described by Daumas-Duport *et al* (1988), are benign mixed glial–neuronal neoplasms characterized by an intracortical location, multinodular architecture, and heterogeneous cellular composition (Prayson and Estes 1999). Most are situated in a temporal lobe, approximately half of them in the medial temporal lobe structures and the other half lateral or anterior to the temporal horn of the lateral ventricle. Series of cases include those of Daumas-Duport *et al* (1988), Kirkpatrick *et al* (1993), Raymond *et al* (1994), and Oxbury *et al* (1995). Common clinical features are:

- Median age at seizure onset is around 9–10 years, with a range between 1 week and 30 years in the series of Raymond *et al* (1994).
- The seizure frequency can be very high, up to >1000/year. The median number was 360/year among the 19 children reported by Oxbury *et al* (1995).
- Abnormal neurologic signs are seen in a small proportion of the patients.
- EEG showed focal epileptiform abnormalities that were concordant with the locus of the pathology in only 23% of the patients reported by Raymond *et al* (1994), and ictal activity was correctly localized in only 50% of those in whom it was recorded.
- On MRI the tumors tend to be hypointense on T1-weighted images with increased signal on T2 (see Chapter 24). They may have some mass effect. They usually have a cortical location and there may be clear

evidence of associated cortical dysplasia that can be remote from the tumor itself. There should not be edema, and the presence of this feature should suggest a different diagnosis. There may be concomitant hippocampal atrophy (dual pathology), especially in a patient with a history of a prolonged convulsion in early childhood, and calvarial erosion may be seen. Between 25% and 50% show calcification that can be very subtle and we have seen one pathologically confirmed case with normal MRI in whom calcification was the only radiologic abnormality.

Overall, around 75% become seizure-free after surgery. The success rate may be even higher with those undergoing surgery in childhood.

GANGLIOGLIOMA

These are described as benign tumors consisting of neoplastic astrocytes (rarely oligodendrocytes) and ganglion cells. Nevertheless, they can spread into the subarachnoid space, apparently without adverse effect on the prognosis, and occasionally they become aggressive (Prayson and Estes 1999). Morris *et al* (1998) reviewed the clinical features of 38 cases of intractable epilepsy associated with ganglioglioma seen at the Cleveland Clinic during the period from 1985. All underwent surgical treatment. The essential preoperative clinical features included:

- Tumor location: 26 temporal lobe, 12 extratemporal (4 frontal).
- Median age at seizure onset was 9.5 years, range <1 to 27 years.
- Median seizure frequency was 13/month, range <1 to 600/month.
- Abnormal neurologic signs were detected in 18%.
- In a small number the EEG showed interictal epileptiform discharges predominantly contralateral to the tumor and/or ictal onset (on extracranial monitoring) apparently from the contralateral side.
- The tumors are usually well-defined on MRI and of low signal on T1-weighted images. Abnormalities included gadolinium enhancement (59%), mass effect (47%), cystic change (31%), and edema (6%). Calcification was seen in around 50% of those that had an abnormal CT scan.
- Cortical dysplasia was found in the excision specimens of 36.8% but had not in any case been detected preoperatively.

Twenty (63%) of the 32 cases of Morris *et al* (1998) were in Engel class I (free from disabling seizures) at 2 years after surgery.

OLIGODENDROGLIOMA AND LOW-GRADE ASTROCYTOMA

Low-grade astrocytoma (grade 1, well-differentiated fibrillary astrocytoma) and oligodendroglioma usually present in early adult or middle life. Epilepsy is one of their common features and they are a common cause of intractable focal epilepsy (Bourekas and Perl 1999). Grade 2 astrocytomas may also present as short-duration intractable epilepsy but they are of a higher degree of malignancy and carry a worse prognosis for long-term survival. Pilocytic astrocytomas are most often found in the cerebellum of a child but they may occur in a cerebral hemisphere in childhood or young adult life and then they too may cause intractable epilepsy. Recurrence after 'total' excision is unusual.

The diagnosis of low-grade glioma is dependent upon neuroimaging (see Chapter 24). It is rarely possible to distinguish with certainty between a dysembryoplastic neuroepithelial tumor or a ganglioglioma on the one hand and a low-grade glioma on the other. For that reason, early surgical intervention is usually advisable in a young person, including a young child, if the tumor is situated in a favorable site.

CAVERNOUS ANGIOMA

A recent review of 2411 publications on this type of vascular anomaly and an analysis of the data contained therein (Moran *et al* 1999) suggested the following.

- 80% are supratentorial. Around 33% of these are situated in a frontal lobe, 30% in a temporal lobe and 21% in a parietal lobe the remainder being occipital, basal ganglia or thalamic, or multilobar in descending order of frequency.
- Around 25% patients had multiple (more than one) cavernomas. Multiplicity was statistically associated with a positive family history of cavernoma.
- Epileptic seizures occurred in 80% of those with a supratentorial cavernoma. The occurrence of epilepsy was not significantly associated with the hemispheric locus of the cavernoma. Generalized seizures, however, were statistically significantly associated with frontal cavernomas.
- Surgical treatment rendered around 85% seizure-free irrespective of the cerebral locus of the cavernoma. The duration of the seizure history was statistically significantly shorter in those who became seizure-free than in those who did not.
- Around 10% of those with epilepsy also experienced an intracerebral hemorrhage. The risk of hemorrhage, manifest by relevant clinical symptoms and radiologic evidence of an acute bleed, was estimated at 0.7% per annum for those who had not previously experienced a hemorrhage. The risk of further hemorrhage may be higher once a first hemorrhage has occurred.

Moran *et al* (1999) point out that there have been no prospective trials of treatment of seizures associated with cavernoma comparing conservative measures with surgery, and that many of the around 85% who became seizure-free postoperatively might have done equally well with medication alone.

HEMICONVULSIONS–HEMIPLEGIA–EPILEPSY SYNDROME

This condition develops in a previously entirely well child usually aged between 6 months and 4 years. An excellent detailed description is given by Chauvel *et al* (1991).

The first feature is a prolonged clonic convulsion involving one side of the body, usually in association with fever such as might be caused by an ear infection. The convulsion is prolonged, almost invariably for more than a half-hour and often for many hours, either because the early period is not noticed (for instance if the child is found in bed convulsing) or because of inadequate acute treatment of the hemiclonic status epilepticus. When the convulsion terminates, the child has a hemiparesis affecting the limbs involved by the convulsion. Unlike a Todd's paresis, this does not resolve within a few hours. Over the subsequent weeks the hemiparesis either converts to a definite spastic hemiplegia or gradually diminishes. As the child grows, the parents become aware of a variable degree of unilateral limb smallness. Some mental retardation is common and can be severe. Serial brain imaging shows the development of a variable degree of unilateral hemisphere atrophy that may be focal or generalized.

The chronic intractable epilepsy begins sometimes within weeks and sometimes not for a number of years. The seizure semeiology varies among patients. Seizures typical of medial temporal lobe onset or of rolandic onset are common. The seizures can be very frequent. Hemispherectomy during childhood is appropriate for those with severe epilepsy, a spastic hemiplegia and little or no useful function of the affected hand. Postoperatively, 50–70% are seizure-free in the long term. Treatment is more difficult for those whose hemiparesis is only mild and who have good hand function.

OTHER CONDITIONS

Other major childhood conditions that are common reasons for hemispherectomy include pre- or perinatal cerebral infarction/hemorrhage (see Chapter 13), Sturge–Weber syndrome (see Chapter 17), and Rasmussen encephalitis (see Chapter 18). All are considered in detail in other chapters and so they are not be described here.

KEY POINTS

1. Certain pathologic conditons, recognizable by neuroradiologic investigation in conjunction with the clinical history, commonly present with intractable focal epilepsy and carry a particularly good prognosis for successful resective surgery.

2. Conditions where removal of the pathology by restricted cerebral excisions should render most patients seizure-free include unilateral severe hippocampal sclerosis, dysembryoplastic neuroepithelioma and ganglioglioma and low-grade glioma, and cavernous angioma. The outcome is best if the pathology can be totally removed.

3. Hemispherectomy for pre- or perinatal stroke, HHE syndrome, Rasmussen encephalitis, and unilateral angiomatosis of Sturge-Weber syndrome will also render the majority of properly selected cases seizure-free.

4. The prognosis for postoperative freedom from seizures is less good with malformations of cortical development, but surgery is appropriate in some cases, especially if the epilepsy is very severe and palliation is an acceptable outcome.

5. Multiple subpial transection may bring about major improvement in at least some cases of Landau-Kleffner syndrome (see Chapter 22).

6. Corpus callosotomy may reduce the frequency of atonic or tonic seizures manifest as drop attack (see Chapter 54).

REFERENCES

Bourekas EC, Perl II J (1999) Imaging tumors in epilepsy. In: Kotagal P, Luders HO (eds) *The Epilepsies: Etiologies and Prevention*, pp 315–335. San Diego: Academic Press.

Bruton CJ (1988) *The Neuropathology of Temporal Lobe Epilepsy* (Institute of Psychiatry Maudsley Monographs 31). Oxford: Oxford University Press.

Cendes F, Cook MJ, Watson C *et al* (1995) Frequency and characteristics of dual pathology in patients with lesional pathology. *Neurology* 45:2058–2064.

Chauvel P, Dravet C, Di Leo M, Roger J, Bancaud J, Talairach J (1991) The HHE syndrome. In: Luders H (ed) *Epilepsy Surgery*, pp 183–196. New York: Raven Press.

Daumas–Duport C, Scheithauser BW, Chodkiewicz JP, Laws ER, Vedrenne C (1988) Dysembryoplastic neuroepithelial tumor: a surgically curable tumor of young patients with intractable partial seizures. *Neurosurgery* 23:545–556.

Falconer MA (1953) Discussion on the surgery of temporal lobe epilepsy: surgical and pathological aspects. *Proceedings of the Royal Society of Medicine* 46:971–975.

Falconer MA (1971) Genetic and related aetiological factors in temporal lobe epilepsy: a review. *Epilepsia* 12:13–31.

Kirkpatrick PJ, Honavar M, Janota I, Polkey CE (1993) Control of temporal lobe epilepsy following en bloc resection of low-grade tumors. *Journal of Neurosurgery* 78: 19–25.

Moran NF, Fish DR, Kitchen N, Shorvon S, Kendall BE, Stevens JM (1999) Supratentorial cavernous angiomas and epilepsy: a review of the literature and case series. *Journal of Neurology, Neurosurgery and Psychiatry*, **66**: 561–568.

Morris HH, Matkovic Z, Estes ML *et al* (1998) Ganglioglioma and intractable epilepsy: clinical and neurophysiologic features and predictors of outcome after surgery. *Epilepsia* 39: 307–313.

Oxbury JM, Squier MV, Adams CBT, Zaiwalla Z, Renowden S, Oxbury SM (1995) Surgical treatment of childhood temporal lobe epilepsy due to dysembryoplastic neuroepithelial tumour. *Epilepsia* 36 (Suppl 3):S23.

Penfield W, Jasper H (1954) *Epilepsy and the Functional Anatomy of the Human Brain*. Boston: Little, Brown.

Prayson RA, Estes ML (1999) Dysembryoplastic neuroepithelial tumor, ganglioglioma, and hamartoma: are they distinct entities? In: Kotagal P, Luders HO (eds) *The Epilepsies: Etiologies and Prevention*, pp 337–347. San Diego: Academic Press.

Raymond AA, Halpin SFS, Alsanjari N *et al* (1994) Dysembryoplastic neuroepithelial tumour. Features in 16 patients. *Brain* 117:461–475.

Raymond AA, Fish DR, Sisodiya SM, Alsanjari N, Stevens JM, Shorvon SD. (1995) Abnormalities of gyration, heterotopias, tuberous sclerosis, focal cortical dysplasia, microdysgenesis, dysembryoplastic neuroepithelial tumour and dysgenesis of the archicortex in epilepsy. Clinical, EEG, and neuroimaging features in 100 adult patients. *Brain* 118:629–660.

Scott CA, Fish DR, Smith SJM *et al* (1999) Presurgical evaluation of patients with epilepsy and normal MRI; role of scalp video-EEG telemetry. *Journal of Neurology, Neurosurgery and Psychiatry* 66:69–71.

Surgical options

CE POLKEY

Modern practice in surgery depends upon the identification of pathology or the recognition of circumscribed pathophysiology as a basis for operative intervention. The various operative interventions, many ingenious or sophisticated, are tailored by the indications for surgery to the needs of any particular patient. Underlying such intervention are certain general principles, such as complete removal of a benign tumor to prevent its recurrence, correction of a circulatory abnormality to improve gaseous exchange or viability of tissue, and so forth. In most surgical operations, including many procedures in general neurosurgery, the principles are not in question but the operative techniques, accessibility, and other factors may be responsible for an imperfect solution or undesirable postoperative effects. However in functional neurosurgery, which includes surgery for movement disorder, pain control, and psychiatric disease, as well as epilepsy surgery, the operative techniques are often fairly simple, although the pathophysiology underlying the disease or the influence of any surgical intervention upon that pathophysiology are ill-understood. Many procedures in this area of neurosurgery may appear to be successful on empirical grounds. It is therefore possible to list the surgical options for the treatment of drug-resistant epilepsy but difficult to explain their mode of action in detail.

THEORETIC BACKGROUND

There is a great deal of experimental work on the pathophysiology of chronic epilepsy and, since the introduction of the concept of kindling (Goddard *et al* 1969), much of this work has been used to try to provide a rationale for epilepsy surgery. However, these animal models do not support in detail the behavior of chronic epilepsy in humans, and in some instances this is fortunate.

The historical development of the investigation of CNS function in humans and animals has at times emphasized some aspects of CNS function at the expense of others. The original descriptions of cerebral localization in humans and animals, such as the localization of voluntary limb movements, were derived from observations of the effects of natural disease and from ablation experiments in animals. Subsequent investigations consisted largely of electrical stimulation and later the recording of electrical potentials in normal and abnormal cerebral function; however, there was considerable neglect of other ways of looking at cerebral function, apart from information about cerebral blood flow. For this reason the longer-term changes in the nervous system mediated by chemical factors other than short-term changes in transmitter substances are poorly understood.

These changes, such as those in protein concentrations associated with learning in frogs (Morrell *et al* 1975), may influence the creation of memory traces. Changes similar to those which occur in laying down memory traces, not only for conscious formal learning but also for social behavior and survival, must play a part in delineating the pathways by which epileptic discharges spread throughout the brain.

Both long-term and short-term changes in cerebral function may prevent or discourage seizures in the normal brain, or permit the occurrence of only certain kinds of seizures in any particular patient. These changes would form the basis of rational surgical intervention, if such information were at our disposal. The experimental neurophysiology of epilepsy has suggested a number of mechanisms by which epileptic seizures and epileptic activity may be propagated through the brain. Two such mechanisms are kindling and secondary epileptogenesis.

Kindling was originally described in the rat, where subthreshold electrical stimuli to the thalami eventually induced seizures that persisted when the stimuli were stopped (Goddard *et al* 1969). Although kindling has been shown in animals to have a seizure-provoking effect, it can also exert a seizure-suppressant effect in certain circumstances that might spread beyond the site of the kindling; Engel and his colleagues have suggested that this might disrupt other cerebral functions (Morrell *et al* 1987). Much has been written about kindling, especially of the medial temporal structures, but little has been shown to be relevant to chronic epilepsy in humans.

Secondary epileptogenesis is a process where injury to a small area of the cortex of an experimental animal induced by cold or the application of noxious chemicals gives rise to a reproducible series of electrophysiologic changes at both the site of injury in the ipsilateral hemisphere, the primary focus, and a homolateral place in the contralateral hemisphere, the secondary focus. These changes give rise to seizures and both the seizures and the electrical foci can be abolished by resection of the primary focus, depending upon the stage that the process has reached. At first, the secondary focus is dependent upon the primary focus and regresses after excision of the primary focus; subsequently it becomes independent both in its discharge pattern and in the fact that it continues after excision of the primary focus. In small mammals, these changes occur predictably and in a very short time period; however, in animals higher up the phylogenetic scale they have a longer time course and are less predictable (Wilder 1982).

It is possible to suspect that a similar process occurs to a limited extent in chronic human epilepsy. General observations regarding the changes in chronic epilepsy show for example that bilateral abnormalities in the scalp EEG are commoner in patients with a long duration of epilepsy

(Hughes and Schlagendorf 1961; Gupta *et al* 1973) and there are also well-documented examples of bilateral EEG changes disappearing after resection of a unilateral lesion (Falconer and Kennedy 1961; Wieser and Yasargil 1982). A detailed analysis was made by Morrell of a particular group of patients from the large Montreal series. Patients with benign unilateral lesions, chiefly in the frontal or temporal lobes, were studied and secondary epileptogenesis identified by neurophysiologic criteria. Evidence of secondary epileptogenesis was found in 36% of 123 patients with temporal lobe lesions and 21% of 57 patients with frontal lobe lesions (Morrell *et al* 1983, 1984; Morrell 1985). Following resection of the primary lesion and focus, i.e. a unilateral resection, two-thirds of these patients showed regression of the secondary focus. Morrell therefore suggests that secondary epileptogenesis exists in humans, as it does in animal models, in a reversible and irreversible form. Irreversibility was associated with a longer duration of epilepsy and a higher seizure frequency. In tumor cases, the likelihood of secondary epileptogenesis was related to the age of seizure onset, with those patients whose seizures began before 25 years of age much more likely to show secondary epileptogenesis (Morrell *et al* 1987). There is now evidence from a number of independent studies of epilepsy due to cavernomas that the number and duration of seizures in these patients significantly influences the outcome following surgery (Cohen *et al* 1995; Zevgaridis *et al* 1996; Cappabianca *et al* 1997). Nevertheless it must be uncommon in human epilepsy for widespread changes to follow the onset of focal epilepsy, otherwise resective surgery would be very unsuccessful. It is difficult to relate these theoretic mechanisms of epilepsy to parameters that can be measured in the patient.

Therefore surgical options have to be exercised on largely empirical grounds. The surgical maneuvers used to treat chronic epilepsy can be divided into two groups. One group aims to resect a locus of seizure origin within the brain, and that locus may be identified in a number of ways. These operations are called resective procedures and are commoner and more successful than those in the other group. Procedures in the second group aim to modify brain function so as to halt the focus or prevent or discourage the spread of epileptic discharges within the brain and are called functional procedures.

RESECTIVE SURGERY

Resective operations are based upon identification of an area within the brain where the seizures commence; if that area can be resected completely then the seizures will cease. A corollary is that the patient should suffer minimal additional physical, intellectual, or psychiatric disability as a result of the resection. Such an area can be identified as a result of a series of clinical inquiries and tests of brain function and these are discussed in detail elsewhere. This evidence includes inquiries regarding any incident in the patient's past medical history that could lead to focal brain damage and a description of the seizures which might indicate a focal origin or locus for the seizures within the brain. Structural brain imaging such as CT and magnetic resonance imaging (MRI), which has become increasingly sophisticated over the last 10 years, can reveal various kinds of lesions. Functional brain imaging, such as magnetic resonance spectroscopy, positron emission tomography, and single-photon emission computed tomography, can reveal focal functional deficits that in some cases, such as the infants described by the Los Angeles group, may be the only, or most obvious, clue to a focal abnormality (Chugani *et al* 1988). Finally a variety of neurophysiologic investigations, both noninvasive and invasive, can be used interictally and ictally; the sophisticated assessment of intellectual function by detailed neuropsychologic tests, including the Wada or intracarotid amobarbital test, may also indicate a focal disorder.

LÜDERS CONCEPTUAL MODEL

An attempt has been made by Lüders and Awad (1992) to rationalize the occurrence and spread of focal epilepsy and relate this to the parameters that we can observe and test. They identify six separate entities and in so doing provide an unambiguous framework for future discussions.

Epileptogenic zone. Region of the cerebral cortex that can generate epileptic seizures. (By definition, total removal or disconnection of the epileptogenic zone is necessary and sufficient for seizure freedom.)

Irritative zone. Region of cortex that generates interictal epileptiform discharges in the scalp EEG.

Pacemaker zone. Region of cortex from which the clinical seizures originate.

Epileptogenic lesion. Structural lesion that is causally related to the epilepsy.

Ictal symptomatogenic zone. Region of cortex that generates the initial seizure symptomatology.

Functional deficit zone. Region of cortex that is functioning abnormally (as judged by neurologic examination, neuropsychologic tests, functional neuroimaging, or nonepileptiform EEG abnormalities).

BROAD PRINCIPLES

The relationship between these definitions can only be described in an anecdotal fashion but with insufficient precision to form a rational basis for resective intervention, which must be made on a more empirical basis. Furthermore any attempt to emphasize one of these defined areas at the expense of another gives a poorer result from the surgery. Therefore, although we can make a series of assertions, as set out below, none of them can be exercised alone with absolute certainty of success.

1. The causal lesion is the origin of the epilepsy and if it can be removed the seizures will be relieved.
2. Complete removal of the causal lesion is necessary for seizure freedom.
3. The epileptogenic zone can be identified precisely and totally, and if removed leads to complete seizure freedom. Apart from the self-fulfilling definition quoted above, this is also difficult to achieve.
4. Certain structures if involved in the epileptic process, for example the medial temporal structures, perpetuate the epilepsy unless removed.
5. Widespread or bilateral neurophysiologic abnormalities may regress after resection of damaged or abnormal tissue.

It has already been noted that none of these assertions is absolutely true. However, there is evidence both in the literature and in practice that in a high proportion of cases such considerations lead to a successful outcome from resective surgery. Let us now look at these in more detail.

Causal lesion is the origin of the epilepsy

Although the early pioneers such as Horsley had no guide except the extent of the lesion, they nevertheless achieved reasonable results in these early cases (Horsley 1886).

Completeness of the removal of the causal lesion

Estimation of the completeness of the removal of the causative lesion in patients undergoing resective surgery is not easy and to some extent depends upon the nature of the lesion. Means of estimating the extent of the removal include the surgeon's observations, which are probably the least reliable, the pathologist's assessment of the specimen, the natural history of the pathologic process under scrutiny, and the results of postoperative structural brain imaging. In this respect the results reported from the Mayo Clinic by Cascino *et al* (1990) for stereotactic lesionectomy used postoperative imaging criteria to judge the completeness of removal. In their patients 56% were in Engel outcome class I (Engel 1987a); however, the results were noticeably different for temporal and extratemporal lesions, only two of nine patients with temporal lobe lesions being free of seizures. By contrast the Yale group report good results from resection of indolent gliomas in which the margin of resection is determined by taking frozen sections until no tumor is seen within them (Boon *et al* 1991). In another study Awad *et al* (1991a), describing a variety of lesions, show that the best chance of seizure relief comes from complete removal of the gross lesion and the worst from resection of the electrical focus without resection of the gross lesion. Fish *et al* (1989, 1991) reported similar poor results from a group of 19 patients where an anterior temporal lobectomy was carried out while leaving a gross lesion in the posterior temporal region. Another powerful instrument for estimating the extent of surgical removal, especially the temporal lobe, and also damage close to the site of surgery is postoperative MRI. For example, the studies by Awad *et al* of outcome and cognitive function showed how they could be related to the amount of tissue removed from various compartments defined on MRI. A study of the Zurich amygdalohippocampectomy patients which showed that outcome depended on the degree of resection of the parahippocampal gyrus, a multicenter study of cognitive outcome after various temporal resections, and a study of the effects of two different techniques of amygdalohippocampectomy have all relied upon postoperative MRI for their resection data (Awad *et al* 1989; Siegel *et al* 1990; Nayel *et al* 1991; Renowden *et al* 1995).

Removal of the lesion leads to seizure relief

In certain instances there is clear evidence that some pathologic tissue can remain, with a high degree of seizure relief in the group as a whole and prolonged seizure relief in individuals. In a series of patients with dysembryoplastic neuroepithelial tumors, we have shown that tumor can remain after surgery with a high rate of seizure relief; this was also shown in the original paper describing this pathology (Daumas-Duport *et al* 1988; Kirkpatrick *et al* 1993).

Definition of the epileptogenic zone

Definition of the epileptogenic zone is a difficult task. If there is evidence of focal neurophysiologic activity after the first resection, then reoperation can remove that activity, often together with residual pathology, and result in freedom from seizures (Wyler *et al* 1989; Awad *et al* 1991b; Awad 1992). In this case it has to be presumed that the epileptogenic zone was not completely removed in the first place.

There is ample evidence that in temporal lobe epilepsy the success rate from resective surgery is better when the medial temporal structures are resected. There are certainly patients in whom a lesionectomy alone in this region does not control the epilepsy, but when the medial temporal structures are removed much better control of the epilepsy is achieved. In the Cascino series referred to above, the temporal lobe patients did worse and Yasargil notes in his justification of selective amygdalohippocampectomy that they found that the removal of lesions alone in the temporal lobe was less effective for seizure relief than an operation which also encompassed the mesial temporal structures. In particular they showed that the extent of removal of the parahippocampal gyrus, which was ostensibly normal, influenced seizure outcome (Yasargil *et al* 1985; Cascino *et al* 1990). Levesque *et al* (1991) describe dual pathology in 54 patients of a series of 178 undergoing temporal lobectomy, where severe cell loss was seen in the mesial temporal structures in addition to another lesion in the temporal lobe. However in many patients this is linked to the fact that the pathology involves these structures to some extent, and the question of whether any subsequent improvement is due to the removal of these structures *per se* or the fact that they may contain pathology is insoluble.

Neurophysiologic abnormalities regress after resection

There is also longstanding evidence that extensive neurophysiologic changes, especially in the scalp EEG, regress after removal of a localized lesion. This has been reported over a wide period of time, for example Falconer and Kennedy (1961) and Wieser and Yasargil (1982).

GENERAL PRINCIPLES

It is apparent that there cannot be hard and fast rules about the surgical options available but rather general principles about which maneuver is most likely to succeed. It is clear in the majority of cases that if a causative lesion can be identified which is clinically and neurophysiologically concordant, then its removal has a high chance of improving seizure control. On the other hand, if a resective seizure is based on neurophysiologic findings or limitations alone, the chances of success are much lower.

The minimalist approach may appear to be the best first line of treatment, although many patients have considerable emotional investment in the first operation, which they may not be prepared to make in a subsequent procedure. The difficulties associated with subsequent surgery, together with the economics involved, probably make this an unviable approach. Reoperation rates vary between centers and for different procedures but are currently between 5 and 10% of first operation series (Polkey *et al* 1993).

Identification and removal of the epileptogenic zone, as defined by Lüders, are more difficult. Other chapters describe the variations and shortcomings of the various neurophysiologic and other methods of seizure identification. In broad terms, the increasing sophistication and complexity of recording methods result in a narrower view of cerebral function in time or space. In relation to the temporal lobe, neurophysiologic investigations lateralize well and localize with some accuracy, although often the final decision regarding the size or nature of the temporal lobe resection is determined by other factors, such as the patient's intellectual profile and the risk of side-effects from surgery. The place of acute corticography in determining the surgical options varies according to the site of the proposed resection. A case can be made in temporal lobe resections for neglecting it altogether and certainly the anatomic boundaries of the resection are more restricting than any other factor. In Yasargil and Wieser's series of selective amygdalohippocampectomy acute corticography was not employed (Wieser 1991), whereas in the standard neocortical removal employed in Dublin corticography was carried out but did not modify the removal (Hardiman *et al* 1988). Similarly, in my personal series of over 150 *en bloc* temporal lobectomies the resection has been modified by the findings at acute corticography in only a minority of cases. An analysis of 76 patients who underwent cerebral resection at the Maudsley Hospital showed that in the 58 who underwent temporal lobe resections the location of the predominant spike focus had no relation to the type or location of pathology or to the outcome (McBride *et al* 1991). In a series of temporal lobe resections for dysembryoplastic neuroepithelial tumor we have found that acute corticography contributed little (Kirkpatrick *et al* 1993). Not all authors share these views and some would argue that when the trouble has been taken to make a detailed preoperative assessment of the neurophysiology using chronic recording with subdural and/or depth electrodes, little more can be gained from the acute recording, which is less extensive in time and space (Talairach and Bancaud 1974). Although Lüders quotes anecdotal examples, he admits that in practice it is difficult to demonstrate the significance of the various zones that he describes and therefore, in both temporal and extratemporal resections, the boundaries of the resection must be relatively arbitrary.

PERIOPERATIVE AND INTRAOPERATIVE CONSIDERATIONS

In addition to options that may emerge from the preoperative investigations and planning, there are also options in the conduct of the operation itself. The choices as to the extent and nature of the cerebral removal are discussed in Chapter 51–53. However, the decision about whether to perform acute corticography and whether, where conditions allow, to conduct the operation under local anesthesia need to be discussed. In the early days of epilepsy surgery, especially in Montreal and centers run by their disciples, local anesthesia was *de rigueur* for most resective surgery. In the development of these techniques there was good reason for this; however, many of these reasons have disappeared. One claim made by the proponents of local anesthesia is that the recorded corticogram is more 'natural.' However, many years of work on the acute corticogram in an attempt to distinguish those spikes important to the persistence of the epilepsy, so-called 'red' spikes, from those which have no such significance, 'green' spikes, has so far been fruitless. We have recently described a method of analysis of the acute corticogram using computer analysis of phase relationships between spiking areas, which identifies areas whose removal is likely to lead to better seizure control (Alarcon *et al* 1997).

The mapping of primary motor, sensory, and speech areas can now be done through implanted mat electrodes, as pioneered in children by Goldring and Gregorie (1984). The determination of speech areas in the dominant hemisphere is another interesting problem. It has been possible to extrapolate, from the work of the early pioneers, that part of the superior temporal gyrus needs to be spared to preserve speech in dominant temporal lobe resections. However there is no proper comparison of the results of such resections under local and general anesthesia. Ojemann and his colleagues, in an elegant series of papers, have shown that the proportion of the middle temporal gyrus resected from the dominant temporal lobe may affect verbal memory and that the area involved can be mapped under local anesthesia in cooperative adults (Ojemann and Dodrill 1985; Ojemann and Engel 1987; Silbergeld and Ojemann 1993). The resection can then be tailored to produce a significant lessening of the verbal memory deficit, with little or no reduction in seizure relief. The amount of middle temporal gyrus involved in such verbal memory function varies from one patient to another, so it is necessary either to map the area in each case or to use a 'fail-safe' technique in which most of the middle temporal gyrus is spared when operating under general anesthesia. Although a basal language area has been described, some suggest that resection of this area does not always produce adverse effects (Krauss *et al* 1996). The developing technology of functional magnetic imaging also allows noninvasive mapping of primary motor and sensory areas together with speech dominance (Cosgrove *et al* 1996).

SEQUELAE

Of equal importance in determining the surgical options are the avoidance or minimization of any physical, intellectual, or psychiatric disability as a result of operation. Clearly, resection of primary motor, sensory, or speech areas has to be avoided or approached deliberately. Experience in this area is sparse even in centers with large numbers of patients. However there is some useful knowledge to be gleaned from the Montreal experience (Rasmussen 1975, 1991). Methods for locating these areas are now more sophisticated and the use of cortical mapping, both to delineate patterns of epileptic activity and to map these areas, is increasing (Ojemann and Engel 1987). As mentioned later, there are now alternative surgical options to resection in these areas. The other major area at risk is vision and the choice of temporal lobe resections to counter this problem is discussed in Chapter 51.

The avoidance of intellectual sequelae from operation is generally a problem in relation to temporal lobe surgery, although it can also be a problem in relation to dominant frontal lobe resections and sometimes in hemispherectomy, depending upon the underlying disease process (Beardsworth and Adams 1988). The possibility of intellectual deficit is principally related to the disease process underlying the epilepsy. With *en bloc* temporal lobectomy we have shown clearly that when the temporal lobe is damaged at a young age there is reorganization of cerebral function that minimizes the effects of lobectomy, in contrast to patients with other lesions where the kind of material-specific deficits reported by Milner (1958, 1975) are seen. These matters are dealt with in detail later.

REOPERATION

The ultimate option in resective surgery is that of reoperation. Many centers are now beginning to consider reoperation in cases of failed resective surgery. Studies of groups in which reoperation has been successful show that the best results are obtained when the original site of resection is involved, and where the resection involves either removal of further epileptogenic tissue or of a structural lesion or both (Awad *et al* 1989, 1991b; Wyler *et al* 1989).

FUNCTIONAL SURGERY

In functional surgery there are a number of possible options available to the surgeon. The choice is more difficult because overall the procedures are less effective than resective operations, and the variety of patients subjected to these operations is wide, so that it is difficult to judge their efficacy.

The mechanisms by which these operations effect their result is ill-understood. The idea that brain lesions can affect the propagation of seizure activity and thus bring about the amelioration of the seizures is an attractive if somewhat simplistic one. However there are no helpful data on these processes in simple experimental models involving a small localized cortical focus, let alone in patients with generalized seizure disorder. Furthermore, although abnormal electrical activity is the easiest parameter to demonstrate, changes in neurotransmitters or other chemicals, such as the protein changes described by Morrell *et al* (1975), may be more important in determining the epileptic activity of these brains. Many of the functional procedures for epilepsy were based on animal experiments in which it could be shown that alterations in EEG could be achieved by stimulation or lesioning of various intracranial structures. Such observations formed the basis for callosotomy and multiple subpial transection as well as cerebellar stimulation. The experimental models were not always matched rigorously to the subsequent procedure; indeed in some circumstances it would not be possible to do this. Exceptions to this are the experimental work carried out by Morrell and the work to justify vagus nerve stimulation.

Following the expansion of epilepsy surgery in the second half of this century there were numerous reports of stereotactic lesioning of the brain to attempt to control both generalized and focal epilepsy. However the indications for these procedures have been difficult to define and since the 1970s they seem to have fallen into disuse, so that by 1975 Ojemann and Ward were dismissive of these techniques and at the First Palm Desert Symposium in 1986 they no longer merited a mention. Two subsequent detailed reviews of epilepsy surgery practice, composed as a result of large and comprehensive international meetings, did not include these procedures (Engel 1987b; Engel 1993). In a comprehensive textbook on epilepsy the emphasis is on three procedures: callosotomy, cerebral stimulation, and multiple subpial transection (Engel and Pedley 1998).

One reason why such procedures have been unpopular is because it has often been difficult to disentangle the results of surgery with regard to the epilepsy from the results of surgery on other parameters. Such a dilemma is typically presented by Narabayashi (1979) on stereotactic lesions in the amygdala or Turner (1982) on temporal lobotomy. Furthermore none of the authors working in the period when such lesioning was popular had the benefit of modern brain imaging to identify the targets or to confirm the sites and size of the subsequent lesions. When stereotactic lesioning has been carried out in centers where resective surgery is also available, it has been shown to be less effective (Talairach and Bancaud 1974); certainly in the temporal lobe a subsequent resective operation may improve seizure control in patients where a stereotactic lesion has failed (Vaernet 1972). Where the seizure onset can be definitely traced to one structure there may be more success. Hood *et al* (1983) describe a single case where stereo-EEG showed a discrete onset in one amygdala and a stereotactic amygdalotomy controlled the seizures. In another report Wieser and Yasargil (1984) note that some 3% of patients explored with stereo-EEG have a purely amygdalar onset for their seizures.

There is also the problem of length of follow-up after operation. Among patients in whom we have implanted depth electrodes in an attempt to identify a seizure focus in the medial temporal structures, two had a seizure-free interval of over 6 months, presumed to be the result of small hematoma formation along the track of the electrodes; similar events have been reported from other centers. In one of our patients the seizures subsequently reappeared. The point is that if follow-up after a stereotactic lesion is relatively short, then there may be a falsely optimistic impression of the outcome.

The use of brain stimulation to control seizures has had a briefer but equally unimpressive role. The method of cerebellar stimulation advocated by Cooper (1973) has been shown to be ineffective when used in a controlled situation (Wright *et al* 1985). Velasquez and his coworkers have described the effects of thalamic stimulation, although this must still be viewed as an experimental procedure (Fisher *et al* 1993). Vagus nerve stimulation is described in detail in Chapter 55. However, there is now a considerable volume of literature describing experimental models which clearly show that epilepsy can be influenced by this stimulation and that the mechanism probably involves permanent changes in the neurochemistry of the nervous system (Lockard *et al* 1990; Woodbury and Woodbury 1990, 1991; McLachlan 1993; Takaya *et al* 1996) In addition, there are also reports of the effect of this treatment in reasonable numbers of patients which suggest that it improves seizure control, although only a small proportion of the patients become seizure-free (Michael *et al* 1993; Anonymous 1995; Murphy *et al* 1995).

The remaining functional maneuver is the transection of fiber tracts to try to restrict the spread of the epileptic discharge. The most popular of these has been callosotomy. In 1940 Erickson described the finding that total division of the corpus callosum in monkeys prevented the spread of afterdischarges from one hemisphere to the other. However the original callosotomies carried out by Van Wagenen and Herren (1940) were based upon the clinical observation that tumor invasion into the corpus callosum reduces seizure frequency. All authors are agreed that the results of callosotomy, either anterior two-thirds or complete, are less effective than resective surgery. Furthermore the indications for the operation are wide and vague. Attempts have been made by various workers, including ourselves, to identify certain neurophysiologic patterns that favor a good outcome but with little success (Marino 1985; Fiol *et al* 1993). The option of partial or complete callosotomy is dealt with in Chapter 55.

The other disconnection procedure was introduced by Morrell *et al* (1989). It is designed to be used in areas where resection would result in an unacceptable neurologic deficit, such as the primary motor or sensory areas. Basically the procedure divides the horizontal connections in the cortex while preserving the vertical ones. The initial report of 25 cases suggested a 50% seizure relief rate. Early results reported by Dogali *et al* (1992) were also quite good. There are now a number of publications on the use of multiple subpial transection. It is often used in combination with resection (Sawhney *et al* 1995; Hufnagel *et al* 1997) or alone (Shimizu *et al* 1991; Rougier *et al* 1996). The results described in these papers show significant benefit but are not as impressive as those originally described by Morrell. Morrell *et al* (1995) also reported good results in treating 14 children with a rare form of epilepsy, Landau–Kleffner syndrome. There are reports of the use of multiple subpial transection in situations where the epileptic disorder is either widespread in one hemisphere or bifrontal, hitherto surgically untreatable problems (Patil *et al* 1997).

Reoperation is also possible following a primary functional procedure. It consists of either completion of the callosotomy, upon which opinion is divided, or a resective procedure. For example, in 30 hemispherectomies, three patients had undergone previous functional operations with little effect.

CONCLUSION

A theoretic basis exists for both resective and functional epilepsy surgery. However, it is not possible to use this information to predict exactly the effects of such surgery. Therefore, the surgery must be conducted on the basis of previous experience, empirical judgments, and using all the modern technical aids available.

KEY POINTS

1. Experimental work on the pathophysiology of epilepsy is extensive, but difficult to apply to the clinical situation and therefore to use as a theoretic basis for epilepsy surgery.
2. Resective surgery is based upon detecting focal pathology and a single onset site for seizures, whereas functional surgery attempts to alter the pathophysiology of epilepsy within the brain.
3. A conceptual model of focal epilepsy and certain broad principles can be used in planning resective procedures.
4. Intraoperative neurophysiologic monitoring and local anesthesia have a decreasing place in resective surgery.
5. A number of functional procedures are less effective and less well understood than resective operations.

REFERENCES

Alarcon G, Garcia Seoane JJ, Binnie CD *et al* (1997) Origin and propagation of interictal discharges in the acute electrocorticogram. Implications for pathophysiology and surgical treatment of temporal lobe epilepsy. *Brain* **120**:2259–2282.

Anonymous (1995) A randomized controlled trial of chronic vagus nerve stimulation for treatment of medically intractable seizures. The Vagus Nerve Stimulation Study Group. *Neurology* **2**:224–230.

Awad IA (1992) Reoperation for intractable seizures. *Clinical Neurosurgery* **39**:125–139.

Awad IA, Katz A, Hahn JF, Kong AK, Ahl J, Lüders H (1989) Extent of resection in temporal lobectomy for epilepsy. I. Interobserver analysis and correlation with seizure outcome. *Epilepsia* **30**:756–762.

Awad IA, Rosenfeld J, Ahl J, Hahn JF, Lüders H (1991a) Intractable epilepsy and structural lesions of the brain: mapping, resection strategies, and seizure outcome. *Epilepsia* **32**:179–186.

Awad IA, Nayel MH, Lüders H (1991b) Second operation after the failure of previous resection for epilepsy. *Neurosurgery* **28**:510–518.

Beardsworth ED, Adams CBT (1988) Modified hemispherectomy for epilepsy. Early results in 10 cases. *British Journal of Neurosurgery* **2**:73–84.

Boon PA, Williamson PD, Fried I *et al* (1991) Intracranial, intraxial, space-occupying lesions in patients with intractable partial seizures: an anatomoclinical, neuropsychological, and surgical correlation. *Epilepsia* **32**:467–476.

Cappabianca P, Alfieri A, Maiuri F, Mariniello G, Cirillo S de, Divitiis E (1997) Supratentorial cavernous malformations and epilepsy: seizure outcome after lesionectomy on a series of 35 patients. *Clinical Neurology and Neurosurgery* **99**:179–183.

Cascino GD, Kelly PJ, Hirschorn KA, Marsh WR, Sharbrough FW (1990) Stereotactic resection of intra-axial cerebral lesions in partial epilepsy. *Mayo Clinic Proceedings* **65**:1053–1060.

Chugani HT, Shewmon DA, Peacock WJ, Shields WD, Mazziotta JC, Phelps ME (1988) Surgical treatment of intractable neonatal-onset seizures: the role of positron emission tomography. *Neurology* **38**:1178–1188.

Cohen DS, Zubay GP, Goodman RR (1995) Seizure outcome after lesionectomy for cavernous malformations. *Journal of Neurosurgery* **83**:237–242.

Cooper I (1973) Chronic stimulation of the paleo-cerebellum in humans. *Lancet* **i**:206.

Cosgrove CR, Buchbinder BR, Jiang H, Rosen BR (1996) Mapping human sensorimotor cortex with functional MRI (abstract). *Acta Neurochirurgica* **138**:632.

Daumas-Duport C, Scheithauer BW, Chodkiewicz J-P, Laws ER, Vedrenne C (1988) Dysembryoplastic neuroepithelial tumor: a surgically curable tumor of young patients with intractable partial seizures. Report of thirty-nine cases. *Neurosurgery* **23**:545–556.

Dogali M, Devinsky O, Luciano D, Perrine K., Beric A (1992) Experiences with multiple subpial cortical transections for the control of intractable epilepsy in exquisite cortex (abstract). *Acta Neurochirurgica* **117**:108.

Engel JJ. (1987a) Outcome with respect to epileptic seizures. In: Engel J (ed) *Surgical Treatment of the Epilepsies*, pp 553–571. New York: Raven Press.

Engel JJ. (1987b) In: Engel JJ (ed) *Surgical Treatment of the Epilepsies*. New York: Raven Press.

Engel JJ (1993) In: Engel JJ (ed) *Surgical Treatment of the Epilepsies*, 2nd edn. New York: Raven Press.

Engel JJ, Pedley TA (1998) In: Engel JJ, Pedley TA (eds) *Epilepsy: A Comprehensive Textbook*. Philadelphia: Lippincott-Raven.

Falconer MA, Kennedy WA (1961) Epilepsy due to small focal temporal lesions with bilateral independent spike-discharging foci. A study of seven cases relieved by operation. *Journal of Neurology, Neurosurgery and Psychiatry* **24**:205–212.

Fiol ME, Gates JR, Mireles R, Maxwell RE, Erickson DM (1993) Value of intraoperative EEG changes during corpus callostomy in predicting surgical results. *Epilepsia* **34**:74–78.

Fish DR, Andermann F, Olivier A (1989) Anterotemporal corticectomy in patients with complex partial seizures and small, relatively inaccessible posterotemporal and extratemporal structural lesions. *Epilepsia* **30**:704.

Fish D, Andermann F, Olivier A (1991) Complex partial seizures and small posterior temporal or extratemporal structural lesions: surgical management. *Neurology* **41**:1781–1784.

Fisher RS, Uthman BM, Ramsay RE *et al* (1993) Alternative surgical techniques for epilepsy. In: Engel J (ed) *Surgical Treatment of the Epilepsies*, 2nd edn, pp 549–564. New York: Raven Press.

Goddard GV, McIntyre DC, Leech CK (1969) A permanent change in brain function resulting from daily electrical stimulation. *Experimental Neurology* **25**:295–330.

Goldring S, Gregorie EM (1984) Surgical management of epilepsy using epidural mats to localise the seizure focus. *Journal of Neurosurgery* **60**:457–466.

Gupta PC, Dharampaul SN, Singh B (1973) Secondary epileptogenic EEG focus in temporal lobe epilepsy. *Epilepsia* **14**:423–426.

Hardiman O, Burke T, Phillips J *et al* (1988) Microdysgenesis in resected temporal neocortex: incidence and clinical significance in focal epilepsy. *Neurology* **38**:1041–1047.

Hood TW, Siegfried J, Wieser HG (1983) The role of stereotactic amygdalotomy in the treatment of behavioral disorders associated with temporal lobe epilepsy. *Applied Neurophysiology* **49**:19–25.

Horsley V (1886) Brain-Surgery. *British Medical Journal* **2**:670–675.

Hufnagel A, Zentner J, Fernandez G, Wolf HK, Schramm J, Elger CE (1997) Multiple subpial transection for control of epileptic seizures: effectiveness and safety. *Epilepsia* **38**:678–688.

Hughes JR, Schlagendorf RE (1961) Electro-clinical correlation in temporal lobe epilepsy with emphasis on the inter-areal analysis of the temporal lobe. *Electroencephalography and Clinical Neurophysiology* **13**:333–339.

Kirkpatrick PJ, Honavar M, Janota I, Polkey CE (1993) Control of temporal lobe epilepsy following *en bloc* resection of low grade gliomas. *Journal of Neurosurgery* **78**:19–25.

Krauss GL, Fisher R, Plate C *et al* (1996) Cognitive effects of resecting basal temporal language areas. *Epilepsia* **37**:476–483.

Levesque MF, Nakasato N, Vinters HV, Babb TL (1991) Surgical treatment of limbic epilepsy associated with extrahippocampal lesions: the problem of dual pathology. *Journal of Neurosurgery* **75**:364–370.

Lockard JS, Congdon WC, DuCharme LL (1990) Feasibility and safety of vagal nerve stimulation in monkey model. *Epilepsia* **31** (Suppl 2): S20–S26.

Lüders H, Awad IA (1992) Conceptual considerations. In: Lüders H (ed) *Epilepsy Surgery*, pp 51–62. New York: Raven Press.

McBride MC, Binnie CD, Janota I, Polkey CE (1991) Predictive value of intraoperative electrocorticograms in resective epilepsy surgery. *Annals of Neurology* **30**:526–532.

McLachlan RS (1993) Suppression of interictal spikes and seizures by stimulation of the vagus nerve. *Epilepsia* **34**:918–923.

Marino R (1985) Surgery for epilepsy. Selective partial microsurgical callosotomy for intractable multiform seizures. Criteria for clinical selection and results. *Applied Neurophysiology* **48**:404–407.

Michael JE, Wegener K, Barnes DW (1993) Vagus nerve stimulation for intractable seizures: one year follow-up. *Journal of Neuroscience Nursing* **6**:362–366.

Milner B (1958) Psychological defects produced by temporal lobe excision. *Research Publications: Association for Research in Nervous and Mental Disease* **36**:244–257.

Milner B (1975) Psychological aspects of focal epilepsy and its surgical management. In: Purpura DP, Penry JK, Walter RD (eds) *Neurosurgical Management of the Epilepsies*, pp 299–332. New York: Raven Press.

Morrell F (1985) Secondary epileptogenesis in man. *Archives of Neurology* **42**:318–335.

Morrell F, Tsuru N, Hoeppner TJ, Morgan D, Harrison WH (1975) Secondary epileptogenesis in frog forebrain: effect of inhibition of protein synthesis. *Canadian Journal of Neurological Science* **2**:407–416.

Morrell F, Rasmussen T, Gloor P, de Toledo-Morrell L (1983) Secondary epileptogenic foci in patients with verified temporal lobe tumors. *Electroencephalography and Clinical Neurophysiology* **54**:26.

Morrell F, Rasmussen T, de Toledo Morrell L, Quesney LF, Gloor P (1984) Frontal lobe epilepsy of neoplastic origin: incidence of secondary epileptogenesis. *Epilepsia* **25**:654–655.

Morrell F, Wada J, Engel J (1987) Appendix III: Potential relevance of kindling and secondary epileptogenesis to the consideration of surgical treatment for epilepsy. In: Engel J (ed) *Surgical Treatment of the Epilepsies*, pp 701–707. New York: Raven Press.

Morrell F, Whisler WW, Bleck TP (1989) Multiple subpial transection. A new approach to the surgical treatment of focal epilepsy. *Journal of Neurosurgery* **70**:231–239.

Morrell F, Whisler WW, Smith MC *et al* (1995) Landau–Kleffner syndrome. Treatment with subpial intracortical transection. *Brain* **118**:1529–1546.

Murphy JV, Hornig G, Schallert G (1995) Left vagal nerve stimulation in children with refractory epilepsy. *Archives of Neurology* **52**:886–889.

Narabayashi H (1979) Long range results of medial amygdalotomy on epileptic traits in adult patients. In: Rasmussen T, Marino R (eds) *Functional Neurosurgery*, pp 243–252. New York: Raven Press.

Nayel MH, Awad IA, Lüders H (1991) Extent of mesiobasal resection determines outcome after temporal lobectomy for intractable complex partial seizures. *Neurosurgery* **29**:55–60.

Ojemann GA, Dodrill CB (1985) Verbal memory deficits after left temporal lobectomy for epilepsy: mechanism and intraoperative prediction. *Journal of Neurosurgery* **62**:101–107.

Ojemann, GA, Engel J (1987) Acute and chronic intracranial recording and stimulation. In: Engel J (ed) *Surgical Treatment of the Epilepsies*, pp 263–288. New York: Raven Press.

Ojemann GA, Ward AA (1975) Stereotactic and other procedures for epilepsy. In: Purpura DP, Penry JK, Walter RD (eds) *Neurosurgical Management of the Epilepsies*, pp 241–264. New York: Raven Press.

Patil AA, Andrews RV, Torkelson R (1997) Surgical treatment of intractable seizures with multilobar or bihemispheric seizure foci (MLBHSF). *Surgical Neurology* **47**:72–77.

Polkey CE, Awad IA, Tanaka T, Wyler AR (1993) The place of reoperation. In: Engel J (ed) *Surgical Treatment of the Epilepsies*, 2nd edn, pp 663–667. New York: Raven Press.

Rasmussen T (1975) Surgery for epilepsy arising in regions other than the frontal or temporal lobes. In: Purpura DP, Penry JK, Walter RD (eds) *Neurosurgical Management of the Epilepsies*, pp 207–226. New York: Raven Press.

Rasmussen T (1991) Surgery for central, parietal and occipital epilepsy. *Canadian Journal of Neurological Sciences* **18**:611–616.

Renowden SA, Matkovic Z, Adams CB *et al* (1995) Selective amygdalo-hippocampectomy for hippocampal sclerosis: postoperative MR appearance. *American Journal of Neuroradiology* **16**:1855–1861.

Rougier A, Sundstrom L, Claverie B *et al* (1996) Multiple subpial transection: report of 7 cases. *Epilepsy Research* **24**:57–63.

Sawhney IMS, Robertson IJA, Polkey CE, Binnie CD, Elwes RD (1995) Multiple subpial transection: a review of 21 cases. *Journal of Neurology, Neurosurgery and Psychiatry* **58**:344–349.

Shimizu H, Suzuki I, Ishijima B, Karasawa S, Sakuma T (1991) Multiple subpial transection (MST) for the control of seizures that originated in unresectable cortical foci. *Japanese Journal of Psychiatry and Neurology* **2**:354–356.

Siegel AM, Wieser HG, Wichmann W, Yasargil MG (1990) Relationship between MR-imaged total amount of tissue removed, resection scores of specific mediobasal limbic subcompartments and clinical outcome following selective amygdalo-hippocampectomy. *Epilepsy Research* **6**:56–65.

Silbergeld DL, Ojemann GA (1993) The tailored temporal lobectomy. *Neurosurgical Clinics of North America* **4**:273–281.

Takaya M, Terry WJ, Naritoku DK (1996) Vagus nerve stimulation induces a sustained anticonvulsant effect. *Epilepsia* **37**:1111–1116.

Talairach J, Bancaud J (1974) Approche nouvelle de la neurochirurgie de l'epilepsie. *Neurochirurgie* **20**:1–12.

Turner EA (1982) Temporal lobe operations. In: Anonymous (ed) *Surgery of the Mind*, pp 126–169. Birmingham, UK: Carver Press.

Vaernet K (1972) Stereotactic amygdalotomy in temporal lobe epilepsy. *Confinia Neurologica* **34**: 176–180.

Van Wagenen WP, Herren RY (1940) Surgical division of commissural pathways in the corpus callosum. *Archives of Neurology and Psychiatry* **44**:740–759.

Wieser HG (1991) Selective amygdalohippocampectomy: indications and follow-up. *Canadian Journal of Neurological Sciences* **4** (Suppl):617–627.

Wieser HG, Yasargil MG (1982) Die 'Selektiv Amygdala-Hippokampektomie' als chirurgische Behandlung du medio-basal Limbischen Epilepsie. *Neurochirurgia* **25**:39–50.

Wieser HG, Yasargil MG (1984) Selective amygdalohippocampectomy as a surgical treatment of mediobasal limbic epilepsy. *Surgical Neurology* 17:445–457.

Wilder BJ (1982) Experimental studies, models, and phylogenetic aspects of secondary epileptogenesis. In: Mayersdorf A, Schmidt RP (eds) *Secondary Epileptogenesis*, 3rd edn, pp 27–43. New York: Raven Press.

Woodbury JW, Woodbury DM (1990) Effects of vagal nerve stimulation on experimentally induced seizures in rats. *Epilepsia* **31** (Suppl 2): S7–S19.

Woodbury JW, Woodbury DM (1991) Vagal stimulation reduces the severity of maximal electroshock seizures in intact rats: use of cuff electrode for stimulating and recording. *Pacing and Clinical Electrophysiology* **14**:94–107.

Wright GDS, McLellan DL, Brice JG (1985) A double-blind trial of chronic cerebellar stimulation in twelve patients with severe epilepsy. *Journal of Neurology, Neurosurgery and Psychiatry* **47**:769–774.

Wyler AR, Hermann BP, Richey ET (1989) Results of reoperation for failed epilepsy surgery. *Journal of Neurosurgery* **71**:815–819.

Yasargil MG, Teddy PG, Roth P. (1985) Selective amygdalo-hippocampectomy. Operative anatomy and surgical technique. In: Symon L (ed) *Advances and Technical Standards in Neurosurgery*, 12th edn, pp 93–123. Wien: Springer-Verlag.

Zevgaridis D, van Velthoven V, Ebeling U, Reulen HJ (1996) Seizure control following surgery in supratentorial cavernous malformations: a retrospective study in 77 patients. *Acta Neurochirurgica* **138**:672–677.

Radiologic evaluation of hippocampal sclerosis

F CENDES

In recent years there has been an extraordinary upsurge of interest in the surgical treatment of temporal lobe epilepsy (TLE). Surgery offers a safe and effective approach capable of greatly reducing the epileptic tendency in some patients (Penfield and Flanigin 1950; Bailey and Gibbs 1951; Penfield and Jasper 1954; Feindel 1991; Gumnit 1991; Engel *et al* 1993a,b; Arruda *et al* 1996; Duchowny *et al* 1997). In the first patients to undergo this form of treatment, the abnormal brain tissue was identified on the basis of gross structural lesions identified on plain skull X-rays and pneumoencephalograms (Penfield and Jasper 1954; Feindel 1991). These methods were, of course, relatively insensitive and were not informative in a large number of patients.

As early as 1938, many patients had surgical excisions of portions of the temporal lobe to control their epileptic attacks (Penfield and Jasper 1954; Feindel 1991). Penfield and Flanigin (1950) reviewed 55 cases, operated between 1938 and 1949, after long-term follow-up. Stimulated by the satisfactory results of surgery on the temporal lobe, and also from reports from other groups including those from Bailey and Gibbs (1951), Penfield and his group focused on trying to elucidate how the temporal lobe might become epileptogenic (Earle *et al* 1953; Feindel and Penfield 1954; Penfield and Jasper 1954). They relied on a unilateral temporal interictal EEG spike focus as the major indication for carrying out anterior temporal lobe resection to treat complex partial seizures. Today, anterior temporal lobe removal is by far the most commonly performed, and generally successful, surgical treatment available for epilepsy (Gumit 1991; Duchowny *et al* 1997; Engel *et al* 1997). Now, approximately 40 years later and using vastly superior technology, we are relying once more on 'structural' abnormalities to help make surgical decisions (Cascino *et al* 1992; Arruda *et al* 1996; Cendes *et al* 1997a; Duchowny *et al* 1997; Engel *et al* 1997; Watson *et al* 1997a).

Presurgical evaluation of patients with refractory partial epilepsy is complex and depends on a multidisciplinary approach. Definition of the cause of the epilepsy and localization of the seizure generator are important, because they play a key role in surgical planning and prognosis. (Engel *et al* 1993a,b, 1997; Arruda *et al* 1996; Hauser *et al* 1996; Cendes *et al* 1997a; Duchowny *et al* 1997). The advent of high-resolution magnetic resonance imaging (MRI) has had a major impact on the evaluation of patients with refractory epilepsy, because MRI can detect many underlying lesions that previously could not be identified *in vivo*. The most common example of this is mesial temporal atrophy associated with neuronal loss and gliosis, which was described as mesial temporal sclerosis (MTS) (Babb and Brown 1987; Bruton 1988; Gloor 1991; Meencke and Veith 1991). MTS is a histopathologic term that indicates neuronal loss and gliosis involving the hippocampus, and often also the amygdala, uncus, and parahippocampal gyrus (Bruton 1988; Gloor 1991; Meencke and Veith 1991). This entity is strongly associated with febrile seizures and other insults during early development (usually under age 4) (Cendes *et al* 1993a,b; Maher and McLachlan 1995; Berg *et al* 1998; Fernandez *et al* 1998; Hamati-Haddad and Abou-Khalil 1998; Shinnar 1998; Sloviter and Pedley 1998), is very likely to produce a mesial temporal ictal onset, and is amenable to treatment by selective mesial temporal resection (Abou-Khalil *et al* 1993; Cendes *et al* 1993b; Arruda *et al* 1996; Hamati-Haddad and Abou-Khalil 1998; Salanova *et al* 1998). The demonstration by MRI of obvious atrophy or altered signal intensity of mesial temporal structures suggesting MTS has greatly streamlined the presurgical evaluation of patients with TLE in whom these abnormalities are present (Kuznicky *et al* 1987; Jack *et al* 1990, 1992a; Berkovic *et al* 1991; Cascino *et al* 1991; Lencz *et al* 1992). Definitive diagnosis requires pathologic evidence of hippocampal sclerosis, preferably with seizure control following surgical removal. However, in patients with the typical clinical picture, the diagnosis can be made with a high degree of confidence by the demonstration of hippocampal atrophy and/or abnormal signal intensity on MRI, a mid-inferomedial temporal ictal EEG onset, and additional evidence of temporal lobe dysfunction from functional imaging and neuropsychology, all on the same side (Kuznicky and Jackson 1995; Cascino *et al* 1996; Cendes *et al* 1997a).

IMAGING OF TEMPORAL LOBE STRUCTURES

The temporal lobes can be divided into two compartments: the neocortex and the medial temporal lobe structures that include the uncus, amygdala, hippocampus, and parahippocampal gyrus. This subdivision follows the clinical-EEG classification of TLE: limbic or medial vs. neocortical.

The lateral temporal cortex can be well evaluated by MRI (Kuznicky and Jackson 1995; Watson *et al* 1997a). The anterior, superior, lateral, and medial aspects are well established, but the posterior end joins the parietal and occipital lobes without any clearly defined boundary, except the inconspicuous temporooccipital incisure (Duvernoy 1991). The superior and inferior temporal sulci divide the lateral surface of the temporal lobe into three gyri: superior, middle, and inferior (Figs 44.1 and 44.2).

The superior temporal gyrus (T1) runs parallel to the lateral fissure. Its anterior end is a part of the temporal pole.

The upper margin of the superior temporal gyrus forms the temporal operculum. It continues into the lateral fissure by a large cortical area, sometimes called the superior surface of the temporal lobe. This surface can only be observed when the superior overlying margin of the lateral fissure has been removed. From front to back the superior surface of the temporal lobe is divided into three parts: the planum polare, the transverse temporal gyri, and the planum temporale. The planum polare is separated from the insula by the inferior circular sulcus (Fig. 44.1b).

The middle temporal gyrus (T2) runs from the temporal pole through the occipital lobe without any clear boundary. The inferior temporal gyrus (T3) is not very visible on the lateral surface and is caudally separated from the occipital lobe by the temporooccipital incisure (Figs 44.1 and 44.2).

The inferior surface of the temporal lobe consists of three gyri: the inferior temporal gyrus (T3), the fusiform gyrus (T4), and the parahippocampal gyrus (T5) (Fig. 44.2). The fusiform gyrus is well delimited by the lateral occipitotemporal sulcus laterally, the collateral or medial occipitotemporal sulcus medially, and the anterior and posterior transverse collateral sulci rostrally and caudally. The fusiform gyrus does not extend to the temporal pole. The parahippocampal gyrus (T5) together with the lingual gyrus form the medial occipitotemporal gyrus. The parahippocampal gyrus is separated from the fusiform gyrus by the collateral sulcus and can be divided into two segments (Figs 44.1 and 44.2): (a) the posterior segment is narrow and its flat surface, or subiculum, is separated from the hippocampus by the uncal sulcus; and (b) the anterior segment is also called the piriform lobe and includes the anterior part of the uncus and the entorhinal area (Amaral and Insausti 1990; Duvernoy 1991).

The anatomy of the medial temporal lobe structures can be studied using high-resolution MRI. Thin coronal slices, obtained perpendicular to the long axis of the hippocampus, provide the optimal images for anatomic details and for determining subtle structural pathologies often associated with TLE (Kuznicky and Jackson 1995; Cascino *et al* 1996; Watson *et al* 1997a). The anatomy of the medial temporal lobe is discussed below.

OPTIMAL TECHNIQUE FOR IMAGING THE MEDIAL TEMPORAL LOBE STRUCTURES

The ideal sequence for MRI acquisition should be that resulting in excellent spatial resolution and contrast in a short period of time. Unfortunately, these are mutually

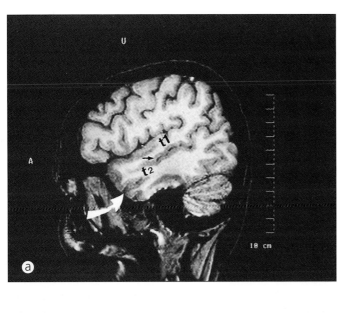
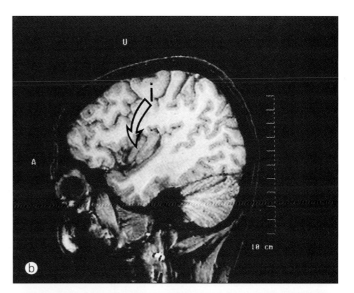
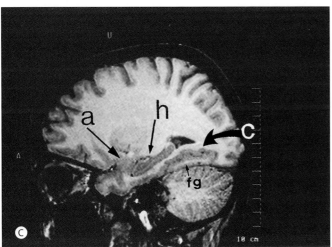
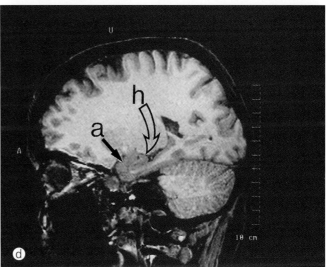

Fig. 44.1 Sagittal images (1-mm thick) obtained with a gradient echo three-dimensional T1-weighted sequence in a normal control subject. (a) Sagittal cut passing through the mid portion of the temporal lateral cortex, showing the superior (small black arrow) and inferior (white arrow) temporal sulci dividing the superior (T1), middle (T2), and inferior (T3) temporal gyri. (b) Sagittal slice 6 mm medially from (a) showing the margin of the planum temporale and planum polare below the insula (i). (c) Sagittal slice 12 mm medially from (b). a, amygdala; h, hippocampus; fg, fusiform gyrus; c, collateral sulcus. (d) Sagittal slice 6 mm medially from (b). Note the amygdala (a) lying anterior and superior to the head of hippocampus (h). The two structures are separated by a white line (alveus).

exclusive due to limitations imposed by physical principles that are beyond the scope of this chapter.

An imaging protocol for the investigation of partial epilepsies should include T1- and T2-weighted sequences in three, or at least two, orthogonal planes using thin slices (Commission on Neuroimaging of the International League Against Epilepsy 1997). Contrast (gadolinium) enhancement is usually not necessary, although it is important to increase specificity in lesional epilepsies. The ideal imaging of temporal lobe structures, particularly the hippocampus, depends on image orientation and sequences optimized to display the anatomy and signal abnormality

of hippocampal sclerosis and other pathologies of the temporal lobe. Nowadays three-dimensional Fourier transformation (3D-FT) imaging is becoming part of the routine for patients with partial seizures (Bastos *et al* 1995; Kuzniecky and Jackson 1995; Commission on Neuroimaging of the International League Against Epilepsy; Watson *et al* 1997a). The advantage of 3D-FT is that, since the entire volume of the image has been acquired, images in any plane can be generated afterwards. Furthermore, the interslice interval is generally very small because it is determined by the space between the voxels. The main disadvantage of three-dimensional imaging is that these

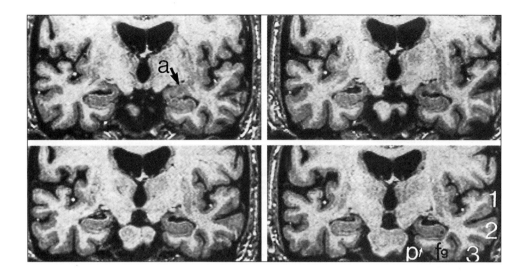

Fig. 44.2 T1-weighted coronal images passing through the head and anterior portion of the body of hippocampi in a normal control subject. These images were reconstructed from a three-dimensional volume acquisition obtained in the sagittal plane. a, amygdala; p, parahippocampal gyrus; fg, fusiform gyrus; 1, 2, and 3 indicate first (T1), second (T2), and third (T3) temporal gyri, respectively. Note the symmetry and oval shape of the healthy hippocampi.

sequences are very time intensive and, because of this, T1-weighted images are the most practical to obtain. Short repetition time (TR) sequences using gradient echo techniques are particularly useful (Sinha *et al* 1998). In the following paragraphs we discuss briefly an example of an MRI protocol for patients with partial epilepsies.

First, T1-weighted sagittal images are acquired covering both hemispheres. Given the characteristics of T1 images, this sequence demonstrates the normal anatomy and allows the visualization of different types of pathology. These sagittal images are also important for ensuring the optimal plane for acquisition of the coronal oblique images (Fig. 44.1).

The second sequence consists of spin-echo (SE) T1-weighted coronal oblique images. These are obtained perpendicular to the long axis of the hippocampi using a sagittal image for planning the acquisition. Slice thickness should be 3 mm or less in order to avoid partial volume and improve definition of anatomic details (Figs 44.2 and 44.3). Some centers routinely use T1-weighted inversion recovery (IR) coronal images for the evaluation of hippocampal pathology. It has been advocated that this sequence may provide information not seen on conventional T1-weighted or three-dimensional images (Kuzniecky and Jackson 1995) because it gives excellent contrast between gray and white matter; acquisition parameters that can be used are: matrix, 256×256 or 256×128; field of view (FOV), 250 mm; echo time (TE), 12–30; TR IR, 1600–3200; inversion time (TI), 428–800 (Figs 44.4 and 44.5).

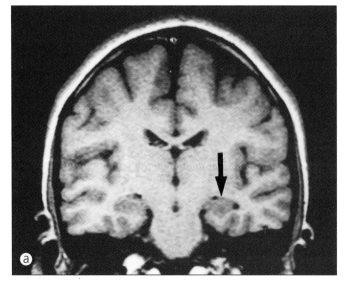
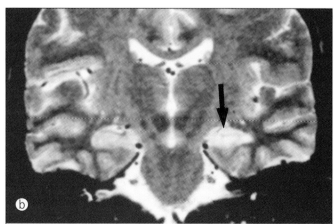

Fig. 44.3 Conventional spin-echo (SE) T1-weighted (a) and SE T2-weighted (b) coronal images in a patient with left temporal lobe epilepsy and left hippocampal atrophy and hyperintense T2 signal (arrows). This patient underwent a left anterior temporal lobe removal and has been seizure-free since surgery.

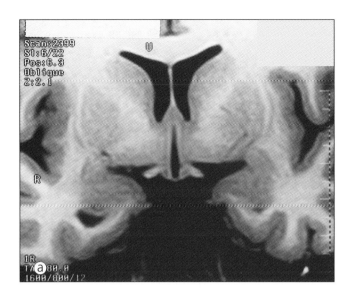
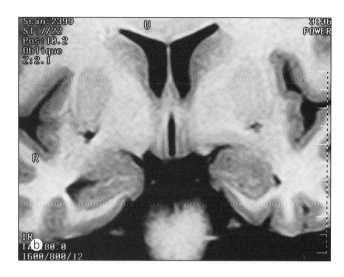
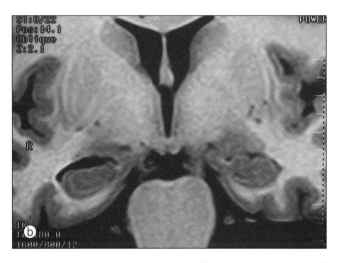
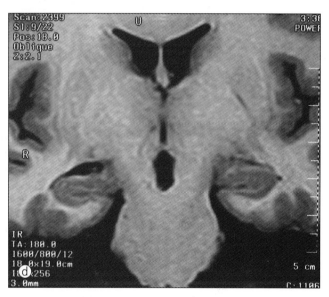

Fig. 44.4 T1-weighted inversion recovery (IR) coronal images (3-mm thick) passing through the anterior segment of the uncus (a, b) and through the head and anterior portion of the body of hippocampi (c, d) in a normal control subject. These images illustrate the excellent contrast between gray and white matter and great definition of anatomic landmarks that can be obtained with IR sequences. The amygdala boundaries can be well delineated on (a–c), above the ventricular horn and separated from the head of hippocampus by the uncal recess of the inferior horn of the ventricle and the alveus covering the hippocampal digitations (b, c) (see also Fig. 44.12). Note the symmetry and oval shape of the healthy hippocampi and the normal (mild) asymmetry of the temporal horns.

The third sequence is a T2-weighted set of images, ideally both in the coronal and axial planes (Figs 44.3, 44.6, and 44.7). This can be obtained using an SE sequence with dual echo, i.e. T2-weighted and proton density images, or a fast SE sequence (FSE) (Fig. 44.7). FSE has replaced conventional SE for T2-weighted scans in many institutions. The shorter imaging times and equal or superior lesion conspicuity of T2 FSE compared with conventional T2 SE has been established by a number of studies (Shaw *et al* 1997; Yousry *et al* 1997; Sinha *et al* 1998). These sequences are important for better definition of dysplastic and tumoral lesions, as well as for the identification

of hyperintense T2 signal often present in hippocampal sclerosis (Jackson *et al* 1993; Kuzniecky and Jackson 1995; Van Paesschen *et al* 1997a,b) (Figs 44.3, 44.6, and 44.7). The acquisition time of T2 FSE such as in Fig. 44.7a is short (less than 4 min).

T1-weighted three-dimensional acquisition, as discussed above, can be implemented as one of the routine acquisitions. This allows for the generation of images in different planes and directions, as well as for quantitative studies, coregistration with other imaging modalities, and automatic segmentation analyses (Collins *et al* 1994; Kuzniecky and Jackson 1995; Sisodiya *et al*

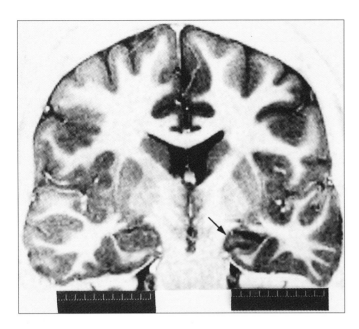

Fig. 44.5 T1-weighted inversion recovery coronal image (3-mm thick) in a patient with left temporal lobe epilepsy showing an atrophic left hippocampus with loss of internal structure (arrow) as well as a smaller temporal lobe on the left side.

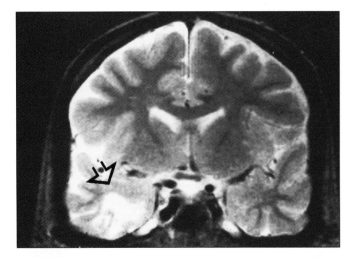

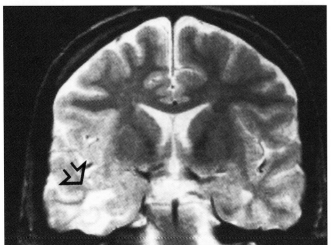

1996; Cendes *et al* 1997a). This can be acquired routinely in every patient; the scanning time should be less than 10–12 min.

MRI FEATURES OF HIPPOCAMPAL SCLEROSIS

Images need to be optimized for the evaluation of features indicating hippocampal pathology. Image orientation is crucial. Coronal slices are mandatory and they need to be obtained on a plane perpendicular to the long axis of the hippocampus guided by a sagittal scout image (Fig. 44.8). The slices need to be thin to allow appreciation of the fine details of the different portions of hippocampal anatomy. Ideally, the slice thickness should be 3 mm or less, and never more than 5 mm. T2-weighted images are important to assess the signal intensity qualitatively, using either conventional SE or FSE sequences (see above). A newer technique

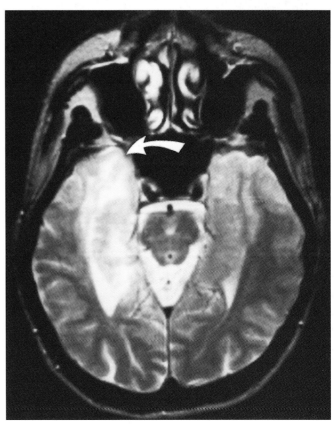

Fig. 44.6 Coronal and axial spin-echo T2-weighted images in a patient with a tumoral lesion (astrocytoma) in the right temporal lobe (arrows).

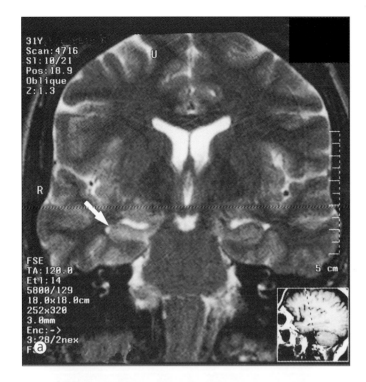

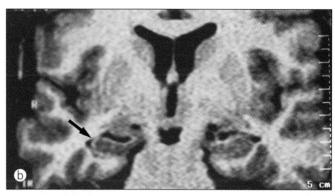

Fig. 44.7 Fast spin-echo (FSE) T2-weighted (a) and T1-weighted inversion recovery (IR) (b) coronal images in a patient with right temporal lobe epilepsy. Note the asymmetry in size and the right hippocampal abnormal signal (arrows), which is brighter than the signal from cerebral cortex and contralateral hippocampus on the FSE T2 image, and darker on the T1 IR image. On the FSE T2 image (a) the signal from within the hippocampus can be well distinguished from the signal of the surrounding cerebrospinal fluid, unlike a conventional SE T2 image shown in Fig. 44.3.

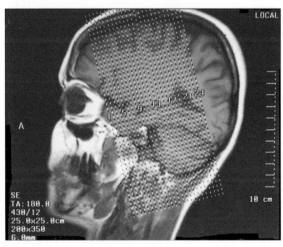

Fig. 44.8 Sagittal image showing the acquisition plane for coronal images (perpendicular to the long axis of the hippocampus).

known as fluid attenuation inversion recovery (FLAIR) can be an alternative (Figs 44.9 and 44.10). A recent evaluation of FLAIR imaging sequences revealed an accuracy of 97% for the demonstration of abnormalities associated with hippocampal sclerosis defined on histopathologic examination (Jack *et al* 1996). To evaluate volume, shape, orientation, and internal structure, high-resolution T1-weighted images, particularly IR, are essential (Figs 44.4, 44.5, and 44.7).

Visual discrimination of a normal from an abnormal hippocampus is straightforward when one is clearly normal and the other is grossly abnormal; however, the visual binary paradigm breaks down in the presence of symmetric bilateral disease or mild unilateral disease (Cendes *et al* 1993c; Free *et al* 1996; Watson *et al* 1997a). Thus absolute quantitative measurements are necessary to determine the presence and severity of hippocampal atrophy in both hippocampi accurately. Preliminary results indicate that the presence and severity of hippocampal sclerosis in both hippocampi may provide useful prognostic information about both postoperative seizure control and memory outcome (Jack *et al* 1992a, 1995; Trenerry *et al* 1993a,b; Berkovic *et al* 1995; Arruda *et al* 1996; Free *et al* 1996; Watson *et al* 1997a).

A majority of patients with hippocampal sclerosis undergoing presurgical evaluation have a clear-cut unilateral atrophic hippocampus with increased signal and a normal-appearing contralateral hippocampus (Figs 44.3, 44.5, 44.7, and 44.10). Several studies have shown volumetric MRI analysis of the hippocampus and amygdala to be very sensitive and specific in the identification of hippocampal sclerosis in this setting (Watson *et al* 1997a). However, simple qualitative visual analysis is also quite sensitive, especially if the images are carefully and properly acquired (Jackson *et al* 1990; Berkovic *et al* 1991; Kuzniecky and Jackson 1995; Watson *et al* 1997a). Measurements of hippocampal volume are unnecessary for clinical purposes in this situation. However, only a few studies have made a direct comparison between quantitative volumetric MRI of the hippocampus and qualitative visual assessment of these same images for

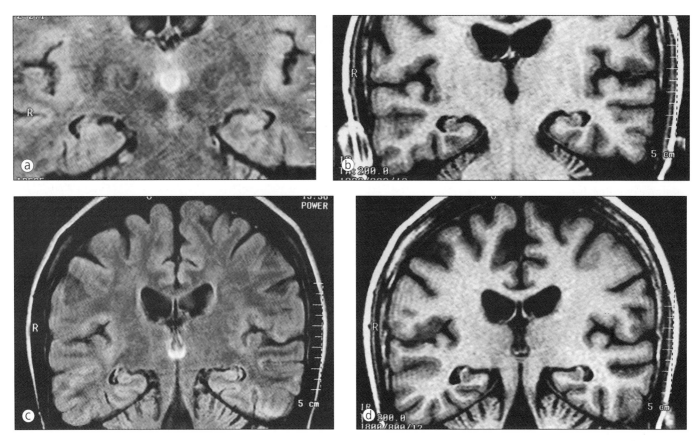

Fig. 44.9 Coronal fluid attenuation inversion recovery (a, c) and T1 inversion recovery (b, d) images showing bilateral, symmetric hyperintense signal and hippocampal atrophy.

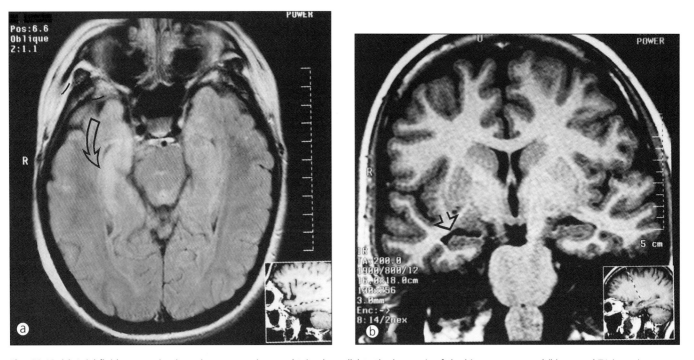

Fig. 44.10 (a) Axial fluid attenuation inversion recovery image obtained parallel to the long axis of the hippocampus and (b) coronal T1 inversion recovery image in a patient with right temporal lobe epilepsy. In (a) a hyperintense signal in the right hippocampus can be observed (arrow); in (b) there is hippocampal atrophy (arrow) as well as atrophy of the right temporal lobe.

signs of hippocampal sclerosis. In the original work by Jack *et al* (1990), volumetric MRI was found to be slightly more sensitive than qualitative image analysis (76 vs. 71%, respectively). However, a more recent investigation using high-resolution techniques found that volumetric MRI measurements had a sensitivity of 92% compared with 56% for qualitative visual inspection blinded to clinical information (Cendes *et al* 1993c). Therefore, volumetric MRI appears to offer a significant improvement in the detection rate of hippocampal abnormalities, particularly bilateral hippocampal volume loss (Jack *et al* 1995; Free *et al* 1996; Watson *et al* 1997a; Ho *et al* 1998). Volumetric MRI is much more time-consuming and must be done correctly to be accurate and reliable. The greatest use for volumetric MRI may be in clinical research (Cendes *et al* 1993d; Jack 1994; Watson *et al* 1997a). MRI-based volumetric studies generate numerical data that permit better comparisons of the degree of medial temporal atrophy in various subgroups of patients. The findings can be statistically correlated with various clinical parameters and thereby lead to better discrimination and understanding of the underlying condition.

The determination of abnormalities of medial temporal structures increases with the experience of the examiner and with knowledge of the anatomic details of the region. The following criteria are important for the visual evaluation of hippocampal sclerosis.

Atrophy of the anterior temporal lobe

When the patient's head is well aligned, the tip of the atrophic temporal lobe starts at a level posterior to the opposite side. The volume of the white matter is reduced compared with the contralateral homologous area. This finding in isolation, which is usually associated with medial temporal atrophy (Figs 44.3, 44.5, and 44.10), is not very sensitive or specific unless it is pronounced because there is much variation in the normal population (Cendes *et al* 1993c,d; Watson *et al* 1997a).

Asymmetry of the temporal horns of the lateral ventricles

This is an indirect sign of hippocampal atrophy, often used in neuroradiologic practice. However, recent studies (Cascino *et al* 1992; Cendes *et al* 1993c) have shown that the size of the temporal horns is extremely variable, both in normals (Figs 44.2 and 44.4) and in patients with hippocampal sclerosis (Figs 44.3, 44.5, and 44.10), which may lead to false lateralization. If the damage occurred early in life there will be atrophy of the temporal structures without dilatation of the ventricular horn (Fig. 44.3). An enlarged ven-

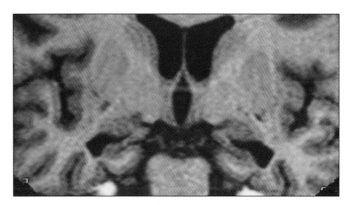

Fig. 44.11 Coronal T1-weighted inversion recovery image at the level of posterior amygdala and head of hippocampus, showing a bilateral symmetric hippocampal atrophy. The hippocampi are flattened and have an abnormal inclination (compare with Figs 44.2 and 44.4).

tricular horn is most often found in patients who sustained medial temporal damage after 4 years of age, particularly in the context of meningoencephalitis, severe head trauma, or hypoxia, and in such cases is often bilateral (Fig. 44.11).

Hippocampal atrophy

This is the most specific and most reliable isolated finding of MTS in patients with TLE. The qualitative diagnosis of hippocampal atrophy is established (qualitatively) by comparing the hippocampal circumference on each side on all available coronal slices. Small asymmetries can be present due to normal variation or a tilted position in the scanner and should not be considered as abnormal. It is important to evaluate the *shape* of the hippocampus as well. A normal hippocampus is oval (Figs 44.2, 44.4, and 44.12). In the presence of hippocampal sclerosis it becomes flattened and usually inclined (Figs 44.5, 44.10, and 44.11). The diagnosis of MTS can be made in most cases on the basis of a significant unilateral or asymmetric hippocampal atrophy (Figs 44.3, 44.5, 44.7, and 44.10), usually associated with other findings, such as loss of internal structure and signal changes. Mild MTS or bilateral symmetric hippocampal atrophy can be missed by visual analysis.

Hyperintense T2-weighted signal

This is usually easy to identify when the atrophy is pronounced, and there is a hypointense T1-weighted signal (Figs 44.3, 44.5, and 44.10). Hyperintense T2-weighted signal alone is not sufficient for the diagnosis of MTS, although FLAIR imaging sequences seem promising for the detection of abnormalities associated with mild hippocampal sclerosis (Jack *et al* 1996). Studies have shown that

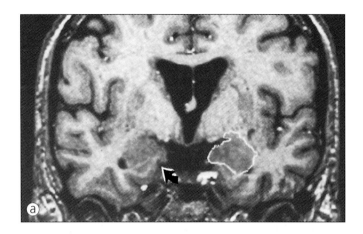

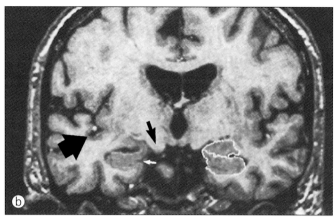

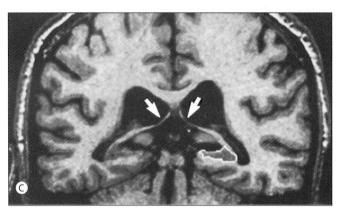

Fig. 44.12 Angled coronal T1-weighted images in a normal control subject. (a) Section through the anterior segment of the uncus with the amygdala outlined on the left side. The arrow indicates the tentorial indentation. (b) Section through the posterior portion of the amygdala (top) and hippocampal head (bottom) outlined on the left side. The large black arrow indicates the circular sulcus of the insula; also seen are the optic tract (small black arrow) and the uncal cleft (small white arrow). (c) Section through the splenium of the corpus callosum with the hippocampal tail outlined on the left side. The arrows indicate the crus of fornix.

quantitative T2 mapping (relaxometry) can improve the diagnosis of hippocampal sclerosis (Jackson *et al* 1993; Kuzniecky and Jackson 1995). Hyperintense T2 signal is caused by an increased concentration of free water in the abnormal tissue, and it has been postulated that this is due to gliosis (Kuzniecky and Jackson 1995). However, a recent study has shown that the hyperintense T2 signal in MTS is not directly correlated with glial cell density and has a different neuropathology to that of hippocampal volume loss (Van Paesschen *et al* 1997b). It is also important to differentiate the intense T2 signal produced by the cerebrospinal fluid and choroid plexus from abnormal signal inside the hippocampus (Jackson *et al* 1993; Kuzniecky and Jackson 1995) (Fig. 44.7).

Loss of internal structure

This is usually associated with atrophy and hyperintense T2 signal. The loss of normal internal hippocampal structure is a consequence of neuronal loss and gliosis, with a collapse of pyramidal cell layers (CA1, CA3, CA4) characteristic of hippocampal sclerosis. This abnormality is better seen on T1-weighted IR images (Figs 44.5, 44.7, and 44.10).

Exceptionally, it can be present without hippocampal atrophy (Jackson *et al* 1994).

MRI VOLUMETRIC STUDIES

TECHNICAL ASPECTS

The histologic hallmarks of hippocampal sclerosis are cell loss and astrogliosis (sclerosis) of the hippocampus and related medial temporal lobe limbic areas (Babb and Brown 1987; Bruton 1988; Gloor 1991; Meencke and Veith 1991). The two principal MRI findings in histologically proven cases of hippocampal sclerosis are hippocampal atrophy and MRI signal changes indicative of increased tissue free water (Kuzniecky *et al* 1987; Jack *et al* 1990, 1992a; Berkovic *et al* 1991; Cascino *et al* 1991; Lencz *et al* 1992; Cendes *et al* 1993b,d; Arruda *et al* 1996; Watson *et al* 1997a). Both MRI properties can be quantified (Jackson *et al* 1993; Watson *et al* 1997a). Hippocampal volumetry is a direct measure of the hippocampal atrophy associated with hippocampal sclerosis. Several studies have demonstrated a close correlation between histologically determined cell loss and atrophy determined through hippocampal volumetric measurements (Cascino *et al* 1991; Lencz *et al* 1992; Cendes *et al* 1993b; Lee *et al* 1995; Watson *et al* 1996a; Van Paesschen *et al* 1997b). MRI-based hippocampal volumetric measurements therefore may be considered a surrogate for pathologic identification of not only the presence but also the relative severity of hippocampal sclerosis in *both* hippocampi (Jack *et al* 1995; King *et al* 1995; Arruda *et al* 1996; Cendes *et al* 1996; Trenerry *et al* 1996; Watson *et al* 1997a).

To maximize the precision and reproducibility of MRI-based hippocampal volume measures, the technical parameters employed when acquiring the images themselves should reflect the following guidelines (Jack 1994; Watson *et al* 1997a).

1. Spatial resolution should be maximized. In practical terms this means that the imaging sections, or slices, should be made as thin as possible, while preserving signal-to-noise ratio, to avoid volume-averaging artifacts in the direction of voxel anisotropy.
2. To display hippocampal boundaries optimally, the signal-to-noise ratios between gray matter, white matter, and cerebrospinal fluid should be high enough to permit reliable discrimination of hippocampal boundaries.
3. The image acquisition time should be short enough (less than 10 min) so that high-quality images free of motion artifact may be acquired in the vast majority of patients.

These criteria lead to two logical choices for the optimum type of imaging sequence to be employed for subsequent volume measurements. The most commonly employed approach is a three-dimensional volumetric pulse sequence. This not only gives an image dataset that is useful for hippocampal volume measurements but also provides whole-head anatomic coverage for routine diagnostic purposes. A potentially attractive alternative to both of these approaches is a three-dimensional FSE approach. Clinically, practical three-dimensional FSE imaging is enabled by the installation of high-performance gradient sets, which have recently been made commercially available by the major manufacturers.

Images acquired in the sagittal plane can be retrospectively reformatted into the coronal plane for hippocampal volume measurement. The advantage of this approach is that the most narrow dimension of the head generally is in the sagittal direction. This in turn permits whole-head anatomic coverage with a three-dimensional volumetric sagittal acquisition composed of 1 or 1.5 mm thick imaging voxels that are essentially isotropic (as opposed to the thicker anisotropic voxels necessary to cover the whole head

if the section selection direction is in the coronal orientation). However, the disadvantage of a sagittal image acquisition is that in order to visually compare the hippocampi for the presence of relative side-to-side atrophy for diagnostic purposes, the images must be secondarily reformatted in the coronal plane. Thus the native or raw images as they are acquired are not suitable for the clinical visual evaluation of hippocampal atrophy. Some authors have actually outlined the hippocampus for volumetric determination in the sagittal plane. While this approach works well for most of the hippocampal borders, portions of the hippocampal border are optimally displayed *only* in the coronal plane not the sagittal plane, particularly the medial subicular–parahippocampal boundary, the medial boundary between the hippocampal head and the amygdala or ambient gyrus, and the posterior border of the hippocampus (Jack 1994; Watson *et al* 1997a).

After the image dataset has been acquired, it must be processed to produce volume measurement information. This step requires great attention to detail in order to produce precise and accurate volume measurements of the hippocampus and amygdala. It is generally done by transferring the images to a computer workstation and manually tracing the borders of the hippocampus and amygdala on serial planimetric slices with a manual interactive device. Manual tracing of these borders creates a volume of interest. The voxels inside the volume of interest are then automatically counted by the computer and multiplied by the number of cubic millimeters per image voxel to generate volumes in cubic millimeters. Discrepancies between the way different software programs handle the counting of border pixels in a traced volume of interest are a likely cause of the variability found by different groups for the 'normal' absolute volumes of the right and left hippocampi and amygdalae in normal subjects. The second likely source of interinstitutional variability in reported 'normal' volumes of the hippocampus and amygdala is the neuroanatomic boundary criteria used to define hippocampal borders (Jack 1994; Watson *et al* 1997a). Rigorous standardized criteria that have a solid neuroanatomic basis must be followed when tracing the borders of the amygdala and hippocampus in order to ensure precise and reproducible volume measurements (Amaral and Insausti 1990; Duvernoy 1991; Watson *et al* 1992, 1997a; Jack 1994).

INTERPRETATION

MRI-based volume measurements of the right and left hippocampus (or amygdala) may be interpreted in two ways, relative or absolute. To date, the relative approach has been employed more commonly: the right and left hippocampus in a given patient are compared with each other by measuring either a right-to-left hippocampal ratio, or the difference between the two sides.

Evaluating hippocampal volume in absolute terms is more complex because a number of different variables affect hippocampal volume in normal individuals, such as head size, age, gender, and hemisphere (Jack *et al* 1989, 1992b; Watson *et al* 1992, 1997a; Cendes *et al* 1994, 1996; Jack 1994; Free *et al* 1996). Ideally, therefore, atrophy of the right or left hippocampus (or both) in any individual should be established by comparing those values to normative percentiles in an age- and gender-matched control population for that hemisphere, and after adjustment for head size. Hippocampal atrophy in any given patient, as a marker of hippocampal sclerosis, would then be expressed in terms of the percentile of adjusted volume in normals. As a rule, studies in epilepsy in which hippocampal volume has been analyzed in absolute terms have not taken into account age effects, because age-related effects on hippocampal volume are found primarily in the very young, due to growth and development, and in older individuals, due to age-related atrophy (Jack *et al* 1989, 1992b; Cendes *et al* 1994, 1996). The effect of gender is small in comparison to that of head size. Therefore, the few studies employing absolute volumetric quantitation in epilepsy have adjusted hippocampal volume only by intracranial volume. This adjustment can take several forms. The two most popular methods are dividing hippocampal volume by total intracranial volume to create a ratio or a covariance approach (Jack *et al* 1989, 1992b; Cendes *et al* 1993d, 1994, 1996; Watson *et al* 1997a) (Table 44.1).

The investigator performing volumetric measurements of the amygdala and hippocampus must have a detailed knowledge of the anatomy of the medial temporal region in order to obtain accurate and reliable results. Also, the structures must be measured consistently according to a predetermined and standardized protocol. Such protocols have been published in detail (Jack *et al* 1989; Watson *et al* 1992, 1996b, 1997a; Cendes *et al* 1993d). When the boundaries of the hippocampus and amygdala are measured

by a knowledgeable investigator following a predetermined and standardized protocol, the accuracy and reproducibility of the measurements are high (Cendes *et al* 1993d, 1997a).

In addition to validating the accuracy and reproducibility of volume measurements, each center must also establish the range of normal values present in their patient and control populations. A number of factors (Jack 1994) enter into the absolute values obtained at each institution, and therefore discrepancies between institutions are to be expected (Jack *et al* 1989, 1990, 1992a,b; Ashtari *et al* 1991; Cascino *et al* 1991; Cook *et al* 1992; Lencz *et al* 1992; Watson *et al* 1992, 1996b, 1997a; Cendes *et al* 1993b,c,d, 1994, 1996; Kuks *et al* 1993; Jack 1994). Therefore each institution must create its own normal database. The following protocol is adapted from that proposed by Watson *et al* (1992, 1996b, 1997a) and Cendes *et al* (1993d).

Volume of the amygdala

The amygdala is an ovoid mass of gray matter situated in the superomedial portion of the temporal lobe, partly above the tip of the inferior horn of the lateral ventricle (Gloor 1997). It occupies the superior part of the anterior segment of the uncus and partially overlies the head of the hippocampus, being separated from that structure by the uncal recess of the inferior horn of the lateral ventricle. The amygdala forms a distinct protrusion on the supermedial surface of the uncus, the semilunar gyrus, which corresponds to the cortical amygdaloid nucleus. It is separated from the ambient gyrus by the semianular or amygdaloid sulcus, which forms the boundary between the amygdala and the entorhinal cortex. The entorhinal cortex extends into the ambient gyrus and forms most of its surface. The amygdala is separated from the substantia innominata by a deep fold, the entorhinal sulcus, which is lined on the amygdaloid side by the medial nucleus of the amygdala. The superior rim of the ambient gyrus, lying in the fundus of the semiannular sulcus, is related to the so-called corticoamygdaloid transition area, which probably represents periamygdaloid cortex. The medial surface of the ambient gyrus often shows a marked indentation, the tentorial indentation, sometimes called the uncal notch (Duvernoy 1991) or the intrarhinal sulcus (Amaral and Insausti 1990), produced by the free edge of the tentorium cerebelli (Figs 44.4 and 44.12).

The anterior end of the amygdala is arbitrarily and consistently measured on the MRI section at the level of the closure of the lateral sulcus to form the entorhinal sulcus. When using thin MRI slices it is possible to determine the outline of the amygdala starting at one or two slices anterior to the closure of the lateral sulcus (Figs 44.4 and

---

Table 44.1 'Normalization' of volumetric MRI measurements of the hippocampal formation (HF) and amygdala (AM).

Obtain the *mean* total intracranial volume (TIV) of the normal control group

'Normalize' the volume of each of the structures measured (e.g. HF or AM) for individual variation in head size, using the formula:

'Normalized' HF (or AM) volume = $R \times$ HF (or AM) volume

where $R = \dfrac{\text{Mean TIV of the controls}}{\text{Patient's TIV}}$

44.12). The medial border of the amygdala is covered by part of the entorhinal cortex which forms the surface of the ambient gyrus in this region. The entorhinal cortex inferior to the tentorial indentation is excluded from the amygdaloid measurement. If the tentorial indentation is poorly defined or not visible in the anterior amygdaloid region, the line of demarcation between the amygdala and the adjacent entorhinal cortex that occupies the ambient gyrus is defined by a line drawn in direct continuation with the inferior and medial border of the amygdala within the substance of the temporal lobe. By proceeding in this manner a small amount of the superior extent of the entorhinal cortex is included in the amygdaloid volume, as is the case when the tentorial indentation is used as the landmark. The inferior and lateral borders of the amygdala are formed by the inferior horn of the lateral ventricle or white matter. To define the superior border of the amygdala, we draw a straight line laterally from the entorhinal sulcus to the fundus of the inferior portion of the circular sulcus of the insula, or just follow the boundaries of the amygdala gray matter when the MRI contrast and resolution allow one to do so. More posteriorly, the optic tract is used as a guide to the lateral extension of the crural cistern into the transverse cerebral fissure. This locates the medial aspect of the posterior amygdala and is used as the point of departure for defining the medial and superior borders of the structure posteriorly (Watson *et al* 1992, 1997a) (Figs 44.4 and 44.12).

At its posterior end, the amygdala occupies the medial half of the roof of the inferior horn of the lateral ventricle, and care must be taken to exclude the tail of the caudate nucleus, the overlying globus pallidus and putamen, and the lateral geniculate body.

Volume of the hippocampus

The hippocampus is a complex structure consisting of an enlarged anterior part that has been called the pes but is perhaps better termed the head of the hippocampus. This portion of the hippocampus exhibits three or four digitations and turns medially to form the posterior segment of the uncus. As it turns medially the hippocampus and the dentate gyrus run in the roof of the uncal cleft [sometimes called the uncal notch, the uncal sulcus (Duvernoy 1991) and, erroneously, the hippocampal sulcus (Watson *et al* 1997a)], the sulcus-like cleft that separates the uncus above from the parahippocampal gyrus below (Fig. 44.12). Once the hippocampus and dentate gyrus reach the medial surface of the uncus, they turn up and form the posterior one-third of the medial and superomedial surface of the uncus. Macroscopically the dentate gyrus is discernible as a narrow

elevation, the band or limbus of Giacomini. This is interposed between the intralimbic gyrus, which forms the posterior pole of the uncus and corresponds to sector CA3 of the hippocampus, and the uncinate gyrus, which extends anterior to the band of Giacomini and corresponds partially to sector CA1 and the subiculum. There is no macroscopically visible border between the uncinate gyrus and the ambient gyrus. The floor of the uncal cleft is formed by the presubiculum (Figs 44.2, 44.4, and 44.12). The body of the hippocampus curves around the upper midbrain and is concave medially (Fig. 44.1). The anatomy in this region is much less complex (Figs 44.2 and 44.12). Posteriorly, the hippocampal body tapers into the tail, which turns medially just anterior to and below the splenium of the corpus callosum (Figs 44.1, 44.2, 44.4, and 44.12). The tail of the hippocampus gives rise to the fasciola cinerea, which ultimately passes around the corpus callosum to continue on its upper surface as the indusium griseum.

It is obviously most difficult to define the boundaries of the hippocampus in its most anterior portion, the hippocampal head (Figs 44.2, 44.4, and 44.12). The most reliable structure separating the head of the hippocampus from the amygdala in this region is the inferior horn of the lateral ventricle (Watson *et al* 1992, 1997a). This is especially true if the ventricular cavity extends into the deep part of the uncus anterior to the head of the hippocampus, thereby forming the uncal recess of the inferior horn. However, portions of the uncal recess are often obliterated, especially medially, and the hippocampal digitations are fused to the amygdala across the ventricular cavity (Duvernoy 1991; Gloor 1997). When this is the case, three guidelines are used to outline the hippocampal head and separate it from the adjacent amygdala (Watson *et al* 1992, 1997a). If an obvious semilunar gyrus is present on the surface of the uncus, a line is drawn connecting the inferior horn of the lateral ventricle to the sulcus at the inferior margin of the semilunar gyrus (i.e. the semianular or amygdaloid sulcus). It is also helpful to use the alveus covering the ventricular surface of the hippocampal digitations to distinguish the hippocampus from the amygdala (Figs 44.4 and 44.12). If neither the semianular sulcus nor the alveus is obvious, a straight horizontal line is drawn connecting the plane of the inferior horn of the lateral ventricle with the surface of the uncus. The inferior margin of the hippocampus is outlined to include the subicular complex and the uncal cleft. The border separating the subicular complex from the parahippocampal gyrus is defined as the angle formed by the most medial extent of those two structures. Unless significant atrophy is present, no attempt is made to outline the gray matter on the superior and inferior banks of the uncal cleft as it is usually quite narrow. The gray matter of the entorhinal cortex or parahippocampal gyrus is excluded from this measurement (Fig. 44.12).

In the hippocampal body, the delineation of the hippocampus includes the subicular complex, hippocampus proper, dentate gyrus, alveus, and fimbria. The border between the subicular complex and the parahippocampal gyrus is defined in the same manner as in the hippocampal head. Therefore, the cortex of the parahippocampal gyrus is once again excluded from the measurement (Figs 44.2, 44.4, and 44.12).

In the hippocampal tail, measurement again includes the subicular complex, hippocampus proper, dentate gyrus, alveus, and fimbria. Excluded at this level are the crus of the fornix, isthmus of the cingulate gyrus, and parahippocampal gyrus. The most posterior section measured is the section with the crus of the fornix clearly separating from the hippocampus and its fimbria when using 3-mm thick slices, or two sections posterior to that when using 1-mm thick slices (Fig. 44.12).

Assuming a total anterior–posterior length of the hippocampus of approximately 40 mm (Amaral and Insausti 1990; Duvernoy 1991; Watson *et al* 1997a), these guidelines should result in a volume measurement of 90–95% of the total hippocampal formation.

CORRELATIONS

Electroencephalography

Since the initial publication on the utility of volumetric MRI measurements of the hippocampus in patients with TLE by Jack *et al* (1990), many studies have illustrated the correlation between EEG lateralization of the epileptogenic region in TLE and the presence of significantly reduced hippocampal volumes (Jack *et al* 1990, 1992a; Ashtari *et al* 1991; Cascino *et al* 1991, 1996; Cook *et al* 1992; Lencz *et al* 1992; Watson *et al* 1992, 1996b; Cendes *et al* 1993b,c,d; Kuks *et al* 1993; Murro *et al* 1993; Spencer *et al* 1993; Jack 1994; Arruda *et al* 1996).

We have analyzed the MRI volumetric measurements (MRIVol) and the clinical and EEG data in 250 consecutive patients with partial seizures (Cendes *et al* 1995a). There were 167 patients with nonlesional TLE, 24 patients with lesional TLE, and 59 patients with partial seizures originating outside the temporal lobe. We found significant atrophy of mesial temporal structures in 83.2% of TLE patients not having foreign tissue lesions. This volume reduction was more pronounced in those with a history of prolonged febrile convulsions in childhood. The EEG lateralization was concordant with the MRIVol in *all* patients with unilateral amygdalohippocampal atrophy. In the 36 patients with bilateral amygdalohippocampal atrophy the predominance of EEG abnormalities was on the more atrophic side in all but four. The 59 patients with extra-TLE had normal amygdalohippocampal volumes (Cendes *et al* 1995a).

Cascino *et al* (1996) recently studied a series of 159 patients with TLE who underwent surgery and had preoperative MRIVol. They compared the MRIVol results with the long-term EEG monitoring and with the results of routine outpatient EEG examinations. They found that patients with unilateral hippocampal atrophy always had concordant lateralization by long-term EEG monitoring and also by routine EEG examinations. In addition, unilateral hippocampal atrophy was correlated with good postoperative outcome. Cascino *et al* (1996) concluded that the results of their study, as well as results from the literature, including our own series (Cendes *et al* 1995a), altered their preoperative strategy of selecting patients with TLE. Patients with a history and ictal semiology consistent with medial TLE may undergo surgical resection of temporal lobe structures if interictal epileptiform discharges recorded during serial routine EEGs or long-term EEG monitoring consistently lateralize to one temporal lobe and these epileptiform discharges are concordant with MRI-identified unilateral hippocampal atrophy, provided that the remainder of the noninvasive presurgical investigation (i.e. neuropsychology and other neuroimaging investigations) do not uncover conflicting evidence for localization or lateralization of the epileptogenic area (Cascino *et al* 1996). Long-term EEG monitoring for recording seizures is mandatory in patients without, or only scarce, interictal epileptiform discharges, bitemporal interictal EEG abnormalities, or patients with a normal quantitative MRI, bilateral hippocampal atrophy, and discordant preoperative studies (Cascino *et al* 1996).

Gambardella *et al* (1995a) reviewed clinical data and scalp EEG findings in 61 consecutive patients with TLE who had atrophy of medial temporal structures by MRIVol; 39 patients had unilateral atrophy, while 22 exhibited bilateral asymmetric atrophy. Spikes were always confined to the temporal regions and were frequently bilateral, without a statistically significant difference between patients with unilateral atrophy (33%) and those with bilateral atrophy (50%). Of 40 EEG foci associated with amygdaloid atrophy 25 had a maximal field over the anterior temporal region. In contrast, all 19 EEG foci associated with isolated hippocampal atrophy were never maximal anteriorly but were maximal over basal and inferomedial temporal regions (zygomatic or sphenoidal electrodes). Secondarily generalized seizures and temporal lobe drop attacks (or 'syncopal' spells; Gambardella *et al* 1994) were correlated with anatomically extensive atrophy, particularly involving the amygdala, confirming previous observations (Cook *et al* 1992; Gambardella *et al* 1994). Prolonged postictal confusion was associated with bilateral atrophy and bitemporal EEG abnormalities. These results help explain some of the variability in the clinical and EEG manifestations in TLE and outline the specific role of amygdaloid involvement in contrast to the more commonly reported involvement of the hippocampus.

Gambardella *et al* (1995b) assessed the significance of EEG background abnormalities and their relationship to spikes and mesial temporal atrophy in a group of 56 patients with TLE; 35 patients had unilateral atrophy, while 21 had bilateral atrophy of medial temporal structures. Trains of delta waves over the temporal regions were observed in over 90% of patients. This focal delta activity was concordant with the side of atrophy and of interictal spikes. Delta waves and spikes occurred together in more than 85% of the cases, and were never discordant with respect to lateralization. These results indicate that in TLE related to medial temporal atrophy, delta transients are a reliable indicator of the epileptogenic focus and presumably reflect the underlying epileptogenic process rather than just structural pathology.

In our experience (Cendes *et al* 1995a, 1996, 1997a; Arruda *et al* 1996; Watson *et al* 1997b), and according to that of others (Jack *et al* 1990; Cook *et al* 1992; Lee *et al* 1995; Cascino *et al* 1996), unilateral hippocampal atrophy always correlated with preponderant ipsilateral EEG lateralization. However, bilateral, even asymmetric, hippocampal atrophy may show discordant EEG lateralization in approximately 10% of patients (Cendes *et al* 1995a, 1996), and preliminary data suggest that this discrepancy is an indicator of poor prognosis (Jack *et al* 1992a, 1995; Arruda *et al* 1996; Cendes *et al* 1996, 1997a; Watson *et al* 1997a).

Intracranial stereotaxic depth EEG

Cascino *et al* (1995) performed a retrospective study of 30 patients with intractable TLE who underwent chronic intracranial EEG monitoring. All patients had previously undergone extracranial ictal EEG monitoring that proved inadequate to localize the epileptogenic zone. A prolonged interhemispheric propagation time ($P < 0.01$) and MRI-identified hippocampal atrophy ($P < 0.01$) correlated with a favorable surgical outcome.

We studied 31 consecutive patients with temporal and extratemporal epilepsy to assess the relationship between amygdaloid and hippocampal atrophy and the location of stereo-EEG seizure onset and stereo-EEG interictal abnormalities (Cendes *et al* 1996). There were 21 patients with temporal lobe seizure onsets and 10 patients with extratemporal seizures according to the stereo-EEG investigation. All patients with extratemporal epilepsy had normal, symmetric volumes of medial temporal structures. The final conclusions of the stereo-EEG investigation coincided with the lateralization obtained by MRI volumetric measurements in the eight patients with significant unilateral atrophy of the amygdala, hippocampus, or both. The seven patients with bilateral asymmetric medial atrophy had bilateral seizure onsets, with predominance from the more atrophic side in four, from the less atrophic side in two, and without predominance in one. The one patient with severe bilateral symmetric atrophy had seizures originating equally from both sides. Our findings also indicate that continuous polymorphic slow waves and decrease or loss of normal fast rhythms may reflect more accurately the degree of hippocampal atrophy than does the frequency of interictal epileptiform discharges.

In another study, King *et al* (1995) documented unilateral or bilateral seizure onset by intracranial EEG in patients with bilateral hippocampal atrophy. They concluded that these seizures may originate ipsilateral or contralateral to the side of predominant atrophy.

Pathology

MTS is found in the histopathologic examination of the majority of patients with drug-resistant TLE undergoing surgical treatment (Bruton 1988; Gloor 1991; Meencke and Veith 1991). This pathologic condition can be identified on MRI as a reduced volume of mesial temporal structures, most often the hippocampus, sometimes associated with changes in signal intensity, in both T2- and T1-weighted sequences (Kuzniecky *et al* 1987; Cendes *et al* 1993c; Kuzniecky and Jackson 1995). High-intensity T2-weighted signals are more frequent in patients with more severe gliosis on postoperative histopathology (Kuzniecky *et al* 1987; Cendes *et al* 1993c); it is not specific for sclerosis since low-grade tumors can present with similar signals (Kuzniecky *et al* 1987; Kuzniecky and Jackson 1995). However there are some patients who have hippocampal sclerosis without volume loss and present with a high-intensity signal on T2-weighted images that correspond to a decreased T1-weighted signal. This has been referred to as 'loss of internal structures' (Kuzniecky and Jackson 1995).

Several studies have correlated hippocampal volumes with pathologic findings after temporal lobe resection (Cascino *et al* 1991; Lencz *et al* 1992; Cendes *et al* 1993a,d; Kim *et al* 1995; Lee *et al* 1995; Watson *et al* 1996a). A strong relationship between the degree of hippocampal volume loss and the severity of hippocampal sclerosis was found in studies that utilized qualitative (Cascino *et al*

1991; Cendes *et al* 1993a,d), semi-quantitative (Watson *et al* 1996a), and quantitative (Lencz *et al* 1992; Lee *et al* 1995) neuropathology. In view of these findings, the severity of hippocampal sclerosis can be predicted preoperatively by MRI volumetric studies.

Neuropsychology

It is well recognized that medial temporal lobe structures such as the hippocampus and amygdala play a critical role in declarative or representational memory function. The same medial temporal lobe structures are involved in other neurologic conditions resulting in memory deficits, such as postanoxic amnesia and Alzheimer's disease. It is not surprising, therefore, that a relationship has been demonstrated between the severity of hippocampal atrophy, as measured by MRI volumetric studies, and memory function using a variety of neuropsychologic tests (Lencz *et al* 1992; Jones-Gotman *et al* 1993a; Loring *et al* 1993; Trenerry *et al* 1993b). Studies have found a significant relationship between left hippocampal volume and verbal memory function (Lencz *et al* 1992; Jones-Gotman *et al* 1993a; Trenerry *et al* 1993b, 1995), as well as a relationship between impaired nonverbal memory function and reduced right hippocampal volumes (Jones-Gotman *et al* 1993a; Trenerry *et al* 1993b). An interesting finding is that patients undergoing left temporal lobectomy with severe left hippocampal atrophy have less verbal memory deficit postoperatively than those with lesser degrees of left hippocampal atrophy (Trenerry *et al* 1993b, 1996). Studies have also shown a correlation between hippocampal atrophy and poor memory function on the intracarotid amobarbital test (Jones-Gotman *et al* 1993b; Loring *et al* 1993).

While outcome following temporal lobectomy is most often thought of in terms of postoperative seizure control, the most common serious cognitive complication of surgery is a postoperative decline in verbally mediated declarative memory following a dominant temporal lobectomy. The clear link between functional and anatomic integrity has led to the evaluation of hippocampal volumetric measurements as a means of predicting *postoperative* memory decline (Jones-Gotman *et al* 1993a, 1997; Trenerry *et al* 1993b, 1995, 1996). The initial studies (Trenerry *et al* 1993b, 1995, 1996; Jones-Gotman *et al* 1997) correlating postoperative memory outcome with hippocampal volumetric measurements indicate that this technique may provide clinically useful prognostic information regarding memory performance. Patients at greatest risk for a decline in verbal memory following a dominant left temporal lobectomy are those with bilaterally symmetric severe atrophy of both the right and left hippocampus. The group at

next greatest risk are patients with volumetrically normal hippocampi bilaterally (i.e. no atrophy). The group at least risk for postoperative verbal memory deficit following a dominant left temporal lobectomy are those with significant unilateral left hippocampal atrophy.

Outcome after surgery

Early EEG and autopsy studies (Bruton 1988; Gloor 1991; Meencke and Veith 1991) indicated that temporal lobe epilepsy is a bilateral condition, with varying degrees of unilaterality. This concept has been supported by recent MRI studies (Jack *et al* 1992a, 1995; King *et al* 1995; Arruda *et al* 1996; Cendes *et al* 1996; Trenerry *et al* 1996; Li *et al* 1997; Watson *et al* 1997a). The spectrum of medial temporal lobe epilepsy can be divided into the following (Jack *et al* 1995; Arruda *et al* 1996; Cendes *et al* 1996; Trenerry *et al* 1996; Li *et al* 1997; Watson *et al* 1997a).

1. Unilateral hippocampal atrophy: hippocampal sclerosis is present unilaterally and the contralateral hippocampus is completely normal.
2. Bilaterally asymmetric hippocampal atrophy: hippocampal sclerosis is present bilaterally but more severely represented on one side.
3. Bilaterally symmetric atrophy: hippocampal sclerosis is present and of equal magnitude in both hippocampi.
4. Volumetrically symmetric normal hippocampi: neither hippocampus has changes of hippocampal sclerosis.

Distinguishing mild hippocampal sclerosis from a normal hippocampus is not straightforward by visual inspection of magnetic resonance images or by qualitative pathologic analysis (Watson *et al* 1997a). These four groups represent conceptual points along a continuous distribution of hippocampal damage, ranging from severe hippocampal sclerosis to anatomic normality, in one or both hippocampi.

An important issue in surgical therapy for seizure control is to predict its outcome. According to general analyses of patients with partial refractory seizures undergoing surgical treatment (Engel *et al* 1993a, 1997; Arruda *et al* 1996), it is estimated that about two-thirds achieve seizure-free status or have a significant reduction in seizure frequency. It is important to know the prognosis for an individual patient, and to determine whether clinical data or the results of complementary examinations can predict a good surgical outcome (Duchowny *et al* 1997; Engel *et al* 1997).

Jack *et al* (1992a) demonstrated a significant relationship between MRI-based hippocampal volumes and outcome after temporal lobe removal. If EEG lateralization was concordant with hippocampal atrophy, 97% of the patients had a favorable outcome (seizure-free or nearly seizure-free).

However, if the hippocampal volumes were not lateralizing, the proportion of patients with a favorable outcome dropped to 42%; if the hippocampal volumes were abnormal on the side opposite the side of surgery, only 33% of patients had a favorable outcome. Similar results have been found in patients requiring depth electrode recordings (Cascino *et al* 1995). Qualitative MRI investigations are also of value in determining the prognosis of temporal lobe resection (Garcia *et al* 1994; Berkovic *et al* 1995).

We recently studied 74 consecutive patients with TLE who were treated surgically and had preoperative volumetric MRI measurements of medial temporal structures (Arruda *et al* 1996). Excellent results (seizure-free or almost seizure-free) were found in 93.6% of the patients with unilateral atrophy; in 61.7% of those with bilateral atrophy; and in 50% of the group with no significant atrophy of mesial temporal structures. In addition, the ratio of hippocampal and amygdalar volumes (ipsilateral or contralateral to the side of surgery) was significantly smaller in those patients who became seizure-free or almost seizure-free than in those with less favorable outcome (classes III or IV; Engel *et al* 1993a). These data, in agreement with other studies (Jack *et al* 1992a; Cascino *et al* 1995), indicate that the degree of asymmetry of medial structures, in those with unilateral and bilateral atrophy, may also be an important factor for postsurgical seizure control in patients with TLE. This suggests that a more atrophic hippocampus in the operated hemisphere, together with a healthier hippocampus on the unresected side, yields the best outcome, a finding that makes intuitive sense for cognitive function as well as for seizure control (Hermann *et al* 1992; Trenerry *et al* 1993b).

In summary, MRI-based volumetric measurement of the amygdala and hippocampus not only aids in the determination of the side of seizure onset in nonlesional TLE but is also an important prognostic tool. For patients with unilateral atrophy, one can expect excellent results in 93–97% of cases. Surgical outcome in those with bilateral atrophy is not as good but still represents a worthwhile option, being best with asymmetric atrophy and worst with symmetric atrophy (Jack *et al* 1992a, 1995; Berkovic *et al* 1995; Arruda *et al* 1996; Watson *et al* 1997a). Patients without significant atrophy have the worst prognosis, and thus remain a major challenge. The likelihood that some of these patients have neocortical temporal lobe epilepsy helps to explain the poorer outcome in this group.

Early childhood insults

Several studies have shown a significant relationship between atrophy of the hippocampus and amygdala, as determined with volumetric MRI, and a history of febrile convulsions in early childhood (Cendes *et al* 1993b; Kuks *et al* 1993; Trenerry *et al* 1993a; Watson *et al* 1997a). The interpretation of this observation remains quite controversial (Abou-Khalil *et al* 1993; Maher and McLachlan 1995; Berg *et al* 1998; Doose 1998; Shinnar 1998; Sloviter and Pedley 1998). One possibility is that the early febrile convulsion damages the hippocampus and is therefore a cause of hippocampal sclerosis (Abou-Khalil *et al* 1993; Berg *et al* 1998; Hamati-Haddad and Abou-Khalil 1998; Kanemoto *et al* 1998; Shinnar 1998; Van Landingham *et al* 1998). However, another possibility is that the child has a prolonged febrile convulsion because the hippocampus was previously damaged due to a prenatal or perinatal insult (Cendes *et al* 1995b; Fernandez *et al* 1998; Sloviter and Pedley 1998). As discussed later, the finding that hippocampal sclerosis is associated more frequently with developmental anomalies such as cortical dysplasia and heterotopias than with other structural lesions may support the second explanation (Raymond *et al* 1994; Cendes *et al* 1995b; Watson *et al* 1997a; Fernandez *et al* 1998; Sloviter and Pedley 1998).

A related question concerns whether hippocampal sclerosis is the cause of repeated seizures or is a consequence of them. Several investigations have shown that no significant relationship exists between atrophy of medial temporal lobe structures and the duration and frequency of seizures (Cendes *et al* 1993a,b, 1995b; Kuks *et al* 1993; Trenerry *et al* 1993a). These studies, along with the febrile convulsion studies mentioned above, suggest that hippocampal sclerosis is caused by an insult early in life that remains relatively stable and that each subsequent seizure does not cause significant additional neuronal cell loss or progressive worsening of hippocampal atrophy. However, further progressive damage over time may be superimposed and other imaging modalities such as magnetic resonance spectroscopy (MRS) may be able to detect this more subtle additional damage (Mathern *et al* 1995; Van Paesschen *et al* 1997a).

SPECIFICITY IN DETECTING HIPPOCAMPAL SCLEROSIS

Several studies have investigated groups of patients with seizures originating in extratemporal and extrahippocampal sites using volumetric MRI as a means of determining if seizures emanating from sites other than the hippocampus and amygdala cause cell loss and subsequent atrophy of those structures, thereby leading to significantly reduced volumes of the hippocampus and amygdala (Cook *et al* 1992; Cascino *et al* 1993; Cendes *et al* 1995b; Gilmore *et al* 1995; Watson *et al* 1996b). In patients with longstanding epilepsy due to extratemporal structural lesions, some studies showed no reduction in hippocampal volumes (Cook *et al* 1992; Watson and Williamson 1994; Cendes *et al* 1995b), and others found a low incidence (6–10.5%) of 'dual pathology,' a condition in which the patient has both a potentially epileptogenic structural lesion and hippocampal sclerosis (Cascino *et al* 1993; Cendes *et al* 1995b; Gilmore *et al* 1995; Watson and Williamson 1995; Watson *et al* 1996b).

BILATERAL TEMPORAL LOBE EPILEPSY

The management of patients with bilateral, independent temporal lobe seizure onset represents one of the greatest challenges in a surgical epilepsy program. Preliminary studies seem to indicate that MRI volumetric studies may be useful in helping to make those surgical decisions (Cascino *et al* 1995; Jack *et al* 1995; King *et al* 1995; Arruda *et al* 1996; Cendes *et al* 1996; Free *et al* 1996). In the presence of bilateral hippocampal atrophy, if the more profoundly atrophic side coincides with the side of more frequent seizure onsets, as determined by extracranial or intracranial video-EEG recording, anterior temporal lobe removal or selective amygdalohippocampectomy may be successful in controlling the patient's seizures (Jack *et al* 1992a, 1995; King *et al* 1995; Arruda *et al* 1996; Cendes *et al* 1996).

T2 RELAXOMETRY

Abnormal T2-weighted signal intensity in the hippocampus may be difficult to detect visually, and T2 mapping provides an objective means of assessing signal abnormality. Jackson *et al* (1993) investigated 50 adult patients suffering from intractable partial epilepsy with MRI optimized to detect hippocampal and cortical gray matter abnormalities, and with T2 relaxation mapping. The range of normal hippocampal T2 relaxation times varied between 99 and 106 ms, and the measurements were reproducible between observers. There were abnormal hippocampal T2 relaxation times in the hippocampus ipsilateral to the site of seizure origin in 70% of patients studied, with the more severe abnormality in the ipsilateral hippocampus in all cases. All hippocampal T2 measurements >116 ms were associated with TLE and histopathologic or MRI evidence of hippocampal sclerosis. Bilateral abnormalities were present in 29% of patients with hippocampal sclerosis.

In another study, Jackson *et al* (1994) studied six patients with MRI and histopathologic evidence of hip-

pocampal sclerosis but no detectable hippocampal atrophy. Loss of normal internal structure and T1- and T2-weighted signal abnormalities allowed the MRI diagnosis of unilateral hippocampal sclerosis when hippocampal volume measurements were normal and symmetric. Although accurate hippocampal volume measurements determine the most severely affected side in most cases, volume measurements or atrophy alone do not always detect all MRI-visible pathology. In patients with TLE and normal hippocampal volumes, additional detailed assessment, such as T2 relaxometry or MRS, may be required before structural abnormality of the hippocampus is excluded (Jackson *et al* 1994; Cendes *et al* 1997a).

T2 quantification appears to be able to detect very mild, bilateral, and progressive hippocampal pathology. Because this technique also provides numerical data, it has great potential for research and for monitoring progression of disease (Jackson *et al* 1994; Kuzniecky and Jackson 1995; Van Paesschen *et al* 1996, 1997a,b). In addition, T2 values can be interpreted in terms of hippocampal pathology, even when the other hippocampus is incomplete or distorted, such as when a lesion is present or after temporal lobe removal (Jackson 1994).

PROTON MAGNETIC RESONANCE SPECTROSCOPY

The MRS signal from ^{1}H (proton MRS) is inherently stronger than that from any other nucleus. Nearly all concentrated metabolites contain ^{1}H nuclei, which in principle could be used to identify them in ^{1}H spectra (Gadian 1995). The signal from ^{1}H nuclei in water is so strong that the much weaker signals from other compounds are hard to detect in its presence. However, techniques for eliminating the water resonance have been successfully applied to living systems (Gadian 1995).

PROTON SPECTRA OF THE HUMAN BRAIN

Water-suppressed, localized magnetic resonance spectra of normal human brain at 'long' echo times (TE 136–272 ms) reveal four major resonances (Gadian 1995) (Fig. 44.13):

1. one at 3.2 ppm, which arises from tetramethylamines (mainly from choline-containing phospholipids) (Cho);
2. one at 3.0 ppm, which arises primarily from creatine and phosphocreatine (Cr);
3. one at 2.0 ppm, which arises from *N*-acetyl groups, mainly *N*-acetylaspartate (NAA);

Right hemisphere

Left hemisphere

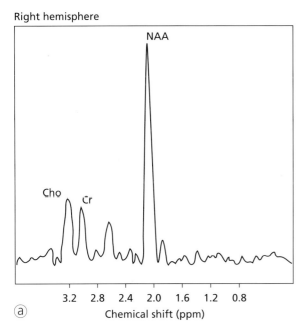
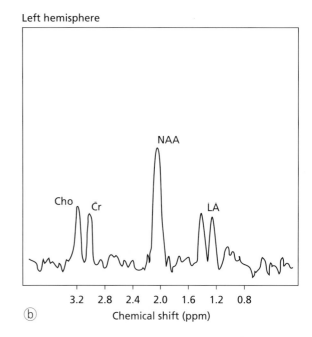

Fig. 44.13 Proton magnetic resonance spectra (TE 272 ms) from the frontocentral regions in a patient with Rasmussen encephalitis presenting with epilepsia partialis continua. The spectra in (b) is from the affected hemisphere: there is a decrease of the *N*-acetylaspartate (NAA) resonance intensity (2.0 ppm) and an abnormally high lactate (LA) peak. Cho, choline-containing compounds; Cr, creatine and phosphocreatine.

4. one at 1.3 ppm, which arises from the methyl resonance of lactate or, in certain pathologic conditions, methyl groups of lipids.

Lipids and other compounds (including inositol, γ-aminobutyric acid, and glutamate) are better observed using much shorter echo times because of short values of T2 and J-modulation effects (Gadian 1995).

Multiple lines of evidence support the use of NAA as a neuronal marker. It is found exclusively in neurons and their processes in the mature brain (Moffett *et al* 1991; Simmons *et al* 1991). In human brain spectra, *in vivo* NAA is reduced in situations known to be associated with neuronal loss, e.g. neuronal degenerative disorders (van der Knaap *et al* 1992), stroke (Duijn *et al* 1992), and glial tumors (Preul *et al* 1996). When decreases in the relative NAA signal arise from neuronal or axonal degeneration, irreversible changes are expected. However, there have been observations of reversible decreases in NAA in a number of conditions, emphasizing that neuronal dysfunction or transient relative volume changes can also lead to decreased NAA (De Stefano *et al* 1995a,b). The ability to quantify neuronal loss or damage specifically is one of the most interesting potential applications of MRS in cerebral disorders.

Changes in the resonance intensity of Cho probably result mainly from increases in the steady-state levels of phosphocholine and glycerol-phosphocholine. These choline-containing membrane phospholipids are released during active myelin breakdown (De Stefano *et al* 1995a). Certain tumors, e.g. meningiomas, may be associated with high steady-state levels of Cho (Preul *et al* 1996).

Total Cr concentration is relatively constant throughout the brain and tends to be relatively resistant to change. However, large changes can be seen with destructive pathology such as malignant tumors (Preul *et al* 1996). It is reasonable to use creatine as an internal standard to normalize resonance intensities of NAA and Cho in order to correct for artifactual variations in signal intensity due to magnetic field and radiofrequency inhomogeneity. However, this must be done with caution (Gadian 1995; Cendes *et al* 1997a,b).

Lactic acid is the endproduct of glycolysis and accumulates when oxidative metabolism cannot meet energy requirements (Duijn *et al* 1992; Ebisu *et al* 1994; De Stefano *et al* 1995a; Preul *et al* 1996). Brain lactate is elevated by seizure activity, as demonstrated by conventional biochemical studies of excised tissue. *In vivo* animal studies using proton MRS allowed more dynamic studies and a better appreciation of how persistent lactate elevation is after even a brief convulsive seizure (Ebisu *et al* 1994; Cendes *et al* 1997c). Selective neuronal injury by kainate-induced status epilepticus in rats was associated with focal reduction of NAA determined by proton MRS imaging, even before T2-weighted MRI changes were observed (Ebisu *et al* 1994).

PROTON MRS STUDIES IN PARTIAL EPILEPSIES

An early use of proton MRS in the context of human epilepsy was for the analysis of extracts of samples from temporal lobe tissue resected for treatment of drug-resistant TLE (Petroff *et al* 1989). This type of *in vitro* study is a useful source of information about concentrations of several human brain metabolites that are observable with *in vivo* MRS studies.

The first observations of an association between a seizure disorder and elevated brain lactate (and also reduced NAA) detected *in vivo* by proton MRS were reported by Matthews *et al* (1990) in two patients with Rasmussen syndrome. Subsequent proton MRS studies have shown focal reductions of NAA signal in patients with nonlesional TLE (Petroff *et al* 1989; Matthews *et al* 1990; Hugg *et al* 1993; Breiter *et al* 1994; Connelly *et al* 1994; Gadian *et al* 1994; Ng *et al* 1994; Vainio *et al* 1994; Cendes *et al* 1995c, 1997a,c; Garcia *et al* 1995a; Hetherington *et al* 1995; Cross *et al* 1996) and extratemporal partial epilepsies (Cendes *et al* 1995d; Garcia *et al* 1995b; Stanley *et al* 1998). Decreases in NAA correlate strongly with EEG abnormalities and severity of cell loss, and may be a more sensitive measure than qualitative or quantitative MRI measures of mesial temporal atrophy. However, the NAA decrease is more widespread than just at the epileptogenic focus, although it appears to be maximal at the site of the seizure generator (Cendes *et al* 1997a). The results of published MRS studies suggest that in patients with partial epilepsy there is a metabolic abnormality throughout the brain, with patterns of asymmetry and focal accentuation that are useful for noninvasive localization of epileptogenic foci

(Petroff *et al* 1989; Matthews *et al* 1990; Hugg *et al* 1993; Breiter *et al* 1994; Connelly *et al* 1994; Gadian *et al* 1994; Ng *et al* 1994; Vainio *et al* 1994; Cendes *et al* 1995c,d, 1997a,c; Garcia *et al* 1995a,b; Hetherington *et al* 1995; Cross *et al* 1996; Stanley *et al* 1998) (Table 44.2).

The initial MRS studies on TLE were limited by two factors. First, the lateralization of the TLE was not always known (Gadian *et al* 1994; Gadian 1995), so that agreement between the spectroscopic data and clinical-EEG lateralization could not be determined. Second, the spectra were obtained from single volumes, the location of which was determined from the MRI prior to acquiring the spectra. Thus, there was no way of knowing whether the spectra were acquired from regions of maximal abnormality, i.e. whether the studies were optimized. The latter uncertainty can be resolved by MRS imaging (MRSI), which allows analysis of the regional distribution of the metabolic abnormality and selection of the volume of maximal abnormality after data acquisition. This should confer an advantage on MRSI over single-voxel MRS techniques (Cendes *et al* 1997a).

We analyzed the findings of proton MRSI and MRIVol in a series of 100 consecutive patients with TLE (Cendes *et al* 1997a). We wished to determine how accurately each of these techniques, and the combination of both, could 'predict' lateralization of TLE as determined after extensive EEG investigation. The NAA/Cr values were abnormally low in at least one temporal lobe in *all but one* patient and were low bilaterally in 54%. The asymmetry between right and left sides with regard to NAA/Cr lateralized 86/93 (92.5%) of patients who had lateralization by ictal EEG. There were seven patients with no clear lateralization by

Table 44.2 Proton MRS studies in temporal lobe epilepsy.

Reference	No. of patients	Ipsilateral decreased NAA	Contralateral decreased NAA	Lateralization in agreement with EEG	Lateralization opposite to the EEG
Breiter *et al* (1994)	7	7 (100%)	0	7 (100%)	0
Cendes *et al* (1997a)	100	100 (100%)	54 (54%)	84 (84%)[a]	2 (2%)[b]
Connelly *et al* (1994)	25[c]	22 (88%)	10 (40%)	15 (60%)	3 (12%)
Cross *et al* (1996)	20[c]	15 (75%)	9 (45%)	11 (55%)	0
Hetherington *et al* (1995)	10	10 (100%)	4 (40%)	10 (100%)	0
Hugg *et al* (1993)	8	8 (100%)	–	8 (100%)	0
Ng *et al* (1994)	25	23 (92%)	3 (12%)	21 (84%)	2 (8%)
Vainio *et al* (1994)	7[c]	7 (100%)	–	7 (100%)	0
Total	202	192 (95.0%)	80 (42.8%)	163 (80.7%)	7 (3.5%)

NAA, *N*-acetylaspartate.
[a]The remaining patients had bilateral MRS abnormalities with no definite lateralization, all of whom had bitemporal EEG abnormalities.
[b]Patients with bitemporal temporal lobe epilepsy; one of them was operated on the side of the EEG lateralization with poor outcome.
[c]Single-voxel MRS.

EEG. The MRSI lateralization was ipsilateral to the EEG in all but two patients, who had bilateral TLE and bilateral amygdalohippocampal atrophy greater on the same side as the MRSI. Of 13 patients with normal MRIVol, 12 had a significant decrease of NAA/Cr within the mesial temporal lobe ipsilateral to the ictal EEG focus. Seven of these underwent surgery and the histopathology showed mild MTS. We concluded that MRSI detects abnormalities in almost all patients with TLE and can lateralize most of these. MRSI also lateralizes most TLE patients with normal MRIVol. Bitemporal abnormalities are detected more frequently by MRSI than by MRIVol. In some patients with bitemporal abnormalities not lateralized by MRSI, MRIVol can provide lateralization. Combination of these two techniques thus improves lateralization of TLE and can reduce the need for costly prolonged hospitalizations and invasive presurgical EEG investigations, as well as providing insights into the pathologic substrate of TLE (Cendes *et al* 1997a).

KEY POINTS

1. Thin coronal MRI slices, perpendicular to the axis of the hippocampus, give the best images for determining hippocampal sclerosis and other subtle pathologies and for ascertaining anatomic detail.

2. MRI features of hippocampal sclerosis, detectable by visual inspection of the images, include:
   (a) hippocampal smallness (atrophy), which is the most specific and reliable feature;
   (b) increased T2 signal, which in isolation may be insufficient to diagnose hippocampal sclerosis;
   (c) loss of internal structure. There may also be asymmetry of the horns of the lateral ventricles, which is variable and may lead to false lateralization, and atrophy of the anterior temporal lobe, which is nonspecific. T2 mapping is an objective method for measuring abnormal T2 signal, which may be difficult to detect visually.

3. Most patients with hippocampal sclerosis undergoing presurgical evaluation have one hippocampus that is clearly smaller than the other on visual inspection and which has increased T2 signal, along with a normal appearing contralateral hippocampus, so that volume measurement is not necessary for clinical purposes. The visual binary paradigm breaks down in the presence of symmetric bilateral atrophy or mild unilateral disease. In these cases volumetric MRI analysis of the hippocampus and the amygdala are very sensitive and specific for identifying hippocampal sclerosis.

4. MRI measurements of hippocampal volumes are a surrogate for histopathologic methods of assessing the presence and severity of neuronal loss in each hippocampus, allowing each to be classed as normal or abnormal. This may give useful prognostic information concerning postoperative seizure control. Surgical treatment of strictly unilateral hippocampal sclerosis should give >90% excellent outcome.

5. Proton MRS lateralizes most cases of TLE with normal MRI and detects bilateral abnormalities more often than does volumetric MRI, although the greater sensitivity of MRS is not invariable.

REFERENCES

Abou-Khalil B, Andermann E, Andermann F, Olivier A, Quesney LF (1993) Temporal lobe epilepsy after prolonged febrile convulsions: excellent outcome after surgical treatment. *Epilepsia* **34**:878–883.

Amaral DG, Insausti R (1990) Hippocampal formation. In: Paxinos G (ed) *The Human Nervous System*, pp 711–755. New York: Academic Press.

Arruda F, Cendes F, Andermann F *et al* (1996) Mesial atrophy and outcome after amygdalohippocampectomy or temporal lobe removal. *Annals of Neurology* **40**:446–450.

Ashtari M, Barr WB, Schaul N, Bogerts B (1991) Three-dimensional fast low-angle shot imaging and computerized volume measurement of the hippocampus in patients with chronic epilepsy of the temporal lobe. *American Journal of Neuroradiology* **12**:941–947.

Babb TL, Brown WJ (1987) Pathological findings in epilepsy. In: Engel J Jr (ed) *Surgical Treatment of the Epilepsies*, pp 511–540. New York: Raven Press.

Bailey P, Gibbs FA (1951) Surgical treatment of psychomotor epilepsy. *Journal of the American Medical Association* **145**:365–370.

Bastos AC, Korah IP, Cendes F *et al* (1995) Curvilinear reconstruction of 3D magnetic resonance imaging in patients with partial epilepsy: a pilot study. *Magnetic Resonance Imaging* **13**:1107–1112.

Berg AT, Darefsky AS, Holford TR, Shinnar S (1998) Seizures with fever after unprovoked seizures: an analysis in children followed from the time of a first febrile seizure. *Epilepsia* **39**:77–80.

Berkovic SF, Andermann F, Olivier A *et al* (1991) Hippocampal sclerosis in temporal lobe epilepsy demonstrated by magnetic resonance imaging. *Annals of Neurology* **29**:175–182.

Berkovic SF, McIntosh AM, Kalnins RM *et al* (1995) Preoperative MRI predicts outcome of temporal lobectomy: an actuarial analysis. *Neurology* **45**:1358–1363.

Breiter SN, Arroyo S, Mathews VP, Lesser RP, Bryan RN, Barker PB (1994) Proton MR spectroscopy in patients with seizure disorders. *American Journal of Neuroradiology* **15**:373–384.

Bruton CJ (1988) *The Neuropathology of Temporal Lobe Epilepsy.* New York: Oxford University Press.

Cascino GD, Jack CR, Parisi JE *et al* (1991) Magnetic resonance imaging-based volume studies in temporal lobe epilepsy: pathological correlations. *Annals of Neurology* **30**:31–36.

Cascino GD, Jack CR Jr, Hirschorn KA, Sharbrough FW (1992) Identification of the epileptic focus: magnetic resonance imaging. *Epilepsy Research* Suppl **5**:95–100.

Cascino GD, Jack CR Jr, Sharbrough FW, Kelly PJ, Marsh WR (1993) MRI assessments of hippocampal pathology in extratemporal lesional epilepsy. *Neurology* **43**:2380–2382.

Cascino GD, Trenerry MR, Sharbrough FW, So EL, Marsh WR, Strelow DC (1995) Depth electrode studies in temporal lobe epilepsy: relation to quantitative magnetic resonance imaging and operative outcome. *Epilepsia* **36**:230–235.

Cascino GD, Trenerry MR, So EL *et al* (1996) Routine EEG and temporal lobe epilepsy: relation to long-term EEG monitoring, quantitative MRI, and operative outcome. *Epilepsia* **37**:651–656.

Cendes F, Andermann F, Gloor P *et al* (1993a) Atropy of mesial structures in patients with temporal lobe epilepsy: cause or consequence of repearted seizures? *Annals of Neurology* **34**:795–801.

Cendes F, Andermann F, Dubeau F *et al* (1993b) Early childhood prolonged febrile convulsions, atrophy and sclerosis of mesial structures and temporal lobe epilepsy: an MRI volumetric study. *Neurology* **43**:1083–1087.

Cendes F, Leproux F, Melanson D *et al* (1993c) MRI of amygdala and hippocampus in temporal lobe epilepsy. *Journal of Computer Assisted Tomography* **17**:206–210.

Cendes F, Andermann F, Gloor P *et al* (1993d) MRI volumetric measurements of amygdala and hippocampus in temporal lobe epilepsy. *Neurology* **43**:719–725.

Cendes F, Andermann F, Gloor P *et al* (1994) Relationship between atrophy of the amygdala and ictal fear in temporal lobe epilepsy. *Brain* **117**:739–746.

Cendes F, Arruda F, Dubeau F, Gotman J, Andermann F, Arnold DL (1995a) Relationship between mesial temporal atrophy and ictal and interictal EEG findings: results in a series of 250 patients (abstract). *Epilepsia* **36** (Suppl 4):23.

Cendes F, Cook MJ, Watson C *et al* (1995b) Frequency and characteristics of dual pathology in patients with lesional epilepsy. *Neurology* **45**:2058–2064.

Cendes F, Andermann F, Dubeau F, Arnold DL (1995c) Proton magnetic resonance spectroscopic imagaging and MRI volumetric studies for lateralization of temporal lobe epilepsy. *Magnetic Resonance Imaging* **13**:1187–1191.

Cendes F, Andermann F, Silver K, Arnold DL (1995d) Imaging of axonal damage *in vivo* in Rasmussen's syndrome. *Brain* **118**:753–758.

Cendes F, Dubeau F, Andermann F *et al* (1996) Significance of mesial temporal atrophy in relation to intracranial ictal and interictal stereo EEG abnormalities. *Brain* **119**:1317–1326.

Cendes F, Caramanos Z, Andermann F, Dubeau F, Arnold DL (1997a) Proton magnetic resonance spectroscopic imaging and magnetic resonance imaging volumetry in the lateralization of temporal lobe epilepsy: a series of 100 patients. *Annals of Neurology* **42**:737–746.

Cendes F, Andermann F, Dubeau F, Matthews PM, Arnold DL (1997b) Normalization of neuronal metabolic dysfunction after surgery for temporal lobe epilepsy. Evidence from proton MR spectroscopic imaging. *Neurology* **49**:1525–1533.

Cendes F, Stanley JA, Dubeau F, Andermann F, Arnold DL (1997c) Proton magnetic resonance spectroscopic imaging for discrimination of absence and complex partial seizures. *Annals of Neurology* **41**:74–81.

Collins DL, Neelin P, Peters TM, Evans AC (1994) Automatic 3D inter-subject registration of MR volumetric data in standardized Talairach space. *Journal of Computer Assisted Tomography* **18**:192–205.

Commission on Neuroimaging of the International League Against Epilepsy (1997) Recommendations for neuroimaging of patients with epilepsy. *Epilepsia* **38**:1255–1256.

Connelly A, Jackson GD, Duncan JS, King MD, Gadian DG (1994) Magnetic resonance spectroscopy in temporal lobe epilepsy. *Neurology* **44**:1411–1417.

Cook MJ, Fish DR, Shorvon SD, Straughan K, Stevens JM (1992) Hippocampal volumetric and morphometric studies in frontal and temporal lobe epilepsy. *Brain* **115**:1001–1015.

Cross JH, Connelly A, Jackson GD, Johnson CL, Neville BGR, Gadian DG (1996) Proton magnetic resonance spectroscopy in children with temporal lobe epilepsy. *Annals of Neurology* **39**:107–113.

De Stefano N, Matthews PM, Antel JP, Preul M, Francis G, Arnold DL (1995a) Chemical pathology of acute demyelinating lesions and its correlation with disability. *Annals of Neurology* **38**:901–909.

De Stefano N, Matthews PM, Arnold DL (1995b) Reversible decreases in *N*-acetylaspartate after acute brain injury. *Magnetic Resonance in Medicine* **34**:721–727.

Doose H (1998) Contradictory conclusions about the possible effects of prolonged febrile convulsions (letter). *Epilepsia* **39**:108–110.

Duchowny MS, Harvey AS, Sperling MR, Williamson PD (1997) Indications and criteria for surgical intervention. In: Engel J Jr, Pedley TA (eds) *Epilepsy: A Comprehensive Textbook*, pp 1677–1685. Philadelphia: Lippincott-Raven.

Duijn JH, Matson GB, Maudsley AA, Hugg JW, Weiner MW (1992) Human brain infarction: proton MR spectroscopy. *Radiology* **183**:711–718.

Duvernoy HM (1991) *The Human Brain: Surface, Three-dimensional Sectional Anatomy and MRI.* Wien: Springer-Verlag.

Earle KM, Baldwin M, Penfield W (1953) Incisural sclerosis and temporal lobe seizures produced by hippocampal herniation at birth. *Archives of Neurology and Psychiatry* **69**:27–42.

Ebisu T, Rooney WD, Graham SH, Weiner MW, Maudsley AA (1994) *N*-Acetylaspartate as an *in vivo* marker of neuronal viability in kainate-induced status epilepticus: ^{1}H magnetic resonance spectroscopic imaging. *Journal of Cerebral Blood Flow and Metabolism* **14**:373–382.

Engel J Jr, Van Ness PC, Rasmussen T, Ojemann LM (1993a) Outcome with respect to epileptic seizures. In: Engel J Jr (ed) *Surgical Treatment of the Epilepsies*, 2nd edn, pp 609–621. New York: Raven Press.

Engel J Jr, Burchfiel J, Ebersole J *et al* (1993b) Long-term monitoring for epilepsy. Report of an IFCN committee. *Eletroencephalography and Clinical Neurophysiology* **87**:437–458.

Engel J Jr, Cascino GD, Shields WD (1997) Surgically remediable syndromes. In: Engel J Jr, Pedley TA (eds) *Epilepsy: A Comprehensive Textbook*, pp 1687–1696. Philadelphia: Lippincott-Raven.

Feindel W (1991) Development of surgical therapy of epilepsy at the Montreal Neurological Institute. *Canadian Journal of Neurological Science* **18**:549–553.

Feindel W, Penfield W (1954) Localization of discharge in temporal lobe automatism. *Archives of Neurology and Psychiatry* **72**:605–630.

Fernandez G, Effenberger O, Vinz B *et al* (1998) Hippocampal malformation as a cause of familial febrile convulsions and subsequent hippocampal sclerosis. *Neurology* **50**:909–917.

Free SL, Li LM, Fish DR, Shorvon SD, Stevens JM (1996) Bilateral hippocampal volume loss in patients with a history of encephalitis or meningitis. *Epilepsia* **37**:400–405.

Gadian DG (1995) *Nuclear Magnetic Resonance and its Applications to Living Systems*, 2nd edn. Oxford: Oxford University Press.

Gadian DG, Connelly A, Duncan JS *et al* (1994) ^{1}H magnetic resonance spectroscopy in the investigation of intractable epilepsy. *Acta Neurologica Scandinavica* Suppl **152**:116–121.

Gambardella A, Reutens DC, Andermann F *et al* (1994) Late-onset drop attacks in temporal lobe epilepsy: a reevaluation of the concept of temporal lobe syncope. *Neurology* **44**:1074–1078.

Gambardella A, Gotman J, Cendes F, Andermann F (1995a) The relationship of spike foci and of clinical seizure characteristics to different patterns of mesial temporal atrophy. *Archives of Neurology* **52**:287–293.

Gambardella A, Gotman J, Cendes F, Andermann F (1995b) Focal intermittent delta activity in patients with mesiotemporal atrophy: a reliable marker of the epileptogenic focus. *Epilepsia* **36**:122–129.

Garcia PA, Laxer KD, Barbaro NM, Dillon WP (1994) Prognostic value of qualitative magnetic resonance imaging hippocampal abnormalities in patients undergoing temporal lobectomy for medically refractory seizures. *Epilepsia* **35**:520–524.

Garcia PA, Laxer KD, Ng T (1995a) Application of spectroscopic imaging in epilepsy. *Magnetic Resonance Imaging* **13**:1181–1185.

Garcia PA, Laxer KD, van der Grond J, Hugg JW, Matson GB, Weiner MW (1995b) Proton magnetic resonance spectroscopic imaging in patients with frontal lobe epilepsy. *Annals of Neurology* **37**:279–281.

Gilmore RL, Childress MD, Leonard C *et al* (1995) Hippocampal volumetrics differentiate patients with temporal lobe epilepsy and extratemporal lobe epilepsy. *Archives of Neurology* **52**:819–824.

Gloor P (1991) Mesial temporal sclerosis: historical background and an overview from a modern perspective. In: Luders H (ed) *Epilepsy Surgery*, pp 689–703. New York: Raven Press.

Gloor P (1997) *The Temporal Lobe and Limbic System*. New York: Oxford University Press.

Gumnit RJ (1991) Cost, accessibility, and quality-of-life issues in surgery for epilepsy. In: Luders H (ed) *Epilepsy Surgery*, pp 47–49. New York: Raven Press.

Hamati-Haddad A, Abou-Khalil B (1998) Epilepsy diagnosis and localization in patients with antecedent childhood febrile convulsions. *Neurology* **50**:917–922.

Hauser WA, Annegers JF, Rocca WA (1996) Descriptive epidemiology of epilepsy: contributions of population-based studies from Rochester, Minnesota. *Mayo Clinic Proceedings* **71**:576–586.

Hermann BP, Wyler AR, Somes G, Berry AD 3rd, Dohan FC Jr (1992) Pathological status of the mesial temporal lobe predicts memory outcome from left anterior temporal lobectomy. *Neurosurgery* **31**:652–656.

Hetherington H, Kuzniecky R, Pan J *et al* (1995) Proton nuclear magnetic resonance spectroscopic imaging of human temporal lobe epilepsy at 4.1 T. *Annals of Neurology* **38**:396–404.

Ho SS, Kuzniecky RI, Gilliam F, Faught E, Morawetz R (1998) Temporal lobe developmental malformations and epilepsy: dual pathology and bilateral hippocampal abnormalities. *Neurology* **50**:748–754.

Hugg JW, Laxer KD, Matson GB, Maudsley AA, Weiner MW (1993) Neuron loss localizes human temporale lobe epilepsy by *in vivo* proton magnetic resonance spectroscopic imaging. *Annals of Neurology* **34**:788–794.

Jack CR Jr (1994) MRI-based hippocampal volume measurements in epilepsy. *Epilepsia* **35** (Suppl 6):S21–S29.

Jack CR Jr, Twomey CK, Zinsmeister AR, Sharbrough FW, Petersen RC, Cascino GD (1989) Anterior temporal lobes and hippocampal formations: normative volumetric measurements from MR images in young adults. *Radiology* **172**:549–554.

Jack CR, Sharbrough FW, Twomey CK *et al* (1990) Temporal lobe seizures: lateralization with MR volume measurements of the hippocampal formation. *Radiology* **175**:423–429.

Jack CR, Sharbrough FW, Cascino GD, Hirschorn KA, O'Brien PC, Marsh WR (1992a) Magnetic resonance image-based hippocampal volumetry: correlation with outcome after temporal lobectomy. *Annals of Neurology* **31**:138–146.

Jack CR Jr, Petersen RC, O'Brien PC, Tangalos EG (1992b) MR-based hippocampal volumetry in the diagnosis of Alzheimer's disease. *Neurology* **42**:183–188.

Jack CR Jr, Trenerry MR, Cascino GD, Sharbrough FW, So EL, O'Brien PC (1995) Bilaterally symmetric hippocampi and surgical outcome. *Neurology* **45**:1353–1358.

Jack CR Jr, Rydberg CH, Krecke KN *et al* (1996) Mesial temporal sclerosis: diagnosis with fluid-attenuated inversion-recovery versus spin-echo MR imaging. *Radiology* **199**:367–373.

Jackson GD (1994) New techniques in magnetic resonance and epilepsy. *Epilepsia* **35** (Suppl 6):S2–S13.

Jackson GD, Berkovic SF, Tress BM, Kalnins RM, Fabinyi GC, Bladin PF (1990) Hippocampal sclerosis can be reliably detected by magnetic resonance imaging. *Neurology* **40**:1869–1875.

Jackson GD, Connelly A, Duncan JS, Grunewald RA, Gadian DG (1993) Detection of hippocampal pathology in intractable partial epilepsy: increased sensitivity with quantitative magnetic resonance T2 relaxometry. *Neurology* **43**:1793–1799.

Jackson GD, Kuzniecky RI, Cascino GD (1994) Hippocampal sclerosis without detectable hippocampal atrophy. *Neurology* **44**:42–46.

Jones-Gotman M, Brulot M, McMackin D *et al* (1993a) World and design list learning deficits related to side of hippocampal atrophy as assessed by volumetric MRI measurements (abstract). *Epilepsia* **34** (Suppl 6):71.

Jones-Gotman M, Brulot M, McMackin D *et al* (1993b) Performance on intracarotid sodium amobarbital memory tests: relationship to hippocampal atrophy as estimated by volumetric MRI (abstract). *Epilepsia* **34** (Suppl 6):94.

Jones-Gotman M, Zatorre RJ, Olivier A *et al* (1997) Learning and retention of words and designs following excision from medial or lateral temporal-lobe structures. *Neuropsychologia* **35**:963–973.

Kanemoto K, Takuji N, Kawasaki J, Kawai I (1998) Characteristics and treatment of temporal lobe epilepsy with a history of complicated febrile convulsion. *Journal of Neurology, Neurosurgery and Psychiatry* **64**:245–248.

Kim JH, Tien RD, Felsberg GJ, Osumi AK, Lee N, Friedman AH (1995) Fast spin-echo MR in hippocampal sclerosis: correlation with pathology and surgery. *American Journal of Neuroradiology* **16**:627–636.

King D, Spencer SS, McCarthy G, Luby M, Spencer DD (1995) Bilateral hippocampal atrophy in medial temporal lobe epilepsy. *Epilepsia* **36**:905–910.

Kuks JB, Cook MJ, Fish DR, Stevens JM, Shorvon SD (1993) Hippocampal sclerosis in epilepsy and childhood febrile seizures. *Lancet* **342**:1391–1394.

Kuzniecky RI, Jackson GD (1995) *Magnetic Resonance in Epilepsy*, pp 107–183. New York: Raven Press.

Kuzniecky R, de la Sayette V, Ethier R *et al* (1987) Magnetic resonance imaging in temporal lobe epilepsy: pathological correlations. *Annals of Neurology* **22**:341–347.

Lee N, Tien RD, Lewis DV *et al* (1995) Fast spin-echo, magnetic resonance imaging-measured hippocampal volume: correlation with neuronal density in anterior temporal lobectomy patients. *Epilepsia* **36**:899–904.

Lencz T, McCarthy G, Bronen RA *et al* (1992) Quantitative magnetic resonance imaging in temporal lobe epilepsy: relationship to neuropathology and neuropsychological function. *Annals of Neurology* **31**:629–637.

Li LM, Cendes F, Watson C *et al* (1997) Surgical treatment of patients with single and dual pathology: relevance of lesion and of hippocampal atrophy to seizure outcome. *Neurology* **48**:437–444.

Loring DW, Murro AM, Meador KJ *et al* (1993) Wada memory testing and hippocampal volume measurements in the evaluation for temporal lobectomy. *Neurology* **43**:1789–1793.

Maher J, McLachlan RS (1995) Febrile convulsions. Is seizure duration the most important predictor of temporal lobe epilepsy? *Brain* **118**:1521–1528.

Mathern GW, Pretorius JK, Babb TL (1995) Influence of the type of initial precipitating injury and at what age it occurs on course and outcome in patients with temporal lobe seizures. *Journal of Neurosurgery* **82**:220–227.

Matthews PM, Andermann F, Arnold DL (1990) A proton magnetic resonance spectroscopy study of focal epilepsy in humans. *Neurology* **40**:985–989.

Meencke HJ, Veith G (1991) Hippocampal sclerosis in epilepsy. In: Luders H (ed) *Epilepsy Surgery*, pp 705–715. New York: Raven Press.

Moffett JR, Aryan MA, Namboodiri MAA, Cangro CB, Neale JH (1991) Immunohistochemical localization of *N*-acetylaspartate in rat brain. *NeuroReport* **2**:131–134.

Murro AM, Park YD, King DW *et al* (1993) Seizure localization in temporal lobe epilepsy: a comparison of scalp-sphenoidal EEG and volumetric MRI. *Neurology* **43**:2531–2533.

Ng TC, Comair YG, Xue M *et al* (1994) Temporal lobe epilepsy: presurgical localization with proton chemical shift imaging. *Radiology* **193**:465–472.

Penfield W, Flanigin H (1950) Surgical therapy of temporal lobe seizures. *Archives of Neurology and Psychiatry* **64**:491–500.

Penfield W, Jasper H (1954) *Epilepsy and the Functional Anatomy of the Human Brain*. Boston: Little, Brown.

Petroff OA, Spencer DD, Alger JR, Prichard JW (1989) High-field proton magnetic resonance spectroscopy of human cerebrum obtained during surgery for epilepsy. *Neurology* **39**:1197–1202.

Preul MC, Caramanos Z, Collins DL *et al* (1996) Accurate, noninvasive diagnosis of human brain tumors by using proton magnetic resonance spectroscopy. *Nature Medicine* **2**:323–325.

Raymond AA, Fish DR, Stevens JM, Cook MJ, Sisodiya SM, Shorvon SD (1994) Association of hippocampal sclerosis with cortical dysgenesis in patients with epilepsy. *Neurology* **44**:1841–1845.

Salanova V, Markand O, Worth R *et al* (1998) FDG-PET and MRI in temporal lobe epilepsy: relationship to febrile seizures, hippocampal sclerosis and outcome. *Acta Neurologica Scandinavica* **97**:146–153.

Shaw DW, Weinberger E, Astley SJ, Tsuruda JS (1997) Quantitative comparison of conventional spin echo and fast spin echo during brain myelination. *Journal of Computer Assisted Tomography* **21**:867–871.

Shinnar S (1998) Prolonged febrile seizures and mesial temporal sclerosis. *Annals of Neurology* **43**:411–412.

Simmons ML, Frondoza CG, Coyle JT (1991) Immunocytochemical localization of *N*-acetyl-aspartate with monoclonal antibodies. *Neuroscience* **45**:37–45.

Sinha U, Sinha S, Lufkin RB (1998) Magnetic resonance image formation. In: Lufkin RB (ed) *The MRI Manual*, 2nd edn, pp 41–99. St Louis: Mosby.

Sisodiya SM, Stevens JM, Fish DR, Free SL, Shorvon SD (1996) The demonstration of gyral abnormalities in patients with cryptogenic partial epilepsy using three-dimensional MRI. *Archives of Neurology* **53**:28–34.

Sloviter RS, Pedley TA (1998) Subtle hippocampal malformation: importance in febrile seizures and development of epilepsy. *Neurology* **50**:846–849.

Spencer SS, McCarthy G, Spencer DD (1993) Diagnosis of medial temporal lobe seizure onset: relative specificity and sensitivity of quantitative MRI. *Neurology* **43**:2117–2124.

Stanley JA, Cendes F, Dubeau F, Andermann F, Arnold DL (1998) Proton magnetic resonance spectroscopic imaging in patients with extratemporal epilepsy. *Epilepsia* **39**:267–273.

Trenerry MR, Jack CR Jr, Sharbrough FW *et al* (1993a) Quantitative MRI hippocampal volumes: association with onset and duration of epilepsy, and febrile convulsions in temporal lobectomy patients. *Epilepsy Research* **15**:247–252.

Trenerry MR, Jack CR Jr, Ivnik RJ *et al* (1993b) MRI hippocampal volumes and memory function before and after temporal lobectomy. *Neurology* **43**:1800–1805.

Trenerry MR, Jack CR Jr, Cascino GD, Sharbrough FW, Ivnik RJ (1995) Gender differences in post-temporal lobectomy verbal memory and relationships between MRI hippocampal volumes and preoperative verbal memory. *Epilepsy Research* **20**:69–76.

Trenerry MR, Jack CR, Cascino GD, Sharbrough FW, So EL (1996) Bilateral magnetic resonance imaging-determined hippocampal atrophy and verbal memory before and after temporal lobectomy. *Epilepsia* **37**:526–533.

Vainio P, Usenius JP, Vapalahti M *et al* (1994) Reduced *N*-acetylaspartate concentration in temporal lobe epilepsy by quantitative ^{1}H MRS *in vivo*. *NeuroReport* **5**:1733–1736.

van der Knaap MS, van der Grond J, Luyten PR, den Hollander JA, Nauta JJ, Valk J (1992) ^{1}H and ^{31}P magnetic resonance spectroscopy of the brain in degenerative cerebral disorders. *Annals of Neurology* **31**:202–211.

Van Landingham KE, Heinz ER, Cavazos JE, Lewis DV (1998) Magnetic resonance imaging evidence of hippocampal injury after prolonged focal febrile convulsions. *Annals of Neurology* **43**:413–426.

Van Paesschen W, Connelly A, Johnson CL, Duncan JS (1996) The amygdala and intractable temporal lobe epilepsy: a quantitative magnetic resonance imaging study. *Neurology* **47**:1021–1031.

Van Paesschen W, Connelly A, King MD, Jackson GD, Duncan JS (1997a) The spectrum of hippocampal sclerosis: a quantitative magnetic resonance imaging study. *Annals of Neurology* **41**:41–51.

Van Paesschen W, Revesz T, Duncan JS, King MD, Connelly A (1997b) Quantitative neuropathology and quantitative magnetic resonance imaging of the hippocampus in temporal lobe epilepsy. *Annals of Neurology* **42**:756–766.

Watson C, Williamson B (1994) Volumetric magnetic resonance imaging in patients with epilepsy and extratemporal lesions. *Journal of Epilepsy* **7**:80–87.

Watson C, Williamson B (1995) Volumetric magnetic resonance imaging in patients with primary generalized epilepsy. *Journal of Epilepsy* **8**:104–109.

Watson C, Andermann F, Gloor P *et al* (1992) Anatomic basis of amygdaloid and hippocampal volume measurement by magnetic resonance imaging. *Neurology* **42**:1743–1750.

Watson C, Nielsen SL, Cobb C, Burgerman R, Williamson B (1996a) Pathological grading system for hippocampal sclerosis: correlation with magnetic resonance imaging-based volume measurements of the hippocampus. *Journal of Epilepsy* **9**:56–64.

Watson C, Cendes F, Andermann F, Dubeau F, Williamson B, Evans A (1996b) Volumetric magnetic resonance imaging in patients with secondary generalized epilepsy. *Journal of Epilepsy* **9**:14–19.

Watson C, Jack CR Jr, Cendes F (1997a) Volumetric magnetic resonance imaging. Clinical applications and contributions to the understanding of temporal lobe epilepsy. *Archives of Neurology* **54**:1521–1531.

Watson C, Cendes F, Fuerst D *et al* (1997b) Specificity of volumetric magnetic resonance imaging in detecting hippocampal sclerosis. *Archives of Neurology* **54**:67–73.

Yousry TA, Filippi M, Becker C, Horsfield MA, Voltz R (1997) Comparison of MR pulse sequences in the detection of multiple sclerosis lesions. *American Journal of Neuroradiology* **18**:959–963.

Invasive neurophysiologic evaluation

RDC ELWES

It is sometimes difficult to localize epileptic foci on the basis of scalp EEG recordings alone. The appearance of epileptiform discharges in the scalp EEG is due to the summation of a cortical abnormality which has to cover an area of about $6\,cm^2$ before it is visible on surface recordings (Cooper *et al* 1965). Well-localized cortical spikes may not, therefore, be apparent on the scalp EEG. In many cases being evaluated for epilepsy surgery, the focus is on the mesial or basal aspect of the hemisphere and not immediately accessible to scalp electrodes placed in the 10/20 system. A further problem with scalp recordings is due to the propagation and rapid spread of epileptiform discharges. By the time the ictal changes are apparent on the scalp EEG the abnormality may be hemispheric, diffuse, or sometimes even falsely localizing.

In order to overcome the limitations of scalp EEG, most epilepsy surgery programs have developed some form of intracranial EEG evaluation. This is carried out by placing recording electrodes in the subdural space or by using stereotactic neurosurgical techniques to implant them directly into brain substance. The procedures are time-consuming, invasive, and require considerable expertise in both their execution and interpretation. Because of this most centers have concentrated on developing one particular technique and detailed descriptions of the various methods of carrying out intracranial EEG are available in a number of specialist publications (Wieser and Elger 1987; Luders 1991; Engel 1993). Rather than attempting to repeat these, this chapter concentrates more on the relative advantages of the different methods of recording intracranial EEG and assessing their overall place in the presurgical evaluation of patients with epilepsy. Particular emphasis is placed on describing their clinical indications and the impact of recent advances in both structural and functional imaging.

HISTORY

Following the development of stereotactic brain atlases in the 1950s, Talairach and Bancaud (1974) in Paris used these techniques to implant EEG electrodes into deep cortical structures in patients being assessed for epilepsy surgery. Initially acute intraoperative EEG recordings were used and the technique was termed stereo-EEG. With the development of chronic postoperative monitoring, great emphasis was placed on a detailed correlation of the EEG features with the clinical characteristics of the epileptic seizures. The implanted electrodes were also used to carry out functional stimulation so as to identify eloquent areas of brain that had to be preserved in any subsequent resective procedure. On the basis of these findings a specific tailored resection was designed for each patient depending on the extent of the epileptogenic zone and the need to avoid neurologic or cognitive deficits. The Paris group have had a major impact on the development of epilepsy surgery in continental Europe. Wieser and Yasargil in Zurich described mesiobasal epilepsy, developed the foramen ovale recording technique and went on to perform an extensive series of selective temporal lobe resections using the trans-sylvian amygdalohippocampectomy (Wieser 1983; Yasargil et al 1985; Yasargill and Wieser 1987). The Continental School has greatly influenced the electroclinical classification of seizures (Commission on Classification and Terminology of the International League Against Epilepsy 1981) and pioneered advances in the treatment of frontal lobe epilepsy (Geier et al 1975; Munari et al 1995a; Chauval et al 1998).

In North America the development of epilepsy surgery followed a different course. Gibbs et al (1948) described patients with psychomotor seizures which were associated with an anterior temporal EEG focus on the scalp EEG. Bailey then performed a series of anterior temporal resections guided by the surface EEG and intraoperative electrocorticography (ECoG) recordings (Bailey and Gibbs 1951). In Montreal, Jasper et al (1951) reported the findings in an extensive series of ECoG recordings and concluded that the most prominent area of electrical involvement was in fact the mesial or basal aspect of the temporal lobe. Crandall et al (1963) in Los Angeles combined stereotactic implantation of EEG electrodes into mesial temporal structures with the technical advances in telemetering biologic signals developed from the space exploration program. This group went on to show with chronic ictal EEG recordings in adults that most temporal lobe seizures do indeed start in the amygdala and hippocampus (Crandall et al 1983).

A separate approach to epilepsy surgery, placing more emphasis on the pathologic substrate of focal seizures, can be traced from the writings of Hughlings Jackson. He described lesions in the uncinate lobe and central areas of the brain in patients with dreamy states and focal motor seizures (Jackson 1870; 1888; 1899). He hypothesized that the lesions caused excessive discharges in the gray matter which gave rise to the symptoms of the seizures, thus providing Horsley (1886) with the rational basis to attempt the surgical removal of an epileptogenic lesion. This work was largely ignored in their own country but generated much enthusiasm in Europe, especially Germany, where interest in epilepsy surgery flourished (Wolf 1991). Penfield worked

with Sherrington in England, Ramon y Cajal in Spain, and Foerster in Germany, before establishing the Montreal Neurological Institute where he and his colleagues pioneered the development of epilepsy surgery. Prior to the discovery of EEG, surgery was largely directed at the removal of a visible lesion seen at the time of craniotomy and great emphasis was placed on the ability to reproduce the symptoms of the seizure by stimulating the surrounding brain. This work culminated in the classic text *Epilepsy and the Functional Anatomy of the Human Brain* (Penfield and Jasper 1954). While the publication of this book was a major landmark, it would appear that the early results of the surgery were conspicuously less successful (Penfield and Jasper 1954). Despite the writings of Hughlings Jackson, surgery on the temporal lobe had to await the invention of the EEG. Falconer (1971) at the Maudsley Hospital then developed the *en bloc* temporal lobectomy and his group went on to show that mesial temporal sclerosis (MTS) was the commonest underlying pathology (Falconer 1974), findings that were concordant with the electrophysiologic studies in Montreal and Los Angeles described above. Falconer went on to conclude that presence of pathology in the resected specimen was an important predictor of successful surgical outcome (Falconer and Serafetinides 1963).

PATHOLOGIC AND ELECTROCLINICAL EVALUATION

It is readily apparent that two divergent schools of thought have influenced the development of epilepsy surgery. The functional approach, typified by the Paris school, places great emphasis on detailed electroclinical evaluation followed by a tailored resection depending upon the limits of the epileptogenic zone and the need to avoid neurologic deficits. As might be expected, extensive use is made of intracranial EEG. A similar approach was used in Montreal, although here greater emphasis was placed on acute ECoG. By contrast the pathologic approach followed by Falconer at the Maudsley was directed toward using standard resections with a view to removing structurally abnormal brain. Neurologic and cognitive deficits were avoided by not extending the resection beyond established anatomic landmarks. A formal evaluation comparing these two techniques has never been undertaken, and the presence of two very divergent philosophies has led to much controversy in the literature which unfortunately has not been resolved to this day.

Successful epilepsy surgery can undoubtedly be carried out in appropriate cases without recourse to intracranial

EEG. This was demonstrated by Falconer long before advances in neuroimaging. He used a combination of meticulous clinical history, detailed interictal surface and sphenoidal EEG, air encephalograms, and additional tests of functional abnormality, such as drug-induced fast activity and neuropsychology, to predict the presence of mesial temporal sclerosis (Engel *et al* 1975). This tradition was carried on by both the Maudsley and Oxford epilepsy surgery programs. It is also likely, however, that when using these techniques a considerable number of cases with bilateral independent EEG abnormalities were inappropriately excluded from surgery and that many of these cases could have been successfully operated upon after intracranial EEG evaluation (Binnie *et al* 1994a).

Now that MTS can be diagnosed on high-resolution magnetic resonance imaging (MRI) presurgical evaluation has become much easier, which has been one of the factors that has led to a major expansion in epilepsy surgery (Sperling *et al* 1992; Kilpatrick *et al* 1997). About one-third of cases with pathologically proven MTS, however, fail following surgery and continue to have intractable seizures (Elwes *et al* 1991). The features that predict a poor outcome include the presence of extratemporal spikes, generalized epileptifom discharges, and frequent convulsive seizures, all of which indicate that the area capable of generating seizures may be much wider than the established pathology would suggest (Bengzon *et al* 1968). The study of human epilepsy immediately suggests that there are patients who have regional, hemispheric, or diffuse areas of epileptogenic brain tissue and it seems naïve to assume that there is one disease entity, called temporal lobe epilepsy, in which the disease process is conveniently confined to the anatomic boundaries of the temporal lobe. Patients being assessed for epilepsy surgery must therefore undergo detailed electroclinical evaluation. If this is nonlocalizing or at variance with the results of structural imaging, then such discrepancies have to be resolved with intracranial EEG. Similarly, patients with nonlesional epilepsy can only undergo surgical treatment after invasive neurophysiologic evaluation. There is an increasing awareness and acceptance of the fact that evaluation must be undertaken by a multidisciplinary team with operative decisions being based upon congruence of information from various diagnostic modalities.

PHASED EVALUATION FOR EPILEPSY SURGERY

The number of presurgical investigations available has increased markedly over the last decade. To take account of this a clear protocol defining the order in which these tests need to be carried out should be defined. This usually involves dividing the evaluation protocol into a series of phases, similar to that proposed by Crandall *et al* (1983). The investigational plan currently used by the Maudsley and King's College Hospitals is shown in Table 45.1.

The principal object of phase Ia is to identify cases with lesional epilepsy, which includes MTS identified on MRI, who can be operated upon without recourse to invasive EEG. In all cases of epilepsy the interictal and ictal surface EEG gives complementary information and the latter is not always of greater localizing value. Due to rapid spread of seizures, the ictal EEG may be nonlocalized while the interictal recording shows an abnormality congruent with the epileptogenic lesion. Considerable emphasis should therefore be placed on obtaining interictal surface records of high technical quality. Because abnormalities fluctuate over a period of hours or days, repeated recordings may have to be carried out which can be conveniently done during telemetry. Focal epileptiform discharges are particularly prone to be activated during sleep. With repeated examinations and sleep activation no more than 15% of cases should have normal or nonspecific findings. If a surgically resectable lesion is present, the clinical features of the epilepsy syndrome and the seizure type are appropriate and the surface EEGs are congruent, then an operation can be performed without intracranial recordings. This philosophy also applies to extratemporal lesions, most commonly those in the frontal lobe. ECoG may have to be used to define the extent of the resection, especially in extratemporal operations. Depending upon locally available facilities or particular research interest some centers would include functional

Table 45.1 Phased evaluation for epilepsy surgery.

Phase Ia Baseline investigations
    Clinical assessment
    High-resolution MRI and FLAIR images
    Routine and sleep EEG
    Scalp telemetry
    Neuropsychology

Phase Ib Further noninvasive investigation
    Quantitative MRI
    Repeated interictal EEGs
    EEG with barbiturate activation
    FDG PET
    Flumazenil PET
    Ictal SPECT

Phase II Carotid amobarbital testing

Phase IIa Telemetry with subdural electrodes
    Foramen ovale electrodes
    Subdural strips

Phase III Telemetry with depth electrodes or subdural mats

imaging such as fluorodeoxyglucose positron emission tomography (FDG PET), ictal single-photon emission computed tomography (SPECT) or postprocessing MRI techniques such as volume measurements in phase Ia. The general principle, however, remains the same. Phase Ia tests should include the cheapest, most widely available, and least invasive investigations.

In a significant proportion of cases, however, the initial tests are either nonlocalizing or the results of imaging and electroclinical evaluation are not congruent. In the experience of the Maudsley and King's College Hospital groups, this occurs in about 20% of cases. If both the electroclinical syndrome and the structural imaging are nonlocalizing then presurgical evaluation is usually abandoned. If, however, the patient has either a clinical syndrome such as complex partial seizures of presumed temporal lobe origin, or a resectable lesion, epilepsy surgery may be possible after intracranial EEG. Before proceeding with invasive physiology, an attempt should be made to clarify the diagnosis using the imaging and electrophysiologic techniques shown in phase Ib. Quantitative MRI techniques using volume measurements of the mesial temporal structures or T2 signal can be of help in the small proportion of cases in whom visual inspection of the images fails to diagnose MTS with certainty. Similarly semiquantitative assessment of regions of interest on functional imaging can clarify the diagnosis in difficult cases. Fluid attenuation inversion recovery (FLAIR) images suppress the signal from cerebrospinal fluid and are particularly useful in identifying peripheral lesions with a high T2 signal and as an aid to the diagnosis of bilateral MTS. The FDG PET scan is a particularly useful test as it often gives localizing information when either the structural imaging or EEG are unhelpful. Another very useful feature of PET scanning is that false-positive results are very rare. The chief drawback is that the area of glucose hypometabolism may be much more extensive than either the pathology or the zone of ictal EEG onset. Initial reports suggest that flumazenil PET scans may be much more helpful in this regard in that areas of reduced benzodiazepine binding are much more localized. It is uncertain if ictal SPECT gives more localizing information over and above MRI and scalp telemetry in cases with complex partial seizures of presumed temporal lobe origin. The principal use of this technique is in the evaluation of extratemporal seizures, especially frontal lobe onsets, when most other imaging techniques may be either normal or unhelpful.

On the basis of the phase Ia and phase Ib tests, a reasonable hypothesis as to the probable site of seizure onset needs to be established. In the first instance, the least invasive tests with recordings from the subdural space using foramen ovale or strip electrodes are used. Only a small pro-portion go on to have phase III tests with the use of depth electrodes or subdural grids or mats. Sodium amobarbital testing is carried out early in the protocol. This test gives very useful localizing information and is crucial in planning decisions concerning invasive EEG. If a resectable lesion is present there is little point in carrying out invasive physiology to prove that the seizures start at this site if any subsequent operative procedure would be contraindicated on the grounds of possible postoperative cognitive deficits.

INDICATIONS FOR INTRACRANIAL EEG EVALUATION

Before undertaking invasive neurologic investigations, a detailed multidisciplinary review of all clinical, EEG, and imaging data should be undertaken along with careful assessment of the neuropsychologic evaluation. On the basis of this review, a specific hypothesis has to be generated concerning the probable site of seizure origin and the most appropriate invasive or intracranial EEG technology is then chosen to answer the questions raised. Intracranial EEG should never be undertaken on a speculative basis or as a last resort if the electroclinical and imaging features are nonlocalizing. This is more often an indication to stop presurgical evaluation.

The indications for intracranial EEG are hard to define precisely as they are to some extent based on negative features or the results of investigations that are inconsistent or do not agree with each other. Furthermore, epilepsy consists of a series of overlapping electroclinical syndromes and has diverse pathologic causes of varying severity. It could be argued that there are as many indications for intracranial EEG as there are different types of epilepsy. Nevertheless, there are a number of situations which occur with sufficient frequency to allow a division into broad groupings, which are summarized in Table 45.2.

Before describing the use of intracranial EEG in specific epilepsy syndromes, a number of general principles should be considered. The great majority of cases with nonlesional epilepsy require intracranial EEG. In the absence of a resectable lesion the scalp EEG rarely gives localizing information of sufficient precision to be of help to the surgeon. Similarly, if the epileptogenic zone is likely to impinge upon eloquent cortex, the accurate delineation of the site of seizure onset and its relationship to the eloquent cortex can usually only be obtained from intracranial EEG. It is universal practice that any resective procedure should always include the structural abnormality. It is incorrect, however, to conclude the reverse and assume that a readily identified

Table 45.2 Principal indications for intracranial EEG.

Nonlesional epilepsy

Nonlocalized structural imaging
  Dual pathology
  Lesions extending beyond standard resection
  Multiple lesions

Atypical electroclinical syndrome

Bilateral independent temporal lobe onsets

Noncongruence of structural imaging, electroclinical data,
and functional abnormalities

Epileptogenic zone impinges on eloquent cortex

Reassessment of operative failures

Table 45.3 Indications for intracranial EEG evaluation in patients with complex partial seizures of presumed temporal lobe origin.

Appropriate electroclinical syndrome but nonlocalizing or noncongruent structural imaging
  Normal MRI
  Extratemporal pathology
  Bilateral mesial temporal sclerosis[a]
  Lesion extending beyond limits of standard temporal resection
  Diffuse or multilobar pathology[a]

Resectable lesion but atypical or noncongruent electroclinical syndrome
Features suggesting diffuse epileptogenic zone
  Lateralized sensory aura
  Unformed visual or auditory aura
  Frequent or exclusive secondarily generalized seizures
  Drop attacks or loss of postural tone during seizures
  Spikes maximal at the sylvian or superior frontal electrodes
  Other extratemporal focus
  Generalized epileptiform discharges
  Regional, hemispheric, or diffuse onset on scalp telemetry
  Localized extratemporal onsets on scalp telemetry
  Multifocal onsets[a]
  Frontal features such as lack of motionless stare, early motor or focal motor attacks, frenetic automatisms, and asymmetric posturing of limbs
Bilateral independent discharges
  Bilateral independent interictal temporal spikes
  Bilateral independent ictal temporal onsets[a]

[a] Usually an indication to stop surgical evaluation.

---

lesion such as a congenital tumor is the cause of a patient's epilepsy. The area of cortex capable of generating seizures may be much more extensive. In every case, therefore, a detailed electroclinical evaluation should be undertaken and unequivocal EEG evidence of the site of seizure onset obtained. In the face of a lack of congruence of noninvasive tests, intracranial EEG remains the final arbiter in determining operative decisions.

COMPLEX PARTIAL SEIZURES OF TEMPORAL LOBE ORIGIN

These cases constitute by far the largest group in all epilepsy surgery series and inconsistencies during evaluation of these patients have been the commonest cause for performing intracranial EEG. It is also true that this is the syndrome in which advances in structural and functional imaging have had the most impact. The indication for intracranial EEG with this syndrome fall into three main groups: nonlesional epilepsy, noncongruence of previous tests, and atypical electroclinical syndromes (Table 45.3).

Nonlocalizing structural imaging

A significant proportion of cases which have the electroclinical syndrome of complex partial seizures of temporal lobe origin have a normal high-resolution MRI. In surgical series this probably accounts for about one-third of cases and it may be a much higher proportion in new-onset temporal lobe epilepsy (van Paesschen *et al* 1997). Enough pathologic or outcome data have not been accumulated to establish whether these cases are truly nonlesional or whether the imaging is merely insensitive. Despite an extensive literature on hippocampal volume measurements in

temporal lobe epilepsy, there are few reports that include pathology. In post-mortem studies hippocampal sclerosis is asymmetric and bilateral in 80% of cases (Margerison and Corsellis 1966), which complicates the interpretation of high-resolution MRI, which depends heavily on comparing the two sides. It would appear that a high proportion of cases have imaging evidence of bilateral disease (Barr *et al* 1997; Quigg *et al* 1997). MTS can undoubtedly occur with normal hippocampal volumes on MRI (Jackson *et al* 1994) and the sensitivity of the test has been reported to vary from 50 to 90% (Berkovic *et al* 1991; Cascino *et al* 1991; Dowd *et al* 1991; Zentner *et al* 1995). Some series that report very high diagnostic rates clearly place great emphasis on MRI in selecting cases, and patients are only operated upon if the MRI is abnormal.

It is difficult to assess the sensitivity of MRI on the basis of these reports, but it is quite clear that it would be most unwise to exclude the patient from further evaluation if the electroclinical syndrome is localizing and the imaging is normal. If either the scalp EEG or FDG PET scan implicates the temporal lobe area, further assessment with carotid amobarbital testing and telemetry using subdural electrodes should be carried out. If the clinical features suggest mesial temporal epilepsy then foramen ovale electrodes are used, but if there are atypical features (see below) or any suggestion of lateral involvement, subdural strips are placed through bilateral temporal burr holes.

Extratemporal pathology

A difficult problem arises when patients have an electroclinical syndrome suggesting complex partial seizures of temporal lobe origin but an extratemporal lesion on MRI. This most commonly occurs with pathology in the frontal or occipital area, such as benign tumors, cortical dysplasia or previous infarcts or contusions. Although it is usual practice for the surgery to be directed at the lesion (Fish *et al* 1991), most groups when assessing a patient with noncongruent electroclinical features would require intracranial EEG evaluation to show that the seizures do indeed start around the area of pathology. This is particularly so if there is any evidence of coexistent MTS. If the lesion is situated mesially and in an inaccessible position, depth electrodes placed using MRI-generated coordinates are used, while subdural recordings are often sufficient around the ipsilateral temporal lobe. Differentiating temporal from frontal onsets is one of the most demanding clinical problems and these usually require depth electrode implantations in both the frontal and mesial temporal areas.

Bilateral mesial temporal sclerosis

Patients with evidence of bilateral MTS are usually excluded early from the epilepsy surgery program, before intracranial EEG is considered. This diagnosis is suggested when the mesial temporal structures appear small or atrophied on visual inspection which is confirmed on hippocampal volume measures. Bilateral increased T2 signal is often better seen using FLAIR images, and bilateral reductions in regional glucose metabolism on FDG PET scan are particularly helpful in establishing the diagnosis. Many cases have extensive neuropsychologic deficits, perform poorly on carotid amobarbital testing, and are excluded from surgery because of the risks of postoperative amnesic deficits.

Dual pathology and extensive lesions

The nature of the pathology also has some bearing on the decision as to whether intracranial EEG should be performed. In general, small indolent tumors tend to be well localized. They often involve the mesial temporal structures (Kirkpatrick *et al* 1993) and detailed intracranial evaluation is not needed. Cavernomas can be removed by MRI-guided stereotactic techniques after acute intraoperative

ECoG. In cortical dysplasia the EEG abnormality is often much greater than that suggested by the pathology seen on the scan (Palmini *et al* 1995) and chronic intracranial EEG recording is more commonly required. Dual pathology is most commonly seen when there is a temporal lesion such as a dysembryoplastic neuroepithelial tumour (DNET) and, in addition, evidence of MTS on MRI. In general, intracranial EEG is not required if both pathologies can be removed by an *en bloc* procedure. Alternatively, intraoperative ECoG can be used to determine the extent of a posterior resection. Multiple areas of pathology are much less common as most are excluded because of coexistent multifocal epilepsy. If presurgical evaluation is pursued in exceptional cases, intracranial EEG is usually needed to determine which lesion is responsible for the site of seizure onset.

A further situation that can give rise to difficulty is that in addition to MTS there may be an atrophic or destructive lesion in the temporal neocortex which extends to the frontal areas or above the sylvian fissure. With increasing use of high-resolution MRI, a not insignificant proportion of cases show loss of gray and white differentiation in the lateral temporal neocortex in addition to MTS. These situations may require detailed intracranial EEG evaluation, often with subdural mats or strips to determine the site of seizure origin. A similar procedure is needed if there is a foreign tissue lesion such as cortical dysplasia or a low-grade tumor which extends to the sylvian fissure and which is likely to impinge directly on eloquent areas of cortex. Detailed functional mapping through subdural mats may then be required before any resective procedure is considered.

Atypical syndrome or electroclinical features

The classical syndrome of mesial temporal epilepsy (French *et al* 1993; Williamson *et al* 1993a) can be easily diagnosed. The patient will have a history of a complicated febrile convulsion and develop epilepsy within the first decade. There may be mild learning difficulties and specific deficits on memory testing but severe or global cognitive deficits are not a feature. The seizures are drug resistant and occur in clusters on a weekly or monthly basis. Patients have simple partial seizures, complex partial seizures and usually less frequent secondarily generalized seizures. Following an appropriate aura there is loss of consciousness with a motionless stare, oroalimentary automatisms and dystonic posturing of the contralateral limbs. The interictal EEG shows spikes of greatest amplitude at the anterior or midtemporal electrode on the 10/20 system or at the superficial or deep sphenoidal electrode. A build-up of rhythmic θ activity is seen in the same distribution on the ictal EEG. The diagnosis is confirmed when MTS is shown on the MRI and there is an area of ipsilateral temporal hypometabolism on the FDG PET scan.

Unfortunately, a significant proportion of cases only have some elements of this syndrome. An etiological factor such as complicated febrile convulsion may not be present and the onset may be late in the second or third decades. Many cases are referred for presurgical evaluation with a presumptive diagnosis of temporal lobe epilepsy. However, after serial EEGs, detailed clinical assessment and scalp telemetry, atypical features are identified. One or more of the classical features of motionless stare, oroalimentary or reactive automatisms may be absent. A common pattern is that there are electroclinical features suggesting that a much more widespread area of brain is involved in the process of generating seizures. At seizure onset there may be a lateralized sensory or unformed visual or auditory symptoms. Abrupt onset of version, asymmetric posturing or frenetic automatisms may implicate the frontal lobes. The interictal EEG can show spikes maximal at the sylvian or frontal electrodes or generalized epileptiform discharges may be present. Similarly, the ictal EEG may be diffuse or nonlocalizing.

Cases with atypical electroclinical syndromes give rise to the greatest difficulty when undertaking presurgical evaluation, and consequently considerable judgment and experience are needed in deciding which ones should be further evaluated with intracranial EEG. If the electroclinical features suggest a lateral or convexity involvement, recordings from the subdural space using strip or mat electrodes may be the most appropriate and least invasive way of further assessment. Differentiating frontal lobe from temporal lobe epilepsy is the most taxing as the discharges can spread very rapidly. The best temporal resolution is obtained by implanting electrodes bilateral into the mesial temporal structures and frontal areas and combining this with subdural electrodes over the orbital frontal, lateral frontal, and temporal areas. This can be conveniently done using the technique described by van Veelen *et al* (1990) where the electrodes are passed through bilateral frontal burr holes.

Bilateral independent temporal discharges

About one-third of cases which have successful resective temporal lobe surgery have bilateral independent interictal temporal lobe discharges on the surface EEG (Jasper *et al* 1951; Gastaut 1953; So *et al* 1989). Because of rapid spread through commissural fibers the ictal EEG may also be bilateral when the discharges first become apparent in surface recordings. In the great majority of these cases, the electroclinical features leave little doubt that the patient suffers from temporal lobe epilepsy although laterality has not been established. Historically these patients have formed the largest group needing intracranial EEG. Engel *et al* (1982) reported that lateralized hypometabolic abnormalities on FDG PET scan were of considerable help in this diagnostic group and that the use of this technique reduced the need to carry out depth recordings. Subsequent advances in high-resolution MRI have shown that the underlying structural basis can usually be established with ease, which has further reduced the need for invasive neurophysiology (Risinger *et al* 1989). It is a common experience that with modern imaging techniques, intracranial EEG is much less commonly needed in temporal lobe epilepsy of uncertain laterality. In nonlesional cases or those with evidence of bilateral but asymmetric disease, foramen ovale or subdural strips recordings, and sometimes stereotactic implants, into both mesial temporal structures, are needed.

COMPLEX PARTIAL SEIZURES OF FRONTAL LOBE ORIGIN.

Considerable advances have been made in defining the electroclinical syndromes of frontal lobe seizures (Williamson *et al* 1985; Morris *et al* 1988; Williamson *et al* 1993b). The spectrum of the disorder is very diffuse with simple absences, complex partial seizures with bizarre automatisms and supplementary motor seizures with lateralized sensory auras, asymmetric dystonic posturing, and retention of consciousness. If an appropriate lesion is present on MRI which does not involve eloquent areas of the brain, a lesionectomy can be undertaken guided by intraoperative ECoG. Greater caution is needed with dysplastic lesions, and if at ECoG the abnormality appears much more diffuse, subdural mats and chronic recordings may be needed.

It is a common experience, however, that in a high proportion of cases with one of the frontal syndromes mentioned above, the high-resolution MRI is normal. Whether these are truly nonlesional cases again remains to be established and in this respect the recent description of familial frontal lobe epilepsy is of some interest (Scheffer *et al* 1995). Many of these patients have very severe and disabling epilepsy with frequent attacks occurring on a daily basis, often with a remarkable lack of associated neuropsychologic or neuropsychiatric deficits. Because the area of brain that has to be sampled is so large and the seizures spread so rapidly, most centers abandon presurgical evaluation in the face of normal structural imaging. FDG and flumazenil PET scanning are not usually of great clinical help in planning depth electrode placements. The only imaging modality which has been consistently reported to be helpful is ictal SPECT (Duncan *et al* 1997) which is technically difficult to perform because of the brevity of the seizures. Notwithstanding these difficulties, some authors using the Paris system of orthogonal electrodes and detailed electroclinical evaluation have reported operative outcomes in this difficult group of patients not dissimilar to lesional temporal lobe surgery (Munari *et al* 1995a; Chauvel *et al* 1998). This represents an important advance in the surgical treatment of epilepsy.

FOCAL MOTOR AND SENSORY SEIZURES

Following the development of multiple subpial transection, surgery can now be considered in cases where the epileptogenic zone encroaches upon the primary motor or sensory areas. For the purposes of intracranial EEG evaluation and surgical treatment, it is more appropriate to combine these cases where the focus involves the pre- or postcentral gyri rather than dividing them on anatomic grounds into frontal and parietal epilepsies. Much has to be learnt concerning the electroclinical features of these cases and it has to be admitted that the classical syndrome of focal motor or sensory Jacksonian seizures is the exception rather than the rule.

The commonest pathologies seen in this area are Rasmussen encephalitis and cortical dysplasia. Both are difficult to manage surgically because of the progressive nature of the former and the frequent diffuse or multifocal involvement of the latter. Even if there is a well-localized lesion, intracranial EEG is usually needed to define precisely the site of seizure onset and its relationship to eloquent areas of brain. As with the more common cases with complex partial seizures of frontal origin, high-resolution MRI may be normal. Intracranial EEG should be considered if there is a single stereotyped seizure type and a well-localized abnormality on the interictal or ictal scalp EEG. The epileptogenic zone and the ictal site of onset is determined by interictal and ictal EEG recordings. Detailed mapping at the motor and sensory areas is then carried out and these may be distorted if there is long-standing congenital pathology such as cortical dysplasia. Lesions or the site of ictal onset that do not involve eloquent areas of cortex can subsequently be biopsied or resected. If the motor or sensory area is involved, multiple subpial transection is performed under ECoG control until the interictal spikes are abolished. As might be expected, these procedures are one of the most demanding and time-consuming of neurosurgical treatments for epilepsy and few surgical series have been published.

LANDAU–KLEFFNER SYNDROME

Remarkable improvements in language function have been reported with this condition following multiple subpial transection. The evaluation protocol described by Morrell *et al* (1995) involves carotid amobarbital testing with EEG control to determine secondary synchrony, as a high proportion of cases have associated electrical status epilepticus during slow-wave sleep. A short-acting general anesthetic can also be used to suppress the generalized discharges leaving the primary focus. Although detailed intracranial evaluation is not usually required, exceptional cases involve the right hemisphere. In this instance, measuring phase relationships from intracranial strip electrodes passed bilaterally can be of help. ECoG is needed to assess the response to subpial transection.

HYPOTHALAMIC HAMARTOMAS

Munari *et al* (1995b) have demonstrated an ictal onset in a hypothalamic hamartoma in a patient with gelastic seizures. Some authors have pointed out that such cases pursue a malignant course not dissimilar to symptomatic generalized epilepsy and suggest that the hamartoma is merely an indicator of a more diffuse cortical involvement (Berkovic *et al* 1988). The striking association of two rare findings, a hypothalamic hamartoma and infantile-onset gelastic seizures, seems so extraordinary that it is difficult to escape a causal relationship. Furthermore, if the lesion is pedunculated, surgical removal may be associated with remission of seizures.

INVASIVE NEUROPHYSIOLOGIC ASSESSMENT IN CHILDREN

A high proportion of patients who undergo resective surgery as adults have experienced intractable epilepsy since childhood. Because of the adverse effects of uncontrolled epilepsy on cognitive and psychosocial development, it is increasingly recognized that wherever possible surgery should be undertaken early in the course of the disorder. In addition there is also some evidence, particularly among cases with foreign tissue as opposed to atrophic lesions, that the outcome following surgery may actually deteriorate with increasing duration of time for which the disease has remained active (Eliashiv *et al* 1997).

Many of the surgical procedures which are predominantly carried out in childhood epilepsy do not require extensive assessment with intracranial EEG.

Hemispherectomy is usually performed when there is clinical and imaging evidence of gross unilateral pathology. The commonest disorders encountered are atrophic or vascular lesions, hemimegalencephaly, Rasmussen syndrome and Sturge–Weber syndrome. In some cases being considered for a major resective procedure, there may be residual function in an upper limb or worries concerning the occurrence of new postoperative deficits such as hemianopia. In these instances a restricted procedure may be performed after mapping the epileptogenic zone and functional stimulation through subdural grids. The exact timing of these procedures can be difficult in patients with Rasmussen syndrome or Sturge–Weber syndrome where there may be a progressing neurologic deficit. Anterior two-thirds callosotomy is predominantly carried out in children with symptomatic generalized epilepsy and disabling drop attacks. Operative decisions are made on the basis of interictal EEG sometimes with carotid amobarbital testing and also intraoperative ECoG to establish desynchronization of bilateral epileptiform discharges. Preoperative evaluation with intracranial EEG is not usually required. Chugani and Conti (1996) have described infants with West syndrome who have focal abnormalities on FDG PET. These are most common posteriorly and can be amenable to resective surgery. The usual pathology is dysplasia, and if there is a clear abnormality on structural and functional imaging then resective procedures can be carried out directly with the guidance of intraoperative ECoG.

In assessing patients for localized resective surgery, it is likely that a higher proportion of children will need intracranial EEG evaluation. In very early childhood the delineation of lesions may be harder on MRI due to incomplete myelination. The electroclinical syndromes are less clearly defined and there is a higher incidence of bilateral or diffuse EEG abnormalities in children with focal epilepsy (Jayakar and Duchowny 1997). In large pediatric series, as many as 50% of cases have dysplastic lesions and there is a higher incidence of extratemporal epilepsy. Both of these groups are harder to evaluate and more frequently require invasive physiologic investigation. Even among patients with temporal lobe epilepsy, there is a greater tendency for the disorder to start in the neocortex, thus requiring detailed neurophysiologic assessment and a tailored resection (Duchowny et al 1997).

Children seem to tolerate intracranial EEG evaluation well. If scalp recordings can be performed in children with attention deficit disorders or cognitive impairment then invasive investigations can usually be undertaken without undue difficulty. For greater safety some form of automatic cable release system is needed. There is a increased theoretical risk of morbidity due to the dangers of blood loss and the production of mass affects or cerebral edema following the implantation of large electrode arrays. Functional mapping may be harder as congenital lesions may distort the normal functional anatomy and it can sometimes be harder to produce a response when stimulating the nervous system which has not undergone full myelination.

METHODS OF INTRACRANIAL EEG EVALUATION

Most patients being considered for epilepsy surgery have complex partial seizures of presumed temporal or frontal lobe origin. The focus is often inaccessible on the mesial or basal parts of the hemisphere and the various techniques used in intracranial EEG reflect an attempt to overcome these anatomic difficulties. If the focus lies over the convexity, it is much more likely to be near eloquent areas of the brain and the evaluation should therefore include a technique that allows detailed mapping of the motor and sensory areas.

FORAMEN OVALE ELECTRODES

Foramen ovale electrodes (Fig. 45.1) were developed by Wieser as a method of recording near the mesial temporal structures without having to implant electrodes through the substance of the brain (Wieser et al 1985). The foramen ovale lies mesially in the middle cranial fossa. The fifth cranial nerve passes up from the brainstem over the petrous temporal bone and the second and third branches exit through it. It is a well-established neurosurgical technique to place a needle within the foramen ovale to carry out coagulation of the trigeminal ganglion for the treatment of tic douloureux. If the needle is advanced further, cerebrospinal fluid (CSF) is obtained as it passes into the subdural space and an electrode can then be passed along the floor of the middle cranial fossa. The wire is usually inserted 3–4 cm and comes to lie along the free edge of the tentorium next to the parahippocampal gyrus. A multicontact electrode is most effective. The electrodes have to be secured at the skin and can usually provide high-quality recordings for a period of a week to 10 days after which they tend to work loose.

In a small proportion of patients with mesial temporal onset, the changes at the foramen ovale electrode may be bilateral by the time the seizure has spread from the hippocampus to the parahippocampal gyrus. Seizures starting in the amygdala may be poorly localized, partly due to the characteristics of the electrical field generated, and also

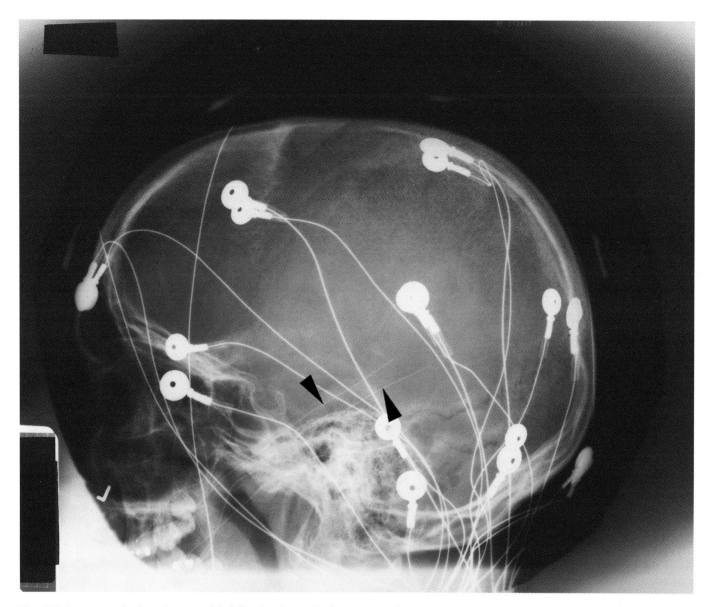

Fig. 45.1 Foramen ovale electrodes. Lateral skull film showing multipolar six-contact foramen ovale electrodes (arrows). After entering the cranium at the base of the middle cranial fossa they follow the edge of the tentorium. The deepest contacts are usually closest to the mesial temporal structures and the more superficial provide recordings from the lateral temporal neocortex.

because this structure is anterior while the foramen ovale electrode comes through the central part of the middle cranial fossa and passes backwards. The technique is probably the safest and least invasive way of establishing, on electroclinical grounds, whether a patient does or does not have mesial temporal epilepsy.

The placement of the needle and wire in the foramen ovale requires considerable skill and should not be performed on an occasional basis. The procedure can be complicated by meningitis and between 1 and 2% of cases have residual numbness or dysthesia over the face, particularly when difficulty has been experienced while inserting the electrodes (Wieser 1991). Cerebral hemorrhage or the development of carotid-cavernous fistulae has been

reported to occur as an exceptional complication (Wieser et al 1993), and the technique should probably not be used if there is anatomic distortion of the mesial temporal structures such as that occurring after previous surgery.

SUBDURAL STRIPS AND MATS

In this form of recording (Fig. 45.2), bilateral burr holes are most commonly made in the temporal areas and the dura opened. A commercially available plastic strip with between four and eight stainless steel or platinum electrodes embedded into it can then be passed directly over the surface of the brain in the subdural space (Goldring and Gregorie, 1984; Wyler et al 1984; Rosenbaum et al 1986).

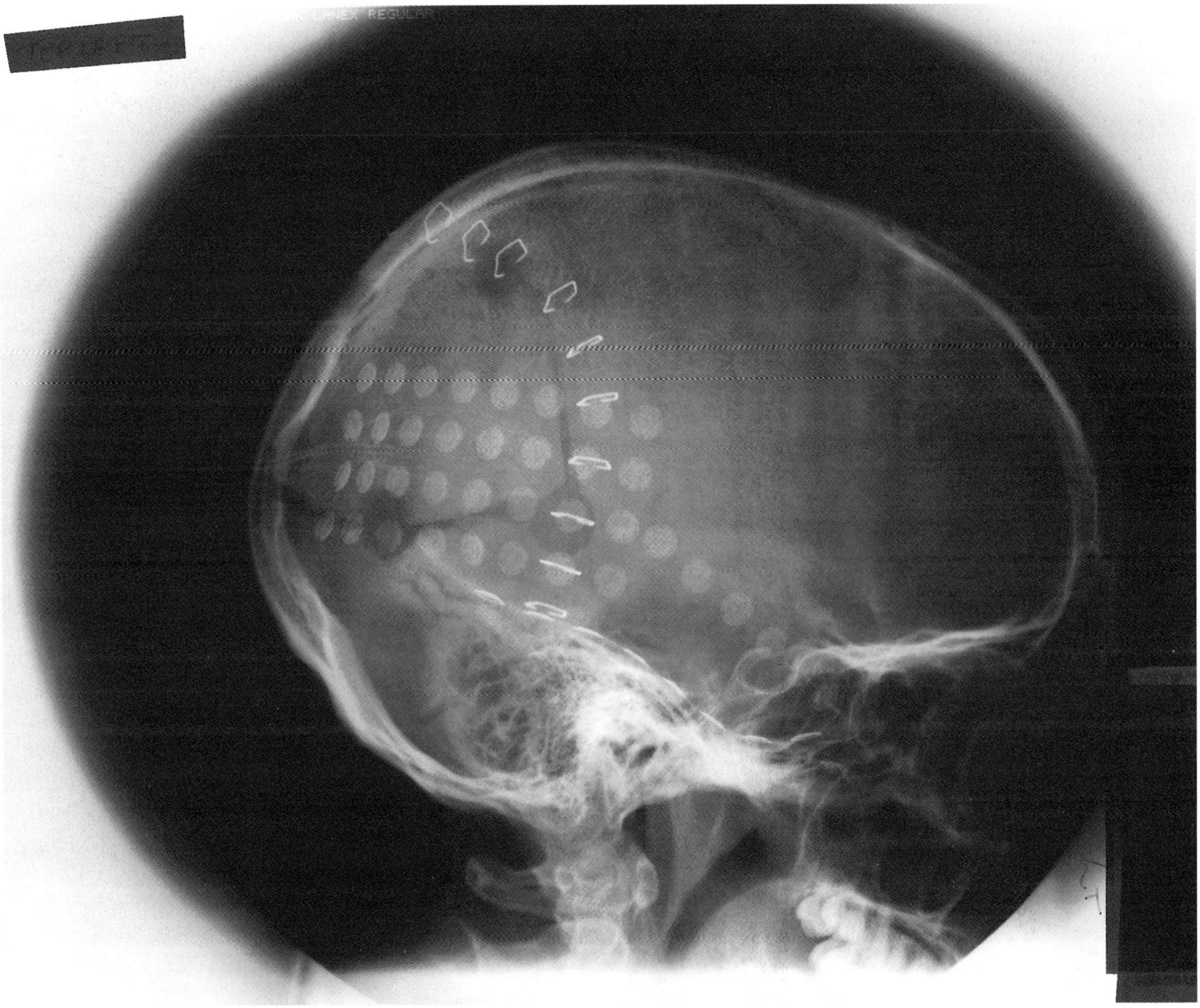

Fig. 45.2 Subdural mats and strips. Lateral skull film showing a 32-contact mat inserted through a left posterior craniotomy and overlying the posterior temporal, parietal, and occipital junction. In addition there is a six-contact strip passing anteriorly toward the left temporal pole and an eight-contact strip on the undersurface of the left temporal lobe.

The passage can be guided inferiorly and mesially such that the most distal contact comes to lie over the parahippocampal gyrus in a similar position to that obtained from foramen ovale recording. Recordings can also be obtained from the lateral neocortex and the sylvian area. Through the same burr hole an electrode can be passed either anteriorly over the frontal lobe or posteriorly toward the occipital area. Through a superior frontal burr hole electrodes can be slid into the interhemispheric fissure, and strips with recording electrodes on both sides can be used so that recordings from both hemispheres can be obtained from one electrode. Through the same burr hole an electrode can pass over the convexity and lateral aspect of the frontal lobe toward the orbital surface.

The electrodes are readily secured and the technical aspects of EEG recording are probably easier than with foramen ovale electrodes. It is, therefore, a simple and robust technique which can supply an answer to many of the problems that arise during phase I evaluation. Although the procedure is less painful than foramen ovale insertion and is well tolerated, it requires more operating time and should probably be considered as being more invasive. Leakage of CSF can occur and there is a greater theoretical risk of infection than with foramen ovale electrodes, due to the greater complexity of the operative procedures and the larger amount of implanted material. Cables should be tunneled under the scalp and exit through a separate wound to reduce the possibility of infection. Subdural hemorrhage can occur from veins which pass through the subdural space and this can be a particular problem with posteriorly placed electrodes or those passing into the interhemispheric fissure.

When subdural mats or grids are used, adequate exposure through a craniotomy is required. A number of commercially available electrode arrays are available and the most commonly used is an eight-by-eight mat which is implanted so that it lies across the central sulcus. The centers of the electrodes lie at 1 cm intervals. When recording over the frontal, temporal, or occipital lobes a smaller mat with eight-by-four or five-by-four electrodes can be used. A double line of electrodes specially curved to fit the contour of the cingulate gyrus is helpful in the assessment of epilepsy of presumed mesial frontal origin. Subdural strips can be slid under the margins of the craniotomy to provide recordings from inaccessible areas, usually on the mesial or basal aspects of the hemisphere. The mats are secured to dura by stitches to stop them moving and the recording wires are again tunneled out through a separate incision. Because the implanted material is more bulky than with strips there is a greater theoretical risk of infection or subdural hematomas and most patients need observation in the high-dependency unit before being transferred for telemetry. Some patients can develop cerebral edema, presumably as a reaction to the foreign material, which is manifest by deteriorating consciousness level. The position of the electrodes can be checked on anteroposterior and lateral skull films. The relationship of individual electrodes to the site of any lesion can also be assessed on MRI.

Maintaining good EEG recordings with so many electrodes can be technically difficult and it is particularly important to secure the connecting cables so that traction on the electrodes does not occur.

DEPTH ELECTRODES

This technique involves passing a recording electrode directly through the substance of the brain so that EEG recordings can be carried out from inaccessible areas of gray matter in the mesial or basal aspects of the hemisphere. The technologies used are the same as those employed in undertaking stereotactic biopsies of the brain. The Paris system used the Talairach atlas combined with standard anatomic marks present on an air encephalogram (Talairach and Bancaud 1974). A preoperative angiogram is also undertaken. Electrodes are then placed through pegs in twist-drill holes and pass orthogonally. The recording electrode has contacts at the distal end which record from deep structures such as the hippocampus or cingulate gyrus, and superficial contacts so that recordings can be also be made from the neocortex.

The sites into which the electrodes are placed are decided individually for each case depending on a detailed noninvasive electroclinical analysis. Further subdural contacts can be obtained by subdural pegs without electrodes passing through substance of the brain. The technique provides particularly good coverage of the mesial and orbital aspects of the frontal lobe which are hard to sample by other methods (Munari *et al* 1994, 1995a; Quesney *et al* 1995).

An alternative approach is to use three-dimensional stereo coordinates obtained from CT or MRI. In this manner particular anatomic regions can be identified with considerable accuracy and electrodes can also be placed near structural abnormalities seen on imaging. There are a number of differing approaches. An electrode may be passed posteriorly from the occipital region so that the mesial temporal structures are sampled by an anteroposterior line of contacts (Spencer *et al* 1993). The method described by van Veelen *et al* (1990) uses bifrontal burr holes. Three electrodes are usually placed symmetrically in the amygdala, anterior and posterior hippocampus and a further depth electrode can go anteriorly into the frontal lobe in the gyrus rectus. The technique should be combined with subdurally placed electrodes, as a number of studies have shown that this improves the diagnostic accuracy compared with using depth electrodes alone (Spencer 1981; Spencer *et al* 1982; Sperling and O'Connor 1989; Privitera *et al* 1990; Binnie *et al* 1994a). The principal complication of depth electrodes is hemorrhage leading to permanent neurologic deficit. The risk is broadly similar to that obtained with the definitive resective procedure and occurs in the order of 1 in 100 cases (Polkey 1996). Most recording electrodes are now MR compatible and the precise localization can be checked postoperatively.

ELECTROCORTICOGRAPHY

ECoG is carried out by placing recording electrodes directly onto the surface of the exposed cortex and carrying out acute recordings during the operation. The system has been most extensively used at the Montreal Neurological Institute where it is used to determine the extent of tailored resections (Rasmussen 1975). A series of 20 flexible silver electrodes with cotton wool pads soaked in saline are used for the recording. For a temporal resection these are usually placed in lines along the inferior, mid, and superior temporal gyrus and some above the sylvian fissure and over the frontal lobe. Flexible electrodes are also passed beneath the margins of the craniotomy toward the frontal pole, the basal aspect of the temporal lobe, and posteriorly. An incision can be made in the temporal lobe and direct recordings made from the hippocampus (Polkey *et al* 1989).

Recordings may also be carried out under local anesthesia to remove drug effects and this can be combined with functional stimulation of the exposed lesion and surrounding cortex (Ojemann and Engel 1987). An injection of a fast-acting barbiturate is often helpful in activating epileptiform discharges (Wyler *et al* 1987).

It is surprising that a technique which has gained such widespread usage has been subjected to so little validation (Fiol *et al* 1991; Binnie *et al* 1994b). In a detailed review of the Maudsley experience, which was undertaken on patients who predominantly had a standard resection, it seemed that the test was of little prognostic significance (McBride *et al* 1991). While an initial low spike rate and the presence of residual postoperative spikes did imply a poor surgical result, there was no obvious correlation with the distribution of spikes and operative outcome. Epileptogenic areas are usually identified by finding the site where the spikes are of greatest amplitude. This assumption may be incorrect. Alarcon *et al* (1994, 1997) have shown that temporal propagation measured by on-line computerized techniques may be a better technique and that identification of the leading zone may also prove to be of greater help in predicting surgical outcome.

The extent to which ECoG is used varies widely between different centers. If a standard *en bloc* temporal lobectomy is performed and detailed imaging and EEG studies have been undertaken, it is uncommon for ECoG measuring amplitude and distribution of spikes to change intraoperative decisions. During a tailored resection the technique can be used to determine the extent of a cortical resection or it can be used to guide the surgeon as to how much cortex should be removed when performing a lesionectomy. There is some evidence that simple lesionectomy as opposed to corticectomy does not give good results, particularly, it seems, if carried out in the temporal lobe (Cascino *et al* 1992). With advances in MRI, more cases with resectable lesions are being identified such as those with cavernomas, cortical dysplasia, and small indolent tumors. Carrying out a resection guided by intraoperative ECoG with or without the use of functional stimulation under local anesthetic is a very cost-effective way of performing epilepsy surgery (Ojemann and Engel 1987). If during craniotomy and ECoG atypical features occur, intracranial mats can be left in place and chronic recordings performed and further functional stimulation carried out. If surgery is being performed in eloquent areas of the brain using multiple subpial transection then ECoG should be used to determine that all areas of spiking have been abolished.

DATA ACQUISITION AND REDUCTION

As with scalp telemetry, continuous 24-hour recording of the EEG with simultaneous video is needed. Of the order of between three and six habitual seizures should be captured which usually necessitates a period of recording of around 1 week and sometimes longer. Multicontact foramen ovale electrodes and subdural strips can be combined with standard scalp electrodes in the 10/20 system so a minimum of 32 channels of EEG is advisable. With depth recordings or subdural mats, 64 EEG channels or more are appropriate. After preamplification the signals are digitized for ease of transmission and the large amount of data generated is stored on standard VHS tape. Commercial systems now allow direct storage of both video and EEG directly onto a computer hard disk which makes subsequent analysis and postprocessing of the EEG much easier.

Seizures are identified by the patient, relative, or attendant staff who activate an event marker. Much useful information such as consciousness level or the presence of dysphasia can be obtained by examining the patient around the time of the seizure. An on-line computerized seizure detection system (Gotman *et al* 1979) is of considerable help in identifying subclinical seizures. Similarly, those cases who have brief complex partial seizures without an aura can be easily missed if undue reliance is placed upon activation of alarm buttons alone.

Prolonged periods of interictal EEG should be reviewed on a daily basis. In addition to electronic storage, hard-paper copies of ictal events are needed for detailed visual inspection. The abnormalities that are often of particular interest are low-voltage fast activity confined to one or two electrodes (see below). These can be seen much more clearly after filtering of slow activity and using a higher gain. The ability to produce a hard copy of simultaneous 64-channel EEG displays is of great help in analyzing the complex patterns of seizure onset and spread that can occur with intracranial EEG. Continuous support from highly trained technicians and nurses are required as well as close cooperation between the neurosurgeon and neurophysiologist on a daily basis. It is important to establish that the seizures observed do indeed correspond to the patient's habitual attacks.

ANTIEPILEPTIC DRUG WITHDRAWAL

Stopping anticonvulsants can undoubtedly influence the results obtained from intracranial EEG recordings (Engel and Crandall 1983). Seizures may spread more rapidly which can make interpretation of the focal onset harder.

The problem is compounded if atypical convulsions or serial seizures occur. Rapid withdrawal can precipitate status epilepticus, especially in patients with extensive brain injury. In exceptional circumstances a new focus which is different from the habitual site of onset can be activated. These difficulties, however, have to be balanced with the need to complete the examination in a reasonable period of time and most telemetry units employ some protocol for drug reduction. In the author's unit, antiepileptic drugs are usually left unchanged for a period of 2–3 days to try and capture habitual seizures on medication. Rapid withdrawal of vigabatrin should be avoided because of postictal psychosis. Phenytoin has a long pharmacokinetic half-life and sodium valproate has a long pharmacodynamic action which makes drug reduction less useful as a means of inducing seizures. Carbamazepine, lamotrigine, and gabapentin can all be safely and rapidly withdrawn and usually precipitate a cluster of habitual seizures within 2–3 days. Rapid withdrawal of the sedating anticonvulsants phenobarbital and benzodiazepines (clobazam and clonazepam) is particularly prone to induce atypical withdrawal convulsions.

DATA ANALYSIS

With implanted electrodes, interictal epileptiform discharges are often seen at multiple and sometimes unexpected sites. While most emphasis should be placed on ictal EEG, the interictal recording can be of great help. During a clinical ictus, localizing information can be obscured by very rapid spread and extensive involvement of the epileptiform discharges. Visual inspection of prolonged periods of recording and the use of a computerized detection system may show subclinical seizures (Gotman *et al* 1979). In temporal lobe epilepsy these are often brief events lasting 1–2 s which can bear a remarkable similarity in terms of morphology and distribution to those occurring at the onset of habitual seizures. While the only study that specifically looked at this phenomenon concluded that they were not of localizing value (Sperling and O'Connor 1990), in the great majority of cases subclinical and habitual seizure did in fact have similar sites of origin. Others have reported that subclinical events are of considerable use in localizing the site of habitual seizure onset (Lieb *et al* 1976; Binnie *et al* 1994a). When recording from the convexity with subdural mats, interictal spikes bear a closer relationship to ictal onset. Dysplastic lesions, which seem to be inherently epileptogenic (Palmini *et al* 1995), may show virtually continuous rhythmic subclinical seizures. The abnormality is often much larger than the MRI-identified lesion and can be multifocal.

In evaluating ictal EEG the first task is to identify the very first behavioral or EEG change. This may not be obvious in simple partial seizures, seizures with subtle changes in behavior or if there is a considerable amount of interictal EEG abnormality. The presence of a generalized decrement in all EEG activity at the onset of seizures is often of great help. Why such a widespread change should occur at the onset of a focal seizure is unclear but the decrement is certainly of great help in identifying ictal onsets. Careful review of the videos in multiple seizures may then reveal some subtle coexisting behavioral change such as movement or opening of the eyes. Following this it is necessary to identify the first new EEG rhythm associated with the ictal onset. This requires careful differentiation from interictal discharges which can sometimes be difficult and the pattern may only become clear after review of multiple seizures. If there is an appreciable delay between ictal onset and the occurrence of the first new EEG rhythm, the possibility of spread from a distant site should be considered. This observation is more likely if the first EEG changes are widespread or regional or consist of a rhythm other than low-voltage fast activity. Considerable clinical judgment may be needed to decide whether this is owing to a sampling error due to the electrodes or whether the onset zone for the seizure is indeed diffuse.

The morphology of EEG waveforms seen at seizure onset with intracranial records is very diverse. Spencer has described the experience of the Yale group and commented on the general paucity of published data (Spencer *et al* 1992). Seizure onset is often heralded by a decrement of interictal activity, including spikes, and the localized appearance of rhythmic low-voltage fast activity (Fig. 45.3). Over a variable period, not uncommonly 10–20 s, the fast activity increases in amplitude and decreases in frequency. This may develop into rhythmic sharpened θ activity. During this period the epileptiform discharges often spread gradually into contiguous areas of gray matter such as passing from amygdala into the anterior and then the posterior hippocampus. In the context of mesial temporal epilepsy, it has often been assumed that low-voltage fast activity correlates with atrophic pathology (Spencer *et al* 1992), although this has been disputed (Lieb *et al* 1981) and may not apply in extratemporal epilepsy. Other rhythms can be seen at onset which include bursts of spikes, rhythmic spike and wave, and also slow activity. Sometimes an interictal abnormality takes on a new morphology or becomes more rhythmic. While published series usually give classical examples, in practice the electrical patterns can be extremely complex. Bursts of slow or epileptiform discharges at one site may be followed by disappearance of all activity only to reappear at distant or multiple sites. The ictal onset patterns may

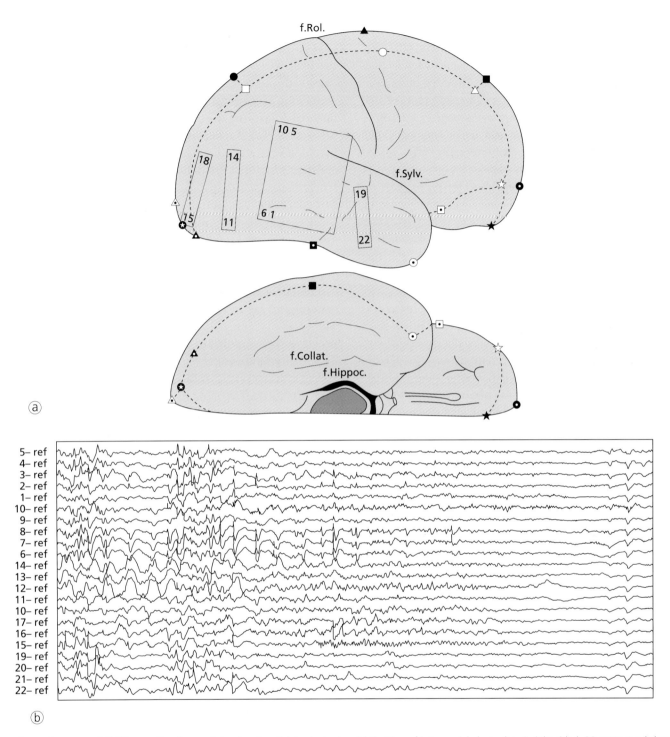

Fig. 45.3 Intracranial EEG recording from subdural mat and strip electrodes. (a) Position of intracranial electrodes. A right-sided, 20-contact subdural mat is placed over the posterior temporal area and adjoining cortex. Two four-contact strips pass over the occipital area and a four-contact electrode is over the anterior temporal region. (b) Preictally there are epileptiform discharges in a wide distribution and the seizure starts focally at electrode 15, the contact nearest the occipital pole. Within 5 s the posterior part of the mat is involved. This 11-year-old girl had intractable complex partial seizures with prominent version to the left and posturing of the left-sided limbs; ictal scalp EEG showed a left posterior temporal onset. Structural imaging was normal but the FDG PET showed a left occipital hypometabolism. On the interictal intracranial EEG (not shown) there were virtually continuous subclinical seizures and the pathology is probably dysplastic. No speech disorder occurred during stimulation at the back of the 20-contact mat.

change throughout the period of recording. The reason for this is uncertain but could be due to the acute effects of the anesthetic, damage related to the electrode implantation, early gliosis along the site of electrode insertion, or drug withdrawal. In other instances there may be inherent variability in the site of ictal onset.

The degree of anatomic resolution identified by the intracranial EEG will depend on the type of electrode used. In mesial temporal epilepsy with implanted depth electrodes, seizure onsets in the amygdala, anterior hippocampus, and posterior hippocampus can be differentiated. If subdural electrodes over the temporal neocortex are simultaneously involved the onset is said to be regional. With foramen ovale electrodes or subtemporal strips placed through a lateral burr hole, the deepest contacts are involved in mesial temporal epilepsy, and the more proximal ones, if there is lateral focus. Because the two recording techniques sample from the parahippocampal gyrus rather than the hippocampus proper, if there is a rapid switch to the contralateral side via commissural pathways, the first EEG changes may be bilateral by the time they have spread into the neocortex. As the degree of asymmetry can vary between seizures, these findings can be misinterpreted as independent bilateral onsets. While clear independent focal onsets in both temporal lobes undoubtedly do occur with low-voltage fast activity and different patterns of seizure spread, they are, in the author's experience, quite unusual.

An attempt should be made to correlate the subsequent patterns of EEG spread with the behavioural features of the seizures (Wieser 1983). Two types of electrical spread can be observed on intracranial EEG. Over a period of seconds, contiguous areas of gray matter may become involved. In mesial temporal epilepsy, the seizure may spread along the limbic structures and then out over the parahippocampal gyrus and into the temporal cortex (Fig. 45.4). In cases with epilepsy arising over the convexity, the spread can be mapped in some considerable detail using subdural grids. As this technique is often combined with functional mapping of motor and sensory areas, a detailed correlation of electrical activity with the behavioral features of the seizure

is possible (Arroyo *et al* 1993). In addition to the above, seizures can spread very rapidly to widely separated areas of the brain through long fiber tracts. In about one-third of cases with mesial temporal epilepsy, the contralateral temporal lobe is involved by commissural spread before the seizure has involved the ipsilateral temporal neocortex (Binnie *et al* 1994a). Rapid spread greatly complicates the interpretation of ictal EEG and is particularly common in frontal epilepsy, where the first EEG changes can be bilateral and synchronous even when recording with intracranial electrodes. Preferential patterns of distant spread can sometimes explain the behavioral features of some seizures, such as the early contralateral version occurring in posterior temporal epilepsy as the seizure spreads to the ipsilateral frontal eye field. While every effort should be made to correlate the site of onset and spread to the behavioral features of the seizures, this can be exceedingly difficult in individual cases. The problem is made greater by limited sampling of the sites involved and heterogenicity of cases. Many of the major behavioral aspects of complex partial seizures such as loss of consciousness, epileptiform dystonia, and automatisms are not accompanied by consistent EEG changes, presumably because they represent spread of electrical activity to deep structures which are not included in routine clinical examinations.

FUNCTIONAL MAPPING AND STIMULATION

Intracranial electrodes can be used to map the function of eloquent areas of cortex using electrical stimulation. This technique is most widely used through subdural mats or

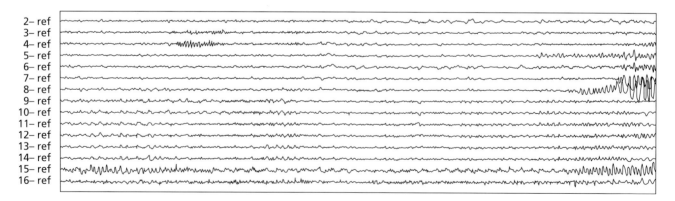

Fig. 45.4 Intracranial recording from subdural strips. Intracranial EEG evaluation using 2 eight-contact subdural strips placed through bilateral temporal burr holes. Channels 2–8 are right-sided with number 8 the deepest lying near the parahippocampal gyrus. Channels 9–16 are on the left in the same distribution. The first EEG changes occur in the deepest contacts on the left. Within 6 s low-voltage fast occurs in the right mesial temporal contacts which rapidly increase in amplitude. The patient had a lesion in the left temporal lobe which was probably dysplastic and the surface interictal and ictal EEGs were nonlocalizing.

grids in cases where a resection is planned close to the motor cortex. Another less widely used technique is to use electrical stimulation to determine the threshold at which habitual seizures can be produced, which may be of help in identifying the epileptogenic zone. This has proved particularly useful in mesial frontal epilepsy where the ictal EEG recordings may be widespread at onset. In mesial temporal epilepsy the threshold may actually be higher on the epileptogenic side, possibly because the sclerosed hippocampus is harder to stimulate (Crandall *et al* 1983). Low-frequency stimulation at 1 cycle s^{-1} may be more effective than the faster frequencies that are often used in clinical practice (Munari *et al* 1993).

Stimulation is usually carried out using biphasic square-wave pulses with a pulse duration of the order of 0.3 ms. The pulse is delivered at 50 cycles s^{-1} and the response assessed during a 3–5 s period. The current is gradually increased from 1 mA up to a maximum of the order of 10–15 mA. It is usually wise to identify the threshold for afterdischarges and the EEG should be monitored from nearby electrodes throughout the procedure. In addition, stimuli that produce after discharges are more likely to spread and can produce falsely localized results. If the technique is carried out through subdural mats it is usual to stimulate across two adjacent electrodes in the anteroposterior direction. Current spread is more likely to occur either superiorly or inferiorly and is less likely to interfere with the identification of the anterior and posterior limits of the motor response. With the pulse duration and current intensity as used above, theoretical side-effects from either hydrolysis and the release of acids, electrolysis of the metal electrodes causing cell damage, or the kindling of new epileptic foci does not seem to be an overt clinical problem. Physiologic responses can usually be obtained in the motor and sensory areas and unformed visual sensations, particularly phosphenes, can be obtained from the posterior occipital cortex. Occasionally the primary auditory cortex is identified. Speech arrest or naming errors occur with stimulation of the anterior and posterior primary language areas and speech arrest can also occur when stimulating the mesial frontal or supplementary motor region.

At the end of the examination it is usually possible to draw up a composite map relating the site of the lesion, the ictal EEG onset, and functionally eloquent areas of the cortex on individual contacts of the subdural mat. In general, resective procedures can be carried out within 1 cm of the functionally eloquent cortex. Areas producing sensory function or motor responses involving the face can be more safely sacrificed than those involved in speech or limb movement. The technique of functional mapping through subdural mats is often followed by a combined operation during which a biopsy or resection is carried out and other eloquent areas of the cortex are treated by multiple subpial transection. The technique can be supplemented by carrying out somatosensory evoked potentials which phase-reverse across the central sulcus. Functional MRI measuring of localized changes in venous hemoglobin saturation in response to voluntary movements, so-called blood oxygen level-dependent (BOLD) imaging, can be used to help identify the motor cortex.

There are still many controversies and difficulties with the techniques of stimulation. Ojemann (1997) has advocated the use of intraoperative functional stimulation immediately prior to resection. Although the technique cannot be carried out in young children or if there are doubts concerning the electroclinical localization, this method does have the considerable advantage of reducing the exposure of the patient to operative and invasive neurophysiologic procedures. The use of short-acting intravenous anesthetics has made the technique much easier and acute ECoG can be performed without possible deleterious effects from inhalational anesthetics. In addition, the motor areas identified are often much more circumscribed and within 0.5 cm of the central sulcus, similar to the classic homunculus described by Penfield and Jasper (1954). In comparison, when using subdural mats it is not unusual for the same motor response to be obtained over distances of 2–3 cm (Uematsu *et al* 1992). During temporal resections, areas of cortex subserving speech may be identified in a number of isolated and unexpected places such as the inferior surface of the temporal lobe. Ojemann (1997) claims that by tailoring the resection to avoid these areas the incidence of postoperative language disorders can be reduced. It is not clear, however, whether these techniques are any more effective than carrying out a standard resection in the dominant temporal lobe and not removing cortex beyond 4 cm from the pole with preservation of the superior temporal gyrus. A further difficulty which is frequently encountered during electrical stimulation is that the lesion or the epileptogenic area may markedly distort the functional motor anatomy. This has received little systematic study. Similarly, there has been little examination of the effects of changing the stimulation parameters. In children under the age of 2, the stimulus threshold is markedly increased, presumably because of incomplete myelination. In addition to increasing current strengths, pulse duration may also have to be prolonged in order to obtain a motor response and reduce the possibility of tissue damage (Jayakar *et al* 1992).

CONCLUSIONS

Because of poor spatial resolution of the scalp EEG, inaccessible areas of cerebral cortex, and rapid spread of epileptiform discharges, it may be necessary to carry out invasive neurophysiologic tests to localize epileptic foci. Advances in neuroimaging have had an important impact on the indications for intracranial EEG. Previously it was most commonly carried out in cases with complex partial seizures of presumed temporal lobe origin in which laterality had not been established. Because MTS and small tumors can be readily diagnosed on MRI, and FDG PET is extremely effective in lateralizing epileptic foci, general experience has shown that a high proportion of these cases can now be operated on without recourse to intracranial EEG. The principal indications for intracranial EEG are now the evaluation of cases with focal epilepsy and normal or nonlocalizing structural imaging, the resolution of discordant data from noninvasive evaluation, and assessment of cases with atypical electroclinical syndromes. A high proportion of extratemporal resections, particularly if they are likely to impinge upon eloquent cortex or if some form of tailored resection is contemplated, will need preoperative assessment with intracranial EEG or detailed intraoperative ECoG.

Many more cases are now being sent for presurgical evaluation and those requiring invasive neurophysiology are much more heterogeneous. Due to the sensitivity of high-resolution MRI and modern functional imaging it is possible to generate a hypothesis as to the probable site of seizure onset in a much higher proportion of cases, many of whom previously might have been considered inoperable. Instead of relying heavily on one particular method of evaluation to examine a frequently occurring problem (namely bitemporal epilepsy), more flexibility is required. A wider range of techniques is needed to answer more complex and diverse problems. It could be argued that subdural recordings with strip electrodes are technically the easiest method and can supply the answer to many of the questions that arise during the initial phases of presurgical evaluation. Depth electrode examinations and cases requiring subdural mats or grids and functional stimulation should probably be assessed in a few specialist centers skilled in these techniques.

KEY POINTS

1. Whenever possible, operations should be carried out on the basis of congruence of noninvasive investigations.
2. Intracranial EEG should only be undertaken to test specific hypotheses and never as a last resort.
3. Between 60% and 80% of cases with temporal lobe epilepsy can be operated without cranial EEG.
4. Intracranial EEG is more often required with extratemporal epilepsy and in children.
5. The most common indications for invasive neurophysiology are nonlocalizing scalp EEG, atypical electroclinical syndromes, normal MRI, dual pathology, lesions extending into the eloquent cortex, and noncongruence of electroclinical syndrome with pathology.
6. Most cases can be evaluated with electrodes in the subdural space, either foramen ovale electrodes, strips, or mats.
7. Insertion of stereotactic depth electrodes may be needed in inaccessible areas, especially the hippocampus and mesial aspects of the hemisphere.
8. Stereo EEG may sometimes be needed to diagnose independent hippocampal onsets and in cases with rapid commissural spread.
9. Failure to use intracranial EEG can lead to inappropriate exclusion of suitable cases, while others may be subjected to unnecessary operations.

REFERENCES

Alarcon G, Guy CN, Binnie CD, Walker SR, Elwes RD, Polkey CE (1994) Intracerebral propagation of interictal activity in partial epilepsy: implications for source localization. *Journal of Neurology, Neurosurgery and Psychiatry* 57:435–449.

Alarcon G, Garcia Seoane JJ, Binnie CD *et al* (1997) Origin and propagation of interictal discharges in the acute electrocortigram. Implications for pathophysiology and surgical treatment of temporal lobe epilepsy. *Brain* 120:2259–2282.

Arroyo S, Lesser RP, Awad IA, Golgring S, Sutherling WW, Resnick TJ (1993) Subdural and epidural grids and strips. In: Engel J (ed.) *Surgical Treatment of the Epilepsies*, pp 377–386. New York: Raven Press.

Bailey P, Gibbs FA (1951) The surgical treatment of psychomotor epilepsy. *Journal of the American Medical Association* 145:365–500.

Barr WB, Ashtari M, Schaul N (1997) Bilateral reductions in hippocampal volume in adults with epilepsy and a history of febrile seizures. *Journal of Neurology, Neurosurgery and Psychiatry* **63**:461–467.

Bengzon AR, Rasmussen T, Gloor P, Dussault J, Stephens M (1968) Prognostic factors in the surgical treatment of temporal lobe epileptics. *Neurology* **18**:717–731.

Berkovic SF, Andermann F, Melanson D, Ethier RE, Feindel W, Gloor P (1988) Hypothalamic hamartomas and ictal laughter: evolution of a characteristic epileptic syndrome and diagnostic value of magnetic resonance imaging. *Annals of Neurology* **23**:429–439.

Berkovic SF, Andermann F, Olivier A *et al* (1991) Hippocampal sclerosis in temporal lobe epilepsy demonstrated by magnetic resonance imaging. *Annals of Neurology* **29**:175–182.

Binnie CD, Elwes RD, Polkey CE, Volans A (1994a) Utility of stereoelectroencephalography in preoperative assessment of temporal lobe epilepsy. *Journal of Neurology, Neurosurgery and Psychiatry* **57**:58–65.

Binnie CD, McBride MC, Polkey CE, Sawhney IM, Janota I (1994b) Electrocorticography and stimulation. *Acta Neurologica Scandinavica* (Suppl) **152**:74–82.

Cascino GD, Jack CR Jr, Parisi JE *et al* (1991) Magnetic resonance imaging-based volume studies in temporal lobe epilepsy: pathological correlations. *Annals of Neurology* **30**:31–36.

Cascino GD, Kelly PK, Sharbrough FW, Hulihan JF, Hirschorn KA, Trenerry MR (1992) Long-term follow-up of stereotactic lesionectomy in partial epilepsy: predictive factors and electroen-cephalographic results. *Epilepsia* **33**:639–644.

Chauvel P, Klienman F, Vignal JP, Chodkiewicz JP, Talairach J, Bancaud J (1998) The clinical signs and symptoms of frontal lobe seizures: phenomenology and classification. In: Jasper HH, Riggio S, Goldman-Rakic PS (eds) *Epilepsy and the Functional Anatomy of the Frontal Lobe*, pp 115–126. New York: Raven Press.

Chugani HT, Conti JR (1996) Etiologic classification of infantile spasms in 140 cases: role of positron emission tomography. *Journal of Child Neurology* **11**:44–48.

Commission on Classification and Terminology of the International League Against Epilepsy (1981) Proposal for revised clinical and electroencephalographic classification of epileptic seizures. *Epilepsia* **22**:489–501.

Cooper R, Winter AL, Crow HJ (1965) Comparison of subcortical, cortical, and scalp activity using chronically indwelling electrodes in man. *EEG Clinical Neurophysiology* **18**:217–228.

Crandall PH, Walter RD, Rand RW (1963) Clinical applications of studies on stereotactically implanted electrodes in temporal lobe epilepsy. *Journal of Neurosurgery* **21**:827–840.

Crandall PH, Engel J, Rausch R (1983) Indications for depth electrode recordings in complex partial epilepsy and subsequent surgical results. In: Rose FC (ed.) *Research Progress in Epilepsy*, pp 507–526. London: Pitman.

Dowd CF, Dillon WP, Barbaro NM, Laxer KD (1991) Magnetic resonance imaging of intractable complex partial seizures: pathologic and electroencephalographic correlation. *Epilepsia* **32**:454–459.

Duncan R, Patterson J, Hadley D, Roberts R (1997) Ictal regional cerebral blood flow in frontal lobe seizures. *Seizure* **6**:393–401.

Duchowny M, Harvey AS, Jayakar P *et al* (1997) The preoperative evaluation of pediatric temporal lobe epilepsy. In: Tuxhorn I, Holthausen H, Boenigk H (eds) *Pediatric Epilepsy Syndromes and Their Surgical Treatment*, pp 261–273. London: John Libbey.

Eliashiv S, Dewer S, Wainwright I, Engel J, Fried I (1997) Long-term follow-up after temporal lobe resection for lesions associated with chronic seizures. *Neurology* **48**:1383–1388.

Elwes RDC, Dunn G, Binnie CD, Polkey CD (1991) Outcome following resective surgery for temporal lobe epilepsy: a prospective follow-up study of 102 consecutive cases. *Journal of Neurology, Neurosurgery and Psychiatry* **54**:949–952.

Engel J Jr (1993) *Surgical Treatment of the Epilepsies*. New York: Raven Press.

Engel J, Crandall PH (1983) Falsely localizing ictal onsets with depth-EEG telemetry during anticonvulsant withdrawal. *Epilepsia* **24**:344–355.

Engel J, Driver MV, Falconer MA (1975) Electrophysiological correlates of pathology and surgical results in temporal lobe epilepsy. *Brain* **98**:129–156.

Engel J, Kuhl DE, Phelps ME, Mazziotta JC (1982) Interictal cerebral glucose metabolism in partial epilepsy and its relation to EEG changes. *Annals of Neurology* **12**:510–517.

Falconer MA (1971) Anterior temporal lobectomy for epilepsy. In: Logue V (ed.) *Operative Surgery*, pp 142–149. London: Butterworths.

Falconer MA (1974) Mesial temporal (Ammon's) sclerosis as a common cause of epilepsy: etiology, treatment and prevention. *Lancet* **ii**:767–770.

Falconer MA, Serafetinides EA (1963) A follow-up study of surgery in temporal lobe epilepsy. *Journal of Neurology, Neurosurgery and Psychiatry* **26**:154–165.

Fiol ME, Gates JR, Torres F, Maxwell RE (1991) The prognostic value of residual spikes in the postexcision electrocortigram after temporal lobectomy. *Neurology* **41**:512–516.

Fish DR, Andermann F, Olivier A (1991) Complex partial seizures and posterior or extratemporal lesions: surgical strategies. *Neurology* **41**:1781–1784.

French JA, Williamson PD, Thadani VM *et al* (1993) Characteristics of medial temporal lobe epilepsy: I. Results of history and physical examination. *Annals of Neurology* **34**:774–780.

Gastaut H (1953) So-called 'psychomotor' and 'temporal'; a critical study. *Epilepsia* **2**:59–76.

Geier S, Bancaud J, Talairach J, Bonis A, Szikla G, Enjelvin M (1975) Clinical note: clinical and tele-stereo-EEG findings in a patient with psychomotor seizures. *Epilepsia* **16**:119–125.

Gibbs EL, Gibbs FA, Fuster B (1948) Psychomotor epilepsy. *Archives of Neurology and Psychiatry* **60**:331–339.

Goldring S, Gregorie EM (1984) Surgical management of epilepsy using epidural recordings to localize the seizure focus. Review of 100 cases. *Journal of Neurosurgery* **60**:457–466.

Gotman J, Ives JR, Gloor P (1979) Automatic recognition of interictal epileptic activity in prolonged EEG recordings. *Electroencephalography and Clinical Neurophysiology* **46**:510–520.

Horsley V (1886) Brain surgery. *British Medical Journal* **2**:675.

Jackson GD, Kuzniecky RI, Cascino GD (1994) Hippocampal sclerosis without detectable hippocampal atrophy. *Neurology* **44**:42–46.

Jackson JH (1870) A study of convulsions. Transactions of the St Andrews Medical Graduate Association, Vol iii. In: Taylor J, Holmes G, Walshe FMR (eds) (1931) *John Hughlings Jackson: Selected Writings Vol I. On Epilepsy and Epileptiform Convulsions*, pp 8–36. Facsimile reproduction published by Monumenta Neurologica ac Psychiatrica (1996) Arts NJM (ed.). Nijmegen: Arts and Boeve.

Jackson JH (1888) On a particular variety of epilepsy (intellectual aura), one case with symptoms of organic brain disease. *Brain* **11**:179–207.

Jackson JH (1899) Epileptic attacks in a patients who had symptoms pointing to gross organic disease of the right temporosphenoidal lobe. *Brain* **22**:534–549.

Jasper H, Tertuisset B, Flanigin H (1951) EEG and cortical electrograms in patients with temporal lobe seizures. *Archives of Neurology and Psychiatry* **65**:272–290.

Jayakar P, Duchowny M (1997) Invasive EEG and functional cortical mapping. In: Tuxhorn I, Holthausen H, Boenigk H (eds) *Pediatric Epilepsy Syndromes and Their Surgical Treatment*, pp 547–556. London: John Libbey.

Jayakar P, Alvarez LA, Duchowny MS, Resnick TJ (1992) A safe and effective paradigm to functionally map the cortex in childhood. *Journal of Clinical Neurophysiology* **9**:288–293.

Kilpatrick C, Cook M, Kaye A, Murphy M, Matkovic Z (1997) Noninvasive investigations successfully select patients for temporal lobe surgery. *Journal of Neurology, Neurosurgery and Psychiatry* **63**:327–333.

Kirkpatrick PJ, Honavar M, Janota I, Polkey CE (1993) Control of temporal lobe epilepsy following *en bloc* resection of low-grade tumors. *Journal of Neurosurgery* **78**:19–25.

Lieb JP, Walsh GO, Babb TL, Walter RD, Crandall PH (1976) A comparison of EEG seizure patterns recorded with surface and depth electrodes in patients with temporal lobe epilepsy. *Epilepsia* **17**:137–160.

Lieb JP, Engel J, Brown WJ, Gevins AS, Crandall PH (1981) Neuropathological findings following temporal lobectomy related to surface and deep EEG patterns. *Epilepsia* **22**:539–541.

Luders H (1991) *Epilepsy Surgery*. New York: Raven Press.

Margerison JH, Corsellis JA (1966) Epilepsy and the temporal lobes. A clinical, electroencephalographic and neuropathological study of the brain in epilepsy, with particular reference to the temporal lobes. *Brain* **89**:499–530.

McBride MC, Binnie CD, Janota I, Polkey CE (1991) Predictive value of intraoperative electrocorticograms in resective epilepsy surgery. *Annals of Neurology* **30**:526–532.

Morrell F, Whisler WW, Smith MC *et al* (1995) Landau–Kleffner syndrome. Treatment with subpial intracortical transection. *Brain* **118**:1529–1546.

Morris HH, Dinner DS, Luders H, Wyllie E, Kramer K (1988) Supplementary motor seizures: clinical and electroencephalographic features. *Neurology* **38**:1075–1082.

Munari C, Kahane P, Tassi L, Fracione S, Hoffmann D, Lo Russo G (1993) Intracerebral low-frequency electrical stimulation: a new tool for the definition of the 'epileptogenic area'? *Acta Neurochirurgica* (Suppl) **58**:181–185.

Munari C, Hoffmann D, Francione S *et al* (1994) Stereo-electroencephalography methodology: advantages and limits. *Acta Neurologica Scandinavica* (Suppl) **152**:56–67.

Munari C, Tassi L, Di Leo M *et al* (1995a) Video-stereo-electroencephalographic investigation of orbitofrontal cortex. Ictal electroclinical patterns. *Advances in Neurology* **66**:273–295.

Munari C, Kahane P, Francione S *et al* (1995b) Role of the hypothalamic hamartoma in the genesis of gelastic fits (a video-stereo-EEG study). *Electroencephalography and Clinical Neurophysiology* **95**:154–160.

Ojemann GA (1997) Intraoperative methods. In: Engel J, Pedley TA (eds) *Epilepsy: A Comprehensive Textbook*, pp 1777–1783. Philadelphia: Lippincott Raven.

Ojemann GA, Engel J (1987) Acute and chronic intracranial recording and stimulation. In: Engel J (ed.) *Surgical Treatment of the Epilepsies*, pp 263–288. New York: Raven Press.

Palmini A, Gambardella A, Andermann F *et al* (1995) Intrinsic epileptogenicity of human dysplastic cortex as suggested by corticography and surgical results. *Annals of Neurology* **37**:476–487.

Penfield W, Jasper H (1954) *Epilepsy and the Functional Anatomy of the Human Brain*. Boston: Little, Brown.

Polkey CE (1996) Complications of epilepsy surgery. In: Shorvon S, Dreifuss F, Fish D, Thomas D (eds) *The Treatment of Epilepsy*, pp 780–793 Oxford: Blackwell Science.

Polkey CE, Binnie CD, Janota I (1989) Acute hippocampal recording and pathology at temporal lobe resection and amygdalohippocampectomy for epilepsy. *Journal of Neurology, Neurosurgery and Psychiatry* **52**:1050–1057.

Privitera MD, Quinlan JG, Yeh HS (1990) Interictal spike detection comparing subdural and depth electrodes during electrocorticography. *Electroencephalography and Clinical Neurophysiology* **76**:379–387.

Quesney LF, Cendes F, Olivier A, Dubeau F, Andermann F (1995) Intracranial electroencephalographic investigation in frontal lobe epilepsy. *Advances in Neurology* **66**:243–258.

Quigg M, Bertram EH, Jackson T, Laws E (1997) Volumetric magnetic resonance imaging evidence of bilateral hippocampal atrophy in mesial temporal lobe epilepsy. *Epilepsia* **38**:588–594.

Rasmussen T (1975) Cortical resection in the treatment of focal epilepsy. In: Purpura DP, Penry JK, Walter RD (eds) *Advances in Neurology*, pp 139–154. New York: Raven Press.

Risinger MW, Engel J Jr, Van Ness PC, Henry TR, Crandall PH (1989) Ictal localization of temporal lobe seizures with scalp/sphenoidal recordings. *Neurology* **39**: 1288–1293.

Rosenbaum TJ, Laxer KD, Vessely M, Smith WB (1986) Subdural electrodes for seizure focus localization. *Neurosurgery* **19**:73–81.

Scheffer IE, Bhatia KP, Lopes Cendes *et al* (1995) Autosomal dominant nocturnal frontal lobe epilepsy. A distinctive clinical disorder. *Brain* **118**:61–73.

So N, Gloor P, Quesney LF, Jones Gotman M, Olivier A, Andermann F (1989) Depth electrode investigations in patients with bitemporal epileptiform abnormalities. *Annals of Neurology* **25**:423–431.

Spencer SS (1981) Depth electroencephalography in selection of refractory epilepsy for surgery. *Annals of Neurology* **9**:207–214.

Spencer SS, Spencer DD, Williamson PD, Mattson RH (1982) The localizing value of depth electroencephalography in 32 patients with refractory epilepsy. *Annals of Neurology* **12**:248–253.

Spencer SS, Guimaraes P, Katz A, Kim J, Spencer D (1992) Morphological patterns of seizures recorded intracranially. *Epilepsia* **33**:537–545.

Spencer SS, So NK, Engel J, Williamson PD, Levesque MF, Spencer DD (1993) Depth electrodes. In: Engel J (ed.) *Surgical Treatment of the Epilepsies*, pp 359–376. New York: Raven Press.

Sperling MR, O'Connor MJ (1989) Comparison of depth and subdural electrodes in recording temporal lobe seizures. *Neurology* **39**: 1497–1504.

Sperling MR, O'Connor MJ (1990) Auras and subclinical seizures: characteristics and prognostic significance. *Annals of Neurology* **28**:320–328.

Sperling MR, O'Connor MJ, Saykin AJ *et al* (1992) A noninvasive protocol for anterior temporal lobectomy. *Neurology* **42**:416–422.

Talairach J, Bancaud J (1974) Stereotaxic exploration and therapy in epilepsy. In: Vinken PJ, Bruyn GW (eds) *Handbook of Clinical Neurology*, pp 758–782. Amsterdam: Elsevier.

Uematsu S, Lesser R, Fisher RS, *et al* (1992) Motor and sensory cortex in humans: topography study with chronic subdural stimulation. *Neurosurgery* **31**:59–72.

van Paesschen W, Duncan JS, Stevens JM, Connelly A (1997) Etiology and early prognosis of newly diagnosed partial seizures in adults: a quantitative hippocampal MRI study. *Neurology* **49**:753–757.

van Veelen CMW, Debets RM, van Huffelen AC (1990) Combined use of subdural and intracerebral electrodes in preoperative evaluation of epilepsy. *Neurosurgery* **26**:93–101.

Wieser HG (1983) *Electroclinical Features of the Psychomotor Seizures*. Stuttgart: Gustav Fischer Verlag.

Wieser HG (1991) Semi-invasive EEG: foramen ovale electrodes. In: Luders H (ed.) *Epilepsy Surgery*. New York: Raven Press.

Wieser HG, Elger CE (1987) *Presurgical Evaluation of Epileptics*. Berlin: Springer-Verlag

Wieser HG, Elger CE, Stodieck SRG (1985) The 'foramen ovale electrode': a new recording method for the preoperative evaluation of patients suffering from mesiobasal temporal lobe epilepsy. *Electroencephalography and Clinical Neurophysiology* **61**:314–322.

Wieser H, Quesney LF, Morris HH (1993) Foramen ovale and PEG electrodes. In: Engel J (ed.) *Surgical Treatment of the Epilepsies*, pp 331–339. New York: Raven Press.

Williamson PD, Spencer DD, Spencer SS, Novelly RA, Mattson RH (1985) Complex partial seizures of frontal lobe origin. *Annals of Neurology* **18**:497–504.

Williamson PD, French JA, Thadani VM *et al* (1993a) Characteristics of medial temporal lobe epilepsy: II. Interictal and ictal scalp electroencephalography, neuropsychological testing, neuroimaging, surgical results, and pathology. *Annals of Neurology* **34**:781–787.

Williamson PD, Van Ness PC, Wieser H, Quesney LF (1993b) Surgically remedial extratemporal syndromes. In: Engel J (ed.) *Surgical Treatment of the Epilepsies*, pp 65–76. New York: Raven Press.

Wolf P (1991) The history of surgical treatment of epilepsy in Europe. In: Luders H (ed.) *Epilepsy Surgery*, pp 9–17. New York: Raven Press.

Wyler AR, Ojemann GA, Lettich E, Ward AA (1984) Subdural strip electrodes for localizing epileptogenic foci. *Journal of Neurosurgery* **60**:1195–1200.

Wyler AR, Richey ET, Atkinson RA *et al* (1987) Methohexital activation of epileptogenic foci during acute electrocorticography. *Epilepsia* **28**:490–494.

Yasargill MG, Wieser HG (1987) Selective microsurgical techniques. In: Wieser HG, Elger CE (eds) *Presurgical Evaluation of Epileptics*, pp 653–658. Berlin: Springer.

Yasargil MG, Teddy PG, Roth P (1985) Selective amygdalohippocampectomy: operative anatomy and surgical technique. In: Symon L (ed.) *Advances and Technical Standards in Neurosurgery*, pp 93–123. Vienna: Springer.

Zentner J, Hufnagel A, Wolf HK *et al* (1995) Surgical treatment of temporal lobe epilepsy: clinical, radiological, and histopathological findings in 178 patients. *Journal of Neurology, Neurosurgery and Psychiatry* **58**:666–673.

Preoperative neuropsychologic assessment

SM OXBURY

Neuropsychologic examination prior to surgery for intractable focal epilepsy is an integral part of the multidisciplinary presurgical evaluation. It comprises both conventional assessment of neuropsychologic abilities and, in some cases, tests of specific functions while part of the brain is temporarily inactivated by sodium amobarbital (see Chapter 47). There are a number of aims:

1. To determine whether the neuropsychologic profile is consistent with the lateralization and localization of the pathology and/or the epileptogenic area to be targeted for surgical excision or suggests, perhaps in addition, dysfunction elsewhere. Consistency or concordance may be based on the finding of clear deficits reflecting the brain area under consideration. Preoperative studies of patients with focal epilepsy, however, have not necessarily revealed deficits as clearly as may have been hoped on the basis of postoperative studies (see, for instance, Chapter 30: section on hippocampal sclerosis and memory). The neuropsychologic contribution is often that of stating that the profile is not actually discordant with the localization based on other investigations. Discordant findings are those which suggest focal dysfunction elsewhere, or give evidence of diffuse damage. The finding of atypical cerebral language dominance will lead to reinterpretation of the results,

possibly resolving apparent anomalies, and it may modify the surgical strategy.

2. To predict the risk to memory and other cognitive function of the proposed surgery. Many psychologists agree that this is a fundamental and crucial aim. The opportunity to relate neuropsychologic change to various preoperative and surgical variables has enabled predictions to be made at least for temporal lobe surgery (see Chapter 60). Among the predictors is preoperative neuropsychologic evidence that the pathology/focus to be excised contains functional tissue. Future work should refine these predictors still further for both temporal lobe and other focal resections.

3. To allow evaluation of neuropsychologic change consequent upon surgery. This is clearly necessary both for clinical purposes and to contribute to knowledge relating to (2) above. Preoperative assessment must therefore be planned with a view to the appropriate postoperative evaluation.

4. To contribute information relevant to psychosocial and/or educational issues. This is achieved using baseline levels, specific abilities and impairments, and also any change over surgery.

5. To contribute to the prediction of seizure outcome. This is seen as an important potential role by some

psychologists (Dodrill *et al* 1993), using multivariate predictors (Dodrill *et al* 1990) or single measures (Chelune *et al* 1998).

6. For audit and research to further knowledge relating to all these issues and to contribute to the evaluation of new developments. Such developments may be in imaging or surgery as well as in neuropsychologic techniques.

GENERAL CONSIDERATIONS

Many publications over the last 20 years or more have described preoperative assessment and the subject has developed enormously during that time (Milner 1975; Taylor 1979; Rausch 1987; Jones-Gotman 1991, 1996; Jones-Gotman *et al* 1993; Loring 1997; Oxbury 1997, 1998; Rausch *et al* 1998). Indeed in 1987, Rausch commented with justification that 'as compared with postoperative neuropsychological studies, neuropsychological research directed toward the preoperative work-up of the epileptic patient is sparse'. The position has certainly improved with respect to temporal lobe excisions (see Chapter 30), the most frequently performed surgery, but less so for frontal lobe excisions which constitute the next most frequent surgery (Chapter 31).

There is general agreement that a wide-ranging assessment is necessary so that the patient's performance on specific localizing tasks can be interpreted both against the background of general cognitive level, and also in relation to any other specific neuropsychologic deficits that may be revealed. For example, impaired language function or visuospatial ability would influence the patient's performance on specific verbal or nonverbal memory tasks. It is also important for evaluation to be sufficiently thorough for evidence of dysfunction elsewhere in the brain to be detected. The preoperative assessment should include tasks that are thought to be valid for *preoperative* evaluation of the cortex that may be removed. It should also include tasks that permit an assessment of *pre-/postoperative* change, bearing in mind that such change may occur in functions not standardly associated with the cortex which is to be removed. For instance, a small proportion of patients who have dominant hemisphere temporal lobe excisions develop some language disturbance, and this impairment could not be evaluated satisfactorily if language function had not been assessed preoperatively.

There are several methodological issues relating to pre-/postoperative evaluation. Repeated exposure to test materials may lead to inflated scores due to a practice effect. For Wechsler intelligence quotient (IQ) tests it is generally accepted that this applies more to Performance IQ than to Verbal IQ, and indeed, a small improvement in Performance IQ is often attributed to a practice effect rather than to genuinely improved function. The problem is more serious in relation to memory and learning tasks where the test paradigms are designed to measure capacity to absorb new material. Re-exposure to material is likely to give a false impression either that the patient has improved or that memory has not altered, whereas in fact it may have deteriorated. It is important, therefore, to use parallel forms of memory and learning tests wherever possible. It is disappointing that many standardized tests do not have alternate forms.

The ontogenetic development of lateralization and localization of specific neuropsychologic functions is not entirely understood. Consequently, methodological difficulties may arise in the preoperative assessment of children when attempts are made to evaluate functions known to be associated with a particular site and side of pathology in adults. Even greater difficulties can arise when attempts are made to plan meaningful pre-/postoperative evaluation of these functions, long term. At the time of surgery the child may be too young to possess functions that would be expected to develop at an older age. The assessments of memory and of executive function are examples.

ASSESSMENT OF ADULTS

GENERAL COGNITIVE MEASURES

The most widely used, as a background measure of overall cognitive ability, is the Wechsler Adult Intelligence Scale – Revised (WAIS-R) (Wechsler 1986). Further knowledge may be gleaned from individual subtest scores, some of which will have a bearing on specific areas such as visuospatial ability, attention, or speed of processing. A new version of this scale is now available, WAIS-III (Wechsler 1999a), and preliminary discussion regarding its use in a neuropsychologic setting has been published by Loring (1997).

In general the Full Scale IQ of patients with focal epilepsy having cortical excisions is in the normal range. An IQ of less than 70 has in the past been considered a contraindication to some types of surgery, but this restriction no longer generally applies (King et al 1993). At this lower range, however, the interpretation of other neuropsychologic tests in terms of localization of function becomes less reliable. Discrepancies between Verbal IQ and Performance IQ should of course be noted and may sometimes be relevant but are not necessarily related to laterality of focus/lesion (Chapter 30).

TESTS OF LANGUAGE FUNCTION

These should include the assessment of naming, comprehension, sentence repetition, reading, writing, and verbal fluency. The tests commonly used include:

Multilingual Aphasia Examination (Benton *et al* 1994) or selected subtests from this scale such as sentence repetition and word association;

Graded Naming Test (McKenna and Warrington 1983; Warrington 1997);

Boston Naming Test (Kaplan *et al* 1983);

Shortened Token Test (De Renzi and Faglioni 1978); Letter fluency, FAS test (Lezak 1995);

Schonell tests of reading and spelling;

Wechsler Objective Reading Dimensions (Wechsler 1993), which despite an upper age limit of 16 can give useful information in older adolescents or young adults for comparing levels of single word reading, spelling, and reading comprehension;

Subtests of Wide Range Achievement Test 3 (Wilkinson 1993).

VISUOSPATIAL AND PERCEPTUAL TASKS

Information about visuospatial constructional ability will be gained from WAIS-R subtests, block design and object assembly, and from the copy of the Rey–Osterrieth figure (Osterrieth 1944). Similarly, visual perceptual problems may be observed or suspected in the patient's performance on naming tests, if difficulty identifying objects is revealed, and on picture completion and picture arrangement subtests of the WAIS-R. Facets of visual perception may be further examined using the Hooper (1983) or the Visual Object and Spatial Perception test (Warrington and James 1991). If there is a risk of surgery creating or extending a visual field defect, as there may be in radical surgery for Rasmussen's syndrome or in posterior hemisphere excisions, it may be prudent to include tests of visual inattention (Behavioral Inattention Test, Wilson *et al* 1987).

ATTENTIONAL AND EXECUTIVE FUNCTION/FRONTAL LOBE TASKS

These include the Wisconsin card sorting test (WCST) (Heaton *et al* 1993), trail making (Lezak 1995), Stroop, Cognitive Estimations (Shallice and Evans 1978), and word association or verbal fluency particularly for left frontal dysfunction. While all these have shown deficits in patients with frontal lobe foci preoperatively, temporal lobe patients may also perform poorly on some tasks including the WCST (Chapters 30 and 31). Baseline performance is nevertheless essential for postoperative comparison, since frontal lobe surgery may be followed by an exacerbation of impairment, whereas temporal lobe surgery patients tend to improve. The Test of Everyday Attention (Robertson *et al* 1994), particularly the subtests addressing divided attention, may have potential for frontal lobe epilepsy patients.

TESTS OF MEMORY AND LEARNING

These are important for all patients, but particularly so for those with temporal lobe foci, who in general perform less well than those with extratemporal dysfunction (Milner 1975; Breier *et al* 1996). Evaluation should include both the verbal and the nonverbal modalities and different test paradigms. Immediate spans, both immediate and delayed recall, learning over several trials and retention of the material are tested. Forms of the Wechsler Memory Scale (WMS) have been much used. The original forms (Wechsler 1945) gave an overall memory quotient combining all subtests and did not include tests of delayed recall. Russell (1975, 1988) adapted parts of the scale to give separate verbal and nonverbal measures and added delayed-recall tests. These scales have the advantage of providing an alternate form so that the practice effect can be avoided. More recent versions of the WMS have since been produced. WMS-R (Wechsler 1987) gives separate verbal and nonverbal indices and tests for delayed recall, but the delayed-memory index does not separate verbal and nonverbal tasks and there is no alternate form. The new WMS-III (Wechsler 1999b) is yet to be tested in epilepsy surgery.

In temporal lobe patients, the WMS verbal subtests have been useful in identifying impairment, but the nonverbal tests are less sensitive. Reproduction of the Rey complex figure has frequently been used as a measure of delayed nonverbal recall with Taylor's (1979) figure as the alternate form. Taylor's figure, however, has been reported as being easier than the Rey figure (Tombaugh and Hubley 1991). The recent updated version of the Rey complex figure test (Meyers and Meyers 1995) uses the Taylor figure in the recognition trial, thus spoiling its use as an alternate form. The Benton Visual Retention Test (Benton 1992) is useful in testing immediate figural recall and provides three alternate forms. Both these figural recall tasks have been criticized as being too easily verbalizable.

The psychologist should consider what areas of memory function should be included and select accordingly. In the verbal domain, tests of immediate span for both digits and sentences, a story recall task with alternate forms if possible and delayed recall of the material after a standard filled interval, and a verbal learning test, are all essential. The latter could be a word list learning task such as the Rey Auditory Verbal Learning Test (RAVLT, Lezak 1995) or the California Verbal Learning Test (CVLT, Delis *et al* 1986) or the selective reminding test (Bushke and Fuld 1974; Spreen and Strauss 1991). The CVLT has only one set of material. The RAVLT is frequently used in one form only, although a parallel form was published by Crawford *et al* (1989). It has recently been extended to three forms by Majdan *et al* (1996) who demonstrated their equivalence on groups of normals. The selective reminding test has four alternate forms that Westerveld *et al* (1994) have shown to be equivalent and reliable and without practice effect. The paired associates from WMS or WMS-R have proved useful in some studies of hippocampal sclerosis. Unfortunately, it has no alternate forms except for the old original WMS. A version with a greater number of pairs allowing a wider spread of scores would be welcome.

In the nonverbal sphere the Corsi block tapping span and the figural recall tasks described above may add useful information about the general status of the patient's memory but are not firmly lateralizing. A design learning task, such as the three versions used by Majdan *et al* (1996), may prove more discriminating (Jones-Gotman 1996). Clinically applicable versions of spatial memory tasks, such as maze learning or incidental spatial memory (Smith and Milner 1981), might also prove to be sensitive preoperatively.

SELF-ASSESSMENT QUESTIONNAIRES

These are used in some centers and may be useful in assessing pre-/postoperative subjective change, which may not entirely reflect changes seen on neuropsychologic assessment (McGlone 1994). The data may also be useful in psychosocial issues and rehabilitation. Several questionnaires have been used in this context (O'Shea *et al* 1996).

The choice of a test battery is important and only when it has been used over a period of time will the neuropsychologist begin to build up experience with different types of patients. So, it is important for an epilepsy surgery center to create a core battery and to stick with it for a reasonable period before determining its usefulness.

ASSESSMENT OF CHILDREN

Children who are candidates for epilepsy surgery span the whole age range, from the first year of life through to adolescence and include those with pathologies of very varying nature and extent. Some have restricted focal pathology, such as a small dysembryoplastic neuroepithelial tumor, and will have excisions similar to adult epilepsy surgery candidates, whereas others may have multilobar pathology or massive hemisphere damage leading to extensive surgery or hemispherectomy. Thus the neuropsychologist must be equipped to evaluate development and cognition over the whole range of childhood, and in children representing a very wide range of ability from severe retardation to normal.

All this will influence the extent to which the aims of neuropsychologic assessment as laid out in the introduction to this chapter are appropriate or can be met. Furthermore, knowledge about neuropsychologic outcome from epilepsy surgery in young children and especially in the long term is only just beginning to accumulate, so relatively few predictions can be made with confidence. The issues and a wide range of suggested tests have been reviewed elsewhere (Jones-Gotman *et al* 1993; Oxbury 1997, 1998). A core battery should include the following:

1. Tests of general developmental level or intelligence
2. Tests of language function
3. Tests of visuospatial ability to supplement the Wechsler Intelligence Scale for Children performance tests
4. Attentional tasks and tests of executive function
5. Memory tests
6. Measurement of educational attainments

Specific tests within these various categories are listed by Oxbury (1998); see Table 46.1.

SPECIFIC SURGERIES, RISKS, AND CONTRAINDICATIONS

The pattern of neuropsychologic function prior to surgery in specific focal epilepsies has been described in Chapters 30, and 31. Interpretation of the results of a comprehensive preoperative assessment as described here must be made in the light of the findings described in those chapters. This is the information that allows us to decide whether the neuropsychologic profile is consistent with the lateralization and localization of the pathology, and/or the epileptogenic area, to be targeted in the proposed surgical excision

Table 46.1 Tests available for the assessment of children.

Test	Age range (years unless stated)	Reference
General developmental and intelligence scales		
Bayley scales of infant development II	1–42 months	Bayley 1993
Uzgiris–Hunt scales		Robinson and Rosenberg 1987
Wechsler scales		
Wechsler Preschool and Primary Scale of Intelligence – Revised	3–7	Wechsler 1989
Wechsler Intelligence Scale for Children – Revised	6–16	Wechsler 1991
British Ability Scales (BAS)	2.6–17.11	Elliott *et al* 1996
Differential Ability Scales (DAS)	2.6–17.11	Elliott 1990
Language		
Verbal development assessment from infant scales		See above
Reynell developmental language scales– second revision	1–7	Reynell and Huntley 1985
Peabody Picture Vocabulary Test – R III	2.6–adult	Dunn and Dunn 1997
British Picture Vocabulary scale 2nd edn	2.6–18	Dunn *et al* 1997
Token Test for Children	3–12	Di Simoni 1978
Test for the Reception of Grammar	4.0–12.11	Bishop 1989
Boston Naming Test	6–12	Halperin *et al* 1989
Expressive one-word picture vocabulary test revised	2–11.11	Gardner 1990a
upper extension	12–15	Gardner 1990b
Receptive one-word picture vocabulary test	2–11.11	Gardner 1992
upper extension	12–15	Brownell 1992
Visuospatial and perceptuomotor		
Developmental test of Visual-motor Integration (VMI)	2–15	Beery 1997
Subtests of infant scales		See above
Constructional tests from other scales e.g. Wechsler block design, object assembly		See above
Memory and learning		
Wide Range Assessment of Memory and Learning	5–17	Sheslow and Adams 1990
Children's Memory Scale	5–16	Cohen 1997
Wechsler Memory Scales (forms I and II)[a]	15+	Wechsler 1945
Children's norms	10–adult	Ivinskis *et al* 1971
WMS paired associate learning test (form I)	6–12	Halperin *et al* 1989
WMS logical memory immediate and delayed recall	10–15	Curry *et al* 1986
Rey Auditory Verbal Learning Test	7–14	Spreen and Strauss 1991
California Verbal Learning Test for Children	5–16.11	Delis *et al* 1993
Buschke Selective Reminding Test[a]	5–8	Morgan 1982
	9–12	Clodfelter *et al* 1987
Story recall (Beardsworth and Bishop)[a]	8–12	Beardsworth and Bishop 1994
Benton Visual Retention Test[a]	8–adult	Benton 1992
BAS/DAS recall of designs		See above
Rey–Osterrieth complex figure	4–adult	Osterrieth 1944
Taylor alternative form		Taylor 1979
Rey complex figure test	6–adult	Meyers and Meyers 1995
Motor ability		
Movement Assessment Battery for Children	4–12	Henderson and Sugden 1992
Purdue peg board	5.0–15.11	Spreen and Strauss 1998
Attention, Frontal and Fluency		
Trail making	8–15	Spreen and Strauss 1998
Wisconsin card sorting test	6–adult	Heaton *et al* 1993
Word fluency	6–12	Halperin *et al* 1989
FAS	6–13	Gaddes and Crockett 1975
Word and design fluency	5–14	Jones-Gotman 1990
Educational attainments		
Wide Range Achievement Test 3	5–adult	Wilkinson 1993

Table 46.1 Continued

Test	Age range (years unless stated)	Reference
Peabody Individual Achievement Test – revised (PIAT-R)	5.0–18.11	Markwardt 1989
Wechsler Objective Reading Dimensions (WORD)	6–16	Wechsler 1993
Neale analysis of reading ability (revised)	6–11.11	Neale 1989
BAS or DAS		See above
Basic number skills		See above
Word reading		See above
Spelling scale		See above
Behavioral and psychosocial		
Child behavior check list and youth self-report	4–18	Achenbach 1991
Vineland adaptive behavior scales	0–18.11	Sparrow et al 1984
Adolescent Psychosocial Seizure Inventory (APSI)	12–19	Batzel et al 1991

[a]Memory and learning tests that have alternate forms.

or suggests dysfunction elsewhere. Neuropsychologic outcome is predicted by combining the results of the preoperative neuropsychologic assessment with knowledge of factors influencing cognitive outcome from surgery, as described in Chapter 60. This may be supplemented by the findings of studies using patients who have been tested postoperatively but not preoperatively. It must be remembered, however, that postoperative studies alone do not tell us whether any observed impairments are consequent upon surgery or were preexisting, nor can they provide information relevant to predicting individual change associated with other preoperative factors, such as magnetic resonance imaging (MRI) findings, suspected pathology, and/or neuropsychologic status.

TEMPORAL LOBE OPERATIONS

Risks to language function and to material-specific memory and associated factors are described in Chapter 60 with emphasis on the functional and structural status of the tissue to be excised. There is a small risk of surgery resulting in a severe global memory deficit when medial structures are excised (Penfield and Milner 1958; Rausch et al 1985; Loring et al 1994). This is associated with preexisting pathology in the contralateral medial structures, particularly the hippocampus (Penfield and Mathieson 1974; Warrington and Duchen 1992). Damage to the contralateral side may be suspected preoperatively if the neuropsychologic findings show memory dysfunction usually attributed to that side, or generally impaired memory raising the question of bilateral damage, or if other investigations are not concordant. Surgery that includes medial structures may then be contraindicated, unless carotid amobarbital studies clearly demonstrate that the not-to-be-operated side can support memory (see Chapter 47). This

situation can be a problem in children aged less than 12 years, as they tolerate amobarbital tests poorly and memory assessment under these conditions tends to be unreliable (Szabo and Wyllie 1993).

Interpretation of other neuropsychologic data must be reevaluated when amobarbital studies show atypical language dominance. This requires caution as it is not safe to assume a simple mirror image or crossover between the hemispheres as Loring's et al (1994) case illustrates (see also Rausch et al 1991).

FRONTAL LOBE SURGERY

Impairment in executive function following frontal lobe surgery is described in Chapter 59. There is inevitably a risk of an aphasic language deficit if the excision approaches Broca's area. Clearly this risk exists particularly for left-hemisphere excisions, but it should be remembered that atypical language representation is not uncommon in people with longstanding epilepsy, even right-handers. Some units would carry out carotid amobarbital tests prior to all right frontal excisions close to the third frontal convolution.

POSTERIOR EXCISIONS

As indicated in Chapter 62, additional preoperative measures may be necessary to tap relevant functions. Functional mapping will be essential in many cases.

HEMISPHERECTOMY

Most of those undergoing this operation are children who have a history of infantile hemiplegia, intractable epilepsy and massive damage to one hemisphere, or children who have acquired Rasmussen's syndrome. Cognitive function has developed in the good hemisphere in the group with early static damage, regardless of side, with most functions represented but usually below the normal range. A Verbal/Performance IQ discrepancy reflecting the side of damage is not usually found. Intractable seizures in these children are not infrequently accompanied by difficult behavior, and both behavior and cognitive function are sometimes deteriorating by the time surgery is considered.

Children with Rasmussen's syndrome have previously been normal and usually present in the first decade of life. The disease progresses over a variable period of time leading to the development of hemiplegia and cognitive deterioration. The cognitive decline usually occurs in both verbal and nonverbal ability, even though the disease is considered to affect one hemisphere only. Language usually develops in the right hemisphere if the pathology has commenced in the left hemisphere before the age of 6 years, but it may make less satisfactory 'transfer' after this age. Apparent transfer of language from left to right hemisphere has, however, been described in an adolescent boy (Taylor 1991). Carotid amobarbital studies are often necessary prior to left-sided surgery to show that the hemisphere is nonfunctional for language. Whether it is best to delay surgery until this point is reached, however, is now debated. Taylor (1991) has described cognitive decline in the condition. He stated clearly the dilemma of whether to proceed to left-hemisphere surgery with the hope of alleviating the continuous seizures before maximum transfer of speech to the right hemisphere, or whether to wait until this has happened while the child suffers further the detrimental effects of the seizures.

CORPUS CALLOSOTOMY

Adults

Preoperatively cognitive ability spans a wide range from normal to considerably impaired, with no particular pattern. Neuropsychologic assessment must include those functions particularly at risk, i.e. speech and language, memory and attention, and motor function. Carotid amobarbital studies are essential to establish cerebral dominance, to determine whether there is bilateral language organization, and to assess the memory function of each hemisphere.

Assessment of the risk of the various complications is a major objective (Pilcher *et al* 1993). Important considerations are: (a) mixed dominance in which language and handedness are localized in opposite hemispheres; (b) bilateral or mixed hemisphere language representation; (c) hemianopia contralateral to the side of language representation; and (d) absence of functional memory in the language-dominant hemisphere.

Children

Neuropsychologic evaluation of children having corpus callosotomy has been described by Lassonde *et al* (1990). Their choice of test battery draws on many different standardized tests depending on the child's developmental level and covers the whole range of cognitive motor and social development. Children operated on under 12 years of age are at less risk of developing the 'split brain' syndromes than older patients (Lassonde *et al* 1986).

KEY POINTS

1. The aims of preoperative neuropsychologic assessment include evaluation of the consistency of the neuropsychologic profile with the results of other investigations, prediction of postoperative cognitive and memory change, and the planning of suitable postoperative assessment to evaluate change.

2. Assessment should be wide ranging and should include tests of general cognitive ability, language function, visuospatial and perceptual function, verbal and nonverbal aspects of memory and learning, attention, and executive function. Appropriate test paradigms known to be sensitive to preoperative cognitive deficits and to pre-/postoperative change should be included. It may be necessary to assess additional functions before specific surgeries, such as posterior hemisphere excisions.

3. In children assessment techniques must cover a wide range of both age and ability. Infant and developmental scales are often called for as well as children's versions of the tasks described for adults. The planning of long-term follow-up should ideally be part of preoperative assessment.

4. Results of intra-arterial sodium amobarbital studies of cerebral language dominance and memory (see Chapter 47) may be essential for the final interpretation of the preoperative profile and the formulation of postoperative predictions. When a significant risk of severe postoperative amnesia is thought to exist medial TL excisions are contraindicated.

REFERENCES

Achenbach TM (1991) *Integrative Guide for the 1991 CBCL/4–18, YSR and TRF Profiles.* Burlington, VT: University of Vermont, Department of Psychiatry.

Batzel LW, Dodrill DB, Dubinsky BL (1991) An objective method for the assessment of psychosocial problems in adolescents with epilepsy. *Epilepsia* 32:202–211.

Bayley N (1993) *Bayley Scales of Infant Development II.* New York: The Psychological Corporation.

Beardsworth ED, Bishop D (1994) Assessment of long-term verbal memory in children. *Memory* 2:129–148.

Beery KE (1997) *The Visual–Motor Integration Test,* 4th edn. Administration, Scoring and Teaching Manual. Austin, TX: Pro-ED.

Benton AL, Hamsher K, Rey JG, Sivan AB (1994) *Multilingual Aphasia Examination,* 3rd edn. Iowa City: AJA Associates.

Benton SA (1992) *Benton Visual Retention Test (BVRT),* 5th edn. New York: The Psychological Corporation.

Bishop DVM (1989) *Test for Reception of Grammar,* 2nd edn. Published by the author; 1989. Available from: Age & Cognitive Performance Research Centre, University of Manchester M13 9PL, UK.

Breier JI, Plenger PM, Wheless JW *et al* (1996) Memory tests distinguish between patients with focal, temporal and extratemporal lobe epilepsy. *Epilepsia* 37(2):165–170.

Brownell R (1992) *ROWPVT.* Odessa, FL: Upper Extension Psychological Assessment Resources.

Bushke H, Fuld P (1974) Evaluating storage, retention and retrieval in disordered memory and learning. *Neurology* 24:1019–1025.

Chelune GJ, Naugle, RI, Hermann BP *et al* (1998) Does presurgical IQ predict seizure outcome after temporal lobectomy? Evidence from the Bozeman Epilepsy Consortium. *Epilepsia* 39(3):314–318.

Clodfelter CJ, Dickson AL, Newton Wilkes C, Johnson RB (1987) Alternate forms of selective reminding for children. *Clinical Neuropsychologist* 1:243–249.

Cohen M (1997) *Children's Memory Scale.* New York: The Psychological Corporation.

Crawford JR, Stewart LE, Moore JW (1989) Demonstration of savings on the AVLT and development of a parallel form. *Journal of Clinical and Experimental Neuropsychology* 16:190–194.

Curry JF, Logue PE, Butler B (1986) Child and adolescent norms for Russell's revision of Wechsler Memory Scale. *Journal of Clinical Child Psychology* 15:214–220.

De Renzi E, Faglioni O (1978) Normative data and screening power of a shortened version of the Token Test. *Cortex* 14:41–49.

Delis DC, Kramer J, Kaplan E, Ober BA, Fridlund A (1986) *California Verbal Learning Test (CVLT) Research Edition.* New York: The Psychological Corporation.

Delis DC, Kramer J, Kaplan E, Ober BA (1993) *California Verbal Learning Test for Children (CVLT-C).* New York: The Psychological Corporation.

Di Simoni F (1978) *The Token Test for Children.* Texas: Allen, DLM Teaching Resource.

Dodrill CB, van Belle G, Wilkus RJ (1990) Stability of predictors of outcome of surgical treatment for epilepsy. *Journal of Epilepsy* 8:29–35.

Dodrill CB, Jones-Gotman M, Loring DW, Sass KJ (1993) Contributions of neuropsychology. In: Engel J Jr (ed.) *Surgical Treatment of the Epilepsies,* 2nd edn, pp 309–312. New York: Raven Press.

Dunn LM, Dunn ES (1997) *Peabody Picture Vocabulary Test – III.* Circle Pines, MN: American Guidance Service.

Dunn LM, Dunn ES, Burley J (1997) *British Picture Vocabulary Scale,* 2nd edn. Windsor: NFER-Nelson.

Elliott CD (1990) *Differential Ability Scales (DAS).* New York: The Psychological Corporation.

Elliott CD, Smith P, McCulloch K (1996) *British Ability Scales,* 2nd edn. Windsor: NFER-Nelson.

Gaddes WH, Crockett DJ (1975) The Spreen–Benton aphasia tests, normative data as a measure of normal language development. *Brain and Language* 2: 257–280.

Gardner MF (1990a) *Expressive One-Word Picture Vocabulary Test – Revised.* Novato, CA: Academic Therapy Publications.

Gardner MF (1990b) *Expressive One-Word Picture Vocabulary Test – Upper Extension.* Novato, CA: Academic Therapy Publications.

Gardner MF (1992) *Receptive One-Word Picture Vocabulary Test (ROWPVT).* Odessa, FL: Psychological Assessment Resources.

Halperin J, Healy J, Zeitschick E, Ludman W, Weinstein L (1989) Developmental aspects of linguistic and mnestic abilities in normal children. *Journal of Clinical and Experimental Neuropsychology* 11(4): 518–528.

Heaton RK, Chelune GJ, Talley JL, Kay GG, Curtiss G (1993) *The Wisconsin Card Sorting Test Manual – Revised and Expanded.* FL: Psychological Assessment Resources.

Henderson SE, Sugden DA (1992) *Movement Assessment Battery for Children.* New York: The Psychological Corporation.

Hooper HE (1983) *Hooper Visual Organization Test.* Los Angeles: Western Psychological Service.

Ivinskis A, Allen S, Shaw E (1971) An extension of Wechsler Memory Scale norms to lower age groups. *Journal of Clinical Psychology* 27:354–357.

Jones-Gotman M (1990) Presurgical psychological assessment in children: special tests. *Journal of Epilepsy* 3(Suppl):93–102.

Jones-Gotman M (1991) Presurgical neuropsychological evaluation for localization and lateralization of seizure focus. In: Luders H (ed.) *Epilepsy Surgery.* New York: Raven Press.

Jones-Gotman M (1996) Psychological evaluation for epilepsy surgery. In: Shorvon S, Dreifuss F, Fish D, Thomas D (eds) *The Treatment of Epilepsy.* Oxford: Blackwell Science.

Jones-Gotman M, Smith M-L, Zatorre RJ (1993) Neuropsychological testing for localizing and lateralizing the epileptogenic region. In: Engel J Jr (ed.) *Surgical Treatment of the Epilepsies,* 2nd edn. New York: Raven Press.

Kaplan EF, Googlass H, Weintraub S (1983) *The Boston Naming Test,* 2nd edn. Philadelphia: Lea and Febiger.

King DW, Olivier A, Spencer SS, Wyllie E (1993) Postscript: exclusion criteria. In: Engel J Jr (ed.) *Surgical Treatment of the Epilepsies,* 2nd edn. New York: Raven Press.

Lassonde M, Sauerwein H, Geoffroy G (1986) Effects of early and late transection of the corpus callosum in children. *Brain* 109:953–967.

Lassonde M, Sauerwein H, Geoffroy G, Decarie M (1990) Long-term neuropsychological effects of corpus callosotomy in children. *Journal of Epilepsy* 3(Suppl 1):279–286.

Lezak MD (1995) *Neuropsychological Assessment,* 3rd edn. New York: Oxford University Press.

Loring DW (1997) Neuropsychological evaluation in epilepsy surgery. *Epilepsia* 38(Suppl 4): S18–S23.

Loring DW, Hermann BP, Meador KJ *et al* (1994) Amnesia after unilateral temporal lobectomy: a case report. *Epilepsia* 35:757–763.

Majdan A, Sziklas V, Jones-Gotman M (1996) Performance of healthy subjects and patients with resection from the anterior temporal lobe on matched tests of verbal and visuoperceptive learning. *Journal of Clinical and Experimental Neuropsychology* 18(3):416–430.

Markwardt FC (1989) *Peabody Individual Achievement Test – Revised.* Circle Pines, MN: American Guidance Service.

McGlone J (1994) Memory complaints before and after temporal lobectomy: do they predict memory performance of lesion laterality? *Epilepsia* 35:529–539.

McKenna P, Warrington EK (1983) *The Graded Naming Test*. Windsor: NFER-Nelson.

Meyers JE Meyers KR (1995) *Rey Complex Figure Test and Recognition Trial (RCFT)*. New York: The Psychological Corporation.

Milner B (1975) Psychological aspects of focal epilepsy and its neurosurgical management. In: Purpura DP, Penry JK, Walter RD (eds) *Advances in Neurology*, Vol 8. New York: Raven Press.

Morgan SF (1982) Measuring long-term memory, storage and retrieval in children. *Journal of Clinical Neuropsychology* 4:77–85.

Neale MD (1989) *Neale Analysis of Reading Ability (Revised)*. Windsor: NFER-Nelson.

O'Shea MF, Saling MM, Bladin PF, Berkovic SF (1996) Does naming contribute to memory self-report in temporal lobe epilepsy? *Journal of Clinical and Experimental Neuropsychology* 18:98–109.

Osterrieth P (1944) Le test de copie d'une figure complex. *Archives of Psychology* 30:206–356.

Oxbury SM (1997) Assessment for surgery. In: Cull C, Goldstein LH (eds) *The Clinical Psychologist's Handbook of Epilepsy*. London: Routledge.

Oxbury SM (1998) Neuropsychological evaluation: children. In: Engel J, Pedley TA (eds) *Epilepsy: a Comprehensive Textbook*. New York: Raven Press.

Penfield W, Mathieson G (1974) Memory: autopsy findings and comments on the role of the hippocampus in experiential recall. *Archives of Neurology* 31:145–154.

Penfield W, Milner B (1958) Memory deficit produced by bilateral lesions in the hippocampal zone. *Archives of Neurology and Psychiatry* 79:475–497.

Pilcher WH, Roberts DW, Flanigan HF *et al* (1993) Complications of epilepsy surgery. In: Engel J (ed.) *Surgical Treatment of the Epilepsies*, 2nd edn, pp 565–581. New York: Raven Press.

Rausch R (1987) Psychological evaluation. In: Engel J (ed.) *Surgical Treatment of the Epilepsies*. New York: Raven Press.

Rausch R, Babb TL, Brown WJ (1985) A case of amnestic syndrome following selective amygdalohippocampectomy. *Journal of Clinical and Experimental Neuropsychology* 7:643.

Rausch R, Boone K, Ary CM (1991) Right-hemisphere language dominance in temporal lobe epilepsy: clinical and neuropsychological correlates. *Journal of Clinical and Experimental Neuropsychology* 13(2):217–231.

Rausch R, Le M-T, Langfitt JT (1998) Neuropsychological evaluation: adults. In: Engel J, Pedley TA (eds) *Epilepsy: a Comprehensive Textbook*. New York: Raven Press.

Reynell J, Huntley M (1985) *Reynell Developmental Language Scales: Second Revision*. Windsor: NFER-Nelson.

Robertson IH, Ward T, Ridgeway V, Nimmo-Smith I (1994) *The Test of Everyday Attention*. Suffolk: Thames Valley Test Company.

Robinson CC, Rosenberg S (1987) A strategy for assessing infants with motor impairment. In: Uzgiris LC, Hunt JMcV (eds) *Infant Performance and Experience: New Findings with Ordinal Scales*, pp 311–319. Urbana/Chicago: University of Illinois Press.

Russell EW (1975) A multiple scoring method for the assessment of complex memory functions. *Journal of Consulting and Clinical Psychology*, 43:800–809.

Russell EW (1988) Renorming Russell's version of the Wechsler Memory Scale. *Journal of Clinical and Experimental Neuropsychology* 10:235–249.

Shallice T, Evans ME (1978) The involvement of the frontal lobes in cognitive estimation. *Cortex* 14: 294–303.

Sheslow D, Adams W (1990) *Wide Range Assessment of Memory and Learning (WRAML)*. New York: The Psychological Corporation.

Smith ML, Milner B (1981) The role of the right hippocampus in the recall of spatial memory. *Neuropsychologia* 19:781–793.

Sparrow SS, Balla DA, Cicchetti DV (1984) *Vineland Adaptive Behavior Scales*. Circle Pines, MN: American Guidance Service.

Spreen O, Strauss E (1991) *A Compendium of Neuropsychological Tests*. New York: Oxford University Press.

Spreen O, Strauss E (1998) *A Compendium of Neuropsychological Tests*. New York: Oxford University Press.

Szabo CA, Wyllie E (1993) Intracarotid amobarbital testing for language and memory dominance in children. *Epilepsy Research* 15:239–246.

Taylor LB (1979) Psychological assessment of neurosurgical patients. In: Rasmussen T (ed.) *Functional Neurosurgery*, pp 165–180. New York: Raven Press.

Taylor LB (1991) Neuropsychologic assessment of patients with chronic encephalitis. In: Andermann F (ed.) *Chronic Encephalitis and Epilepsy, Rasmussen's Syndrome*, pp 111–121. Boston: Butterworth-Heinemann.

Tombaugh TN, Hubley AM (1991) Four studies comparing the Rey–Osterrieth and Taylor complex figures. *Journal of Clinical and Experimental Neuropsychology* 13: 587–599.

Warrington EK (1997) The Graded Naming Test: a restandardization. *Neuropsychological Rehabilitation* 7(2):143–146.

Warrington EK, Duchen LW (1992) A reappraisal of a case of persistent global amnesia following right temporal lobectomy: a clinicopathological study. *Neuropsychologia* 30:437–450.

Warrington EK, James M (1991) *Visual Object and Space Perception Battery (VOSP)*. Suffolk: Thames Valley Test Co.

Wechsler D (1945) A standardized memory scale for clinical use. *Journal of Psychology* 19:87–95.

Wechsler D (1986) *Wechsler Adult Intelligence Scale – Revised UK Edition (WAIS-R UK)*. New York: The Psychological Corporation.

Wechsler D (1987) *Manual for the Wechsler Memory Scale – Revised*. New York: The Psychological Corporation.

Wechsler D (1989) *Wechsler Preschool and Primary Scale of Intelligence – Revised*. New York: The Psychological Corporation.

Wechsler D (1991) *Wechsler Intelligence Scale for Children*, 3rd edn. New York: The Psychological Corporation.

Wechsler D (1993) *Wechsler Objective Reading Dimensions (WORD)*. New York: The Psychological Corporation.

Wechsler D (1999a) *Wechsler Adult Intelligence Scale*, 3rd edn. New York: The Psychological Corporation.

Wechsler D (1999b) *Wechsler Memory Scale*, 3rd edn. New York: The Psychological Corporation.

Westerveld M, Sass KJ, Sass A, Henry HG (1994) Assessment of verbal memory in temporal lobe epilepsy using the Selective Reminding Test: equivalence and reliability of alternate forms. *Journal of Epilepsy* 7:57–63.

Wilkinson GS (1993) *Wide Range Achievement Test 3 (WRAT3)*. New York: The Psychological Corporation.

Wilson BA, Cockburn J, Halligan P (1987) *Behavioral Inattention Test (BIT)*. Suffolk: Thames Valley Test Co.

Carotid amobarbital testing and other amobarbital procedures

S BAXENDALE

Patients who undergo unilateral removal of the mesial temporal lobe structures may suffer material-specific memory decline postoperatively but pure amnesic syndromes are rare (Baxendale 1998). Postoperative memory function in these patients critically depends on both the functional adequacy of the tissue removed and the functional reserve of the remaining contralateral structures (Chelune 1995). All the available evidence from the unilateral temporal lobectomies that have resulted in amnesia to date seems to support Milner's (1966) contention that only patients with contralateral hippocampal damage are liable to become amnesic after a unilateral temporal lobectomy. It is therefore crucial to ensure preoperatively that the memory capacity of the contralateral temporal lobe alone is adequate to maintain useful memory functions postoperatively.

The intracarotid sodium amobarbital test (ISA), or Wada test (named after Juhn Wada (1949) who introduced it to establish the side of language dominance), is used for this purpose in epilepsy surgery programs worldwide and is an integral part of the preoperative evaluation for temporal lobectomy in most centers. It is an extremely effective test for language lateralization (Loring *et al*, 1991b) and is currently used as the 'gold standard' against which newer techniques, such as functional magnetic resonance imaging (FMRI), are evaluated (Desmond *et al* 1995; Binder *et al* 1996; Bahn *et al* 1997; Hertz-Pannier *et al* 1997). However, the primary role of the ISA in the presurgical evaluation of temporal lobe epilepsy patients is to identify individuals who may be at risk of a postoperative amnesic syndrome.

RATIONALE

The standard ISA typically involves the injection of sodium amobarbital ('amobarbital') into a single carotid artery through a catheter placed via the femoral artery. This functionally inactivates a variable part of the ipsilateral hemisphere for up to 10 min. It is presumed that anesthetizing the mesial temporal lobe structures temporarily mimics the potential mnestic effects of the proposed surgery, albeit in a fairly crude way. Contralateral hemiplegia and ipsilateral EEG slowing provide information that the amobarbital is active. During this time the patient is presented with a number of items to name and remember. Memory is usually tested in both recall and recognition formats. Normal memory function is expected when the side ipsilateral to the seizure focus is injected. When the hemisphere contralateral to the seizure focus is anesthetized, patients with medial temporal lobe pathology are typically impaired on memory tasks because of reduced mnestic capacity consequent upon the cerebral pathology underlying the seizure focus (see Fig. 47.1).

Asymmetric memory performance on ISA has therefore been proposed as a measure of lateralized temporal lobe dysfunction (Engel *et al* 1981; Wyllie *et al* 1991a; Dodrill 1993; Kneebone *et al* 1997). In epilepsy surgery centers today, results from ISA are used to lateralize language functions, to screen for postoperative amnesic risk, to predict postoperative memory change (Wyllie *et al* 1991b; Jones-Gotman 1992; Kneebone *et al* 1995) and seizure control (Loring *et al* 1994a; Sperling *et al* 1994; Perrine *et al* 1995b); and to lateralize seizure foci (Wyllie *et al* 1991a; Perrine *et al* 1995b; Kneebone *et al* 1997) and pathology (Davies *et al* 1996).

PREPARATION

Although all patients (or their legal guardians) will sign a consent form and should understand the purpose of and rationale for ISA in the context of their evaluation for surgery, centers vary widely in the amount of detailed information given to the patient prior to the test. In some programs, patients are explicitly told about the temporary hemipareses and speech and language difficulties that are expected following each injection. In others, these details are withheld from the patients in order to incorporate their recall of these disturbances into the overall memory assessment. Each approach has advantages and disadvantages. Memory for factors such as arm weakness, speech disturbance, or visual defect may be used as a mnestic sign, but

some patients may become worried by an unexpected hemiparesis or speech loss and this distress can occasionally interfere with the test.

It is important to ensure that the patient can 'pass' both the language and the memory components of the test under normal conditions prior to the procedure. This is particularly important for children and intellectually limited patients who should be thoroughly familiar with the testing requirements prior to the actual procedure, since time does not allow prolonged instructions or explanations during the test itself. For these patients, 'dry runs' with practice materials should be conducted as a matter of course.

NEURORADIOLOGY

ANGIOGRAPHY

Perfusion patterns following an injection into the internal carotid artery vary from patient to patient and as a function of a number of factors including differences in the vascular anatomy and the injection technique (see below). Therefore, angiography is undertaken routinely prior to ISA in over 90% of epilepsy surgery centers (Rausch *et al* 1993). Injection of 2–3 ml of contrast medium, at the same rate as the subsequent amobarbital injection, should outline the areas that the latter will reach. Machine injections or rapid manual injections using a larger contrast volume may outline a greater area and/or induce crossflow and interference with capillary bed regulation. Slower injections may show incomplete opacification because of dilution of the contrast medium and deficient perfusion of distal vessels or capillaries (Silfvenius *et al* 1997). Many centers adjust the injection

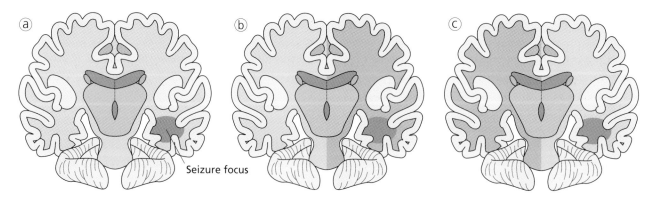

Fig. 47.1 Diagrammatic representation of the intracarotid amobarbital procedure. When the side ipsilateral to the seizure focus is injected, normal memory functioning is expected (b). When the hemisphere contralateral to the side of the suspected seizure focus is injected (c), the memory capacities of the patient are typically impaired due to the disruptive effects of the seizure focus and the contralateral hemisphere anesthesia.

and drug parameters in ISA to minimize any effects of crossflow or other interfering factors that are seen on angiography. The true perfusion pattern of the amobarbital is, however, unknown. Even when the angiogram and the ISA studies are using identical parameters, the amobarbital may be perfusing differently, since at least 10% contrast is needed in angiographic studies (Rausch *et al* 1993). To overcome these problems, fluorodeoxyglucose positron emission tomography (FDG-PET) and single-photon emission computed tomography (SPECT) studies have been used to examine the distribution of amobarbital in the vascular territories during ISA. Wieser *et al* (1997) found that while PET studies showed a rather widespread and bilateral amobarbital-induced decrease of metabolism, SPECT studies confirmed the selective distribution of tracer (injected immediately before the amobarbital) in the expected vascular territories.

Centers vary in the perfusion patterns that they consider important. Individual differences in arterial perfusion patterns mean that the posterior cerebral artery (PCA) territory may not be perfused. Theoretically, this may contribute to a false 'pass' as the mesial temporal structures may not be adequately anesthetized. However, although some have related the extent of the memory deficit to the extent of the PCA filling (Morton *et al* 1996), others have found that the latter is not reliably predictive and is less contributory than the injection side and the seizure laterality (Perrine *et al* 1995a). Angiographic studies should also be examined for basilar tip and bilateral posterior cerebral artery perfusion. Although rare, this can cause a transient cortical blindness, which would obviously invalidate much of the ISA testing.

SELECTIVE PROCEDURES

In response to some of these problems, Jack *et al* (1988, 1989) developed a more selective amobarbital procedure where memory is assessed following injection directly into the *PCA*. This procedure has theoretical and practical advantages over the standard ISA in that the amobarbital is delivered more directly to the ipsilateral hippocampal formation and memory testing can usually be conducted immediately after the injection without the confounding effects of aphasia and/or decreased consciousness. Other selective procedures have been inspired by selective surgical procedures such as selective amygdalohippocampectomy (Yasargil *et al* 1985; Wieser 1988). The *anterior amytal tests* (Wieser 1991; Wieser *et al* 1997) are based on the fact that branches of the anterior choriodal artery (AChA) supply the amygdala, the anterior hippocampus, and the fascia dentata, which are structures removed in a selective

amygdalohippocampectomy. Methods include the temporary balloon occlusion of the internal carotid artery distal to the origin of the AChA with subsequent amobarbital inactivation of the territories of the AChA, the PCA, and the ophthalmic artery; the selective catheterization and injection of amobarbital into the AChA; and the selective catheterization and injection into the P_2 segment of the PCA. Although these selective procedures model the effects of temporal lobectomy and selective amygdalohippocampectomy more closely, problems still arise from the variability of the vascular territory of the AChA. The anterior third of the hippocampus and the amygdala can be supplied by branches of the PCA and not by the AChA. Thus neither the selective PCA nor AChA approach will entirely model a mesial temporal lobe resection.

Selective amobarbital procedures are neuroradiologically more complex than standard ISA and therefore carry at least the potential for greater morbidity. The survey of practice with respect to amobarbital testing at 68 epilepsy surgery centers reported by Rausch *et al* (1993) revealed that 12 used selective procedures, mostly only infrequently. Around 50% of the 68 centers conducted more than 25 ISA procedures each year, but only one conducted more than 10 selective procedures. Most centers (79%) reported less than 1% morbidity from ISA. In contrast, 3 of the 12 centers using selective procedures had experienced a higher morbidity. Two US centers reported no longer using the selective PCA procedure. One of them was the Mayo Clinic where, after 59 cases had been examined, it was concluded that the benefits arising from the major advantages of the test did not outweigh the risks (Jones-Gotman *et al* 1993).

The PCA procedure has been used more often than the other selective procedures (Rausch *et al* 1993). It does not enable language lateralization to be established reliably and so could not replace ISA. It may, however, have a place in the repeat assessment of patients who have unambiguously failed the standard ISA and who otherwise appear to be good surgical candidates.

Selective amobarbital procedures should only be carried out by neuroradiologists with an ongoing experience of interventional neuroradiological techniques with an established low complication rate.

DOSE

The administration of the amobarbital in the standard ISA procedure can vary across a number of parameters. Some centers inject a single bolus at a preset dose for all patients, while others increase the dose incrementally until a specific behavioral marker, normally a dense hemiparesis, is observed. In their 1992 survey of 68 epilepsy centers,

Rausch *et al* (1993) found wide variations in the dose used in the standard procedure, ranging from 60 to 200 mg with 125 mg the most frequently reported. However centers using an incremental administration have reported doses of between 400 and 600 mg for some patients (Baxendale *et al* 1996, 1997). In some centers, men are given slightly larger doses than women because the adult male brain is heavier and this higher dose may equate the effects (Dodrill 1993). There is also significant variation in the concentration of the solution and the speed of the manual injection. Rausch *et al* (1993) found ranges from 10 cc at 1 cc s^{-1} to 1.25 cc at 3–5 cc s^{-1}. All these variables influence the behavioral effects of the amobarbital and the subsequent validity of the test. Low doses may decrease some of the undesirable sedative effects that can invalidate the test. They may not be sufficient, however, to suppress medial temporal lobe function adequately. The combination of the speed of injection and drug concentration will influence both the pattern of the arterial perfusion and the subsequent intensity or longevity of the drug effect.

LANGUAGE TESTING

As with every other aspect of the ISA, there is considerable variability across centers in the methods used to determine language representation. These range from the qualitative comparison of clinical impressions of speech arrest and dysphasic responses following the injection into each hemisphere, to rigid quantitative indices of language function. This has resulted in significant between-center differences in the relative proportion of right and left hemisphere-dominant patients that each purports to evaluate. For example, reports of left hemisphere language dominance in left-handed patients range from 38% (Serafetinides *et al* 1965) to 70% (Rasmussen and Milner 1977). These wide variations are partly due to a lack of universally applied objective criteria. In particular, there are no clear guidelines for the classification of patients with bilateral language representation.

Benbadis *et al* (1995a) evaluated three different criteria for reporting language dominance based purely on the duration of speech arrest, and recommended the adoption of a laterality index that takes into account both the side-to-side difference and the absolute duration of speech arrest. The index provides a graded continuous variable for language lateralization analogous to some handedness questionnaires. However, a number of factors unrelated to language dominance can influence the duration of speech arrest, including altered states of arousal or attention, aki-netic mutism, and other more general sedative effects. In addition, this approach is based purely upon the duration of speech arrest and does not take into account the many other forms of language disturbance that can result from amobarbital perfusion of the dominant hemisphere, for example, comprehension difficulties, anomias, and dysphasic errors. Although FMRI correlates of comprehensive ISA language assessments have been recorded (Binder *et al* 1996), the duration of speech arrest is not related to changes in hemispheric blood flow recorded with FMRI (Benbadis *et al* 1998).

Adopting a more qualitative approach, Ravdin *et al* (1997) assessed the pattern of language recovery following injection. They found that recovery from a dominant injection followed a typical progression, with the gradual return of naming and comprehension skills following the resumption of vocalization. Repetition errors and paraphasic responses persisted the longest. While some patients were rendered mute following an injection into the non-dominant hemisphere, all language functions tended to return simultaneously with vocalization. The progressive nature of the recovery following the contralateral injection was not evident. While universally accepted criteria for the classification of language dominance via ISA have yet to be developed, the way forward may lie in the innovative combination of these qualitative and quantitative approaches.

MEMORY TESTING

The basic test procedure is illustrated in Fig. 47.2. The testing protocols used in individual centers, however, can differ in a number of important respects, a fact rarely acknowledged in the comparative literature. Composite 'memory' scores for each hemisphere can be derived from a number of different memory tests. Theoretically, recall or recognition for material presented immediately following the amobarbital injection should be tested while the amobarbital is still having an effect, since this condition most closely imitates the anticipated postoperative state. Intervening tasks, or the presentation of distracter objects prior to the recall or recognition test, must be given as it is possible for amnesic patients to retain new information over a short period of time with rehearsal if no interfering tasks are given.

The physical constraints of the procedure can make the presentation and subsequent testing of material during the action of the amobarbital problematic. Firstly, the effects of the amobarbital are most potent immediately after the injection and gradually wear off over the next 10 min

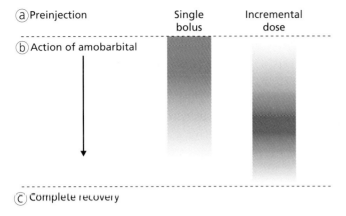

ⓐPreinjection   Single   Incremental
                               bolus   dose

ⓑAction of amobarbital

ⓒComplete recovery

Fig. 47.2 Amobarbital test structure. Memory for material presented prior to the injection (a) can be tested during the action of the amobarbital (b), and upon recovery (c). Memory for material presented during the action of the amobarbital (b) can also be tested in the same phase (b) and upon recovery (c).

(Fig. 47.2). Presentation of memory stimuli earlier during hemispheric anesthesia yields results that are more sensitive to lateralized temporal lobe pathology than does presentation of items later during the procedure (Lesser *et al* 1986; Carpenter *et al* 1996; Loring *et al* 1997a). Dysphasia complicates testing recall while the amobarbital is still acting after dominant hemisphere injection. Furthermore, individual differences in vascular architecture and pharmacokinetics make it difficult to predict precisely the potency and duration of the amobarbital effects on an individual patient. The levels of sedation achieved and the subsequent rate of recovery vary widely between patients. Therefore, memory for material presented immediately after the injection is often tested once the patient has recovered and the effects of the amobarbital are no longer apparent.

Such a testing paradigm does not strictly imitate the postoperative state. This is because the patient has access to the mesial temporal lobe structures of both hemispheres when memory is tested, even though only one set of temporal lobe structures was available to lay down the memory when material was presented immediately after the injection. Nevertheless, the testing paradigm is thought to be reasonable for assessing the risk of severe amnesia postoperatively, since it appears to be the ability to retain new memories that is lost in the temporal lobe amnesic syndrome. Significant retrograde amnesia is not a feature. Consequently, intact memory for material presented *prior* to the injection, while the amobarbital is still active during ISA, should not be relied upon as a sign that the patient is not at risk of severe amnesia postoperatively. Recent evidence also suggests that a relatively stable representation of events is achieved within seconds of encoding (Gleissner *et al* 1997).

ISA is not a single standardized procedure and a variety of protocols have been developed, each with their own advantages and disadvantages. Between-center comparisons of these protocols are problematic since patient characteristics, selection criteria, and ISA parameters differ enormously. However, by combining the key aspects of three different ISA protocols into a single procedure, Dodrill and Ojemann (1997) compared the three protocols in 172 adults. The *Montreal procedure* involves the presentation of five items during the period of the drug effect with recognition testing after the drug has dissipated. In the *Seattle procedure*, the patient is presented with a continuously recycling three-part task: (a) object naming, (b) reading, and (c) recall – the recall of the object named before the reading card was presented. In the *interview procedure*, the patient's recall for five basic events that occurred during the period of the drug effect is evaluated after the drug has dissipated and the patient has returned to normal. These events are the presence or absence of speech arrest, motor weakness, naming errors, reading errors, and recall errors (during the Seattle procedure). While some similarities existed, Dodrill and Ojemann found that the three procedures were in agreement in only one-third of the cases. The Montreal and Seattle procedures were most in agreement with a 70% concordance in pass or fail classification. Since the procedures evaluate different types of memory (recognition vs. recall) at different points in time (during vs. post-drug activation), it is not surprising that there is some disagreement. In addition to the procedure, the side of proposed surgery and language dominance also influenced concordance rates.

The value of each procedure in predicting postoperative memory function was also examined. The findings suggest that the Seattle procedure probably evaluates verbal memory skills, since failures were routinely greatest when the injection was into the language-dominant hemisphere regardless of whether it was the side of the seizure focus. The interview procedure may be a more sensitive measure of nonverbal memory and other factors since passes were consistently lowest on the nondominant side, while the Montreal procedure may be more mixed with respect to verbal and visual spatial memory. Overall, these results suggest that these amobarbital procedures might be used in a complementary manner, with the results interpreted to answer specific questions for individual patients.

MATERIALS

The materials used in ISA are governed to some extent by the constraints of the protocol employed. Common household objects, plastic animals, color photographs, and pictures and line drawings are frequently used, as are modified items from standard neuropsychologic tests such as the Warrington recognition memory test and the de Renzi token test (Rausch *et al* 1993; Carpenter *et al* 1995, 1996; Baxendale *et al* 1996). The type of stimuli employed in the test may affect the results. Real objects are superior to line drawings in discriminating right from left temporal lobe epilepsy groups (Loring *et al* 1997b). Rausch and MacDonald (1997) examined memory for three types of visual stimuli (pictures of common objects, words, and abstract forms) after right and left hemisphere injections. They found that selective deficits, specific to stimulus type, occurred following the perfusion of each hemisphere. Perrine *et al* (1993) used a combination of line drawings, faces, maths problems, shapes, words, and abstract forms. They found that the material-specific memory appropriate to the hemisphere contralateral to the seizure focus remained intact, but wider representation may occur for stimuli normally associated with the ipsilateral hemisphere. The stimuli used as foils in a recognition memory test are also important. While verbal recall is generally better following object presentation to an intact left rather than right hemisphere, Kaplan *et al* (1994) found that only the right hemisphere could discriminate original objects from the same name foils. They suggested that the left temporal lobe has an advantage in encoding the verbal representation of an object, while the right is critical for the memory of specific visual attributes.

The results of ISA should always, therefore, be interpreted with reference to the type of stimuli used and its relation to the side of the seizure focus and the laterality of language dominance.

TESTING SCHEDULE

In most centers, memory and language abilities are tested following an injection into the hemisphere ipsilateral to the suspected seizure focus, and following recovery, an injection into the contralateral hemisphere. This enables relative judgments about hemispheric memory function in addition to any absolute pass or fail criteria. Some groups routinely administer the first injection ipsilateral to the seizure focus (Baxendale *et al* 1996; Dodrill and Ojemann 1997). Others sequentially alternate the order of injection regardless of the laterality of seizure focus (Loring *et al* 1993a; Selwa *et al* 1997) or counterbalance for sex, seizure focus, and hand preference (Smith *et al* 1993). Both sides may be examined on the same day (Loring *et al* 1993a; Kneebone *et al* 1995; Baxendale *et al* 1996; Selwa *et al* 1997). It is important,

however, to leave an interval of at least 45 min between injections and to note that electrographic recovery appears to be slower following the injection of the nonepileptogenic hemisphere (Selwa *et al* 1997). Other centers examine the two sides on different days (Carpenter *et al* 1995; Helmstaedter *et al* 1997). This approach has the advantage of avoiding any confounding residual effects of the amobarbital from the previous injection, but might increase the morbidity risks associated with the puncturing of the femoral artery and placing the catheter which must be done twice. See also Meador and Losing (1999).

SPECIAL CONSIDERATIONS FOR CHILDREN

ISA can be used to assess language and memory function in pediatric populations and has been conducted on children as young as 5 years old (Szabo and Wyllie 1993). However, it is primarily used to determine language dominance in children aged less than 12 years, and the assessment of memory skills may be unreliable at less than 13 years (Williams and Rausch 1992; Szabo and Wyllie 1993). Extra pretest teaching, emotional preparation, adjusted amobarbital dose, and simplified test items, tailored to the child's abilities, should be employed.

RELIABILITY AND VALIDITY

Although ISA as a test of language is fairly robust, doubts have been raised about its reliability and validity in predicting postoperative amnesia, an event that has an extremely low occurrence (Saling 1989; Loring *et al*, 1990, 1991a, 1992b, 1994b; Trenerry and Loring 1995). Many factors, unrelated to the functional integrity of the temporal lobe can contribute to an impression of memory failure during ISA.

Functional disturbance in other structures within the hemisphere may be responsible for test errors. Perseverative responses are frequently seen when frontal lobe function is compromised. This may lead to the patient becoming inaccessible to further tests if they perseverate responses from the previous task. Perseverative responses may be more common following injection of the language-dominant hemisphere (Kurthen *et al* 1992). Perceptual difficulties can also interfere with memory testing when more posterior parts of the brain are affected (Fedio *et al* 1997).

Dosage and the level of sedation can affect the pass or fail outcome (Loring *et al* 1992b; Baxendale *et al* 1996). Novelly and Williamson (1989) found that 21 of 25 (84%) patients who had previously failed the amobarbital test passed on a second occasion when a lower dose was used. Baxendale *et al* (1996) did not find a significant effect of dose *per se* on ISA scores, but two indices of the level of sedation induced by the dose were related to memory scores. These were (a) the time taken to respond to simple verbal commands, and (b) the total time taken to regain normal limb power. A number of other studies have also found that ISA memory scores may be affected by the patients' level of consciousness during the procedure (Malmgren *et al* 1992; Meador *et al* 1997). Blum *et al* (1997) found that patients with evidence of mesial temporal sclerosis on MRI were more than twice as likely to experience excessive sedation than were equivalently dosed patients with normal MRI or nonatrophic lesions. Similarly, mixed-dominance patients and those with full-scale intelligence quotient (IQ) less than 80 were more likely to become oversedated following a standard dose of 125 mg. A number of studies have reported greater levels of sedation following injection into the language-dominant hemisphere (Baxendale *et al* 1996; Blum *et al* 1997; Meador *et al* 1997).

Although rare, extreme emotional reactions, both positive and negative, can occur following amobarbital perfusion (Kurthen *et al* 1991; Calverie and Rougier 1994). Severe dysarthria and other physiologic disturbances including teeth chattering and occasional violent shivers are sometimes seen. All of these responses can interfere with the administration and scoring of the memory tasks.

It is difficult to test the validity of ISA in predicting those at risk of an amnesic syndrome following surgery, since patients who fail the test are usually excluded from the surgical program. Nevertheless, the relatively high percentage of failures remains at variance with the rare incidence of the amnesic syndrome, suggesting a low specificity for the test (Dasheiff *et al* 1993). Loring *et al* (1990) reported a series of 10 patients who had failed to remember items presented early, late, or throughout the procedure, but who nonetheless proceeded to surgery. None of these patients developed a serious anterograde amensia postoperatively. The authors concluded that ISA falsely identified those at risk of an amnesic syndrome. They suggested that, to minimize the possibility of the unnecessary exclusion of patients from a viable therapeutic option, the results from ISA should be interpreted in the context of all the other data when evaluating candidacy for temporal lobectomy. In a more recent study, Loring *et al* (1994a) reported the case of a young man who became densely amnesic following a dominant temporal lobectomy. On ISA he had failed to remember the items presented immediately after the injection. However, four other patients in their series demonstrated an identical deficit and did not become amnesic following surgery. Doubts about the validity of the test have also been raised by studies of memory function following perfusion of the hemisphere contralateral to the epileptic focus, since a high rate of memory test passes (59%) have been reported to occur under these conditions (Jones-Gotman 1987).

Histologically verified neuronal loss has been used to validate the role of ISA in assessing the functional integrity of the hippocampi. Rausch *et al* (1989) found that a severely damaged hippocampus was unable to support memory when sodium amobarbital is injected into the contralateral hemisphere. Five of their six patients with 80% or more neuronal loss in the hippocampal subfields failed the memory component of the ISA following injection contralateral to the pathology. However, marked cell loss that was limited to either the anterior or the posterior plane of the hippocampus was not sufficient to predict a memory failure, and consistent failures were only observed in those patients with marked damage extending throughout the hippocampus. Similarly, Sass *et al* (1991) found a significant correlation between the raw memory scores obtained following injection contralateral to the seizure focus and cell loss in the CA3 subfield. Other studies, however, have failed to replicate this finding. O'Rourke (1993) found that the degree of unilateral memory impairment ipsilateral to the seizure focus was significantly correlated with decreased neuronal densities in the hilar and dentate granule regions but not in the CA1, CA2, and CA3 regions.

THE FUTURE OF THE SODIUM AMOBARBITAL TEST

In addition to these methodological difficulties, ISA has a number of other disadvantages. It is an invasive test that is uncomfortable for the patients and both expensive and labor intensive. Over the last decade a variety of more sophisticated methods have been developed to evaluate the structural and functional integrity of the temporal lobes. Intraoperative hippocampal cooling, stereotactic depth electrode EEG, transcranial magnetic stimulation, PET, and SPECT studies have all been examined in relation to ISA (Perrine 1994; Benbadis *et al* 1995b; McMakin *et al* 1997; Wieser *et al* 1997). The real hopes lie in noninvasive measures of both structural and functional integrity. A number of studies have reported significant relationships between structural measures of hippocampal integrity and functional measures using traditional neuropsychologic tests of memory functioning (Lencz *et al* 1992; Loring *et al* 1993a; Trenerry *et al* 1993; Baxendale 1995; Baxendale *et al* 1998). Wada memory asymmetries have also been associated with hippocampal volume asymmetries recorded on MRI (Loring *et al* 1993a; Baxendale *et al* 1997).

At present, the results suggest that the combination of functional measures from ISA and structural MRI indices increases the localizing power of both and thus their value in the preoperative evaluation for epilepsy surgery. A number of FMRI paradigms have been developed to localize language function (Desmond *et al* 1995; Binder *et al* 1996; Bahn *et al* 1997; Hertz-Pannier *et al* 1997). It is hoped that similar paradigms for memory assessment are just on the horizon.

SUMMARY

ISA has traditionally fulfilled two roles in the presurgical assessment of patients with temporal lobe epilepsy. It is an extremely effective test of language lateralization. It is also used to screen for postoperative amnesic risk. However, doubts have been raised about its reliability and validity in predicting postoperative amnesia. The testing protocol, choice of behavioral stimuli, dose and administration of the amobarbital, and a host of factors related to the individual's reaction to the injection can interfere with the results. FMRI protocols for determining language dominance are promising. It is hoped that the innovative combination of structural and FMRI techniques together with baseline neuropsychologic measures may eventually supersede ISA in the presurgical assessment of temporal lobe epilepsy patients.

KEY POINTS

1. The primary roles of ISA before epilepsy surgery are firstly, to lateralize language function, which may be particularly important when planning both temporal lobe and extratemporal excisions, and secondly, to identify the risk that a severe amnesic syndrome might follow temporal lobe surgery.

2. ISA may also assist in the prediction of lesser degrees of memory decline following temporal lobe surgery and it may give corroborative evidence of unilateral medial temporal lobe dysfunction.

3. No single standardized procedure is available for assessing either language or memory. Different centers use different techniques which vary in many respects (e.g. amobarbital dose, which side is examined first and whether or not both sides are examined on the same day, time after injection when memory items are presented, test material used, etc.).

4. ISA is a robust test of the lateralization of language function but, although widely used, its reliability for predicting postoperative severe amnesia is unestablished. The false-positive (memory failure) rate is probably high and could lead to unnecessarily withholding surgery from some patients.

5. ISA may be able to establish the language-dominant side in children aged less than 12 years, but assessment of memory function below that age is unreliable.

REFERENCES

Bahn MM, Lin W, Silbergeld DL *et al* (1997) Localization of language cortices by functional MR imaging compared with intracarotid amobarbital hemispheric sedation. *American Journal of Roentgenology* **169**(2):575–579.

Baxendale SA (1995) The hippocampus: functional and structural correlations. *Seizure* **4**:105–117.

Baxendale S (1998) Amnesia in temporal lobectomy patients: historical perspective and review. *Seizure* **7**:15–24.

Baxendale SA, Thompson PJ, Savvy L, Bhattarcharya J, Shorvon SD (1996) Dose effects on intracarotid amobarbital test performance. *Journal of Epilepsy* **9**:135–143.

Baxendale SA, Van Paesschen WV, Thompson PJ, Duncan JS, Shorvon

SD, Connelly A (1997) The relation between quantitative MRI measures of hippocampal structure and the intracarotid amobarbital test. *Epilepsia* **388**(9):998–1007.

Baxendale SA, Van Paesschen WV, Thompson PJ, Connelly A, Duncan JS, Harkness WF, Shorvon SD (1998) The relationship between quantitative MRI and neuropsychological functioning in temporal lobe epilepsy. *Epilepsia* **39**(2):158–166.

Benbadis SR, Dinner DS, Chelune GJ, Piedmonte, Luders HO (1995a) Objective criteria for reporting language dominance by intracarotid amobarbital procedure. *Journal of Clinical and Experimental Neuropsychology* **17**(5):682–690.

Benbadis SR, So NK, Antar MA, Barnett GH, Morriss HH (1995b) The value of PET scan (and MRI and Wada test) in patients with bitemporal epileptiform abnormalities. *Archives of Neurology* **52**(11):1062–1068.

Benbadis SR, Binder JR, Swanson SJ *et al* (1998) Is speech arrest during Wada testing a valid method for determining hemispheric representation of language? *Brain and Language* **65**(3): 441–446.

Binder JR, Swanson SJ, Hammeke TA *et al* (1996) Determination of language dominance using functional MRI: a comparison with the Wada test. *Neurology* **46**:978–984.

Blum DE, Bortz JJ, Ehsan T (1997) Factors affecting degree of sedation after intracarotid amytal injection. *Journal of Epilepsy* **10**(1):42–46.

Calverie B, Rougier A (1994) Positive emotional reactions in intracarotid sodium amytal (Wada) procedures. *Journal of Epilepsy* **7**:137–143.

Carpenter K, Berti A, Oxbury S, Molyneux AJ, Bisiach E, Oxbury JM (1995) Awareness of and memory for arm weakness during intracarotid sodium amytal testing. *Brain* **118**(1):243–251.

Carpenter K, Oxbury JM, Oxbury S, Wright GD (1996) Memory for objects presented early after intracarotid sodium amytal: a sensitive clinical neuropsychological indicator of temporal lobe pathology. *Seizure* **5**(2):103–108.

Chelune GJ (1995) Hippocampal adequacy versus functional reserve: predicting memory functions following temporal lobectomy. *Archives of Clinical Neuropsychology* **10**(5):413–432.

Dasheiff RM, Shelton J, Ryan C (1993) Memory performance during the amytal test in patients with nontemporal lobe epilepsy. *Archives of Neurology* **50**(7):701–705.

Davies KG, Hermann BP, Foley KT (1996) Relation between intracarotid amobarbital memory asymmetry scores and hippocampal sclerosis in patients undergoing anterior temporal lobe resections. *Epilepsia* **37**(6):522–525.

Desmond JE, Sum JM, Wagner AD (1995) Functional MRI measurement of language lateralization in Wada-tested patients. *Brain* **118**:1411–1419.

Dodrill CB (1993) Preoperative criteria for identifying eloquent brain: intracarotid amobarbital for language and memory testing. *Neurosurgery Clinics of North America* **4**:211–216.

Dodrill CB, Ojemann GA (1997) An exploratory comparison of three methods of memory assessment with the intracarotid amobarbital procedure. *Brain Cognition* **33**(2):210–223.

Engel J Jr, Rausch R, Lieb J *et al* (1981) Correlation of criteria used for localizing epileptic foci in patients considered for surgical therapy of epilepsy. *Annals of Neurology* **9**:215–224.

Fedio P, August A, Patronas N, Sato S, Kufta C (1997) Semantic, phonological and perceptual changes following left and right intracarotid injection (Wada) with a low amytal dosage. *Brain and Cognition* **33**(1):98–117.

Gleissner U, Helmstaedter C, Kurthen M, Elger CE (1997) Evidence of very fast memory consolidation: an intracarotid amytal study. *Neuroreport* **8**(13):2893–2896.

Helmstaedter C, Kurthen M, Linke DB, Elger CE (1997) Patterns of language dominance in focal left and right hemisphere epilepsies: relation to MRI findings, EEG, sex and age of onset of epilepsy. *Brain and Cognition* **33**(3):135–150.

Hertz-Pannier L, Gaillard WD, Mott SH *et al* (1997) Noninvasive assessment of language dominance in children and adolescents with functional MRI. *Neurology* **48**:1003–1012.

Jack C, Nichols D, Sharbrough F, Marsh WR, Petersen R (1988) Selective posterior cerebral artery amytal tests for evaluating memory function before surgery for temporal lobe seizures. *Neuroradiology* **168**:787–793.

Jack CR Jr, Nichols DA, Sharbrough FW *et al* (1989) Selective posterior cerebral artery injection of amytal: a new method of preoperative memory testing. *Mayo Clinic Proceedings* **64**(8):965–975.

Jones-Gotman M (1987) Commentary: psychological evaluation – testing hippocampal function. In: Engel J Jr (ed.) *Surgical Treatment of the Epilepsies*, p 203. New York: Raven Press.

Jones-Gotman M, Barr WB, Dodrill CB *et al* (1993) Controversies concerning the use of intra-arterial amobarbital procedures. In: Engel J Jr (ed.) *Surgical Treatment of the Epilepsies*, 2nd edn, pp 445–449. New York: Raven Press.

Kaplan RF, Meadows ME, Verfaellie M *et al* (1994) Lateralization of memory for the visual attributes of objects: evidence from the posterior cerebral artery amobarbital test. *Neurology* **44**(6):1069–1073.

Kneebone AC, Chelune GJ, Dinner DS, Naugle I, Awad IA (1995) Intracarotid amobarbital procedure as a predictor of material-specific memory change after anterior temporal lobectomy. *Epilepsia* **36**(9):857–865.

Kneebone AC, Chelune GJ, Luders HO (1997) Individual patient prediction of seizure lateralization in temporal lobe epilepsy: a comparison between neuropsychological memory measures and the intracarotid amobarbital procedure. *Journal of the International Neuropsychology Society* **3**(2):159–168.

Kurthen M, Linke DB, Reuter BM, Hufnagel A, Elger CE (1991) Severe negative emotional reactions in intracarotid sodium amytal procedures: further evidence for hemispheric asymmetries? *Cortex* **27**:333–337.

Kurthen M, Linke DB, Elger CE, Schramm J (1992) Linguistic perservation in dominant-side intracarotid amobarbital tests. *Cortex* **28**(2):209–219.

Lencz T, McCarthy G, Bronen RA *et al* (1992) Quantitative magnetic resonance imaging in temporal lobe epilepsy: relationship to neuropathology and neuropsychological function. *Annals of Neurology* **31**:629–637.

Lesser RP, Dinner DS, Luders H, Morris HH (1986) Memory for objects presented soon after intracarotid amobarbital sodium injections in patients with medically intractable complex partial seizures. *Neurology* **36**:895–899.

Loring DW, Lee GP, Meador KJ *et al* (1990) The intracarotid amobarbital procedure as a predictor of memory failure following unilateral temporal lobectomy. *Neurology* **40**:605–610.

Loring DW, Lee GP, Meador KJ, King DW (1991a) Controversies in epileptology: does memory assessment during amobarbital testing predict postsurgical amnesia? *Journal of Epilepsy* **4**:19–24.

Loring DW, Meador KJ, Lee GP *et al* (1991b) Cerebral language lateralization: evidence from carotid amobarbital testing. *Neuropsychologia* **28**:831–838.

Loring DW, Meador KJ, Lee GP (1992) Amobarbital dose effects on Wada memory testing. *Journal of Epilepsy* **5**:171–174.

Loring DW, Murro AM, Meador MD *et al* (1993a) Wada memory testing and hippocampal volume measurements in the evaluation for temporal lobectomy. *Neurology* **43**:1789–1793.

Loring DW, Meador KJ, Lee GP (1993b) Motor strength and lateralized temporal lobe dysfunction: a sodium amobarbital study. *Journal of Epilepsy* **6**:1399–1441.

Loring DW, Meador KJ, Lee GP *et al* (1994a) Wada memory performance predicts seizure outcome following anterior temporal lobectomy. *Neurology* **44**(12):2322–2324.

Loring DW, Hermann BP, Meador KJ *et al* (1994b) Amnesia after unilateral temporal lobectomy: a case report. *Epilepsia* **35**(4):757–763.

Loring DW, Meador KJ, Lee GP *et al* (1997a) Wada memory and timing of stimulus presentation. *Epilepsy Research* **26**(3):461–464.

Loring DW, Hermann BP, Perrine K, Plenger PM, Lee GP, Meador KJ (1997b) Effect of Wada memory stimulus type in discriminating lateralized temporal lobe impairment. *Epilepsia* **38**(2):219–224.

Malmgren K, Biltin M, Hagberg I, Hedstrom A, Silfvenious H, Starmark JE (1992) A compound score for estimating the influence of inattention and somnolence during the intracarotid amobarbital test. *Epilepsy Research* **12**(3):253–259.

Meador KJ, Loring DW (1999) The Wada test: controversies, concerns, and insights. *Neurology* **52**:1535–1536.

Meador KJ, Loring DW, Lee GP, Nichols ME, Moore EE, Figueroa RE (1997) Level of consciousness and memory during the intracarotid sodium amobarbital procedure. *Brain and Cognition* **33**(2):178–188.

Milner B (1966) Amnesia following operation on the temporal lobes. In: Whitty CMW, Zangwill OL (eds) *Amnesia*, pp 109–133: London: Butterworths.

McMackin D, Dunbeau F, Jones-Gotman M *et al* (1997) Assessment of the functional effect of the intracarotid sodium amobarbital procedure using coregistered MRI/HMPAO-SPECT and SEEG. *Brain and Cognition* **33**(1):50–70.

Morton N, Polkey CE, Cox T, Morris RG (1996) Episodic memory dysfunction during sodium amytal testing of epileptic patients in relation to posterior cerebral artery perfusion. *Journal of Clinical and Experimental Neuropsychology* **18**(1):24–37.

Novelly RA, Williamson PD (1989) Incidence of false-positive memory impairment in the intracarotid amytal procedure (abstract). *Epilepsia* **30**:711.

O'Rourke DM, Saykin AJ, Gilhool JJ, Harley R, O'Connor MJ, Sperling MR (1993) Unilateral hemispheric memory and hippocampal neuronal density in temporal lobe epilepsy. *Neurosurgery* **32**(4):574–581.

Perrine K (1994) Future directions for functional mapping. *Epilepsia* **35**(6):90–102.

Perrine K, Gershengorn J, Brown ER, Choi IS, Luiciano DJ, Devinsky O (1993) Material-specific memory in the intracarotid amobarbital procedure. *Neurology* **43**(4):706–711.

Perrine K, Devinsky O, Luciano DJ, Choi IS, Nelson PK (1995a) Correlates of arterial-filling patterns in the intracarotid amobarbital procedure. *Archives of Neurology* **52**(7):712–716.

Perrine K, Westerveld M, Sass KJ *et al* (1995b) Wada memory disparities predict seizure laterality and postoperative seizure control. *Epilepsia* **36**(9):851–856.

Rasmussen T, Milner B (1977) The role of early left brain injury in determining lateralization of cerebral speech functions. *Annals of the New York Academy of Science* **299**:355–369.

Rausch R, MacDonald K (1997) Effects of hemisphere speech dominance and seizure focus on patterns of behavioral response errors for three types of stimuli. *Brain and Cognition* **33**(2):161–177.

Rausch R, Babb TL, Engel J Jr, Crandall PH (1989) Memory following IAP contralateral to hippocampal damage. *Archives of Neurology* **46**:783–788.

Rausch R, Silfvenius H, Weiser HG, Dodrill CB, Meador KJ, Jones-Gotman M (1993) Intra-arterial amobarbital procedures. In: Engel J Jr (ed.) *Epilepsies*, 2nd edn, pp 341–357. New York: Raven Press.

Ravdin LD, Perrine K, Haywood CS, Gershengorn J, Nelson PK, Devinsky O (1997) Serial recovery of language during the intracarotid amobarbital procedure. *Brain and Cognition* **33**(2):151–160.

Saling MM (1989) The Wada test: is it necessary? In: Vajda FJ, Berkovic SF, Donnan DA (eds) *Epilepsy update*. Proceedings of the 4th Biannual Epilepsy Workshop, pp 55–57.

Sass KJ, Lencz T, Westerveld M, Novelly RA, Spencer DD, Kim JH (1991) The neural substrate of memory impairment demonstrated by the intracarotid amobarbital procedure. *Archives of Neurology* **48**:48–52.

Selwa LM, Buchtel HA, Henry TR (1997) Electrocerebral recovery during the intracarotid amobarbital procedure: influence of interval between injections. *Epilepsia* **12**:1294–1299.

Serafetinides EA, Hoare RD, Driver MV (1965) Intracarotid sodium amobarbitone and cerebral dominance for speech and consciousness. *Brain* **88**:107–130.

Silfvenius H, Fagerlund M, Saisa J, Olivecrona M, Christianson SA (1997) Carotid angiography in conjunction with amytal testing of epilepsy patients. *Brain and Cognition* **33**:33–49.

Smith IM, McGlone J, Fox AJ (1993) Intracarotid amobarbital memory protocol: muteness, dysphasia and variations in arterial distribution of the drug do not affect recognition results. *Journal of Epilepsy* **6**:75–84.

Sperling MR, Saykin AJ, Glosser G *et al* (1994) Predictors of outcome after anterior temporal lobectomy: the intracarotid amobarbital test. *Neurology* **44**(12):2325–2330.

Szabo CA, Wyllie E (1993) Intracarotid amobarbital testing for language and memory dominance in children. *Epilepsy Research* **15**(3):239–246.

Trenerry MR, Loring DW (1995) Intracarotid amobarbital procedure: the Wada test. *Neuroimaging* **5**(4):721–728.

Trenerry MR, Jack CR, Ivnik RJ *et al* (1993) MRI hippocampal volumes and memory function before and after temporal lobectomy. *Neurology* **43**:1800–1805.

Wada J (1949) A new method for the determination of the side of cerebral speech dominance. A preliminary report on the intracarotid injection of sodium amytal in man (in Japanese). *Igaku to seibutsugaki* **14**:221–222.

Wieser HG (1988) Selective amygdalohippocampectomy for temporal lobe epilepsy. *Epilepsia* **29**(Suppl 2):S100–S113.

Wieser HG (1991) Anterior cerebral artery amobarbital test. In: Luders H (ed.) *Epilepsy Surgery*, pp 515–523. New York: Raven Press.

Wieser HG, Mueller S, Schiess R, Khan N *et al* (1997) The anterior and posterior selective temporal lobe amobarbital tests: angiographic, clinical, electroencephalographic, PET, SPECT findings, and memory performance. *Brain and Cognition* **33**(1):71–97.

Williams J, Rausch R (1992) Factors in children that predict performance on the intracarotid amobarbital procedure. *Epilepsia* **33**(6):1036–1041.

Wyllie E, Naugle R, Chelune G, Luders H, Morris H, Skibinski C (1991a) Intracarotid amobarbital procedure: II. Lateralizing value in evaluation for temporal lobectomy. *Epilepsia* **32**(6):865–869.

Wyllie E, Naugle R, Awad I *et al* (1991b) Intracarotid amobarbital procedure: I. Prediction of decreased modality-specific memory scores after temporal lobectomy. *Epilepsia* **32**(6):857–864.

Yasargil MG, Teddy PJ, Roth R (1985) Selective amygdalohippocampectomy: operative anatomy and surgical techniques. *Advances in Technical and Standard Neurosurgery* **12**:93–123.

Functional imaging of epilepsy

AC NOBRE AND A RAO

Methodologies that allow noninvasive visualization of the physiology of the human brain have begun to transform the diagnosis and treatment of neurologic disorders such as epilepsy. Methods continue to be developed and refined that enable fine-grained inspection of neural anatomy, pathology, chemical milieu, blood flow, metabolism, electrical activity, and neurochemical signaling with improving spatial and temporal resolution.

In particular, recent developments of variants of the technology of nuclear magnetic resonance have provided especially accessible and versatile measures of neural function with which to localize epileptogenic tissue, study its pathophysiology, and plan effective and safe surgical procedures to relieve medically intractable conditions. Structural magnetic resonance imaging (MRI) provides high-precision anatomic information with which lesions, developmental malformations, regional atrophy, and tissue damage can be identified. Magnetic resonance spectroscopy (MRS) measures signals from magnetic nuclei (e.g. ^1H, ^{31}P, ^{13}C, ^{17}O) in many organic compounds, thereby providing chemically specific information relevant to the neuropathology and neurochemistry of epilepsy. Functional MRI (FMRI) involves adaptations of MRI to measure dynamic signals linked to neural activity. FMRI has become increasingly useful for localizing critical brain areas involved in sensory, motor, and cognitive functions, so that surgery may be planned accordingly. FMRI may also become a useful noninvasive method with which to localize the seizure focus and chart its pattern of spread.

More invasive functional methods that rely on radioactive tracers continue to play an important role in the diagnosis and investigation of epilepsy. Single-photon emission computed tomography (SPECT) following the injection of metabolic tracers during an epileptic seizure remains the most accessible and reliable method to lateralize the ictal focus. Images of metabolism obtained with positron emission tomography (PET), even interictally, also provide reliable data for localizing the epileptogenic area. SPECT and PET data can be especially critical in cases where the structural or pathologic data from nuclear magnetic resonance are not conclusive. PET carries the additional potential for studying neurochemical alterations during epilepsy quantitatively.

IMAGING PATHOLOGY

STRUCTURAL MAGNETIC RESONANCE IMAGING

MRI provides images of the living human brain based upon the differential distribution and environment of hydrogen nuclei (protons) in water molecules. Images can be obtained with different parameters in order to optimize the signal and contrast that originates from blood, cerebrospinal fluid, white matter, and gray matter. Structural images reveal neuroanatomic detail that was previously only possible with autopsy. Lesions or structural malformations associated with epilepsy can be identified with high accuracy and spatial resolution, including malformations of cortical development, vascular malformations, tumors, and other acquired cortical damage. MRI has thus become an essential tool for the diagnosis of the underlying *regional* pathology associated with epilepsy (see Duncan 1997 for a review).

MRI also highlights *neuronal* pathology associated with epilepsy. Hippocampal sclerosis resulting from neuronal death is highly correlated with medically intractable temporal lobe epilepsy (TLE). Successful means to measure decreases in hippocampal volumes in TLE patients have evolved in many centers (Jack *et al* 1990; McCarthy and Luby 1994). Despite the significant variability in hippocampal volumes in the normal population, and the many technical considerations that need to be taken into account, hippocampal volumetrics has become a key component of the diagnostic work-up of epileptic patients (see Chapter 44). Positive findings of lateralized hippocampal sclerosis are a clear marker of unilateral TLE, and rarely lead to false localization of the pathologic tissue. The regional pattern of sclerosis along the hippocampus does not always coincide with the site of seizure onset or predict its pattern of spread as measured with invasive intracranial EEG (King *et al* 1997; Spanedda *et al* 1997). The relationship between hippocampal sclerosis and epileptogenicity in tissue at the microscopic level therefore remains to be elucidated. At present, however, hippocampal sclerosis is among the best macroscopic markers of TLE, although additional information is often necessary for a complete and reliable diagnosis (Spencer 1998). Occasionally, nonatrophic medial temporal lobes can be epileptogenic (Jack *et al* 1994; King *et al* 1997), and the existence of additional pathologies cannot be ruled out. Relative hippocampal volume measures also provide useful prognostic information about the effectiveness of surgical treatment (Berkovic *et al* 1995; Cascino *et al* 1996; Gilliam *et al* 1997; Li *et al* 1999).

Neuronal pathology can also be assessed with novel MRI sequences sensitive to the T2 relaxation time in tissue. In addition, measures can be improved using sequences that attenuate signals from cerebrospinal fluid (fluid attenuated inversion recovery, FLAIR; Bergin *et al* 1995; Cascino *et al* 1996). Abnormalities of hippocampal T2 signals and T2-relaxation times (HCT2) are also reliably found in the pathologic tissue in TLE. The HCT2 and measures of hippocampal sclerosis from volumetrics are thought to convey complementary information regarding neuronal pathology in the hippocampal region (Van Paesschen *et al* 1995, 1997). Signal change in T2 and measures of hippocampal atrophy occasionally give discrepant findings (Bronen *et al* 1995), and using information from either method alone could be misleading. In some studies that have compared the sensitivity of different MRI methods directly, HCT2 showed inferior sensitivity to quantified volume-based methods (Kuzniecky *et al* 1997). However, the relative advantages of one method over another are often still influenced by specific technical optimizations within different centers.

MAGNETIC RESONANCE SPECTROSCOPY

Many nuclei have resonance frequencies, which are modulated by their chemical milieu. Spectra of signal intensity against frequency measure the concentrations of common compounds containing the resonant nucleus. The most abundant nucleus is hydrogen and therefore proton MRS has the best signal-to-noise ratio and yields the most reliable results. There have been numerous reviews of MRS and its increasing application to epilepsy diagnosis and research (see Prichard 1994, 1997; Garcia *et al* 1995; Novotny 1995; Duncan 1997; Laxer 1997).

The proton spectrum contains signals from many common compounds. Of particular importance for assessing neuronal pathology are the signals from *N*-acetylaspartate (NAA), creatine (Cr), and choline (Cho). NAA is located primarily within neurons and precursor cells; consequently, decreases in this signal can be used to mark neuronal loss. Cr and Cho are more highly concentrated in glial cells than neurons. Decreases in NAA have been shown to be sensitive to medial temporal lobe sclerosis (Connelly *et al* 1994; Gadian *et al* 1994). The ratio of NAA to Cr and/or Cho is an especially sensitive measure (Gadian *et al* 1994; Ende *et al* 1997), as reactive gliosis often occurs in sclerotic hippocampi, resulting in increased levels of Cr and Cho (Cross *et al* 1996). Decreased NAA levels are highly correlated with complementary measures of neuronal loss obtained by hippocampal volumetrics (Cendes *et al* 1995). When compared with other methods for localizing neuronal pathology, proton MRS has been found to be a sensitive and accurate measure (Thompson *et al* 1998).

MRS data can be acquired in two modes. In earlier studies, spectra were obtained over a prespecified region of interest. More recently, it has been possible to acquire proton MRS spectra over individual cubic voxels of the brain volume. Results can be displayed as MRS images (MRSI) that plot the intensity of signal from a given compound (or ratio between compounds) across the brain. MRSI involves longer acquisition times and diminishes the signal-to-noise ratio, but the anatomic resolution gained is very informative (Prichard 1997). MRSI can be used to identify the side of TLE pathology accurately (Cendes *et al* 1997a; Ende *et al* 1997). In addition, it has revealed that neuronal abnormalities can be widespread, although the abnormalities at the seizure focus are more pronounced (Garcia *et al* 1995; Hetherington *et al* 1995a,b). Accurate localization of pathology has also been observed for patients with extratemporal epilepsy (Stanley *et al* 1998) and in cases of malformation of cortical development (Li *et al* 1998).

IMAGING NEURAL ACTIVITY

The defining feature of epilepsy is not any particular type of lesion or malformation that affects the structural anatomy of the brain. Instead, the disorder is characterized by abnormal control and propagation of neural activity. Therefore, methods for visualizing neural activity with high spatial resolution are of critical relevance to the investigation and diagnosis of epilepsy.

The ideal method would yield pictures of brain activity before, during, and after epileptic seizures, with real-time resolution and high anatomic precision noninvasively. At present, we rely on converging measures that provide temporal resolution and spatial resolution separately. Images of the baseline interictal state of the epileptic brain, as well as images during or just following ictal events, have been extremely useful in charting the abnormalities of brain activity underlying epilepsy.

In order to evaluate functional abnormalities relative to individuals' neuroanatomy, functional brain images from any method need to be coregistered with high-resolution structural anatomic images from MRI (see Duncan 1997; Duncan and Fish 1998). Methods for automated image coregistration and quantitation applied to epilepsy are improving rapidly (see Wright *et al* 1995; Koepp *et al* 1996; Richardson *et al* 1996, 1997). It can be difficult to evaluate results between groups of patients and normal controls, or between distinct groups of patients, since the underlying anatomy may differ between groups because of pathology. For instance, partial-volume effects resulting from regional atrophy need to be taken into account and corrected. Observer bias can also pose problems, especially in methods that do not offer the possibility of quantitative analysis.

POSITRON EMISSION TOMOGRAPHY

PET images the location of radioactive tracers within the brain volume. Coincident γ-rays emitted as a consequence of the decay of the radioactive nuclei are sensed by circular arrays of detectors. Signal can therefore be obtained from any radioisotope that can be introduced safely and that has a relatively short decay half-life, so that the integrated measures correspond to a particular brain state at a known time. PET is primarily a functional brain-imaging technique. Most common are studies of blood flow, using ^{15}O, and studies of glucose metabolism, using 2-deoxy-2-[^{18}F]fluoro-D-glucose (FDG). PET also enables the performance of relatively noninvasive studies of functional neurochemistry *in vivo*. The quality and impact of such studies increases as specific radiolabeled neurochemical agonists and antagonists are developed.

For obvious reasons, PET has not been a very practical method for studying neural activity associated with ictal events. Brain imaging with PET or MRI cameras requires head immobilization, a prerequisite that is difficult to satisfy when seizures involve muscle contractions. Seizures also need to be frequent enough to allow for a reasonable probability of occurrence during the PET examination. Fast-decaying isotopes are usually produced on-line at high costs, so that it is not economic to keep patients idle in a scanner for long periods of time. Even under optimal conditions, the time resolution of most PET methods may not be sufficient for capturing a pure ictal event. The temporal resolution of the method is mainly dictated by the decay half-life of the radioactive nucleus. Metabolic images using FDG have a temporal resolution of about 30 min, too long for capturing most ictal events without contamination from the postictal state (see Engel *et al* 1983a,b). Images of regional cerebral blood flow (rCBF) using ^{15}O have a temporal resolution of about 30–90 s, and are better suited to the task. However, in addition to considerations about the half-life of the tracer, time needs to be allowed for the arrival of the tracer to the brain area, another 30 s or so, depending on the subject. Therefore catching an ictal event while the subject is lying on a scanner and being able to image it without contamination from postictal factors is a rare and lucky happening.

PET studies during seizures have been carried out in patients with extended ictal states or in those whose seizures can be reliably triggered by an external event. In a study of epilepsia partialis continua (Franck *et al* 1986), ictal ^{15}O-PET revealed frontal increases in rCBF, increases in O_2 metabolism, and decreases in the O_2 extraction fraction that were more severe in the hemisphere contralateral to the clonus. Imaging of complex partial seizures has been achieved by inducing seizures with pentylenetetrazole (Theodore *et al* 1996) and measuring rCBF with ^{15}O. EEG was measured continuously during PET scanning. In one case a spontaneous seizure event was captured. Ictal changes in rCBF were found to be widespread, also for the spontaneous seizure, suggesting that both seizure onset and spread were imaged with this method. The method may also have underestimated blood-flow changes because of the brain permeability limitation of water at very high flow rates. The widespread image of blood-flow changes is less useful for localizing the seizure focus than alternative structural and functional methods. PET studies of naturally occurring complex partial seizures have not been carried out systematically. The method therefore is of limited clinical validity compared with other diagnostic imaging tools.

Interictal PET studies, on the other hand, have been extremely valuable. PET is the most sensitive functional imaging method for visualizing the alterations in baseline brain activity due to epilepsy. Metabolic studies using FDG have been more reliable than blood-flow studies. Measures of metabolism and cerebral perfusion can be uncoupled in the same patients, and measures of glucose metabolic rate are more sensitive (Gaillard et al 1995). PET images of metabolism obtained interictally can be subjected to quantitative analysis, since the glucose metabolism is at steady state.

FDG-PET in TLE patients has consistently revealed a region of hypometabolism centered over the epileptic focus (Kuhl et al 1980; Henry et al 1993a; Gaillard et al 1995). The reproducibility of these findings is such that negative metabolic PET findings can call a diagnosis into question (Spencer 1998). However, the relationship between metabolic deficits and structural pathology is not always one to one. The region of hypometabolism is often larger than the region of underlying structural pathology (Engel et al 1982). Hypometabolism often extends into the lateral temporal lobes, even when the seizure focus is limited to medial structures as evidenced by EEG or atrophy measured with MRI (Henry et al 1993b). In some cases, metabolism can also be decreased in areas outside the temporal lobes, such as the thalamus or the frontal cortex (Henry et al 1993c). Areas of decreased metabolism outside the seizure focus have been difficult to interpret. Inhibition or deafferentation of neurons surrounding the epileptic tissue may be involved. Another possibility is that these regions represent projection zones of the affected tissue and therefore their activity levels are decreased as a consequence of hypometabolism of one of their main afferent structures. Lateral temporal hypometabolism has been observed to resolve after medial temporal surgical resection, and has been linked to the resolution of seizures (Swartz et al 1989; Wieser et al 1992).

FDG-PET has also been used to study metabolic disturbances in frontal lobe epilepsy (FLE). Findings can range from no abnormal regions of hypometabolism, small focal regions of hypometabolism, to diffuse regional hypometabolism in one hemisphere (Engel et al 1995). The method therefore is not as useful clinically for FLE as it is for TLE. Nevertheless, it can help in certain cases, especially when other methods fail to provide definitive diagnosis. Unlike TLE, focal metabolic changes in FLE can localize completely with the underlying structural pathology, without hypometabolism extending beyond the lesion boundaries. While patients with TLE often (about 30%) have reduced frontal metabolism, those with FLE do not have frontal hypometabolism outside the ictal region (Engel et al 1995). These focal metabolic and structural disturbances accurately localize the ictal region (Theodore et al 1986; Henry et al 1991; Swartz et al 1991). These findings demonstrate that the metabolic consequences of focal FLE and TLE can be very different. FLE seems to cause less disruption to cerebral metabolism in other regions. FDG-PET has also recently been used to help localize seizure foci in patients for whom other methods failed to provide sufficient diagnostic information (Theodore et al 1997). The method was judged to provide useful information that could diminish the need for invasive intracranial EEG monitoring.

SINGLE-PHOTON EMISSION COMPUTED TOMOGRAPHY

SPECT produces images of rCBF following the injection of radiolabeled tracers. Currently the most commonly used tracer is ^{99m}Tc-hexamethylpropylenamine oxime (^{99m}Tc-HMPAO), which has a 70% uptake in 1 min and yields a stable image for about 6 hours. SPECT is less costly and more widely available than PET. However, the method has an inferior spatial resolution to PET (7–8 mm) and does not allow for fully quantitative data analysis.

SPECT has been probably the most useful functional brain imaging method for revealing changes in neural activity associated with the ictal event. The blood-flow tracer can be injected at the time of seizure, without the need for the patient to be immobilized in a scanner, and imaging can take place hours later. The resulting image has a temporal resolution of about 30–60 s. Depending on the duration of the seizure and the time of the injection, postictal events may therefore also contribute. Accurate interpretation of ictal SPECT requires careful records and concomitant EEG and video monitoring (see Duncan 1997; Duncan and Fish 1998). In TLE, ictal SPECT reveals focal regions of hypermetabolism in the epileptic temporal lobe with high sensitivity and accuracy (Newton et al 1994; Devous et al 1998). Reference interictal SPECT can be useful as a baseline for comparison and may aid in more quantitative analysis of the results (Devous et al 1998). In a prognostic study of TLE, results from ^{99m}Tc-HMPAO SPECT were categorized into typical temporal hyperperfusion, temporal hyperperfusion plus additional posterior involvement, bilateral hyperperfusion, and atypical cases in which the surgical specimen did not show abnormality. The surgical outcome, measured over 2 years, was similar for all cases except those with atypical results. Lack of abnormality was correlated with a worse level of remission (33%) than otherwise (60–69%). This study also showed that the extent of hyperperfusion does not correlate with the outcome of TLE surgery, suggesting that the more widespread signal changes reflect seizure spread rather than intrinsically epileptogenic tissue. In addition to changes of different extent within the temporal lobes in TLE, changes can also be seen in other brain regions. Decreases in rCBF were consistently noted in the frontal cortex of patients with TLE (Rabinowicz *et al* 1997). The reason for such remote and apparently compensatory changes are unclear. They may reflect 'plumbing' limitations of blood within the brain or intrinsic aspects of TLE ictal pathology. Ictal foci for nontemporal epilepsy can also be imaged with ^{99m}Tc-HMPAO SPECT. Occipital hyperperfusion was correlated with six cases of occipital seizures, with two cases showing parallel hyperperfusion of the mesial temporal lobe (Duncan *et al* 1997). These results were consistent with complementary EEG.

Interictal SPECT images on their own have not maintained a prominent role in effective epilepsy diagnosis. Interictal measures of blood flow offer less reliable indices of disrupted neural activity than images of glucose metabolism, as seen with PET. The less quantitative nature and the lower resolution of SPECT make its interictal measures of blood flow even less reliable. The results can reveal reduced regional blood flow associated with the seizure focus, but not always reliably (see Duncan 1997 for review).

FUNCTIONAL MAGNETIC RESONANCE IMAGING

Physiologic measures can be obtained with adaptations of MRI. The most well-developed technique is known as blood oxygenation level-dependent (BOLD) imaging (Bandettini *et al* 1992; Kwong *et al* 1992; Ogawa *et al* 1992). BOLD images are sensitive to the level of deoxygenated hemoglobin, which serves as an endogenous paramagnetic tracer in the blood. Many factors may contribute to changes in the blood signal, such as changes in blood flow and oxygen extraction. Overall, brain regions of increased neural activity have shown concomitant increases in the BOLD signal with a lag of 2–5 s. Ultra-fast image acquisition is often used, enabling imaging of brain slices within tens of milliseconds. Functional images can be obtained using magnet strengths available in typical clinical scanners (1.5 T).

FMRI is thus in an excellent position to join other nuclear magnetic resonance methodologies in becoming an integral part of the preoperative evaluation of epileptic patients. So far, there have been few applications of this new method and no consistent protocol exists for examining patterns of abnormal brain activity related to epileptic seizures. With additional clinical investigations and the continuous improvements in technology, the scenario is likely to change soon.

For the same reasons as described for PET, evaluation of ictal activity with FMRI is not likely to be very practical. Head movements are a great source of artifact in FMRI. In addition, the signal-to-noise ratio of FMRI is relatively low and reliable results necessitate many scans in each condition of interest. Seizures would have to be frequent and reproducible to permit investigation.

One successful case of localization of seizure activity has been reported (Jackson *et al* 1994; Connelly 1995). A young boy with frequent partial seizures on the right side was imaged with conventional FMRI, using a sequence sensitive to the BOLD effect. Images obtained during clinical seizures were compared with images obtained in the absence of seizures. The functional activations colocalized with regions of structural abnormality and with abnormal metabolism imaged with ictal SPECT.

FMRI may be able to localize the source and spread of ongoing abnormal neural activity evident in the EEG as interictal spikes. The first step toward this possibility was the development of MRI-compatible and safe methods for measuring the EEG during MRI scanning. Methods using fiberoptics or increased electrode resistances have made EEG measurement during MRI safe (Ives *et al* 1993; Lemieux *et al* 1997), and methods are becoming commercially available. The quality of the MRI signals are not significantly compromised and ultra-fast FMRI permits monitoring of the EEG between image acquisition (Ives *et al* 1993). Warach *et al* (1996) combined EEG and FMRI to study changes in neural activity triggered by interictal spikes in two patients. Images obtained following spikes were compared with baseline images that were not triggered by spikes. In both cases focal changes in signals were observed. Additional studies, with convergent information about seizure localization, are necessary before the method is fully validated.

Methods for acquisition and analysis in FMRI are improving at a rapid pace. Event-related FMRI methods should soon enable visualization of changing brain activations triggered by single events. Functional interactions between brain regions can be modeled to assess changes in influences among brain regions. The improved temporal resolution of FMRI and the ability to look at the activity of brain networks should have direct applicability to the understanding of the functional pathologies in epilepsy.

IMAGING NEUROCHEMISTRY

Functional brain imaging methods may soon allow the non-invasive measurement of the dynamics of specific chemicals involved in neurotransmission and neuromodulation and may have a role in investigating the mechanisms underlying neurologic pathology. Many endeavors to image specific receptors in the human brain are underway, both with PET and MRS.

POSITRON EMISSION TOMOGRAPHY

The most widely studied receptor complex in epilepsy has been the γ-aminobutyric acid (GABA) A receptor. GABA is the major inhibitory neurotransmitter in the mammalian brain. Dysfunctions in GABA have been associated with epilepsy, and many antiepileptic drugs act by increasing GABA levels in the brain.

The GABA$_A$ receptor complex is an intricate structure and includes the benzodiazepine receptor (BZR) complex. Flumazenil labeled with ^{11}C is a highly specific BZR antagonist and has excellent properties for functional imaging with PET. Flumazenil readily crosses the blood–brain barrier, has low affinity for peripheral BZRs, and little nonspecific binding. It does not affect GABA$_A$ currents and therefore does not interfere with the physiologic process being measured. At the dosages required, the ligand has no significant pharmacologic or physiologic effects.

In TLE, ^{11}C-flumazenil PET has consistently revealed significant decreases in the binding of BZRs in the medial temporal lobe containing the seizure focus (Savic et al 1988). Individual analysis has shown that the responses do not result from partial-volume effects, but resist correction for atrophy and coregistration with structural anatomic scans (Henry et al 1993b). Measures of BZR binding correlate strongly with the degree of atrophy of the medial temporal structures and with measures of cell death in surgically excised tissue (Burdette et al 1995). Thus, BZR binding by ^{11}C-flumazenil provides an indirect but extremely accurate measure of neuronal pathology in medial temporal lobe structures. The extent of signal abnormality is more restricted than the metabolic images obtained with other functional PET measures, such as

interictal glucose metabolism measured with FDG (Savic et al 1993). In this sense, a functional marker for a specific neurochemical receptor complex can serve as a more general structural marker for cell loss in epileptic tissue.

In addition to marking general neuronal pathology, PET images of ^{11}C-flumazenil also indicate neurochemical disruptions in epilepsy. Using fully automated means to correct for partial-volume effects and to coregister functional and anatomic scans of patients with those of control populations (Koepp et al 1996), Koepp and colleagues (1997) showed that the levels of BZR binding were reduced over and above the loss of brain volume. Similar conclusions were obtained from an autoradiographic study where more detailed analysis of BZR binding was possible (Hand et al 1997).

The use of ^{11}C-flumazenil PET has been extended to nontemporal lobe epilepsies. During generalized tonic–clonic seizures decreased BZR binding was found in the thalamus, while elevated levels were obtained in the cerebellar nuclei, with no significant alterations elsewhere. The results implicated an abnormality in the cerebellar–thalamic–cortical loop in the epileptic condition (Savic et al 1994). Focal signal decreases have been obtained in patients with frontal seizures, including those without abnormalities in MRS measures (Savic et al 1995). Regions of larger signal abnormality were observed with functional FDG scans. In these cases, more detailed studies will need to assess the relative contributions of neuronal loss and specific GABAergic pathology.

The introduction of novel radiolabeled ligands with high specificity and affinity for neurotransmitters and neuromodulators allows the exploration of the many signaling systems within the human brain (see Henry 1996). Three PET ligands have been developed that have differential affinity profiles for the different subclasses of opiate receptors (μ, κ, and δ). Imaging opiate ligands interictally in TLE has shown increases in the μ opiate receptor concentration over lateral and inferior temporal neocortex and decreases in the amygdala (Frost et al 1988; Mayberg et al 1991). These complex alterations cannot be explained simply by regional neuronal or synaptic loss. Their source and significance remain to be elucidated. Methods for measuring serotonin synthesis capacity (Chugani et al 1998) and muscarinic acetylcholine receptors (Pennell et al 1995, 1999) have also been developed.

MAGNETIC RESONANCE SPECTROSCOPY

MRS signals from nuclei with different resonance frequencies can be used selectively to image abundant neurochemicals. A method based on proton MRS has been developed for measuring GABA concentrations (Rothman *et al* 1993). GABA levels were measured in regions of interest placed over occipital cortex, and agreed with the levels measured in surgically excised human tissue. Values of GABA were found to be elevated by GABA-modulating antiepileptic medications in a dose-dependent manner, but were shown to plateau at a certain dose (Petroff *et al* 1995, 1996). Development of additional MRS methods to target other common neurotransmitters would offer great clinical potential, not only for understanding and diagnosing epilepsy but also for monitoring the efficacy of medical treatments.

IMAGING ELOQUENT CORTEX NONINVASIVELY

A final role for functional imaging during the preoperative evaluation of epileptic patients is delineating the sensory, motor, or cognitive functions of the cortex in or near the epileptic focus. Planning effective neurosurgery that minimizes potential debilitating behavioral deficits cannot proceed without such information.

Functional assessment of cortex that may be implicated in the neurosurgical resection has traditionally relied on highly invasive and somewhat primitive procedures. Hemispheric specialization for language and memory functions is assayed by injecting an anesthetic into each carotid artery that irrigates one cerebral hemisphere. Motor and cognitive capacities are probed during the time window when the hemisphere is dormant. The procedure carries risk and does not permit extensive testing and retesting of multiple functions. More specific localization of function within each hemisphere has relied on intraoperative cortical stimulation during simple tasks, such as speaking, reading, or object naming. Eloquent cortex is defined as an area that upon stimulation either interferes with task performance, such as producing speech arrest, or elicits movements or sensations, such as visual phosphenes, auditory sounds, somatosensory feelings, or memories. Using such cortical stimulation procedures, many cortical areas remain 'silent.' This probably reflects the poverty of the testing methods that can be employed under intraoperative conditions and the fact that many brain areas involved in cognitive functions are not essential for their operation. By using methods to visualize the brain areas involved in tasks, and a greater variety of sensorimotor and cognitive tasks, many more cortical areas would become eloquent and tell us about their functional specializations. In some cases it would still be necessary to assess the critical nature of the area's involvement in a task using more invasive cortical stimulation. However, the amount of invasive testing required would be diminished and the procedures would be much more targeted.

FMRI provides the method of choice for charting the specializations of cortical areas for preoperative planning. The method has resolution at the single-subject level, and functional results can be readily integrated with structural anatomic scans obtained during the same imaging session. Even though FMRI has been around for less than a decade, there has already been an explosion of experiments using this technique and findings on all kinds of behavioral tasks, from the simplest sensorimotor tasks to the most high-level cognitive operations such as planning or theory of mind. Reviewing the range of possible experiments is well beyond the scope of this chapter. For a sample of the field, the reader may wish to consult the published abstracts from the most recent meeting of the Society for Human Brain Mapping.

Sensory and motor cortex have been mapped reliably in patients being evaluated for neurosurgery (see Plate 4 and Puce *et al* 1995). Rao *et al* (1995) have replicated the hemispheric and topographic organization of primary motor cortex by assessing activations during finger, elbow, and toe movements. The activations in individuals were found to follow the gyral anatomy and were restricted to the cortical ribbon. Puce *et al* (1995) used both sensory and motor tasks to locate sensory and motor cortices in normal volunteers and in four presurgical patients with lesions impinging upon sensorimotor areas. Reliable activations were obtained in all cases at the individual level. More importantly, the activations in the patients colocalized with sensory-evoked potential localization of sensory cortex obtained intraoperatively as well as with cortical stimulation results. Fried *et al* (1995) showed that reliable activation of motor and visual cortices was possible in patients, even using conventional scanning sequences available in clinical machines. The location of the activations was checked against functional studies using PET.

Localization of higher-level cognitive functions, such as language and memory, using FMRI has developed more slowly (see Plate 5). Large networks of brain regions are typically activated during cognitive tasks, such as those involving language and memory. Lateralization of the activations is rarely complete. Simple and reliable tasks for identifying critical cognitive areas are therefore still under development. Results from PET suggest that the endeavor is worthwhile. Activations during language tasks have been shown to correlate with localization using subdural electrical recordings (Bookheimer *et al* 1995) and cortical stimulation (Bookheimer *et al* 1997). Bookheimer *et al* (1997) confirmed that in addition to activations that coregistered with critical areas identified using cortical stimulation, additional activation foci are obtained during visual or auditory naming tasks. Desmond *et al* (1995) demonstrated that it is possible to use FMRI successfully to lateralize critical language functions. Activations of the inferior frontal gyrus were found to provide lateralizing information and correlated well with results from invasive intracarotid amobarbital testing. This general approach has recently been adapted for lateralizing language functions in children (Hertz-Pannier *et al* 1997), where validating information was obtained with the intracarotid amobarbital test or intraoperative cortical stimulation. Testing of other cognitive functions whose integrity may be compromised by epilepsy or surgical procedures is also being developed. Detre *et al* (1998) have applied memory tasks involving recollection of complex visual scenes in the study of medial temporal lobe function. These tasks have been shown to activate medial temporal lobe structures. Asymmetry ratios of medial temporal activation were calculated in both normals and patients using a region-of-interest approach. In normals the values obtained were nearly symmetric, while in patients the activations were significantly skewed and concurred with findings using the intracarotid amobarbital test.

Functional mapping in the presurgical evaluation of epilepsy has therefore already started in some centers. Most FMRI studies remain confirmatory at this stage and the method has not superseded the more traditional invasive methods. In the near future many more functional studies of cognition are likely to play a role in the clinical evaluation and prognosis of epileptic patients.

CONCLUSIONS

During the last decade or so, there has been a huge increase in the use of brain-imaging techniques in the field of epilepsy diagnosis and prognosis. Structural and functional imaging together reveal the underlying pathology of the condition. Lesions or tissue malformations are readily observable. Neuronal pathology in the absence of structural lesions can be evident as regional atrophy, measured with MRI volumetrics. Markers of neuronal activity provide parallel accurate information, such as NAA imaged with proton MRS or concentrations of widespread receptors (e.g. BZR) using PET. Increasingly detailed information of the pathology should become available as additional specific high-affinity ligands for receptors implicated in epilepsy are developed for PET investigation, and as methods for imaging additional compounds implicated in epilepsy are developed for MRS. Improvements in techniques for functional imaging of neural activity will also guide important advances in basic research and clinical applications. At present, it is possible to measure the baseline metabolic state of the brain interictally using PET and to observe reliable focal increases in rCBF correlated with the ictal event using SPECT. FMRI may provide improved methods with which to observe the focus and spread of abnormal brain activity associated with subclinical epileptic events. Event-related FMRI methods should greatly improve the temporal resolution with which we can visualize changes in brain activity. Such methods should provide significantly improved complementary information to the most direct measure of epileptic activity, the EEG, which has real-time resolution but lacks in spatial resolution. Dynamic studies of brain activity should be possible and the consequences of abnormal activity within cortical networks may be revealed. The relationship between pathologic activity and the functioning of sensorimotor and cognitive brain networks will also provide vital information for diagnosis and prognosis of epilepsy conditions. Surgery can be planned to minimize behavioral deficits. In addition, the neuropsychologic consequences of epilepsy may be better understood.

KEY POINTS

1. Methods are available for the noninvasive visualization of brain anatomy, pathology, chemistry and metabolism, and blood flow; and for localizing areas critical for both function and epileptic seizures.
2. In TLE:
   (a) decreased levels of NAA compared with Cr and/or Cho as measured by MRS and decreased binding of BZRs as measured by flumazenil PET, are especially sensitive indices of medial temporal lobe sclerosis;
   (b) the epileptic focus is consistently associated with interictal ipsilateral temporal lobe hypometabolism on FDG-PET;
   (c) ictal SPECT reveals temporal lobe hypermetabolism ipsilateral to the seizure onset.
3. Both FMRI and PET require head immobilization and so, given

KEY POINTS

current technology, are impractical for studying neural activity associated with seizures involving muscle contractions.

4. FMRI should become the method of

choice for plotting the location of 'eloquent' cortical areas responsible for important cortical functions prior to excisional surgery. It should replace both intracarotid

amobarbital testing and preexcisional cortical mapping by electrical stimulation.

REFERENCES

Bandettini P, Wong E, Hinks R, Tikofsky R, Hyde J (1992) Time course EPI of human brain function during task activation. *Magnetic Resonance in Medicine* **25**:390–397.

Berkovic AJ, Rowley HA, Andermann F (1995) MR in partial epilepsy: value of high-resolution volumetric techniques. *American Journal of Neuroradiology* **16**:339–343.

Bergin PS, Fish DR, Shorvon SD, Oatridge A, deSouza NM, Bydder GM (1995) Magnetic resonance imaging in partial epilepsy: additional abnormalities shown with the fluid attenuated inversion recovery (FLAIR) pulse sequence. *Journal of Neurology, Neurosurgery and Psychiatry* **58**:439–443.

Bookheimer S, Zeffiro TA, Blaxton T *et al* (1995) Regional cerebral blood flow changes during object naming and word reading. *Human Brain Mapping* **3**:93–106.

Bookheimer SY, Zeffiro TA, Blaxton T *et al* (1997) A direct comparison of PET activation and electrocortical stimulation mapping for language localization. *Neurology* **48**:1056–1065.

Bronen RA, Fulbright RK, Kim JH, Spencer SS, Spencer DD, al Rodhan NR (1995) Regional distribution of MR findings in hippocampal sclerosis. *American Journal of Neuroradiology* **16**:1193–1200.

Burdette D, Sakurai S, Henry T *et al* (1995) Temporal lobe central benzodiazepine binding in unilateral mesial temporal lobe epilepsy. *Neurology* **45**:934–941.

Cascino GD, Trenerry MR, So EL *et al* (1996) Routine EEG and temporal lobe epilepsy: relation to long-term EEG monitoring, quantitative MRI, and operative outcome. *Epilepsia* **37**:651–656.

Cendes F, Andermann F, Dubeau F, Arnold DL (1995) Proton magnetic resonance spectroscopic images and MRI volumetric studies for lateralization of temporal lobe epilepsy. *Magnetic Resonance Imaging* **13**:1187–1191.

Cendes F, Caramanos Z, Andermann F, Dubeau F, Arnold D (1997a) Proton magnetic resonance spectroscopic imaging and magnetic resonance imaging volumetry in the lateralization of temporal lobe epilepsy: a series of 100 patients. *Annals of Neurology* **42**:737–746.

Chugani DC, Muzik O, Chakraborty P *et al* (1998) Human brain serotonin synthesis capacity measured *in vivo* with alpha-(C-11) methyl-l-tryptophan. *Synapse* **28**:33–43.

Connelly A (1995) Ictal imaging using functional magnetic resonance. *Magnetic Resonance Imaging* **13**:1233–7.

Connelly A, Jackson GD, Duncan JS, King MD, Gadian DG (1994) Magnetic resonance spectroscopy in temporal lobe epilepsy. *Neurology* **44**:1411–1417.

Cross JH, Connelly A, Jackson GD, Johnson CL, Neville BG, Gadian DG (1996) Proton magnetic resonance spectroscopy in children with temporal lobe epilepsy. *Annals of Neurology* **39**:107–113.

Desmond JE, Sum JM, Wagner AD et al (1995) Functional MRI measurement of language lateralization in Wada-tested patients. *Brain* **118**:1411–1419.

Detre JA, Maccotta L, King D *et al* (1998) Functional MRI lateralization of memory in temporal lobe epilepsy. *Neurology* **50**:926–932.

Devous MD Sr, Thisted RA, Morgan GF, Leroy RF, Rowe CC (1998) SPECT brain imaging in epilepsy: a meta-analysis. *Journal of Nuclear Medicine* **39**:285–293.

Duncan JS (1997) Imaging and epilepsy. *Brain* **120**:339–377.

Duncan JS, Fish DR (1998) Integration of structural and functional data. *Current Opinion in Neurology* **11**:119–122.

Duncan R, Biraben A, Patterson J *et al* (1997) Ictal single photon emission computed tomography in occipital lobe seizures. *Epilepsia* **38**:839–843.

Ende GR, Laxer KD, Knowlton RC *et al* (1997) Temporal lobe epilepsy: bilateral hippocampal metabolite changes revealed at proton MR spectroscopic imaging. *Radiology* **202**:809–817.

Engel J Jr, Kuhl DE, Phelps ME (1982) Patterns of human local cerebral glucose metabolism during epileptic seizures. *Science* **218**:64–66.

Engel J Jr, Kuhl DE, Phelps ME (1983a) Regional brain metabolism during seizures in humans. *Advances in Neurology* **34**:141–148.

Engel J Jr, Kuhl DE, Phelps ME, Rausch R, Nuwer M (1983b) Local cerebral metabolism during partial seizures. *Neurology* **33**:400–413.

Engel J Jr, Henry TR, Swartz BE (1995) Positron emission tomography in frontal lobe epilepsy. *Advances in Neurology* **66**:223–238.

Franck G, Sadozt B, Salmon E (1986) Regional cerebral blood flow and metabolic rates in human focal epilepsy and status epilepticus. *Advances in Neurology* **44**:935–948.

Fried I, Nenov V, Ojemann S, Woods R (1995) Functional MR and PET imaging of rolandic and visual cortices for neurosurgical planning. *Journal of Neurosurgery* **83**:854–861.

Frost J, Mayberg H, Fisher R et al (1988) Mu-opiate receptors measured by positron emission tomography are increased in temporal lobe epilepsy. *Annals of Neurology* **23**:231–237.

Gadian DG, Connelly A, Duncan JS *et al* (1994) 1H magnetic resonance spectroscopy in the investigation of intractable epilepsy. *Acta Neurologica Scandinavica Suppl* **152**:116–121.

Gaillard WD, Fazilat S, White S *et al* (1995) Interictal metabolism and blood flow are uncoupled in temporal lobe cortex of patients with complex partial epilepsy. *Neurology* **45**:1841–1847.

Garcia PA, Laxer KD, van der Grond J, Hugg JW, Matson GB, Weiner MW (1995) Proton magnetic resonance spectroscopic imaging in patients with frontal lobe epilepsy. *Annals of Neurology* **37**:279–281.

Gilliam F, Bowling S, Bilir E *et al* (1997) Association of combined MRI, interictal EEG, and ictal EEG results with outcome and pathology after temporal lobectomy. *Epilepsia* **38**:1315–1320.

Hand K, Beain V, Van Paesschen W et al (1997) Central benzodiazepine receptor autoradiography in hippocampal sclerosis. *British Journal of Pharmacology* **122**:358–364.

Henry TR (1996) Functional neuroimaging with positron emission tomography. *Epilepsia* **37**:1141–1154.

Henry TR, Sutherling WW, Engel J Jr *et al* (1991) Interictal cerebral metabolism in partial epilepsies of neocortical origin. *Epilepsy Research* **10**:174–182.

Henry TR, Engel J Jr, Mazziotta JC (1993a) Clinical evaluation of interictal fluorine-18-fluorodeoxyglucose PET in partial epilepsy. *Journal of Nuclear Medicine* **34**:1892–1898.

Henry TR, Frey KA, Sackellares JC et al (1993b) *In vivo* cerebral metabolism and central benzodiazepine-receptor binding in temporal lobe epilepsy. *Neurology* **43**:1998–2006.

Henry TR, Mazziotta JC, Engel J Jr (1993c) Interictal metabolic anatomy of mesial temporal lobe epilepsy. *Archives of Neurology* **50**:582–589.

Hertz-Pannier L, Gaillard WD, Mott SH et al (1997) Noninvasive assessment of language dominance in children and adolescents with functional MRI: a preliminary study. *Neurology* **48**:1003–1012.

Hetherington H, Kuzniecky R, Pan J et al (1995a) Proton nuclear magnetic resonance spectroscopic imaging of human temporal lobe epilepsy at 4.1 T. *Annals of Neurology* **38**:396–404.

Hetherington HP, Kuzniecky RI, Pan JW, Vaughan JT, Twieg DB, Pohost GM (1995b) Application of high field spectroscopic imaging in the evaluation of temporal lobe epilepsy. Magnetic Resonance *Imaging* **13**:1175–1180.

Ives J, Warach S, Schmitt F, Edelman R, Schomer D (1993) Monitoring the patient's EEG during echo planar MRI. *Electroencephalography and Clinical Neurophysiology* **87**:417–420.

Jack CR Jr, Sharbrough FW, Twomey CK et al (1990) Temporal lobe seizures: lateralization with MR volume measurements of the hippocampal formation. *Radiology* **175**:423–429.

Jack CR Jr, Mullan BP, Sharbrough FW et al (1994) Intractable nonlesional epilepsy of temporal lobe origin: lateralization by interictal SPECT versus MRI. *Neurology* **44**:829–836.

Jackson GD, Connelly A, Cross JH, Gordon I, Gadian DG (1994) Functional magnetic resonance imaging of focal seizures. *Neurology* **44**:850–856.

King D, Bronen RA, Spencer DD, Spencer SS (1997) Topographic distribution of seizure onset and hippocampal atrophy: relationship between MRI and depth EEG. *Electroencephalography and Clinical Neurophysiology* **103**:692–697.

Koepp M, Richardson M, Brooks D et al (1996) Cerebral benzodiazepine receptors in hippocampal sclerosis. An objective in vivo analysis. *Brain* **119**:1677–1687.

Koepp MJ, Richardson MP, Labbe C et al (1997) ^{11}C-flumazenil PET, volumetric MRI, and quantitative pathology in mesial temporal lobe epilepsy. *Neurology* **49**:764–773.

Kuhl D, Engel JJ, Phelps M, Selin C (1980) Epileptic patterns of local cerebral metabolism and perfusion in human determined by positron emission tomography of 18-FDG and 13-NH₃. *Annals of Neurology* **8**:348–360.

Kuzniecky RI, Bilir E, Gilliam F et al (1997) Multimodality MRI in mesial temporal sclerosis: relative sensitivity and specificity. *Neurology* **49**:774–778.

Kwong K, Belliveau J, Chesler D et al (1992) Dynamic magnetic resonance imaging of human brain activity during primary sensory stimulation. *Proceedings of the National Academy of Sciences USA* **89**:5675–5679.

Laxer KD (1997) Clinical applications of magnetic resonance spectroscopy. Epilepsia **38** (Suppl 4):S13–S17.

Lemieux L, Allen P, Franconi F, Symms M, Fish D (1997) Recording of EEG during fMRI experiments: patient safety. *Magnetic Resonance in Medicine* **38**:943–952.

Li LM, Cendes F, Bastos AC, Andermann F, Dubeau F, Arnold DL (1998) Neuronal metabolic dysfunction in patients with cortical developmental malformations: a proton magnetic resonance spectroscopic imaging study. *Neurology* **50**:755–759.

Li LM, Cendes F, Andermann F et al (1999) Surgical outcome in patients with epilepsy and dual pathology. *Brain* **122**:799–805.

McCarthy G, Luby M (1994) Imaging the structural changes associated with human epilepsy. *Clinical Neuroscience* **2**:82–88.

Mayberg HS, Sadzot B, Meltzer CC et al (1991) Quantification of mu and non-mu opiate receptors in temporal lobe epilepsy using positron emission tomography. *Annals of Neurology* **30**:3–11.

Newton MR, Berkovic SF, Austin MC, Rowe CC, McKay WJ, Bladin PF (1994) Ictal, postictal and interictal single-photon emission tomography in the lateralization of temporal lobe epilepsy. *European Journal of Nuclear Medicine* **21**:1067–1071.

Novotny JE (1995) The role of NMR spectroscopy in epilepsy. *Magnetic Resonance Imaging* **13**:1171–1173.

Ogawa S, Tank D, Menon R et al (1992) Intrinsic signal changes accompanying sensory stimulation: functional brain mapping with magnetic resonance imaging. *Proceedings of the National Academy of Sciences USA* **89**:5951–5955.

Pennell PB, Henry TR, Koeppe R, Kilbourn M, Frey K (1995) PET imaging of benzodiazepine and muscarinic receptor loss in mesial temporal lobe epilepsy. *Epilepsia* **36** (Suppl 4):24.

Pennell PB, Burdette DE, Ross DA (1999) Muscarinic receptor loss and presentation of presynaptic cholinergic terminals in hippocampal sclerosis. *Epilepsia* **40**:38–46.

Petroff O, Pleban L, Spencer D (1995) Symbiosis between *in vivo* and *in vitro* NMR spectroscopy: the creatine, N-acetylaspartate, glutamate, and GABA content of the epileptic human brain. *Magnetic Resonance Imaging* **13**:1197–1211.

Petroff O, Rothman D, Behar K, Mattson R (1996) Human brain GABA levels rise after initiation of vigabatrin therapy but fail to rise further with increasing dose. *Neurology* **46**:1459–1463.

Prichard JW (1994) Nuclear magnetic resonance spectroscopy of seizure states. *Epilepsia* **35** (Suppl 6):S14–S20.

Prichard L (1997) New nuclear magnetic resonance data in epilepsy. Current *Opinion in Neurology* **10**:98–102.

Puce A, Constable RT, Luby ML et al (1995) Functional magnetic resonance imaging of sensory and motor cortex: comparison with electrophysiological localization. *Journal of Neurosurgery* **83**:262–270.

Rabinowicz AL, Salas E, Beserra F, Leiguarda RC, Vazquez SE (1997) Changes in regional cerebral blood flow beyond the temporal lobe in unilateral temporal lobe epilepsy. *Epilepsia* **38**:1011–1014.

Rao S, Binder J, Hamneke T et al (1995) Somatotopic mapping of human primary motor cortex with functional magnetic resonance imaging. *Neurology* **45**:919–924.

Richardson MP, Koepp MJ, Brooks DJ, Fish DR, Duncan JS (1996) Benzodiazepine receptors in focal epilepsy with cortical dysgenesis: an ^{11}C-flumazenil PET study. *Annals of Neurology* **40**:188–198.

Richardson MP, Friston KJ, Sisodiya SM et al (1997) Cortical grey matter and benzodiazepine receptors in malformations of cortical development. A voxel-based comparison of structural and functional imaging data. *Brain* **120**:1961–1973.

Rothman D, Petroff O, Behar K, Mattson R (1993) Localized (1)H NMR measurements of gamma-aminobutyric acid in human brain in vivo. *Proceedings of the National Academy of Sciences USA* **90**:5662–5666.

Savic I, Persson A, Roland P, Pauli S, Sedvall G, Widen L (1988) In-vivo demonstration of reduced benzodiazepine receptor binding in human epileptic foci. *Lancet* **ii**:863–866.

Savic I, Ingvar M, Stone Elander S (1993) Comparison of ^{11}C]flumazenil and ^{18}F]FDG as PET markers of epileptic foci. *Journal of Neurology, Neurosurgery, and Psychiatry* **56**:615–621.

Savic I, Pauli S, Thorell JO, Blomqvist G (1994) In vivo demonstration of altered benzodiazepine receptor density in patients with generalised epilepsy. *Journal of Neurology, Neurosurgery and Psychiatry* **57**:797–804.

Savic I, Thorell J, Roland P (1995) [(11)C]Flumazenil positron emission tomography visualizes frontal epileptogenic regions. *Epilepsia* **36**:1225–1232.

Spanedda F, Cendes F, Gotman J (1997) Relations between EEG seizure morphology, interhemispheric spread, and mesial temporal atrophy in bitemporal epilepsy. *Epilepsia* **38**:1300–1314.

Spencer SS (1998) Substrates of localization-related epilepsies: biologic implications of localizing findings in humans. *Epilepsia* **39**:114–123.

Stanley JA, Cendes F, Dubeau F, Andermann F, Arnold DL (1998) Proton magnetic resonance spectroscopic imaging in patients with extratemporal epilepsy. *Epilepsia* **39**:267–273.

Swartz BE, Halgren E, Delgado Escueta AV *et al* (1989) Neuroimaging in patients with seizures of probable frontal lobe origin. *Epilepsia* **30**:547–558.

Swartz H, Chen K, Hu H, Hideg K (1991) Contrast agents for magnetic resonance spectroscopy: a method to obtain increased information in in vivo and in vitro spectroscopy. *Magnetic Resonance in Medicine* **22**:372–377.

Swartz BE, Tomiyasu U, Delgado Escueta AV *et al* (1992) Neuroimaging in temporal lobe epilepsy: test sensitivity and relationships to pathology and postoperative outcome. *Epilepsia* **33**:624–634.

Theodore WH, Holmes MD, Dorwart RH *et al* (1986) Complex partial seizures: cerebral structure and cerebral function. *Epilepsia* **27**:576–582.

Theodore WH, Balish M, Leiderman D, Bromfield E, Sato S, Herscovitch P (1996) Effect of seizures on cerebral blood flow measured with ^{15}O-H$_2$O and positron emission tomography. *Epilepsia* **37**:796–802.

Theodore WH, Sato S, Kufta CV, Gaillard WD, Kelley K (1997) FDG-positron emission tomography and invasive EEG: seizure focus detection and surgical outcome. *Epilepsia* **38**:81–86.

Thompson JE, Castillo M, Kwock L (1998) MR spectroscopy in the evaluation of epilepsy. *Magnetic Resonance Imaging Clinics of North America* **6**:21–29.

Van Paesschen W, Sisodiya S, Connelly A *et al* (1995) Quantitative hippocampal MRI and intractable temporal lobe epilepsy. *Neurology* **45**:2233–2240.

Van Paesschen W, Revesz T, Duncan JS, King MD, Connelly A (1997) Quantitative neuropathology and quantitative magnetic resonance imaging of the hippocampus in temporal lobe epilepsy. *Annals of Neurology* **42**:756–766.

Warach S, Ives JR, Schlaug G *et al* (1996) EEG-triggered echo-planar functional MRI in epilepsy. *Neurology* **47**:89–93.

Wieser H, Swartz B, Delgado Escueta A *et al* (1992) Differentiating frontal lobe seizures from temporal lobe seizures. *Advances in Neurology* **57**:267–285.

Wright I, McGuire P, Poline J, Travere J, Murray R, Frith C (1995) A voxel-based method for the statistical analysis of gray and white matter density applied to schizophrenia. *Neuroimage* **2**:244–252.

Presurgical psychosocial evaluation

GA BAKER AND A JACOBY

Epilepsy can be a cause of major disability and handicap in the 20–30% of people whose seizures are intractable. Advances in medical technology have enabled an increasing number of such patients to be rendered seizure-free through surgery, and both the number of centers offering such treatment and the number of operations being performed have been increasing significantly. Engel *et al* (1993) have conducted two worldwide surveys of the outcome of epilepsy surgery. These include data on almost 10 000 patients and show marked improvement in clinical outcome as measured by the number of patients rendered seizure-free. Surgery is generally considered appropriate for those patients whose seizures have a significant impact on their quality of life (Engel and Sherman 1993). According to Dreiffus (1987), the ideal candidate for surgical treatment of epilepsy is one whose seizures represent the sole or predominant factor preventing normal quality of life. Certainly, a major aim of surgery is to significantly improve the patient's degree of independence or functional capacity. Nevertheless, it is important to note that despite recognition that epilepsy surgery can have a positive influence on psychosocial functioning and quality of life, the precise degree of its impact remains largely undefined (Taylor 1987; Spencer 1994).

Surgical treatment is an expensive option, involving lengthy and costly preoperative evaluation in addition to the cost of the operation itself. It is vital to establish the costs and benefits of epilepsy surgery if the benefits derived from increasingly limited health care resources are to be maximized (Sculpher 1993). Identification of the patients most likely to benefit from the procedure requires extensive presurgical assessment not only of primarily clinical issues but also of others beyond, including preoperative psychiatric status, neuropsychologic functioning, psychosocial functioning, and the patients' and their families' expectations of the surgical outcome.

Given that the ultimate aim of epilepsy surgery is improved quality of life, assessments of its outcome need to be widened beyond the traditional clinical ones to include patient-based measures (Hermann *et al* 1992; Vickrey *et al* 1992). This point is amply illustrated by the finding from one recent study (Wilson *et al* 1998) that just as not all those who continued to have seizures judged surgery a failure, so neither did all patients who became seizure-free judge it a success. Historically, however, there has been a dearth of scientifically rigorous measures of the outcome of epilepsy care (Berg 1994). They have only recently begun to be developed (Baker *et al* 1991; Vickrey *et al* 1992; Jacoby *et al* 1993; Devinsky *et al* 1995).

FACTORS TO BE CONSIDERED IN THE PRESURGICAL PSYCHOSOCIAL EVALUATION

In determining whether a patient is likely to be a good candidate for the surgery program, a number of questions should be considered:

1. Is the patient refractory to antiepileptic drug treatment?
2. Is the patient likely to benefit from surgery?
3. Do the patient and the family understand the risks and benefits associated with surgery and are their expectations of the outcome realistic?
4. Do they have the necessary support to cope postoperatively?
5. Are there any psychologic or psychiatric factors that are contraindicators to surgery?

Polkey and Binnie (1993), on the basis of their extensive experience with the surgical program at the Maudsley Hospital, have devised a list of criteria for admission to an epilepsy surgery program (see Table 49.1). They make explicit the need to consider a number of psychosocial factors, including the degree of disability associated with the seizures; the patient's emotional resources; and the patient's previous and current psychologic and psychiatric status. In the authors' experience, psychosocial variables are likely to heavily influence the outcome of the surgical intervention. Polkey (1989) has also suggested four possible criteria on which the success of surgery can be judged: (a) freedom from or significant control of seizures; (b) complications of surgery, including intellectual and behavioral changes; (c) mortality short and long term; and (d) social and behavioral improvements. To date, however, there has been relatively little research on the impact of surgery on the latter. Most studies have been small and have focused on limited measures of functioning, psychiatric assessment, and personality profiles (Taylor 1987; Seidman-Ripley et al 1993). They have not generally addressed the patients' perception of the impact of the epilepsy, nor have they considered their expectations of surgery.

What is abundantly clear from the available literature is that patients who are rendered seizure-free by surgery exhibit significantly greater improvements in self-reported emotional and psychosocial outcome compared with those who are not rendered seizure-free (Rausch and Crandall 1982; Hermann and Wyler 1989; Bladin 1992; Hermann et al 1992; Guldvog 1994). Further, the most significant predictor of a patient's postoperative psychosocial

Table 49.1 Preoperative assessment program. (Reproduced, with kind permission, from Polkey and Binnie 1993.)

Criteria for admission
1. (a) Reliable diagnosis for intractable epilepsy
   (b) Attacks are epileptic, no pseudoseizures[a]
   (c) Failure of appropriate medication
   (d) Patient is compliant[a]
2. Seizures of such a frequency and nature that they are disabling, having regard to the patient's lifestyle[a]
3. No other contradictions, for example a coagulation defect

Criteria for investigation for resective surgery
1. Partial seizures, whether or not secondarily generalized
2. Full-scale IQ not less than 70 points
3. Age not more than 55 years
4. Patient has the emotional resources to withstand the procedures, including the possibility of being found inoperable[a]

Note (a) A single EEG focus is not a requirement
     (b) Psychiatric or behavioral disorder are not automatic exclusion criteria[a]

[a]Requires assessment of disability, handicap, and psychiatric and psychosocial status.

adjustment is the adequacy of their preoperative adjustment (Hermann et al 1992). This confirms earlier research of Taylor and Falconer (1968), who demonstrated that a positive preoperative psychologic status predicted a positive mental status postoperatively.

PRESURGICAL IMPACT OF EPILEPSY

An understanding of the presurgical impact of epilepsy on a patient's day-to-day functioning, as perceived by the patient, is critical if a realistic assessment of their postoperative adjustment is to be estimated. As a great number of studies have illustrated only too clearly, epilepsy has the potential to impact on a patient's physical, psychologic, social and vocational status. A range of mediating factors either increase or decrease the magnitude of this impact. Such factors include: (a) the severity of the condition and the burden of the symptoms associated with it; (b) the adequacy of the clinical management; (c) the meaning attached to the illness by the patient and their family; (d) the patient's innate coping abilities; and (e) the level of the social support and the extent of the resources which can be mobilized to deal with it. All these factors will contribute to the patient's perception of the impact and hence to their adjustment to epilepsy. Studies of the impact of epilepsy on the quality of life of people with intractable epilepsy are reviewed in detail in Chapter 33. There are also several other helpful reviews of the literature on the impact of epilepsy (see, for example, Levin et al 1988; Cramer 1994), for which reason their key messages are only briefly summarized here.

First, and at its most extreme, epilepsy is associated with increased mortality, in some cases due to its underlying causes, in others because of the associated increased risk of accident and injury (Hauser *et al* 1980). Though the evidence suggests that increased mortality is not uniform across all groups of people with epilepsy, it appears nonetheless to be a matter of genuine concern to many of those affected (Mittan 1986). Less dramatically, people with epilepsy experience seizure-related injuries of varying severity (Buck *et al* 1997; Sonnen 1997) and have to contend with the side-effects of their medications, which may be both physical and cognitive and are more common with polytherapy. Undesirable antiepileptic drug side-effects may be a key factor in noncompliance, which in turn may contribute to the problem of seizure intractability (Schachter 1993).

There is incontrovertible evidence that there are not only increased physical risks for people with epilepsy, but also psychologic ones (Whitman and Hermann 1986). Anxiety and depression are the problems most commonly cited; they frequently coexist (Robertson *et al* 1987). People with epilepsy may also experience low self-esteem (Collings 1990) and a poor sense of mastery (Matthews and Barabas 1981). Other more serious psychiatric morbidity has also been documented among people with epilepsy (Fenwick 1987; Trimble 1988, 1991). Attempts to disentangle the relative influences of clinical, medication, and social factors on psychopathology in epilepsy (Hermann and Whitman 1986; Hermann *et al* 1990) have been inconclusive, but as is stated in Chapter 33, there does appear to be a clear, even if not perfectly linear, relationship between psychopathology and increased seizure frequency.

Epilepsy also has implications for the psychologic well-being of other family members. It has been shown that the families of children with epilepsy are significantly less cohesive, have lower levels of esteem and communication, and have reduced levels of social support compared with those of children with other chronic conditions (Ferrari *et al* 1983; Austin 1988). The presence of a child with epilepsy in the family seems to have important repercussions for all its members, particularly for mothers and siblings (Rutter *et al* 1970; Bagley 1971; Hoare 1984), both of whom appear to be at greater risk of psychiatric disturbance. Sillanpaa (1973) reported higher rates of divorce among the parents of children with epilepsy.

Social withdrawal and isolation are commonly reported among people with epilepsy (Lechtenberg 1984), and are factors which in turn contribute to their lower rates of marriage and fertility when compared with the general population (Dansky *et al* 1980; Lechtenberg 1984). Both under- and unemployment are more common in people with epilepsy, because of a range of factors including educational underachievement (Elwes *et al* 1991), the failure to achieve seizure control, the presence of multiple neurologic or nonneurologic handicaps (Hauser and Hesdorffer 1990), the disabling side-effects of antiepileptic medication, and the prejudice of potential employers (Espir and Floyd 1986). The importance of the statutory restrictions on driving should not be minimized, particularly in societies such as our own, where the car is a taken-for-granted mode of transport.

It seems that any presurgical assessment should aim to elicit an understanding of these various potential consequences of epilepsy at the individual level, since patients' decisions about whether or not to pursue the surgical option are likely to be based on an algorithm which includes them all (Berg 1994).

COPING WITH EPILEPSY PRE- AND POSTSURGICALLY

How people cope with their lives presurgically is a good indicator of their likely coping ability postsurgically. As part of any presurgical assessment, it is important to try to establish the ways in which people cope with their epilepsy by asking questions such as:

1. How do they manage when they have seizures?
2. Who supports them?
3. What arrangements do they make?
4. How does the family cope with the seizures?
5. Is there anything the affected person does to prevent a seizure occurring?
6. How do the seizures affect day-to-day functioning?
7. How would their life be different if the patient were seizure-free?
8. How would their life be if they continued to have seizures?

From probing patients' answers to questions such as these, it is possible to gain valuable insights into how well or badly they will cope with the outcomes of surgery. One important piece of research, and also clinical anecdotal evidence, suggests that for some individuals being rendered seizure-free constitutes a significant life event, in response to which their coping abilities prove at least temporarily inadequate. For example, Bladin (1992) documents how, for a significant number of patients, the sudden acquisition of seizure-free status demands a radical restructuring of family dynamics and relearning of lifestyles and adaptation to what he refers to as the 'burden of normality'. Thus, it appears that those whose operations are successful may be in as much need of support and counseling pre- and postoperatively as those in whom they fail.

PATIENT AND FAMILY EXPECTATIONS OF THE OUTCOMES OF SURGERY

Both people with epilepsy and their families have goals and priorities which they hope will be met as a result of their surgery (Bladin 1992). They often, for example, express their desires for the outcome in terms of the person with epilepsy getting married, having children, finding employment and living a less dependent lifestyle – in other words, leading a 'normal' life. Since being rendered seizure-free does not necessarily guarantee success in any of these areas, this outcome, successful though it may be in clinical terms, can become the source of great stress in psychosocial terms. The failure to realize their expectations may help to account for the relatively high incidence of depression in patients postsurgically.

Determining patients' and their families' expectations of surgery should therefore be considered an important prerequisite of assessing whether they are suitable candidates for the surgery program. In a recent study, Wilson *et al* (1998) examined patients' expectations of the outcome of anterior temporal lobectomy (ATL). Using a standardized semistructured clinical interview, 11 categories of expectations were identified including issues relating to practical aspects of

daily living, such as driving and employment, issues relating to clinical factors, and issues relating to personal factors such as improved self-esteem (Table 49.2).

The authors have examined the distribution of patients' presurgical expectations in relation to their perceptions of the outcome of the surgery, and reported that those who saw the operation as a success had primarily had expectations that led to a practical or clearly identifiable end result – for example, gaining seizure freedom, a driving license or employment, or being able to initiate new activities. In contrast, the group that reported an unsuccessful outcome had a combination of expectations which included both the practical and the psychosocial (such as increased personal independence and improvement in family dynamics), as well as a nonspecific belief that the operation would generally enhance their quality of life. Their less practical expectations, it is suggested, then predisposed them to a greater degree of uncertainty about the outcome. Wilson *et al* (1998) conclude that patients being considered for epilepsy surgery need to be psychologically prepared through a process of 'clear and detailed counselling about the types of gains that can realistically be expected postoperatively'.

This point is reiterated by Wheelock *et al* (1998), who report that despite the evidence that surgery results in complete elimination of seizures in only around 70–80% of

Table 49.2 Patients' expectations of epilepsy surgery. (Reproduced with kind permission from Wilson *et al* 1998.)

Expectation	Definition	Example
Seizure ablation	The complete abolition of epileptic seizures	'To get rid of my turns'
Driving	Attainment of a license	'To get my drivers license'
Employment	Attainment of employment or improvement of employment opportunities, including training or further education	'To return back to school and repeat year 12' 'So I can return to work'
Family	The presence of family pressure to have the operation or a perceived need to change the family dynamics	'To have children' 'Because of the family shame about my seizures'
Social	The perception of seizures as socially disabling or a desire to change the social milieu	'To go out more and not be embarrassed.' 'To improve my social life'
Relationships	The perception that the operation provides a chance to improve current relationships or develop new ones	'To perhaps get married and have children in the future'
Independence	A desire to become independent of family members or friends, so as not to be a burden upon them	'To lift the extra burden on my life and my family' 'Not to rely on others'
Medication	The desire to decrease or cease the intake of antiepileptic drugs	'To eventually decrease my medication'
Self-change	The perception that the operation provides a chance for self-change, including personality or cognitive abilities	'Maybe to improve my memory and concentration' 'Hopefully to improve my confidence'
General improvements	A nonspecific notion that the operation will provide the patient with a general improvement in his/her quality of life	'To make my life happier' 'To improve my lifestyle'
New activities	The perception that the operation provides a chance to take up new hobbies or travel	'To take up ten-pin bowling' 'To take off and travel around Australia'

patients, almost all subjects in their study placed themselves, presurgically, in the successful-outcome group, apparently choosing to ignore the possibility of continuing seizures postsurgically. As a result, subjects who achieved seizure freedom reported high satisfaction with the outcome and a marked improvement in quality of life, while those who failed to do so reported low satisfaction and little change in quality of life. These authors make the point that because seizure reduction, however substantial, does not result in the same quality of life gains as seizure elimination, patients need careful counseling about the benefits that may, nonetheless, accrue from this less than perfect clinical outcome.

PSYCHIATRIC STATUS OF THE SURGICAL CANDIDATE

A number of studies have established the presence of a serious psychiatric disorder as a contraindication to surgery (Spencer and Katz 1990) and psychotic symptoms as an outcome (Guldvog et al 1991; Mace and Trimble 1991). Bladin (1992) found that 64% of patients rendered seizure-free by surgery nevertheless experienced postoperative psychiatric problems, including anxiety, depression, and psychosis. Personality disorders are not uncommon in patients with complex partial seizures. While surgical treatment may result in an improvement, even a fully successfully outcome may not ameliorate such disorders where they are long-established. Patients with fixed or chronic schizophreniform disorders do not appear to benefit from surgical treatment as far as their psychosis is concerned. Some centers have been reluctant to offer epilepsy surgery to patients with fixed interictal psychosis. A recent publication from the Montreal Neurological Institute (Reutens et al 1997), however, has pointed out that with appropriate psychiatric input, patients with chronic psychosis and refractory epilepsy can undergo surgery successfully, and that freedom from seizures improved their integration into psychiatric treatment facilities. Likewise, self-limiting and benign psychotic episodes, particularly those associated with temporal lobe epilepsy, do not constitute a contraindication to surgery, although it has been recommended that surgical treatment should not proceed before remission (Jensen and Larsen 1998). In the view of Polkey and Binnie (1993), a careful and complete psychiatric history should be taken prior to the decision as to whether the patient is a suitable candidate, and particular care should be taken to distinguish between those psychiatric complaints which are known to be associated with chronic epilepsy and those that are independent.

METHODS OF ASSESSMENT

PSYCHIATRIC MEASURES

Although surgery for partial epilepsy more often than not results in favorable outcomes, there is, nonetheless, a need to consider treatment failures, particularly with regard to psychiatric status. The 1986 Palm Desert Conference on the Surgical Treatment of Epilepsy (Engel and Sherman 1993) reported that the standard of psychiatric assessments in centers offering such treatment varied significantly, with most units conducting little or no clinical review pre- or postsurgically. A consensus group convened specifically to consider this issue recommended the possible use of the following psychiatric assessment tools: the present state examination (PSE); the Hamilton or Beck depression inventory; and Neppe's temporal lobe symptom profile. The group also suggested that a diagnosis should always be given using one of the international diagnostic classifications. They proposed that an assessment be conducted by a trained psychiatrist preoperatively, three times in the first postoperative year and at longer intervals thereafter. They also recommended a detailed assessment of sexuality pre- and postoperatively. In those centers where no such psychiatric expertise exists, use of the psychiatric symptom questionnaire or the Goldberg clinical information schedule was recommended. Four years on, the consensus of the 1992 Palm Desert Conference was still that there was a need for a common psychiatric assessment protocol, but no agreement could be reached about what standardized questionnaires should be used. There was, however, general consensus that each patient should have a social and psychiatric care program with set goals determined prior to surgery, and that these should be monitored postsurgically.

Blumer et al (1998) have also argued for the use of a pre- and postsurgery psychiatric evaluation developed specifically to reflect the characteristics of patients with epilepsy. This would include an epilepsy questionnaire, neurobehavioral inventory, and a semistructured interview, with data obtained from both the patient and their next of kin. Using such a battery, the authors were able to conclude from a recent study that some psychiatric complications could not have been avoided by selecting only psychiatrically stable surgical candidates.

PSYCHOSOCIAL AND QUALITY OF LIFE MEASURES

So far, there has been no systematic use of psychosocial or quality of life measures to assess the outcomes of epilepsy surgery. A review conducted by Vickrey *et al* (1993) of those centers attending the 1992 Palm Desert Conference revealed little consistency in the application of such measures. The most common assessment was the Washington psychosocial inventory (WPSI) (Dodrill *et al* 1980), used in 66% of those epilepsy centers participating in the conference. This is despite the fact that the WPSI was not specifically devised to address the outcome of surgical procedures, and so may need to be complimented with more sensitive measures to assess their impact fully. Vickrey is herself the author of a measure developed specifically to assess quality of life in this group of people with epilepsy, the epilepsy surgery inventory (ESI-55) (Vickrey *et al* 1992) which is described in Chapter 33. Based on the generic health status measure, the SF-36 (Ware and Sherbourne 1992), it also includes items to address issues of relevance to epilepsy surgery patients including cognitive function and memory problems. The ESI-55 is gaining increasing popularity as an outcome measure. In a recently reported study, Vickrey *et al* (1995) demonstrated that quality of life was significantly improved for seizure-free patients, but also to a lesser extent for patients having auras only, when compared with those with ongoing seizures postoperatively.

Other psychosocial measures that have been used to assess the outcome from epilepsy surgery include the SF-36 itself (Ware and Sherbourne 1992), the hospital anxiety and depression scale (Zigmond and Snaith 1983), and the sickness impact profile (Bergner *et al* 1976). Kellett *et al* (1997) have applied the Liverpool quality of life battery to assessing surgical outcomes. One problem with all the studies so far reported is that the assessments are retrospective and the measures have been used simply to discriminate between groups at a single time-point. Although the fact that they do so is reassuring, their ability to detect within-patient changes over time cannot automatically be assumed (Juniper *et al* 1996). A possible alternative to structured measures such as these is the patient-generated approach developed by Trimble *et al* (see Chapter 33), which they have recently begun to use with epilepsy surgery patients (Selai and Trimble 1998).

CONCLUSIONS

Presurgical psychosocial evaluations serve a number of important purposes: (a) to identify those who are most and least likely to benefit from surgery; (b) to predict likely postoperative outcome; (c) to provide a baseline measurement against which the achieved outcome can be measured; and (d) to determine the required level of postoperative rehabilitiation. Currently, there are a number of unresolved problems in carrying out such assessments, including the lack of consensus about presurgical protocols, a continuing failure to recognize the importance of nonclinical measures, the lack of well-validated epilepsy-specific outcome measures, and inconsistency in their use. This last is problematic in as much as psychosocial data from the various studies so far reported cannot be easily pooled. It is difficult, therefore, to derive statements that are strongly based in evidence about the outcomes of epilepsy surgery. However, the authors think the importance of presurgical psychosocial evaluations is now firmly established on the clinical and research agendas.

KEY POINTS

1. Epilepsy surgery can have a positive influence on psychosocial functioning, and indeed the ultimate aim is an improved quality of life, but the precise degree of the impact of surgery in this domain remains largely undefined.

2. Psychosocial variables should be carefully assessed preoperatively because they are likely to influence the broad outcome of the surgery, and preoperative psychosocial adjustment is the most significant predictor of the postoperative adjustment.

3. Patients who are rendered seizure-free by surgery report significantly better emotional and psychosocial outcome than do those who are not rendered seizure-free even to the extent of only having isolated auras.

4. Freedom from seizures does not guarantee success in psychosocial domains such as gaining employment, and some patients initially have difficulty coping with being seizure-free postoperatively.

REFERENCES

Austin JK (1988) Childhood epilepsy: child adaption and family resources. *Journal of Childhood and Pediatric Neurology* **1**:18–24.

Bagley C (1971) *The Social Psychology of the Child with Epilepsy.* London: Routledge and Kegan Paul.

Baker GA, Smith DF, Dewey M, Morrow J, Crawford PM, Chadwick DW (1991) The development of a seizure severity scale as an outcome measure in epilepsy. *Epilepsy Research* **18**:245–251.

Berg AT (1994) Evaluating the outcomes of epilepsy surgery. *Clinical Neuroscience* **2**:10–16.

Bergner M, Bobbitt RA, Pollard WE (1976) The sickness impact profile: validation of a health status measure. *Medical Care* **14**:57–67.

Bladin PF (1992) Psychosocial difficulties and outcome after temporal lobectomy. *Epilepsia* **33**:898–907.

Blumer D, Wakhlu S, Davies K, Hermann B (1998) Psychiatric outcome of temporal lobectomy for epilepsy: incidence and treatment of psychiatric complications. *Epilepsia* **39**:478–486.

Buck D, Baker GA, Jacoby A, Smith DF, Chadwick D (1997) Patients' experiences of injury as a result of epilepsy. *Epilepsia* **6**:87–93.

Collings JA (1990) Epilepsy and well-being. *Social Science and Medicine* **31**:165–170.

Cramer JA (1994) Quality of life for people with epilepsy. *Neurology Clinics* **12**(1):1–13.

Dansky LV, Andermann E, Andermann F (1980) Marriage and fertility in epileptic patients. *Epilepsia* **21**:261–271.

Devinsky O, Vickrey BG, Cramer J et al (1995) Development of the quality of life in epilepsy inventory. *Epilepsia* **36**:1089–1104.

Dodrill CB, Batzel LW, Queisser HR, Temkin NR (1980) An objective method for the assessment of psychological and social problems among epileptics. *Epilepsia* **21**:123–135.

Dreiffus FE (1987) Goals of surgery for epilepsy. In: Engel J (ed.) *Surgical Treatment of the Epilepsies,* pp 31–50. New York: Raven Press.

Elwes RDC, Marshall J, Beattie A, Newman PK (1991) Epilepsy and employment: a community-based survey in an area of high unemployment. *Journal of Neurology, Neurosurgery and Psychiatry* **54**:200–203.

Engel J, Sherman DA, (1993) Who should be considered a surgical candidate? In: Engel J (ed.) *Surgical Treatment of the Epilepsies,* 2nd edn. New York: Raven Press.

Engel J, Van Ness PC, Rasmussen TB, Ojemann LM (1993) Outcome with respect to epileptic seizures. In: Engel J (ed) *Surgical Treatment of the Epilepsies,* pp 609–621. New York: Raven Press.

Espir M, Floyd M (1986) Epilepsy and recruitment. In: Edwards F, Espir M, Oxley J (eds), *Epilepsy and Employment: a Medical Symposium on Current Problems and Best Practices.* London: Royal Society of Medicine.

Fenwick P (1987) Epilepsy and psychiatric disorders. In: Hopkins A (ed.) *Epilepsy.* London: Chapman and Hall.

Ferrari M, Matthews WS, Barabas G (1983) The family and child with epilepsy. *Family Process* **22**:53–59.

Guldvog B (1994) Patient satisfaction and epilepsy surgery. *Epilepsia* **35**:579–584.

Guldvog B, Loyning B, Hauglie-Hanseen E et al (1991) Surgical versus medical treatment of epilepsy. II. Outcome related to social areas. *Epilepsia* **32**:477–486.

Hauser WA, Hesdorffer DC (1990) Employment. In: Hauser WA, Hesdorffer DC (eds). *Epilepsy: Frequency, Causes and Consequences.* Maryland: Epilepsy Foundation of America.

Hauser WA, Annegers JF, Elveback LR (1980) Mortality in patients with epilepsy. *Epilepsia* **21**:339–412.

Hermann BP, Whitman S (1986) Psychopathology in epilepsy: a multi-etiological model. In: Whitman S, Hermann BP (eds) *Psychopathology in Epilepsy: Social Dimensions.* Oxford: Oxford University Press.

Hermann BP, Wyler AR (1989) Depression, locus of control, and the effects of epilepsy surgery. *Epilepsia* **30**:332–338.

Hermann BP, Whitman S, Wyler AR, Anton MT, Vanderzwagg R (1990) Psychosocial predictors of psychopathology in epilepsy. *British Journal of Psychiatry* **156**:98–105.

Hermann BP, Wyler AR, Somes G (1992) Preoperative psychological adjustment surgical outcomes are determinants of postoperative psychosocial status after anterior temporal lobectomy. *Journal of Neurology, Neurosurgery and Psychiatry* **55**:491–496.

Hoare P (1984) Psychiatric disturbance in the families of epileptic children. *Developmental Medicine and Child Neurology* **26**:14–19.

Jacoby A, Baker GA, Smith DF, Dewey M, Chadwick DW (1993) Measuring the impact of epilepsy: the development of a novel scale. *Epilepsy Research* **16**:83–88.

Jensen I, Larsen JK (1998) Mental aspects of temporal lobe epilepsy. Follow-up of 74 patients after a resection of a temporal lobe. *Journal of Neurology, Neurosurgery and Psychiatry* **42**:256–265.

Juniper EF, Guyatt GH, Jaeschke R (1996) How to develop and validate a new health-related quality of life instrument. In: Spilker B (ed.) *Quality of Life and Pharmacoeconomics in Clinical Trials,* pp 49–55. Philadelphia: Lippincott-Raven.

Kellet MW, Smith DF, Baker GA, Chadwick DW (1997) Quality of life after epilepsy surgery. *Journal of Neurology, Neurosurgery and Psychiatry* **63**:52–58.

Lechtenberg R (1984) *Epilepsy and the Family.* Cambridge, MA: Harvard University Press.

Levin R, Backs S, Beng B (1988) Psychosocial dimensions of epilepsy: a review of the literature. *Epilepsia* **29**:805–816.

Mace CJ, Trimble MR (1991) Psychosis following temporal lobe surgery: a report of six cases. *Journal of Neurology, Neurosurgery and Psychiatry* **54**:639–644.

Matthews WS, Barabas G (1981) Suicide and epilepsy: a review of the literature. *Psychosomatics* **22**:515–524.

Mittan RJ (1986) Fear of seizures. In: Whitman S, Hermann B (eds) *Psychopathology in Epilepsy: Social Dimensions.* Oxford: Oxford University Press.

Polkey CE (1989) Surgical treatment of chronic epilepsy. In: Trimble MR (ed.) *Chronic Epilepsy: its Prognosis and Management.* Chichester: John Wiley.

Polkey CE, Binnie CD (1993) Neurosurgical treatment of epilepsy. In: Laidlaw J, Richens A, Chadwick D (eds) *A Textbook of Epilepsy,* 4th edn, pp 561–612. London: Churchill Livingstone.

Rausch R, Crandall PH (1982) Psychological status related to surgical control of temporal lobe seizures. *Epilepsia* **23**:191–202.

Reutens DC, Savard G, Andermann F, Dubeau F, Olivier A (1997) Results of surgical treatment in temporal lobe epilepsy with chronic psychosis. *Brain* **120**:1929–1936.

Robertson MM, Trimble MR, Townsend HRA (1987) Phenomenology of depression in epilepsy. *Epilepsia* **28**:364–372.

Rutter M, Graham P, Yule W (1970) A neuropsychiatric study in childhood. In: *Clinics in Developmental Medicine Nos 35/36.* London: Spastics International and Heinemann Medical.

Schachter SC (1993) Advances in the assessment of refractory epilepsy. *Epilepsia* **34**:S24–S30.

Sculpher M (1993) *A Snip at the Price? A Review of the Economics of Minimal Access Surgery.* HERG Discussion Paper No. 11. London: Brunel University, Health Economics Research Group.

Seidman-Ripley JG, Bound VK, Andermann F, Olivier A, Gloor P, Feindel WH (1993) Psychosocial consequences of postoperative seizure relief. *Epilepsia* **34**:248–254.

Selai CE, Trimble MR (1998) Quality of life before and after temporal lobectomy (abstract). *Epilepsia* **39**(2):63.

Sillanpaa M (1973) Medicosocial prognosis of children with epilepsy. *Acta Paediatrica Scandinavica* **237** (Suppl.):3–104.

Sonnen AEH (1997) *Risks of Accidents in Daily Life in Epilepsy,* p 11. The Netherlands: International Bureau for Epilepsy.

Spencer SS (1994) Evolving indications and applications of epilepsy surgery. *Clinical Neuroscience* **2**:3–9.

Spencer SS, Katz A (1990) Arriving at the surgical options for intractable seizures. *Seminars in Neurology* **4**:422–430.

Taylor DC (1987) Psychiatric and social issues in measuring the input and outcome of epilepsy surgery. In: Engel J (ed.) *Surgical Treatment of the Epilepsies,* pp 485–503. New York: Raven Press.

Taylor DC, Falconer MA (1968) Clinical, socioeconomic and psychological changes after temporal lobectomy for epilepsy. *British Journal of Psychiatry* **114**:1247–1261.

Trimble MR (1988) The psychoses of epilepsy. In: Laidlaw J, Richens A, Oxley J (eds) *A Textbook of Epilepsy,* 3rd edn. Edinburgh: Churchill Livingstone.

Trimble MR (1991) Epilepsy and behavior. *Epilepsy Research* **10**:71–79.

Vickrey BG, Hays RD, Graber J, Rausch R, Engel J, Brook RH (1992) A health-related quality of life instrument for patients evaluated for epilepsy surgery. *Medical Care* **30**(4):299–319.

Vickrey BG, Hays RD, Hermann BP, Bladin PF, Batzel LW (1993) Outcomes with respect to quality of life. In: Engel J (ed.) *Surgical Treatment of the Epilepsies,* pp 623–635. New York: Raven Press.

Vickrey BG, Hays RD, Engel J *et al* (1995) Outcome assessment for epilepsy surgery: the impact of measuring health-related quality of life. *Annals of Neurology* **37**:158–166.

Ware JE, Sherbourne CD (1992) The MOS 36-item Short-Form Health Survey (SF-36). I. Conceptual framework and item selection. *Medical Care* **30**(6):473–483.

Wheelock I, Peterson C, Buchtel HA (1998) Presurgery expectations, postsurgery satisfaction, and psychosocial adjustment after epilepsy surgery. *Epilepsia* **39**:487–494.

Whitman S, Hermann BP (eds) (1986) *Psychopathology in Epilepsy: Social Dimensions.* Oxford: Oxford University Press.

Wilson SJ, Saling MM, Kincade P, Bladin PF (1998) Patient expectations of temporal lobe surgery. *Epilepsia* **39**:167–174.

Zigmond AS, Snaith RP (1983) The hospital anxiety and depression scale. *Acta Psychiatrica Scandinavica* **67**:361–370.

Rational preoperative investigation programs and patient selection

CE POLKEY, CD BINNIE, JM OXBURY, AND M DUCHOWNY

Selection for epilepsy surgery depends upon a number of factors including, inevitably, the spectrum of surgical treatments available, and our perception of them. It is useful to discuss how various methodologies have controlled and changed the selection criteria, the place of theoretic schemata in rational selection and finally the problem of redundancy, specificity, and sensitivity in preoperative selection.

Any scheme of rational selection for surgery must include the costs of the investigations to the institution and the dangers to the patient, attempting to minimize both. The dangers to the patient of invasive intracranial monitoring are significant, and although the risk decreases with experience and volume of work, nevertheless hemorrhage, significant neurologic deficit and infection are recorded in the literature as 2–3%.

These risks must also be balanced against the eventual benefit from the subsequent resection. Thus, if the use of depth electrodes in a patient with temporal lobe epilepsy will justify a resection with a 70% chance of seizure remission, then the risk is justified. If, on the other hand, the chance of seizure remission were less than 30%, then the risk of investigation might not be justified.

The selection criteria in children differ from those in adults because severe and chronic drug-resistant epilepsy may interfere with normal physical and cognitive development and also blight education and prevent normal social integration. To derive a practical guide to selection for surgery from all these considerations is a complex, but not impossible task.

HISTORY

The surgical treatment of epilepsy has gone through a number of changes since it first became a practical and serious proposition towards the end of the nineteenth century. At that time the pioneering operations were undertaken on the basis of recently acquired knowledge about the functioning of the nervous system and observations of the typical features of focal seizures. Such a case is that described by Horsley (1886). The advent of EEG meant that seizure origin and generation could now be recorded and documented, resulting in an era of neurophysiologic investigation and selection. However, through the two decades from 1950 to 1970, it became clear that discrete pathology played a crucial part in the outcome from resective surgery. Finally, the next two decades, 1970–1990, saw the development of direct brain imaging of such pathology and functional neuroimaging, adding two more dimensions to the selection process. Different strengths in individual institutions and correlations between new and old knowledge, including outcome data and neuropathologic studies, have led to diverse and varied claims for the best methods of selection.

OVERALL SELECTION

Selection for resective surgery depends mostly upon proving the discrete pathology that can be removed without causing unacceptable neurologic or cognitive deficits. Various theoretic schemata, based upon the identification of different components in the generation of seizures, can be visualized. Examination of the outcome from resective surgery suggests that this is clearly related to the identification and complete removal of discrete pathology. The case of unilateral hemisphere disease is a special one in which it is clear that a number of operative procedures which combine resection and disconnection give roughly equivalent results whose ultimate effectiveness may depend upon the completeness of the functional removal rather than any other factor.

In functional operations, there are various theoretic models and concepts which are described in detail elsewhere (see Chapter 43). These theoretic considerations are not sufficient to be used as selection criteria which are therefore derived from known outcomes. The basis of this chapter is a staged management process, in which the patient proceeds through a series of phases of investigation. These phases become more complex, dangerous, and costly with the option to quit or perform surgery as each phase is passed. These phases, and their implications, are described below.

PHASE 1a – BASIC INVESTIGATIONS

This phase is devoted to characterizing the patient's epilepsy and examining the possibilities of various surgical options. The elements of this phase are as follows.

CLINICAL HISTORY

This is of paramount importance, as the semeiology of the focal seizures is necessary to establish the origin of the epilepsy from one part of the brain, or to connect it with a known structural abnormality. Such information has to be obtained with patience and care and must include descriptions from independent witnesses as well as the patient. The use of clinical terms such as 'petit mal' and 'temporal lobe fit' by lay persons should be interpreted with care and

circumspection, but without giving offence. In addition to the seizure history, the patient's other medical history, especially in childhood, is of great importance for many reasons. Not only may it give a positive clue to the underlying pathology, but it may also indicate multiple pathology, or in a negative sense it may eliminate one pathology or suggest another. The usefulness of such information, typified by the observations of Ounsted *et al* (1966) in their original group of 100 children with temporal lobe epilepsy, is dealt with in detail in other chapters.

NEUROPHYSIOLOGY

Focal EEG changes can be seen on routine scalp recordings in a proportion of patients, although there are many caveats to the usefulness of the interictal EEG in presurgical assessment. Such abnormalities are seen more readily if sufficient technical standards are maintained, if the registration includes a sleep phase, and if the recordings are repeated.

NEUROIMAGING

The gold standard is undoubtedly magnetic resonance imaging (MRI), whose specificity and sensitivity for structural lesions is very high. Here, more than anywhere else, standards are easy to define and maintain. An examination which does not comprise the relevant number of sequences in the correct planes, or is marred by movement, may give information which is useless or even misleading. Such an examination must include sequences which will detect and describe temporal lobe disease accurately and also reflect pathology including multiple pathology or multifocal occurrence of one pathology. In the authors' view, mesial temporal sclerosis, in all its variants, is a lesion and therefore nonlesional cases are relatively rare. Careful examination may reveal dual pathology in up to 20% of patients.

NEUROPSYCHOLOGY

A basic battery of tests is required to quantify verbal and nonverbal intelligence quotient (IQ), memory function, and frontal lobe function. In children, different test batteries may be needed. In infants and young children, various developmental scales may be appropriate. Although important in preoperative assessment, and especially if they are carried out sequentially in indicating deterioration, these tests are equally important in predicting cognitive outcome from the proposed intervention.

QUALITY OF LIFE AND NEUROPSYCHIATRY

These tests are not standard, even in the authors' own institution. There are now good, well-validated tests of quality of life which have enabled proper assessment of the effects of resective surgery to be made (Vickrey *et al* 1992, 1994, 1995). They are now a good tool of clinical research but are not a predictor of surgical outcome and therefore are not a useful test for selection of patients for surgery.

DECISION

At this point candidates may be selected for lesionectomy, hemispherectomy, or the functional procedures such as VNS or callosotomy. Patients proceeding beyond this point are presumed to be possible candidates for cortical resection which may be either temporal, extratemporal, or multilobar.

PHASE 1b

In this phase, the emphasis is on further demonstration of the presence and nature of pathology with the use of videotelemetry to delineate seizure semeiology. It is debatable whether some of the more complex aspects of structural MRI should be included in this phase as they may be necessary only to elaborate details of temporal lobe disease. At the end of this phase the majority of patients suitable for surgery, both resective and functional surgery, will have been identified.

NEUROPHYSIOLOGY – VIDEOTELEMETRY AND SPECIAL ELECTRODES

Videotelemetry is an essential tool in clarifying seizure semeiology and the electrographic characteristics of seizures. This investigation is particularly useful in revealing consistent seizure patterns and in permitting detailed analysis of very brief seizures such as those that originate in the frontal lobes. It is also considered by some that any patient who is a potential candidate for epilepsy surgery should have videotelemetry in order to identify patients with nonepileptic attacks. The authors have not taken that view if the other information about the patient is consistent with epilepsy.

Videotelemetry may suggest that seizures have a mesial temporal or orbital frontal origin, in which case information obtained may be increased by the use of special electrodes such as sphenoidal wires, foramen ovale electrodes, epidural peg electrodes, etc. At King's College Hospital it is the custom to use foramen ovale electrodes in investigating temporal lobe foci if wishing to confirm a mesiobasal onset for the patient's seizures. Many other groups, including the Oxford group, will use sphenoidal electrodes for the same purpose. Such confirmation is especially important when other data are noncongruent, or if there is no clear EEG focus, or if the procedure proposed is a selective amygdalo-hippocampectomy.

There are two circumstances in which foramen ovale recording is not used. The first is when an extratemporal origin for the seizures, such as from the adjacent frontal lobe, is suspected. In these circumstances, exploration with subdural strips may be necessary, even if these are a prelude to more complex intracranial invasive recording in phase 2. The second is when the insertion of foramen ovale electrodes has proved difficult or impossible, or if the patient has had a previous temporal lobe operation. In either of these circumstances subdural strips are used. In addition, other maneuvers such as drug withdrawal and sleep deprivation, may be necessary to elicit sufficient seizures.

There are certain cortical areas, such as the mesial surface of the frontal lobe, where it is impossible to detect seizure origin from scalp recordings alone, and major invasive intracranial electrodes may be the next step, even if scalp recordings have demonstrated seizures with appropriate semeiology.

NEUROIMAGING

Special MRI protocols

It could be debated as to which sequences from structural MRI examinations should be reserved for this phase. It is probable that volumetric measurements of hippocampal structures should be included. It is generally agreed that a difference between left and right giving a ratio of 0.8, or less, is detectable by eye and that the normal variation lies between 0.85 and 1.0. However, to be certain, or to detect bilateral hippocampal sclerosis, or sclerosis which may be mild in the presence of an extrahippocampal lesion, volumetric measurement is necessary. Therefore, if no asymmetry is apparent on visual inspection but if it is suspected for other reasons, such as a history of an atypical febrile convulsion, that mesial temporal sclerosis may be present, then volume measurements may be helpful. It must also be recalled that hippocampal shrinkage is not necessarily uniform and volume measurements may reveal a profile which is not evident from visual inspection.

The use of T2 measurements may also be useful, as may be the use of fluid attenuation inversion recovery

(FLAIR) sequences. These FLAIR sequences may also reveal other pathology or make it more evident on further scrutiny of the original examination. Finally, there is the possibility of 3-D reconstruction of scan sequences to reveal anomalies of the gyral pattern; such anomalies are often associated with neuronal cortical migration disorders. As a positive target these may be more important in infants and children, where they form a higher proportion of the pathology in patients with intractable focal epilepsy, although in adults this examination may reveal areas of neuronal migration disorder which account for a failure of respective surgery.

Functional brain imaging

At present there are three modalities available: MRI in the form of magnetic resonance spectroscopy and functional MRI mapping; positron emission tomography (PET) imaging which is interictal; and single-photon emission computed tomography (SPECT) imaging whose chief virtue is seen in ictal imaging.

Magnetic resonance spectroscopy is currently still untried as a localizing test. The chief reason for this is twofold, firstly because it seems to reveal information about the proportion of gliotic cells in brain regions. Such gliosis may be bilateral, especially in the case of mesial temporal sclerosis, and not related to seizure onset (della-Rocchetta *et al* 1995; Duncan 1996). Secondly, the techniques of acquiring these spectra vary from manufacturer to manufacturer, making comparison difficult.

The use of functional MRI in delineating motor cortex and speech areas is increasing and becoming more useful as an indication of the anatomic relationship between lesions and these vital areas, and thus improving preoperative planning.

It is now clear that interictal PET using HMPAO indicates blood flow and is not useful in identifying epileptic foci. However, there is a solid literature indicating that FDG-PET and more recently flumazenil-PET are very good lateralizing tests in temporal lobe epilepsy. They therefore tend to be used in this phase. By contrast it has been clearly shown that SPECT, which again measures blood flow, if used ictally and compared with the interictal scan in the same patient, will show temporal lobe foci with a high degree of specificity (Rowe *et al* 1989, 1991; Newton *et al* 1992; Swartz *et al* 1992a). The use of SPECT in examining frontal lobe foci is more difficult, probably because these seizures are notoriously brief. Recently, a ligand has been developed which can be premixed and this may give better results because it can be injected sooner.

NEUROPSYCHOLOGY

Standard and selective carotid amobarbital tests

The determination of speech dominance, and memory distribution and reserve, is the chief neuropsychologic concern in phase 1b. The commonest way to do this is using the classical WADA test in which sodium amobarbital is injected under radiographic and EEG control into first one and then the other internal carotid artery. This was first proposed by Milner *et al* (1962) and has been used with various modifications since. There have been a number of criticisms of this test in spite of which, for most subjects, its conclusions seem to be valid and are a reasonable guide to the outcome of surgery, in all parts of the hemisphere with regard to speech and for temporal lobe surgery with regard to memory. Selective amobarbital tests have been described and there are a few occasions when such tests are justified. Details of their use and results can be found elsewhere (see Chapter 47).

It should also be mentioned that speech dominance can be determined noninvasively by using functional PET, functional MRI, and transcranial magnetic stimulation. Determining memory reserve with functional MRI is currently being explored experimentally. Magnetoencephalography is advocated, by some, both for the localization of deep epileptic foci and for the identification of functional cortical areas, especially when coregistered with MRI (see Chapter 29).

DECISION

At this point those patients who are suitable for temporal or extratemporal resections should have been identified, except in those cases where the possible site of resection needs to be identified using a neurophysiologic hypothesis requiring intracranial electrodes. At this point it is also possible to consider whether patients rejected for resective surgery would benefit from a functional procedure.

PHASE 2

Phase 2 is devoted almost entirely to neurophysiologic investigations, involving major invasive intracranial procedures using subdural or depth electrodes or a combination of both. The purpose of such interventions is twofold, primarily to localize seizure onset and origin. The second purpose is to map cerebral function especially in eloquent areas such as the speech and primary motor and sensory cortices, so as to minimize neurologic or cognitive deficit. Although this information can be obtained to some extent using functional MRI, it is felt that mapping through implanted electrodes is more accurate, currently allows more functions to be mapped than MRI, and can be used in subjects who would be uncooperative in the MRI scanner. However, these techniques are not without their dangers for the patient and are expensive in materials and manpower in their execution. Intracranial electrodes, especially intracerebral depth electrodes, sample activity from a very small volume of cerebral tissue. Therefore, because the investigation is limited in time and space, care must be taken to advance a suitable hypothesis for each individual patient which the invasive electrodes have to answer.

In the authors' practice, neither subdural grids and strips nor stereotactically placed depth electrodes have been used exclusively, but sometimes one technique and sometimes the other depending upon the information which is required to be derived from the exploration. As one might expect, in general, subdural grids and strips are used to address problems around the primary motor and sensory cortices and depth electrodes for problems in the temporal or frontal lobe.

Both methods of exploration carry the risk of major complications. In the case of the subdural electrodes, there is a risk of hemorrhage into the extradural or subdural space and of infection. It is often important to know the precise position of subdural grids and the problems associated with brain shrinkage and attempts at coregistration can mean that results from these investigations may be difficult to implement in practice. The literature suggests that the incidence of complications in the use of these electrodes is around 1–2%, approximately 1 in 1000 electrodes. In the authors' own group of 33 patients in whom these electrodes have been used, hemorrhage has occurred in 6% and infection – sufficient to need removal of the bone flap – in another 6%.

In the case of the depth electrodes there is a risk of intracerebral hemorrhage, with its attendant neurologic consequences, and of infection. Although it can be shown that the risk of hemorrhage varies with the approach even the most conservative figures would suggest that it occurs with clinical significance in 2–3%. These figures, however, can be extremely variable. Van Veelen *et al* (1990) had no complications using a combination of subdural and depth electrodes in 40 patients, whereas the authors had two episodes of hemorrhage and one of ischemia, with significant neurologic effects, in 60 patients.

It is generally agreed that the effect of these invasive methods is to increase the number of patients to whom surgery can be offered with a significant chance of seizure relief and a reasonably accurate prediction of the possible side-effects, especially in operating in eloquent areas. In the authors' material they were able to offer temporal lobe surgery to 59.5% of patients undergoing depth electrode exploration, with a seizure-free outcome in 25% and an improvement in seizure control in a further 25%. In the patients with a good outcome, 81% had a proven pathology in the resected specimen.

DECISION

At this point patients can be divided into two groups. A group in which the hypothesis is confirmed and a local resection is possible; and a second group divided into two subgroups, one of which merits no further surgical treatment and the other who may be suitable for a functional operation.

PRACTICAL IMPLICATIONS

The process described above aims to separate potential candidates for surgery into several groups. At each stage a patient may be identified as suitable for a resective operation, a functional operation, no operation, or further investigation. Although it is necessary to discuss in outline the methods available for identifying such candidates, it is now appropriate to turn the process on its head and look at the practical implications of using these methods to select patients. In this respect one must look at a number of different areas. In effect these are:

1. Invasive vs. noninvasive neurophysiologic recording in selecting candidates for temporal lobe resections, and to a lesser extent frontal lobe resections.
2. The value of neuroimaging, and especially structural neuroimaging, in identifying candidates for temporal lobe resections, and to a lesser extent frontal lobe resections.
3. The selection of patients with unilateral hemisphere disease for major resections or hemispherectomy.
4. The selection of patients who would benefit from multiple subpial transection.
5. The selection of patients who would benefit from callosal section.
6. The selection of patients who would benefit from vagus nerve stimulation.

CANDIDATES FOR TEMPORAL OR EXTRATEMPORAL EXCISIONS

Invasive vs. noninvasive recording

The authors' own experience suggests that it is reasonable to proceed to temporal lobe resection when all the evidence from 'simple' investigations is congruent. An example is a patient with a history of a severe atypical febrile convulsion followed by a Todd's paresis, and of the subsequent development of complex partial seizures with an epigastric aura and appropriate ictal dystonia; they have the appropriately lateralized features of mesial temporal sclerosis on an MRI scan and interictal changes on a sleep EEG, and have a concordant neuropsychologic profile. However, if there is any doubt about the nature of the seizures, or the seizure semeiology, then scalp telemetry should be performed.

It was evident from the authors' early work (Polkey 1994), that patients can be selected effectively using noninvasive tests alone. This has also been shown by Sperling et al (1992) and others. The use of invasive neurophysiologic recording in these patients has diminished in the last 10 years (Engel and Ojemann 1993) and many authors report good results using noninvasive recording alone, although this often includes videotelemetry with scalp recording. Thus Adler et al (1991) and Erba et al (1992) report good results in both temporal and extratemporal cases using long EEG monitoring. The group at Duke University examined the neurophysiologic data as a predictor of outcome in 116 cases operated on between 1980 and 1989. They looked at EEG localization, ranking the investigations hierarchically and using the results accordingly, so that if the patient had had invasive intracranial recording, the results of this were used even if they had also had ictal scalp monitoring and interictal EEGs. However, if a patient had only undergone interictal EEGs then the results of these were used. In the same way, because imaging technology was changing, localized abnormalities were counted whether they were detected by pneumoencephalography, CT, or MRI. They found that there were three predictors of outcome: EEG activity from the site of resection, a localized imaging abnormality, and lack of use of invasive neurophysiologic recording (Armon et al 1996). Spencer et al (1993) note that the best predictors of outcome in their temporal lobe series were the presence of mesial temporal sclerosis, presumably detected by MRI, but confirmed by examination of the resected material, and the absence of secondary generalization of the seizures.

A similar report has been given by Thadani et al (1995), who reported good results in patients operated on without invasive recording. Interestingly, Sperling et al (1992) found, not only that a majority of patients could be offered surgery on the basis of noninvasive investigations, but also that the results in those eventually operated on after further invasive studies were less favorable.

What then, is the case for invasive recording? The ability to identify the epileptogenic zone still remains a cornerstone of resective surgery. If this zone, and its probable inclusion within the resection, cannot be inferred from noninvasive findings, then invasive recording may have a place to answer a specific question. However, Spencer et al (1997) estimated that in 10% of their patients with known temporal lobe pathology, there was discordance between MRI and EEG findings, and in half of these patients successful surgery was undertaken after further investigation with invasive recordings. Likewise, Sperling et al (1996) describe the need to use intracranial recording in 31 of 89 patients undergoing temporal lobe resections, with no apparent difference in outcome once the decision to operate was made. Depth electrodes are also useful in excluding patients from surgery as shown by Spencer (1981), where 18% of patients were rejected for this reason.

Frontal lobe epilepsy, especially in the absence of a demonstrated lesion, is equally challenging. Toczek et al (1997) claim to have located a focus in seven of nine patients with mesial frontal epilepsy. Biraben et al (1997) claim good results, even in nonlesional frontal lobe patients, using a combination of careful consideration of seizure semeiology and stereo-EEG.

In other extratemporal epilepsies, subdural grids or mats are used to map function but their effectiveness in revealing the epileptogenic zone is less evident. Masuoka and Spencer (1993) showed that seizure onset was difficult to define or to correlate with a known lesion. In separate papers, Awad et al (1991) and Jennum et al (1993) describe the use of interictal activity to try to define the epileptogenic zone, but the results of surgery based upon these considerations were poor.

The value of neuroimaging, and especially structural neuroimaging

The place of imaging is also well established, and it has been shown that volume measurements of the hippocampus when they are concordant with EEG findings correlate well with outcome from surgery (Jack et al 1992). Swartz et al (1992b), however, suggest that there is no correlation between the type of MRI abnormality, pathologic substrate, or surgical outcome, in spite of the good outcome where 67% of patients were seizure-free and 94% were within

Engel's groups 1–3A. Kuzniecky *et al* (1993) are clear that an abnormal MRI on visual inspection is associated with a good outcome and this view is confirmed by Oliver and Russi (1994). Berkovic *et al* (1995) have used an actuarial method to correlate pathology detectable by MRI with outcome, finding that outcome was worse in those patients with a normal MRI. Similar results have been shown with frontal lobe lesions (Goldensohn 1992; Fish *et al* 1993).

The special case of resections from the central, parietal, and occipital regions has also to be considered. However, there is not the experience or necessity to deal with them in detail here. Clearly, because of the need to map eloquent cortex, and to study the seizure semeiology carefully, there will be more need for videotelemetry with invasive recording in these patients. Furthermore, especially in children, the pathologic substrate is most likely to be some form of cortical neuronal migration disorder, which does not always present a neat appearance, from the surgical point of view, on structural MRI.

UNILATERAL HEMISPHERE DISEASE

These patients present a special problem of selection for a number of reasons. They will often have multiple seizure types, varying in their occurrence with the underlying pathology. The changes on structural and functional neuroimaging will be widespread. The effects of the underlying disease on cognitive function are also of major importance. Furthermore, the neurophysiologic changes will often be more obvious in the unaffected hemisphere (Carmant *et al* 1995). The feasibility of a major resection or one of the variations of hemispherectomy or hemispherotomy will often depend upon the likely changes in neurologic function, especially of the primary motor, sensory, and speech functions, and less frequently upon major changes in the field of vision. This in turn will depend upon the size and nature of the hemispheric insult and the age at which it was sustained. Sometimes, in assessing these patients, it may be necessary to go to sophisticated lengths to show seizure origin, either to justify unilateral surgery in patients whose seizure semeiology might suggest more widespread disease, or to justify a lesser resection in patients where there is some preservation of the primary functions described above. In general, the guidelines for hemispherectomy are simple.

1. Intractable epilepsy with a focal motor component.
2. A hemiplegia, either a fixed deficit from major pathology, or a functional deficit from uncontrolled epilepsia partialis continuans.

These matters are dealt with in more detail in Chapter 60.

FUNCTIONAL PROCEDURES

Multiple subpial transection

The rationale of this technique is essentially physiologic and therefore the criteria for its use must also be physiologic. There are two applications, either to reduce epileptic discharge from eloquent cortex, or to control those rare epileptic syndromes which arise as a consequence of secondary epileptogenesis.

In the first instance, the decision is part of a complex decision, usually in relation to a demonstrated structural lesion, where contiguous cortex that is thought to be participating in the epileptogenic zone has essential function.

The second situation is much less common. There have been a number of reports from one group (Patil *et al* 1997), describing the use of multiple subpial transection in patients with multilobar epilepsy. These patients were selected for surgery using both neurophysiologic investigations, structural MRI, PET scanning, and Wada tests. However, the commonest use of this application is in Landau–Kleffner syndrome where the indications are much better known. As well as the appropriate clinical criteria, it has to be shown that the bilateral EEG abnormalities (ESES) are driven from one hemisphere. This can be done using the Wada test or in some cases by carrying out intracranial recording and using a phase analysis.

Callosal section

The criteria for this procedure are almost entirely empirical and based upon experience of previous practice. These empirical indications include patients in whom resective surgery is not appropriate and those who suffer generalized seizures associated with falling and injury, principally atonic seizures, but also tonic–clonic seizures. There are no positive neurophysiologic or imaging criteria for this procedure.

Vagus nerve stimulation

The criteria for this procedure are equally empirical. It has been applied to almost every kind of epilepsy, including patients with multiple seizure types. Contraindications are few but include respiratory disease or swallowing difficulties. The early papers described its use in adults with partial complex seizures (Handforth *et al* 1998). Significant improvements in seizure control have also been reported in other seizure types and in children. These matters are dealt with in more detail in Chapter 55.

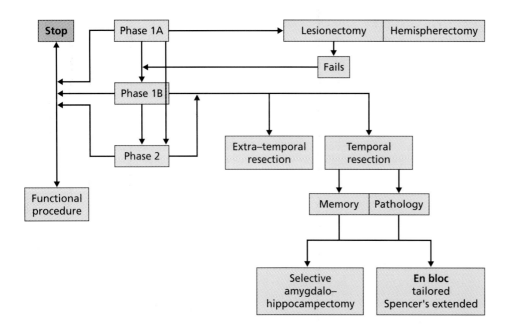

Fig 50.1 Phased management of selection for epilepsy surgery

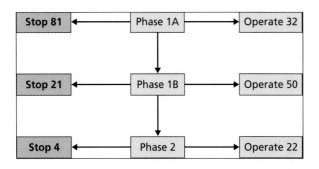

Fig 50.2 Fate of 210 adults admitted to the Kings/Maudsley epilepsy surgery assessment program.

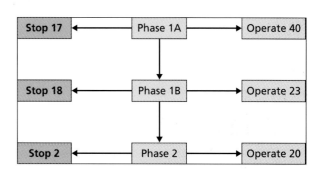

Fig 50.3 Fate of 100 children admitted to the Kings/Maudsley epilepsy surgery assessment program.

CONCLUSION

Patients with chronic intractable drug-resistant epilepsy can be assessed for surgical treatment by a staged process of investigation. This process is outlined in Fig. 50.1 and can be applied to both adults and children. The results of passing a cohort of patients through this process in the epilepsy program at the Maudsley Hospital and King's College Hospital between 1990 and 1995 are shown in Figs 50.2 and 50.3.

KEY POINTS

1. History has shown that a number of different techniques have been used successively to select patients for epilepsy surgery.
2. Selection now depends upon clinical review and neurophysiologic, neuroimaging, and neuropsychologic findings and these modalities are used in
    phases of increasing complexity, expense, and risk.
3. At the completion of each phase, patients are assigned either to surgery, further investigation, or rejection from the surgical program.
4. The three phases are identified as phase 1a, phase 1b, and phase 2.
5. The practical implications of using this
    method are described in relation to resective procedures (temporal lobe and extratemporal surgery, major resections, and hemispherectomy).
6. In the same way, selection for the functional procedures of multiple subpial transection, callosal section, and vagus nerve stimulation is made.

REFERENCES

Adler J, Erba G, Winston KR, Welch K, Lombroso CT (1991) Results of surgery for extratemporal partial epilepsy that began in childhood. *Archives of Neurology* 2:133–140.

Armon C, Radtke RA, Friedman AH, Dawson DV (1996) Predictors of outcome of epilepsy surgery: multivariate analysis with validation. *Epilepsia* 37:814–821.

Awad IA, Rosenfeld J, Ahl J, Hahn JF, Luders H (1991) Intractable epilepsy and structural lesions of the brain: mapping, resection strategies, and seizure outcome. *Epilepsia* 32:179–186.

Berkovic SF, McIntosh AM, Kalnins RM *et al* (1995) Preoperative MRI predicts outcome of temporal lobectomy: an actuarial analysis. *Neurology* 45(7):1358–1363.

Biraben A, Scarabin JM, Vignal JP, Chauvel P (1997) Stereo-EEG (SEEG) exploration in frontal lobe epilepsy – rationale and results. In: Tuxhorn I, Holthausen H, Boenigk H (eds) *Paediatric Epilepsy Syndromes and Their Surgical Treatment*, pp 696–708. London: John Libbey.

Carmant L, Kramer U, Riviello JJ *et al* (1995) EEG prior to hemispherectomy: correlation with outcome and pathology. *Electroencephalography and Clinical Neurophysiology* 94:265–270.

della-Rocchetta AI, Gadian DG, Connelly A *et al* (1995) Verbal memory impairment after right temporal lobe surgery: role of contralateral damage as revealed by ^{1}H magnetic resonance spectroscopy and T2 relaxometry. *Neurology* 45:797–802.

Duncan JS (1996) Magnetic resonance spectroscopy. *Epilepsia* 37:598–605.

Engel J Jr, Ojemann GA (1993) The next step. In: Engel J (ed.) *Surgical Treatment of the Epilepsies*, 2nd edn, pp 319–329. New York: Raven Press.

Erba G, Winston KR, Adler JR, Welch K, Ziegler R, Hornig GW (1992) Temporal lobectomy for complex partial seizures that began in childhood. *Surgical Neurology* 38:424–432.

Fish DR, Smith SJ, Quesney LF, Andermann F, Rasmussen T (1993) Surgical treatment of children with medically intractable frontal or temporal lobe epilepsy: results and highlights of 40 years' experience. *Epilepsia* 34:244–247.

Goldensohn E (1992) Structural lesions of the frontal lobe. Manifestations, classification, and prognosis. *Advances in Neurology* 57:435–447.

Handforth A, DeGiorgio CM, Schachter SC *et al* (1998) Vagus nerve stimulation therapy for partial-onset seizures: a randomized active-control trial. *Neurology* 51:48–55.

Horsley V (1886) Brain surgery. *British Medical Journal* 2:670–675.

Jack CRJ, Sharbrough FW, Cascino GD, Hirschorn KA, O'Brien PC, Marsh WR (1992) Magnetic resonance image-based hippocampal volumetry: correlation with outcome after temporal lobectomy. *Annals of Neurology* 31:138–146.

Jennum P, Dhuna A, Davies K, Fiol M, Maxwell R (1993) Outcome of resective surgery for intractable partial epilepsy guided by subdural electrode arrays. *Acta Neurologica Scandinavica* 87:434–437.

Kuzniecky R, Burgard S, Faught E, Morawetz R, Bartolucci A (1993) Predictive value of magnetic resonance imaging in temporal lobe epilepsy surgery. *Archives of Neurology* 50:65–69.

Masuoka LM, Spencer SS (1993) Seizure localization using subdural grid electrodes. *Epilepsia* 34(Suppl 6):8.

Milner B, Branch C, Rasmussen T (1962) Study of short-term memory after the intracarotid injection of sodium amytal. *Transactions of the American Neurological Society* 87:224–226.

Newton MR, Berkovic SF, Austin MC, Reutens DC, McKay WJ, Bladin PF (1992) Dystonia, clinical lateralization, and regional blood flow changes in temporal lobe seizures. *Neurology* 42:371–377.

Oliver B, Russi A (1994) What is needed for resective epilepsy surgery from a neurosurgical point of view? *Acta Neurologica Scandinavica* 152(Suppl):187–189.

Ounsted C, Lindsay J, Norman J (1966) *Biological Factors in Temporal Lobe Epilepsy*. London: Heinemann.

Patil AA, Andrews RV, Torkelson R (1997) Surgical treatment of intractable seizures with multilobar or bihemispheric seizure foci (MLBHSF). *Surgical Neurology* 47:72–77; discussion 77–78.

Polkey CE (1994) Epilepsy surgery: noninvasive versus invasive focus localization. What is needed from the neurosurgical point of view. *Acta Neurologica Scandinavica* 152(Suppl):183–186.

Rowe CC, Berkovic SF, Sia STB *et al* (1989) Localization of epileptic foci with postictal single photon emission computed tomography. *Annals of Neurology* 26:660–668.

Rowe CC, Berkovic SF, Austin MC, McKay WJ, Bladin PF (1991) Patterns of postictal cerebral blood flow in temporal lobe epilepsy: qualitative and quantitative analysis. *Neurology* 41:1096–1103.

Spencer SS (1981) Depth electroencephalography in selection of refractory epilepsy for surgery. *Annals of Neurology* 9:207–214.

Spencer SS, Spencer DD, Berg A (1993) Predictors of remission 1 year after resective epilepsy surgery: a multivariate analysis. *Epilepsia* 34(Suppl 6):27.

Spencer SS, Sperling MR, Shewmon DA (1997) Intracranial electrodes. In: Engel J, Pedley TA (eds) *Epilepsy: A Comprehensive Textbook*, pp 1719–1747. Philadelphia: Lippincott-Raven.

Sperling MR, O'Connor MJ, Saykin AJ *et al* (1992) A noninvasive protocol for anterior temporal lobectomy. *Neurology* 42:416–422.

Sperling MR, O'Connor MJ, Saykin AJ, Plummer C (1996) Temporal lobectomy for refractory epilepsy. *Journal of the American Medical Association* 276:470–475.

Swartz BE, Theodore WH, Sanabria E, Fisher RS (1992a) Positron emission and single photon emission computed tomographic studies in the frontal lobe with emphasis on the relationship to seizure foci. *Advances in Neurology* 57:487–497.

Swartz BE, Tomiyasu U, Delgado Escueta AV, Mandelkern M, Khonsari A (1992b) Neuroimaging in temporal lobe epilepsy: test sensitivity and relationships to pathology and postoperative outcome. *Epilepsia* 33:624–634.

Thadani VM, Williamson PD, Berger R *et al* (1995) Successful epilepsy surgery without intracranial EEG recording: criteria for patient selection. *Epilepsia* 36:7–15.

Toczek MT, Morrell MJ, Risinger MW, Shuer L (1997) Intracranial ictal recordings in mesial frontal lobe epilepsy. *Journal of Clinical Neurophysiology* 14:499–506.

Van Veelen CMW, Debets C, Van Huffelen AC *et al* (1990) Combined use of subdural and intracerebral electrodes in preoperative evaluation of epilepsy. *Neurosurgery* 26:93–101.

Vickrey BG, Hays RD, Graber J, Rausch R, Engel JJ, Brook RH (1992) A health-related quality of life instrument for patients evaluated for epilepsy surgery. *Medical Care* 30:299–319.

Vickrey BG, Hays RD, Rausch R, Sutherling WW, Engel J Jr, Brook RH (1994) Quality of life of epilepsy surgery patients as compared with outpatients with hypertension, diabetes, heart disease, and/or depressive symptoms. *Epilepsia* 3:597–607.

Vickrey BG, Hays RD, Engel J Jr *et al* (1995) Outcome assessment for epilepsy surgery: the impact of measuring health-related quality of life. *Annals of Neurology* 37(2):158–166.

Temporal lobe resections

CE POLKEY

Since the surgical treatment of epilepsy became accepted the temporal lobe structures have been common surgical targets. In the past such procedures have included not only unilateral resections of various kinds but also bilateral resections and stereotactic procedures. In modern times the principal procedures have been unilateral resections of temporal lobe structures and the chief controversies have been over the selection methods and the site and extent of the subsequent resection. The field is further enhanced by the knowledge of temporal lobe functions and pathology in humans revealed by the study of temporal lobe epilepsy and the consequences of surgery. There is a considerable variation in the types of procedures that patients are offered between one center and another. Modern anesthesia and neurosurgical technique have made temporal lobe surgery more versatile while remaining safe. The advent of MRI, and its development into an accurate structural tool, has made it possible to examine and quantify the site and amount of tissue removed by the surgeon and thereby to assess the efficacy of the surgery objectively.

Disregarding the bilateral resections, which were abandoned early because of the unacceptable effects on recent memory (Scoville and Milner 1957) and stereotactic interventions, which will be dealt with later, temporal lobe resections have passed through a series of distinct but overlapping phases. The early resections were virtually all superficial corticectomies, although the early reports of Meyer and colleagues (Meyer *et al* 1954) showed the importance of pathology and led to the development of the 'en bloc' lobectomy. Before that it had been shown that superficial removals gave unsatisfactory results with regard to seizure outcome, and removal of the deep structures by suction was added (Penfield and Paine 1955). Bailey in Illinois also began by removing only superficial temporal cortex, sparing the deep structures (Bailey 1961), but by 1956 Green, one of Bailey's pupils, was resecting hippocampus. Between the mid-1950s and the 1980s, most temporal lobe resections involved varying degrees of removal of the superficial and deep structures, the latter usually by suction without preserving them for pathologic examination. It had been suspected that the deep mesial temporal structures played a key part in the genesis of temporal lobe seizures and in 1958 Niemeyer had described removal of the deep structures by a transcortical route (Niemeyer 1958). In the early 1980s Wieser and Yasargil, described a trans-sylvian route (Wieser and Yasargil, 1984; Yasargil *et al* 1985) and other groups have revived Niemeyer's transcortical route (Olivier 1987). Two useful and significant modifications of the temporal lobectomy have been described. Ojemann and his colleagues described the use of memory testing under local anesthesia to tailor dominant resections (Ojemann and Dodrill 1985, Walsh and Ojemann 1992; Silbergeld and Ojemann, 1993). Spencer observed that, in some patients explored by depth electrodes, the onset of seizures was quite posterior in the hippocampus and described a technique in which the cortical removal was relatively restricted but the removal of the hippocampal structures was extended posteriorly (Spencer *et al* 1984). The final influence on temporal lobe surgery has been the ability of MRI to categorize pathology before operation, thus improving both the selection of patients and the planning of operative procedures, and of postoperative MRI to indicate the importance of adequate removal of both pathology and the mesial temporal structures.

SELECTION

The principles of concordance, established in the course of phased investigation discussed elsewhere, naturally apply to selection for temporal lobe surgery.

Phase 1A includes the past medical history and seizure semeiology. The previous history suggests the nature of the underlying pathology, within broad limits, and the ictal history suggests the likely site of origin of the seizures. A syndrome of mesial temporal lobe epilepsy (MTLE), described and defined by Wieser and Engel, can be distinguished by its clinical, neurophysiologic, and other features. Wieser and Engel suggest that mesial temporal sclerosis (MTS) produces a distinct pathophysiology involving an amplifier mechanism between the hippocampus and the parahippocampal gyrus, which determines the clinical and neurophysiologic characteristics associated with this syndrome (Wieser *et al* 1993).

The clinical features of MTLE include an increased familial incidence of epilepsy and febrile convulsions. In 80% of patients there is a history of a complicated febrile convulsion, usually lasting 20–30 minutes or more, in whom the pathology is subsequently shown to be MTS. Babb has shown that the occurrence of hippocampal sclerosis and the clinical syndrome associated with it, together with the seizure relief secured by operation, can be related to the absence or presence of an initial precipitated injury. Those patients who experienced repetitive nonprolonged seizures with their initial precipitated injury showed the shortest latent period and earliest age of onset of temporal lobe epilepsy (TLE) (Mathern *et al* 1995). Gil-Nagel *et al*, analyzing 35 patients who had a successful outcome from temporal lobe surgery, noted that patients with MTS had a prior history of febrile convulsions and were more likely to have oral automatisms (Gil-Nagel and Risinger 1997). Other events can also lead to mesial temporal damage. Davies and colleagues have described 13 patients, 1.9% of their patients undergoing craniotomy for intractable epilepsy, who had suffered meningitis as the presumed cause of their brain damage. In 11 of these patients seizure

onset was shown to be in the temporal lobe; of the 12 patients who underwent temporal lobectomy, 10 (83%) were seizure-free (Davies *et al* 1996). They also described 11 patients who suffered viral encephalitis. The pathology was varied, but the four patients who had MTS did well after surgery (Davies *et al* 1995). Lancman *et al* analyzed the relationship between central nervous system infection and outcome from surgery. They found that 48.2% of their patients had unilateral mesial temporal lobe epilepsy, 16.1% had bilateral mesial temporal lobe epilepsy, and 35.7% had neocortical epilepsy. The patients with unilateral complete mesial temporal lobe epilepsy had the same outcome from surgery as others without a history of viral encephalitis. (Lancman and Morris 1996).

Although in some patients the chronic epilepsy soon follows the febrile convulsions, in other patients there may be simple partial seizures that are unrecognized or the initial seizures may be easily controlled so that the patient has a period of remission. However, in late childhood or early adolescence, the seizures invariably reappear and are then difficult to control.

In other patients where the origin of the seizures is different, the history of febrile convulsions will be absent, the onset of the seizures is often later, and the patients are of normal intellectual and educational attainment. Comparisons of this kind were first made by Ounsted (Ounsted *et al* 1996) and confirmed by a later longitudinal follow-up of children with temporal lobe epilepsy (Ounsted *et al* 1987).

To some extent, elements in the seizure pattern may distinguish between the pathology within the temporal lobe and also between partial seizures of temporal lobe and frontal lobe origin. It has previously been noted that the aura of seizures of temporal lobe origin, especially mesial temporal origin, tend to be of a visceral type or fear, whereas other lesions tend to produce *déjà vu*, taste, or smell auras. Partial complex seizures with a focal origin within the temporal lobe may often be confined to the temporal lobe structures before spreading to other parts of the brain; this can be demonstrated with intracranial electrodes. Wieser and Engel note that this slow progression is often associated with the MTLE syndrome. Sometimes the seizure is aborted at an early stage and rarely becomes secondarily generalized. After the warning or aura phenomenon, the seizure proceeds to a motionless stare with arrest of activity, then there may be lip-smacking or chewing, manual automatisms, and dystonic posturing (Kotagal *et al* 1989; Elwes *et al* 1993). There are often postictal automatisms. Where the seizures are not of mesial temporal origin there may often be rapid secondary generalization. Brockhaus and Elger studied seizures of temporal lobe origin in a small series of 29 children aged 18 months to

16 years. In children less than 6 years of age, atypical semeiology with symmetric motor phenomena, posturing similar to that seen in frontal lobe seizures, and head nodding may be seen (Brockhaus and Elger 1995).

Complex partial seizures may be accompanied by speech disturbance. Murray Falconer described speech arrest during the seizure, or dysphasia afterwards, when the dominant temporal lobe was involved, and speech automatisms when the nondominant temporal lobe was involved (Serafetidines and Falconer 1963). Privitera *et al* asked patients undergoing video-telemetry to read a test phrase aloud as soon as a seizure was detected and found that this may detect patients with unusual cerebral speech dominance (Privitera *et al* 1996). Yen and colleagues evaluated the speech manifestations in 68 patients who subsequently underwent anterior temporal lobectomy. Cerebral speech dominance had been established using the Wada test. Some form of ictal speech was identified in 47.1% of the patients. Ictal verbalization lateralized to the nondominant hemisphere in 90% of patients with this manifestation. They also observed that bilingual patients used their mother tongue in 72.2% of seizures with verbalization (Yen *et al* 1996).

A significant number of partial complex seizures may be of extratemporal origin, usually from the frontal lobe. These have particular characteristics as described by Williamson *et al* (1987) They occur frequently and cluster, and the seizures are brief (less than 30 seconds) and tend to be of sudden onset and recovery with minimal postictal confusion.

Finally, appropriate enquiry should be made about the educational and psychiatric history.

The next part of Phase 1A is the structural imaging of the temporal lobes. Older methods of neuroimaging are of low sensitivity and specificity. MRI is now the gold standard. Appropriate sequences and volumetric measurements of the hippocampus and amygdala are necessary to make full use of this technique. These sequences should include T2 and FLAIR (fluid attenuation inversion recovery) sequences. These examinations can be long and tedious and some patients may require general anesthesia to obtain an adequate examination. Bergin *et al* showed that the FLAIR sequence revealed additional lesions in 11 of 20 patients; some of these lesions were in the hippocampus or amygdala (Bergin *et al* 1995). Typical of the findings in patients with intractable complex partial seizures are those in the following two series. Lee and his colleagues described a retrospective study of the MRI imaging in 186 patients who underwent temporal lobectomy. MRI imaging showed 93% sensitivity and 83% specificity in detecting abnormalities of the hippocampus or amygdala and they found that an abnormally high signal on T2-weighted sequences has a sensitivity of 93% and a specificity of 74%

in detecting mesial temporal sclerosis. For temporal lobe 'tumors', the sensitivity was 83% and the specificity was 93%. This was based, however, both on abnormal signal and on mass effect (Lee *et al* 1998). Another recent study of 222 patients with temporal lobe epilepsy showed that 180 patients (81%) had MRI-detectable abnormalities, with 55% having hippocampal sclerosis, 7.2% developmental abnormalities, 6.8% tumors, 5% scars, 4.5% cavernous angiomas, and miscellaneous abnormalities in 7.2% (Lehericy *et al* 1997). A further account is found in a review by Cascino (1997).

The diagnosis of MTS on structural MRI depends upon several factors. The size of the hippocampus can be judged by eye or by volumetric measurements. There are many papers that demonstrate relationships between hippocampal volume, MTS quantified by neuronal counts, and outcome from surgery (Jackson *et al* 1990; Cascino *et al* 1992a, 1993b; Kuzniecky *et al* 1993). Lee *et al* have shown that absolute hippocampal volume can demonstrate bilateral hippocampal atrophy where visual comparison cannot and also correlates with neuronal density in resected temporal lobes (Lee N *et al* 1995). Oppenheim *et al* have shown that in 22 patients out of 24 patients with histologically proven MTS the normal digitations of the hippocampal head were not visible. This finding had a sensitivity of 92% and a specificity of 100% (Oppenheim *et al* 1998). Kuzniecky and associates examined the place of various sequences in detecting mesial temporal sclerosis. Inversion recovery (IR) and T1-weighted volume acquired images would lateralize the side of surgery in 93% of patients with visual inspection and 97% of patients with quantitative volumetric figures. Prolongation of T2 was present in 79% (Kuzniecky *et al* 1997). Kim and colleagues investigated the distribution of sclerosis in individual hippocampi and in their sample of 29 patients the process was diffuse; 81% of these patients were seizure-free (Kim *et al* 1995b). Similar findings have been reported by Quigg *et al* (1997). The same group showed that, although unilateral asymmetry of the fornix and mamillary bodies could be shown on MRI in association with severe hippocampal sclerosis, the finding was not sufficiently robust to be useful in affecting surgical outcome (Kim *et al* 1995a). Clearly, MTS can be reliably detected by MRI and shown to be either unilateral or bilateral in any particular patient.

Modern brain imaging, especially high-quality structural MRI, will often reveal that pathology such as dysplasia or MTS may be multiple or bilateral, or they may occur together as 'dual pathology.' Some would regard this as a contraindication to surgery, whereas others have said that if the patient's seizures can be located to the demonstrated pathology then surgery may be justified. In 27 patients with a principal diagnosis of hippocampal sclerosis, Prayson *et al* found five patients with coexistent cortical dysplasia, and 93% had white-matter neuronal heterotopia. Twenty-two of these patients, including the five with cortical dysplasia, were seizure-free after surgery (Prayson *et al* 1996). However, a retrospective examination of the MRI scans of patients from the National Hospital, Queens Square, who had mesial temporal sclerosis revealed extrahippocampal abnormalities in 14 patients, 10 of whom did not become seizure-free after surgery, compared with 13 patients without such abnormalities, 11 of whom became seizure-free (Sisodiya *et al* 1997). Li and colleagues from the Montreal Neurological Institute (MNI) have reported 10 patients with bilateral periventricular heterotopia. Six were investigated with depth electrodes, which demonstrated hippocampal onset in three patients, regional temporal onset in two patients, and occipital-temporal onset in the remaining patient. In all 10 patients some form of temporal lobe resection was carried out, but in only one patient was the heterotopia resected. None of these patients became seizure-free (Li *et al* 1997).

Ho *et al* have examined the relationship between developmental malformations and dual pathology in the temporal lobe. The MRI scans of patients with unilateral developmental malformations in the temporal lobe were examined visually and by volume measurements to assess the occurrence of amygdalar and hippocampal atrophy. Visual inspection revealed bilateral hippocampal atrophy in 2 of 30 patients and unilateral hippocampal atrophy in 21 of 30 patients; volume measurements showed hippocampal atrophy in 26 patients, bilateral in 17, and amygdalar atrophy in 18 patients, bilateral in 15 of these patients. By contrast, in 92 patients with pure hippocampal sclerosis it was bilateral in only 18% (Ho *et al* 1998).

Magnetic resonance spectroscopy has been reported to be abnormal in the temporal lobes of patients with temporal lobe epilepsy, especially those with mesial temporal sclerosis (Kuzniecky *et al* 1992; Breiter *et al* 1994).

Laxer has reviewed the clinical applications of magnetic resonance spectroscopy. Although the decrease in the ratio, or absolute value, of the NAA (*N*-acetyl aspartate) signal in the temporal lobe, especially with hippocampal sclerosis is now recognized, his summary indicates that a decrease contralateral to the affected side is seen in 20% of patients and he considered it to be a false lateralization in 6% (Laxer 1997). Hugg and colleagues, reporting from Alabama, describe normalization of an abnormal Cr/NAA ratio in the unoperated temporal lobe 1 year after temporal lobectomy (Hugg *et al* 1996). Thompson *et al* have carried out a comparative study of magnetic resonance spectroscopy in control volunteers and patients subsequently operated for unilateral temporal epilepsy. They found decreased NAA in the hippocampus of seizure patients compared with controls at a significant level (Thompson *et al* 1998). della Rochetta, examining patients retrospectively who had undergone temporal lobectomy, found that an abnormal ratio seemed to relate to poor cognitive function, suggesting a minor degree of hippocampal sclerosis in the remaining temporal lobe.

The place of neurophysiologic investigations in this noninvasive Phase 1A is clear. Interictal EEGs should consist of long recordings with appropriate placement of the scalp electrodes, and natural or drug-induced sleep. If a structural abnormality has been demonstrated by MRI or CT, and the other findings, including seizure semeiology, are concordant with that lesion, then the interictal scalp EEG findings, provided they are localized to some degree, may be accepted. Foldvary and colleagues claim that it is possible to distinguish between patients with mesial temporal onset and neocortical temporal epilepsy by the frequency and distribution of lateralized rhythmic activity on EEG as well as their previous history and seizure semeiology (Foldvary *et al* 1997). There is good evidence in the literature that patients with clear unilateral lesions may have bilateral scalp EEG abnormalities that resolve after the lesion is removed, and the seizures cease, although such resolution may take up to a year (Falconer and Kennedy 1961; Wieser and Yasargil 1982). However, if the findings are not concordant then the patient must move on to the next phase of management (Sperling *et al* 1992; Rausch *et al* 1993).

Basic neuropsychologic testing should also be carried out at this stage but should be interpreted with caution for two reasons. Cerebral dominance must be considered since this may influence the interpretation of the results. Secondly, a bland but low-level score must not be taken as indicating the absence of a lateralizing lesion, since both Ounsted (Ounsted *et al* 1966) and Powell (Powell *et al* 1985) have shown that early cerebral damage may be masked by subsequent brain reorganization. Chelune and colleagues have shown a relationship between preoperative IQ and the outcome from temporal lobectomy in 1034 patients. Patients who continued to have seizures had a small but significantly reduced overall IQ. If a structural lesion, other than MTS, was present and patients had an IQ of 75 or less, then the chances of continuing seizures were increased fourfold (Chelune *et al* 1998). A number of papers from Seidenberg and colleagues in Chicago have shown that verbal memory decline is less after left-sided surgery in patients with mesial temporal lobe epilepsy, in whom the pathology is likely to be hippocampal sclerosis (Seidenberg *et al* 1997). Trenerry *et al* investigated patients considered to have evidence of bilateral hippocampal atrophy. The effects of temporal lobe surgery on verbal memory seemed to be related to the side of operation as much as the severity of atrophy (Trenerry *et al* 1996). Baxendale and colleagues have reported postoperative decline in verbal recall with excision of either the left or right hippocampus if they were relatively intact. However, neuronal densities in the CA1 subfield correlated with preoperative scores on immediate and delayed recall of stories (Baxendale *et al* 1998). These findings emphasize the importance of pathology in determining neuropsychologic status and outcome following surgery. Again, if there is a clear neuropsychologic deficit, consistent with cerebral speech dominance and the patient's clinical history, then there may be no need for an intracarotid amytal test.

At this stage it may be impossible to decide whether a temporal lobe resection is appropriate, or which of the various techniques should be used. Therefore the next stage of management, Phase 1B, consisting of minor invasive tests, must now be entered.

The most important neurophysiologic investigation in Phase 1B is the use of video-telemetry, either with or without minor invasive electrodes. This technique is important in detecting nonepileptic seizures and in providing an objective picture of the patient's seizure semeiology. Henry *et al* examined the results of long-term video monitoring in 145 patients who had temporal interictal EEG spikes and appropriate seizure semeiology; 12 of these patients (8%) had nonepileptic seizures (Henry and Drury 1997). Ebersole reviewed the ictal scalp-recorded EEGs of 93 patients and correlated the patterns seen in these recordings with the results of intracranial recording and MRI. They concluded that it was possible to distinguish between hippocampal and neocortical onset and thus select patients for intracranial recording (Ebersole and Pacia 1996). For minor invasive recording there are a number of electrode techniques that can be used. Many centers use sphenoidal electrodes for this purpose. Some question whether sphenoidal electrodes are superior to appropriately placed scalp electrodes, variously described as anterior temporal placements or superficial sphenoidal placements (Binnie *et al* 1989). Both Fenton and Kanner claim that fluoroscopically placed sphenoidal electrodes are more likely to record meaningfully (Fenton *et al* 1997; Kanner and

Jones 1997). Ictal sphenoidal recording can identify unilateral temporal lobe onsets of seizures and can be used to select patients for surgery (Falconer, 1971a; So *et al.* 1994; Sirven *et al* 1997a Sirven *et al* 1996). Although there is minimal morbidity associated with sphenoidal electrodes, their disadvantages are that they record remote from the source of the seizures and, because they are extracranial, they are more prone to artifact. Wieser first described electrodes placed through the foramen ovale so as to lie adjacent to the mesial temporal structures in 1985, validating them against depth electrodes, and in 1988 described a multicontact version. (Siegfried *et al* 1985; Wieser and Moser 1988). He and Siegel reported the results of foramen ovale investigation and selective amygdalohippocampectomy in 77 patients and showed that the same kind of neurophysiologic characteristics that are associated with depth electrode exploration were true of this population (Wieser and Siegel 1991). Awad and Kuzniecky have both reported effective selection of patients using foramen ovale electrodes (Kuzniecky *et al* 1990; Awad *et al* 1991a). Complications are rare; probably only 1–2% are serious or persistent. Schuler has reported brain stem lesions in two patients, one of whom had undergone previous temporal surgery (Schuler *et al* 1993). It is probably unwise to use these electrodes to investigate patients who have had previous surgery. Foramen ovale electrodes are used to confirm a mesiobasal onset for the patient's seizures, especially when other data is noncongruent or if there is no clear neurophysiologic focus. There are two circumstances in which foramen ovale recording is not used: if an extratemporal origin for the seizures is suspected, such as in the adjacent frontal lobe, or if insertion of foramen ovale electrodes has proved difficult or impossible. In either of these circumstances subdural strips are preferable.

Before major invasive neurophysiologic recording is considered, there are three tests that would identify the 'functional deficit zone' proposed by Luders and Awad (1992). These are PET and SPECT, and the intracarotid sodium amytal or Wada test (Wada 1949).

In the data collected by Engel, 19 of 30 centers had access to PET, whereas 4 did not (Engel 1993); the ILAE survey showed that about half of the centers responding mentioned PET and among those responders 30–40% used it in their assessment of patients for surgery (Anonymous 1997b).

FDG-PET will show lateralized hypometabolism in 60–90% of patients with refractory mesial temporal lobe epilepsy. In 37 patients studied at UCLA with the mesial TLE syndrome, in whom the extracranial EEG and FDG-PET studies were concordant, depth electrode studies never contradicted the findings, and similar findings have been reported from the Cleveland Clinic (Engel *et al* 1990; Chee *et al* 1991). Interictal hypoperfusion contralateral to the seizure onset established by depth electrode studies is very rare and probably iatrogenic (Engel *et al* 1990).

Debets and his colleagues examined the role of ^{11}C-flumazenil PET, FDG-PET, and ^{123}I-iomazenil SPECT in assessing 23 patients for temporal lobe surgery. They concluded that these examinations had a useful place in patients where the MRI or EEG were unhelpful. ^{11}C-Flumazenil PET was not superior to FDG-PET in this role. There was no relation to the pathology found in the resected specimen. They also found that interictal ^{123}I-iomazenil was highly inaccurate in lateralizing the lobe for surgery (Debets *et al* 1997). A similar result has been described by Lamusuo *et al* (1997). Sperling *et al* described two patients in whom FDG-PET was falsely localizing, probably because of subclinical seizure activity producing hypermetabolism (Sperling *et al* 1995a). Theodore *et al* examined the relationship between seizure focus revealed by invasive EEG and FDG-PET findings in patients where the surface video-telemetry was not localizing. In 26 patients with unilateral temporal FDG-PET hypometabolism, there was a congruent focus on intracranial EEG; 23 of these patients were operated and 18 were seizure-free. Five patients had unilateral frontotemporal hypometabolism and an intracranial focus and three of these patients were seizure-free after surgery. Fourteen patients had no lateralization on FDG-PET. However, there was no discordance between patients with MRI lateralization in the form of increased signal or decreased volume and FDG-PET lateralization (Theodore *et al* 1997).

The data collected by Engel, and the ILAE study indicate a similar level of use for SPECT and PET. Most recent SPECT studies have used HMPAO, which measures cerebral blood flow. Many of the early studies were confused by apparently contradictory results. There were two reasons for this: first the variations in technique used, and secondly the relationship of the examination to the patient's last seizure. Rowe's group first showed that interictal SPECT measurements had limited usefulness (Rowe *et al* 1991b). They subsequently showed that the time of injection of the ligand in relation to seizure onset was important, and if these peri-ictal scans were studied carefully there were reliable changes, which were consistent with seizure onset in 72% of 25 patients studied using the depth electrodes (Rowe *et al* 1989). Duncan showed that such changes could be found in 93% of 28 patients they investigated and that 22 of 23 patients subsequently operated achieved a significant seizure reduction (Duncan *et al* 1993). Furthermore, Rowe's group showed that peri-ictal scans gave

correct localization in 69% of patients with a unilateral EEG focus (Rowe *et al* 1991a). Further work by Newton *et al* showed that only 6 of 63 patients subjected to temporal surgery had atypical patterns, and that these six patients had nonspecific pathology in the specimens and only 33% were seizure-free compared with 60–70% of those with the other patterns (Ho *et al* 1997). They were able to relate the pattern of ictal SPECT to temporal lobe pathology (Ho *et al* 1996).

The intracarotid sodium amytal test was first described by Wada in 1949 as a test of cerebral speech dominance (Wada 1949) and was proposed by Milner as a test of recent memory in 1962 (Milner *et al* 1962). Dashieff *et al* applied the test to patients with frontal lobe and generalized epilepsy and concluded that the test was of low specificity (Dasheiff *et al* 1993). A number of selective amytal tests have been described, which have their advantages and disadvantages (Jack *et al* 1988; Wieser *et al* 1989). These matters are dealt with in detail in another chapter, but whatever form is used the test appears to give meaningful results. Powell *et al* examined 27 patients who had undergone the classical carotid amytal test. A lower proportion, 63% instead of 83%, had speech totally in the left hemisphere; 51% had their memory completely, or almost so, in one temporal lobe; and 22% could not sustain memory with either hemisphere (Powell *et al* 1987). Perrine and colleagues have examined the relationship between memory disparities revealed by the Wada test and outcome from temporal lobe surgery. Seizure outcome and laterality were correctly predicted in 70 left speech-dominant patients, where significant difference between hemispheres was found in 71.4% of these patients and correctly predicted the side for surgery in 98%. It also predicted correctly the 80% of patients who became seizure-free at 1 year (Perrine *et al* 1995). Lancman reported similar findings (Lancman *et al* 1998). Baxendale *et al* have shown that there is a relationship between MRI measures of hippocampal asymmetry and a measure of functional asymmetry derived from the difference scores in the intracarotid amytal test (Baxendale *et al* 1997). It is therefore reasonable to assert that the intracarotid amytal test is a reliable predictor both of a nonfunctioning temporal lobe and of surgical outcome.

If it is still not possible to make a decision regarding the site of seizure onset, and the matter is still worth pursuing, then management must proceed to Phase 2. This involves determination of the side or site of seizure onset using gross invasive neurophysiology. In 1993 Spencer suggested that depth electrode utilization varied from 25% to 50% (Spencer *et al* 1993a). In 1992, So noted that bitemporal discharges were seen in the extracranial EEG recordings of 20–35% of their patients and that in 44% of these patients an exclusively unilateral onset for their seizures could be demonstrated by depth recording, and a predominantly unilateral onset in another 36% (So, 1992). Sperling used intracranial recording in 31 of his 89 patients undergoing temporal lobe resections, with no apparent difference in outcome once the decision to operate was made (Sperling *et al* 1996). Some believe that equally valid information can be obtained using subdural strip electrodes; however, they admit that such electrodes may not necessarily demonstrate the true onset of seizures that begin in the deep mesial temporal structures (Sperling and O'Connor 1989; Wyler *et al* 1993). The Bonn group have described a postictal slow focus that can be identified on ictal recordings from subdural electrodes. This focus is commoner in seizures of temporal origin and in electrographic seizures lasting more than 32 seconds. Frequent occurrence of such a focus in one temporal lobe was strongly correlated with a successful outcome from surgery directed to that temporal lobe (Hufnagel *et al* 1995). Sperling and O'Connor investigated 21 patients using subdural and depth electrodes simultaneously; in all the patients who had localized partial complex seizures, the seizures first appeared at the depth electrodes and subsequently at the subdural electrodes. In three patients with rapid bilateral seizure spread, the seizure onset could be seen in the depth electrodes but not in the subdural electrodes (Sperling and O'Connor 1989). Spencer *et al* (1991) agree that subdural electrodes are less sensitive than depth electrodes. There is not doubt that, because depth electrodes penetrate the cerebral substance, they carry risks that are not seen with the use of subdural electrodes. Van Veelen and his colleagues proposed the use of combined subdural and depth electrodes to minimize this risk (Van Veelen *et al* 1990; Spencer *et al* 1991).

Cascino and his group made a retrospective study of 30 patients who underwent depth electrode implantation, and 25 of these patients had a predominantly or exclusively unilateral temporal lobe onset of their seizures. Nine patients (43%) had an Engel Class 1 outcome and a total of 12 patients (57%) had a significant seizure reduction. Factors for a favorable outcome were a prolonged interhemispheric propagation time and the presence of hippocampal atrophy on MRI (Masada *et al* 1996). Holmes *et al* reported the results of operation in 44 patients who required intracranial monitoring because of bitemporal independent interictal epileptiform discharges, and who were subsequently offered surgery. Twenty-two (50%) were seizure-free and 36 (82%) had a significant improvement in their seizure control. Three factors contributed to a good result: concordance of MRI abnormality and side of operation, a history of febrile seizures, and lateralization of all seizure onsets to the side of operation (Holmes *et al* 1997). Sirven *et al* describe the

results of operation in 15 patients who were offered surgery from a group of 28 who were shown to have independent bilateral temporal lobe partial complex seizures as a result of depth electrode exploration. Ten of these 15 patients became seizure-free. Favorable factors were a lateralized result on a Wada test, or unilateral hippocampal sclerosis on MRI (Sirven *et al* 1997b). Cendes and colleagues described 31 patients who were evaluated with SEEG because their ictal or interictal scalp EEG, including sphenoidal recordings, had shown bilateral abnormalities. All of the patients had volumetric MRI; in eight of them there was clear unilateral atrophy of the amygdala or hippocampus and in these patients more than 75% of the seizures, and in some cases all of the seizures, originated from the atrophic side. In seven patients in whom the atrophy was bilateral but asymmetrical, more than 70% of seizures originated from the more atrophied side in four patients. In the remaining three patients, and one patient with bilateral astrophy the seizures had various origins. In five patients without atrophy on MRI, a unilateral onset was found in four patients. Patient with strictly unilateral atrophy were more likely to be free of seizures after surgery than those with bilateral atrophy or no atrophy (Cendes *et al* 1996).

Spencer and his colleagues have also investigated the relationship between EEG findings, from both surface and depth recordings, and the presence of hippocampal atrophy as defined by MRI volumetric studies. They were able to identify 119 patients with hipocampal atrophy, unilateral in 97, bilateral in 13, and in 9 patients hippocampal atrophy coexisted with a mass lesion. Of the 63 patients with isolated unilateral hippocampal atrophy who underwent surgery, 82% had ictal depth onsets concordant with the side of atrophy and 72% of ictal surface EEG onsets were concordant. Whereas four patients with concordant ictal onset and atrophy failed to achieve seizure control, there were three patients in whom resection of the hippocampus of ictal onset produced a good seizure outcome even though the remaining hippocampus was sclerosed. Four of the nine patients with lesions achieved good seizure control from lesionectomy alone (King *et al* 1997). Another publication from the same group indicates that they identified bilateral hippocampal atrophy, at least in the posterior part, in 5 of 53 patients. Surgery was performed on the side of ictal onset, identified by intracranial recording, in all five patients and four of them have been seizure-free for more than 2 years (King *et al* 1995). An interesting finding by the same group is that if the seizure recorded intracranially terminates close to its site of onset, then there is more chance that the patient will remain seizure-free (Spencer and Spencer 1996). Depth electrodes are also useful in excluding patients from surgery as shown by Spencer and colleagues, where 18% of patients were rejected for this reason (Spencer 1981).

The use of invasive neurophysiologic recording has diminished in the last ten years (Engel and Ojemann 1993) and many authors report good results using noninvasive recording alone, although this often includes video-telemetry with scalp recording. It was evident from our early work (Polkey 1994), and it has also been shown by Sperling (Sperling *et al* 1992) and others, that patients can be selected effectively using noninvasive tests alone. Patients selected by the noninvasive methods, which comprise Phase 1A and Phase 1B in our scheme, do better than those selected using intracranial recordings. Careful scrutiny of the papers quoted in the previous paragraph shows that results in patients explored with depth electrodes were best in those patients who had some other reason for a good outcome, such as an identifiable lesion on MRI. Holmes compares 28 patients who did not require intracranial recording with 29 who did. Whereas 92.9% of nonmonitored patients had a significant reduction in their seizure frequency, only 63% of the monitored patients had a similar result. However, those monitored patients who had a strictly unilateral anterior to midtemporal interictal discharge had a similar outcome to the nonmonitored patients, with 88.8% experiencing a significant reduction in their seizure frequency (Holmes *et al* 1996).

At the conclusion of these investigations, three questions must be asked in the case of any particular patient:

- Has the pathology been identified if possible?
- Has the source of the seizures been identified?
- Is there sufficient information to allow an accurate assessment of the risks of surgery, and of which temporal lobe resection is the most appropriate for that patient.

PRINCIPLES OF TEMPORAL LOBE SURGERY

The first important principle is to select the appropriate surgical technique for the demonstrated pathology. Complete removal of the pathology is most productive in terms of seizure relief. Therefore, once pathology has been detected, the surgery should at least encompass the pathology wherever possible. However, there is also a relationship between the hippocampus and the temporal neocortex, especially the parahippocampal gyrus, in line with Wieser and Engel's 'amplifier' hypothesis, which make it desirable to remove both in order to obtain a good result, as was found by Wieser in selective amygdalohippocampectomy (Siegel *et al*

1990). In all cases serious consideration must be given to including these structures in the resection even if they are not thought to contain gross pathology. In addition, the possibility of dual pathology must be considered. It is estimated that in cases with clear extrahippocampal pathology there may be additional hippocampal pathology in 10–30% of cases (Levesque *et al* 1991; Nakasato *et al* 1992; Cascino *et al* 1993b; Jay *et al* 1993; Cendes *et al* 1995).

The intellectual consequences of temporal lobe resections, especially on recent memory, can be influenced by technique and predicted, in part, from the preoperative investigations. It is known from very early surgical experience that bilateral removal of the medial temporal structures leads to an unacceptable amnesic syndrome (Scoville and Milner 1957). It subsequently emerged that the healthier temporal lobe might be the electrically more active and so be removed, again leading to a gross amnesic syndrome. However, even when the other temporal lobe was apparently completely healthy, there could still be memory problems following standard unilateral temporal lobectomy, and these material-specific deficits were first described by Milner in 1958. However, the severity of such memory disorders is related to the nature of the pathology within the temporal lobe and the age of onset of that pathology. In patients with mesial temporal sclerosis, cerebral reorganization may have occurred at an early age, so that there is no memory function within the affected temporal lobe, and therefore no penalty for removing it (Powell *et al* 1985). The memory function of each temporal lobe can be assessed to some degree using the intracarotid sodium amytal test, and therefore it is possible to assess the likely effect of temporal lobe resection, preoperatively, in any particular patient.

There are well-described psychiatric consequences of temporal lobe resections, although they cannot be predicted in the same way as the intellectual changes.

Techniques are available to allow intraoperative tailoring of temporal lobe resections; these are acute electrocorticography and operation under local anesthesia to allow mapping of speech and memory areas.

Acute electrocorticography is limited in space and time, allowing only recording from those areas that can be reached at operation, and revealing the cerebral activity during the recording. Because the anatomic boundaries of temporal lobectomy are set to minimize neurologic deficits, especially speech and visual field defects, variations in the resection are limited. Findings from ECoG will sometimes allow the surgeon to spare small areas of cortex, but, there are equally frequent occasions when spiking areas have to be left unresected. In the Palm Desert Survey, although 68% of centers used acute ECoG, only 56% of these claimed to modify the operation as a result of the ECoG findings (Spencer and Ojemann 1993). It is possible to use acute electrocorticography to decide whether to carry out a selective amygdalohippocampectomy or a temporal lobectomy (Polkey et al 1989). Although there is a general correlation between spikes in the postresection corticogram for temporal lobectomy and seizure outcome (Bengzon et al 1968), others have found no such correlation (Wyllie et al 1987). Tran and colleagues reported 47 patients who had preresection and postresection recordings and could find no relationship between residual spikes and outcome (Tran et al 1995). Schwartz and colleagues analyzed the results of pre- and postoperative ECoG in 29 patients undergoing temporal lobectomy with a pathologic diagnosis of MTS. They observed no relationship between their findings and seizure outcome (Schwartz et al 1997). Cascino et al also found no connection between the topography of ECoG spikes, hippocampal volume, or extent of lateral resection in 165 patients undergoing temporal lobe surgery (Cascino et al 1995). Kanner et al report a group of patients in whom amygdala and hippocampus were spared at resection because they showed no epileptiform activity during depth electrode recording or intraoperative depth recording. Their seizure outcome was not worse as a consequence (Kanner et al 1995). A new method of analyzing the ECoG at operation, developed by Alarcon, that depends upon the phase relations between recorded spikes suggests that it may be possible to identify leading regions whose removal improves seizure outcome (Alarcon et al 1997).

Operation under local anesthesia has become rarer for a number of reasons. It was realized first that precise mapping of the speech areas was not necessary, and secondly that cerebral activity recorded under light general anesthesia was as useful as that recorded under local anesthesia. Ojemann's work has shown that it is possible to minimize the verbal memory defect at dominant temporal lobectomy by mapping memory areas under local anesthesia (Ojemann and Dodrill 1985), but such information can be obtained using chronic subdural mat recording. In the Palm Desert Survey only 30% of centers routinely mapped language at temporal lobectomy, whereas another 33% would use this method in selected cases (Spencer and Ojemann 1993).

G.P. Lee and colleagues have described the use of intraoperative cooling to try to demonstrate whether this was a practical means of discovering whether the hippocampus could be resected. Although they were able to resect hippocampus in 11 patients where the test suggested there was adequate contralateral support for memory without disadvantage to the patient, they nevertheless felt the test was too difficult to recommend for routine use (Lee GP et al 1995a,b)

PREOPERATIVE PREPARATION AND PERIOPERATIVE CARE

Patients are covered with an antibiotic from the anesthetic room to 4 days after operation; steroids are not used routinely. Premedication should be used according to local custom; the precise formula is unimportant, but if acute ECoG is used routinely then the premedication should be consistent, so as to make the results of that examination easy to interpret. Postoperative care is that afforded to any patient after craniotomy; the general complications of craniotomy must be watched for and dealt with appropriately on the rare occasions when they arise. The common neurologic complications of temporal lobe surgery will be described in detail in the section on outcome.

Seizures in the postoperative period occur for two reasons. Some patients, either because of a proclivity to generalized seizures or because of temporary loss of anticonvulsant medication, some of which cannot be given parenterally, may have such seizures in the immediate postoperative period. These are best dealt with in the usual way. Other patients may be afflicted with appropriately localized focal motor seizures in the first few days after surgery. Again they are easily controlled and have no long-term prognostic significance.

Finally, it goes without saying that informed consent for the procedure must be obtained. Details of what should be considered can be gathered from the outcome section later in this chapter. It is particularly important to emphasize that surgery can be expected to improve the seizure control in the majority of patients fulfilling the selection criteria, but absolute freedom from seizures and discontinuance of their antiepileptic medication is more difficult to achieve.

AVAILABLE TEMPORAL LOBE RESECTIONS AND TECHNIQUES

Except where specifically referred to, the outcome of temporal lobe resections and their complications are remarkably uniform and will be treated collectively. Although there are minor variations in detail temporal lobe resections can be divided into four groups:

(a) Neocorticectomy and lesionectomy
(b) Combined removal of neocortical and mesial structures
(c) Selective removal of the mesial temporal structures including the parahippocampal gyrus
(d) Nonsurgical destruction of the mesial temporal structures

NEOCORTICECTOMY AND LESIONECTOMY

Neocorticectomy was virtually abandoned during the early evolution of temporal lobe surgery, mainly because it was relatively inefficient in relieving epilepsy. In the only modern series, from Dublin, a standard removal of a block of neocortex was performed (Hardiman *et al* 1988).

Murray Falconer described two cases of removal of a posterior temporal lesion to control seizures in 1962 (Falconer *et al* 1962). Cascino has reported poor results when lesionectomy was carried out in the temporal lobe (Cascino *et al* 1992b). He subsequently notes that 3 of the 15 patients who underwent lesionectomy in the temporal lobe proved to have dual pathology, and were helped by the temporal lobectomy (Cascino *et al* 1993a).

Casazza described the typical dilemma in reporting the results of lesionectomy in 54 patients; 36 of these patients had slow-growing tumors, the remaining 18 had cavernous hemangiomas. The patients could be divided into two groups: in one the seizures were controlled, in the other group they were not. Eight of the patients had an amygdalohippocampectomy in addition to the lesionectomy because of the uncontrolled seizures. Six patients required reoperation for persistent tumor (Casazza *et al* 1997). Lombardi and colleagues from Geneva described 22 patients with low-grade gliomas consisting of seven patients in whom they were extratemporal, eight in whom they were extrahippocampal but in the temporal lobe, and seven in whom they had invaded the amygdala or hippocampus. The eight patients with extrahippocampal lesions underwent lesionectomy, but four of them subsequently required removal of hippocampus and amygdala. In two of these cases the hippocampal atrophy was identifiable on MRI and these both did well. All of the patients with invasion of the mesial temporal structures were treated with temporal lobectomy and did well (Lombardi *et al* 1997).

COMBINED REMOVAL OF TEMPORAL NEOCORTEX AND MESIAL TEMPORAL STRUCTURES

The data from the Palm Desert participants show a considerable variation in the amount of temporal lobe tissue removed. In the nondominant temporal lobe it varied from 2 to 7 cm with a median of 5.5 cm, in the dominant hemisphere from 2 to 6 cm with a median of 4.5 cm. The amount of hippocampus removed also varied from 1 to 3.5 cm, the median was 3 cm (Spencer and Ojemann 1993). It seems likely, allowing that there are broad anatomic

restrictions on temporal lobe resection and that the best attempt is made to remove the pathology, that the effects of these minor variations on seizure relief and complications are insignificant. The position has been summarized by Olivier (1991). It was shown early in the MNI programme that removal of the hippocampus and uncus improved seizure outcome (Penfield and Jasper 1954). He notes that in this group of epileptics the seizure discharges usually involve these medial structures. From the same source there is a description of the effects of different temporal lobe resections in two groups of 100 patients studied over a similar period of time. Each patient underwent lateral neocortical resection of similar proportions, but in one group there was a major resection of the amygdala nucleus with minimal hippocampal removal, whereas in the other group there was a more extensive hippocampal removal (Feindel and Rasmussen 1991). The seizure relief rates were almost identical in the two groups, with 21% absolutely seizure-free (Engel outcome group 1A) and 53–55% virtually seizure-free (Engel outcome group 1). Awad notes that freedom from seizures was related primarily to the extent of the resection of the mesial temporal structures and secondarily to the completeness of the removal of any structural lesion (Nayel *et al* 1991).

There are variations in the technique of anterior temporal lobectomy. The structures may be removed 'en bloc' as described by Falconer (1971b) or the superficial cortex may be removed first and then the deep structures resected (Olivier 1991). The availability of the ultrasonic dissector (CUSA) and the operating microscope has improved the dissection of the mesial temporal structures.

To highlight the technical problems, a brief description of the 'en bloc' lobectomy will be given, but before this two significant variations must be mentioned. Ojemann and Dodrill have described a method of intraoperative tailoring in dominant (left) resections that minimizes the damage to verbal memory (Ojemann and Dodrill 1985). This method has not come into general use. Spencer describes an extended resection (Spencer *et al* 1984) in which they gain access to the temporal horn by a 4 cm neocortical resection and then carry out a radical removal of the hippocampus and parahippocampal gyrus. Babb has shown that the best result is obtained when all the sclerosed hippocampus is removed (Babb *et al* 1984) and this extended hippocampal removal is clearly a significant advance. In 1995, Wyler *et al* confirmed this in reporting results from extending the hippocampal resection more posteriorly; those with a more posterior removal had a better seizure outcome, 69% being seizure-free compared with 38% of the group with the less extensive removal (Wyler *et al* 1995).

Technical description of 'en bloc' lobectomy

The head should be positioned so that the lateral surface of the temporal lobe is more or less horizontal but there is sufficient 'head up' to prevent undue venous congestion and the neck is not under undue stress, which generally means propping up the trunk into an oblique position. The external landmarks necessary for an adequate exposure are the external angular groove that marks the floor of the anterior fossa and the root of the zygoma, which marks the floor of the middle fossa. The most convenient scalp incision is a 'question mark' shape. The osteoplastic craniotomy flap is fashioned in the same way using burrholes at the levels described to mark the base. The inferior margin of the craniotomy is rongeured away to reach as close as possible to the temporal pole; typically one can get to within 5–10 mm and down to the floor of the middle cranial fossa. In patients with mesial temporal sclerosis and temporal lobe atrophy, the mastoid air cells may come up higher than usual and be entered. They should immediately be patched over using pericranium sutured to the dura and the nearby muscle, otherwise there is danger of local infection, which proved difficult to eradicate in some patients early in our series. This preliminary work is important because otherwise the deep dissection becomes difficult, especially in patients with a shallow middle fossa, which in this position of the head becomes a relatively deep, narrow space.

The cerebral resection is commenced by making a vertical incision in the middle temporal gyrus between 5.5 cm and 6.5 cm from the pole. In children, the height of the temporal lobe at the midpoint of the sylvian fissure is used as the distance from the pole at which the incision to the ventricle is made. This vertical incision is deepened until the ventricle is entered, giving a clear view of the choroid plexus medially and the surface of the hippocampus laterally.

In the nondominant, usually right, temporal lobe the cortical incision is taken vertically up to the sylvian fissure and then passes along the upper margin of the superior temporal gyrus. In the dominant, usually left, temporal lobe the path of the incision is along the junction between the middle temporal gyrus and the superior temporal gyrus until a point about 1.5–2.0 cm from the pole, where the incision then crosses the superior temporal gyrus to come to the edge of the sylvian fissure. Alternatively, a uniformly curved incision is used situated more posteriorly in the nondominant hemisphere as noted in the Palm Desert Survey (Spencer and Ojemann 1993). The incision is brought forward along the sylvian fissure, peeling the temporal lobe off the insula by subpial dissection and thus protecting the middle cerebral artery and its branches. Inferiorly the dissection is continued until the insular cortex recurves and the temporal stem of white matter is encountered. This process first extends the dissection forwards and then returns again along the sphenoid ridge to the beginning of the free edge of the tentorium; this position is marked using a small pattie.

On returning to the surface, the posterior part of the cortical incision is extended backward to join up with the incision down to the ventricle. This incision is then entered and, using the choroid plexus as a medial boundary, the incision is extended forward again. It passes through the amygdala, which may be tough or the site of a benign tumor or hamartoma, and eventually the marker pattie is found.

One travels posteriorly again, this time in the choroid fissure. The hippocampus is drawn laterally and the dissection is subpial so as to protect the structures lying within the tentorial hiatus, in particular the posterior cerebral artery and its branches, the third (oculomotor) nerve and the basal vein and brain stem. This pial boundary is often respected by pathology and many benign lesions in the hippocampus do not extend across it. Such a lesion may be so large as to obscure the landmarks, and in that case it is better to continue posteriorly, leaving some of the mass to be removed separately when there is more room. Now, the hippocampus is marked where it is to be divided by a transverse cut.

Next a coronal section from the inferior margin of the ventricular incision is made through the cortex down to the floor of the middle fossa and toward the free edge of the tentorium, until the transverse incision in the hippocampus is encountered; this is then incorporated into the resection edge. Finally, the structures are retracted laterally over the free edge of the tentorium and the pia arachnoid and any vessels definitely going to the specimen are divided. At this stage the main trunk of the posterior cerebral artery is most at risk and care must be taken to identify it and preserve if from injury. Except for a few superficial veins, the specimen should now be free and can be removed. It is worth being careful with these veins since if they are torn from their connections into the floor of the middle fossa considerable bleeding may occur. Excessive diathermy on the floor of the middle fossa may cause temporary damage to the fifth nerve, with corresponding transient facial numbness.

Now the resection of any residual lesions within the tentorial hiatus, usually dysembryoplastic neuroepithelial tumor or low-grade tumors, should be performed. If this becomes hazardous, small portions of the lesion may be left behind; if they are isolated from functioning temporal lobe tissue, as is usually the case, they do not affect the prognosis, as noted in a survey of our material (Kirkpatrick *et al*

1993). At this stage a further ECoG can be carried out and any further resection achieved with ease. Thereafter it is merely a case of ensuring hemostasis and closing the craniotomy in the usual fashion.

The principal points of difference in Spencer's extended lobectomy are that the neocortical removal is less, around 4 cm from the pole, and that the position of the head is more akin to that used for amygdalohippocampectomy by the trans-sylvian route, so that the temporal horn is almost vertical and the surgeon works down into the depths of it. An operating microscope is recommended (Spencer *et al* 1984).

SELECTIVE REMOVAL OF THE MESIAL TEMPORAL STRUCTURES INCLUDING THE PARAHIPPOCAMPAL GYRUS

The management decisions that govern the use of this procedure are relatively complex and have been discussed in an article devoted to amygdalohippocampectomy (Polkey 2000). This selective removal of the mesial structures may be used in patients where there is a discrete pathologic abnormality within those structures that is the cause of the epilepsy and that can be completely encompassed within the resection. It may also be used in patients with no gross structural lesion but in whom the neurophysiologic findings indicate that the origin of the seizures is unilateral and within the mesial temporal structures. It may be proposed in patients where there is significant preservation of memory function within the target temporal lobe. The converse of these indications would preclude a selective medial removal or be in favor of a more gross anterior temporal lobectomy.

The preoperative and perioperative considerations are those already mentioned but it is not practical to conduct these procedures under local anesthesia and many centers find ECoG unhelpful. The operating microscope is essential for accurate and safe surgery in this area with its restricted access.

The approach is either trans-sylvian or transventricular, entering the temporal horn through the lateral neocortex as first proposed by Niemeyer in 1958. As yet there is no published series from any one center of patients subjected to one approach or the other. Stereotactic amygdalohippocampectomy using the Kelly–Goerst system has been described. The trajectory varies; in some cases a posterior temporal-occipital approach has been used (Cascino *et al* 1990), in others an approach through the lateral neocortex (Kratimenos *et al* 1992). These approaches have been described and discussed by Renella (1989b). Wieser and Yasargil claim that with the trans-sylvian approach more

frontal fibers are divided, and Goncalves Ferreira notes that the trans-sylvian route is the longest to these structures but disrupts the minimal amount of neural tissue (Goncalves-Ferreira *et al* 1994). The transcortical approach to the ventricle has been described by the Montreal group. Olivier initially used an approach through the superior temporal gyrus but latterly through the middle temporal gyrus; for ease of access such incisions should be horizontal (Olivier 1987). Vajkoczy has described a novel microsurgical approach to the mesial temporal structures in 32 patients. The basis of the surgery is a wide opening of the sylvian fissure and identification of the structures around the tentorial hiatus before 'en bloc' resection of the amygdala, anterior hippocampus, parahippocampal gyrus, and subiculum (Vajkoczy *et al* 1998). Park reports a subtemporal approach through the parahippocampal gyrus that avoids the possibility of injury to the fusiform gyrus and the lateral temporal neocortex (Park *et al* 1996). Smith has described an infraoccipital approach for posterior medial temporal lesions. The majority of these were low-grade tumors. Six of their seven patients were seizure-free and there was no morbidity; a viewing wand for intraoperative navigation was found helpful (Smith and Spetzler 1995).

Selective medial resections, technical details

For the transventricular approach the position described for 'en bloc' lobectomy is appropriate. If the trans-sylvian approach, described by Yasargil, is used, the head must be tilted 30° away from the side of operation with the malar as the highest point, so that the sylvian fissure is vertical; otherwise, the resection becomes extremely difficult. The other details of the trans-sylvian approach are described by Yasargil (Yasargil *et al* 1985).

Yasargil's approach precludes the use of the ultrasonic aspirator (CUSA) because of the restricted access. In Yasargil's approach the amygdala is encountered first, on the way to the temporal horn, and its partial removal facilitates the visualization of the temporal horn and hippocampus. The amygdala, which may appear gray or grayish-brown, is removed piecemeal and in the medial or mediobasal direction the optic tract is eventually encountered. Olivier notes that in the transventricular approach the amygdala is visualized after the main hippocampal specimen has been removed and can be removed dorsally up to the middle cerebral artery. A vital step in the hippocampal removal is the identification of the hippocampal sulcus, called sulcus choroideus by Yasargil, and the Ammon's horn artery or arteries that run into the hippocampus and may originate from both the anterior choroidal artery and the posterior choroidal arteries. Yasargil commences his hippocampal removal at this point anteriorly, where the anterior choroidal artery and the posterior choroidal arteries. Yasargil commences his hippocampal removal at this point anteriorly, where the anterior choroidal artery is identified and safeguarded. Only the lateral branches from the artery are divided. Papaverine may be applied locally to the anterior choroidal trunk after the dissection in this area has been completed to minimize spasm. The dissection proceeds posteriorly from this point until the hippocampus is divided across its tail, usually at the end of the P2 portion of the posterior cerebral artery. The dissection then proceeds anteriorly but laterally at the level of the collateral sulcus and including the parahippocampal gyrus until passing around the pes hippocampus it joins the starting point and the specimen can then be removed. In the trans-sylvian approach it is neither possible nor prudent to put brain retractors inside the cortical incision. Although Yasargil and Teddy describe removal of up to 4 cm of hippocampus, in our cases between 1.5 and 2 cm is removed; this may be because a higher proportion of our patients have hippocampal sclerosis. It is possible, having removed the bulk of the hippocampus, to remove more from the distal stump before concluding the removal. After the resection is complete, careful hemostasis is carried out in the cavity; a light pack of cotton wool and patience are best.

When the procedure is carried out under stereotactic guidance, presumably the boundaries of the resection are determined by the brain imaging.

Vascular injury is the most important complication of this operation. In the trans-sylvian approach the M1 portion of the middle cerebral artery is at risk, especially with the limited access. It has to be protected from retraction, accidental injury, and trauma associated with diathermy of adjacent vessels. Similarly, in dissecting the hippocampus free, the vessels in the ambient cistern must be identified positively, and care taken in dealing with the small vessels that pass to the hippocampus to avoid damage to more major vessels. Schaller studied 20 patients undergoing trans-sylvian amygdalohippocampectomy with ultrasound to determine the blood flow within basal cerebral arteries before and after the surgery. The commonest reaction was an ipsilateral or bilateral increase in flow velocities seen in 14/18 patients, no reaction in 4 patients, and a paradoxical reaction in two patients. There was no mortality or morbidity (Schaller and Zentner 1998).

CLOSED AND NONSURGICAL METHODS OF DESTROYING THE MESIAL TEMPORAL STRUCTURES

The use of various stereotactic methods of destroying or lesioning the hippocampus and amygdala are dealt with in detail in the section on Functional Surgery. However, there are two methods applied particularly to the mesial temporal structures that should be mentioned here.

There are anecdotal accounts of stereotactic thermocoagulation of the hippocampus. Patil and colleagues imaged the amygdala–hippocampus complex using CT and then used a thermocoagulation electrode to destroy the targeted volume. In six of the seven patients the destructive lesion was preceded by multiple subpial transection of the lateral temporal cortex, and in some cases other areas. There were no complications referable to the lesioning and all the patients improved; about half of them were seizure free (Patil et al 1995).

Stereotactic radiosurgery has been used for many years in the treatment of small, inaccessible lesions in the brain and there is a large and informative literature about the use of this treatment and its technical details and possible complications (Anonymous 1997a). The use of stereotactic radiosurgery in the treatment of focal epilepsy, and especially temporal lobe epilepsy, was first proposed in the 1980s and there were sporadic reports of its efficiency (Barcia-Salorio et al 1992; Heikkinen et al 1992; Barcia-Salorio et al 1994). These reports were of cases with space-occupying lesions treated before the advent of modern brain imaging, and in particular sophisticated MRI, which has allowed the accurate identification of pathology in the temporal lobe. More recently, Regis has published details of this treatment in patients with pure unilateral mesial temporal sclerosis (Regis et al 1995). As described by Regis and others, the sequence of events in patients treated with radiosurgery is as follows. The radiation is administered as a single dose and, except in isolated cases, nothing happens for about 8 months. Then, over a period of about 1 month, the patient has an increased frequency of simple partial seizures followed by a cessation of all seizures. A similar sequence of events was described by Barcia-Solario (Barcia-Salorio et al 1994). The radiologic evidence of the action of radiosurgery suggests that the process is a gradual one occurring over 1–2 years, but the precise mechanism of action of stereotactic radiosurgery in this situation is not known. Because seizure cessation occurs before MRI changes and in some patients the mesial temporal structures appear to return to normal after 2 years, it is thought that a nondestructive process is concerned. There is a minimal dose, probably around 20–25 Gy, below which the effect is only partial and takes a long time to appear. Currently, Regis is using a 50% dose of 24 Gy to a lateral nonconforming target with a maximum volume of 7000 mm^3 (J. Regis, personal communication).

PATHOLOGIC SUBSTRATES

The advent of direct brain imaging, especially MRI, and the increase in the number of patients operated have resulted in a better documentation of the pathologic substrates encountered in specimens from temporal lobe resection. The distribution of these substrates differs between adults and children. In Table 51.1 (see later) the distribution of pathology from our own series is shown.

SYNOPSIS OF PATHOLOGIC SUBSTRATES

Mesial temporal sclerosis

This entity is well recognized, having first been described in the early 19th century (Bouchet and Cazauvieihl 1825). Margerison and Corsellis showed, in a group of chronic epileptic's coming to autopsy, that characteristic changes could be seen in the hippocampus. These changes were exclusively unilateral in only 34% of cases, although severe sclerosis involving hippocampus was seen unilaterally in 28% of cases and bilaterally in 11% cases. About 75% of their cases with hippocampal sclerosis had either unilateral or predominantly unilateral changes (Margerison and Corsellis 1966). This is in line with MRI estimates of bilateral hippocampal sclerosis at 15–20%. Bilateral hippocampal sclerosis is not necessarily a bar to surgery, but it is difficult to identify the operable side and the outcome is not so good as when pathology is unilateral.

Cortical neuronal migration disorder

This entity was first described in surgical specimens by Taylor et al (1971). MRI has allowed identification of these lesions, and the results are good when 80% or more of the lesion can be removed. This was commonly the case when the lesions were in the temporal lobe (Olivier et al 1996; Palmini et al 1996). In one MNI report, 55% of the lesions in 85 patients were in the temporal lobe (Olivier et al 1996). In 18 of our patients, who were all less than 16 years old at operation, there are only two with lesions in the temporal lobe. Patients with widespread cortical dysplasia will not respond well to temporal lobe resections; Chugani et al have described 18 infants with infantile spasms and bitemporal FDG-PET hypometabolism in whom the outcome when followed up for some years was very poor, suggesting that these patients would not have benefited from cortical resection (Chugani et al 1996).

It is now clear that the lesion described as dysembryoplastic neuroepithelial tumor (DNT or DNET) is a form of cortical neuronal migration disorder (Daumas-Duport et al 1988). Raymond et al found 21 DNET lesions in 100 patients with some form of cortical neuronal migration disorder (Raymond et al 1995). They also examined the features of DNET lesions in their 16 operated patients. The lesion involved the temporal lobe in 15 of these 16 patients and was close to the mesial structures in 11 of 14 patients; 12 of the 14 patients available for follow-up were seizure-free (Raymond et al 1994). Prayson et al (1993) reported changes of cortical dysplasia close to astrocytic tumors. There is a report of DNET lesions associated with neurofibromatosis type 1 in two children, but this association is probably fortuitous (Lellouch-Tubiana et al 1995). DNET lesions tend to be discrete and easy to excise, unless they are in eloquent cortex, and therefore the outcome from surgery is good.

Other pathologic lesions

Benign astrocytic tumors are found in the temporal lobe, as are mixed tumors such as gangliogliomas, and a variety of other lesions such as angiomas, cavernous hemangiomas, and others. Sometimes the first manifestation of Rasmussen disease is in the temporal lobe.

Dual pathology

Cendes et al described the occurrence of dual pathology in 167 patients with identifiable lesions. Dual pathology it was commonest in association with neuronal migration disorder (25%), and in 25 patients (15%) it was hippocampal sclerosis (Cendes et al 1995). Ho et al found hippocampal formation atrophy unilaterally in 87% of patients with temporal lobe developmental malformations; it was bilateral in 57% of the patients (Ho et al 1998). Another report described 14 patients with extrahippocampal structural abnormalities among 27 patients with hippocampal sclerosis who failed surgery (52%) (Sisodiya et al 1997). In 20 children reported from Toronto, dual pathology in the form of hippocampal sclerosis was commonly associated with cortical disorders or the overlap with tuberose sclerosis (Jay et al 1993).

In 1987 Babb and Jann-Brown reported that the hippocampal cell loss in patients with extrahippocampal pathology was less severe than in patients with hippocampal sclerosis alone (Babb and Jann-Brown 1987). Nakasato et al showed that patients with the combination of even mild hippocampal sclerosis and extrahippocampal pathology were more likely to have residual seizures after a standard temporal lobectomy (Nakasato et al 1992). A previous paper showed that in 13 patients with heterotopia the hippocampal cell loss tended to be severe, whereas in 12 patients with glioma the cell loss was mild (Levesque *et al* 1991).

OUTCOME

The effects of the surgery have to be viewed from a wider perspective than that of seizure relief alone, even though chronic intractable epilepsy was the reason for the inclusion of patients in the surgical program. Indeed, some outcome measures, such as that proposed by Rougier, recognize that fact (Rougier *et al* 1992). The outcome will be discussed in terms of seizure relief, mortality and nonneurologic complications; neurologic, intellectual, and psychiatric sequelae; and an assessment of psychosocial outcome. King *et al* (1997) have used a Markov model to show that anterior temporal lobectomy is probably a cost-effective use of medical resources.

SEIZURE RELIEF

The results of surgery from early series are difficult to compare and for the sake of retrospective analysis it is difficult for any particular center to change their method of assessing seizure relief. In 1985 Engel proposed an outcome scale as a result of the First Palm Desert Symposium and this is now in more general use (Engel 1987). In the early series of temporal lobe resections the results were not divided according to the underlying pathologic substrate (Jensen 1975b; Engel 1987; Engel *et al* 1993; Anonymous 1997b). The first literature survey by Jensen in 1975 showed considerable variation in seizure outcome, the proportion of patients becoming seizure-free varying between 28% and 62% (Jensen 1975b). In the pooled results from the First Palm Desert Symposium in 1987, the proportion of seizure-free patients varied between 26% and 80% (Engel 1987). In the Second Palm Desert Symposium in 1993, the data was presented according to procedure but, from 3579 anterior temporal lobectomies, 67.9% were seizure-free as were 68.8% of 413 amygdalohippocampectomies (Engel *et al* 1993).

More recent series have been analyzed according to underlying pathology, showing that there is a relationship between the nature of the pathology and seizure outcome. Hippocampal sclerosis or another recognized pathology were two of the three factors predicting a 1-year remission in Spencer's analysis of 105 patients undergoing temporal lobe surgery (Spencer *et al* 1993b). Schulz *et al* (1995) reported 65 temporal lobe resections: 33 of their patients

had MTS and the remaining 32 some other pathology. The majority of these patients (70.9%) were seizure-free and 92.3% had a significant improvement. Berkovic reported the results of 135 consecutive temporal lobectomies. At 2 years, 80% of patients with foreign tissue lesions, 62% of patients with hippocampal sclerosis, and 36% of patients with a normal MRI were seizure-free, although some have suffered early seizures. In all the groups 'rundown' seizures were seen and only in those with hippocampal sclerosis was late recurrence of seizures seen (Berkovic *et al* 1995). Morris *et al* have described the outcome in 38 patients with intractable epilepsy and ganglioglioma. There were 28 temporal resections. Overall, 79% of the 38 patients were in Engel group 1 at 6 months but this had decreased to 63% at 2 years. Good outcome was associated with lower age at operation, absence of generalized seizures and no epileptiform discharges on a postoperative EEG (Morris *et al* 1998). Thadani has reported 22 patients, followed up for 4 years, in whom operation was performed without intracranial recording. MTS was identified on MRI in 18 of these patients and histologically in 20. Eighteen of these patients (82%) became seizure-free (Thadani *et al* 1995). Arruda *et al* examined the results of anterior temporal lobectomy and selective amygdalohippocampectomy in 74 patients divided into three groups: those with clear unilateral mesial temporal atrophy, those with bilateral atrophy, and those with no atrophy at all. Seizure outcome of grade 1 or 2 by Engel's classification was achieved in 93.6% of those with unilateral atrophy, in 61.7% of those with bilateral atrophy, and in only 50% in those with no atrophy. The two resective techniques were equally effective (Arruda *et al* 1996). Jack *et al* (1992) showed that outcome was related to the preoperative volume of hippocampus. Nakasato *et al* described a careful analysis of the relationship between the degree of hippocampal sclerosis and outcome. Those patients who had only hippocampal sclerosis obtained good result in 90% of those with severe cell loss, defined as greater than 30% cell loss, whereas only 65% obtained a good result when the cell loss was less severe. Those patients with extrahippocampal lesions showed no difference in the outcome whether the hippocampal cell loss was mild or severe (Nakasato *et al* 1992). Nayel *et al* found that seizure relief was related to the extent of the resection of mesial temporal structures in 94 patients undergoing temporal lobectomy from the Cleveland Clinic (Nayel *et al* 1991). Wieser and colleagues analyzed the extent and size of resection in 30 patients selected from their series of 204 amygdalohippocampectomies. Seizure outcome was related both to the size and to the site of the resection; radical resection of the parahippocampal gyrus was associated with good outcome (Siegel *et al* 1990).

Therefore, if it is assumed that MRI-demonstrated atrophy is equivalent to the presence of hippocampal sclerosis, when this pathologic substrate is severe, and unilateral, the seizure relief from appropriate temporal lobe resection is good. It can be difficult, even in modern series, to unravel the relationship between this observation and those of Awad and Wieser that the overall size of a resection and the extent of mesial resection are both good indicators of excellent seizure relief. Perhaps this indicates that it is difficult, even with modern neuroimaging techniques, to be certain of the extent of the involvement of the hippocampus and parahippocampal gyrus is these pathologic processes.

A seminal paper by Adelson et al (1992) describes the results of temporal lobe surgery in 33 children, and also summarizes the early literature, from which it is clear that in many of those reports the proportion of patients with tumors is much higher than in adults. The seizure relief is very good, varying between 65% and 100%. Their own series includes 16 patients (48%) with tumors, a further 13 patients (39%) with some form of cortical migrational neuronal disorder, and only one patient with hippocampal sclerosis. Wyllie describes 14 patients operated before the age of 12 years in the Cleveland Clinic; 10 of these patients had either low-grade tumors or cortical dysplasia and only 4 had mesial temporal sclerosis (Wyllie et al 1993). Blume et al described the results of temporal lobectomy, without invasive recording, in 14 children aged 12 years or less at the time of surgery. In 13 patients the seizures began with a simple partial component. The pathology consisted of low-grade tumors in 8, MTS was present in 7 but was the sole pathology in only one of these, 5 others had cortical developmental abnormalities, and one had Sturge–Weber syndrome. With time all these patients became seizure-free (Blume et al 1997). In a series of 73 children operated in Montreal between 1940 and 1980, tumors having been excluded, 25 patients had no clear pathology in the resective specimen. Among remaining patients mesial temporal sclerosis, or febrile convulsion, was found in 26 patients. Forty-three of these 73 patients (59%) had an Engel class 1 outcome (Fish et al 1993). Falconer and Davidson, assessing the result of surgery in 40 children, suggested that early surgery would be beneficial (Davidson and Falconer 1973). Goldstein et al also describe 33 patients subjected to temporal lobe resections and note that certain features in their patients were associated with a good outcome. These include younger age at seizure onset, and at surgery, and shorter duration of epilepsy. This would indicate that patients with favorable features such as a localized unilateral temporal lesion, absence of generalized seizures, absence of mental retardation, or a significant prior history should be offered early surgery at least for the sake of seizure outcome if not for other reasons (Goldstein et al 1996).

A number of other factors have to be considered when looking at seizure outcome. Consideration must also be given to the preoperative seizure type. The work of Spencer and others shows that seizures with a consistent aura, especially if this is accompanied by indications that the seizure remains localized in one temporal lobe for some time, are associated with a good outcome. There is also a relationship between persisting seizures and preoperative seizure type. Fried has examined the relationship between auras, pathology, and outcome. The semeiology of the auras was related to the location, but not lateralization, of the pathology. Thus epigastric, gustatory, and olfactory were associated with hippocampal sclerosis and vertigo or dizziness with extratemporal lesions. Persisting auras were seen in 18.9% of the patients with hippocampal sclerosis, but in only 2.6% of patients with other lesions, some of which were located extratemporally (Fried et al 1995). The group in London, Ontario, have described the changes in seizure pattern seen in 26 of 100 patients who failed to respond completely to temporal lobe resection. In addition to eliminating or reducing the number of complex partial seizures, surgery also simplified or eliminated the aura features of the residual complex partial seizures. Nineteen of 20 patients with only simple partial seizures postoperatively ultimately obtained a better than 90% reduction in their seizure frequency and seven became seizure-free (Blume and Girvin 1997). Specht and colleagues found a relationship in 78 patients between seizure outcome, the occurrence of generalized seizures within 2 years of surgery, and the presence of significant cerebellar atrophy. Whereas 87.5% of patients were seizure-free if neither feature was present, this figure fell to 30% when both were present (Specht et al 1997).

The development of nonepileptic seizures after temporal lobectomy has been described by Taylor. Recently Ney and his colleagues described 5 patients among 96 who had undergone surgery for epilepsy in whom new nonepileptic seizures had developed. Three risk factors were identified: preoperative psychopathology, low preoperative IQ, and major surgical complications (Ney et al 1998).

Patrick and colleagues have examined postoperative EEGs and outcome following epilepsy surgery. There were 78 patients with MTS and 47 patients with low-grade tumors; seizures persisted in 24% of the patients with MTS and 27% of the patients with tumors. All of the MTS patients with normal EEGs were seizure-free and only one of the tumor patients with a normal EEG had persistent seizures. The type of EEG abnormality was significant only in the MTS patients, and in those the significant abnormalities were focal slowing and epileptiform discharges (Patrick *et al* 1995).

The majority of patients after temporal lobe resection will not maintain absolute freedom from seizures. In the acute, postoperative phase, two kinds of seizures may be seen. Focal seizures involving the face or mouth, and speech in dominant hemisphere operations, have been described in the past and attributed, probably correctly, to local edema; in our practice they have become much less frequent in recent years. They have, in our experience, no prognostic value. Secondly, if the patient's anticonvulsant medication is missed in the postoperative period, or if the patient suffers some vascular, infective, or metabolic disturbance, then generalized seizures may occur. Beyond the immediate postoperative period, persistent or recurrent seizures may have a number of causes, some of which will be easy to identify and others that will remain obscure. In general, patients who have a significant improvement in their seizure control at 2 years after surgery will maintain it. The interpretation of the long-term outcome after surgery depends upon the method of seizure recording, the commonest method being conventional seizure counting. In the 65 patients described by Schulz, there were 25 patients with persisting seizures, 10 relapsed when their medication was reduced, in 6 patients the removal was incomplete, and in 9 patients the course was not clear. Ten of these patients were controlled with medication or reoperation (Schulz *et al* 1995). Cascino's group have analyzed seizure frequency and time after surgery. In 184 patients the only significant changes were seen between years 3 and 4, and this seemed to be due to patients changing their status as a result of discontinuing antiepileptic medication. (So *et al* 1997). Sperling *et al* followed up 89 patients for 5 years after anterior temporal lobectomy. After 5 years, 70% of these patients were seizure-free and only 6% had an unfavorable outcome; 4% died, all of whom had persistent seizures. Fifty-five percent of the seizure recurrences occurred within 6 months and 93% within 2 years of surgery. In 90 patients submitted to 'en bloc' temporal lobectomy, at least 60 patients had been followed up for 5 years and the maximum follow-up period was 12 years. Although 58% of these patients were in Engel group 3A or better, only 25% remained constantly seizure-free (Polkey and Scarano 1993). Actuarial analysis has been used to examine the outcome in 102 patients who underwent temporal lobectomy. The probability of achieving 1-year remission was 57% by 1 year, 70% by 2 years, and 77% by 7 years. If the patient achieved 1 year of remission the probability of remaining seizure-free was 90%; with two consecutive years the probability rose to 94% (Elwes *et al* 1991).

Finally, an analysis of the outcome of our temporal resections carried out in the Maudsley/King's Neurosurgical Unit between 1976 and 1998 is provided as a series of tables. In Table 51.1 the pathology in 377 temporal lobe resections is presented; 85 of these patients were aged less than 16 years at surgery, the remaining 292 were older. MTS was found in the 58.9% of the adults compared with 47% of children. Over such a long period of time changes in brain imaging might affect selection. In Table 51.2 the percentage of pathology in children and adults is presented for the periods 1976–1986 and 1986–1996. There is little difference between them. In Table 51.3 the outcome in 46 children and 193 adults with at least 2 years follow-up is presented. The outcome in the children is much better. Finally, in Table 51.4 the outcome at 2 years and 5 years after surgery is presented for various pathologic substrates.

Table 51.1 Pathology in specimens from 377 temporal lobe resections performed between 1976 and 1998.

	Age at surgery	
Pathology	<16 years	>16 years
Total	85	292
AVM[a]	0	2
CD[a]	3	7
DNET[a]	8	9
Hamartoma	6	8
Malformation	1	2
Tumor	21	28
Other	3	19
All positive pathology	42	75
MTS[a]	40	172
Nonspecific	3	45

[a]AVM, arteriovenous malformations; CD DNET, dysembryoplastic neuroepithelial tumor; MTS, mesial temporal lobe sclerosis.

Table 51.2 Comparison of pathology in two series between adults and children.

	n	MTS[a]	Other	Nonspecific
1976–86				
Children	21	18.9%	36.7%	None
Adults	68	81.8%	63.3%	100%
1986–96				
Children	34	10.6%	30.3%	2.9%
Adults	195	89.4%	69.7%	97.1%

[a]Mesial temporal lobe sclerosis.

Table 51.3 Comparison of results in children and adults 1976–1996.

Result	Children (n = 46)	Adults (n = 193)
1A, absolutely seizure-free	52%	25.9%
1, seizure-free (Engel 1)	76.1%	53.4%
Improved (Engel 3A or better)	95.6%	83.9%
Not improved (Engel 3B or worse)	4.4%	16.1%

Table 51.4 Outcome from temporal lobe resections between 1976 and 1996. Outcome in respect of pathology at 2 years follow-up and 5 years follow-up.

Outcome	Follow-up (years)	All (n = 289, 125)	MTS[a] (n = 134, 79)	Tumour (n = 63, 30)	Nonspecific (n = 26, 15)
Absolutely	2	32.3%	23.9%	46%	15.4%
seizure-free	5	29.6%	24%	40%	13.3%
(Engel 1A)					
Seizure-free	2	57.7%	54.5%	68%	27%
(Engel 1)	5	62.4%	58.2%	66.7%	33%
Improved	2	86.2%	87.3%	90.4%	46%
(better than	5	91.2%	89.9%	93.3%	46.7%
Engel 3A)					
Not improved	2	13.8%	12.7%	9.6%	54%
(worse than	5	8.8%	10.1%	6.7%	53.3%
Engel 3B)					

[a]Mesial temporal lobe sclerosis.

MORTALITY AND NONNEUROLOGIC MORBIDITY

Jensen, in her original survey, found a mortality of around 1% (Jensen 1975b); at the First Palm Desert Symposium it was around 0.39% (Van Buren 1987); and in the latest review it is less than 1%, with some centers, such as the MNI, reporting no deaths in 526 cases (Pilcher *et al* 1993). In our 305 consecutive lobectomies there have been only two perioperative deaths; one patient developed a DVT and then hemorrhaged as a result of anticoagulant therapy, and another suffered unexplained brain swelling at the end of uneventful surgery. Other general neurosurgical complications are low; the commonest is postoperative infection, which is given at 0.5% in the Second Palm Desert Symposium (Pilcher *et al* 1993). Generally, these complications do not lead to any permanent disability or change in the overall prognosis from the surgery.

Late mortality in patients subjected to temporal lobe surgery is a different matter. Jensen notes that there is an excess mortality among chronic epileptics, around 59.4 deaths per 1000 patients, and that suicide was a common cause of death in this group. There were 50 late deaths in 2282 patients, 21.9 per 1000 or around 2%, and 31 of these were either suicide or epilepsy and tended to be those patients who had not benefited from surgery (Jensen 1975a). Taylor and Marsh reported 37 (19%) deaths in 193 patients operated by Falconer and 23 of these deaths were either in circumstances that related to epilepsy or by suicide, half the suicides occurring in patients who were seizure-free (Taylor and Marsh 1977). In our 305 consecutive temporal lobe resections there were 17 other deaths, 13 of which were epilepsy-related, and 6 of which were sudden and unexpected with no cause found at autopsy (SUDEP). It is

clear that surgery reduces the excess mortality among drug-resistant epileptics, but does not remove it completely.

Resections are similar, and since the beginning of temporal lobe surgery the complication rate has fallen. At an early stage resection of the insular cortex, to remove spikes, was found to have a high risk of hemiparesis, called manipulation hemiplegia, probably because of manipulation of branches of the middle cerebral artery, without any increased improvement in seizure relief (Penfield *et al* 1961). The commonest neurologic sequelae to temporal lobe resection are a contralateral hemiparesis or hemiplegia, a contralateral visual field defect, and a homolateral third-nerve palsy or paresis. Jacobson and colleagues have described a transient fourth-nerve paresis in 14% of their patients following temporal lobectomy (Jacobson *et al* 1995). An unusual complication of cerebellar hemorrhage in four cases of temporal lobectomy has been described by Toczek *et al* (1996). There is a report of a middle fossa cyst presenting as a mass lesion 2 years after lobectomy. It was successfully treated by shunting (Weaver *et al* 1996). There is a single report of a Kluver–Bucy syndrome following left temporal lobectomy for an oligodendroglioma in a woman aged 70 years, with no lesion in the opposite temporal lobe MRI (Ghika-Schmid *et al* 1995). Jensen provides a good summary of the experience up to 1975 (Jensen 1975b) and subsequent results are to be found in the two Palm Desert Symposia (Van Buren 1987; Pilcher *et al* 1993). The avoidance of hemiplegia or hemiparesis must be related mainly to vascular causes, especially in selective mesial resections. In combined resections the risk varies between zero and 1–2%, being lower in larger series, and in selective amygdalohippocampectomy varies between less than 0.5% in the Zurich series to 2% in our series, with two transient hemiparesis (3.2%) in Renella's series (Renella 1989a). McLachan *et al* have shown that neurologic complications are not more common in patients operated after 45 years of age (McLachlan *et al* 1992).

The size of the visual field defect depends upon the size of the resection, that is, the length of temporal lobe taken measured from the temporal pole. Falconer and Wilson showed that this was due to the course of the visual fibers around the temporal horn (Falconer and Wilson, 1958). Such visual field defects relate to the disruption of the fibers in the roof of the temporal horn (Dodrill *et al* 1993). Awad and his colleagues suggest that a visual field defect is correlated with resection in their central quadrant, showing that the more lateral the resection the more likely it was to produce a deficit, although there was no close correlation between the size of the resection and the severity of the visual field defect (Katz *et al* 1989). The size of the defect cannot be predicted with resections of less than 7.5 cm (Pilcher *et al* 1993). Spencer's extended lobectomy does not produce more visual field defects than the standard operation (Spencer *et al* 1984). Rarely, visual field defects may result from vascular causes, although neither Yasargil nor Renella report any hemianopia following selective amygdalohippocampectomy.

INTELLECTUAL SEQUELAE

It has been known since the beginning of temporal lobe surgery that bilateral temporal excision will result in global amnesia (Scoville and Milner 1957). It subsequently became clear that if there was insufficient memory reserve in the unoperated temporal lobe then global amnesia could also be a result. However, the amnestic effect of a subsequent catastrophe in a patient who has undergone temporal lobectomy has only recently been reported (Oxbury *et al* 1997).

In general, the postoperative intellectual changes relate to the nature of the underlying pathology in the temporal lobe and the type of resection performed. Van Buren notes serious memory deficit in seven cases (0.37%) (Van Buren 1987) and the last Palm Desert assessment states that global amnesia is less than 1% (Pilcher *et al* 1993). Another review in the same volume treats the matter in more detail (Dodrill *et al* 1993). A number of studies have shown that patients with predominantly unilateral sclerotic lesions of the temporal lobe tend to suffer less change in their intellectual performance as a result of anterior temporal lobectomy than those with other pathology or nonspecific changes in the temporal lobe (Powell *et al* 1985; McMillan *et al* 1987). Davies *et al* have shown that patients with left MTS suffer less decline in their naming ability after left temporal lobectomy (Davies *et al* 1998). The Bonn group found that significant deterioration in verbal memory was related to age

at surgery, with no patients less than 15 years of age suffering a deterioration whereas 61% of patients aged more than 30 years at surgery suffered a deterioration. It is not clear how this is related to the pathology in these patients. In a previous paper they note that left temporal lobectomy can lead to a new impairment in verbal memory (Helmstaedter and Elger 1996, 1998). The work of Ojemann and Dodrill in limiting verbal memory loss by mapping under local anesthesia has already been described (Ojemann and Dodrill 1985). Krauss *et al* have investigated the effect of removal of the basal temporal language area in 25 patients where this had been mapped with stimulation. There was no significant difference in verbal IQ for recognition memory for words and verbal learning between patients who had resection of this area and those who did not, although there was some persistent decrease in naming ability (Krauss *et al* 1996). Koike and colleagues have shown that musical ability can be preserved following right temporal lobectomy (Koike *et al* 1996).

It was hoped that selective amygdalohippocampectomy would minimize the intellectual sequelae of temporal lobe resection. There are now early and late reports from Zürich (Wieser 1988, 1991) and also from Renella (Renella 1989a). Renella noted slight deterioration in all aspects of intellectual performance in his small group of patients when they had left-sided operations, and the converse following right-sided operations. Wieser described two factors influencing improvement, when the function examined was subserved by the nonoperated side and freedom from seizures (Wieser 1988). A later report by Nadig (Wieser 1991) suggests that right-sided operations result in an improvement in learning and memory, whereas left-sided operations have the converse effect, the same findings as Renella. A multicenter study of the cognitive outcome of neocortical resection, amygdalohippocampectomy, and classical temporal lobectomy failed to show any clear advantage of one of these techniques over the others. There may be a number of reasons for this, including variations in the pathology and in the structural results of each operative technique (Jones-Gotman *et al* 1997). Renowden *et al* described the results of transcortical and trans-sylvian amygdalohippocampectomy. Seven patients operated by the transcortical route and 10 patients operated by the trans-sylvian route were compared with anterior temporal lobectomy and there was no difference in seizure outcome. Patients who underwent left amygdalohippocampectomy fared better in terms of verbal IQ than those undergoing left anterior lobectomy. Examination of the changes in the white matter suggested that there was probably more secondary damage in the temporal lobe after amygdalohippocampectomy than has previously been realized (Renowden *et al* 1995).

Improvement in cognitive function after operation is also related to improvement in seizure control (Novelly *et al* 1984) and Lieb showed that the predictors of poor seizure control are also predictors of poor cognitive function after surgery (Lieb *et al* 1982). Awad, using quantitative analysis of postresection MRI scans, attempted to correlate resection with intellectual changes. In contrast to Ojemann's experience they were unable to correlate the extent of lateral cortical resection with memory loss in the dominant temporal lobe, but the decrease in verbal memory correlated with the extent of resection in the mesial and basal quadrants, and a similar correlation was found with nonverbal memory and right-sided resections (Katz *et al* 1989). This is consistent with the earlier descriptions of material-specific deficits by Milner in 1958. An investigation of self-report and behavioral memory in patients undergoing either temporal lobectomy or selective amygdalohippocampectomy showed similar effects from both operations (Bidzinski *et al* 1992; Goldstein and Polkey 1992). Subsequently, 42 patients undergoing either operation, all left hemisphere dominant, were studied (Goldstein and Polkey 1993). If seizures persisted then there was a poor performance in the material-specific tasks performed by the target temporal lobe, a finding similar to those reported by others. Selective amygdalohippocampectomy had less effect on the functions of the target temporal lobe than anterior temporal lobectomy but the converse was true of the nontarget temporal lobe. The numbers in our series with nonspecific changes in the resected specimen and persisting seizures was too small for formal analysis, but they all suffered considerable deterioration in cognitive function after operation, as suggested by Wieser and his colleagues. (Wieser 1988). Wyler *et al* reported results for extending the hippocampal resection more posteriorly in otherwise comparable groups of patients undergoing temporal lobectomy; there was no difference in neuropsychologic effects (Wyler *et al* 1995).

It is difficult to summarize this information. There is probably a hierarchical organization of cognitive function so that verbal functions are more fragile than nonverbal functions and more likely to suffer. Martin *et al* has shown that there is a substantial variation in memory change after anterior temporal lobectomy and that selected aspects of verbal and visual memory can be affected by both right- and left-sided operations (Martin *et al* 1998). Selective amygdalohippocampectomy is probably better, all other things being equal, when there is residual memory in the target temporal lobe and operation should probably be avoided in those patients with no structural lesion and a substantial amount of memory in the target temporal lobe.

PSYCHIATRIC CONSEQUENCES AND SOCIAL OUTCOME

Behavioral changes in patients undergoing temporal lobe surgery are well documented and the patients can be divided into two groups: those who have an aggressive behavior disorder before surgery and those who are subject to psychosis, either before surgery or as a consequence of surgery.

Behavior disorder in patients selected for surgery does not seem to be as prevalent now as it was in some of the earlier series; for example, in the series described by Falconer (Taylor and Falconer 1968; Falconer 1973) only a small proportion of the patients were considered to be normal prior to operation, with a significant proportion improving as a result of operation. In a world survey, Jensen found that only 6.2% of patients were psychiatrically normal before operation, whereas 23.5% were normal after surgery and a further 40.9% were improved (Jensen 1975b), and in 74 patients from Denmark, none of whom was normal before surgery, 39% were in employment afterwards (Jensen 1976). The origin of such behavioral changes is complex. Ferguson and Rayport suggest that they fall into two groups: those whose behavior relates to increased ictal activity and those whose behavior is a reaction to chronic uncontrolled epilepsy (Ferguson and Rayport 1988). If the surgery controls the seizures, the behavior will improve. Ounsted, in his longitudinal survey of children, noted that all the operated children had a satisfactory behavioral and social outcome, whereas the unoperated children, in spite of intensive treatment, remained handicapped (Ounsted *et al* 1987). Manchanda *et al* examined the pattern of psychiatric morbidity in 300 consecutive patients admitted to an epilepsy surgery assessment program; there were 231 with a temporal lobe focus. Surprisingly, 47.3% of these 300 patients emerged with a psychiatric diagnosis. The commonest diagnosis was anxiety disorder (10.7%), but a schizophrenia-like psychosis was seen in 4.3% of patients. No significant differences were found between the temporal and nontemporal groups of patients, nor with regard to laterality of seizure focus (Manchanda *et al* 1996).

Psychosis supervening upon chronic epilepsy is usually a late event. Serafetidines and Falconer (1962) and Jensen (Jensen and Larsen 1979) showed that the temporal lobe resection had no effect upon such a psychosis. Temporal lobe surgery, at any rate resective surgery, can produce a schizophreniform psychosis often associated with left-sided resections, or a depressive illness more often associated with right-sided operations. In the patients reported by Taylor (1975) or those described by Jensen and Larsen (1979), the incidence of schizophreniform illness was relatively high, 15% and 12%, respectively. In more recent material the incidence has been much lower; in our series around 2–3%. We have not been able to confirm the connection with left-handed females who had alien tissue lesions described by Taylor and Bruton (Taylor 1975). Mace and Trimble (1991) note that both left-sided and right-sided operations may be followed by psychosis.

Detection of a depressive illness following temporal lobe surgery requires long and careful follow-up because it does not necessarily occur immediately after surgery, and may require careful questioning to elicit the symptoms. Taylor noted that the patients subjected to temporal lobe surgery already have a high loading of factors that predispose to suicide (Taylor and Marsh 1977). In our own material, suicide is relatively rare—two known cases in 300 operations—but depression is much commoner; an informal survey suggests around 35%, almost exclusively in nondominant, usually right-sided, resections. We have found that it is rare after amygdalohippocampectomy and in children, although one 12-year-old child with a large resection developed clinical depression requiring treatment. Other groups have begun to report depression following right-sided operations (Hefner et al 1993; Stagno et al 1993). Blumer et al have described the incidence of psychiatric disorders in a group of 50 consecutive patients, 44 of whom underwent temporal lobectomy. Before surgery, 57% of the 44 patients who underwent temporal lobe surgery had dysphoric disorders. These dysphoric disorders contain elements equivalent to the irritability and aggression described earlier by Falconer and others. After surgery, 39% experienced 'de novo' psychiatric disorders, six psychotic disorders, six dysphoric disorders, and two depressive episodes. In three other patients there was an exacerbation of the preoperative dysphoric disorder. Finally, 8 of the previously intact 19 patients developed dysphoric disorders in relation to recurrent seizures. Except those patients who had recurrent seizures, all the psychiatric disorders occurred in the first 2 months after surgery (Blumer et al 1998). There is a report from Naylor et al of the psychiatric morbidity following amygdalohippocampectomy in 37 patients operated between 1987 and 1991. Five of these patients developed depressive symptoms, which where a new illness in three. No paranoid-hallucinatory psychoses were seen. There was no relation with lateralization, cerebral dominance, or pathology (Naylor et al 1995).

There is thus no doubt that temporal lobe surgery, for whatever reason, can produce significant psychiatric disorders.

SOCIAL OUTCOME

The early papers from Falconer and Taylor (Taylor and Falconer 1968) and Jensen (Jensen 1976) suggested that the social outcome was largely beneficial, although Taylor, reviewing the matter in 1987, notes that the gains were small and left many of the patients some distance from the 'well-adjusted' score (Taylor 1987). By comparison Ounsted's group were very impressed with the changes in lifestyle seen in the children treated surgically (Ounsted et al 1987). A preliminary study from the University of Washington Regional Epilepsy Center suggests that the gains are slight and that, although a patient's status within his employment group may be improved, movement from one group to another is less evident (Fraser et al 1993). Guldvog published a very detailed account of the social outcome following epilepsy surgery. He compared equally matched groups of around 200 patients who had been treated medically and surgically and who had been followed for up to 20 years (Guldvog et al 1991). Significant improvement in their work situation occurred only in those patients who were in full-time education or employment prior to surgery. In recent years, objective measurements of quality of life (QOL) after epilepsy surgery have been described. Such scales have been applied by Vickrey and colleagues to 248 patients with epilepsy, 202 of whom had undergone some form of resective surgery. Although the operated patients had higher QOL scores, this was not reflected in employment status or prospectively assessed quality of life (Vickrey et al 1995). McLachlan et al examined QOL before and after epilepsy surgery, comparing patients with medically treated patients; their conclusions were similar to those of Guldvog. At 2 years, those patients who were seizure-free, or who had a 90% reduction in their seizure frequency, reported significant improvements in health-related quality of life. This was true of the surgical and medical groups, but surgery was more likely to give control of seizures in the group as a whole (McLachlan et al 1997). Although complete freedom from seizures (Engel 1A) brings the best improvement in QOL, significant improvement in seen with lesser degrees of seizure control, including simple partial seizures (Vickrey et al 1992; Kellett et al 1997; Malmgren et al 1997). Reeves and colleagues have examined the factors affecting work outcome after temporal lobectomy. They investigated 134 patients and found that significantly more patients were independent in activities of daily living, or were able to drive. Income from work was also increased. The factors associated with full-time work after surgery were being a student or having full-time work a year before surgery, no disability benefits before surgery, low postsurgical seizure frequency, excellent or improved seizure control after surgery, driving after surgery, and further education after surgery (Reeves et al 1997). Rose and colleagues examined 47 patients before and after temporal lobectomy. They note that the best improvement in health-related quality-of-life scores was found in those patients with low or medium preoperative scores. They therefore conclude that postoperative improvement must be related to preoperative status as well as the postoperative seizure control (Rose *et al* 1996). Occupational outcome after temporal lobectomy has been examined in 86 patients by Sperling *et al*; 73 of these patients qualified for work before and after surgery. Unemployment rates declined from 25% before surgery to 11% after surgery and underemployment also diminished. Improvement in occupational status was clearly related to postoperative seizure control. Patients with seizures in each year of surgery fared worst, with increased unemployment after surgery. Employment gains came slowly; unemployed patients took up to 6 years to find work. In those patients who were seizure-free there was reduced mortality and improved employment (Sperling *et al* 1995b, 1996). Kellett *et al* found that 80% of patients who were seizure-free and 53% of those having less than 10 seizures per year were gainfully employed postoperatively, compared with 28% of those having more than 10 seizures per year and 27% of those unsuitable for surgery (Kellett *et al* 1997). They, and others, suggest that one possible explanation for the failure of surgery to improve social outcome lies with the low profile given to postoperative rehabilitation.

REOPERATION

Reoperation in epilepsy surgery is undertaken either to use a resection to achieve a better result when a functional operation has failed, or to carry out a further resection because the first was considered inadequate or sometimes was performed for an inappropriate reason, such as biopsy of a lesion. In temporal lobe surgery, further resection is the usual form of reoperation, although in Vaernet's series of patients treated with stereotactic lesions in the hippocampus a significant proportion subsequently underwent anterior temporal lobectomy with benefit (Vaernet 1972). Further resections are usually undertaken either because the original procedure has failed to encompass the pathology or to remove sufficient of the mesial temporal structures. The means of demonstrating the justification for reoperation are those employed in the original assessment, although Awad and his colleagues have described a specific method of subdural recording appropriate to patients who had already undergone temporal lobe resection (Awad *et al* 1992). The possibility of dual pathology, which can be either extratemporal or comprise dual lesions within the temporal lobe, has to be considered. In the Maudsley series of patients undergoing epilepsy surgery, the reoperation rate is 3.6%; half of these were temporal resections, two had been preceded by occipital resections, one by a parietal resection, and the remaining

three were temporal reoperations. These reoperations resulted in freedom from seizures (Engel's group 1) in four patients and significant improvement in the other two patients. Two patients who underwent amygdalohippocampectomy had larger resections and such operations were needed in 5% of the Zurich series (H.G. Wieser, personal communication). Adelson *et al* (1992) note that reoperation was necessary in 3 of their 33 children undergoing temporal lobe surgery. Results from the MNI reported by Germano describe 40 patients who underwent further temporal lobe surgery. In all cases there were residual mesial temporal structures and in four cases there was pathology other than gliosis of the mesial temporal structures. Seizure control after the second operation was good. The overall reoperation rate was about 5% (Germano *et al* 1994). Awad and colleagues also describe 10 patients who had epileptogenic lesions in residual temporal structures, mesial in six of them, lateral in the remaining four (Awad *et al* 1991b). The literature indicates that reoperation brings the best results in those patients with focal seizures arising from the original operation site (Tanaka *et al* 1989; Awad *et al* 1991b; Guldvog *et al* 1991). If resective reoperation is considered as a whole, further resection is more effective in the temporal lobe than elsewhere, with 55.7% seizure-free and only 16.5% not improved.

STEREOTACTIC SURGERY

Unilateral or bilateral temporal lobe lesions made by stereotactic means were originally proposed on neurophysiologic grounds and often carried out in order to ameliorate behavior as well as to relieve seizures. Narabayashi, as a result of work carried out in the 1950s and 1960s, reported beneficial results on both seizure frequency and aggression (Narabayashi and Shima 1973; Narabayashi 1979). European workers subsequently reported similar results, especially with unilateral epileptic foci and unilateral lesions (Talairach and Bancaud 1974; Mundinger *et al* 1976). Mempel and his colleagues, describing a substantial group of patients evaluated with SEEG and then having lesions performed in the mesial temporal structures, reported that 11% were seizure-free and 74% improved. Some of the patients had multiple lesions made (Mempel *et al* 1980). As pointed out by Fisher and others, it is difficult to evaluate the results of past experience with stereotactic lesions (Fisher *et al* 1993). Until an experienced group has carried out a proper evaluation of these techniques, it will be difficult to give advice to patients and their referring physicians about these techniques.

KEY POINTS

1. Historically, temporal lobe surgery evolved from superficial removals to deep resections based on pathology and the known origin of seizures.

2. Selection for surgery depends upon concordance between seizure semeiology, neurophysiology, neuroimaging, and neuropsychology.

3. The surgery is based upon removal of pathology, which is usually synonymous with removal of the seizure focus. The resection is tailored to minimize physical and intellectual sequelae.

4. Neocorticectomy, lesionectomy, combined removal of superficial and deep structures have all been used; the combined removals are the most effective. There are noninvasive methods of treating temporal lobe epilepsy, such as thermocoagulation and stereotactic radiosurgery, which are currently under review.

5. Pathologic substrates in temporal lobe epilepsy fall into well-defined groups of which the commonest two are MTS and cortical neuronal migration disorder.

6. Seizure relief relates to pathology, but overall 60% are in Engel group 1 and results are better in children because of the different pathology.

7. Mortality and morbidity are less than 1–2%, intellectual and psychiatric sequelae are at an acceptable level.

8. Quality of life improvement is seen in patients who become completely seizure-free, Engel group 1A, but some improvement is seen with lesser degrees of seizure control. This improvement is not always reflected in employment or other social factors.

REFERENCES

Adelson PD, Peacock WJ, Chugani HT *et al* (1992) Temporal and extended temporal resections for the treatment of intractable seizures in early childhood. *Pediatric Neurosurgery* **18**:169–178.

Alarcon G, Garcia Seoane JJ, Binnie CD, *et al* (1997) Origin and propagation of interictal discharges in the acute electrocorticogram. Implications for pathophysiology and surgical treatment of temporal lobe epilepsy. *Brain* **120**:2259–2282.

Anonymous (1997a) In: Ganz JC (ed) *Gamma Knife Surgery*, 2nd edn. New York: Springer-Verlag.

Anonymous (1997b) A global survey on epilepsy surgery, 1980–1990: a report by the Commission on Neurosurgery of Epilepsy, the International League Against Epilepsy. *Epilepsia* **38**:249–255.

Arruda F, Cendes F, Andermann F *et al* (1996) Mesial atrophy and outcome after amygdalohippocampectomy or temporal lobe removal. *Annals of Neurology* **40**:446–450.

Awad IA, Assirati JA Jr, Burgess R, Barnett GH, Luders H (1991a) A new class of electrodes of 'intermediate invasiveness': preliminary experience with epidural pegs and foramen ovale electrodes in the mapping of seizure foci. *Neurological Research* **13**:177–183.

Awad IA, Nayel MH, Luders H (1991b) Second operation after the failure of previous resection for epilepsy. *Neurosurgery* **28**:510–518.

Awad IA, Wingkun EC, Nayel MH, Luders H (1992) Surgical failures and reoperations. In: Luders H (ed) *Epilepsy Surgery* pp 679–685. New York: Raven Press.

Babb TL, Jann-Brown W (1987) Pathological findings in epilepsy. In: Engel J (ed) *Surgical Treatment of the Epilepsies*, pp 511–540. New York: Raven Press.

Babb TL, Brown WJ, Pretorius J, Davenport C, Lieb JP, Crandall PH (1984) Temporal lobe volumetric cell densities in temporal lobe epilepsy. *Epilepsia* **25**:729–740.

Bailey P (1961) Surgical treatment of psychomotor epilepsy. Five year follow-up. *Southern Medical Journal* **54**:299–301.

Barcia-Salorio JL, Barcia JA, Hernandez G, Lopez-Gomez L (1994) Radiosurgery of epilepsy. Long-term results. *Acta Neurochirurgica Supplementum* **62**:111–113.

Barcia-Salorio JL, Barcia JA, Hernandez G, Lopez-Gomez L, Roldan P (1992) Radiosurgery of epilepsy. *Acta Neurochirugica* **117**:109(Abstract)

Baxendale SA, Van Paesschen W, Thompson PJ, Duncan JS, Shorvon SD, Connelly, A (1997) The relation between quantitative MRI measures of hippocampal structure and the intracarotid amobarbital test. *Epilepsia* **38**:998–1007.

Baxendale SA, Van Paesschen W, Thompson PJ, Duncan JS, Harkness WF, Shorvon SD (1998) Hippocampal cell loss and gliosis: relationship to preoperative and postoperative memory function. *Neuropsychiatry, Neuropsychology, and Behavioral Neurology* **11**:12–21.

Bengzon AR, Rasmussen T, Gloor P, Dussault J, Stephens M (1968) Prognostic factors in the surgical treatment of temporal lobe epileptics. *Neurology* **18**:717–731.

Bergin PS, Fish DR, Shorvon SD, Oatridge A, deSouza NM, Bydder GM (1995) Magnetic resonance imaging in partial epilepsy: additional abnormalities shown with the fluid attenuated inversion recovery (FLAIR) pulse sequence. *Journal of Neurology, Neurosurgery and Psychiatry* **4**:439–443.

Berkovic SF, McIntosh AM, Kalnins RM *et al* (1995) Preoperative MRI predicts outcome of temporal lobectomy: an actuarial analysis [see comments]. *Neurology* **45**:1358–1363.

Bidzinski J, Bacia T, Ruzikowski E (1992) The results of the surgical treatment of occipital lobe epilepsy. *Acta Neurochirurgica Wien* **114**:128–130.

Binnie CD, Marston D, Polkey CE (1989) Distribution of temporal spikes in relation to the sphenoidal electrode. *Electroencephalography and Clinical Neurophysiology* **73**:403–409.

Blume WT, Girvin JP (1997) Altered seizure patterns after temporal lobectomy. *Epilepsia* **38**:1183–1187.

Blume WT, Girvin JP, McLachlan RS, Gilmore BE (1997) Effective temporal lobectomy in childhood without invasive EEG. *Epilepsia* **38**:164–167.

Blumer D, Wakhlu S, Davies K, Hermann B (1998) Psychiatric outcome of temporal lobectomy for epilepsy: incidence and treatment of psychiatric complications. *Epilepsia* **39**:478–486.

Bouchet, Cazauvieihl (1825) De l'epilepsie consideree dans ses rapportes avec l'alienation mentale. *Archives de General Médecine* 9:510–542.

Breiter SN, Arroyo S, Mathews VP, Lesser RP, Bryan RN, Barker PB (1994) Proton MR spectroscopy in patients with seizure disorders. . *American Journal of Neuroradiology* 15:373–384.

Brockhaus A, Elger CE (1995) Complex partial seizures of temporal lobe origin in children of different age groups. *Epilepsia* 36:1173–1181.

Casazza M, Avanzini G, Ciceri E, Spreafico R, Broggi G (1997) Lesionectomy in epileptogenic temporal lobe lesions: preoperative seizure course and postoperative outcome. *Acta Neurochirurgica Supplementum* 68:64–69.

Cascino GD (1997) Structural brain imaging. In: Engel J, Pedley TA (eds) *Epilepsy: A Comprehensive Textbook*, pp 937–946. Philadelphia: Lippincott-Raven.

Cascino GD, Kelly PJ, Hirschorn KA, Marsh WR, Sharbrough FW (1990) Stereotactic resection of intra-axial cerebral lesions in partial epilepsy. *Mayo Clinic Proceedings* 65:1053–1060.

Cascino GD, Jack CRJ, Parisi JE *et al* (1992a) MRI in the presurgical evaluation of patients with frontal lobe epilepsy and children with temporal lobe epilepsy: pathologic correlation and prognostic importance. *Epilepsy Research* 11:51–59.

Cascino GD, Kelly PJ, Sharbrough FW, Hulihan JF, Hirschorn KA, Trenerry MR (1992b) Long-term follow-up of stereotactic lesionectomy in partial epilepsy: predictive factors and electroencephalographic results. *Epilepsia* 33:639–644.

Cascino GD, Jack CR, Jr, Parisi JE *et al* (1993a) Operative strategy in patients with MRI-identified dual pathology and temporal lobe epilepsy. *Epilepsy Research* 14:175–182.

Cascino GD, Jack CR Jr, Parisi JE, *et al* (1993b) Operative strategy in patients with MRI-identified dual pathology and temporal lobe epilepsy. *Epilepsy Research* 2:175–182.

Cascino GD, Trenerry MR, Jack CR Jr *et al* (1995) Electrocorticography and temporal lobe epilepsy: relationship to quantitative MRI and operative outcome. *Epilepsia* 36:692–696.

Cendes F, Cook MJ, Watson C *et al* (1995) Frequency and characteristics of dual pathology in patients with lesional epilepsy. *Neurology* 45:2058–2064.

Cendes F, Dubeau F, Andermann F *et al* (1996) Significance of mesial temporal atrophy in relation to intracranial ictal and interictal stereo EEG abnormalities. *Brain* 119:1317–1326.

Chee MWL, Morris HH, Antar M, Van Ness PC, Dinner DS (1991) Concordant interictal temporal spikes and FDG-PET hypometabolism can accurately lateralise the epileptogenic focus in temporal lobe epilepsy. *Epilepsia* 32:S103.

Chelune GJ, Naugle RI, Hermann BP *et al* (1998) Does presurgical IQ predict seizure outcome after temporal lobectomy? Evidence from the Bozeman Epilepsy Consortium. *Epilepsia* 39:314–318.

Chugani HT, Da Silva E, Chugani DC (1996) Infantile spasms: III. Prognostic implications of bitemporal hypometabolism on positron emission tomography. *Annals Neurology* 39:643–649.

Dasheiff RM, Shelton J, Ryan C (1993) Memory performance during the Amytal test in patients with non-temporal lobe epilepsy. *Archives of Neurology* 50:701–705.

Daumas-Duport C, Scheithauer BW, Chodkiewicz J-P, Laws ER, Vedrenne C (1988) Dysembryoplastic neuroepithelial tumor: a surgically curable tumor of young patients with intractable partial seizures report of thirty-nine cases. *Neurosurgery* 23:545–556.

Davidson S, Falconer MA (1973) Outcome of surgery in 40 children with temporal lobe epilepsy. *Lancet* 1260–1263.

Davies KG, Hermann BP, Wyler AR (1995) Surgery for intractable epilepsy secondary to viral encephalitis. *British Journal of Neurosurgery* 9:759–762.

Davies KG, Hermann BP, Dohan FC Jr, Wyler AR (1996) Intractable epilepsy due to meningitis: results of surgery and pathological findings. *British Journal of Neurosurgery* 10:567–570.

Davies KG, Bell BD, Bush AJ, Hermann BP, Dohan FC Jr, Jaap AS (1998) Naming decline after left anterior temporal lobectomy correlates with pathological status of resected hippocampus. *Epilepsia* 39:407–419.

Debets RM, Sadzot B, van Isselt JW *et al* (1997) Is ^{11}C-flumazenil PET superior to [18]FDG PET and ^{123}I-iomazenil SPECT in presurgical evaluation of temporal lobe epilepsy? *Journal of Neurology, Neurosurgery and Psychiatry* 62:141–150.

Dodrill CB, Hermann BP, Rausch R, Chelune G, Oxbury S (1993) Neuropsychological testing for assessing prognosis following epilepsy surgery. In: Engel J (ed) *Surgical Treatment of the Epilepsies*, 2nd edn, pp 263–271. New York: Raven Press.

Duncan R, Patterson J, Roberts R, Hadley DM, Bone I (1993) Ictal/postictal SPECT in the pre-surgical localisation of complex partial seizures. *Journal of Neurology, Neurosurgery and Psychiatry* 56:141–148.

Ebersole JS, Pacia SV (1996) Localization of temporal lobe foci by ictal EEG patterns. *Epilepsia* 37:386–399.

Elwes RD, Dunn G, Binnie CD, Polkey CE (1991) Outcome following resective surgery for temporal lobe epilepsy: a prospective follow up study of 102 consecutive cases. *Journal of Neurology, Neurosurgery and Psychiatry* 54:949–952.

Elwes RD, Sawhney IMS, Binnie CD, Polkey CE (1993) Lateralised ictal automatisms during complex partial seizures. *Epilepsia* 34:S181.

Engel J (1987) Outcome with respect to epileptic seizures. In: Engel J (ed) *Surgical Treatment of the Epilepsies*, pp 553–571. New York: Raven Press.

Engel J (1993) Appendix II Presurgical evaluation protocols. In: Engel J(ed) *Surgical Treatment of the Epilepsies*, 2nd edn, pp 707–754. New York: Raven Press.

Engel J Jr, Ojemann GA (1993) The next step. In: Engel J (ed) *Surgical Treatment of the Epilepsies*, 2nd edn, pp 319–329. New York: Raven Press.

Engel J, Henry TR, Risinger MW *et al* (1990) Presurgical evaluation for partial epilepsy: relative contributions of chronic depth-electrode recordings vs FDG-PET and scalp-sphenoidal ictal EEG. *Neurology* 40:1670–1677.

Engel J, Van Ness PC, Rasmussen T, Ojemann LM (1993) Outcome with respect to epileptic seizures. In: Engel J. (ed) *Surgical Treatment of the Epilepsies*, 2nd edn, pp 609–622. New York: Raven Press.

Falconer MA (1971a) Genetic and related aetiological factors in temporal lobe epilepsy. *Epilepsia* 12:13–31.

Falconer MA (1971b) Anterior temporal lobectomy for epilepsy. In: Logue V (ed) *Operative Surgery*, Vol 14 *Neurosurgery*, pp 142–149. London: Butterworths.

Falconer MA (1973) Reversibility by temporal lobe resection of the behavioural abnormalities of temporal lobe epilepsy. *New England Journal of Medicine* 289:451–455.

Falconer MA, Kennedy WA (1961) Epilepsy due to small focal temporal lesions with bilateral independent spike-discharging foci. A study of seven cases relieved by operation. *Journal of Neurology, Neurosurgery and Psychiatry* 24:205–212.

Falconer MA, Wilson JL (1958) Visual field changes following anterior temporal lobectomy: their significance in relation to 'Meyer's loop' of the optic radiation. *Brain* 81:1–14.

Falconer MA, Driver MV, Serafetidines EA (1962) Temporal lobe epilepsy due to distant lesions: two cases relieved by operation. *Brain* 85:521–534.

Feindel W, Rasmussen T (1991) Temporal lobectomy with amygdalectomy and minimal hippocampal resection: review of 100 cases. *Canadian Journal of Neurological Sciences* 18:603–605.

Fenton DS, Geremia GK, Dowd AM, Papathanasiou MA, Greenlee WM, Huckman MS (1997) Precise placement of sphenoidal electrodes via fluoroscopic guidance. *American Journal of Neuroradiology* 18:776–778.

Ferguson SM, Rayport M (1988) A multidimensional approach to the understanding and management of behavior disturbance in epilepsy. In: Howells, JG (ed) *Modern Perspectives in Clinical Psychiatry*, pp 302–330. New York: Brunner/Mazel.

Fish DR, Smith SJ, Quesney LF, Andermann F, Rasmussen T (1993) Surgical treatment of children with medically intractable frontal or temporal lobe epilepsy: results and highlights of 40 years' experience. *Epilepsia* **34**:244–247.

Fisher RS, Uthman BM, Ramsay RE *et al* (1993) Alternative surgical techniques for epilepsy. In: Engel J (ed) *Surgical Treatment of the Epilepsies*, 2nd edn, pp 549–564. New York: Raven Press.

Foldvary N, Lee N, Thwaites G *et al* (1997) Clinical and electrographic manifestations of lesional neocortical temporal lobe epilepsy. *Neurology* **49**:757–763.

Fraser RT, Gumnit RJ, Thorbecke R, Dobkin BH (1993) Psychosocial rehabilitation: a pre- and postoperative assessment. In: Engel J (ed) *Surgical Treatment of the Epilepsies*, 2nd edn, pp 669–677. New York: Raven Press.

Fried I, Spencer DD, Spencer SS (1995) The anatomy of epileptic auras: focal pathology and surgical outcome. *Journal of Neurosurgery* **83**:60–66.

Germano IM, Poulin N, Olivier A (1994) Reoperation for recurrent temporal lobe epilepsy. *Journal Neurosurgery* **81**:31–36.

Ghika-Schmid F, Assal G, de Tribolet N, Regli F (1995) Kluver–Bucy syndrome after left anterior temporal resection. *Neuropsychologia* **33**:101–113.

Gil-Nagel A, Risinger MW (1997) Ictal semiology in hippocampal versus extrahippocampal temporal lobe epilepsy. *Brain* **120**:183–192.

Goldstein LH, Polkey CE (1992) Everyday memory after unilateral temporal lobectomy or amygdalo-hippocampectomy. *Cortex* **28**:189–201.

Goldstein LH, Polkey CE (1993) Short-term cognitive changes after unilateral temporal lobectomy or unilateral amygdalo-hippocampectomy for the relief of temporal lobe epilepsy. *Journal of Neurology, Neurosurgery and Psychiatry* **56**:135–140.

Goldstein R, Harvey AS, Duchowny M *et al* (1996) Preoperative clinical, EEG, and imaging findings do not predict seizure outcome following temporal lobectomy in childhood. *Journal of Child Neurology* **11**:445–450.

Goncalves-Ferreira A, Miguens J, Farias JP, Melancia JL, Andrade M (1994) Selective amygdalohippocampectomy: which route is the best? An experimental study in 80 human cerebral hemispheres. *Stereotactic and Functional Neurosurgery* **63**:182–191.

Guldvog B, Loyning Y, Hauglie-Hanssen E, Flood S, Bjornaes H (1991) Surgical versus medical treatment for epilepsy. II. Outcome related to social areas. *Epilepsia* **32**:477–486.

Hardiman O, Burke T, Phillips J *et al* (1988) Microdysgenesis in resected temporal neocortex: Incidence and clinical significance in focal epilepsy. *Neurology* **38**:1041–1047.

Hefner G, Elger CE, Burr W, Hufnagel A, Zentner J, Schramm J (1993) Psychosocial and psychiatric outcome after temporal lobe resections in epileptic patients. *Epilepsia* **34**:S67(Abstract).

Heikkinen ER, Heikkinen MI, Sotaniemi K (1992) Stereotactic radiotherapy instead of conventional epilepsy surgery. A case report. *Acta Neurochirurgica Wien* **119**:159–160.

Helmstaedter C, Elger CE (1996) Cognitive consequences of two-thirds anterior temporal lobectomy on verbal memory in 144 patients: a three-month follow-up study. *Epilepsia* **37**:171–180.

Helmstaedter C, Elger CE (1998) Functional plasticity after left anterior temporal lobectomy: reconstitution and compensation of verbal memory functions. *Epilepsia* **39**:399–406.

Henry TR, Drury I (1997) Non-epileptic seizures in temporal lobectomy candidates with medically refractory seizures [see comments]. *Neurology* **48**:1374–1382.

Ho SS, Berkovic SF, McKay WJ, Kalnins RM, Bladin PF (1996) Temporal lobe epilepsy subtypes: differential patterns of cerebral perfusion on ictal SPECT. *Epilepsia* **37**:788–795.

Ho SS, Newton MR, McIntosh AM *et al* (1997) Perfusion patterns during temporal lobe seizures: relationship to surgical outcome. *Brain* **120**:1921–1928.

Ho SS, Kuzniecky RI, Gilliam F, Faught E, Morawetz R (1998) Temporal lobe developmental malformations and epilepsy: dual pathology and bilateral hippocampal abnormalities. *Neurology* **50**:748–754.

Holmes MD, Dodrill CB, Ojemann LM, Ojemann GA (1996) Five-year outcome after epilepsy surgery in nonmonitored and monitored surgical candidates. *Epilepsia* **37**:748–752.

Holmes MD, Dodrill CB, Ojemann GA, Wilensky AJ, Ojemann LM (1997) Outcome following surgery in patients with bitemporal interictal epileptiform patterns. *Neurology* **48**:1037–1040.

Hufnagel A, Poersch M, Elger CE, Zentner J, Wolf HK, Schramm J (1995) The clinical and prognostic relevance of the postictal slow focus in the electrocorticogram. *Electroencephalography and Clinical Neurophysiology* **94**:12–18.

Hugg JW, Kuzniecky RI, Gilliam FG, Morawetz RB, Fraught RE, Hetherington HP (1996) Normalization of contralateral metabolic function following temporal lobectomy demonstrated by ^{1}H magnetic resonance spectroscopic imaging. *Annals of Neurology* **40**:236–239.

Jack CR, Nichols DA, Sharbrough FW, Marsh WR, Petersen RC (1988) Selective posterior cerebral amytal test for evaluating memory function before surgery for temporal lobe seizure. *Radiology* **168**:787–793.

Jack CRJ, Sharbrough FW, Cascino GD, Hirschorn KA, O'Brien PC, Marsh WR (1992) Magnetic resonance image-based hippocampal volumetry: correlation with outcome after temporal lobectomy. *Annals of Neurology* **31**:138–146.

Jackson GD, Berkovic SF, Tress BM, Kalnins RM, Fabinyi GC, Bladin PF (1990) Hippocampal sclerosis can be reliably detected by magnetic resonance imaging. *Neurology* **40**:1869–1875.

Jacobson DM, Warner JJ, Ruggles KH (1995) Transient trochlear nerve palsy following anterior temporal lobectomy for epilepsy. *Neurology* **45**:1465–1468.

Jay V, Becker LE, Otsubo H, Hwang PA, Hoffman HJ, Harwood-Nash D (1993) Pathology of temporal lobectomy for refractory seizures in children. Review of 20 cases including some unique malformative lesions. *Journal of Neurosurgery* **79**:53–61.

Jensen I (1975a) Temporal lobe epilepsy. Late mortality in patients treated with unilateral temporal lobe resections. *Acta Neurologica Scandinavica* **52**:374–380.

Jensen I (1975b) Temporal lobe surgery around the world. Results, complications, mortality. *Acta Neurologica Scandinavica* **52**:354–373.

Jensen I (1976) Temporal lobe epilepsy: Social conditions and rehabilitation after surgery. *Acta Neurologica Scandinavica* **54**:22–44.

Jensen I, Larsen JK (1979) Mental aspects of temporal lobe epilepsy: follow-up of 74 patients after resection of a temporal lobe. *Journal of Neurology, Neurosurgery and Psychiatry* **42**:256–265.

Jones-Gotman M, Zatorre RJ, Olivier A *et al* (1997) Learning and retention of words and designs following excision from medial or lateral temporal-lobe structures. *Neuropsychologia* **35**:963–973.

Kanner AM, Jones JC (1997) When do sphenoidal electrodes yield additional data to that obtained with antero-temporal electrodes? *Electroencephalography and Clinical Neurophysiology* **102**:12–19.

Kanner AM, Kaydanova Y, de Toledo-Morrell L *et al* (1995) Tailored anterior temporal lobectomy. Relation between extent of resection of mesial structures and postsurgical seizure outcome. *Archives of Neurology* **52**:173–178.

Katz A, Awad IA, Kong AK *et al* (1989) Extent of resection in temporal lobectomy for epilepsy. II. Memory changes and neurologic complications. *Epilepsia* **30**:763–771.

Kellett MW, Smith DF, Baker GA, Chadwick DW (1997) Quality of life after epilepsy surgery. *Journal of Neurology, Neurosurgery and Psychiatry* **63**:52–58.

Kim JH, Tien RD, Felsberg GJ, Osumi AK, Lee N (1995a) Clinical significance of asymmetry of the fornix and mamillary body on MR in hippocampal sclerosis. AJNR. *American Journal of Neuroradiology* **16**:509–515.

Kim JH, Tien RD, Felsberg GJ, Osumi AK, Lee N, Friedman AH (1995b) Fast spin-echo MR in hippocampal sclerosis: correlation with pathology and surgery. AJNR. *American Journal of Neuroradiology* **16**:627–636.

King D, Spencer SS, McCarthy G, Luby M, Spencer DD (1995) Bilateral hippocampal atrophy in medial temporal lobe epilepsy. *Epilepsia* **36**:905–910.

King D, Spencer SS, McCarthy G, Spencer DD (1997a) Surface and depth EEG findings in patients with hippocampal atrophy. *Neurology* **48**:1363–1367.

King JT, Jr Sperling MR, Justice AC, O'Connor MJ (1997b) A cost-effectiveness analysis of anterior temporal lobectomy for intractable temporal lobe epilepsy. *Journal of Neurosurgery* **87**:20–28.

Kirkpatrick PJ, Honavar M, Janota I, Polkey CE (1993) Control of temporal lobe epilepsy following en bloc resection of low grade gliomas. *Journal of Neurosurgery* **78**:19–25.

Koike A, Shimizu H, Suzuki I, Ishijima B, Sugishita M (1996) Preserved musical abilities following right temporal lobectomy. *Journal of Neurosurgery* **85**:1000–1004.

Kotagal P, Luders H, Morris HH *et al* (1989) Dystonic posturing in partial complex seizures of temporal lobe onset: a new lateralising sign. *Neurology* **39**:196–201.

Kratimenos GP, Pell MF, Thomas DG, Shorvon SD, Fish DR, Smith SJ (1992) Open stereotactic selective amygdalo-hippocampectomy for drug resistant epilepsy. *Acta Neurochirurgica Wien* **116**:150–154.

Krauss GL, Fisher R, Plate C *et al* (1996) Cognitive effects of resecting basal temporal language areas. *Epilepsia* **37**:476–483.

Kuzniecky R, Faught E, Morawetz R (1990) Surgical treatment of epilepsy: initial results based upon epidural electroencephalographic recordings. *Southern Medical Journal* **83**:637–639.

Kuzniecky R, Elgavish GA, Hetherington HP, Evanochko WT, Pohost GM (1992) In vivo ^{31}P nuclear magnetic resonance spectroscopy of human temporal lobe epilepsy. *Neurology* **42**:1586–1590.

Kuzniecky R, Murro A, King D *et al* (1993) Magnetic resonance imaging in childhood intractable partial epilepsies: pathologic correlations. *Neurology* **43**:681–687.

Kuzniecky RI, Bilir E, Gilliam F *et al* (1997) Multimodality MRI in mesial temporal sclerosis: relative sensitivity and specificity. *Neurology* **49**:774–778.

Lamusuo S, Ruottinen HM, Knuuti J *et al* (1997) Comparison of [^{18}F] FDG-PET, [^{99m}Tc]-HMPAO-SPECT, and [^{123}I]-iomazenil-SPECT in localising the epileptogenic cortex. *Journal of Neurology, Neurosurgery, and Psychiatry* **63**:743–748.

Lancman ME, Morris HH 3rd (1996) Epilepsy after central nervous system infection: clinical characteristics and outcome after epilepsy surgery. *Epilepsy Research* **25**:285–290.

Lancman ME, Benbadis S, Geller E, Morris HH (1998) Sensitivity and specificity of asymmetric recall on WADA test to predict outcome after temporal lobectomy. *Neurology* **50**:455–459.

Laxer KD (1997) Clinical applications of magnetic resonance spectroscopy [Review]. *Epilepsia* **38** (Suppl 4):S13–17.

Lee DH, Gao FQ, Rogers JM *et al* (1998) MR in temporal lobe epilepsy: analysis with pathologic confirmation. *American Journal of Neuroradiology* **19**:19–27.

Lee GP, Loring DW, Smith JR, Flanigin HF (1995a) Intraoperative hippocampal cooling and Wada memory testing in the evaluation of amnesia risk following anterior temporal lobectomy. *Archives of Neurology* **52**:857–861.

Lee GP, Smith JR, Loring DW, Flanigin HF (1995b) Intraoperative

thermal inactivation of the hippocampus in an effort to prevent global amnesia after temporal lobectomy. *Epilepsia* **36**:892–898.

Lee N, Tien RD, Lewis DV *et al* (1995) Fast spin-echo, magnetic resonance imaging-measured hippocampal volume: correlation with neuronal density in anterior temporal lobectomy patients. *Epilepsia* **36**:899–904.

Lehericy S, Semah F, Hasboun D *et al* (1997) Temporal lobe epilepsy with varying severity: MRI study of 222 patients. *Neuroradiology* **39**:788–796.

Lellouch-Tubiana A, Bourgeois M, Vekemans M, Robain O (1995) Dysembryoplastic neuroepithelial tumors in two children with neurofibromatosis type 1. *Acta Neuropathologica* **90**:319–322.

Levesque MF, Nakasato N, Vinters HV, Babb TL (1991) Surgical treatment of limbic epilepsy associated with extrahippocampal lesions: the problem of dual pathology. *Journal of Neurosurgery* **75**:364–370.

Li LM, Dubeau F, Andermann F *et al* (1997) Periventricular nodular heterotopia and intractable temporal lobe epilepsy: poor outcome after temporal lobe resection. *Annals of Neurology* **41**:662–668.

Lieb JP, Rausch R, Engel J (1982) Changes in intelligence following temporal lobectomy: relationship to EEG activity, seizure relief and pathology. *Epilepsia* **23**:1–13.

Lombardi D, Marsh R, de Tribolet N (1997) Low grade glioma in intractable epilepsy: lesionectomy versus epilepsy surgery. *Acta Neurochirurgica Supplementum* **68**:70–74.

Luders H, Awad IA (1992) Conceptual considerations. In: Luders H (ed) *Epilepsy Surgery*, pp 51–62. New York: Raven Press.

Mace CJ, Trimble MR (1991) Psychosis following temporal lobe surgery: a report of six cases. *Journal of Neurology, Neurosurgery and Psychiatry* **54**:639–644.

Malmgren K, Sullivan M, Ekstedt G, Kullberg G, Kumlien E (1997) Health-related quality of life after epilepsy surgery: a Swedish multicenter study. *Epilepsia* **38**:830–838.

Manchanda R, Schaefer B, McLachlan RS *et al* (1996) Psychiatric disorders in candidates for surgery for epilepsy. *Journal of Neurology, Neurosurgery and Psychiatry* **61**:82–89.

Margerison JH, Corsellis JAN (1996) Epilepsy and the temporal lobes. A clinical, electroencephalographic and neuropathological study of the brain in epilepsy, with particular reference to the temporal lobes. *Brain* **89**:499–534.

Martin RC, Sawrie SM, Roth DL *et al* (1998) Individual memory change after anterior temporal lobectomy: a base rate analysis using regression-based outcome methodology. *Epilepsia* **39**:1075–1082.

Masada T, Itano T, Fujisawa M *et al* (1996) Protective effect of vagus nerve stimulation on forebrain ischaemia in gerbil hippocampus. *Neuroreport* **7**:446–448.

Mathern GW, Babb TL, Vickrey BG, Melendez M, Pretorius JK (1995) The clinical-pathogenic mechanisms of hippocampal neuron loss and surgical outcomes in temporal lobe epilepsy. *Brain* Pt 1, 105–118.

McLachlan RS, Chovaz CJ, Blume WT, Girvin JP (1992) Temporal lobectomy for intractable epilepsy in patients over age 45 years. *Neurology* **42**:662–665.

McLachlan RS, Rose KJ, Derry PA, Bonnar C, Blume WT, Girvin JP (1997) Health-related quality of life and seizure control in temporal lobe epilepsy. *Annals of Neurology* **41**:482–489.

McMillan T, Powell GE, Janota I, Polkey CE (1987) Relationship between neuropathology and cognitive functioning in temporal lobe patients. *Journal of Neurology, Neurosurgery and Psychiatry* **50**:167–176.

Mempel E, Witkiewicz B, Stadnicki R *et al* (1980) The effect of medial amygdalotomy and anterior hippocampectomy on behavior and seizures in epileptic patients. *Acta Neurochirurgica Supplementum Wien* **30**:161–167.

Meyer A, Falconer MA, Beck C (1954) Pathological findings in temporal lobe epilepsy. *Journal of Neurology, Neurosurgery and Psychiatry* **17**:276–285.

Milner B (1958) Psychological defects produced by temporal lobe excision. *Research Publication of the Association for Research in Nervous and Mental Disease* 36:244–257.

Milner B, Branch C, Rasmussen T (1962) Study of short-term memory after the intracarotid injection of sodium Amytal. *Transactions of the American Neurological Association* 87:224–226.

Morris HH, Matkovic Z, Estes ML *et al* (1998) Ganglioglioma and intractable epilepsy: clinical and neurophysiologic features and predictors of outcome after surgery. *Epilepsia* 39:307–313.

Mundinger F, Becker P, Grolkner E (1976) Late results of stereotactic surgery of epilepsy predominantly temporal lobe type. *Acta Neurochirurgica* S23:177–182.

Nakasato N, Levesque MF, Babb TL (1992) Seizure outcome following standard temporal lobectomy: correlation with hippocampal neuron loss and extrahippocampal pathology. *Journal of Neurosurgery* 77:194–200.

Narabayashi H (1979) Long range results of medial amygdalotomy on epileptic traits in adult patients. In: Rasmussen T, Marino R (eds) *Functional Neurosurgery*, pp. 243–252. New York: Raven Press.

Narabayashi H, Shima F (1973) Which is the better amygdalar target, the medial or lateral nuclei? (For behaviour problems and paroxysms in epileptics). In: Laitinen LV, Livingstone KE (eds) *Surgical Approaches in Psychiatry*, pp 129–134. Lancaster: MTP.

Nayel MH, Awad IA, Luders H (1991) Extent of mesiobasal resection determines outcome after temporal lobectomy for intractable complex partial seizures. *Neurosurgery* 29:55–60.

Naylor AS, a Rogvi-Hansen B, Kessing LV, Kruse-Larsen C, Bolwig TG, Dam M (1995) Psychiatric morbidity in connection with surgical treatment of epilepsy. A short-term follow-up of patients with amygdalohippocampectomy [in Danish]. *Ugeskrift for Laeger* 157:5245–5250.

Ney GC, Barr WB, Napolitano C, Decker R, Schaul N (1998) New-onset psychogenic seizures after surgery for epilepsy. *Archives of Neurology* 55:726–730.

Niemeyer P (1958) The transventricular amygdala-hippocampectomy in temporal lobe epilepsy. In: Baldwin M, Bailey P (eds) *Temporal Lobe Epilepsy*, pp. 461–482. Springfield: Charles C. Thomas.

Novelly RA, Augustine EM, Mattson RH (1984) Selective memory improvement and impairment in temporal lobectomy for epilepsy. *Annals of Neurology* 15:64–67.

Ojemann GA, Dodrill CB (1985) Verbal memory deficits after left temporal lobectomy for epilepsy: mechanism and intraoperative prediction. *Journal of Neurosurgery* 62:101–107.

Olivier A (1987) Commentary: Cortical resections. In: Engel J (ed) *Surgical Treatment of the Epilepsies*, pp 405–416. New York: Raven Press.

Olivier A (1991) Relevance of removal of limbic structures in surgery for temporal lobe epilepsy. *Canadian Journal of Neurological Sciences* 18:628–635.

Olivier A, Andermann F, Palmini A, Robitaille Y (1996) Surgical treatment of the cortical dysplasias. In: Guerrini R, Andermann F, Canapicchi R, Roger J, Zifkin BG, Pfanner P (eds) *Dysplasias of the Cerebral Cortex and Epilepsy*, pp 351–366. Philadelphia: Lippincott-Raven.

Oppenheim C, Dormont D, Biondi A (1998) Loss of digitations of the hippocampal head on high-resolution fast spin-echo MR: a sign of mesial temporal sclerosis. *American Journal of Neuroradiology* 19:457–463.

Ounsted C, Lindsay J, Norman J (1966) *Biological Factors in Temporal Lobe Epilepsy.* London: Heinemann.

Ounsted C, Lindsay J, Richards P (1987) *Temporal Lobe Epilepsy. A Biographical Study 1948–1986.* Oxford: Blackwell Scientific.

Oxbury S, Oxbury J, Renowden S, Squier W, Carpenter K. Severe amnesia: usual late complication after temporal lobectomy. *Neuropsychologia* 1997, 35:975–988.

Palmini A, Gambardella A, Andermann F *et al* (1996) Outcome of

surgical treatment in patients with localized cortical dysplasia and intractable epilepsy. In: Guerrini R, Andermann F, Canapicchi R, Roger J, Zifkin BG, Pfanner P (eds) *Dysplasias of the Cerebral Cortex and Epilepsy*, pp 367–374. Philadelphia: Lippincott-Raven.

Park TS, Bourgeois BF, Silbergeld DL, Dodson WE (1996) Subtemporal transparahippocampal amygdalohippocampectomy for surgical treatment of mesial temporal lobe epilepsy. Technical note. *Journal of Neurosurgery* 85:1172–1176.

Patil AA, Andrews R, Torkelson R (1995) Stereotactic volumetric radiofrequency lesioning of intracranial structures for control of intractable seizures. *Stereotactic and Functional Neurosurgery* 64:123–133.

Patrick S, Berg A, Spencer SS (1995) EEG and seizure outcome after epilepsy surgery. *Epilepsia* 36:236–240.

Penfield W, Jasper H (1954) *Epilepsy and the Functional Anatomy of the Human Brain.* Boston: Little, Brown.

Penfield W, Paine K (1955) Results of surgical therapy for focal epileptic seizures. *Canadian Medical Association Journal* 73:515–530.

Penfield W, Lende RA, Rasmussen T (1961) Manipulation hemiplegia, an untoward complication in the surgery of focal epilepsy. *Journal of Neurosurgery* 18:769–776.

Perrine K, Westerveld M, Sass KJ *et al* (1995) Wada memory disparities predict seizure laterality and postoperative seizure control. *Epilepsia* 36:851–856.

Pilcher WH, Roberts DW, Flanigin HF *et al* (1993) Complications of epilepsy surgery. In: Engel J (ed) *Surgical Treatment of the Epilepsies*, 2nd edn, pp. 565–581. New York: Raven Press.

Polkey CE (1994) Epilepsy surgery: non-invasive versus invasive focus localization. What is needed from the neurosurgical point of view. *Acta Neurologica Scandinavica Supplementum* 152:183–186.

Polkey CE (2000) Amygdalo-hippocampectomy for drug-resistant temporal lobe epilepsy. In: Schmidek HH, Sweet WH (eds) *Operative Neurosurgical Techniques. Indications, Methods, Results*, 4th edn, in press. Philadelphia: Saunders.

Polkey CE, Scarano P (1993) The durability of the result of anterior temporal lobectomy for epilepsy. *Journal of Neurosurgical Sciences* 37:141–148.

Polkey CE, Binnie CD, Janota I (1989) Acute hippocampal recording and pathology at temporal lobe resection and amygdalo-hippocampectomy for epilepsy. *Journal of Neurology, Neurosurgery and Psychiatry* 52:1050–1057.

Powell GE, Polkey CE, McMillan TM (1985) The new Maudsley series of temporal lobectomy I: Short term cognitive effects. *British Journal of Clinical Psychology* 24:109–124.

Powell GE, Polkey CE, Canavan AGM (1987) Lateralisation of memory function in epileptic patients by the use of the sodium amytal (WADA) technique. *Journal of Neurology, Neurosurgery and Psychiatry* 50:665–672.

Prayson RA, Estes ML, Morris HH (1993) Coexistence of neoplasia and cortical dysplasia in patients presenting with seizures. *Epilepsia* 34:609–615.

Prayson RA, Reith JD, Najm IM (1996) Mesial temporal sclerosis. A clinicopathologic study of 27 patients, including 5 with coexistent cortical dysplasia. *Archives of Pathology and Laboratory Medicine* 120:532–536.

Privitera M, Kohler C, Cahill W, Yeh HS (1996) Postictal language dysfunction in patients with right or bilateral hemispheric language localization. *Epilepsia* 37:936–941.

Quigg M, Bertram EH, Jackson T (1997) Longitudinal distribution of hippocampal atrophy in mesial temporal lobe epilepsy. *Epilepsy Research* 27:101–110.

Rausch R, Silfvenius H, Wieser HG, Dodrill CB, Meador KJ, Jones-Gotman M (1993) Intraarterial amobarbital procedures. In: Engel J (ed) *Surgical Treatment of the Epilepsies*, 2nd edn, pp 341–358. New York: Raven Press.

Raymond AA, Halpin SF, Alsanjari N *et al* (1994) Dysembryoplastic neuroepithelial tumor. Features in 16 patients. *Brain* **117**:461–475.

Raymond AA, Fish DR, Sisodiya SM, Alsanjari N, Stevens JM, Shorvon SD (1995) Abnormalities of gyration, heterotopias, tuberous sclerosis, focal cortical dysplasia, microdysgenesis, dysembryoplastic neuroepithelial tumour and dysgenesis of the archicortex in epilepsy. Clinical, EEG and neuroimaging features in 100 adult patients. [Review]. *Brain* **118**:629–660.

Reeves AL, So EL, Evans RW, Cascino GD *et al* (1997) Factors associated with work outcome after anterior temporal lobectomy for intractable epilepsy. *Epilepsia* **38**:689–695.

Regis J, Peragui JC, Rey M *et al* (1995) First selective amygdalohippocampal radiosurgery for 'mesial temporal lobe epilepsy'. *Stereotactic and Functional Neurosurgery* **64**(suppl 1):193–201.

Renella RR (1989a) Outcome of surgery. In: *Microsurgery of the Temporal Region*, pp 158–164. Wien: Springer-Verlag.

Renella RR (1989b) *Microsurgery of the Temporo-Medial Region*. Wien: Springer-Verlag.

Renowden SA, Matkovic Z, Adams CB (1995) Selective amygdalohippocampectomy for hippocampal sclerosis: postoperative MR appearance. *American Journal of Neuroradiology* **16**:1855–1861.

Rose KJ, Derry PA, Wiebe S, McLachlan RS (1996) Determinants of health-related quality of life after temporal lobe epilepsy surgery. *Quality of Life Research* **5**:395–402.

Rougier A, Dartigues J-F, Commenges D, Claverie B, Loiseau P, Cohadon F (1992) A longitudinal assessment of seizure outcome and overall benefit from 100 corticectomies for epilepsy. *Journal of Neurology, Neurosurgery and Psychiatry* **55**:762–767.

Rowe CC, Berkovic SF, Sia STB *et al* (1989) Localisation of epileptic foci with postictal single photon emission computed tomography. *Annals of Neurology* **26**:660–668.

Rowe CC, Berkovic SF, Austin MC, McKay WJ, Bladin PF (1991a) Patterns of postictal cerebral blood flow in temporal lobe epilepsy: qualitative and quantitative analysis. *Neurology* **41**:1096–1103.

Rowe CC, Berkovic SF, Austin MC *et al* (1991b) Visual and quantative analysis of interictal SPECT with technetium-99m-HMPAO in temporal lobe epilepsy. *Journal of Nuclear Medicine* **32**:1688–1694.

Schaller C, Zentner J (1998) Vasospastic reactions in response to the transsylvian approach. *Surgical Neurology* **49**:170–175.

Schuler P, Neubauer U, Schulemann H, Stefan H (1993) Brain-stem lesions in the course of a presurgical re-evaluation by foramen-ovale electrodes in temporal lobe epilepsy. *Electroencephalography and Clinical Neurophysiology* **86**:301–302.

Schulz R, Ebner A, Schuller M *et al* (1995) Analysis of postoperative seizure recurrence after 65 temporal lobe partial resections [in German]. *Nervenarzt* **66**:901–906.

Schwartz TH, Bazil CW, Walczak TS, Chan S, Pedley TA, Goodman RR (1997) The predictive value of intraoperative electrocorticography in resections for limbic epilepsy associated with mesial temporal sclerosis. *Neurosurgery* **40**:302–309; discussion 309–311.

Scoville WB, Milner B (1957) Loss of recent memory after bilateral hippocampal lesions. *Journal of Neurology, Neurosurgery and Psychiatry* **20**:11–21.

Seidenberg M, Hermann BP, Schoenfeld J, Davies K, Wyler A, Dohan FC (1997) Reorganization of verbal memory function in early onset left temporal lobe epilepsy. *Brain and Cognition* **35**:132–148.

Serafetinides EA, Falconer MA (1962) The effects of temporal lobectomy in epileptic patients with psychosis. *Journal of Mental Science* **108**:584–593.

Serafetinides EA, Falconer MA (1963) Speech disturbances in temporal lobe seizures: a study in 100 epileptic patients submitted to anterior temporal lobectomy. *Brain* **86**:333–346.

Siegel AM, Wieser HG, Wichmann W, Yasargil MG (1990) Relationship between MR-imaged total amount of tissue removed, resection scores

of specific mediobasal limbic subcompartments and clinical outcome following selective amygdalo-hippocampectomy. *Epilepsy Research* **6**:56–65.

Siegfried J, Wieser HG, Stodieck SRG (1985) Foramen ovale electrodes: A new technique enabling presurgical evaluation of patients with mesiobasal temporal lobe seizures. *Applied Neurophysiology* **48**:408–417.

Silbergeld DL, Ojemann GA (1993) The tailored temporal lobectomy. *Neurosurgery Clinics of North America* **4**:273–281.

Sirven JI, Sperling MR, French JA, O'Connor MJ (1996) Significance of simple partial seizures in temporal lobe epilepsy. *Epilepsia* **37**:450–454.

Sirven JI, Liporace JD, French JA, O'Connor MJ, Sperling MR (1997a) Seizures in temporal lobe epilepsy: I. Reliability of scalp/sphenoidal ictal recording. *Neurology* **48**:1041–1046.

Sirven JI, Malamut BL, Liporace JD, O'Connor MJ, Sperling MR (1997b) Outcome after temporal lobectomy in bilateral temporal lobe epilepsy. *Annals of Neurology* **42**:873–878.

Sisodiya SM, Moran N, Free SL *et al* (1997) Correlation of widespread preoperative magnetic resonance imaging changes with unsuccessful surgery for hippocampal sclerosis. *Annals of Neurology* **41**:490–496.

Smith KA, Spetzler RF (1995) Supratentorial-infraoccipital approach for posteromedial temporal lobe lesions. *Journal of Neurosurgery* **82**:940–944.

So EL, Ruggles KH, Ahmann PA, Trudeau P, Weatherford K (1994) Yield of sphenoidal recording in sleep-deprived outpatients. *Journal of Clinical Neurophysiology* **11**:226–230.

So EL, Radhakrishnan K, Silbert PL, Cascino GD, Sharbrough FW, O'Brien PC (1997) Assessing changes over time in temporal lobectomy: outcome by scoring seizure frequency. *Epilepsy Research* **27**:119–125.

So NK (1992) Depth electrodes studies in mesial temporal epilepsy. In: Luders, H (ed) *Epilepsy Surgery*, pp 371–393. New York: Raven Press.

Specht U, May T, Schulz R *et al* (1997) Cerebellar atrophy and prognosis after temporal lobe resection. *Journal of Neurology, Neurosurgery and Psychiatry* **62**:501–506.

Spencer DD, Ojemann GA (1993) Overview of therapeutic procedures. In: Engel, J (ed) *Surgical Treatment of the Epilepsies*, 2nd edn, pp 455–471. New York: Raven Press.

Spencer DD, Spencer SS, Mattson RH, Williamson PD, Novelly RA (1984) Access to the posterior medial temporal structures in the surgical treatment of temporal lobe epilepsy. *Neurosurgery* **15**:667–671.

Spencer SS (1981) Depth electroencephalography in selection of refractory epilepsy for surgery. *Annals of Neurology* **9**:207–214.

Spencer SS, Spencer DD (1996) Implications of seizure termination location in temporal lobe epilepsy. *Epilepsia* **37**:455–458.

Spencer SS, Spencer DD, Williamson PD, Mattson R (1991) Combined depth and subdural electrode investigation in uncontrolled epilepsy. *Neurology* **40**:74–79.

Spencer SS, So NK, Engel J, Williamson PD, Levesque MF, Spencer DD (1993a) Depth electrodes. In: Engel, J (ed) *Surgical Treatment of the Epilepsies*, 2nd edn, pp 359–376. New York: Raven Press.

Spencer SS, Spencer DD, Berg A (1993b) Predictors of remission one year after resective epilepsy surgery: a multivariate analysis. *Epilepsia* **34**(Suppl 6):27.

Sperling MR, O'Connor MJ (1989) Comparison of depth and subdural electrodes in recording temporal lobe seizures. *Neurology* **39**:1497–1504.

Sperling MR, O'Connor MJ, Saykin AJ (1992) A noninvasive protocol for anterior temporal lobectomy. *Neurology* **42**:416–422.

Sperling MR, Alavi A, Reivich M, French JA, O'Connor MJ (1995a) False lateralization of temporal lobe epilepsy with FDG positron emission tomography. *Epilepsia* **36**:722–727.

Sperling MR, Saykin AJ, Roberts FD, French JA, O'Connor MJ (1995b)

Occupational outcome after temporal lobectomy for refractory epilepsy. *Neurology* **45**:970–977.

Sperling MR, O'Connor MJ, Saykin AJ, Plummer C (1996) Temporal lobectomy for refractory epilepsy. *JAMA* **276**:470–475.

Stagno SJ, Naugle RI, Roca C, Dechman J, Morris H (1993) Neuropsychiatric disorders occurring in patients after surgery for epilepsy. *Epilepsia* **34**:S67 (Abstract).

Talairach J, Bancaud J (1974) Approche nouvelle de la neurochirugie de l'epilepsie. *Neurochirugie* **20**:1–12.

Tanaka T, Yonemasu Y, Olivier A, Andermann F (1989) Clinical analysis of reoperation in cases of complex partial seizures. *Neurological Surgery* **17**:933–937.

Taylor DC (1975) Factors influencing the occurrence of schizophrenia-like psychosis in patients with temporal lobe epilepsy. *Psychological Medicine* **5**:249–254.

Taylor DC (1987) Psychiatric and social issues in measuring the input and outcome of epilepsy surgery. In: Engel J (ed) *Surgical Treatment of the Epilepsies*, pp 485–503. New York: Raven Press.

Taylor DC, Falconer MA (1968) Clinical, socio-economic and psychological changes after temporal lobectomy for epilepsy. *British Journal of Psychiatry* **114**:1247–1261.

Taylor DC, Marsh SM (1977) Implications of long-term follow-up studies in epilepsy: With a note on the cause of death. In: Penry JK (ed) *Epilepsy. The Eighth International Symposium*, pp 27–34. New York: Raven Press.

Taylor DC, Falconer MA, Bruton CJ, Corsellis JAN (1971) Focal dysplasia of the cerebral cortex in epilepsy. *Journal of Neurology, Neurosurgery and Psychiatry* **34**:369–387.

Thadani VM, Williamson PD, Berger R *et al* (1995) Successful epilepsy surgery without intracranial EEG recording: criteria for patient selection. *Epilepsia* **36**:7–15.

Theodore WH, Sato S, Kufta CV, Gaillard WD, Kelley K (1997) FDG-positron emission tomography and invasive EEG: seizure focus detection and surgical outcome. *Epilepsia* **38**:81–86.

Thompson JE, Castillo M, Kwock L, Walters B, Beach R (1998) Usefulness of proton MR spectroscopy in the evaluation of temporal lobe epilepsy. *American Journal of Roentgenology* 771–776.

Toczek MT, Morrell MJ, Silverberg GA, Lowe GM (1996) Cerebellar hemorrhage complicating temporal lobectomy. Report of four cases. *Journal of Neurosurgery* **85**:718–722.

Tran TA, Spencer SS, Marks D, Javidan M, Pacia S, Spencer DD (1995) Significance of spikes recorded on electrocorticography in nonlesional medial temporal lobe epilepsy. *Annals of Neurology* **38**:763–770.

Trenerry MR, Jack CR, Jr, Cascino GD, Sharbrough FW, So EL (1996) Bilateral magnetic resonance imaging-determined hippocampal atrophy and verbal memory before and after temporal lobectomy. *Epilepsia* **37**:526–533.

Vaernet K (1972) Stereotactic amygdalotomy in temporal lobe epilepsy. *Confinia Neurologica* **34**:176–180.

Vajkoczy P, Krakow K, Stodieck S, Pohlmann-Eden B, Schmiedek P (1998) Modified approach for the selective treatment of temporal lobe epilepsy: transsylvian-transcisternal mesial en bloc resection. *Journal of Neurosurgery* **88**:855–862.

Van Buren JM (1987) Complications of surgical procedures in the treatment and diagnosis of epilepsy. In: Engel J (ed) *Surgical Treatment of the Epilepsies*, pp 465–475. New York: Raven Press.

Van Veelen CMW, Debets C, Van Huffelen AC *et al* (1990) Combined use of subdural and intracerebral electrodes in preoperative evaluation of epilepsy. *Neurosurgery* **26**:93–101.

Vickrey BG, Hays RD, Graber J, Rausch R, Engel JJ, Brook RH (1992) A health-related quality of life instrument for patients evaluated for epilepsy surgery. *Medical Care* **30**:299–319.

Vickrey BG, Hays RD, Rausch R *et al* (1995) Outcomes in 248 patients who had diagnostic evaluations for epilepsy surgery. *Lancet* **8988**:1445–1449.

Wada J (1949) A new method for the determination of the side of cerebral speech dominance. A preliminary report on the intra-carotid injection of sodium amytal in man. *Medicine and Biology* **14**:221–222.

Walsh AR, Ojemann GA (1992) Anterior temporal lobectomy for epilepsy. *Clinical Neurosurgery* **38**:535–547.

Weaver JP, Phillips C, Horowitz SL, Benjamin S (1996) Middle fossa cyst presenting as a delayed complication of temporal lobectomy: case report. *Neurosurgery* **38**:1047–1050; discussion 1050–1051.

Wieser HG (1988) Selective amygdalo-hippocampectomy for temporal lobe epilepsy. *Epilepsia* **29**:S100–S113.

Wieser HG (1991) Selective amygdalohippocampectomy: indications and follow-up. *Canadian Journal of Neurological Sciences* **4** (Suppl): 617–627.

Wieser HG, Moser S (1988) Improved multipolar foramen ovale elctrode monitoring. *Journal of Epilepsy* **1**:13–22.

Wieser HG, Siegel AM (1991) Analysis of foramen ovale electrode-recorded seizures and correlation with outcome following amygdalo-hippocampectomy. *Epilepsia* **32**:838–850.

Wieser HG, Yasargil MG (1982) Die 'Selektiv Amygdala-Hippokampektomie' also chirugische Behandlung du medio-basal Limbischen Epilepsie. *Neurochirugia* **25**:39–50.

Wieser HG, Yasargil MG (1984) Selective amygdalohippocampectomy as a surgical treatment of mediobasal limbic epilepsy. *Surgical Neurology* **17**:445–457.

Wieser HG, Valvanis A, Roos A, Isler P, Renella RR (1989) "Selective" and "superselective" temporal lobe Amytal tests: I Neuroradiological, neuroanatomical and electrical data. In: Manelis J (ed) *Advances in Epileptology*, Vol 17, pp 20–27. New York: Raven Press.

Wieser HG, Engel J, Williamson PD, Babb TL, Gloor P (1993) Surgically remediable temporal lobe syndromes. In: Engel J (ed) *Surgical Treatment of the Epilepsies*, 2nd edn, pp. 49–63. New York: Raven Press.

Williamson PD, Wieser HG, Delgado-Escueta AV (1987) Clinical characteristics of partial complex seizures. In: Engel J (ed) *Surgical Treatment of the Epilepsies*, pp 101–120. New York: Raven Press.

Wyler AR, Wilkus RJ, Blume WT (1993) Strip electrodes. In: Engel J (ed) *Surgical Treatment of the Epilepsies*, 2nd edn, pp. 387–397. New York: Raven Press.

Wyler AR, Hermann BP, Somes G (1995) Extent of medial temporal resection on outcome from anterior temporal lobectomy: a randomized prospective study. *Neurosurgery* **37**:982–990; discussion 990–991.

Wyllie E, Luders H, Morris HH (1987) Clinical outcome after complete or partial cortical resection for intractable epilepsy. *Neurology* **37**:1634–1641.

Wyllie E, Chee M, Granstrom ML *et al* (1993) Temporal lobe epilepsy in early childhood. *Epilepsia* **34**:859–868.

Yasargil MG, Teddy PG, Roth P (1985) Selective amygdalo-hippocampectomy. Operative anatomy and surgical technique. In: Symon L (ed) *Advances and Technical Standards in Neurosurgery*, 12th edn, pp. 93–123. Wien: Springer-Verlag.

Yen DJ, Su MS, Yiu CH *et al* (1996) Ictal speech manifestations in temporal lobe epilepsy: a video-EEG study. *Epilepsia* **37**:45–49.

Extratemporal cortical excisions for epilepsy

H SILFVENIUS

In the early practice of epilepsy surgery (ES) extratemporal (ET) structural lesions were often excised after peroperative electrical stimulation of the brain (Penfield and Jasper 1954). The diagnostic facilities available at this time were plain radiography (XR), ventriculography, angiography, EEG, and ECoG. The seizures were often due to lesions in eloquent cortex and concordance between seizures and peroperative findings was crucial, because most of this surgery was carried out under local anesthesia, neurologic deficits were minimized. Over 100 epilepsy surgery publications mirror the interest in extratemporal intervention before the 1950s, when anterior temporal lobectomy (ATL) became an epilepsy surgery procedure (Penfield and Flanigin 1950). Currently, extratemporal epilepsy surgery (ETES) designates a removal within any lobe outside the temporal lobe, an excision that may extend beyond one lobe.

Proposals to carry out extratemporal resections may raise concern about the creation of a neurologic deficit, or increase in an existing deficit, and so create prejudice against the procedure. Undue concern should not delay investigations or extratemporal operations in selected candidates. The results of epilepsy surgery on seizure outcome are evaluated using widely accepted scales (Engel et al 1993). The outcome of these extratemporal operations cannot equal that of anterior temporal lobectomy because there are often multiple or multifocal lesions, diagnosis of the epileptogenic focus and underlying pathology is more complex, and the extent of any surgical intervention is restricted by the need to preserve eloquent cortex. But, even a partial improvement is worthwhile and may allow improved education and better use of rehabilitation facilities, thereby improving quality of life. The chances and risks of extratemporal surgery can only be assessed accurately by using appropriate preoperative and peroperative tests. The risks of surgery should be balanced against the manifest consequences of not operating, which in the future often include poor psychosocial situation and untimely death. The clinical evaluation should take place at an early stage and, as is the case with patients being assessed for anterior temporal lobectomy, it should be viewed in a broad perspective, where morbidity, quality of life, and life expectancy are assessed (Taylor and Falconer 1968; Augustine et al 1984; Dodrill et al 1986; Fraser 1988). ETES has recently been reviewed by Comair et al (1997).

CANDIDATES FOR EXTRATEMPORAL EPILEPSY SURGERY

Both infants and adults with drug-resistant partial, extratemporal epilepsy may be candidates for surgery. Early investigations are urgent when seizures interfere with language, cognition, and motor functions and patients with intractable extratemporal focal epilepsy should wait no longer than patients with temporal lobe seizures before being evaluated for epilepsy surgery. Pediatric epilepsy surgery is advisable early in children younger than 5 years, who are better able to recover command of language and gain improvement in behavior, mental capabilities, and sensorimotor (SM) functions. Adults, with neurologic deficits from early lesions, or with late onset of intractable partial epilepsy due to microsopic structural lesions, would benefit from presurgical investigations within 2 years of failing, adequate antiepileptic drug (AED) therapy. Magnetic resonance imaging (MRI) and functional MRI (fMRI) provide accurate diagnosis in cases who had been deemed unsuitable for epilepsy surgery using previous investigation methods. Magnetic resonance spectroscopy (MRS) is a new tool for detecting cerebral metabolic changes (Connelly 1997; Laxer 1997). To localize superficial and deep-seated extratemporal epileptogenic lesions, which may present considerable diagnostic difficulty, one may require SPECT, PET, invasive video-EEG, functional mapping, and even magnetoencephalography (MEG) (Hari 1993).

ETIOLOGY

The 'classical' histopathologic findings in extratemporal epilepsy surgery will be mentioned in the appropriate text section. There is a new awareness, revealed by MRI, of developmental disturbances, cortical dysplasias, microdysgeneses, dysembryoplastic neuroectodermal tumor, and slowly growing neocortical gliomas and cavernous angiomas as etiologies in candidates for epilepsy surgery (Britton *et al* 1994; Fried *et al* 1994; Dubeau *et al* 1995; Prayson and Estes 1995; Raymond *et al* 1995; Brännström *et al* 1996; Guerrini *et al* 1996; Mihara *et al* 1997). Coexisting mental retardation does not necessarily contraindicate evaluation and extratemporal epilepsy surgery.

THE FRONTAL LOBES

The frontal lobe extends to the central sulcus, in front of which is the motor cortex (area 4). From a practical point of view, the frontal lobe stops at the precentral sulcus. The lobe is divided into the polar, intermedial dorsolateral, intermedial mediofrontal, and orbitofrontal regions. The orbitofrontal cortex extends to the depth of the optic chiasm region. The frontal convexity contains the superior, middle, and inferior frontal gyri. On the mesial aspect are the superior frontal and the cingulate gyri. Some areas are surgically noteworthy: the premotor cortex (area 6), the supplementary sensorimotor area (SSMA, area 6) and, below it, the anterior cingulate area (1–2 gyri, area 24) adjacent to the corpus callosum (CC), and laterally the 2nd–3rd convolutions of the inferior frontal gyrus by the sylvian fissure, the operculum. On the speech-dominant side, these gyri enharbor Broca's area. The frontal gyri run in bends, turn deep, and may hide epileptogenic sites diagnostically undefinable from the surface.

The surgical problem is the extent and technique of invasive investigation/therapeutic excision. Fiber connections involved in seizure projections may complicate the clinical diagnosis. The corpus callosum is relevant to the appearance of bilateral synchronous epileptic discharges. The uncinate fasciculus links the anterior frontal and temporal lobes, and participates in complex partial seizures (CPS) of frontal origin. The superior longitudinal fasciculus may interlink frontoparietooccipital epileptic discharges.

One should consider briefly the vascular supply of the frontal lobe. The two upper frontal gyri are perfused via the anterior cerebral artery (ACA), the inferior gyrus by the middle cerebral artery (MCA). Hemodynamic variations or vascular aberrations should be kept in mind when evaluating dominant hemisphere lesions, impaired speech, or unusual or inconsistent results from the intracarotid amytal test (IAT) (Chapter 48). The surgeon should be well-versed with the interpretation of the IAT, particularly in dealing with lesions interfering with language.

SEIZURES AND DIAGNOSIS

The nature of auras or clinical seizures of frontal lobe origin can be derived from their semeiology, imaging, and electrophysiology. Interictal behavior may be described in neuropsychologic terms. Seizure patterns are described in detail by several authors (Penfield and Jasper 1954; Engel

1987; Rasmussen 1963, 1970, 1975a, 1983a; Bancaud and Talairach 1992; Lüders 1992; Engel *et al* 1993; Engel and Pedley 1997) (Chapter 6). Structural lesions, evident on MRI, may be from a number of diverse etiological sources including those of a postinfectious, traumatic, or encephalitic nature, a cavernous angioma, tuberous sclerosis, Sturge–Weber malformation, glial tumor, porencephalic cyst, cortical dysplasia, encephalomalacia, etc. (Kazemi *et al* 1997). The etiology of frontal seizures studied in 100 patients remained unknown in 37%, was due to neonatal anoxia in 18%, to encephalitis in 15%, to postnatal traumatic in 15%, and to miscellaneous causes in 15% (Talairach *et al* 1992a). Rasmussen (1983a) described the histopathology of 40 patients as follows: meningocerebral cicatrix in 50%; cicatrix or gliosis in 33%; hamartoma or dysplasia in 8%; 10% had no findings. An account of the Montreal Neurological Institute (MNI) findings in nonneoplastic surgical specimens from 180 frontal cases was specified as follows: meningocerebral cicatrix 33%; neuronal loss and gliosis 33%; cortical dysgeneses 15%; contusions 11%; gliosis 4%; meningoencephalitides 3%; miscellaneous 3%; and abscess 1% (Robitaille *et al* 1992).

PET in frontal epilepsy may show hypometabolism, at times spatially discordant with the epileptogenic region (Henry *et al* 1992). SPECT investigations have been published (Swartz *et al* 1992) (Chapter 26). Neuropsychology is an integral part of the work-up (Chapter 26). The electrophysiology of frontal lobe epilepsy can be clarified with scalp EEG (Quesney 1992). Invasive recordings, often bilateral are now common (Talairach *et al* 1992b) (Chapter 22). Video-EEG of ictal activity preceding the clinical seizures is performed. Monitoring with invasive electrodes also allows repeated electrical stimulation and studies of auras, seizures, and cerebral functions.

Invasive video-EEG is carried out with electrodes placed under general anesthesia epidurally, subdurally, or intracerebrally. Intraosseal peg electrodes may also be used. The antiepileptic drugs are reduced cautiously. Laterohorizontal frontal stereotactic implantation of multipolar electrodes into one or both cerebral hemispheres was described by Talairach *et al* (1958). Several reports refer to this stereotaxic EEG (SEEG) technique, practised before invasive surface recording (Wyler *et al* 1984). Clinical, angiographic, and scalp EEG data originally guided the electrode positioning. Now SEEG incorporates MRI and digital subtraction angiography, and achieves high resolution 3-D images for exact electrode placement, at times supplemented by SPECT or PET data (Olivier 1992). New image-guided investigations accurately direct the electrode placements or assist in planning the extratemporal epilepsy surgery

(Olivier et al 1996). Epidural strip or grid electrodes can be positioned using a craniotomy without causing meningeocortical adhesions. Peroperative epidural ECoG and functional mapping, inferior in precision to subdural mapping, may be carried out. Pain fibers along dural arteries should be cut before stimulation. The implants are photographed and the anchored wires are tunneled out. CT or MRI images of electrode positions are used for EEG or SEEG localization and functional mapping. Subdural strips are inserted through burr holes on the lateromesial surfaces, and can be curved subfrontally. The placement may be unilateral or bilateral, parasagittal or laterofrontal, or both. Additional strips may be placed through other burr holes on and beneath the temporal lobes, in case of patients with complex partial seizures.

The midline exposure for subdural recording is often unilateral and allows the placement of mesial grids or alternatively, strips with bilateral contacts, recording from both the ipsilateral mesial cortex directly and the contralateral mesial cortex through the falx; alternatively, strips can be placed on either side of the falx. They can be stabilized by anchoring them to the dura, and ECoG and functional mapping can be carried out before closure. The intraoperative findings may be compared with those of video-EEG, and of spontaneous and electrically evoked discharges. Mapping of speech and SM cortices is possible in the cooperative patient using systematic stimulation of each electrode contact (monopolarly against cranial bone, and with bipolar switching polarity). Video-EEG will localize Broca's area, from where aphasia or dysphasia is evoked. A fractionated, comprehensive functional mapping may need several hours to accomplish. Patients have been described with drop attacks and bilateral synchronous epileptic EEG abnormality who, after anterior callosotomy, may then show a unilateral frontal focus, possibly with an excisable lesion; but this is probably an uncommon and therefore relatively infrequent occurrence (Turmel *et al* 1992).

EXCISIONS AND RESULTS

If they have not been previously reduced, antiepileptic drugs should not be reduced until the day before surgery, so as to minimize the risk of severe seizures. The operation may be carried out under local or special general anesthesia. The medial incision of a frontotemporal skin flap should follow the midline, or be 1 cm across it, extending far enough posteriorly that there is access to mesial frontal and SM cortices. Under local anesthesia, SM functions and speech may be studied; under general anesthesia, movements can also be elicited by functional mapping of the motor gyrus, and somatosensory evoked potentials (SEPs) elicited from the gyral crest, or from hidden banks of microsurgically exposed SM sulci (Lüders *et al* 1987). Under general anesthesia ECoG can be run for 5–15 minutes during reduced nitrous oxide flow. Droperidol and fentanyl loadings are checked. Spontaneous ictal and interictal epileptic discharges may be localized. Attention is paid to the background activity, frequently impaired in an epileptogenic region. If ECoG activity is sparse then, intravenous methohexital (25–50 mg) may provoke or enhance epileptic activity (Wyler *et al* 1987). Intermittent electrical stimulation of the cortex for a few seconds (mono-/bipolar 0.5–5 mA, 1–2 ms pulses, 60 Hz) may evoke low-threshold epileptic afterdischarges. Stimulation should not be repeated until the afterdischarges have receded. Occasionally, a clinical seizure occurs but usually fades away by itself. Functional mapping (< 15 mA) locates the SM cortex in relation to planned excision. Too short a pulse will not excite the cortex, as has been clearly shown in children (Jayakar *et al* 1992). Absence of mapping responses should be regarded cautiously: they could reflect cortical depression (Lüders *et al* 1992). The sites of the functional mapping can be marked with letters, the epileptogenic area with numbers, and encircled with a black thread. The exposure, with a transparent millimeter scale, is photographed.

Structural and epileptogenic lesions, at some distance from each other, leave it to the surgeon to choose what to excise. It has been suggested that priority should be given to the lesion (Clarke *et al* 1996). The epileptogenic region determines the size and nature of the resection and guides whether it is a gyrectomy, a topectomy, or a partial or full lobectomy. Respect for arteries and veins must be exercised; the excisions should be performed with the least traumatic technique under visual magnification; use should be made of thermocoagulation and neat subpial suction with a small bore metal sucker, or an ultrasound aspirator. Gyri are excised after a longitudinal coagulation and truncated neatly. The excision should expose, but not intrude into, the white matter in the gyral troughs. A mesial excision should similarly extend to the white matter, either along the sulcus of the superior frontal gyrus, the anterior cingulate area, or close to the corpus callosum, respecting the pericallosal artery. Branches of the frontopolar or callosomarginal arteries may be coagulated, provided they do not head toward the motor cortex. A mesial excision may include either the supplementary sensorimotor area or the anterior cingulate area, or both (see later). An orbitofrontal excision may extend to the internal carotid artery, but in the speech-dominant hemisphere must curve in front of Broca's area, sheltering it by a 1–2 cm rim (Rasmussen 1975a). An exci-

sion along a portion of the premotor gyrus necessitates great care. Also on the mesial surface, the excision may extend posteriorly to the primary motor gyrus. Where the pathology produces cortical toughness, piecemeal thermocoagulation, scissors, a hook or microdissector, or an ultrasound aspirator may prove advantageous. Traction on the white matter should be avoided. Postresection ECoG recording helps to evaluate whether the excision has achieved complete or partial abolition of the epileptogenic area. An exposed frontal horn is covered with a cellulose patch and the final excision is photographed. A sizable excision will reduce the bulk of the anterior corpus callosum, evident on later imaging. Beneficial excisions can be made in either frontal lobe; correctly performed, they will not harm the patient.

The outcome of extratemporal epilepsy surgery in regard to seizures does not generally match that of anterior temporal lobectomy (Olivier 1992) (Chapter 16). Despite that, excision is recommended where preoperative studies suggest an accessible focus and especially if a well-delineated epileptogenic lesion can be removed. The outcome of frontal lobe excisions reported from the MNI, and the Hôpital Sainte-Anne (HSA), Paris, are as follows: of the 257 MNI patients operated, 26% became seizure-free, 30% obtained a marked reduction, and 40% a lesser reduction in seizure tendency (Rasmussen 1975a). The outcome of excisions for nontumoral lesions in 239 patients was described as 17% seizure-free (Rasmussen 1983a). Later, the outcome of 253 cases was correlated with the anatomic location of the excision. An anterior frontal excision rendered 47% seizure-free, while a parasagittal removal was the least favorable, 18% of the patients becoming seizure-free (Rasmussen 1991).

The overall success of excisions in 100 HSA patients was 55%. Patients with epileptogenic regions correctly delineated by SEEG had the best chances, 85% of them benefiting from surgery. The outcome was: seizure-free 23%; 32% had rare seizures; and 21% were markedly improved. In relation to the anatomic location of the resected tissue, 45% of the prefrontal excisions were successful, 35% of the intermediofrontal, 14% of the frontotemporal, and 49% of the medial frontal excisions (Talairach *et al* 1992a). Improved seizure control was usually accompanied by behavioral improvement, with neuropsychologic improvement in 40%. However, a behavioral disorder could persist despite the disappearence of seizures. Turmel *et al* (1992) reported the surgical outcome of 21 cases, 38% becoming seizure-free. An additional survey of frontal extratemporal epilepsy surgery reported up to the year 1997 traced 15 reports (Van Ness 1992; Rougier *et al* 1992; Cascino *et al* 1992, 1994; Davies and Weeks 1993; Salanova *et al* 1993, 1994; Laskowitz *et al* 1995; Lorenzo *et al* 1995; Olivier 1995; Zentner *et al* 1996a; Cukiert *et al* 1996; Kazemi *et al* 1997; Comair *et al* 1997). To mention but a few, successful outcome was achieved in 25% of the Lorenzo *et al* study, 67% in the Laskowitz *et al* sample, and 70% of the Kazemi *et al* follow-up. Reoperation in 39 cases studied by Salanova *et al* (1994) rendered 20% of the patients seizure-free.

SURGICAL COMPLICATIONS

The complications of extratemporal epilepsy surgery are reported here by area of excision. Rasmussen (1963) reported no mortality in 117 MNI patients operated after 1945. A global survey of the complications of extratemporal epilepsy surgery listed no mortality among 432 cases, and a morbidity in 2% (Van Buren 1987). The HSA frontal lobe material included no diagnostic complications, a mortality of 5%, and a morbidity of 32%, consisting of infection or inflammation, aphasia, reduced verbal fluency, accentuated motor deficit, akinesia, or increased sensory deficit (Talairach *et al* 1992a). Turmel *et al* (1992) reported that most of their patients presented a morbidity or an aggravation of existing deficits, or new neuropsychologic deficits, despite a marked reduction in seizures. Cascino *et al* (1994) studied complications in mainly frontal extratemporal epilepsy surgery, noting at least one adverse event in 13 of 29 cases.

BIFRONTAL LESIONS

At times, unfortunate patients with epilepsy, bilateral lesions—usually posttraumatic or infectious in origin—and mental retardation are referred for extratemporal epilepsy surgery evaluation. These patients can be offered a palliative bifrontal resection, especially if the lesions are polar. Section of the corpus callosum or a vagal nerve stimulation are alternative procedures.

PERSONAL EXPERIENCE

As at the end of 1996, the author had performed local frontal excisions in 43 children and adults (left 25; right 18). The etiologies were similar to those already mentioned (21% glial tumors). One-third of the patients had a reoperation for continued postoperative seizures. The seizure outcome, including that of reoperation, was class I 34.9%, class II 9.3%, and class III 16.3%.

THE CINGULATE AREA

SEIZURES, DIAGNOSIS, EXCISIONS, AND RESULTS

Anterior cingulum seizures may be expressed as fear, screaming, aggression, emotion, complex motor behavior, or partial loss of consciousness (Chauvel *et al* 1992; Munari and Bancaud 1992). Such seizures may fit the description of two functional areas of the cingulate cortex: an executive and an evaluative one (Vogt *et al* 1992; Devinsky *et al* 1995). Mazars (1970) reported a successful excision in about one-half of the cases. Talairach *et al* (1992a) reported the outcome from patients studied with SEEG, who subsequently had excisions in the 'intermediate frontal (area) on the medial surface.' They had the least favorable outcome of all frontal cases, 18% success rate. Olivier (1995) stated that 'paramedian' resections are included in certain frontal excisions. The surgical outcome in his 27 patients was excellent in 44%. Comair *et al* (1996), in a series of 15 mesial cases, reported cingulate area removal in two. Complications from cingulate area extratemporal epilepsy surgery seem rare.

THE CONVEXITY SENSORIMOTOR CORTEX

SEIZURES AND DIAGNOSIS

Focal epileptogenic lesions within the SM cortex may produce seizures starting somewhere within the SM homunculus (Chapter 6). Postictally there may be a transient paresis (Rasmussen 1975b; Olivier 1992). A long-standing structural epileptogenic lesion in the SM cortex may have caused a neurologic deficit in the face, hand, arm, or leg. In spite of that, the lesion may not be documented radiologically. If so, microdysgenesis can be suspected (Guerrini *et al* 1996). Simple partial seizures starting from the SM gyral crests may differ from those of gyral banks, because of different modality-specific organizations. Sutherling *et al* (1992) investigated the cortical S-representation of the human hand, noting deviations from the classical homunculus. Sophisticated MRI, with high resolution and 3-D rendering, can detect minute lesions in the SM strip, allowing precise semeiology, and their subsequent location using the new image-guided technology screens, such as the Magic Wand. Accurate MRI identification of the rolandic sulcus is possible in relation to the corpus callosum, and the forward slope of the SM cortex, by various means such as fMRI, ictal SPECT, and PET (Levesque *et al* 1992; Uematsu *et al* 1992). Meyer *et al* (1996) found the mean ratio of cortical thickness of the motor:sensory gyri to be 1.54; the motor gyrus should thus appear thicker than the sensory gyrus on MRI. Jack *et al* (1994) reported presurgical mapping to match fMRI and invasive mapping. Yetkin *et al* (1995) reviewed fMRI and MRI localizations of the SM cortex, concluding that in the majority of studies the anatomically defined central sulcus coincided exactly or approximately with the activated SM cortex. In tumor cases with SM cortex displaced, it can still be defined by functional mapping. Lehman and Kim (1995) utilized a callosal grid system, with superposition of other data for localization of seizure onsets. Yetkin *et al* (1997) compared the spatial accuracy of fMRI and peroperative functional mapping, noting it in all instances to be less than 2 cm, and in 87% of sites less than 1 cm. Morioka *et al* (1995), evaluating presurgical MEG, fMRI, and motor-evoked potentials in sensorimotor localization, found MEG to be the most reliable method, and this agrees with the MEG study of Smith *et al* (1994). Other preoperative diagnostic SM studies have been published (Puce 1995; Roberts and Darcey 1996; Cosgrove *et al* 1996; Devaux *et al* 1996). Patil *et al* (1995) reported a patient successfully treated by stereotactic targeting and excision of seizure focus identified by using Xe-enhanced CT.

If noninvasive studies fail to localize the epileptogenic lesion, the region should be explored. If the intraoperative investigation remains inconclusive, a chronic study is conducted in the cooperating patient, evaluating video-EEG, movements, SEPs, and electrically evoked afterdischarges. The region from which the patient's habitual seizures, or similar seizures, are evoked by low-intensity stimulation is assumed to be the epileptogenic region.

EXCISIONS AND RESULTS

Bearing in mind the basic functional neuronal network of modality-specific cortical afference–integration–efference (Chapter 46), delicate surgical excisions will cause little functional loss. This is especially relevant in established functional plasticity (Hedström *et al* 1996). The ranking in respect of SM functions can be listed as the hand–arm–foot–leg–trunk–face. At times, compromises resulting in functional postoperative losses must be made, in order to achieve cessation or significant reduction in the frequency of severe seizures whose continuation may be accompanied by significant ictal or postictal neurologic dysfunction.

If surgery is carried out under general anesthesia and the motor cortex is to be stimulated, a short-acting muscle relaxant should be used. In epilepsy surgery under local anesthesia, the sensory cortex is explored first, the patient reporting the sensations elicited (Olivier 1992). The identification of the motor cortex is done after ECoG, often in combination with electrical stimulation to elicit afterdischarges. The subdivisions of the SM cortex are defined with monopolar stimulation using the bone or the ECoG stand as the reference, or bipolar stimulation with a space between the contacts of 5–10 mm. The mapping is made with precision, registering contralateral twitches or movements. Functional mapping of the sensory cortex under general anesthesia can utilize SEPs from peripheral nerves in the arms or legs. Once the epileptogenic lesion and the SM cortex have been marked with numbers or letters, the exposure is photographed.

The risks of functional loss following SM excisions is reduced if arterial branches and small draining veins remain intact. Careful subpial suction, peeling off of cortex, and neat gray-matter truncation should be done toward bordering cortex. A lesion involving the tongue–face area may be excised, possibly causing a transient paralysis (Olivier 1992). The upper limit of an excision should be the lower border of the M-thumb area. A premotor excision, anterior to the M-face area can be made in the nondominant hemisphere and exceptionally, in the dominant hemisphere (see later). It is particularly important to be aware of the results of any amytal test (intracarotid or superselective) in planning excisions adjacent to the suprasylvian SM cortex. An excision within other parts of the SM cortex will usually lead to a permanent neurologic deficit, the degree of which is related to the size and function of the somatotopic division removed or interfered with. If the patient has voluntary finger–hand–arm movements, an excision within this part of the 'motor homunculus' is not recommended, except in cases of epilepsia partialis continua, which by definition usually renders the M cortex involved practically useless. Removals from the M cortex serving trunk or leg areas are avoided, except when the seizures are too heavy a burden for the patient. A hidden structural lesion in the M cortex can be removed microsurgically with minimal sequelae, via a minute crossgyral corticotomy. A lesion in the premotor gyrus above the face area may be excised with extreme care. The subpial excision then extends to the depth of the premotor sulcus, leaving the sulcal pia-arachnoidea of the M cortex intact, and carefully respecting its gray and white matter. The technical success of such a removal can be checked intraoperatively by electrically stimulating the exposed white matter of the premotor cortex, the sulcal M cortex, and the crest of the M gyrus. If the movements elicited from each spot are identical to those elicited before the excision with identical stimulation parameters, the patient suffers no harm.

Cortical excisions in the sensory cortex outside the face area should be carried out carefully and within restricted areas. This applies especially to the sensory hand area, which will lose extero- and proprioceptive capacities related to the size of removal (Olivier 1992). The intraoperative electrical stimulation of the motor cortex, and neighboring regions, may then be altogether negative, even on high-intensity stimulation, because of basic chronaxie problems as discussed by Jayakar *et al* (1992).

A large paracentral lesion may, in addition to the SM cortex, involve parts of the frontal, temporal, or parietal areas. The excision will be extensive or multilobar depending on whether the lesion is located in the speech-dominant hemisphere or not. Multiple subpial transection (MST) is a surgical alternative (Chapter 46).

A survey of the literature on epilepsy surgery to the convexity SM area revealed four reports in addition to the 15 already referred to in the text (Uematsu *et al* 1992; Lehman *et al* 1994; Zentner *et al* 1996a). Olivier *et al* (1996) underscored the helpfulness of interactive image-guided procedures in a large number of operations.

At the MNI, 151 excisions in the SM area had been performed up to 1981 (Rasmussen 1987b). Pooled results of resections from the central, parietal, and occipital regions in 203 patients revealed that 34% had become seizure-free, and 23% almost seizure-free or markedly improved. Lehman *et al* (1994) published the outcome in patients with seizure onset in the SM face area. Six of 20 cases had a reoperation, 18 had at least a moderate improvement. All the five patients of Lehman and Kim (1995) became seizure-free. Complications from SM cortex excisions are related to the location of the excision; complete or partial motor and sensory impairment may follow as referred to above. The author's personal experience is five cases.

THE SUPPLEMENTARY SENSORIMOTOR AREA

SEIZURES AND DIAGNOSIS

The supplementary sensorimotor area (SSMA) comprises the mesial parasagittal cortex in front of the SM area proper, turning around the vertical edge of the cerebral hemisphere. Epileptic seizures may start from the mesial portion of the SM foot area, from cortex in front of that, from the SSMA, or from the mesial parietooccipital cortex.

A comprehensive analysis of SSMA seizures and their surgical treatment has been published (Lüders 1996). Invasive bilateral video-EEG or SEEG monitoring in combination with functional mapping can be employed. Munari *et al* (1996) reported on nine patients studied with SEEG in whom the seizures originated in SSMA. In all cases except one, the seizure activity spread to neighboring areas. Laich *et al* (1997) studied ictal SPECT in SSMA seizures, noting two perfusion patterns: in one there was ipsilateral involvement of the SSMA and the dorsal premotor cortex; in the other they saw bilateral asymmetrical mesial frontal propagation. Study of SSMA seizures in children has required prolonged EEG or invasive recordings (Bass *et al* 1995).

EXCISIONS AND RESULTS

Experience with SSMA excisions has been elegantly described by Comair *et al* (1996). Bleasel and Morris (1996) reported on the outcome after mesial frontal epilepsy surgery due to seizures or a tumor presenting with seizures in 10 patients, 6 of whom had a normal neurologic outcome. Mihara *et al* (1996) reported the results of cortical removal in 5 of 16 patients with foci in the SSMA studied invasively. All were clinical successes in regard to seizures, and they all had a transient hemiparesis, which was persistent in one case. Smith and King (1996) reported a successful outcome in 8 of 12 SSMA patients. Olivier's (1996) material consisted of 28 cases, 47% obtaining complete or a better than 90% seizure relief. Spencer and Schumacher (1996) reported on 8 patients of whom 4 obtained excellent outcome in regard to seizures. Comair *et al* (1996) reported no permanent morbidity in 15 cases. Zentner *et al* (1996b) analyzed in particular the morbidity in 28 SSMA cases, concluding that it was usually transient.

THE INSULAR CORTEX

SEIZURES AND EXCISIONS

Excisions of structural epileptogenic lesions in the hidden insular cortex are sometimes carried out without an ATL (Roper *et al* 1993). In connection with a frontal excision, or an ATL, when a part of the insula is exposed, its cortex should not be removed because it increases the risk of a deficit without increasing the chances of seizure relief (Silfvenius *et al* 1964).

THE LANGUAGE CORTICES

The Broca and the Wernicke language areas are surgically sacrosanct. Occasionally, an MST and, even more rarely, an excision is carried out within or near them. Such a procedure relies on the demonstration of intrahemisphere or interhemisphere transfer of speech and/or language comprehension, the precise location of language areas, and the nature of the lesion (Schaffler *et al* 1996). The IAT will clarify whether the language capacities of the two hemispheres are equal or whether one hemisphere is preponderant. If speech is bilaterally represented, and an IAT does not induce aphasia, then a patient with a low lateral frontal lesion could have it excised from either side (Milner *et al* 1996). Preoperative, chronic functional mapping on the side of planned surgery would remove all doubts about cortical speech representation (cf. Loring *et al* 1992). If aphasia is produced by intracarotid amytal injection on both sides, then an excision in the Broca/Wernicke areas, or their homologs, should not be performed without additional penetrating analysis. At times, an early lesion in the speech-dominant hemisphere may exhibit minimal or no clinical symptoms. Hinz *et al* (1994), in pediatric patients, correlated the IAT results for speech dominance with intraoperative functional mapping, noting a strong correlation between left-handedness and atypical speech lateralization, but also between right-sided hemiparesis and atypical speech (see also Tuxhorn *et al* 1997).

BROCA AREA

Seizures and diagnosis

The surgical options vary for an excision of a lesion indenting or profusely invading Broca's area, or its immediate surroundings. Chronic functional speech mapping allows exact investigation of Broca's area, and its spatial relation to the suprasylvian SM cortex. Combining it with video-EEG, spontaneous or induced ictal sequences can be recorded. The positions of the implanted electrode contacts through which changes in speech were evoked are noted and compared with other diagnostic data.

Excisions and results

Tradition recommends that epilepsy surgery near Broca's area should respect a safety zone 1–3 cm above the sylvian fissure and in front of the motor–tongue–face area. Whereas invasive glial tumors can often be only partially excised, with less chance of seizure relief, well-demarcated, indenting glial tumors can be excised without detriment to the vascular bed. Small cavernous angiomas can be excised under the microscope with excellent outcome. If hidden, a transgyral slit will expose the angioma and its yellowish epileptogenic border zone. Intraoperative ultrasound localization can be used to improve excision of angiomas. Sometimes the results of invasive diagnostic tests will define the possible postoperative speech impairment with sufficient accuracy to preclude resection at that site. Haglund *et al* (1992) tested sophisticated optical imaging of functional activity in Broca's and Wernicke's areas. The next personal case illustrates an unexpected response evoked during chronic functional speech mapping.

Illustrative case 1

The patient was a 53-year-old right-handed woman with a 6-year history of simple partial motor seizures involving the right face, accompanied with transient dysphasia. Routine EEGs as well as CT scans were normal. MRI, 5 years after onset of seizures, revealed a glial tumor in the left frontal operculum (Plate 6).

Instead of an IAT, functional cortical mapping was performed after subdural strips had been placed across and adjacent to the glial tumor (Plate 6a). Postoperative mapping under ECoG control defined the Broca area. The tumor was adjacent to it. An unexpected, behavioral response was that, in addition to becoming aphasic from stimulation, the patient became emotionally upset. Asked why she wept, she replied that she heard her mother blaming her as a child for some wrong-doing. When the same spot was stimulated while the patient was silent, the emotional memory was not elicited. ECoG did not record any afterdischarges. The mapping phenomenon was interpreted as induced projected activity from the operculum via the uncinate fasciculus to the temporal lobe. Removal of the oligodendroglioma caused no speech disturbance and rendered her seizure-free, which she has been for 8 years (Plate 6b). Postoperative radiotherapy was given, but there has been tumor recurrence.

WERNICKE AREA

Seizures and diagnosis

An early lesion may have displaced or rearranged the Wernicke area, a fact that reduces or removes the surgical risk. The IAT should correctly evaluate the changes in language in relation to the areas perfused by the MCA or the posterior cerebral artery (Silfvenius *et al* 1997) (Chapter 39). Intraoperative and chronic cortical mapping provides exact definition of the Wernicke area. The inferior temporal border of Wernicke's area is not identical as defined by functional mapping and by excision (Penfield and Roberts 1959).

Excisions and results

When extratemporal epilepsy surgery in the dominant temporoparietooccipital region is contemplated, consideration must be given to Wernicke's area. Some guidance about the safe borders of surgery in this area can be derived from the ATL literature (Chapter 43). Epilepsy surgery in or around the Wernicke area is planned with the same considerations and techniques that were discussed in relation to resection in Broca's area. Epilepsy surgery can be performed under local or general anesthesia (Gorecki *et al* 1992; Silbergeld *et al* 1992; Müller and Morris 1993). The border of the suprasylvian Wernicke area, as defined functionally, is 3–4 cm down from the turn of the parasagittal cortex, and 3–5 cm anterior to the occipital pole (Crandall 1987). Both chronic and intraoperative functional mapping provide precise information about the extent and organization of the Wernicke area. An excision can be combined with MST (Chapter 46). Microsurgical excisions of arteriovenous malformations (AVM) in language areas can be performed successfully with either no impairment or only subtle language impairment, for example, in the use of one but not of the other language in a bilingual patient (Gomez-Tortosa *et al* 1995; Hojo *et al* 1995). Case 2 is a personal one illustrating epilepsy surgery in the Wernicke area.

Illustrative case 2

The patient was a 29-year-old right-handed man whose father had an inoperable cerebral 'von Hippel–Lindau malformation.' The patient's simple partial seizures (vague sound) started at age 19 years, at times secondarily generalized. Speech was slightly neologistic, and he had a right facial weakness. CT scans and conventional and MRI angiography identified a large, posterior left temporal cavernous angioma surrounded by gliosis (Fig. 52.1).

An IAT established left hemisphere language dominance. A transgyral 5 mm corticotomy made it possible to remove the angioma microsurgically. Postoperatively, for a few days, he had a just appreciable transient receptive dysphasia. He has been seizure-free for 3 years.

LANDAU–KLEFFNER SYNDROME

Seizures, diagnosis, and excisions

The Landau–Kleffner syndrome is an acquired aphasia in epileptic children with a poor prognosis for speech recovery (Chapter 16). When caused by a tumor, a resection of it may result in improvement (Nass *et al* 1993). Nontumoral cases are successfully operated with MST (Chapter 54). Heschl's gyri are hidden in the sylvian fissure and structural lesions in this area in the speech-dominant hemisphere have been excised successfully for seizures (Silbergeld 1997).

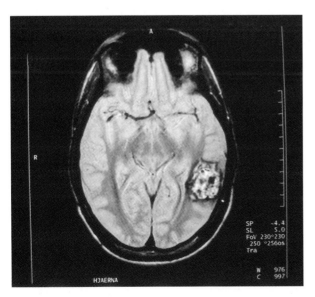
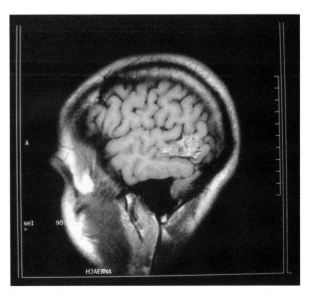

Fig. 52.1 Case 2. MRI of a large cavernous angioma in the Wernicke area, microsurgically removed.

THE PARIETAL LOBE

SEIZURES AND DIAGNOSIS

Epileptic lesions in the nondominant parietal lobe can be clinically 'silent,' i.e., the seizures may be symptomatic of the adjacent lobes (Chapter 6). Salanova *et al* (1995a) reported the clinical aspects of 82 nontumoral cases. Dominant parietal lobe seizures may interfere with language and cognitive capacities. Structural etiologies mentioned include atrophic cysts, cortical dysplasia, glial tumors, tuberous sclerosis, cavernous angiomas, AVM, gliosis, Sturge–Weber malformation, etc. (Morris *et al* 1993; Prayson and Estes 1995; Salanova *et al* 1995b). The microdysgeneses should be kept in mind (Guerrini *et al* 1996). Ictal SPECT can be a helpful localizing method (Ho *et al* 1994). Invasive video-EEG monitoring may become necessary in the language-dominant lobe and superselective amytal testing of adjacent arteries may need to be carried out.

EXCISIONS AND RESULTS

Excisions in the nondominant parietal lobe may be radical and extend posteriorly from the sensory cortex, without causing neurologic deficits, except for visual field defects that may occur if the resection involves the underlying temporoparietal white matter. (Olivier 1992). The SM cortex is defined prior to the excision. The medial portion of the parietal cortex may be excised, respecting the large bridging veins. On the speech-dominant side, the excision must not encroach upon the lower parietal cortex below the motor thumb–finger area (Crandall 1987). The intraparietal sulcus has been suggested as the lower lateral boundary for an excision (Olivier 1992). Williamson *et al* (1992) reported on the outcome in 11 patients with a circumscribed lesion; 10 became seizure-free. Cascino *et al* (1993a) performed lesionectomy in 10 patients, 9 of whom became seizure-free. In their series of nontumoral cases, Salanova *et al* (1995a) described a complete or nearly complete cessation of seizures in 65% of cases. The neurologic deficits and complications from parietal lobe excisions are reported to be minor and transient. Extensive, nondominant inferior parietal excisions did occasionally cause disturbances of body image and postoperative sensory deficits when the excision extended into the sensory cortex. Another study of Salanova *et al* (1995b), of 28 tumoral patients, described complete freedom from seizures in 32% of these cases, with a postoperative sensory deficit developing in 12% of the 28 patients. No Gerstmann syndrome evolves if the excision is outside the posterior language zone (Rasmussen 1987b). The author has experience of eight parietal cases; one is described in detail. Figure 52.2 shows a microsurgical excision in the presumed speech-dominant parietal lobe.

Illustrative Case 3

A 16-year-old right-handed, neurologically normal boy had drug-resistant partial seizures that occasionally generalized, since the age of 4 years. The fits occurred 2–4 times daily and consisted of short 'absences' hardly seen by others, except the family. He reported an ictal sensation of a rhythm in his head. He wished to be operated on in order to get a driver's license. Neuroradiologically, there was a small nodule in the left parietal region at the trigone, invading the cortex. The EEG showed left temporoparietal abnormality with some spiking. Since a microsurgical excision was planned, no IAT was performed, although the lesion was located in the presumed posterior language zone. A stereotactic CT adapter localization (Laitinen *et al* 1985) of the lesion was obtained preoperatively with the assistance of Dr M. Hariz (Fig. 52.2a,b). A CT scan was repeated under general anesthesia to guide the insertion of plastic tubing through a drill hole and the correct position was confirmed (Fig. 52.2c). The patient was taken back to the operating room and a parietooccipital craniotomy was made. ECoG showed sparse interictal spiking. A depth electrode was inserted freehand into the track of the removed tubing, and to the same depth. The deepest contact showed vigorous epileptic activity. A 1-cm subsylvian corticotomy was made and the structural lesion was removed microsurgically (Fig. 52.2d). Postoperatively there were no deficits. Histopathology showed the lesion to be tuberous sclerosis. After surgery the patient is seizure-free.

THE OCCIPITAL LOBE

SEIZURES AND DIAGNOSIS

Nontumoral epileptic occipital lobe lesions constituted 5% of the extratemporal epilepsy surgery carried out at the MNI between 1928 and 1970 (Rasmussen 1979) and another MNI analysis reported lesions in 1% of cases (Rasmussen 1987b). The expanded MNI series of 42 cases has been described (Salanova *et al* 1992). In addition, Palmini *et al* (1993) reported on SEEG studies in eight occipitotemporal patients. Bidzinski *et al* (1992), from Warsaw, reported that 2% of their series had occipital lesions. Fried *et al* (1994) described, inter alia 12

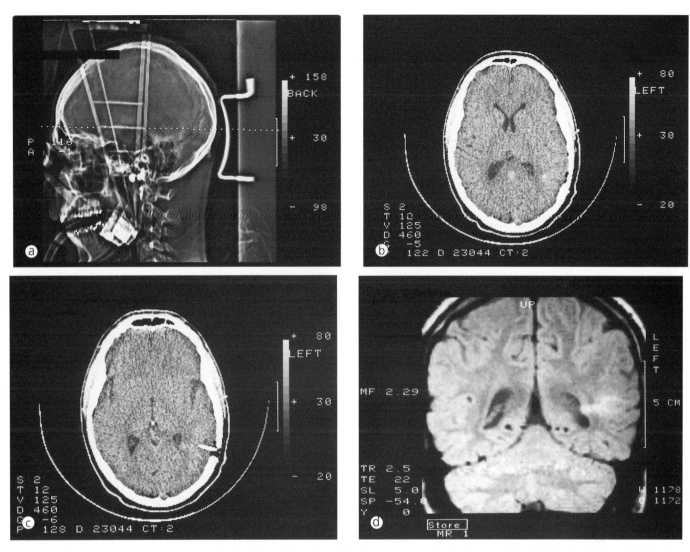

Fig. 52.2 Case 3. Diagnostic CT scans and MRI. (a) A lateral view of the CT-adapted tomography for intracranial localization (Laitinen *et al* 1985). (b) The small subcortical nodular tuber in the left parietal trigonum. (c) The intraoperative CT scan and the location of the plastic tubing inserted through a burr hole. (d) A coronal MRI of the lesion.

patients with seizures from clinically indolent occipital glial tumors, and Davies and Weeks (1993) also presented some cases. Clinical seizures are described in Chapter 6. Even in unilateral parietooccipital focal epilepsies, the epileptic activity may become bilateral. The superior and inferior longitudinal fasciculi may project occipital discharges to the frontotemporal regions, increasing the diagnostic complexity. The etiology of epileptogenic lesions was listed as birth trauma, anoxia, postnatal trauma, postinflammatory scarring, tumor and vascular lesion, multiple potential factors, miscellaneous, and unknown (Rasmussen 1979).

EXCISIONS AND RESULTS

A lateral occipital exploration near the midline gives ECoG access to the lateral, mesial, and basal surfaces, and to

functional mapping (SM responses). A radical nondominant excision leads to contralateral hemianopia and so the patient must be warned that new visual skills must be learnt, with turning of the head, to recognize events on the anopic side. An excision involving the visual radiation to the superior calcarine cortex will cause a contralateral lower-quadrant hemianopia; one involving the inferior radiation will cause an upper-quadrant hemianopia. Excision of lesions in the speech-dominant hemisphere is possible, but the resection must usually be made posterior to the Wernicke's area, defined functionally, in order to avoid dysphasia or dyslexia. Well-localized lesions (glial tumors, cavernous angiomas, etc) and surrounding epileptogenic area may be excised. A complete nondominant occipital lobe resection, as for a large Sturge–Weber malformation, is carried out by clipping the lobar arteries; dividing the lateral cortex in or near the parietal region; coagulating parasagittal, basal, and sigmoidal bridging veins, or leaving them embedded in a remnant of parasagittal cortex; and opening the occipital horn and removing the lobe after cutting the splenium of the corpus callosum. A large excision may require ventriculoperitoneal shunting.

Recent MNI experience has been described with 37 cases in whom an occipital excision alone was done, and 14 cases with inclusion of parietotemporal regions (Salanova *et al* 1992). When five other cases with a temporal excision are included, 46% of the cases became seizure-free. In the Bidzinski *et al* 1992 series, 10 of 11 patients became free from seizures. A summary of the results of central, parietal, and occipital extratemporal epilepsy surgery in 203 MNI patients with nontumoral epileptogenic lesions revealed that 34% had become seizure-free, and 23% markedly improved (Rasmussen 1987b). The author has experience from five occipital excisions. The next personal case illustrates the surgical effect on the visual field.

Illustrative case 4

The patient was a 31-year-old, right-handed woman who had suffered from partial epilepsy since the age of 3 years. As a child she would complain about lightning, occasionally followed by a generalized seizure. She now described her seizures as lightning in her left visual field as if she were driving along an avenue of trees. If the lightning spread to the right visual field, she lost consciousness. Visual examination revealed a left homonymous, medial, lower-quadrant field defect. Neuroradiologic investigations disclosed a small glial right mesial-parasagittal tumor. Scalp EEG showed a nonspecific, right-sided, frontotemporal abnormality. The IAT showed the patient was left hemisphere-dominant for speech. Subdural video-EEG recording from the right centroparietooccipital lobe showed short ictal discharges concomitant with the patient's visual experiences arising from the occipital region. A right craniotomy disclosed a superficial glial tumor in planum occipital, 3 cm from the midline. ECoG showed some local sharp waves. The tumor removed was a grade II astrocytoma. She has a complete left lower-quadrant hemianopia, her seizure outcome is class I (Engel *et al* 1993). Figure 52.3a and Plate 7 show the postexcision finding and Fig. 52.3b preoperative (thin line) and postoperative (thick line) visual field defects.

SPECIAL ENTITIES

GELASTIC SEIZURES

Diagnosis, surgery, and results

Gelastic seizures, at times associated with dyscrinia, behavioral, and mental problems, suggest the presence of a hypothalamic hamartoma. Munari *et al* (1995) studied the epileptogenicity of the hamartoma itself. Valdueza *et al* (1994) surveyed 12 cases of hamartoma resection, adding two cases of their own. Four out of 14 (28%) cases became seizure-free, 3 improved. Pallini *et al* (1993) published a case report on the outcome of anterior callosal section for generalized seizures. Maccado *et al* (1991) reported a case in which the lesion was resected. Cascino *et al* (1993b) reported a multicenter study of which 9 of 12 cases had other conventional epilepsy surgery interventions based on EEG findings; however, none of these patients became seizure-free. These two surveys include 21 cases treated with different surgical strategies. A partial or complete hamartoma excision gave better results than EEG-guided epilepsy surgery. Valdueza *et al* (1994) emphasized that only pendulous hamartomas are suitable for resection, otherwise there are high risks of complications. Kuzniecky *et al* (1997) reported a single case in which a right frontal lobectomy was only of temporary help. A later intratumoral stereotaxic thermocoagulation, preceded by intratumoral SEEG and functional stimulation, relieved the patient's seizures and ameliorated the behavioral problems. Surgery of gelastic epilepsy could thus be either removal of a pendulous hamartoma or a stereotaxic intrahamartomal electrocoagulation of sessile one. Nishio *et al* (1994) reported a successful outcome in a child after hamartoma removal.

CHRONIC ENCEPHALITIS

Seizures, diagnosis, and excisions

A book on chronic encephalitis was published in honour of Dr Theodore Rasmussen, the first physician to describe this severe epileptic condition (Andermann 1991) (Chapter 15). A surgical report of 39 such cases showed that 69% had a frontal, or a combined extrafrontal excision. The removals did not influence the course of the disease.

EPILEPSIA PARTIALIS CONTINUA

Seizures, diagnosis, and excisions

Patients with partial status epilepticus, epilepsia partialis continua of Kojewnikov, may have seizures continuing for days or longer. This severe clinical problem has been discussed in

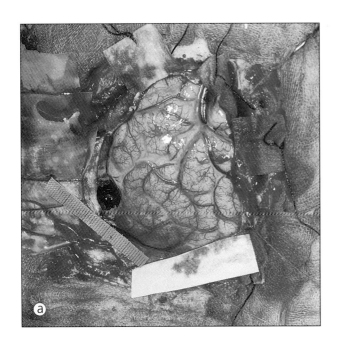

Fig. 52.3 Case 4. (a) A postexcision photograph of the exposed right occipital lobe after removal of a small mesioparasagittal astrocytoma (see Plate 7). (b,c) The preoperative (narrow lines) and postoperative (thick line) visual fields.

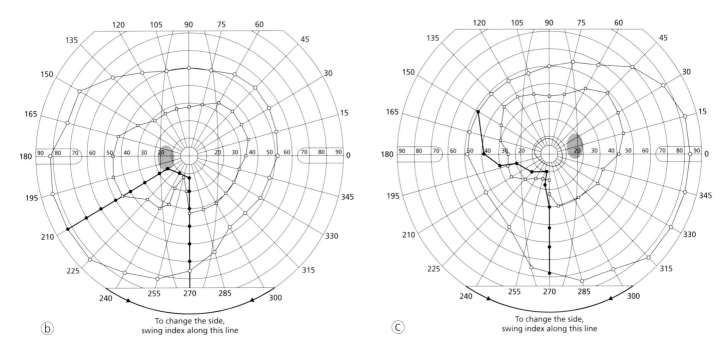

depth by Chauvel *et al* (1992), reporting SEEG analyses of 14 cases, and a mediocre surgical outcome in half of them (Talairach *et al* 1992a). If the excision was limited to the motor cortex, 1 out of 7 patients became seizure-free.

NEURONAL DEVELOPMENTAL DISTURBANCES

Chapter 7 focuses on neuronal developmental disturbances. Palmini *et al* (1992) studied the epileptogenicity of dysplastic cortex and presented aspects on the use of

ECoG during surgery. Dubeau *et al* (1995) presented a study on subcortical or periventricular heteropia in 52 patients. Seven of them were operated, two became seizure-free, or were significantly improved. Brännström *et al* (1996) described 22 extratemporal epilepsy surgery cases with mild cortical dysplasia, 46% becoming seizure-free and 9% almost seizure-free. Mihara *et al* (1997) reported on 25 patients operated for focal cortical dysplasia: 11 out of 14 became seizure-free. Palmini *et al* (1996) reported that a complete or near-complete (>80%) removal of the imaged lesion resulted in a favourable outcome in 55% of cases.

REOPERATIONS

Reoperation is carried out for extratemporal epilepsy. Rasmussen (1963) reported results of frontal excisions in 250 cases. Thirty-two cases were reoperated: two-thirds of them became seizure-free or markedly improved. Salanova *et al* (1994) studied the role of reoperation in 39 frontal lobe patients, 14% of all frontal lobe cases. One-fifth of them became seizure-free and 31% had a significant seizure reduction. Lehman *et al* (1994) reported reoperation in 6 of 20 patients with lower SM area seizures: 5 of the 6 patients became seizure-free or had rare seizures or more than 50% seizure reduction.

MULTILOBAR EXCISIONS

Large epileptogenic lesions extending beyond any one lobe require bilobar or multilobar removals, i.e., frontotemporocentral, frontocentroparietal, or frontoperisylvian excisions (Rasmussen 1987c; Chapter 45). The limits of the excisions are set by respect for eloquent cortices.

EXTRATEMPORAL EXCISIONS IN CHILDREN

Extratemporal epilepsy surgery can successfully be carried out in infants or children, as can hemispherectomies or hemispherotomies (Chapter 45). A lesion secondary to an intrauterine injury may lead to neurologic deficits, with or without mental retardation. If surgery is carried out soon after the onset of drug-resistant epilepsy, the excision will have the best chance of a good outcome, and cause the least neurologic deficits. Rasmussen (1977) reported the proportion of children (<16 years) who had undergone excisions in extratemporal areas; frontal 18%, sensorimotor cortex 41%, parietal 23%, and large destructive lesions in 50%. He also

reported the surgical outcome of 368 children (Rasmussen 1983b): there were 127 children with nontumoral epileptic lesions in the suprasylvian region, of whom 43% became seizure-free. Goldring (1987) reported extratemporal epilepsy surgery in 41 children, of whom 63% had a good outcome. A textbook on pediatric epilepsy surgery has recently been published (Tuxhorn *et al* 1997). The author has experience of local extratemporal epilepsy surgery in 32 children.

RADIOSURGERY FOR EPILEPSY

Huang *et al* (1995) reported on the radiosurgical management of epilepsy from arteriovenous malformations. Seizure control was obtained in about 77% of the 90 patients studied.

SUMMARY

Extratemporal epilepsy surgery can safely be carried out, but it is essential to define the chance of seizure relief and the risks to neurologic and cognitive function. On the whole, the clinical seizures are indicative of the laterality, location, and extent of the epileptogenic lesion. Imaging usually detects the lesion. Neuropsychology evaluates the patient's pre- and postsurgical capabilities. Invasive EEG or SEEG analysis and functional cortical mapping will supply detailed information for extratemporal epilepsy surgery. The outcome with regard to seizures is less favorable than after ATL because of restrictions imposed by the need to avoid damage to vital cortices. Frontal excisions lead to freedom from seizures in 20–50% and resections from other extratemporal regions leads to freedom from seizures in about 35%. Engel *et al* (1993) reported that extratemporal epilepsy surgery in 805 patients accomplished freedom from seizures in about 45%. The ILAE 1980–1990 Global Survey on Epilepsy Surgery (ILAE 1997) collected 566 extratemporal epilepsy surgery cases, of whom about 42% became seizure-free. The operative mortality is 0–5%, the morbidity 2–30%. The most frequent surgical complications, at times transient, are hemiparesis, dysphasia, and visual-field deficits. The outcome of extratemporal epilepsy surgery and the risks associated with these interventions should be balanced against the long-term outcome of intractable extratemporal epilepsy treated medically.

KEY POINTS

1. Extra temporal epilepsy surgery (ETES) is less frequent than anterior temporal lobectomy (ATL). Infants and adults with drug resistant partial epilepsy may be ETES candidates.
2. The classical histopathological ETES etiologies are well known. Development disturbances, cortical dysplasias, microdysgeneses, cavernous angiomas etc are recent etiologies disclosed by MRI.
3. Frontal lobe epilepsy surgery is the most common form of ETES. It utilizes 'state-of-the-art' diagnostics. A local excision, or a lobectomy, as reported in large patient series, will lead to freedom from seizures in 17–55%. A global survey on ETES complications listed no mortality, and a 2% morbidity.
4. Sensorimotor cortical epilepsy demands expert management. Excisions will cause little functional loss, if supported by neuronal plasticity. Pooling the central, parietal and occipital surgical results of some 200 patients, revealed that 34% were rendered seizure-free.
5. A comprehensive study of supplementary sensorimotor area (SSMA) seizures and their surgical treatment has recently been published. Invasive diagnostics with functional mapping prior to SSMA excisions in 28 cases resulted in 47% freedom from seizures. No, or transient morbidity was reported.
6. The language areas are surgically sacrosanct. Occasionally, an excision for epilepsy is carried out under precaution, within/near them, after exquisite diagnostics.
7. Non-dominant parietal lobe epileptic lesions can be clinically "silent", i.e. the seizures are symptomatic of the adjacent lobes. Dominant parietal lobe seizures may intefere with language and cognition and necessiate invasive diagnostics. Non-dominant parietal lobe excisions posterior to the S-cortex, may at times cause minor diagnostics. Extensive excisions may create disturbances of body image and sensory deficits. A speech-dominant excision must be carefully planned and executed. Parietal lobe excisions result in 45-65% freedom from seizures.
8. Nontumoral epileptic occipital lobe lesions consitute up to 5% of the ETES. Diagnostics should give access to the occipital surfaces for functional mapping. A radical non-dominant excision creates contralateral hemianopia. Excisions involving the visual radiations will cause contralateral quadrant hemianopias. Excising lesions on the speech-dominant side must be made posterior to the defined Wernicke area. Surgical experience has described 46% of the patients seizure-free.
9. ETES also involves surgery for: gelastic seizures, cingulate area seizures, Landau-Kleffner syndrome, chronic encephalitis, epilepsia partialis continua, insular area seizures, etc.
10. Reoperations may produce freedom from seizures in 20-65%.

REFERENCES

Andermann F (ed) (1991) *Chronic Encephalitis and Epilepsy: Rasmussen's Syndrome*. Montavle: Butterworths Heinemann.

Augustine EA, Novelly RA, Mattson RH *et al* (1984) Occupational adjustment following surgical treatment of epilepsy. *Annals of Neurology* 15:68–72.

Bancaud J, Talairach J (1992) Clinical semiology of frontal lobe seizures. In: Chauvel P, Delgado-Escueta AV, Halgren E *et al* (eds) *Frontal Lobe Seizures and Epilepsies* (Advances in Neurology, Vol 57), pp. 3–58. New York: Raven Press.

Bass N, Wyllie E, Comair Y *et al* (1995) Supplementary sensorimotor area seizures in children and adolescents. *Journal of Pediatrics* 126:537–544.

Bidzinski T, Bacia T, Rusikowski E (1992) The results of surgical treatment of occipital lobe epilepsy. *Acta Neurochirurgica* 114:128–130.

Bleasel AF, Morris HH III (1996) Supplementary sensorimotor area epilepsy in adults. *Advances in Neurology*. 70:271–284.

Britton JW, Cascino GD, Sharbrough FW *et al* (1994) Low-grade glial neoplasms and intractable partial epilepsy: efficacy of surgical treatment. *Epilepsia* 35:1130–1135.

Brännström T, Silfvenius H, Olivecrona M (1996) The range of disorders of cortical organization in surgically treated epilepsy patients. In: Guerrini R, Andermann F, Canapicchi R *et al* (eds) *Dysplasias of Cerebral Cortex and Epilepsy*, pp. 57–64. Philadelphia: Lippincott-Raven.

Cascino GD, Jack CR Jr, Parisi JE *et al* (1992) MRI in the presurgical evaluation of patients with frontal lobe epilepsy and children with temporal lobe epilepsy: pathologic correlation and prognostic importance. *Epilepsy Research* 1:51–59.

Cascino GD, Hulihan JF Sharbrough FW *et al* (1993a) Parietal lobe lesional epilepsy: electroclinical correlation and operative outcome. *Epilepsia* 34:522–527.

Cascino GD, Andermann F, Berkovic SF *et al* (1993b) Gelastic seizures and hypothalamic hamartomas: evaluation of patients undergoing chronic intracranial EEG monitoring and outcome of surgical treatment. *Neurology* 43:747–750.

Cascino GD, Sharbrough FW, Trenerry MR *et al* (1994) Extratemporal cortical resections and lesionectomies for partial epilepsy: complications of surgical treatment. *Epilepsia* 35:1085–1090.

Chauvel P, Delgado-Escueta AV, Halgren E *et al* (eds) (1992) *Frontal*

Lobe Seizures and Epilepsies (Advances in Neurology, Vol 57). New York: Raven Press.

Clarke DB, Olivier A, Andermann F *et al* (1996) Surgical treatment of epilepsy: the problem of lesion/focus incongruence. *Surgical Neurology.* **46**:579–585, discussion 585–586.

Comair YG, Hong SC, Bleasel AF (1996) Invasive investigation and surgery of the supplementary motor area. The Cleveland experience. In: Lüders HO (ed) *Supplementary Sensorimotor Area*, pp 369–378. Philadelphia: Lippincott-Raven.

Comair YG, Ha YC, Van Ness P (1997) Neocortical resections. In: Engel J Jr, Pedley TA (eds) *Epilepsy: A Comprehensive Textbook*, pp. 1819–1828. Philadelphia: Lippincott-Raven.

Connelly A (1997) Proton magnetic resonance spectroscopy (MRS) in epilepsy. *Epilepsia* **38** (Suppl 10): 33–38.

Cosgrove GR, Buchbinder BR, Jiang H (1996) Functional magnetic resonance imaging for intracranial navigation. *Neurosurgery Clinics of North America* **7**:313–322.

Crandall PH (1987) Cortical resections. In: Engel J Jr (ed) *Surgical Treatment of the Epilepsies*, pp. 377–404. New York: Raven Press.

Cukiert A, Olivier A, Andermann F (1996) Post traumatic frontal lobe epilepsy with structural changes: excellent results after cortical resection. *Canadian Journal of Neurological Sciences* **23**:114–117.

Davies KG, Weeks RD (1993) Cortical resections for intractable epilepsy of extratemporal origin: experience with seventeen cases over eleven years. *British Journal of Neurosurgery* **7**:343–353.

Devaux B, Meder JF, Missir O *et al* (1996) [The rolandic line: a simple baseline for the identification of the central region. An MRI study and functional validation]. *Journal of Neuroradiology* **23**:6–18.

Devinsky O, Morrel MJ, Vogt BA (1995) Contributions of anterior cingulate cortex to behaviour. *Brain* **118**:279–306.

Dodrill CB, Wilkus RJ, Ojemann GA *et al* (1986) Multidisciplinary prediction of seizure relief from cortical resection surgery. *Annals of Neurology* **20**:2–12.

Dubeau F, Tampieri D, Lee N *et al* (1995) Periventricular and subcortical nodular heterotopia. A study of 33 patients. *Brain* **118**:1273–1287.

Engel J Jr (1987) Outcome with respect to epileptic seizures. In: Engel J Jr (ed) *Surgical Treatment of the Epilepsies*, pp.553–72. New York: Raven Press.

Engel J Jr, Pedley TA (eds) (1997) *Epilepsy: A Comprehensive Textbook*, Vol III. Philadelphia: Lippincott-Raven.

Engel J Jr, Van Ness PC, Rasmussen TB *et al* (1993) Outcome with respect to epileptic seizures. In: Engel J Jr (ed) *Surgical Treatment of the Epilepsies*, 2nd edn, pp. 609–621. New York: Raven Press.

Fraser A (1988) Improving functional rehabilitation outcome following epilepsy surgery. *Acta Neurologica Scandinavica* **78**(Suppl 117):122–128.

Fried I, Kim JH, Spencer DD (1994) Limbic and neocortical gliomas associated with intractable seizures: a distinct clinicopathological group. *Neurosurgery* **34**:815–823, discussion 823–824.

Goldring S (1987) Surgical management of epilepsy in children. In: Engel J Jr (ed) *Surgical Treatment of the Epilepsies*, pp. 445–464. New York: Raven Press.

Gomez-Tortosa E, Martin EM, Gaviria M *et al* (1995) Selective deficit of one language in a bilingual patient following surgery in the left perisylvian area. *Brain and Language* **48**:320–325.

Gorecki JP, Smith RR, Wee AS (1992) Excision of arteriovenous malformation in sensorimotor and language related neocortex using stimulation mapping and corticography under local anesthesia. *Stereotactic and Functional Neurosurgery* **58**:89.

Guerrini R, Andermann F, Canapicchi R *et al* (eds) (1996) *Dysplasias of Cerebral Cortex and Epilepsy*. Philadelphia: Lippincott-Raven.

Haglund MM, Ojemann GA, Hochman DW (1992) Optical imaging of epileptiform and functional activity in human cerebral cortex. *Nature* **358**:668–671.

Hari R (1993) Magnetoencephalography as a tool of clinical neurophysiology. In: Niedermeyer E, Lopez da Silva (eds) *Electroencephalography. Basic Principles, Clinical Applications and Related Fields*, pp. 1035–61. Baltimore: Williams & Wilkins.

Hedström A, Malmgren K, Hagberg I *et al* (1996) Cortical reorganisation of sensory, motor and language functions due to early cortical damage. *Epilepsy Research* **23**:157–167.

Henry TR, Mazziotta JC, Engel J Jr (1992) The functional anatomy of frontal lobe epilepsy studied with PET. In: Chauvel P, Delgado-Escueta AV Halgren E *et al* (eds) *Frontal Lobe Seizures and Epilepsies* (Advances in Neurology Vol 57), pp 449–463. New York: Raven Press.

Hinz AC, Berger MS, Ojemann GA *et al* (1994) The utility of the intracarotid Amytal procedure in determining hemispheric speech lateralization in pediatric epilepsy patients undergoing surgery. *Child's Nervous System* **10**:239–243.

Ho SS, Berkovic SF, Newton MR *et al* (1994) Parietal lobe epilepsy: clinical features and seizure localization by ictal SPECT. *Neurology* **44**:2277–2284.

Hojo M, Miyamoto S, Nakahara I *et al* (1995) [A case of arteriovenous malformation successfully treated with functional mapping of the language area by PET activation study]. *No Shinkei Geka* **23**:537–541.

Huang CF, Somaza S, Lunsford LD *et al* (1995) Radiosurgery in the management of epilepsy associated with arteriovenous malformations. In: Kondziolka D (ed) *Radiosurgery*, pp. 195–200. Basel: Karger.

ILAE (1997) Global Survey on Epilepsy Surgery, 1980–1990: A Report by the Commission on Neurosurgery of Epilepsy. *Epilepsia* **38**:249–256.

Jack CR Jr, Thompson RM, Butts RK *et al* (1994) Sensory motor cortex: correlation of presurgical mapping with functional MR imaging and invasive cortical mapping. *Radiology* **190**:85–92.

Jayakar P, Alvarez LA, Duchowny MS *et al* (1992) A safe and effective paradigm to functionally map the cortex in childhood. *Journal of Clinical Neurophysiology* **9**:288–293.

Kazemi NJ, So EL, Mosewich RK *et al* (1997) Resection of frontal encephalomalacias for intractable epilepsy: outcome and prognostic factors. *Epilepsia* **38**:670–677.

Kuzniecky R, Guthrie B, Mountz J *et al* (1997) Intrinsic epileptogenesis of hypothalamic hamartomas in gelastic epilepsy. *Annals of Neurology* **42**:60–67.

Laich E, Kuzniecky R, Mountz J *et al* (1997) Supplementary sensorimotor area epilepsy. Seizure localization, cortical propagation and subcortical activation pathways using ictal SPECT. *Brain* **120**:855–864.

Laitinen LV, Liliequist B, Fagerlund *et al* (1985) An adapter for computed tomography-guided stereotaxis. *Surgical Neurology* **23**:559–566.

Laskowitz DT, Sperling MR, French JA *et al* (1995) The syndrome of frontal lobe epilepsy: characteristics and surgical management. *Neurology* **45**:780–787.

Laxer KD (1997) Clinical applications of magnetic resonance spectroscopy. *Epilepsia* **38**(Suppl 4):S13–17.

Lehman RM, Kim HI (1995) Partial seizures with onset in central area: use of the callosal grid system for localization. *Acta Neurochiraurgica Wien Supplementum* **64**:79–82.

Lehman R, Andermann F, Olivier A *et al* (1994) Seizures with onset in the sensorimotor face area: clinical patterns and results of surgical treatment in 20 patients. *Epilepsia* **35**:1117–1124.

Levesque MF, Sutherling WW, Crandall PH (1992) Surgery of central sensory motor and dorsolateral frontal lobe seizures. *Stereotactic and Functional Neurosurgery* **58**:168–171.

Lorenzo NY, Parisi JE, Cascino GD *et al* (1995) Intractable frontal lobe epilepsy: pathological and MRI features. *Epilepsy Research* **20**:171–178.

Loring DW, Meador KJ, Lee GP *et al* (1992) (eds) *Amobarbital Effects and Lateralized Brain Function. The Wada Test.* New York: Springer-Verlag. pp. 1–138.

Lüders HO (ed) (1992) *Epilepsy Surgery*. New York: Raven Press.

Luders HO (ed) (1996) *Supplementary Sensorimotor Area* (Advances in Neurology Vol 70). Philadelphia: Lippincott-Raven.

Lüders H, Lesser R, Dinner DS *et al* (1987) Commentary: Chronic intracranial recording and stimulation with subdural electrodes. In: Engel J Jr (ed) *Surgical Treatment of the Epilepsies*, pp 297–321. New York: Raven Press.

Lüders HO, Lesser RP, Dinner DS *et al* (1992) A negative motor response elicited by electrical stimulation of the human frontal cortex. In: Chauvel P, Delgado-Escueta AV, Halgren E *et al* (eds) *Frontal Lobe Seizures and Epilepsies* (Advances in Neurology, Vol 57), pp 149–158. Philadelphia: Lippincott-Raven.

Maccado HR, Hoffman HJ, Hwang PA (1991) Gelastic seizures treated by resection of a hypothalamic hamartoma. *Child's Nervous System* 7:462–465.

Mazars G (1970) Criteria for identifying cingulate epilepsies. *Epilepsia* 11:41–48.

Meyer JR, Roychowdhury S, Russell EJ *et al* (1996) Location of the central sulcus via cortical thickness of the precentral and postcentral gyri on MR. *American Journal of Neuroradiology* 17:1699–1706.

Mihara T, Tottori T, Inoue Y *et al* (1996) Surgical strategies for patients with supplementary sensorimotor area epilepsy. The Japanese experience. *Advances in Neurology* 70:405–414.

Mihara T, Matsuda K, Tottori T *et al* (1997) [Focal cortical dysplasia and epilepsy surgery]. *No To Hattatsu* 29:134–144.

Milner B, Branch C, Rasmussen T (1966) Evidence for bilateral speech representation in some non right handers. *Transactions of the American Neurological Association* 91:306–308.

Morioka T, Yamamoto T, Mizushima A *et al* (1995) Comparison of magnetoencephalography, functional MRI, and motor evoked potentials in the localization of the sensory motor cortex. *Neurological Research* 17:361–367.

Morris HH, Estes ML, Gilmore R *et al* (1993) Chronic intractable epilepsy as the only symptom of primary brain tumor. *Epilepsia* 34:1038–1043.

Müller WM, Morris GL III (1993) Intraoperative and extraoperative identification of eloquent brain using stimulation mapping. *Neurosurgery Clinics of North America* 4:217–222.

Munari C, Bancaud J (1992) Electroclinical symptomatology of partial seizures of orbital frontal origin. In: Chauvel P, Delgado-Escueta AV, Halgren E *et al* (eds) *Frontal Lobe Seizures and Epilepsies* (Advances in Neurology, Vol 57), pp. 257–266. New York: Raven Press.

Munari C, Kahane P, Francione S (1995) Role of the hypothalamic hamartoma in the genesis of gelastic fits. *Electroencephalography and Clinical Neurophysiology* 95:154–160.

Munari C, Quarato PP, Di Leo M *et al* (1996) Surgical strategies for patients with supplementary motor area epilepsy. The Grenoble experience. *Advances in Neurology* 70:379–403.

Nass R, Heier L, Walker R (1993) Landau Kleffner syndrome: temporal lobe tumor resection results in good outcome. *Pediatric Neurology* 9:303–305.

Nishio S, Morioka T, Fukui M *et al* (1994) Surgical treatment of intractable seizures due to hypothalamic hamartoma. *Epilepsia* 35:514–519.

Olivier A (1992) Extratemporal cortical resections: principles and methods. In: Lüders HO (ed) *Epilepsy Surgery*, pp. 559–568. New York: Raven Press.

Olivier A (1995) Surgery of frontal lobe epilepsy. *Advances in Neurology* 66:321–348, discussion 348–352.

Olivier A (1996) Surgical strategies for patients with supplementary sensorimotor area epilepsy. The Montreal experience. *Advances in Neurology* 70:429–443.

Olivier A, Alonso Vanegas M *et al* (1996) Image guided surgery of epilepsy. *Neurosurgery Clinics of North America* 7:229–243.

Pallini R, Bozzini V, Colichio G *et al* (1993) Callosotomy for generalized seizures associated with hypothalamic hamartoma. *Neurological Research* 15:139–141.

Palmini A, da Costa JC, Andermann I *et al* (1992) Focal electographic ictal activity during acute cortical recording over dysplastic lesions in humans. *Epilepsia* 33:75.

Palmini A, Andermann F, Dubeau F *et al* (1993a) Occipitotemporal epilepsies: evaluation of selected patients requiring depth electrodes studies and rationale for surgical approaches. *Epilepsia* 34:84–96.

Palmini A, Gambordella A, Andermann F *et al* (1996) Outcome of surgical treatment in patients with localized cortical dysplasia and intractable epilepsy. In: Guerrini R, Andermann F, Canapicchi R *et al* (eds) *Dysplasias of Cerebral Cortex and Epilepsy*, pp. 367–374. Philadelphia: Lippincott-Raven.

Patil AA, McConnel JR, Torkelson RD (1995) Stereotactic location and excision of seizure focus with Xenon enhanced CT. *American Journal of Neuroradiology* 16:644–646.

Penfield W, Flanigin H (1950) Surgical therapy of temporal lobe seizures. *AMA Archives of Neurology and Psychiatry* 64:491–500.

Penfield W, Jasper HH (1954) *Epilepsy and the Functional Anatomy of the Human Brain*. Boston: Little Brown.

Penfield W, Roberts L (1959) *Speech and Brain Mechanisms*. Princeton: Princeton University Press.

Prayson RA, Estes ML (1995) Cortical dysplasia: a histopathologic study of 52 cases of partial lobectomy in patients with epilepsy. *Human Pathology* 26:493–500.

Puce A (1995) Comparative assessment of sensorimotor function using functional magnetic resonance imaging and electrophysiological methods. *Journal of Clinical Neurophysiology* 12:450–459.

Quesney LF (1992) Extratemporal epilepsy: clinical presentation, preoperative EEG localization and surgical outcome. *Acta Neurologica Scandinavica* 86(Suppl 140):81–94.

Rasmussen T (1963) Surgical therapy of frontal lobe epilepsy. *Epilepsia* 4:181–198.

Rasmussen T (1970) Surgical therapy of frontal lobe epilepsy. *Epilepsia* 11:27–28.

Rasmussen T (1975a) Surgery of frontal lobe epilepsy. In: Purpura DP *et al* (eds) *Advances in Neurology*, Vol 8, pp. 197–205. New York: Raven Press.

Rasmussen T (1975b) Surgery of epilepsy arising in regions other than the temporal and frontal lobes. In: Purpura DP *et al* (eds) *Advances in Neurology*, Vol 8, pp 207–226. New York: Raven Press.

Rasmussen TB (1977) Surgical aspects. In: Braw ME (ed), *Topics in Child Neurology*, pp. 143–157. Toronto: Spectrum Publications.

Rasmussen T (1979) Cortical resection for medically refractory focal epilepsy: results, lessons, and questions. In: Rasmussen T, Marino R (eds) *Functional Neurosurgery*, pp 253–269. Raven Press: New York.

Rasmussen T (1983a) Characteristics of a pure culture of frontal lobe epilepsy. *Epilepsia* 24:482–493.

Rasmussen T (1983b) Cortical resection in children with focal epilepsy. In: Parsonage M *et al* (eds) *Advances in Epileptology* XIVth Int. Epilepsy Symp, pp. 249–254. New York: Raven Press.

Rasmussen T (1987a) Commentary: Extratemporal cortical excisions and hemispherectomy. In: Engel J Jr (ed) *Surgical Treatment of the Epilepsies*, pp. 417–424. New York: Raven Press.

Rasmussen T (1987b) Focal epilepsies of nontemporal and nonfrontal origin. In: Wieser HG, Elger CE (eds) *Presurgical Evaluation of Epileptics*. pp. 300–305. Berlin: Springer Verlag.

Rasmussen T (1987c) Cortical resection for multiple epileptogenic lesions. In: Wieser HG, Elger CE (eds) *Presurgical Evaluation of Epileptics*. pp. 344–351. Berlin: Springer Verlag.

Rasmussen T (1991) Tailoring of cortical excisions for frontal lobe epilepsy. *Canadian Journal of Neurological Sciences* 18:606–610.

Raymond AA, Fish DR, Sisodiya SM *et al* (1995) Abnormalities of gyration, heterotopias, tuberous sclerosis, focal cortical dysplasia, microdysgenesis, dysembryoplastic neuroepithelial tumour and dysgenesis of the archicortex in epilepsy. Clinical, EEG and neuroimaging features in 100 adult patients. *Brain* 118:629–660.

Roberts DW, Darcey TM (1996) The evaluation and image guided surgical treatment of the patient with a medically intractable seizure disorder. *Neurosurgery Clinics of North America* 7:215–227.

Robitaille Y, Rasmussen T, Dubeau F *et al* (1992) Histopathology of non neoplastic lesions in frontal lobe epilepsy: review of 180 cases with recent MRI and PET correlations. In: Chauvel P, Delgado-Escueta AV, Halgren E *et al* (eds) *Frontal Lobe Seizures and Epilepses* (Advances in Neurology, Vol 57), pp 499–514. Philadelphia, Raven Press.

Roper SN, Levesque MF, Sutherling WW *et al* (1993) Surgical treatment of partial epilepsy arising from the insular cortex. Report of two cases. *Journal of Neurosurgery* 79:266–269.

Rougier A, Dartigues JF, Commenges D *et al* (1992) A longitudinal assessment of seizure outcome and overall benefit from 100 cortectomies for epilepsy. *Journal of Neurology, Neurosurgery and Psychiatry* 55:762–767.

Salanova V, Andermann F, Olivier A *et al* (1992) Occipital lobe epilepsy: electroclinical manifestations, electrocorticography, cortical stimulation and outcome in 42 patients treated between 1930 and 1991. Surgery of occipital lobe epilepsy. *Brain* 115:1655–1680.

Salanova V, Morris HH III, Van Ness PC *et al* (1993) Comparison of scalp electroencephalogram with subdural electrocorticogram recordings and functional mapping in frontal lobe epilepsy. *Archives of Neurology* 50:294–299.

Salanova V, Quesney LF, Rasmussen T *et al* (1994) Reevaluation of surgical failures and the role of reoperation in 39 patients with frontal lobe epilepsy. *Epilepsia* 35:70–80.

Salanova V, Andermann F, Rasmussen T *et al* (1995a) Parietal lobe epilepsy. Clinical manifestations and outcome in 82 patients treated surgically between 1929 and 1988. *Brain* 118:607–627.

Salanova V, Andermann F, Rasmussen T *et al* (1995b) Tumoural parietal lobe epilepsy. Clinical manifestations and outcome in 34 patients treated between 1934 and 1988. *Brain* 118:1289–1304.

Schaffler L, Lüders HO, Beck GJ (1996) Quantitative comparison of language deficits produced by extraoperative electrical stimulation of Broca's, Wernicke's, and basal temporal language areas. *Epilepsia* 37:463–475.

Silbergeld DL (1997) Tumors of Heschl's gyrus: report of two cases. *Neurosurgery* 40:389–392.

Silbergeld DL, Mueller WM, Colley PS *et al* (1992) Use of propofol (Diprivan) for awake craniotomies: technical note. *Surgical Neurology* 38:271–272.

Silfvenius H, Gloor P, Rasmussen T (1964) Evaluation of insular ablation in surgical treatment of temporal lobe epilepsy. *Epilepsia* 5:307–320.

Silfvenius H, Fagerlund M, Säisä J *et al* (1997) Carotid angiography in conjunction with amytal testing of epilepsy patients. *Brain and Cognition* 33:33–49.

Smith JR, King DW (1996) Surgical strategies for patients with supplementary sensorimotor area epilepsy. The Medical College of Georgia experience. *Advances in Neurology* 70:415–427.

Smith JR, Gallen CC, Schwartz BJ (1994) Multichannel magnetoencephalographic mapping of sensorimotor cortex for epilepsy surgery. *Stereotactic and Functional Neurosurgery* 62:245–251.

Spencer DD, Schumacher J (1996) Surgical management of patients with intractable supplementary motor area seizures. The Yale experience. *Advances in Neurology* 70:445–450.

Sutherling WW, Levesque MF, Baumgartner C (1992) Cortical sensory representation of the human hand: size of finger regions and nonoverlapping digit somatotopy. *Neurology* 42:1020–1028.

Swartz BE, Theodore WH, Sanabria E *et al* (1992) Positron emission and single photon emission computed tomographic studies in the frontal lobe with emphasis on the relationship to seizure foci. In: Chauvel P, Delgado-Escueta AV, Halgren E *et al* (eds) *Frontal Lobe Seizures and Epilepsies* (Advances in Neurology, Vol 57), pp 487–497. New York: Raven Press.

Talairach J, David M, Toumoux P (eds) (1958) *L'exploration chirurgicale stéréotaxique et technique chirurgicale.* Paris: Masson.

Talairach J, Bancaud J, Bonis A *et al* (1992a) Surgical therapy for frontal epilepsies. In: Chauvel P, Delgado-Escueta AV, Halgren E *et al* (eds) *Frontal Lobe Seizures and Epilepsies.* (Advances in Neurology, Vol 57), pp 707–732. New York: Raven Press.

Talairach J, Toumoux P, Musolino A *et al* (1992b) Stereotaxic exploration in frontal epilepsy. In: Chauvel P, Delgado-Escueta AV, Halgren E *et al* (eds) *Frontal Lobe Seizures and Epilepsies* (Advances in Neurology, Vol 57), pp 651–688. New York: Raven Press.

Taylor DC, Falconer MA (1968) Clinical, socio-economic, and psychological changes after temporal lobectomy. *British Journal of Psychiatry* 114:1247–1261.

Turmel A, Giard N, Bouvier G *et al* (1992) Frontal lobe seizures and epilepsy: Indications for cortectomies or callosotomies. In: Chauvel P, Delgado-Escueta AV, Halgren E *et al* (eds) *Frontal Lobe Seizures and Epilepsies* (Advances in Neurology, Vol 57), pp. 689–706. New York: Raven Press.

Tuxhorn I, Holthausen H, Boenigk H (eds) (1997) *Paediatric Epilepsy Syndromes and Their Surgical Treatment.* London. John Libbey.

Uematsu S, Lesser R, Fisher RS *et al* (1992) Motor and sensory cortex in humans: topography studied with chronic subdural stimulation [see comments]. *Neurosurgery* 31:59–71, discussion 71–72.

Valdueza JM, Cristante L, Dammann O *et al* (1994) Hypothalamic hamartomas: with special reference to gelastic epilepsy and surgery. *Neurosurgery* 34:949–958, discussion 958.

Van Buren JM (1987) Complications of surgical procedures in the diagnosis and treatment of epilepsy. In: Engel J Jr. (ed) *Surgical Treatment of the Epilepsies*, pp. 465–475. New York: Raven Press.

Van Ness PC (1992) Surgical outcome of neocortical (extrahippocampal) focal epilepsy. In: Lüders HO (ed) *Epilepsy Surgery*, pp. 613–624. New York: Raven Press.

Vogt B, Finch D, Olson C (1992) Functional heterogeneity in the cingulate cortex: the anterior executive and posterior evaluative regions. *Cerebral Cortex* 2:435–443.

Williamson PD, Boon PA, Thadani VM *et al* (1992) Parietal lobe epilepsy: diagnostic considerations and results of surgery. *Annals of Neurology* 31:193–201.

Wyler AR, Ojemann GA, Lettich E *et al* (1984) Subdural strip electrodes for localizing epileptogenic foci. *Journal of Neurosurgery* 60:1195–1200.

Wyler AR, Richey ET, Atkinson RA *et al* (1987) Methohexital activation of epileptogenic foci during acute electrocorticography. *Epilepsia* 28:490–494.

Yetkin FZ, Papke RA, Mark LP *et al* (1995) Location of the sensorimotor cortex: functional and conventional MR compared. *American Journal of Neuroradiology* 16:2109–2113.

Yetkin FZ, Mueller WM, Morris GL *et al* (1997) Functional MR activation correlated with intraoperative cortical mapping. *American Journal of Neuroradiology* 18:1311–1315.

Zentner J, Hufnagel A, Ostertun B *et al* (1996a) Surgical treatment of extratemporal epilepsy: clinical, radiologic, and histopathologic findings in 60 patients. *Epilepsia* 37:1072–1080.

Zentner J, Hufnagel A, Pechstein U *et al* (1996b) Functional results after resective procedures involving the supplementary motor area. *Journal of Neurosurgery* 85:542–549.

Hemispherectomy

GF TUITE, CE POLKEY, AND W HARKNESS

BACKGROUND

Hemispherectomy refers to a variety of operations that functionally isolate the cerebral cortex of one hemisphere from the rest of the nervous system. Hemispherectomy accounted for 7.9% of operations at the Maudsley Hospital and around 5% of operations in other surgical units (Anonymous 1997). It is useful for a subset of patients with medically refractory epilepsy originating from a globally disturbed hemisphere with multiple seizure foci. It has recently gained wider acceptance as a safe and effective treatment option for selected patients with medically refractory epilepsy, but its origins can be traced to tumor surgery nearly 70 years ago.

In 1928, Dandy and L'Hermitte each described their use of complete hemisphere removal as a radical treatment for diffuse infiltrative glioma (Dandy 1928; L'Hermitte 1928). The operation was well-tolerated, but it eventually proved futile because of inevitable tumor recurrence. Ten years later, K.G. MacKenzie performed the first hemispherectomy for seizures, but its use failed to gain wide acceptance (MacKenzie 1938). In 1950, Krynauw reported hemisphere removal in the treatment of 12 patients with infantile hemiplegia and uncontrollable seizures (Krynauw

1950). Excellent seizure control with minimal morbidity and mortality were encouraging, but he was also impressed by the striking and lasting behavioral improvement after surgery.

Hemispherectomy waned in popularity during the 1960s as more effective anticonvulsants became available and significant long-term complications of the operation became apparent. The most striking of these was the occurrence of a slow neurologic and intellectual deterioration and death, which was estimated by Oppenheimer and Griffith as 17% in the Oxford series (Oppenheimer and Griffith 1966) and by Falconer and Wilson as 22% in the Guy's–Maudsley series (Falconer and Wilson 1969). The reason for this perplexing decline was eventually elucidated by Oppenheimer and Griffith (1966). They recognized that delayed hemorrhage was responsible for the deterioration, resulting in hemosiderosis of the remaining brain and ventricles, leading to mass effect or hydrocephalus and eventual decline.

For the past 30 years, surgeons have developed techniques that remove or isolate epileptogenic cortex from the remainder of the nervous system while minimizing the dead space created by an anatomic hemisphere removal. Rasmussen's subtotal hemispherectomy lessened the incidence of hemosiderosis, but seizure control was disappointingly poor (Rasmussen 1973). To improve seizure control, a modification was employed that disrupts all white-matter connections while leaving the frontal and occipital lobes intact. This functional hemispherectomy has improved seizure control while maintaining a low incidence of hemosiderosis (Rasmussen 1983). Similarly, Hoffman's hemispheric corticectomy removes all epileptogenic tissue on the affected side without removing the underlying tissue, thus minimizing dead space (Villemure *et al* 1993). The Oxford modification takes a different approach, by removing the entire hemisphere but isolating the intracranial compartments from each other, eliminating the dead space by tacking the dural leaves over the remaining cavity (Adams 1983). Delalande and colleagues and Schramm and colleagues have developed the procedure of hemispherotomy, providing a functional hemispheric disconnection with minimal brain tissue removal (Delalande *et al* 1993; Schramm *et al* 1995).

Because each modification produces a functional disconnection of the affected hemisphere's cortex, they are likely to prove similarly effective in seizure control, and the outcome may also be related to the pathology in the affected hemisphere. The improved safety of these modifications, coupled with the improvements in neuroimaging and neurophysiologic monitoring, has made hemispherectomy a more attractive and useful treatment for a subset of patients with medically refractory epilepsy. It is also of interest that this sequence of events has led to an operation that is mostly a disconnection since the amount of tissue removed in recent Montreal functional hemispherectomies is much less than in the original description of the operation.

PATHOLOGY OF UNILATERAL HEMISPHERE DISEASE

Patients with major or diffuse hemispheric injury and intractable seizures are usually considered for surgery during childhood. They suffer from a wide variety of conditions, which may be divided into three groups based on the mode of onset of the disease and tempo of its progression (Wilson 1970; Polkey 1990). The first group consists of patients with a sudden, massive insult that results in a fixed neurologic deficit. These are usually children with infantile hemiplegia, but those with posttraumatic brain injury or vascular insults of various etiologies may also be included. The second group is made up of patients with congenital conditions such as Sturge–Weber syndrome or neuronal migrational disorders such as hemimegalencephaly, whose neurologic manifestations often have a later onset and may be progressive. The final group consists of diseases with a

delayed presentation and a progressive course, such as Rasmussen encephalitis (Table 53.1).

VASCULAR INSULTS

Extensive hemispheric injury can occur as the result of vascular disease from a variety of causes. Most patients are classified as infantile hemiplegia, usually the result of a prenatal, birth, or neonatal injury. The precise etiology is often unknown, and the diagnosis of a vascular injury is presumptive, based on the extensive damage to the hemisphere, most often in the middle cerebral artery distribution (Cairns 1951; McKissock 1953). Prior to the introduction of modern antibiotics and aggressive hydration in the treatment of infectious disease, many patients had diffuse hemispheric injury related to infarction after severe dehydration. While this form of ischemic injury is becoming more unusual, cerebral infarction related to severe hypotension is not uncommon. This latter group consists primarily of patients who undergo cardiac surgery or those treated with extracorporeal membranous oxygenation (ECMO). Children only rarely suffer injury to the hemisphere as a result of vascular malformations or aneurysms, but these conditions can similarly result in diffuse hemispheric injury.

Patients with infantile hemiplegia usually have a severe unilateral injury resulting in a dense contralateral spastic hemiplegia and homonymous hemianopsia. Because injury usually occurs at a young age, language function is localized to the contralateral hemisphere (Krynauw 1950; Cairns 1951; White 1961; Wilson 1970; Verity and Strauss 1982; Goodman and Williamson 1985). The commonest injury is infarction in the middle cerebral artery territory, producing relative sparing of the frontal lobe. On other occasions, hypotensive hemispheric infarction may result in unilateral injury in a watershed distribution, sparing the occipital lobe. The severity of the hemiparesis is variable and visual function may be intact. The degree of language impairment

Table 53.1 Diseases affecting patients chosen for hemispherectomy. Comparison of an early and contemporary series.

Pathology	Late series (Maudsley) (n = 34)		Early series (Wilson)[a] (n = 48)	
	No	(%)	No	(%)
Neonatal injury	15	(44%)	27	(54%)
Rasmussen disease	13	(38%)		
Unclear			15	(30%)
Hemimegalencephaly	4	(12%)		
Sturge–Weber	2	(6%)	6	(12%)

[a]Wilson PJE (1970).

depends on the age at the time of insult and whether the insult was to the dominant hemisphere (Rasmussen and Milner 1977). Injury from vascular anomalies present with widely variable neurologic signs. Structural imaging reflects the severity of the disease, and may be manifested as atrophy, porencephalic cysts, and diffuse atrophy.

HEMIMEGALENCEPHALY AND OTHER NEURONAL MIGRATIONAL DISORDERS

Neuronal migrational disorders can vary in severity from lissencephaly to focal cortical dysplasias. They produce variable neurologic deficits with a variety of different seizure disorders. Patients with medically refractory epilepsy and focal cortical dysplasia may be candidates for focal resections, but hemimegalencephaly is the most common neuronal migrational disorder considered for hemispherectomy (Palmini et al 1994).

Patients with hemimegalencephaly present with an early onset of seizures, psychomotor retardation, hemiparesis, and often a hemianopia (King et al 1985; Pelayo and Barasch 1994). They sometimes have a large head and an associated skin disorder such as linear nevus sebaceus or chronic linear nevi (Clancy and Kurtz 1985). There is an early seizure onset, and a propensity for partial motor seizures. Structural imaging shows a markedly enlarged hemisphere, with a disrupted and thickened cortical mantle (Kalifa and Chiron 1987; Osborn and Byrd 1988; Kuzniecky 1994; Renowden and Squier, 1994; Yuh and Nguyen 1994). Their characteristic EEG shows hemihypsarrhythmia on the affected side, with a high-frequency background and almost continuous spikes, sharp waves, and spike waves. Pathologically, there is pachygyria with poorly represented white matter on gross inspection. Microscopically, a loss of cortical lamination, giant neurons, neuronal heterotopia, and gliosis are typical (Dambska and Wisniewski 1984; Robain et al 1988).

Neurologic deficits are variable, and those with significant preservation of function may be candidates for focal resection or multiple subpial transection (King et al 1985; Vigevano et al 1989; Vigevano and Di 1990; Koelfen and Freund 1993). However, before surgery can be considered, the EEG findings must be predominantly localized to the side with the major structural abnormality.

STURGE–WEBER SYNDROME

Sturge–Weber syndrome is characterized by a facial port-wine stain and pial angiomatosis (Falconer and Rushworth 1959). Patients develop progressive hemiparesis, seizures, and mental retardation. A variety of seizure types may develop, but the radiographic appearance is quite specific. CT and plain films show extensive hemispheric calcification. Gadolinium-DTPA enhanced MRI demonstrates pial angiomatosis (Marti-Bonmati and Menor 1993). PET shows focal metabolic changes, and can be useful for following disease progression (Chugani and Mazziotta 1989; Rintahaka et al 1993).

The syndrome can initially produce minimal symptoms, but patients show progressive calcification and venous changes resulting in a decline in neurologic function, seizure control, and cognitive ability. The syndrome can vary between focal changes and more diffuse change, and in the speed of its progression. When the change is focal, the patients tend to have normal intellectual function. When it is diffuse, they are often retarded and may deteriorate rapidly. Those with focal disease may be suitable for local resection and in some cases, if the neurologic deficit is not complete and the predominant seizure type is atonic or drop attacks, then callosotomy may be successful in controlling them. If the initial procedure is not successful in controlling the seizures, hemispherectomy may be a later option. Hoffman described 22 patients with Sturge–Weber disease (Hoffman et al 1979). In 11 of these patients there was localized disease that responded to a local resection in 10 patients, 8 of whom were seizure-free. The remaining 11 patients underwent hemispherectomy or hemidecortication and 10 of these became seizure-free. All the patients undergoing local resections were of normal intelligence and their seizures began after 2 years of age; among the patients undergoing hemispherectomy or hemidecortication, 5 of the 8 patients who were assessed were mentally retarded (unpublished data).

RASMUSSEN ENCEPHALITIS

In 1958 Rasmussen first described a chronic childhood encephalitis that leads to intractable epilepsy and progresses to severe neurologic and cognitive deficits (Rasmussen et al 1958; Vining et al 1993). Approximately half of his patients had a preceding viral illness, but a clear viral etiology has not been established (Malaclan and Girvin 1993). The etiology of this disease is unclear, but studies in recent years have linked it to various viruses, including cytomegalic viruses, and others have suggested that it has an autoimmune basis (Power et al 1990; Asher and Gajdusek 1991; Grenier et al 1991; Coates et al 1992; Farrell et al 1995). McNamara and Andrews have reported the possibility that autoantibodies to the GluR3 receptor are responsible (McNamara and Andrews 1995). Focal motor, partial complex, or generalized tonic clonic seizures are the usual presenting signs. Drop attacks are uncommon, but over 50% of patients develop epilepsia partialis continua (Malaclan and Girvin 1993).

Structural and functional imaging reflect the progressive, unilateral nature of the disease. CT and MRI are initially nondiagnostic, but documentation of slowly progressive unilateral hemispheric atrophy is characteristic. Functional imaging shows diffuse hypometabolism on the affected side, with focal areas of increased uptake (Adams *et al* 1992).

Unlike in Sturge–Weber syndrome, there are no specific physical, neurophysiologic, or imaging findings that confirm the diagnosis of Rasmussen disease. Without pathologic confirmation from brain tissue obtained for biopsy, the diagnosis can only be made by exclusion. Perivascular lymphocyte cuffing and gliosis characterize the microscopic findings (Rasmussen *et al* 1958; Malaclan and Girvin 1993).

PREOPERATIVE ASSESSMENT

SEIZURE TYPE AND NEUROLOGIC EXAMINATION

Candidates for hemispherectomy may present with widely varied seizure types and severity. Diffuse hemispheric injury often causes drop attacks, and a sudden startle tends to precipitate seizures (Oguni *et al* 1998). There is no seizure type that characterizes the different hemispheric syndromes, but there are some general trends (Rasmussen *et al* 1958; Rasmussen 1983; Chugani *et al* 1988; Davies *et al* 1993). Patients with hemimegalencephaly have a propensity for focal motor seizures. Rasmussen disease may begin with partial complex seizures or generalized seizures, but 50% of the patients eventually develop epilepsia partialis continua.

Patients considered for hemispherectomy usually have a contralateral spastic hemiparesis and hemineglect. Motor function is most severely affected in the distal upper and lower extremities, with functionally impaired fine finger, wrist, or foot movements. Gross sensory deficits and sympathetic changes are often undetectable. A contralateral homonymous hemianopia is often present, but in patients with watershed infarctions, Rasmussen encephalitis, or more localized disease, there may be only a partial visual field defect or none at all.

The patient's language function depends on the severity of the disease and whether the dominant hemisphere is affected. The most important determinant of language function in patients with dominant hemisphere disease is the age at the time of hemisphere damage. The younger the patient at the time of injury, the less likely it is for language function to be affected. The exact age when the human brain becomes unable to transfer language function is unknown, but it is generally accepted that injury after 10 years of age will result in language impairment (Annet 1973; Chi and Dooling 1977; Rasmussen and Milner 1977; Woods and Teuber 1978).

Preoperative hemispheric language localization is not necessary in most patients considered for hemispherectomy, but the older child with good language function and left hemisphere disease should have language function lateralized. Amytal testing has long proved useful, but the dichotic listening test and transcranial magnetic stimulation may provide reliable, noninvasive alternatives to language lateralization (Wada 1949; Kimura 1967; Geffen and Quinn 1984; Jennum and Friberg 1994).

DETERMINING MEDICAL INTRACTABILITY

Patients should only be considered for hemispherectomy after they have had maximal medical treatment. Just as the seizure characteristics can be quite variable, the response to medication is similarly unpredictable. Trials of many drugs, alone or in combination, can be an arduous task, with variable responses and complications. However, surgical options should only be addressed after a thorough effort for medical seizure control has been made by a neurologist who is comfortable with complex anticonvulsant management strategies. In 2 of our 11 hemispherectomies for Rasmussen disease, the operation has had to be undertaken as an emergency in patients with uncontrolled epilepsia partialis continua requiring ventilation. In Rasmussen disease there are a number of anti-inflammatory measures including steroids and antiviral drugs such as acyclovir and gancyclovir, which have proved useful in a few cases, but the responses have either been transient or occurred in only some of the treated patients (Dulac *et al* 1991). In addition, the recent reports of an autoimmune basis have suggested the use of plasma exchange (McNamara and Andrews 1995).

STRUCTURAL AND FUNCTIONAL NEUROIMAGING

Structural imaging with CT and MRI are now the mainstays of the surgical evaluation of the hemispherectomy candidate. MRI readily demonstrates structural changes in the cortex, white matter, and ventricles. It is quite useful in demonstrating the extent of leptomeningeal angiomatosis in Sturge–Weber syndrome. MRI evaluation should be thorough and consistent. General epilepsy protocols, including T2 and T1 inversion recovery sequences at right angles to the hippocampus, give good whole-brain views while providing hippocampal detail. T2 relaxation mapping effectively delineates hippocampal pathology, but it is less useful for most hemispherectomy candidates (Jackson and Connelly 1993; Gadian and Connelly 1994). Dix *et al* looked at magnetic resonance images from 23 patients with cerebral atrophy. In 9/11 of this group who had a history of childhood febrile convulsions there was mesial temporal sclerosis (MTS), whereas only one of the remaining 12 patients without MTS had such a history (Dix and Cail 1997). Patients with Sturge–Weber syndrome should also have postcontrast sequences and MR angiography to further delineate the vascular anatomy. MR spectroscopy is currently used as a research tool but it may eventually elucidate further methods for lateralizing seizure foci (Connelly *et al* 1994).

As the information MRI provides has expanded, the role of CT in the preoperative assessment has diminished. CT remains superior to MRI in the reliable demonstration of calcium, particularly in Sturge–Weber syndrome. CT is still an effective tool for postoperative assessment and follow-up. Angiography is only necessary in the rare cases of vascular malformation.

While the quality of structural imaging has improved dramatically, functional imaging has also emerged as a powerful tool (Chugani and Shields 1990; Adams *et al* 1992; Rintahaka *et al* 1993). SPECT scanning is readily available and provides information about cerebral blood flow. PET scanning using $H_2^{15}O$ provides more detailed and quantitative cerebral blood flow data. 2-Deoxy-2-^{18}F-fluoro-D- glucose PET provides such data about cerebral metabolism. These functional studies play an important role in patients without asymmetry on CT or MRI, by allowing lateralization and EEG corroboration. In those with structural lesions, functional studies can confirm EEG localization and further localize the abnormal area within the hemisphere.

Because changes in blood flow and metabolism can indicate seizure foci, functional imaging complements EEG. Recent evidence suggests that PET findings in the contralateral hemisphere, like EEG findings, may be a good indicator of bilateral disease and may predict poorer seizure outcome after hemispherectomy (Chiron *et al* 1991; Rintahaka *et al* 1993).

NEUROPHYSIOLOGY

For 50 years, EEG was the principal tool used in hemisphere localization prior to hemispherectomy. However, with the rapid advance in structural and functional imaging technology, radiographic localization has supplanted EEG as the mainstay for surgical planning. Modern imaging allows the search for the epileptic focus to be narrowed to specific areas, and EEG is useful for confirming the site as epileptogenic.

The primary goal of EEG in the hemispherectomy candidate is to lateralize the disease to the radiologically and clinically affected hemisphere and to assess independent or secondary involvement of the contralateral hemisphere. A thorough investigation with ictal and interictal recordings should be performed. This may necessitate lengthy recording times and a temporary reduction in antiepileptic drugs.

EEG patterns vary with the nature of the seizure disorder and the anatomic injury. On the affected hemisphere, the normal rhythm is often replaced by a tracing with a reduced amplitude and excessive slow waves (Smith *et al* 1991). Seizure foci in the affected hemisphere show spike and wave configurations that may be multiple and independent. Similar abnormalities may be seen on the contralateral side, making the distinction difficult. Abnormal background activity and bilateral synchrony of epileptiform discharges in the contralateral hemisphere are not associated with a poor outcome after hemispherectomy. A recent study of 12 patients from Boston has shown that a good outcome from hemispherectomy is associated with the following EEG features: suppression of activity over the affected hemisphere, absence of contralateral slowing, absence of generalized discharges or bilateral spiking, and the detection of ipsilateral ictal discharges (Carmant *et al* 1995). However, when there are bilateral independent foci, the prognosis for seizure control is worse, but hemispherectomy may not be contraindicated if one hemisphere is clearly the source of the majority of seizures (Smith *et al* 1991; Quirk and Kendall 1993).

In most cases the EEG complements the structural imaging, but both studies are important to confirm the laterality of the seizure foci. In addition, EEG has a critically important role in the evaluation of patients with no radiographic lateralization. If EEG is unable to lateralize the abnormality in these patients, corticography or depth electrodes may be indicated.

NEUROPSYCHOLOGY AND BEHAVIORAL ASSESSMENT

Most hemispherectomy candidates have a diffuse cerebral injury that causes some degree of behavioral and intellectual disability. The degree and type of disturbance is multifactorial, depending on the age at the time of insult and the extent and progression of the disease. Very early injury often allows patients to compensate but bilateral injury may lead to severe disturbances.

Regardless of the etiology, severe behavioral and intellectual impairment are sources of major handicap for these patients. Nearly all patients considered for hemispherectomy have some element of behavioral disturbance, ranging from impairments in interpersonal skills to outbursts of rage and violence. The patients usually have intellectual impairment, with most having an intelligence quotient (IQ) less than 90. When the seizure disorder is uncontrolled or when the disease is progressive, behavioral and intellectual function may show progressive decline (Ounsted *et al* 1987). A particular problem arises when Rasmussen disease appears relatively late in the dominant hemisphere and speech functions may not transfer so readily in the unaffected hemisphere. In some of our patients with Rasmussen disease, this has lead to considerable incapacity following left hemispherectomy.

Thorough preoperative psychologic and behavioral testing develops a solid baseline and can be helpful in documenting deterioration. Psychologic testing should include measures of intelligence, memory, and frontal lobe function. Behavioral studies should address aggressiveness, impulsivity, and judgment.

An important adjunct is the psychiatric assessment of both the patient and their family before surgery. This, coupled with family counseling, ensures that realistic goals are set for general outcome and seizure control after surgery.

SURGICAL TIMING

Hemispherectomy candidates with a progressive underlying disease, such as Rasmussen encephalitis, should be considered for surgery early in the disease process (Vining *et al* 1993). However, many patients considered for hemispherectomy had a sudden, dramatic early insult that resulted in a static clinical condition. In these patients, the timing of surgery is controversial and the risks and benefits of early or late surgery must be weighed in each case.

Early surgery offers the advantages of seizure reduction while maximizing the compensatory abilities of the immature nervous system. There is evidence that prolonged seizures in the immature nervous system can result in psychiatric disease and long-term deficits in intelligence, behavior, learning, and memory (Davidson and Falconer 1973; Dikman and Matthews 1975; Lindsay and Ounsted 1979). Additionally, surgery in early childhood allows maximization of the neuronal compensatory mechanisms. There is no definite period beyond which the human brain will not compensate for a functional deficit. However, it is generally agreed that, within the first decade of life, the less

mature the brain at the time of injury the greater is the ability to compensate for injury; after the first decade, the compensation for cerebral injury is quite variable (Annet 1973; Chi and Dooling 1977; Woods and Teuber 1978; Shields *et al* 1993).

The possible benefits of early operation in maximizing compensation and to minimize brain injury must be weighed against the risk of operating before the permanency and laterality of the seizure disorder is established. In patients with a static lesion, such as an infantile hemispheric insult, probably the only absolute indication for hemispherectomy is the onset of dementia, whereas in Rasmussen disease, hemimegalencephaly, and possibly Sturge–Weber syndrome, the physician's hand may be forced by epilepsia partialis continua.

As mentioned earlier, determining seizure intractability can be difficult because of the multitude of medications and patient noncompliance. Additionally, there are a number of benign, self-limiting partial seizure disorders that can be mistaken for intractable seizures (Heigbel and Blom 1975; Dalla and Chiamenti 1985; Matheson *et al* 1993).

Delaying surgery often provides greater opportunities to determine true intractability while allowing additional time to establish an etiology and localize the problem to a specific hemisphere. In some cases, only prolonged observation and testing establish the seizures to be just one manifestation of any number of neurodegenerative or metabolic conditions whose fatal outcome may preclude surgery (Harding and DePhil 1990).

OPERATIVE TECHNIQUES

There are a number of techniques available for performing a hemispherectomy, and which operative technique is employed will depend upon a number of factors. First consideration is given to the pathology. Among the various pathologic substrates encountered in gross unilateral hemispheric disease only two, Rasmussen disease and Sturge–Weber syndrome, might be considered to constitute a risk of further epilepsy or disease if they were left *in situ*. In fact there is no evidence that either of these conditions will progress in a way that has a practical consequence in the patient. There are no reports suggesting that continued deterioration is seen following functional hemispherectomy compared with other techniques. Although examples of bilateral occurrence of both conditions are described, it appears from experience that even Rasmussen disease, which often fails to respond to anything less than an hemispherectomy, does not usually progress after that procedure.

Andermann reports one case in 48 patients with Rasmussen disease where brain stem symptoms supervened, leading to the death of the patient (Andermann *et al* 1991). For reasons that will become apparent later, it is easier to carry out an anatomic hemispherectomy on patients with gross hemiatrophy.

The second consideration is the ability to achieve a complete disconnection. The skill and experience of the operator and the extent and nature of the pathology will have a considerable influence on this. However, it should be evident that a complete disconnection is inevitable with anatomic hemispherectomy but difficult to ensure with hemispherotomy. It is clear from the experience of the Montreal group that removal or disconnection of the insula is necessary. Otherwise, if the patient suffers persistent seizures the surgical team will not know whether these arise from the insular remnant (Villemure and Mascott 1995).

The third consideration, especially in infants, is the length and severity of the procedure. The chief acute dangers are hemorrhage, air embolism, cooling, and tissue destruction, which will determine the length and difficulty of the convalescence. Clearly, those operations that require only minimal access will be more favorable for these candidates.

The final consideration is the occurrence of late complications, in particular the cerebral hemosiderosis that occurs after anatomic hemispherectomy. However, this complication is also seen after functional hemispherectomy, reported in 3/27 patients by Peacock *et al* (1996) and after hemidecortication (Hoffman 1997).

For the purposes of this discussion the available techniques can be divided into four groups: modifications of anatomic hemispherectomy, functional hemispherectomy, hemidecortication, and hemispherotomy.

Perioperative management

The anesthetic should be given by an experienced neuroanesthetist with appropriate monitoring and adequate vascular access. At all stages in the operation, and especially in infants and young children, the danger of hemorrhage, especially major venous hemorrhage and less likely the possibility of air embolism, must be borne in mind. A central venous line is desirable, especially in younger children for whom intraoperative blood loss is a potentially life-threatening situation. Prophylactic antibiotics are given during the procedure and anticonvulsant regimes are continued but possibly adjusted so as to allow intravenous or nasogastric administration of the drugs. Intraoperative blood loss should be anticipated and where possible replaced with fresh whole blood. End-tidal CO_2 should be carefully monitored, especially when there is increased hazard of air embolism. The patient should be reversed from the anesthesia and intensive postoperative monitoring should be carried out. However, in infants and younger children, a period of elective ventilation lasting between 12 and 24 hours may be desirable after the operation. A swinging pyrexia may be encountered during the first week. Sources for sepsis should be eliminated, but this pyrexia is probably due to blood in the hemicranium. Hydrocephalus has been reported as both an immediate and a delayed postoperative complication.

ANATOMIC HEMISPHERECTOMY

The technique that will be described is Adams' modification of the classical hemispherectomy (Adams 1983). This will also suffice as a description of the classical hemispherectomy, although this is now much less commonly used and the only difference is in the closure, which in the classical operation is simply a standard craniotomy closure with reconstitution of the dura in its normal position. The general conduct of the procedure is the same whatever the underlying pathology in the diseased hemisphere, but in operating on a hemimegalencephalic hemisphere there can be difficulty in finding the landmarks owing to distortion and especially in being sure that the correct lateral ventricle is being entered; sometimes there can also be problems with access and exposure that may force the surgeon to perform the operation piecemeal.

Craniotomy for access

Because it is necessary at one point to move the head from the lateral to a vertical position and later to move it back again, it is not appropriate to secure the head with a pin headrest. The movement should be carried out before the patient is draped to ensure that the endotracheal tube will not be dislodged and to make sure that the anesthetist is comfortable with the maneuver. The patient is then draped and the marked skin incision is infiltrated according to the local custom. The skin incision starts in the midline anteriorly and around the level of the lambdoid suture turns vertically to end behind the ear.

An osteoplastic bone flap is based on the temporalis muscle; the base is at the level of the anterior fossa as marked by the external angular groove and the floor of the middle fossa as judged from the root of the zygoma. The most anterior burr hole is governed by the frontal sinus, which may be greatly enlarged on the atrophied side. The posterior limit of the flap is determined by the most posterior burr hole that can be made. The bone may be very thick. If a series of burr holes is being made, those in the midline should be made last and these areas cut with the Gigli saw last. A piece of muscle should be taken from the temporalis muscle at this point. This is needed for two purposes: first, to block the foramen of Monroe; secondly, it may be useful if a venous bleeder has to be oversewn. The dura is then opened either in a stellate fashion or with the usual dural flap based upon the superior sagittal sinus superiorly and coming as close as possible to the margin of the craniotomy in order to make the greatest area of dura available for the subsequent closure.

Clipping of the middle cerebral artery

In the usual way, the internal carotid artery is exposed and is followed up beyond the bifurcation into the sylvian fissure to expose the M1 portion just below the trifurcation, thereby sparing any deep branches. The artery is dissected free from the surrounding tissue. Because most neuroimaging departments will no longer image patients with any form of metal clip, it is possibly wise to use some form of plastic clip for this purpose. Such clips are available for use in general surgery. Two Ligaclips are placed above this and the vessel is coagulated and divided below them.

The formal corticectomy

The head is turned from the lateral to an almost vertical position. The dissection is begun in the frontal region by dividing the bridging veins and retracting the hemisphere medially. At this point, two principles must be applied. The first is to divide the veins close to the cortical surface so that if there is any subsequent problem it is possible to recoagulate the vein without damage to the sinus. The second is to respect the medial surface of the healthy hemisphere by dissecting the damaged hemisphere in a subpial manner. From the midfrontal region, working posteriorly, the surgeon will soon come to the corpus callosum, which should be exposed posteriorly as far as practical at this stage.

The lateral ventricle is entered through the corpus callosum, which is not divided in the midline but lateral to the ipsilateral anterior cerebral artery. It is wise to preserve the anterior cerebral trunk for a substantial portion of its course because occasionally it supplies both hemispheres. This approach also ensures that the body of the lateral ventricle is entered off the midline, making it likely that the correct ventricle will be entered and also preserving the septum pellucidum, which will be visible medially. The callosal incision is now extended forward and the genu is divided, and the anterior dissection of the frontal lobe is continued so that the operator comes down along the course of the anterior cerebral artery above the optic apparatus to the carotid bifurcation.

The surgeon now returns to the ventricle in the region of the trigone and unroofs the temporal horn of the ventricle from above, proceeding forward. At the same time, an incision must be made through the region of the internal capsule to separate the basal ganglia, leaving them as medial structures, so as to detach the insular cortex. Now the temporal lobe is separated in the choroid fissure from in front, working backward along the free edge of the tentorium. The P2 portion of the posterior cerebral artery is not deliberately divided; those branches that are passing laterally to structures that will be included in the specimen, such as the hippocampus and posterior part of the parahippocampal gyrus, are divided individually. Eventually, at the posterior end of this maneuver the individual cortical branches coming out over the tentorial edge are also divided.

Next the splenium of the corpus callosum is divided, the remainder of the hemisphere is separated, and the white matter at the trigone is also divided. Particular care is needed at the posterior limit of this dissection in the tentorial hiatus near the midline because there are venous tributaries draining into the Great vein of Galen or the straight sinus that, if torn, can cause embarrassing venous bleeding.

At this stage, the only structures tethering the hemisphere are the draining veins posteriorly, which tend to drain either into the superior sagittal sinus or the transverse sinus. An assistant therefore holds the specimen while as far as is possible these veins are divided in a careful and controlled fashion. When this has been done, the hemisphere can be lifted out.

Hemostasis and dural closure

At this stage some attention to the veins and sinuses is needed, but patience, use of Surgicel and the occasional oversewing will achieve the necessary hemostasis. With the systolic blood pressure at a suitable level, hemostasis on the stump of the basal ganglia is obtained. These structures and the exposed medial frontal cortex are usually covered with a sheet of Surgicel. It is usual to coagulate the whole of the choroid plexus within the lateral ventricle to discourage CSF formation in what will become a subdural compartment. Finally, a plug of muscle is placed in the foramen of Monroe to block the operation cavity off from the rest of the ventricular system as recommended by Adams.

The dural flap is now brought down and positioned so that it can be secured to the most anterior part of the falx/tentorial hiatus gap. It may be necessary to incise into the base of this flap to mobilize it sufficiently. The flap is secured around the falx/tentorial hiatus with individual

Vicryl sutures. It is necessary to avoid damaging to the opposite hemisphere or provoking bleeding from veins, especially around the posterior end of the tentorial hiatus. In the last few cases we have taken to using Tiseel to seal the dural edge and reduce the number of sutures needed. Closure of the extradural space using a Zenoderm graft has been described by Dunn *et al* (1995).

Extradural closure

Extradural closure is not difficult. Hemostasis, especially venous hemostasis, is obtained. The sutures that were used to retract the dural edge close to the edge of the craniotomy are now used to hitch this dura up to the pericranium. The bone flap is secured by whatever means is usually adopted. The scalp is closed in two layers. Care must be taken in the use of drains. Following a tragedy in which excessive suction from a presuctioned drain caused sufficient shift to infarct part of the healthy hemisphere, we no longer use these drains. For the same reason, although less likely than with the classical hemispherectomy, the patient should be nursed with the operation side upward for 12–24 hours to avoid shift of structures.

In some patients there may be evidence within the first week after operation of increasing hydrocephalus. If it is necessary to insert a shunt into the remaining lateral ventricle, it should be placed anteriorly since, if it is placed in the more usual posterior position, there is a remote chance of producing a contralateral hemianopia that would render the patient blind.

FUNCTIONAL HEMISPHERECTOMY

The procedure of functional hemispherectomy was first described by Rasmussen, who noticed that patients undergoing multilobar resections did not appear to suffer any of the complications associated with a classical anatomic hemispherectomy. He attributed this to the buttressing effect of the residual cortex, which prevented chronic small movements of the remaining hemisphere that, it was felt, were responsible for the bleeding (Rasmussen 1987). He therefore proposed an anatomically incomplete hemispherectomy in which the residual cerebral cortex was disconnected, thereby producing a functionally complete hemispherectomy. This improved the seizure outcome from the subtotal hemispherectomy, which they had used between 1968 and 1974 to avoid the late complications of classical anatomic hemispherectomy while avoiding those complications. Since then, Villemure and others have modified this procedure to reduce the

amount of resected tissue while preserving the functionally complete isolation of the hemisphere. As we have already noted, outcome is more likely to be related to pathology than to technique, but it may be that one technique will prove more appropriate than another in certain age groups or pathologies.

Craniotomy for access

The patient is positioned supine on the operating table with the head in the almost true lateral position and the vertex at the same level as the external auditory meatus. The head is fixed with the Mayfield clamp. During the course of the procedure it may be necessary to raise or lower the head, but there should be no need to readjust the Mayfield clamp. A limited head shave is performed such that a strip about 2 cm wide down the midline is joined by a vertical limb coming up from the zygoma. This allows a T-shaped incision to be marked and prepared.

The skin incision is made with the diathermy micropoint Colorado needle, which reduces blood loss to a minimum because of the excellent hemostasis that it affords. The pericranium is lifted with the scalp flap and the vertical element of the T-shaped incision is taken down through the temporalis muscle to the zygoma. The two leaves of the T are then opened to expose a large portion of the frontal and temporal bones. A free bone flap is then elevated, placing the burr holes sufficiently close to each other to allow the dura to be stripped easily. The bone dust is saved, and moistened with a small quantity of blood from the arterial line to keep it fresh. The dura is opened with an H-shaped incision, the superior limb is hinged on the superior sagittal sinus, and the inferior limb is hinged so as to allow access to the middle cranial fossa.

Temporal lobectomy

This is a standard extended temporal lobectomy; a subpial dissection of the superior temporal gyrus is carried out to preserve the branches of the middle cerebral artery as they lie on the insula. At all intracerebral stages of the operation the difficulty of the operation will be related to the underlying pathologic process, being relatively easy in a patient with gross hemisphere atrophy and a large porencephaly and difficult and demanding in a patient with hemimegalencephaly. The temporal lobe may be removed 'en bloc,' or the neocortex and deep structures may be removed separately depending upon the preference and custom of the surgeon, provided an adequate removal of the amygdala and hippocampus is achieved.

Central resection

The central sulcus is now identified in the suprasylvian region. A subpial dissection is once again performed above the sylvian fissure, identifying the branches of the middle cerebral artery where they lie on the insula. A resection of a vertical strip of cortex, 5–6 cm wide, is performed from above the sylvian fissure to the margin of the hemisphere adjacent to the superior sagittal sinus. The veins passing from the cerebral hemisphere to the sinus should be treated with great respect and coagulated close to the cortex wherever possible, bearing in mind the risks of hemorrhage and air embolism associated with dealing with these particular vessels. If there are a number of engorged veins it may be more sensible to extend the subpial dissection through the hemisphere, parallel to the sinus, until the pia of the medial surface is reached. The remnant of cortex can either be removed later with the ultrasonic aspirator (CUSA) or simply left.

The two incisions are then taken down medially until the corpus callosum is encountered and the ipsilateral lateral ventricle is entered at this stage. The frontal and occipital incisions are then deepened so that this central cortex hinges laterally and at its base the subpial dissection is completed through the corona radiata, allowing this specimen of central cortex to be delivered for histology.

Corpus callosum section and isolation of the residual cortex

The removal of the central cortex begins the section of the corpus callosum, which is then extended both anteriorly and posteriorly, either from within the ventricle or in the hemispheric fissure. The latter is easier, and also allows good visualization of the ipsilateral pericallosal artery. By keeping lateral to this vessel, any damage both to itself and, probably of more importance, to the contralateral pericallosal vessel is avoided. The residual frontal and parieto-occipital cerebral cortex and the insular cortex are still connected by their white-matter tracts. These areas are isolated by dividing the white-matter tracts as they enter the corona radiata. Because in some of the Montreal series in whom the insular cortex was not undercut there were persisting seizures, Rasmussen recommended that this be done. Therefore the insular cortex is undercut at this stage, ensuring preservation of the overlying vessels.

Closure

Hemostasis is secured with Surgicel and the whole cavity is irrigated. The dura is closed in a watertight fashion and peripheral and central hitching stitches are placed. The bone flap is replaced, secured using a heavy dissolvable suture. The scalp is closed in a single layer using either clips or a reabsorbable suture. A subperiosteal drain is used, with only gravity rather than suction. A light dressing is placed on the wound.

HEMIDECORTICATION

This technique was first described in 1968 by Ignelzi and Bucy and consists of removing only the cortex, preserving the white matter and thereby avoiding entrance into the ventricular system. The chief proponents of this procedure have been Hoffman in Toronto and the group at the Johns Hopkins in Baltimore. There is no evidence that this technique is superior to the others described and it may even be accompanied by a higher incidence of hydrocephalus than other techniques and possibly involves a greater hemodynamic disturbance (Brian *et al* 1990; Hoffman 1997).

HEMISPHEROTOMY

There are two variations of this procedure, one described by Schramm that involves a temporal or perisylvian approach similar to that described for functional hemispherectomy, and that described by Delalande in which the hemisphere is approached through the lateral ventricle superiorly and the whole of the disconnection is achieved through this minimal approach. The Schramm approach is really very similar to the functional hemispherectomy described by Villemure (Villemure and Mascott 1995), which is itself a minimization of the original functional hemispherectomy described by Rasmussen (Schramm *et al* 1995). This procedure therefore begins with a central craniotomy, which allows access to the temporal or sylvian region from which, either by temporal resection or by sylvian resection, access is obtained to the lateral ventricle from where the relevant deafferentation can be achieved by performing a transventricular callosotomy and other relevant fiber tract divisions. One group has described the use of ultrasound to locate the relevant structures while performing a functional hemispherectomy (Kanev *et al* 1997).

By contrast, Delalande's procedure approaches the ventricle from above, entering into the lateral ventricle either through the gross pathology or by creating a small window in the posterior frontal region superiorly. Once access to the ventricular system has been gained, it is possible to carry out a similar deafferentation totally from within the lateral ventricle, dividing the corpus callosum, transecting the white matter anterior to the thalamus, and completing the transection posteriorly so as to disconnect the temporal structures. Delalande makes the point that the whole procedure can be carried out within white matter, thereby reducing hemorrhage to almost none (Delalande *et al* 1993).

Reoperation is not common in hemispherectomy candidates. However, Peacock *et al* report that further disconnection was necessary in 5/27 of their functional hemispherectomies (Peacock *et al* 1996).

CONCLUSION

The choice of operative procedure is clearly not simple. It depends upon the experience of the surgeon, the age of the patient, and the pathology. Sometimes a second procedure will be necessary and may not be the same as the first one.

SEIZURE AND NEUROLOGIC OUTCOME

SEIZURE OUTCOME

With proper patient selection and operative technique, large series report some degree of seizure control in 100% of patients undergoing hemispherectomy. Seventy-five percent of these patients are seizure-free, with their anticonvulsant use significantly reduced and simplified. Some patients are seizure-free and off all anticonvulsants, but this proportion varies widely between 6% and 72% of all those who have surgery. Comparisons of seizure outcome are difficult because standardized outcome measures have not been employed in previous series. Use of a seizure outcome scale such as the Engel classification in future studies will prove very useful in comparing results in different surgical series (Engel 1987). Application of Engel's grading scheme to previous publications is limited by ambiguities in reporting. However, roughly 75% will have a class 1 Engel outcome and fewer than 10% a class 4 outcome (French and Johnson 1955; Wilson 1970; Ameli 1980; Verity and Strauss 1982; Lindsay and Ounsted 1987; Beardsworth and Adams 1988; Tinuper and Andermann 1988; Winston *et al* 1992; Davies *et al* 1993; Di Rocco and Caldarelli 1993; Villemure *et al* 1993). The results of a retrospective multicenter study coordinated at the Bielefeld meeting devoted to pediatric epilepsy surgery in 1995 have been published. A total of 333 patients had been surveyed and the results were carefully analyzed by Holthausen. The series included patients treated over 20 years; the perioperative mortality was 1.5%, which Holthausen thought was probably an underestimate. The overall seizure relief rate was 70.4% seizure-free, but he

also found that there were significant differences between operative techniques, with the best result from hemispherotomy (85.7%) and the worst from hemidecortication (60.7%). However, these differences could be attributed both to the long period of time over which the patients had been treated and the different proportions of the various etiologies in the individual series. By contrast, there was a clear difference in the outcome with different pathologies, the best being with Sturge–Weber syndrome (82.1%) and the worst with dysplastic lesions (56.6%). The poor results in hemimegalencephaly may be due to technical difficulties at operation, or to the presence of dysplastic tissue elsewhere in the brain; there is evidence that some of these patients may have bilateral abnormalities (Jahan *et al* 1997; Villemure *et al* 1993). There was no significant relationship between seizure outcome and preoperative EEG findings, preoperative seizure type, or frequency and age at surgery (Holthausen *et al* 1997a). This Bielefeld series included patients from Baltimore and UCLA who have been reported separately elsewhere (Peacock *et al* 1996; Vining *et al* 1997).

NEUROLOGIC OUTCOME

The neurologic effects of hemispherectomy depend on the age at initial insult and on the degree of the preoperative deficits. The typical patient who presents with an abrupt onset of hemiplegia and hemianopia at a young age usually has no long-term change in motor, sensory, or visual function after surgery. Most patients with preservation of motor, sensory, or visual function in the affected hemisphere before surgery will have neurologic decline after hemispherectomy. Distal fine motor function is more severely affected, with the arm more significantly affected than the leg. Those without preoperative visual loss can expect a dense homonymous hemianopia. These visual changes will not improve, but some recovery of proximal motor function, particularly in the leg, can be expected. Because these neurologic changes can be quite severe, more focal resections should be considered carefully in the patient with preserved hemispheric function. Worsening of motor function is noted immediately after surgery, particularly in the face and hands, but this may improve over several weeks. It can take up to a month to get patients walking comfortably again. A marked reduction in hypertonicity immediately after surgery usually persists; this often proves functionally advantageous. Holthausen, in studying patients operated in Bielefeld, noted that if the disease was present before birth the patient was more likely to retain relatively sophisticated movements of the upper limb. His conclusion was that if the insult was suffered before myelination was complete then the patient was less likely to show a severe spastic hemiplegia (Holthausen *et al* 1997b).

Language function after hemispherectomy has attracted great interest because of the minimal effects of surgery, even after the left hemisphere is removed. There are no reported cases of chronic mutism following right or left hemispherectomy, providing support for the concept of equipotentiality of hemispheric function in the immature nervous system. However, the true plasticity of the brain in hemispherectomized patients is difficult to assess because most patients suffered a hemispheric insult prior to surgery. Conclusions about hemispheric adaptability are also limited by the lack of longitudinal studies of language function in these patients (McFie 1961; Wilson 1970; Vargha-Khadem and Polkey 1993).

Despite the reported success of language transfer, there has been great interest in the more subtle language deficits that occur in left hemispherectomized patients. A multitude of studies have concluded that patients with isolated right hemispheres have difficulties in verbal fluency, in the manipulation of grammatical structure, in analyzing words in relation to their phonetic features, and in comprehending abstract words (Dennis and Cohen 1975; Dennis and Whitaker 1976; Zaidel 1977, 1978; Dennis 1980; Dennis and Lovett 1981; Vargha-Khadem and Polkey 1993). A study of four patients from New Zealand has suggested that the hemispheres are equipotential in infancy but that the left hemisphere becomes more specialized in spelling (Ogden 1996). Vargha-Khardem and Mishkin have recently reviewed this topic extensively. Their conclusions are that before the age of 5 or 6 years the hemispheres are equipotential, but that after that age the left hemisphere usually begins to dominate speech and language. Although there is a direct effect of left-hemisphere injury on speech and language after the age of 5 years, in addition, there is an indirect effect if severe damage to either hemisphere is sufficient to reduce overall IQ. Finally, the rate at which the right hemisphere will adapt following left-hemisphere damage will be influenced by the frequency and severity of epileptic seizures because these may interfere with the functioning of the undamaged hemisphere (Vargha-Khadem and Mishkin 1997).

Just as language function has been studied extensively in left-hemispherectomized patients, visuospatial functions have been scrutinized in right-hemispherectomized patients with conflicting results. Damasio and Gott found these patients to have no deficits in tests to right-hemisphere function such as spatial orientation, visuospatial construction, or face perception (Gott 1973; Damasio and Lima 1975). However, Villemure reported a 13-year-old patient who had a dense prosapagnosia after right

hemispherectomy (Villemure *et al* 1991). Further studies have addressed more subtle right-hemisphere function with the Weinstein/Semmes Personal Orientation Test, the Porteus Maze Test, and the WISC Maze Test. These studies have shown that the gross visuospatial function in right-hemispherectomized patients is unaffected, but these patients have greater difficulty with demanding visuospatial tasks (Ogden 1989; Kohn and Dennis 1974; Vargha-Khadem and Polkey 1993). There have been a number of studies of 'blind-sight' in hemispherectomized patients suggesting that they have some residual visual ability but that it is at a subcortical level (King *et al* 1996a, 1996b; Tomaiuolo *et al* 1997; Wessinger *et al* 1996a,b). There is also some evidence for preservation of auditory spatial localization, again at a subcortical level, in right-hemispherectomized patients (Zatorre *et al* 1995).

PSYCHOLOGIC AND BEHAVIORAL OUTCOME

Improvements in intelligence, memory, and behavior after hemispherectomy can be quite gratifying for the patient and family. These long-recognized benefits have been directly attributed to the surgery, but they may actually represent a combination of the effects of reducing or eliminating the seizures and/or the antiepileptic drugs.

NEUROPSYCHOLOGIC AND COGNITIVE CHANGES

The effect of hemispherectomy on patient IQ is variable, but in the majority of published studies 40–70% of cases show a 10-point or greater increase in IQ after surgery (Lindsay and Ounsted 1979; Verity and Strauss 1982; Beardsworth and Adams 1988). A smaller number of patients (10–25%) show a decline of 10 points or greater (Lindsay and Ounsted 1979; Verity and Strauss 1982; Beardsworth and Adams 1988; Vargha-Khadem and Polkey 1993).

Despite improvements in postoperative intellectual function, the majority of patients remain significantly impaired, with intelligence quotients significantly below normal (Lindsay and Ounsted 1979; Verity and Strauss 1982; Beardsworth and Adams 1988). It is generally recognized that intellectual improvement is more likely in patients with a late onset of seizures, a shorter duration and less severe preoperative disease, and a long postoperative disease-free follow-up. Patients with Rasmussen encephalitis usually improve less than other patients because of the late onset of their disease (Taylor 1991; Vargha-Khadem and Polkey 1993; Vining *et al* 1993).

It has been suggested that two cooperating hemispheres are necessary for normal short-term memory, but thorough investigation of hemispherectomized patients' memory abilities has been limited. In 1973, Gott studied patients who had right and left hemispherectomies and found that verbal memory and processing abilities measured on the Wechsler Memory Scale were low, significantly less than predicted from IQ (Gott 1973). In 1988 Ogden also found his patients to have impaired memory, but their impairment was similar to that predicted by IQ (Ogden 1988). Despite these differences, it is clear that verbal and nonverbal memory are markedly impaired in patients who undergo right or left hemispherectomy (Dikman and Matthews 1975; Ogden 1988; Vargha-Khadem and Polkey 1993). Again, these changes are usually a manifestation of the disease rather than a consequence of the surgery.

BEHAVIORAL CHANGES

Improvements in aggressiveness and social function are often dramatic following hemispherectomy. Krynauw recognized this as a significant benefit to the patient and the family several decades ago (Krynauw 1950). In a 17-year follow-up study by Davies *et al*, function improved enough for their patients to achieve substantial social and financial independence and for 63% to be employable (Davies *et al* 1993). Caplan has described four patients undergoing right hemispherectomy for Rasmussen disease in whom there were improvements in social communication and language related to the age of onset and duration of their disease, and reversibility of preoperative PET hypometabolism (Caplan *et al* 1996).

COMPLICATIONS

OPERATIVE AND PERIOPERATIVE COMPLICATIONS

All variations of hemispherectomy can pose significant intraoperative risks, specifically related to air embolism and excessive hemorrhage. Hemispherectomy in all its forms requires extensive dissection, which can lead to significant blood loss, particularly for the very young child. An analysis of 10 hemispherectomies carried out on children in Boston showed that there can be sudden and precipitous hemorrhage, and arterial and venous pressure lines are essential to cope with this possibility (Matheson *et al* 1993). Blood loss can be particularly problematic with hemimega-

lencephalic patients because of the technical challenges posed by such a large hemisphere. Significant hemorrhage can also occur in Sturge–Weber syndrome when the angioma involves the scalp. If life-threatening hemorrhage is encountered during surgery, a staged procedure should be considered.

Meningitis, sepsis, wound infection, acute hydrocephalus, and cerebral edema can all occur in the early postoperative period. These problems, along with hemorrhagic complications during surgery, led to a 6–8% perioperative death rate in early series (Smith *et al* 1991; Villemure *et al* 1993). This mortality is probably less in more modern series; Holthausen reports 1.5% mortality in his multicenter series; Peacock reports one death in 58 patients; but Vining had four deaths in 58 patients (Peacock *et al* 1996; Vining *et al* 1997). In our series of 46 hemispherectomies there has been only one death (2.2%). Advances in anesthetic care, surgical technique, and perioperative care have reduced the complication rate, but the operation may still cause devastating complications (Brian *et al* 1990). Schramm and Delalande both note that one of the advantages of hemispherotomy is the reduced risk of blood loss and other potential vascular complications, especially in infants (Schramm *et al* 1995; Delalande *et al* 1993).

HYDROCEPHALUS

Hemispherectomy acutely reduces the functional absorptive area of the subarachnoid space, sometimes leading to acute hydrocephalus postoperatively. Its presentation may also be delayed, possibly secondary to acquired acqueductal stenosis or as a manifestation of hemosiderosis. This can sometimes occur very late after the original hemispherectomy (Kalkanis *et al* 1996). Regardless of the tempo of its presentation, it can have deleterious effects. The original Montreal series of anatomic hemispherectomy produced a 52% hydrocephalus rate, with approximately two-thirds related to hemosiderosis. Operative variations on anatomic hemispherectomy, such as the Oxford modification, have effectively reduced the rate of this complication (Villemure *et al* 1993). In the Maudsley series of 46 hemispherectomies, only four patients have needed shunts (8.7%). Series describing both functional hemispherectomy and hemidecortication indicate that some of these patients also require shunting for hydrocephalus (Peacock *et al* 1996; Vining *et al* 1997; Hoffman 1997).

The development of more advanced imaging techniques has had a greater impact on reducing the hydrocephalus-related morbidity than variations in operative technique. Diagnosing hydrocephalus was difficult when the operation was first introduced, leading to significant morbidity and mortality (Falconer and Wilson 1969).

HEMOSIDEROSIS

Oppenheimer and Griffith first described this condition in a group of patients who had a long trouble-free period after anatomic hemispherectomy but later developed an insidious, slow deterioration to eventual death. Autopsy showed superficial hemosiderosis over the brain and spinal cord with a lining histologically indistinguishable from a chronic subdural membrane. The remaining ventricle was lined by ventricular ependymitis. It is believed that this membrane forms as a result of blood products generated at the time of surgery. This membrane is friable and prone to repeated hemorrhages, which in turn lead to superficial hemosiderosis and granular ependymitis. These changes then lead to a recurrence of seizures, hydrocephalus, and an eventual rise in intracranial pressure (Oppenheimer and Griffith 1966).

Its incidence was very high in the original series of anatomic hemispherectomy, occurring in approximately 30% of patients in the long term (Falconer and Wilson 1969; Wilson 1970). Each modification of hemispherectomy was devised to minimize the incidence of this complication. While the long-term follow-up is limited, it seems that each modification has effectively reduced the incidence of and the morbidity associated with hemosiderosis (Villemure et al 1993).

However, although the risk is now much less, it is still important to remain aware of this complication as a possible source of gradual, delayed deterioration (Verity and Strauss 1982). It becomes symptomatic an average of 8 years after surgery, but it has been recognized as early as 4 years and as late as 20 years postoperatively (Villemure et al 1993). With CT scanning, treatment can be tailored to the specific manifestation. Chronic fluid collections usually resolve with burr-hole drainage. Craniotomy is indicated for large acute hematomas or for chronic fluid cavities that develop septations. Hydrocephalus should be treated with prompt shunting. Regardless of the treatment, early recognition remains the key to a good outcome (Verity and Strauss 1982).

ALTERNATIVE TREATMENTS

While hemispherectomy is now safer than originally reported, complications still occur and more limited operations are indicated whenever possible. When there is an isolated seizure focus within the hemisphere, a focal cortical resection is the treatment of choice.

Patients with diffuse hemispheric involvement and preserved neurologic function in the affected hemisphere may be candidates for corpus callosotomy or amygdalectomy as alternatives to hemispherectomy. In 1970, Luessenhop et al reported the successful treatment of two patients with infantile hemiplegia by corpus callosotomy (Luessenhop et al 1970). Since then, other authors have also reported similarly gratifying results using this procedure for intractable seizures associated with infantile hemiplegia (Wilson et al 1975; Avila and Radvany 1980; Goodman 1986). However it must be recalled that this procedure does not render more than 5% of patients seizure-free, compared with 70–80% with hemispherectomy. The principal indication for callosal section in potential candidates for hemispherectomy is where there is some useful preserved motor or sensory function in the limbs served by the diseased hemisphere, and the chief problem is atonic or drop attacks. In 1975, Balasubramanian and colleagues described a method of creating a chemical or thermal stereotactic lesion in the amygdala; all patients had cessation or near-cessation of their seizures (Balasubramanian and Kanaka 1975). There is one account of a patient in whom embolization was used as a treatment for hemimegalencephaly. The patient's seizures were controlled for one year and it was felt that blood loss at the subsequent hemispherectomy was less than it otherwise would have been (Mathis et al 1995). EEG showed diffuse excess rhythmic activity over the left hemisphere with ictal and interictal spike waves, particularly over the parietal and occipital lobes. Ictal SPECT showed hyperperfusion in the left parietal and temporal lobes, with interictal SPECT showing hyperperfusion in a similar area.

Where there are predominantly focal seizures from the affected hemisphere, with preserved function, as is sometimes seen in Rasmussen disease, then Morrell's technique of multiple subpial transection (MST) may be employed (Morrell et al 1989). Among the 10 patients undergoing hemispherectomy for Rasmussen disease at the Maudsley Hospital, two had previous MST and resection but in two others this maneuver controlled the seizure disorder, avoiding hemispherectomy. The choice of hemispherectomy techniques, including hemispherotomy, make it feasible to operate on very young or very ill patients and therefore callosal section or MST should only be used when there is a desire to preserve primary motor or sensory function.

CLINICAL EXAMPLES

PATIENT 1

This 3-year-old girl was born by a normal spontaneous vaginal delivery after a pregnancy complicated by preeclampsia. She had her first seizure at 3 weeks of age, consisting of generalized tonic flexions of the neck and extremities. These were diagnosed as infantile spasms and she was treated with ACTH and phenobarbital. She began having more frequent seizures and thereafter underwent an exhaustive trial of anticonvulsant polytherapy. Even with the combination of phenytoin and clobazam providing optimal seizure control, she continued to have three episodes of generalized stiffness and staring per day, lasting approximately 3 minutes.

During her 3-year evaluation and treatment period, she was noted to have a right hemiparesis and right hemianopsia. Her head circumference was on the 97th centile from birth, and remained at this level throughout her evaluation. Her language development was significantly delayed, but there were no behavioral disturbances.

Brain MRI showed a markedly larger left hemisphere with generalized thickening of the cortex. with occasional bouts of serial attacks. In 1988, at the age of 10 years, she had a spastic right hemiparesis with some preservation of finger movements, and a complete right homonymous hemianopia.

Even with optimal seizure control, her epilepsy was felt to be significantly affecting her development. Structural, functional, and neurophysiologic investigations suggested left hemimegalencephaly as the source of her seizure disorder. She underwent a left functional hemispherectomy without complication and made an uncomplicated postoperative recovery. There was no change in her neurologic examination postoperatively. She remained seizure-free during the first 6 postoperative months, while on anticonvulsants. When she was slowly weaned from the medications, she developed occasional seizures that were similar to those seen before surgery. She was placed back on antiepileptic medications, at lower doses than were used before surgery, with no recurrence of seizures. Her developmental progress has been good, albeit slightly behind her peers.

PATIENT 2

Hannah is a left-handed child with a right infantile hemiplegia who suffered from epilepsy from the age of 7 years. She was one of undiagnosed twins; the other was born dead and probably died *in utero* 2 weeks before delivery. Hannah was born of healthy nonconsanguineous parents; she has one healthy younger brother, and there is no family history of epilepsy. There appeared to be no further problems until the age of 6 months, when she was noticed to be using her right hand less than she should and it subsequently became clear that she had a spastic right hemiparesis. However, she remained in mainstream education and developed normally.

Her seizures began at the age of 7 years and could be provoked by a startle or a trip. The seizures themselves were brief, lasting at most 20 seconds, during which, after calling out, her right arm and both legs would extend and she would fall to the ground. She would average one fit per day prior to operation.

Her scalp EEG showed bilateral abnormalities, but with frequent epileptiform discharges over the left hemisphere. Her neuropsychologic profile showed a Verbal IQ of 97 with a Performance IQ of 92 and a reading age corresponding to her chronological age. A CT scan showed a marked left hemiatrophy with almost all of the cortical mantle destroyed except for a small remnant as the frontal lobe. An anatomic total hemispherectomy, using Adams' modification, was carried out when she was 10 years old. The specimen showed changes consistent with major circulatory damage late in intrauterine life.

Immediately after operation it was noted that she retained her clumsy finger movements and that her gait had been unaltered by the surgery. There has been complete cessation of seizures and her antiepileptic drugs were withdrawn 2 years after operation. When she was last seen 5 years after surgery, there was no change in her situation.

CONCLUSION

In spite of its chequered history, hemispherectomy and all its variations, including hemispherotomy, remain procedures that are now safe and effective for a small number of patients with intractable epilepsy.

KEY POINTS

1. Severe unilateral hemisphere disease can cause intractable drug-resistant epilepsy. Etiologies include intrauterine or neonatal damage, Rasmussen disease and hemimegalencephaly.

2. The original procedure of anatomic hemispherectomy has been modified because of the late-delayed complications associated with hemosiderosis, which caused late mortality in up to 30% of cases.

3. Surgical procedures involving first hemispheric removal and subsequently combinations of disconnection and removal has been developed to overcome this problem.

4. There is currently a choice of procedures from which the individual epilepsy surgery center can select an appropriate operation, avoiding major surgery in young children, the effects of hemosiderosis, and having regard to the underlying pathology.

5. Seizure relief is probably related to the underlying etiology varying between 80% for atrophy and 60% for hemimegalencephaly.

6. Mortality and morbidity are around 1–2% and certainly less than 5%.

REFERENCES

Adams C, Hwang PA, Gilday DL, Armstrong DC, Becker LE, Hoffman HJ (1992) Comparison of SPECT, EEG, CT, MRI, and pathology in partial epilepsy. *Pediatric Neurology* **8**:97–103.

Adams CBT (1983) Hemispherectomy – a modification. *Journal of Neurology, Neurosurgery and Psychiatry* **46**:617–619.

Ameli N (1980) Hemispherectomy for the treatment of epilepsy and behavior disturbance. *Journal Canadien des Sciences Neurologiques* 7(1):33–38.

Andermann F, Rasmussen TB, Oguni H (1991) The natural history of the syndrome of chronic encephalitis and epilepsy: A study of the MNI series of 48 cases. In: Andermann F (ed) *Chronic Encephalitis and Epilepsy*, pp 7–35. Boston: Butterworth-Heinemann.

Annet M (1973) Laterality of childhood hemiplegia and the growth of speech and intelligence. *Cortex* **9**:4–49.

Anonymous (1997) A global survey on epilepsy surgery, 1980–1990: a report by the Commission on Neurosurgery of Epilepsy, the International League Against Epilepsy. *Epilepsia* **38**:249–255.

Asher DM, Gajdusek DC (1991) Virologic studies in chronic encephalitis. In: Andermann A (ed) *Chronic Encephalitis and Epilepsy*, pp 147–158. Boston: Butterworth-Heinemann.

Avila J, Radvany J (1980) Anterior callosotomy as a substitute for hemispherectomy. *Acta Neurochirugica* **30**:S137–S143.

Balasubramanian V, Kanaka T (1975) 'Why hemispherectomy?'. *Applied Neurophysiology* **38**:197–205.

Beardsworth ED, Adams CBT (1988) Modified hemispherectomy for epilepsy. Early results in 10 cases. *British Journal of Neurosurgery* **2**:73–84.

Brian JE, Jr, Deshpande JK, McPherson RW (1990) Management of cerebral hemispherectomy in children. *Journal of Clinical Anesthesia* **2**:91–95.

Cairns H (1951) Hemispherectomy in the treatment of infantile hemiplegia. *Lancet* 411–415.

Caplan R, Curtiss S, Chugani HT, Vinters HV (1996) Pediatric Rasmussen encephalitis: social communication, language, PET and pathology before and after hemispherectomy. *Brain and Cognition* **32**:45–66.

Carmant L, Kramer U, Riviello JJ *et al* (1995) EEG prior to hemispherectomy: correlation with outcome and pathology. *Electroencephalography and Clinical Neurophysiology* **94**:265–270.

Chi J, Dooling E (1977) Gyral development of the human brain. *Annals of Neurology* **1**:86–93.

Chiron C, Raynaud C, Jambaque I, Dulac O, Zilbovicius M, Syrota A (1991) A serial study of regional cerebral blood flow before and after hemispherectomy in a child. *Epilepsy Research* **8**:232–240.

Chugani HT, Mazziotta JC (1989) Sturge–Weber syndrome. A study of cerebral glucose utilization with positron emission tomography. *Journal of Pediatrics* **114**:244–253.

Chugani HT, Shields WD (1990) Infantile spasms: I. PET identifies focal cortical dysgenesis in cryptogenic cases for surgical treatment. *Annals of Neurology* **27**:406–413.

Chugani HT, Shewmon DA, Peacock WJ, Shields WD, Mazziotta JC, Phelps ME (1988) Surgical treatment of intractable neonatal-onset seizures: the role of positron emission tomography. *Neurology* **38**:1178–1188.

Clancy R, Kurtz M (1985) Neurologic manifestations of the organoid nevus syndrome. *Archives of Neurology* **42**:236–240.

Coates P, Honavar M, Janota I, Polkey CE (1992) Polymerase chain reaction studies in Rasmussen's encephalitis. *Neuropathology and Applied Neurobiology* **18**:310.

Connelly A, Jackson GD, Duncan JS, Grunewald RA, King MD, Gadian GD (1994) Magnetic resonance spectroscopy in temporal lobe epilepsy. *Neurology* **44**:1411–1417.

Dalla B, Chiamenti C (1985) Benign partial epilepsies with effective symptoms (benign psychomotor epilepsy). Epilepsy syndromes in infancy, childhood and adolescence. *Eurotext* 171–175.

Damasio A, Lima A (1975) Nervous function after right hemispherectomy. *Neurology* **25**:89–93.

Dambska M, Wisniewski K (1984) An autopsy case of hemimegalencephaly. *Brain and Development* **6**:60–64.

Dandy W (1928) Removal of the right cerebral hemisphere for certain tumors with hemiplegia: preliminary report. *Journal of the American Medical Association* **90**:823–825.

Davidson S, Falconer MA (1975) Outcome of surgery in 40 children with temporal lobe epilepsy. *Lancet* **1**:1260–1263.

Davies KG, Maxwell RE, French LA (1993) Hemispherectomy for intractable seizures: long-term results in 17 patients followed for up to 38 years. *Journal of Neurosurgery* **78**:733–740.

Delalande O, Pinard JM, Basdevant C, Plouin P, Dulac O (1993)

Hemispherotomy: a new procedure for hemispheric disconnection. *Epilepsia* **34**:140 (Abstract).

Dennis M (1980) Capacity and strategy for syntactic comprehension after right or left hemidecortication. *Brain and Language* **10**:287–317.

Dennis M, Cohen B (1975) Comprehension of syntax in infantile hemiplegics after cerebral hemidecortication: left hemisphere superiority. *Brain and Language* **2**:472–482.

Dennis M, Lovett M (1981) Written language acquisition after right or left hemidecortication in infancy. *Brain and Language* **12**:54–91.

Dennis M, Whitaker H (1976) Language acquisition following hemidecortication: linguistic superiority of the left over the right hemisphere. *Brain and Language* **3**:404–433.

Di Rocco C, Caldarelli M (1993) Surgical indication in children with congenital hemiparesis. *Childs Nervous System* **9**:72–80.

Dikman S, Matthews C (1975) Effect of early versus late onset of major motor epilepsy upon cognitive-intellectual performance. *Epilpesia* **16**:73–81.

Dix JE, Cail WS (1997) Cerebral hemiatrophy: classification on the basis of MR imaging findings of mesial temporal sclerosis and childhood febrile seizures. *Radiology* **203**:269–274.

Dulac O, Robain O, Chiron C et al (1991) High-dose steroid treatment of epilepsia partialis continuans due to chronic focal encephalitis. In: Andermann A (ed) *Chronic Encephalitis and Epilepsy*, pp 193–200. Boston: Butterworth-Heinemann.

Dunn LT, Miles JB, May PL (1995) Hemispherectomy for intractable seizures: a further modification and early experience. *British Journal of Neurosurgery* **9**:775–783.

Engel J (1987) Outcome with respect to epileptic seizures. In: Engel J (ed) *Surgical Treatment of the Epilepsies*, pp. 553–571. New York: Raven Press.

Falconer MA and Rushworth R (1959) Treatment of encephalotrigeminal angiomatosis (Sturge–Weber disease) by hemispherectomy. *Journal of Neurosurgery* 443–447.

Falconer MA and Wilson PJE (1969) Complications relating to delayed haemorrhage after hemispherectomy. *Journal of Neurosurgery* **30**:413–426.

Farrell MA, Droogan O, Secor DL, Poukens V, Quinn B, Vinters HV (1995) Chronic encephalitis associated with epilepsy: immunohistochemical and ultrastructural studies. *Acta Neuropathologica* **89**:313–321.

French L, Johnson D (1955) Cerebral hemispherectomy for the control of intractable convulsive seizures. *Journal of Neurosurgery* **12**:154–164.

Gadian DG, Connelly A (1994) ^{1}H magnetic resonance spectroscopy in the investigation of intractable epilepsy. *Acta Neurologica Scandinavica* **152**:116–121.

Geffen G, Quinn K (1984) Hemispheric specialization and ear advantage in processing speech. *Psychological Bulletin* **96**:273–291.

Goodman R (1986) Hemispherectomy and its alternatives in the treatment of intractable epilepsy in patients with infantile hemiplegia. *Developmental Medicine and Child Neurology* **28**:251–258.

Goodman R, Williamson P (1985) Interhemispheric commissurotomy for congenital hemiplegics with intractable epilepsy. *Neurology* **35**:1351–1354.

Gott P (1973) Cognitive abilities following right and left hemispherectomy. *Cortex* **9**:266–274.

Grenier Y, Antel JP, Osterland CK (1991) Immunologic studies in chronic encephalitis of Rasmussen. In: Andermann A (ed) *Chronic Encephalitis and Epilepsy*, pp. 125–134. Boston: Butterworth-Heinemann.

Harding B, DePhil B (1990) Progressive neuronal degeneration of childhood with liver disease (Alpert–Hutenlocher syndrome): a personal review. *Journal of Child Neurology* **5**(4):273–287.

Heigbel J, Blom J (1975) Benign epilepsy of children with centrotemporal EEG foci: a study of incidence rate in out-patient care. *Epilepsia* **16**:657–664.

Hoffman HJ (1997) Hemispherectomy. In: Tuxhorn I, Holthausen H, Boenigk H (eds) *Paediatric Epilepsy Syndromes and Their Surgical Treatment*, pp. 739–742. London: John Libbey.

Hoffman HJ, Hendrick EB, Dennis M, Armstrong D (1979) Hemispherectomy for Sturge–Weber syndrome. *Childs Brain* **3**:233–248.

Holthausen H, May TW, Adams CBT et al (1997a) Seizures post hemispherectomy. In: Tuxhorn I, Holthausen H, Boenigk H (eds) *Paediatric Epilepsy Syndromes and Their Surgical Treatment*, pp 749–773. London: John Libbey.

Holthausen H, Strobl K, Pieper T, Teixeira VA, Oppel F (1997b) Prediction of motor functions post hemispherectomy. In: Tuxhorn I, Holthausen H, Boenigk H (eds) *Paediatric Epilepsy Syndromes and Their Surgical Treatment*, pp. 785–798. London: John Libbey.

Ignelzi RJ, Bucy PC (1968) Cerebral hemidecortication in the treatment of infantile cerebral hemiatrophy. *Journal of Nervous and Mental Disease* **147**:14–30.

Jackson GD, Connelly A (1993) Detection of hippocampal pathology in intractable partial epilepsy: increased sensitivity with quantitative magnetic resonance T2 relaxometry. *Neurology* **43**:1793–1799.

Jahan R, Mischel PS, Curran JG, Peacock WJ, Shields DW, Vinters HV (1997) Bilateral neuropathologic changes in a child with hemimegalencephaly. *Pediatric Neurology* **17**:344–349.

Jennum P, Friberg L (1994) Speech localisation using repetitive transcranial magnetic stimulation. *Neurology* **44**:269–273.

Kalifa GL, Chiron C (1987) Hemimegalencephaly: MR imaging in five children. *Radiology* **165**:29–33.

Kalkanis SN, Blumenfeld H, Sherman JC, et al (1996) Delayed complications thirty-six years after hemispherectomy: a case report. *Epilepsia* **37**:758–762.

Kanev PM, Foley CM, Miles D (1997) Ultrasound-tailored functional hemispherectomy for surgical control of seizures in children. *Journal of Neurosurgery* **86**:762–767.

Kimura K (1967) Functional assymetry of the brain in dichotic listening. *Cortex* **3**:157–178.

King M, Stephenson JBP, Tiervogel M, Doyle D, Galbraith S (1985) Hemimegalencephaly – a case for hemispherectomy? *Neuropaediatrics* **16**:46–55.

King SM, Azzopardi P, Cowey A, Oxbury J, Oxbury S (1996a) The role of light scatter in the residual visual sensitivity of patients with complete cerebral hemispherectomy. *Visual Neuroscience* **13**:1–13.

King SM, Frey S, Villemure JG, Ptito A, Azzopardi P (1996b) Perception of motion-in-depth in patients with partial or complete cerebral hemispherectomy. *Behavioural Brain Research* **76**:169–180.

Koelfen W, Freund M (1993) Hemimegalencephaly. Therapy with hemispherectomy. *Monatsschrift für Kinderheilkunde* **141**:300–302.

Kohn B, Dennis M (1974) Selective impairments of visuo-spatial abilities in infantile hemiplegics after right hemidecortication. *Neuropsychologica* **12**:505–512.

Krynauw RA (1950) Infantile hemiplegia treated by removing one cerebral hemisphere. *Journal of Neurology, Neurosurgery and Psychiatry* **13**:243–267.

Kuzniecky RI (1994) Magnetic resonance imaging in developmental disorders of the cerebral cortex. *Epilepsia* **35**(Suppl 6):544–556.

L'Hermitte J (1928) L'ablation complete de l'hemisphere droit dans le cas de tumeur cerebrale localisee compliquee d'hemiplegie: la decerebration suprathalamique unilaterale chez l'homme. *Encephal* **23**:314–323.

Lindsay J, Ounsted C (1979) Longterm outcome in children with temporal lobe seizures I: Social outcome and social factors. *Developmental Medicine and Child Neurology* **21**:630–636.

Lindsay J, Ounsted C (1987) Hemispherectomy for childhood epilepsy:

a 36 year study. *Developmental Medicine and Child Neurology* **29**:592–600.

Luessenhop AJ, Dela-Cruz TC, Fairchild DM (1970) Surgical disconnection of the cerebral hemispheres for intractable seizures. Results in infancy and childhood. *Journal of the American Medical Association* **213**:1630–1636.

MacKenzie K (1938) The present status of a patient who had the right cerebral hemisphere removed. *Proceedings of the American Medical Association*, Chicago **111**:618.

Malaclan R, Girvin JP (1993) Rasmussen's chronic encephalitis in adults. *Archives of Neurology* **50**:269–274.

Marti-Bonmati L, Menor F (1993) The Sturge–Weber syndrome: correlation between clinical status and radiological CT and MRI findings. *Childs Nervous System* **9**:107–109.

Matheson JM, Truskett P, Davies MA, Vonau M (1993) Hemispherectomy: a further modification using omentum vascularized free flaps. *Australian and New Zealand Journal of Surgery* **8**:646–650.

Mathis JM, Barr JD, Albright AL, Horton JA (1995) Hemimegalencephaly and intractable epilepsy treated with embolic hemispherectomy. *American Journal of Neuroradiology* **16**:1076–1079.

McFie J (1961) The effects of hemispherectomy on intellectual function in cases of infantile hemiplegia. *Journal of Neurology, Neurosurgery and Psychiatry* **24**:240–249.

McKissock W (1953) Infantile hemiplegia. *Proceedings of the Royal Society of Medicine* **46**:431–434.

McNamara JO, Andrews PI (1995) Autoimmune epilepsy: aspects of the pathogenesis of Rasmussen's encephalitis. *Epilepsia* **36**(Suppl 3):S172.

Morrell F, Whisler WW, Bleck TP (1989) Multiple subpial transection. A new approach to the surgical treatment of focal epilepsy. *Journal of Neurosurgery* **70**:231–239.

Ogden J (1988) Language and memory functions after long recovery periods in left hemispherectomised subjects. *Neuropsychologia* **26**:645–659.

Ogden J (1989) Visuo-spatial and other 'right hemispheric' functions after long recovery periods in left hemispherectomised subjects. *Neuropsychologia* **27**:765–776.

Ogden JA (1996) Phonological dyslexia and phonological dysgraphia following left and right hemispherectomy. *Neuropsychologia* **34**:905–918.

Oguni H, Hayashi K, Usui N, Osawa M, Shimizu H (1998) Startle epilepsy with infantile hemiplegia: report of two cases improved by surgery. *Epilepsia* **39**:93–98.

Oppenheimer DR, Griffith HB (1966) Persistent intracranial bleeding as a complication of hemispherectomy. *Journal of Neurology, Neurosurgery and Psychiatry* **29**:229–240.

Osborn RE, Byrd SE (1988) MR imaging of neuronal migration disorders. *American Journal of Neuroradiology* **9**:1101–1106.

Ounsted C, Lindsay J, Richards P (1987) *Temporal Lobe Epilepsy. A Biographical Study, 1948–1986*. Oxford: Blackwell Scientific.

Palmini A, Gambardella A, Andermann F et al (1994) Operative strategies for patients with cortical dysplastic lesions and intractable epilepsy. *Epilepsia* **35**(Suppl 6):S57–71.

Peacock WJ, Wehby-Grant MC, Shields WD et al (1996) Hemispherectomy for intractable seizures in children: a report of 58 cases. *Childs Nervous System* **12**:376–384.

Pelayo R, Barasch E (1994) Progressively intractable seizures, focal alopecia and hemimegalencephaly. *Neurology* **44**:969–971.

Polkey CE (1990) The place of hemispherectomy and major cortical resection in the control of drug resistant epilepsy [Review]. *Acta Neurochirurgica Supplementum* **50**:131–133.

Power C, Poland SD, Blume WT, Girvin JP, Rice GPA (1990) Cytomegalovirus and Rasmussen's encephalitis. *Lancet* **336**:1282–1284.

Quirk J, Kendall B (1993) EEG features of cortical dysplasia in children. *Neuropediatrics* **24**:193–199.

Rasmussen T (1973) Post-operative superficial hemosiderosis of the brain, its diagnosis, treatment and prevention. *American Neurological Association* **98**:133–137.

Rasmussen T (1983) Hemispherectomy for seizures revisited. *Canadian Journal of Neurological Sciences* **10**:71–78.

Rasmussen T (1987) Cortical resection for multilobe epileptogenic lesions. In: Wieser HG, Elger CE (eds) *Presurgical Evaluation of Epileptics*, pp. 344–351. Berlin: Springer-Verlag.

Rasmussen T, Milner B (1977) The role of early left brain damage in determining the lateralisation of cerebral speech functions. *Annals of the New York Academy of Sciences* **299**:355–369.

Rasmussen T, Obozewski J, Lloyd-Smith D (1958) Focal seizures due to chronic localised encephalitis. *Neurology* **8**:435–445.

Renowden SA, Squier M (1994) Unusual magnetic resonance and neuropathological findings in hemimegalencephaly: report of a case following hemispherectomy. *Developmental Medicine and Child Neurology* **4**:357–361.

Rintahaka PJ, Chugani HT, Messa C, Phelps ME (1993) Hemimegalencephaly: evaluation with positron emission tomography. *Pediatric Neurology* **9**:21–28.

Robain O, Floquet CH, Heldt N, Rozenberg F (1988) Hemimegalencephaly: a clinicopathological study of four cases. *Neuropathology and Applied Neurobiology* **14**:125–135.

Schramm J, Behrens E, Entzian W (1995) Hemispherical deafferentation: an alternative to functional hemispherectomy. *Neurosurgery* **36**:509–515; discussion 515–516.

Shields WD, Duchowny MS, Holmes GL (1993) Surgically remediable syndromes of infancy and early childhood. In: Engel, J (ed) *Surgical Treatment of the Epilepsies*, 2nd edn, pp 35–48. New York: Raven Press.

Smith SJ, Andermann F, Villemure JG, Rasmussen T, Quesney LF (1991) Functional hemispherectomy: EEG findings, spiking from isolated brain postoperatively, and prediction of outcome. *Neurology* **41**:1790–1794.

Taylor LB (1991) Neuropsychological assessment of patients with chronic encephalitis. In: Andermann, F. (ed) *Chronic Encephalitis and Epilepsy: Rasmussen's Syndrome*, pp. 111–121. Boston: Butterworth-Heinemann.

Tinuper P, Andermann F (1988) Functional hemispherectomy for treatment of epilepsy associated with hemiplegia: rationale, indications, results, and comparison with callosotomy. *Annals of Neurology* **24**:27–34.

Tomaiuolo F, Ptito M, Marzi CA, Paus T, Ptito A (1997) Blindsight in hemispherectomized patients as revealed by spatial summation across the vertical meridian. *Brain* **120**:795–803.

Vargha-Khadem F, Mishkin M (1997) Speech and language outcome after hemispherectomy in childhood. In: Tuxhorn I, Holthausen H, Boenigk H (eds) *Paediatric Epilepsy Syndromes and Their Surgical Treatment*, pp 774–784. London: John Libbey.

Vargha-Khadem F, Polkey CE (1993) A review of cognitive outcome after hemidecortication in humans. In: Rose FD, Johnson DA (eds) *Recovery from Brain Damage. Reflections and Directions*, pp 137–152. New York: Plenum Press.

Verity C, Strauss E (1982) Long-term follow-up after cerebral hemispherectomy: neurophysiologic, radiologic, and psychological findings. *Neurology* **32**:629–639.

Vigevano F, Di RC (1990) Effectiveness of hemispherectomy in hemimegalencephaly with intractable seizures. *Neuropediatrics* **21**:222–223.

Vigevano F, Bertini E, Boldrini R et al (1989) Hemimegalencephaly and intractable epilepsy: benefits of hemispherectomy. *Epilepsy* **30**:833–843.

Villemure JG, Mascott CR (1995) Peri-insular hemispherotomy: surgical principles and anatomy. *Neurosurgery* **37**:975–981.

Villemure JG, Andermann F, Rasmussen T (1991) Hemispherectomy for the treatment of epilepsy due to chronic encephalitis. In: Andermann

F (ed) *Chronic Encephalitis and Epilepsy: Rasmussen's Syndrome*, pp 235–241. Boston: Butterworth-Heinemann.

Villemure JG, Adams CBT, Hoffman HJ, Peacock WJ (1993) Hemispherectomy. In: Engel J (ed) *Surgical Treatment of the Epilepsies*, 2nd edn, pp 511–518. New York: Raven Press.

Vining EP, Freeman JM, Brandt J, Carson BS, Uematsu S (1993) Progressive unilateral encephalopathy of childhood (Rasmussen's syndrome): a reappraisal. *Epilepsia* **34**:639–650.

Vining EP, Freeman JM, Pillas DJ *et al* (1997) Why would you remove half a brain? The outcome of 58 children after hemispherectomy – the Johns Hopkins experience: 1968 to 1996. *Pediatrics* **100**:163–171.

Wada J (1949) A new method for the determination of the side of cerebral speech dominance. A preliminary report on the intra-carotid injection of sodium amytal in man. *Medicine and Biology* **14**:221–222.

Wessinger CM, Fendrich R, Gazzaniga MS, Ptito A, Villemure JG (1996a) Extrageniculostriate vision in humans: investigations with hemispherectomy patients. *Progress in Brain Research* **112**:405–413.

Wessinger CM, Fendrich R, Ptito A, Villemure JG, Gazzaniga MS (1996b) Residual vision with awareness in the field contralateral to a partial or complete functional hemispherectomy. *Neuropsychologia* **34**:1129–1137.

White H (1961) Cerebral hemispherectomy in the treatment of infantile hemiplegia. *Confinia Neurologicala* **21**:1–50.

Wilson DH, Culver C, Waddington M, Gazzaniga M (1975) Disconnection of the cerebral hemispheres. An alternative to hemispherectomy for the control of intractable seizures. *Neurology* **12**:1149–1153.

Wilson PJE (1970) Cerebral hemispherectomy for infantile hemiplegia: a report of fifty cases. *Brain* **93**:147–180.

Winston KR, Welch K, Adler JR, Erba G (1992) Cerebral hemicorticectomy for epilepsy [see comments]. *Journal of Neurosurgery* **77**:889–895.

Woods BT, Teuber HL (1978) Changing patterns of childhood aphasia. *Annals of Neurology* **3**:273–280.

Yuh WT, Nguyen HD (1994) MR of fetal central nervous system abnormalities. *AJNR American Journal of Neuroradiology* **15**:459–464.

Zaidel E (1977) Unilateral auditory language comprehension on the Token Test following cerebral commissurotomy and hemispherectomy. *Neuropsychologia* **15**:1–15.

Zaidel E (1978) Auditory language comprehension in the right hemisphere following cerebral commissurotomy and hemispherectomy: a comparison with child language and aphasia. In: *Language Acquisition and Language Breakdown: Parallels and Divergencies*, pp 229–275. Baltimore: Johns Hopkins University Press.

Zatorre RJ, Ptito A, Villemure JG (1995) Preserved auditory spatial localization following cerebral hemispherectomy. *Brain* **118**:879–889.

Functional surgery for epilepsy

54

CE POLKEY

INTRODUCTION

The early surgical treatment of epilepsy was directed towards the identification and removal of structural abnormality once the irrational 'witchcraft' treatments of skull trepanation had been superseded by the scientific age of surgery. The identification of the motor cortex in animals and humans enabled pioneers in epilepsy surgery such as William McEwan and Victor Horsley to reflect pathology from such areas in patients with appropriate seizures. The work of the Montreal Neurological Institute in developing early epilepsy surgery originated from Penfield's work on scar maturation with Foerster. However, although based at the outset on stimulation to identify seizure origin and very soon after that on direct cortical recording at surgery, the philosophy was nevertheless one of resective surgery in which an area of cortex thought to be responsible for the epilepsy was removed. With the refinement and improvements in structural and functional brain imaging and the acquisition of considerable and complex knowledge of the pathophysiology of epilepsy, both in experimental models and in human disease, the rationale and treatment of resective surgery has been improved but it remains the same process. These surgical principles underlie the majority of

interventions for the surgical relief of epilepsy, at least that currently reported in the refereed world literature, and it is interesting that in successive reviews of epilepsy surgery (1975, 1987, 1993, 1997), the functional methods of treatment have received less and less attention (Ojemann and Ward 1975; Spencer 1987; Fisher *et al* 1993; Morrell 1997).

However, there have been developments in our understanding of the pathophysiology of epilepsy within the brain. The adaptation of the brain to the physiologic consequences of chronic epilepsy has been greatly helped by the studies of experimental epileptogenesis, in particular the concepts of kindling and secondary epileptogenesis (Goddard *et al* 1969; Morrell 1985; Morrell *et al* 1987). The information from these studies is not sufficient to plan operative procedures. There has been a finite limit to the spatial and temporal resolution of electrophysiologic studies in patients and in comparison with the lower phylogenetic orders the development of these processes of secondary epileptogenesis in higher primates and humans is less certain and less crisp. For this reason the various functional procedures available to treat medically intractable epilepsy are either empirical or based on scanty scientific premises.

The procedures used in functional surgery for epilepsy fall into three broad groups. First, stereotactic lesioning to abolish or modify the spread of epileptic discharges through patients derived some benefit, but in four cases it was insufficient, and the patients proceeded to hemispherectomy within some weeks to 1 year. However, in two patients, one of whom had a frontal resection as well, seizure control within Engel group 1 was achieved and has been maintained for 2 or 3 years (Sawhney *et al* 1995).

Outcome in Landau–Kleffner syndrome

Here different criteria must apply. In Morrell's series of 14 patients reported in 1995 all had been mute for 2 years, and in the author's series of seven patients all had been mute for over six months (Morrell *et al* 1991). The natural history of the condition is for the patient to make a slow and imperfect recovery. Deonna *et al* (1989) followed seven patients into adulthood: only one regained normal speech, one had profound dyslexia, one a profound receptive problem, and the others were more severely affected. The literature suggests that if the patient has been mute for more than 1 year then a severe and permanent language disability will follow (Van Harskamp *et al* 1978). There are three criteria for improvement in these patients. The first is improvement in language function, the second is concomitant improvement in behavior, and the last is improvement in the EEG. Although the publication in 1995 described 14 patients, a more recent paper (Grote *et al* 1999) indicates that 18 patients have now been treated in Chicago. Four of these patients failed to improve and one of the author's seven patients came into the same category; in retrospect all of these patients were bad selections. The patients in the Rush series comprised seven boys and seven girls; their ages at surgery varied between 5.1 and 13.1 years with a mean age of 4 years. Nine patients were operated on the left side and five on the right. Follow-up varied between 6 months and 6 years. Three patients required two operations. The author's own series was similar with five left-sided operations and two right-sided operations. In that series, one patient required reoperation. In the Rush series, there was improvement in speech and behavior, language became normal in six patients and improved in another five.

Recently the results of preoperative and postoperative language testing in the Rush patients have been published. Neuropsychologists used two tests, the revised versions of the Peabody Picture Vocabulary Test (PPVT-R) which tests receptive vocabulary and the Expressive One Word Picture Vocabulary Test (EOWPVT-R) which tests expressive vocabulary. Comparison was made between preoperative and postoperative scores using a paired *t*-test and the operation was shown to have produced significant improvement. Two factors were associated with this. One was the time between testing and operation; the later the test was given after surgery the better was the result. The second factor was the time between language deterioration and surgery; the shorter this period the greater the improvement (Grote *et al* 1999). Generally the EEG abnormalities resolve after surgery. In Morrell's patients, two of the patients with improvement continued to have abnormal EEGs and the four patients who had not improved, and were clearly a poor selection on other grounds, also failed to shown improvement in their EEG. In the author's patients there were four who showed a transient deterioration some months after surgery with increased seizures, deterioration or halting of language improvement and deterioration in EEG. Three of these patients improved after a short time, one required restoration of anticonvulsant medication, the other patient underwent reoperation. This condition is rare, and the number of patients treated is small, but provided the selection is rigorous then 70% or more will benefit, especially if the surgery is carried out fairly promptly.

Outcome from multilobar and multifocal epilepsy

At present this application of multiple subpial transection has been published only by Patil and colleagues. They have therefore accepted, as Morrell himself speculated, that multiple subpial transection could be used as an initial treatment for drug-resistant epilepsy. They described intervention in 19 patients where previous investigations using the methods described above identified multiple cortical areas which were epileptogenic zones. The technique of multiple subpial transection was employed with four passes over each area. If this failed to remove the spikes then small cortical resections (topectomies) were carried out. In most of these areas the pathologist described gliosis, but in one there was heterotopia. In two patients the operations were bilateral. Three patients had a contralateral weakness which resolved after 1–8 months. The effects of the operations on seizure control were not immediate but became maximum at 9 months after surgery. There were nine patients in whom the seizures were either completely controlled or they had less than five seizures per year (47%) and a further eight patients who were in Engel group 3a (41%) (Grote *et al* 1999). Recently Palmini has also described the use of this technique in a smaller group of similar patients with good results (personal communication). Patil has also described the application of this technique to six patients with autistic epileptiform regression.

CONCLUSION

The technique of multiple subpial transection is an innovative method for the treatment of drug-resistant epilepsy which has a permanent effect on seizure control with an acceptable morbidity.

BRAIN STIMULATION

The indications for stimulation, the techniques, complications, and outcomes are discussed in Chapter 55.

GENERAL CONCLUSION

All of these function interventions are less efficient at reducing epilepsy than resective operations. There are a number of reasons for this. The patient population is seldom as uniform and frequently suffers with multiple seizure types. The neurophysiologic basis for these interventions is much less certain and virtually impossible to demonstrate or test in humans and probably cannot be influenced to great change. Nevertheless they have a place in controlling epilepsy and improving quality of life for the patients and their carers with acceptably low morbidity and mortality.

KEY POINTS

1. Functional procedures for epilepsy attempt to alter the way in which the brain deals with the epileptic discharge, rather than trying to identify a focal origin for the epilepsy and to remove that origin by resective surgery.

2. Such procedures are generally less efficient at relieving epilepsy with seizure free outcomes of around 5–10%, compared with seizure-free outcomes of 60% or more from patients subjected to resective operations after careful selection.

3. Functional procedures depend upon dividing connections, usually in the form of fibre tracts, sometimes in destroying grey matter, as in stereotactic amygdalotomy or in brain stimulation.

4. At present there are only two procedures of practical interest apart from stimulation which is dealt with in chapter 56. These two procedures are callostomy and multiple subpial transection.

5. Callosotomy is appropriate for patients with multiple seizure types, but some seizure types are more responsive than others, and it is best used for 'drop' attacks. Its role in patients with multiple seizure types which include generalized seizures, as for example in Lennox-Gastaut syndrome, may well be supplanted by vagus nerve stimulation.

6. Multiple subpial transection is now of proven value in focal epilepsy and Landau-Kleffner syndrome. It may be helpful in other multifocal epilepsies.

REFERENCES

Aicardi J (1994) The place of neuronal migration abnormalities in child neurology. *Canadian Journal of Neurological Sciences* **3**:185–193.

Alarcon G, Garcia Seoane JJ, Binnie CD *et al* (1997) Origin and propagation of interictal discharges in the acute electrocorticogram. Implications for pathophysiology and surgical treatment of temporal lobe epilepsy. *Brain* **120**:2259–2282.

Ambrosetto G, Antonini L (1995) Anterior corpus callosotomy: effects in a patient with congenital bilateral perisylvian syndrome and oromotor seizures. *Italian Journal of Neurological Sciences* **16**:311–314.

Avila J, Radvany J (1980) Anterior callosotomy as a substitute for hemispherectomy. *Acta Neurochirurgica* **30**:S137–S143.

Awad IA, Wyllie E, Luders H, Ahl J (1990) Intraoperative determination of the extent of corpus callosotomy for epilepsy: two simple techniques. *Neurosurgery* **26**:102–105.

Balasubramanian V, Kanaka T (1975) 'Why hemispherectomy?' *Applied Neurophysiology* **38**:197–205.

Bogen JE (1999) The neurosurgeon's interest in the corpus callosum. In: Greenblatt SH (ed.) *A History of Neurosurgery in its Scientific and Professional Contexts*, pp 489–498. Park Ridge, IL: American Association of Neurosurgeons.

Cendes F, Ragazzo PC, da Costa V, Martins LF (1993) Corpus callosotomy in treatment of medically resistant epilepsy: preliminary results in a pediatric population. *Epilepsia* **34**:910–917.

Chadan N, Sautreaux JL, Giroud M *et al* (1992) MRI assessment of anterior callosotomy in the treatment of pharmacoresistant epilepsy. *Journal of Neuroradiology* **19**:98–106.

Collins SD, Walker JA, Barbaro N, Laxer KD (1989) Corpus callosotomy in the treatment of Lennox–Gastaut syndrome. *Epilepsia* **30**:689–690.

Deonna T, Peter CL, Ziegler A (1989) Adult follow-up of the acquired aphasia-epilepsy syndrome in childhood. A report of seven cases. *Neuropediatrics* **20**:132–138.

Devinsky O, Perrine K, Vazquez B, Luciano DJ, Dogali M (1994)

Multiple subpial transections in the language cortex. *Brain* **117**:255–265.

Editorial (1986) Cerebral dominance and epilepsy surgery. *Lancet* **2**:1318–1319.

Editorial (1997) A global survey on epilepsy surgery, 1980–1990: a report by the Commission on Neurosurgery of Epilepsy, the International League Against Epilepsy. *Epilepsia* **38**(2):249–255.

Engel J (1987) Outcome with respect to epileptic seizures. In: Engel J (ed.) *Surgical Treatment of the Epilepsies*, pp 553–571. New York: Raven Press.

Engel J, Van Ness PC, Rasmussen T, Ojemann LM (1993) Outcome with respect to epileptic seizures. In: Engel J (ed.) *Surgical Treatment of the Epilepsies*, 2nd edn, pp 609–622. New York: Raven Press.

Erickson TC (1940) Spread of the epileptic discharge. An experimental study of the after-discharge induced by electrical stimulation of the cerebral cortex. *Archives of Neurology and Psychiatry* **43**:429–452.

Fiol ME, Gates JR, Mireles R, Maxwell RE, Erickson DM (1993) Value of intraoperative EEG changes during corpus callosotomy in predicting surgical results. *Epilepsia* **34**:74–78.

Fisher RS, Uthman BM, Ramsay RE et al (1993) Alternative surgical techniques for epilepsy. In: Engel J (ed.) *Surgical Treatment of the Epilepsies*, 2nd edn, pp 549–564. New York: Raven Press.

Fuiks KS, Wyler AR, Hermann BP Somes G (1991) Seizure outcome from anterior and complete corpus callosotomy [see comments]. *Journal of Neurosurgery* **74**:573–578.

Garcia-Flores E (1994) Surgical treatment of complex partial seizures: 20 years' experience. *Stereotactic and Functional Neurosurgery* **62**:216–221.

Gates JR, Mireles R, Maxwell R, Sharbrough F, Forbes G (1986) Magnetic resonance imaging, electroencephalogram, and selected neuropsychological testing in staged corpus callosotomy. *Archives of Neurology* **11**:1188–1191.

Gates JR, Wada JA, Reeves AG et al (1993) Reevaluation of corpus callosotomy. In: Engel J (ed.) *Surgical Treatment of the Epilepsies*, 2nd edn, pp 637–648. New York: Raven Press.

Gates JR, Rosenfeld WE, Maxwell RE, Lyons RE (1987) Response of multiple seizure types to corpus callosum section. *Epilepsia* **28**:28–34.

Gilliam F, Wyllie E, Kotagal P, Geckler C, Rusyniak G (1996) Parental assessment of functional outcome after corpus callosotomy. *Epilepsia* **37**:753–757.

Goddard GV, McIntyre DC, Leech CK (1969) A permanent change in brain function resulting from daily electrical stimulation. *Experimental Neurology* **25**:295–330.

Goodman R (1986) Hemispherectomy and its alternatives in the treatment of intractable epilepsy in patients with infantile hemiplegia. *Developmental Medicine and Child Neurology* **28**:251–258.

Grote CL, Van Slyke P, Hoeppner JB (1999) Language outcome following multiple subpial transection for Landau–Kleffner syndrome. *Brain* **122**:

Guerrini R, Dravet C, Raybaud C et al (1992) Neurological findings and seizure outcome in children with bilateral opercular macrogyric-like changes detected by MRI. *Developmental Medicine and Child Neurology* **8**:694–705.

Harbaugh RE, Wilson DH, Reeves AG, Gazzaniga MS (1983) Forebrain commissurotomy for epilepsy. Review of 20 consecutive cases. *Acta Neurochirurgica* **68**:263–275.

Heimburger RF, Small IF, Small JG, Milstein V, Moore D (1978) Stereotactic amygdalotomy for convulsive and behavioral disorders. Long-term follow-up study. *Applied Neurophysiology* **41**:43–51.

Hood TW, Siegfried J, Wieser HG (1983) The role of stereotactic amygdalotomy in the treatment of behavioral disorders associated with temporal lobe epilepsy. *Applied Neurophysiology* **49**:19–25.

Hubel DH, Wiesel TN (1962) Receptive fields, binocular interaction and functional architecture in the cat's visual cortex. *Journal of Physiology* **160**:106–154.

Hufnagel A, Zentner J, Fernandez G, Wolf HK, Schramm J, Elger CE

(1997) Multiple subpial transection for control of epileptic seizures: effectiveness and safety. *Epilepsia* **38**:678–688.

Jones-Gotman M, Zatorre RJ, Cendes F et al (1997) Contribution of medial versus lateral temporal lobe structures to human odor identification. *Brain* **120**:1845–1856.

Joseph R (1986) Reversal of cerebral dominance for language and emotion in a corpus callosotomy patient. *Journal of Neurology, Neurosurgery and Psychiatry* **49**:628–634.

Kuzniecky R, Andermann F, Guerrini R (1994) The epileptic spectrum in the congenital bilateral perisylvian syndrome. CBPS Multicenter Collaborative Study. *Neurology* **44**:379–385.

Landau WM, Kleffner FR (1957) Syndrome of acquired aphasia with convulsive disorder in childhood. *Neurology* **7**:523–530.

Landy HJ, Curless RG, Ramsay RE, Slater J, Ajmone Marsan C, Quencer RM (1993) Corpus callosotomy for seizures associated with band heterotopia. *Epilepsia* **34**:79–83.

Lassonde M, Sauerwein C (1997) Neuropsychological outcome of corpus callosotomy in children and adolescents. *Journal of Neurosurgical Sciences* **41**:67–73.

Liu Z, Zhao Q, Li S, Tian Z, Cui Y, Feng H (1995) Multiple subpial transection for treatment of intractable epilepsy. *Chinese Medical Journal* **108**:539–541.

Luczywek E, Mempel E, Olsnes K (1978) Effect of amygdalotomy on behavior disorders in epileptics. *Neurologia i Neurochirurgia Polska* **12**(2):145–150.

Luders H, Bustamante LA, Zablow L, Goldensohn ES (1981) The independence of closely spaced discrete experimental spike foci. *Neurology* **31**:846–851.

Luessenhop AJ (1970) Interhemispheric commissurotomy (the split brain operation) as an alternate to hemispherectomy for the control of intractable seizures. *American Surgeon* **36**:265–268.

Luessenhop AJ, Dela-Cruz TC, Fairchild DM (1970) Surgical disconnection of the cerebral hemispheres for intractable seizures. Results in infancy and childhood. *Journal of the American Medical Association* **213**:1630–1636.

Lutsep HL, Wessinger CM, Gazzaniga MS (1995) Cerebral and callosal organization in a right hemisphere-dominant 'split brain' patient. *Journal of Neurology, Neurosurgery and Psychiatry* **59**:50–54.

Marino R (1985) Surgery for epilepsy. Selective partial microsurgical callosotomy for intractable multiform seizures. Criteria for clinical selection and results. *Applied Neurophysiology* **48**:404–407.

Marossero F, Ravagnati L, Sironi VA et al (1980) Late results of stereotactic radiofrequency lesions in epilepsy. *Acta Neurochirurgica Supplementum* **30**:145–149.

Mempel E, Witkiewicz B, Stadnicki R et al (1980) The effect of medial amygdalotomy and anterior hippocampotomy on behavior and seizures in epileptic patients. *Acta Neurochirurgica Supplementum* **30**:161–167.

Morrell F (1959) Secondary epileptogenic lesions. *Epilepsia* **1**:538–560.

Morrell F (1961) Microelectrode studies in chronic epileptic foci. *Epilepsia* **2**:81–88.

Morrell F (1985) Secondary epileptogenesis in man. *Archives of Neurology* **42**:318–335.

Morrell F (1997) Multiple subpial transections and other interventions. In: Engel JJ, Pedley TA (eds) *Epilepsy: A Comprehensive Textbook*, pp 1877–1890. Philadelphia: Lippincott-Raven.

Morrell F, Hanbery JW (1969) A new surgical technique for the treatment of focal cortical epilepsy. *Electroencephalography and Clinical Neurophysiology* **26**:120.

Morrell F, Whisler WW (1996) Multiple subpial transection. In: Shorvon S, Dreifuss FE, Fish D, Thomas DG (eds) *The Treatment of Epilepsy*, pp 739–751. Oxford: Blackwell Science.

Morrell F, Tsuru N, Hoeppner TJ, Morgan D, Harrison WH (1975) Secondary epiletogenesis in frog forebrain: effect of inhibition of protein synthesis. *Canadian Journal of Neurological Science* **2**:407–416.

Morrell F, Wada J, Engel J (1987) Appendix III: Potential relevance of kindling and secondary epileptogenesis to the consideration of surgical treatment for epilepsy. In Engel J (ed.) *Surgical Treatment of the Epilepsies*, pp 701–707. New York: Raven Press.

Morrell F, Whisler WW, Bleck TP (1989) Multiple subpial transection. A new approach to the surgical treatment of focal epilepsy. *Journal of Neurosurgery* 70:231–239.

Morrell F, Whisler WW, Smith MC (1991) Multiple subpial transection in Rasmussen's encephalitis. In: Andermann F (ed.) *Chronic Encephalitis and Epilepsy: Rasmussen's Syndrome*, pp 219–233. Boston: Butterworth-Heinemann.

Morrell F, Whisler WW, Smith MC *et al* (1995) Landau–Kleffner syndrome. Treatment with subpial intracortical transection. *Brain* 118:1529–1546.

Mountcastle VB (1957) Modality and topographic properties of single neurons of cat's somatic sensory cortex. *Journal of Neurophysiology* 20:408–434.

Mundinger F, Becker P, Grolkner E (1976) Late results of stereotactic surgery of epilepsy predominantly temporal lobe type. *Acta Neurochirugica* S23:177–182.

Murro AM, Flanigin HF, Gallagher BB, King DW, Smith JR (1988) Corpus callosotomy for the treatment of intractable epilepsy. *Epilepsy Research* 2:44–50.

Narabayashi H (1979) Long-range results of medial amygdalotomy on epileptic traits in adult patients. In: Rasmussen T, Marino R (eds) *Functional Neurosurgery*, pp 243–252. New York: Raven Press.

Narabayashi H, Shima F (1973) Which is the better amygdalar target, the medial or lateral nuclei? (For behavior problems and paroxysms in epileptics). In: Laitinen LV, Livingstone KE (ed.) *Surgical Approaches in Psychiatry*, pp 129–134. Lancaster: MTP.

Narabayashi H, Nagao T, Sato Y (1963) Stereotactic amygdalotomy for behavior disorder. *Archives of Neurology* 9:1–16.

Nordgren RE, Reeves AG, Viguera AC, Roberts DW (1991) Corpus callosotomy for intractable seizures in the pediatric age group. *Archives of Neurology* 48:364–372.

Oguni H, Olivier A, Andermann F, Comair J (1991) Anterior callosotomy in the treatment of medically intractable epilepsies: a study of 43 patients with a mean follow-up of 39 months. *Annals of Neurology* 30:357–364.

Ojemann GA, Ward AA (1975) Stereotactic and other procedures for epilepsy. In: Purpura DP, Penry JK, Walter RD (eds) *Neurosurgical Management of the Epilepsies*, pp 241–264. New York: Raven Press.

Olsnes K, Luczywek E, Mempel E (1976) Effect of amygdalectomy on memory and learning in patients treated surgically for epilepsy [Polish]. *Neurologia i Neurochirurgia Polska* 10:775–780.

Pallini R, Aglioti S, Tassinari G, Berlucchi G, Colosimo C, Rossi GF (1995) Callosotomy for intractable epilepsy from bihemispheric cortical dysplasias. *Acta Neurochirurgica* 132:79–86.

Palmini A, Andermann F, Aicardi J *et al* (1991) Diffuse cortical dysplasia, or the 'double cortex' syndrome: the clinical and epileptic spectrum in 10 patients. *Neurology* 41(10):1656–1662.

Papo I, Quattrini A, Provinciali L *et al* (1990) Callosotomy for the treatment of drug-resistant generalized seizures. *Acta Neurochirurgica Supplementum* 50:134–135.

Papo I, Quattrini A, Ortenzi A *et al* (1997) Predictive factors of callosotomy in drug-resistant epileptic patients with a long follow-up. *Journal of Neurosurgical Sciences* 41:31–36.

Patil AA, Andrews R, Torkelson R (1995) Stereotactic volumetric radiofrequency lesioning of intracranial structures for control of intractable seizures. *Stereotactic and Functional Neurosurgery* 64:123–133.

Patil AA, Andrews RV, Torkelson R (1997) Surgical treatment of intractable seizures with multilobar or bihemispheric seizure foci (MLBHSF). *Surgical Neurology* 47:72–77.

Pendl G, Grunert P, Graf M, Czech T (1990) Surgical treatment of epilepsy. *Neurochirurgia* 33(Suppl 1):27–29.

Penfield W, Jasper H (1954) *Epilepsy and the Functional Anatomy of the Human Brain*. Boston: Little, Brown.

Phillips J, Sakas DE (1996) Anterior callosotomy for intractable epilepsy: outcome in a series of 20 patients. *British Journal of Neurosurgery* 10:351–356.

Pinard JM, Delande Jambaque I, Chiron C, Plouin P, Dulac O (1991) Anterior and total callosotomy in epileptic children: prospective one-year follow-up study. *Epilepsia* 32 (Suppl 1):54.

Pressler R, Binnie CD, Polkey CE, Elwes RDC (1998) Return of generalized discharges and seizures after callosotomy. In: Stefan H, Andermann F, Shorvon S, Chauvel P (eds) *Plasticity and Epilepsy* pp 171–182. New York: Lippincott-Raven.

Purves SJ, Wada JA, Woodhurst WB *et al* (1988) Results of anterior corpus callosum section in 24 patients with medically intractable seizures. *Neurology* 38:1194–1201.

Quattrini A, Papo I, Cesarano R *et al* (1997a) EEG patterns after callosotomy. *Journal of Neurosurgical Sciences* 41:85–92.

Quattrini A, Del Pesce M, Provinciali L *et al* (1997b) Mutism in 36 patients who underwent callosotomy for drug-resistant epilepsy. *Journal of Neurosurgical Sciences* 41:93–96.

Ramani SV, Yap JC, Gumnit RJ (1980) Stereotactic fields of Forel interruption for intractable epilepsy. *Applied Neurophysiology* 43:104–108.

Reichental E, Hocherman S (1977) The critical cortical area for development of penicillin-induced epilepsy. *Electroencephalography and Clinical Neurophysiology* 42:248–251.

Reutens DC, Bye AM, Hopkins IJ *et al* (1993) Corpus callosotomy for intractable epilepsy: seizure outcome and prognostic factors. *Epilepsia* 34:904–909.

Ritter FJ, Gates JR, Maxwell RE, Jacobs MP (1989) Seizure outcome after corpus callosotomy in Lennox–Gastaut syndrome. *Epilepsia* 30:658.

Roberts DW (1995) Section of the corpus callosum for epilepsy. In: Schmidek HH, Sweet WH (eds) *Operative Neurosurgical Techniques. Indications, Methods, Results*, 3rd edn, pp 1351–1358. Philadelphia: WB Saunders.

Roberts DW (1997) Corpus callosotomy. In: Engel J, Pedley TA (eds) *Epilepsy: A Comprehensive Textbook*, pp 1851–1858. Philadelphia: Lippincott-Raven.

Rossi GF, Colicchio G, Marchese E, Pompucci A (1996) Callosotomy for severe epilepsies with generalized seizures: outcome and prognostic factors. *Acta Neurochirurgica* 138:221–227.

Rougier A, Sundstrom L, Claverie B *et al* (1996) Multiple subpial transection: report of seven cases. *Epilepsy Research* 24:57–63.

Sakaki T, Nakase H, Morimoto T, Hoshida T, Tsunoda S (1991) Partial corpus callosotomy beneficial for Lennox–Gastaut syndrome – report of two cases. *Neurol Med Chir Tokyo* 31:226–232.

Sakas DE, Phillips J (1996) Anterior callosotomy in the management of intractable epileptic seizures: significance of the extent of resection. *Acta Neurochirurgica* 138:700–707.

Sass KJ, Spencer SS, Spencer DD, Novelly RA, Williamson PD, Mattson RH (1988) Corpus callosotomy for epilepsy. II. Neurologic and neuropsychological outcome. *Neurology* 38:24–28.

Sawhney IM, Robertson IJ, Polkey CE, Binnie CD, Elwes RD (1995) Multiple subpial transection: a review of 21 cases. *Journal of Neurology, Neurosurgery and Psychiatry* 58(3):344–349.

Shimizu H, Suzuki I, Ishijima B, Karasawa S, Sakuma T (1991) Multiple subpial transection (MST) for the control of seizures that originated in unresectable cortical foci. *Japanese Journal of Psychiatry and Neurology* 2:354–356.

Small IF, Heimburger RF, Small JG, Milstein V, Moore DF (1977) Follow-up of stereotaxic amygdalotomy for seizure and behavior disorders. *Biological Psychiatry* 12:401–411.

Smith MC (1998) Multiple subpial transection in patients with extratemporal epilepsy. *Epilepsia* 39 (Suppl 4):S81–S89.

Sonnen AE, Manen JV, van Dijk B (1976) Results of amygdalotomy and fornicotomy in temporal lobe epilepsy and behavior disorders. *Acta Neurochirurgica* **S23**:215–219.

Sorenson JM, Wheless JW, Baumgartner JE *et al* (1997) Corpus callosotomy for medically intractable seizures. *Pediatric Neurosurgery* **27**:260–267.

Spencer DD (1987) Postscript: Should there be a surgical treatment of choice and if so how should it be determined? In: Engel J (ed.) *Surgical Treatment of the Epilepsies*, pp. 477–484. New York: Raven Press.

Spencer SS, Spencer DD (1991) Corpus callosotomy in chronic encephalitis. In: Andermann F (ed) *Chronic Encephalitis and Epilpesy: Rasmussen's Syndrome*, 19th edn, pp 213–218. Boston: Butterworth-Heinemann.

Spencer SS, Spencer DD, Williamson PD, Sass K, Novelly RA, Mattson RH (1988) Corpus callosotomy for epilepsy. I. Seizure effects. *Neurology* **38**:19–24.

Spencer SS, Spencer DD, Sass K, Westerveld M, Katz A, Mattson R (1993) Anterior, total, and two-stage corpus callosum section: differential and incremental seizure responses. *Epilepsia* **34**:561–567.

Sperry RW, Miner N (1955) Pattern perception following insertion of mica plates into the visual cortex. *Journal of Comp Physiology and Psychology* **48**:463–469.

Sperry RW, Miner N, Myers RE (1955) Visual pattern perception following subpial slicing and tantalum wire implantations in visual cortex. *Journal of Comp Physiology Psychology* **48**:50–58.

Talairach J, Bancaud J (1974) Approche nouvelle de la neurochirugie de l'epilepsie. *Neurochirugie* **20** (Suppl 1):205–213.

Tien RD, Ashdown BC, Lewis DVJ, Atkins MR, Burger PC (1992) Rasmussenen's encephalitis: neuroimaging findings in four patients. *American Journal of Roentgenology* **158**:1329–1332.

Turmel A, Giard N, Bouvier G *et al* (1992) Frontal lobe seizures and epilepsy: indications for corticectomies or callosotomy. *Advances in Neurology* **57**:689–706.

Van Harskamp F, Van Dongen HR, Loonen MCB (1978) Acquired aphasia with convulsive disorder in children: a case study with a seven-year follow-up. *Brain Lang* **6**:141–148.

Vaernet K (1972) Stereotaxic amygdalotomy in temporal lobe epilepsy. *Confinia Neurologica* **34**:176–180.

Van Wagenen WP, Herren RY (1940) Surgical division of commissural pathways in the corpus callosum. *Archives of Neurology and Psychiatry* **44**:740–759.

Williams BA, Abbott KJ, Manson JI (1992) Cerebral tumors in children presenting with epilepsy. *Journal of Child Neurology* **7**:291–294.

Wilson DH, Reeves A, Gazzaniga M, Culver C (1977) Cerebral commissurotomy for control of intractable seizures. *Neurology* **27**:708–715.

Wilson DH, Reeves AG, Gazzaniga M (1982) 'Central' commissurotomy for intractable generalized: series two. *Neurology* **32**:687–697.

Yang TF, Wong TT, Kwan SY, Chang KP, Lee YC, Hsu TC (1996) Quality of life and life satisfaction in families after a child has undergone corpus callosotomy. *Epilepsia* **37**:76–80.

Yoshii N (1977) Follow-up study of epileptic patients following forel-H-tomy. *Applied Neurophysiology* **40**:1–12.

Brain stimulation for epilepsy

CE POLKEY

The notion that brain stimulation could improve cerebral malfunction is well recognized, and such techniques have been applied to the treatment of chronic pain and movement disorder in the past. A great deal has been learned from such applications about the technical aspects of this treatment and also about the place of patient selection and the inherent difficulties of stimulation. As is the case with its use for the treatment of pain and movement disorder, the anatomic and neurophysiologic background of such treatment relies upon observations made from the effects of lesioning in the brain, a matter that is dealt with in more detail in Chapter 59.

Of the three areas where stimulation has been used, the underlying anatomic and pathophysiologic substrates are probably least understood in epilepsy, as was pointed out by Bancaud in 1974 (Talairach and Bancaud 1974):

> L'idée qui sans doute animee la plupart des opérateurs est celle de réaliser dans l'épilepsie une intervention prenant sons modèle dans la chirugie dede la maladie de Parkinson. L'espoir est de perturber à un endroit précis un système fonctionnel sous-cortical qui jouerait un rôle essentiel dans l'initiation et surtout la propagation (ou la généralisation) des décharges critiques.

Without doubt most surgeons are driven by the idea that they can perform an intervention in epilepsy modeled upon the surgical treatment of Parkinson disease. It is hoped that the functional subcortical system, which plays an essential role in the initiation, and above all the propagation (or generalization) of the crucial discharges, could be disrupted by intervention at a precise point.

Furthermore, it is becoming clear that investigating the influence of such stimulation in the human subject is not at all easy. In some circumstances the stimulator could not be activated when tests could be made, such as using MRI scanning, specifically functional MRI (fMRI). In others, such as PET, repeated testing has radiation exposure implications; and in yet others, such as magnetic source imaging or EEG dipole modeling, the validation of the methods is not universally accepted. To this must be added the undoubted observation that the effect of stimulation on epilepsy may improve with time, so that repeated testing may be necessary to detect an effect.

The difficulties of running double-blind controlled trials of such stimulation are immediately apparent. If the stimulation has side-effects, as is the case with vagus nerve stimulation, then the patient will know when the stimulus is being applied. This is a particular anxiety to governmental agencies who wish to obtain evidence about the cost-effectiveness of these treatments.

The debate over lesioning versus stimulation has not been conducted vigorously in the same way as that over the surgical treatment of Parkinson disease because the procedures do not have equivalence in epilepsy surgery. However, it is still valid to rehearse some of these arguments. Lesioning produces a permanent change in the brain, and if this is ineffective then the lesion has to be enlarged or another lesion produced elsewhere. Because making a lesion involves destruction of brain tissue, there is a small but significant risk of neurologic or other consequences from hemorrhage or mislocation. In treating Parkinson disease, it is clear that bilateral lesions may produce speech and cognitive difficulties apart from the unilateral effects of each lesion. On the other hand lesioning involves a small number of procedures with a definite end point. Stimulation, by contrast, is a potentially reversible treatment whose effects can be reversed if they are ineffective or undesirable. Furthermore, if the patient's circumstances change, then the locus and parameters of stimulus can be changed. However, placement and setting up of stimulation is more complex and may require a considerable degree of continuous supervision. The devices themselves are relatively expensive and failure of various components may cause additional surgery and expense, especially if the patient lives at some distance from the center. Most devices are made by commercial enterprises and failure of the components is rare, but other factors such as disconnection, migration of the electrodes, infection, or wound hematomas can occur. At present they are battery-driven and the generators require replacement every 3–5 years. Responsibility for the device, and the anxiety it engenders, may not be acceptable to some patients or their carers.

At present there are three main scenarios for the use of stimulation in epilepsy: stimulation of the left vagus nerve, of the centromedian nucleus of the thalamus, and last the cerebellum, although the last has now been discredited.

GENERAL THEORETIC PRINCIPLES

There are a number of points for discussion. The first is the mechanism of stimulation and its local effects. Of particular concern is whether certain modes would cause local tissue destruction. There is no good evidence from experience with stimulators used in other circumstances that the electrodes cause any problems other than those due to the original implantation. In theory, microelectrolytic lesions could occur at the site of stimulation, but there is little evidence in the literature, either from therapeutic stimulation or when depth electrodes are used for stimulation, that such changes are of importance. Work on vagus nerve stimulation has shown that both in experimental animals and in humans there is probably a permanent change in the nervous system, possibly of a neurochemical nature, as a result of the chronic stimulation (Ben-Menachem 1996; Woodbury and Woodbury 1990). It has also been demonstrated that changes in the nerve to which the electrode has been applied are related more to the mechanical stresses

rather than to the electrolytic effects of the chronic stimulation (Agnew and McCreery 1990).

Another concern is whether stimulation, especially deep brain stimulation, will induce epilepsy. Because of the known effect of kindling (Goddard et al 1969), this has to be a very reasonable suspicion. However, it is also known that the epileptogenic properties of kindling depend upon a number of conditions that are probably rare in humans. First, the site of stimulation usually favored in experimental situations is the hippocampus, which is known to be more epileptogenic than other regions of the brain. Secondly, there is a clear phylogenetic influence on the occurrence of kindling, which can be produced more certainly and more quickly the lower the animal is on the phylogenetic scale. Thirdly, the stimulus parameters are adjusted to produce afterdischarges in a nervous system that is ostensibly normal. There is no experimental work on inhibiting stimulation. There is little clinical evidence for the occurrence of kindling in patients subjected to stimulation for other reasons such as chronic pain. There is, for example, an account of a seizure occurring 1 month after implantation of deep brain electrodes in the pallidum for Parkinson's disease (Galvez-Jimenez et al 1998). However there are a number of other possible reasons for such a seizure and persistent seizures from deep brain stimulating electrodes appear to be very rare. Transcranial magnetic stimulation of the brain has been applied to patients with epilepsy. Conflicting accounts of the effect exist; thus one group describes no effect on electrophysiologic recordings, including recordings from foramen ovale electrodes (Steinhoff et al 1993), whereas another group describes seizure provocation by such stimulation, dependent upon the stimulation interval (Chen et al 1997). The theoretic basis on which current stimulation programs is based varies and therefore will be described with each method.

Although the treatments are best described separately, the techniques have some features in common, especially with regard to technical problems and the complications of implantation. All of the systems are of virtually the same kind, with electrodes implanted at the appropriate site and then connected subcutaneously to a generator device that is usually battery-driven. Communication with the device is usually by means of a radio link and there is also usually a simple means of adjustment, available to the patient using a magnet. The principal complication of implantation is infection. It is associated with the usual factors, which include hemorrhage into the wounds, length of surgery, and noncompliance of patients. Antibiotic cover at the time of surgery is advisable; once infection occurs attempts can be made to treat it conservatively with culture of the wound and appropriate antibiotics. However, this will often not succeed unless the device, which is foreign material, is removed.

CEREBELLAR STIMULATION

The original inspiration for Cooper's proposal of cerebellar stimulation was Snider's observations that stimulation of the cerebellum could modify the EEG in experimental models of epilepsy (Cooke and Snider 1955). However, although a number of similar observations suggested that cerebellar stimulation, both of the cortical surface and of the deep nuclei, could decrease or abolish seizures or seizure activity in these animal models, there were other reports suggesting that such stimulation was ineffective. This matter has recently been reviewed by Fisher (Fisher *et al* 1997). Consideration also has to be given to the fact that in many patients with epilepsy there may be changes in the cerebellum, and especially in the Purkinje cell population, because of previous anticonvulsant treatment. In truth, the varying effects of stimulation on the structures in the cerebellum and the possible changes in effect produced by varying the frequency and other stimulation parameters are complex and have not been sufficiently explored to exclude a rational explanation for the observed effects.

INDICATIONS

As originally applied by Irving Cooper, the indications were both partial complex seizures and generalized seizures. Some of his patients had a warning, and the system was so designed that the patient could interpolate an additional stimulus. Subsequently, the technique has been applied by a number of groups to similar patients. Many of these patients had multifocal EEG abnormalities and by the neuroimaging tests available were free of focal structural abnormality specific neurophysiologic indications.

TECHNIQUE

The electrodes consisted of plastic strip electrodes with four contacts and one of each was laid on the superior surface of the cerebellum. A small posterior fossa craniectomy was made and the electrodes were inserted through small incisions in the dura and then connected to an appropriate driving apparatus. The stimuli were delivered, in Cooper's series, to both electrodes simultaneously but for periods of 10 seconds on and 10 seconds off. The frequency of the pulse trains was 10 Hz with a voltage of 10 V, giving currents of 1–3 mA, each pulse having a duration of 1 ms. The

other substantial series, described in the literature by Davis and colleagues, employed frequencies between 0 and 30 Hz. They were very particular about the current, believing that the correct charge density was crucial to determining the appropriate effect, suggesting that it should be between 0.7 and 1.6 μC cm^{-2} per phase (Davis and Gray 1980).

COMPLICATIONS

The literature regarding complications is not very forthcoming. Clearly, some patients succumbed to seizures, especially when the treatment was not particularly effective. Davis states that CSF leaks were often seen but does not say how frequent they were. Technical problems with the apparatus were not uncommon, as might be expected at that stage in the development of the technology, and included lead fracture. Hematomas in the posterior fossa were also seen, and this was the cause of death in one of Cooper's patients; another is reported as occurring spontaneously 5 years after implantation of the electrode array (Zuccarello *et al* 1986). It is also clear from various accounts in the literature that the electrodes become surrounded by an area of gliosis after implantation, although Davis states that this only occurred to two of their electrodes because of their design. He also produces evidence from his own series and the descriptions of others to indicate that when there is a high current density, either as a consequence of therapy or for some other reason, there may be considerable damage (Fisher *et al* 1993). Infection was clearly a problem, Davis, describing 318 patients implanted with cerebellar stimulators, mostly for spasticity, report infection in 4.4%. In half, the infecting organism was *Staphylococcus aureus* and the infection became apparent within 1 month of surgery; infection by *S. epidermidis* could occur up to 2 years after implantation. In 12 of the 14 patients affected, the system was removed completely and the infection resolved. In the remaining two patients the cerebellar electrodes were left in place, but in one patient they had to be removed to obtain resolution of the infection (Davis *et al* 1982).

OUTCOME

The results of cerebellar stimulation in regard to seizure control are in dispute. As summarized by Fisher, there are 11 reports in the literature of uncontrolled series in which some 25% are rendered seizure-free and a further 50% are improved in that their seizure frequency is reduced by more than half, leaving about one-quarter unaffected (Fisher *et al* 1997). However, there are only two controlled series in the literature, one comprising five patients described by Van

Buren and a further nine patients described by Wright (Van Buren *et al* 1978; Wright *et al* 1985). In neither of these series was convincing benefit derived from stimulation.

CONCLUSION

Fisher concludes, because of the larger number of patients who may have benefited from this treatment and the small number in whom controlled trials have been conducted, that the question whether cerebellar stimulation for epilepsy is useful still has to be resolved by proper double-blind controlled trials (Fisher *et al* 1997).

STIMULATION OF THE CAUDATE NUCLEUS AND THALAMUS

There is some evidence from experimental models of epilepsy that low-frequency stimulation of the caudate nucleus can produce changes that might have therapeutic value. Reports document modulation of cerebellar activity in the cat (Hablitz and Wray 1977) and inhibition of a rhinencephalic focus (Mutani 1969), but complex results were obtained in another instance where both continuous and alternating stimuli were used to modulate a focus on the motor cortex of a monkey (Oakley and Ojemann 1982).

The evidence in respect of the thalamic nuclei is more robust. Dempsey and Morison described the recruiting response resulting from low-frequency stimulation of the nonspecific nuclei of the thalamus (Dempsey and Morison 1942). Desynchronization of the EEG can be produced by high-frequency stimulation of these structures and seizures have been terminated in a primate model by thalamic stimulation (Monnier *et al* 1960; Wilder and Schmidt 1965). Penfield and Jasper proposed the idea of centrencephalic epilepsy involving the same structures (Penfield and Jasper 1954). In other circumstances, stimulation of the thalamic nuclei can produce seizures. Mirski and colleagues have suggested a circuit involving the posterior hypothalamus and the anterior thalamic nuclei (Mirski and Fisher 1994).

INDICATIONS

Stimulation of these deep nuclei has been used in an empirical fashion for several different groups of patients. Sramka and Chkhenkeli had described the use of low-frequency stimulation of the caudate nucleus, but their patient population is not clear. The same group have described the use of caudate stimulation in status epilepticus (Chkhenkeli 1978;

Chkhenkeli and Sramka 1989). Cooper also described the use of electrodes in the anterior thalamus in patients with multiple seizure types (Cooper and Upton 1985; Cooper *et al* 1980). However, the major work in this area has been carried out by Velasco and Velasco. They have applied the technique to patients with generalized seizures (Velasco *et al* 1995) as well as patients with partial and motor seizures (Velasco *et al* 1989). Subsequently, they have reported patients with Lennox–Gastaut syndrome (Velasco *et al* 1993a). In 1993 they summarized their experience with 23 patients whose main seizure types were generalized tonic–clonic seizures (9 cases), partial motor seizures (3 cases), complex partial seizures (5 cases) and tonic–clonic seizures associated with the Lennox–Gastaut syndrome (6 cases) (Velasco *et al* 1993b). Fisher and colleagues then carried out a pilot controlled trial of thalamic stimulation for which they selected seven patients, six of whom had generalized seizures. In both the Velasco and the Fisher series the aim was to apply stimulation for 3 months and then assess the patients over a poststimulation period for persistent effects on seizure control.

TECHNIQUE

Both the Russian experience and that of the Velasco brothers involved attempts to identify areas that might respond to stimulation by using chronic depth recording. It was an important feature of the patients treated in Mexico City that the stimulation locus was partly determined by the ability to obtain a recruiting response at low frequency (6 Hz) and desynchronization of the EEG at higher frequency (60 Hz) (Velasco *et al* 1993b). Stimulation alternated between left and right electrodes in a 1-minute train with a 4-minute interval between them. These stimuli were applied for 2 hours each day for 3 months. In the Fisher series, the stimulation frequency was higher at 65 Hz and the individual square waves were briefer, lasting only 0.1 ms compared with 1 ms in the Velasco series. The stereotactic techniques employed by the two groups were different; in the Velasco series stereotactic location was by using pneumoencephalography, whereas in the Fisher series CT and MRI were used. There are number of other reasons for believing that the site and nature of the stimulus were different between the two series, as explained by Velasco in 1993 (Velasco *et al* 1993b).

COMPLICATIONS

Both Velasco and Fisher admit that the complications were infrequent and minor. In the Velasco series, there was one patient who sustained a scalp hematoma and another in whom there was transient swelling of the internal capsule due to mislocation of an electrode. There were three other instances of mislocation of electrodes and seven instances of external failure of leads and generators. In the Fisher group of patients, there was one patient who had a generator failure and another with an asymptomatic hematoma adjacent to one of the depth electrodes (Fisher *et al* 1992).

OUTCOME

In respect of the caudate nucleus stimulation, the results of Chkhenkeli and his colleagues are relatively inaccessible but they describe good results from low-frequency stimulation of the caudate nucleus alone or in combination with other structures.

The outcome in the Velasco series is much clearer. Looking at their four different groups of patients, those with partial motor seizures (group B, Rasmussen's type) and those with generalized tonic-clonic seizures (group D, LGS type) showed improvement (Velasco *et al* 1993b). A subsequent analysis also suggested that generalized tonic-clonic seizures, independent of Lennox-Gastaut syndrome, also responded well and were accompanied by a decrease in interictal paroxysmal discharges (Velasco *et al* 1995). They were also able to demonstrate significant improvements in cognitive function and background EEG waveforms in three of their four groups (Velasco *et al* 1993c). In contrast, the Fisher study showed no benefit to seizure control but also suggested that the treatment caused no gross deterioration.

CONCLUSION

The conclusion has to be that expressed by Fisher that further work is needed before this procedure can be either validated or abandoned (Fisher *et al* 1992).

VAGUS NERVE STIMULATION

The theoretic basis of vagus nerve stimulation is complex and incompletely understood and rests upon a number of premises. The first is the anatomic premise that the afferent inputs from the vagus nerve have a very wide distribution both directly and indirectly through the nucleus solitarus that projects to the hypothalamus, amygdala, thalamus, and insular cortex, all of which are sites involved in epilepsy.

The second factor is the effect of stimulation of these vagal afferents. Clearly, this effect is related to the frequency and intensity of stimulation, which will determine which fibers in the nerve are affected by the stimulus. It has been shown that stimulation of the vagus nerve in experimental models can produce evoked potentials in various parts of the central nervous system; the evidence has been reviewed in detail by Rutki (1990).

The third observation is that vagus nerve stimulation can produce changes in the EEG. Thus, stimulation of the nerve in a cat model can produce EEG desynchronization and block sleep spindles in the slow wave sleep (Zanchetti *et al* 1952). Stimulation of the nucleus solitarius will produce synchronous EEG discharges at low frequency (1–16 Hz) and desynchronization at high frequency (> 30 Hz) (Magnes *et al* 1961). A number of experiments by Chase and colleagues have suggested that adjusting the stimulus parameters, which will determine whether myelinated or unmyelinated fibres are stimulated, can produce different effects on the EEG. Desynchronization was produced by fibers that conduct at <15 ms^{-1} (Chase *et al* 1966, 1967; Chase and Nakamura 1968). Stimulation of both the vagus nerve and the nucleus solitarius can produce slow-wave sleep (Puizillout and Foutz 1976; Piuzillout 1986). Recent observations have also shown that the effects of vagus nerve stimulation on epilepsy are dependent upon the integrity of the locus cæruleus (Krahl *et al* 1998). There is no detectable effect on the EEG in humans from clinical vagus nerve stimulation (Salinsky and Burchiel 1993).

The fourth observation is that in experimental models of epilepsy, such as those using strychnine spikes, the spikes can be affected by vagus nerve stimulation, being suppressed or enhanced depending upon the stimulus characters (Stoica and Tudor 1967, 1968). The work that immediately preceded the clinical application of vagus nerve stimulation was carried out by Woodbury and by Zabara. These workers showed that in various experimental models vagus nerve stimulation would suppress experimentally induced seizures (Woodbury and Woodbury 1990). It has also been shown that pretreatment with vagus nerve stimulation can suppress seizures provoked with pentylenetetrazol. Recent work using rat models has shown that there is a persistent anticonvulsant effect from vagus nerve stimulation dependent upon the cumulative duration of the stimulus (Takaya *et al* 1996). Details of seminal studies in rats have been reviewed by Woodbury and Woodbury (Woodbury and Woodbury 1990), and in monkeys by Lockard *et al* (1990).

A number of animal studies have shown a metabolic effect for vagus nerve stimulation. Thus, the expression of *fos*, which is an indicator of neuronal activity, is increased in the limbic structures by stimulation of the vagus (Naritoku *et al* 1995). Studies of 2-deoxyglucose have shown a

excluded from the random trials. The early reports of this treatment were encouraging (Penry and Dean 1990; Trenerry *et al* 1993; Uthman *et al* 1993; Ben-Menachem *et al* 1994) and the first random controlled trial (E03) was published in 1995. This comprised 114 patients allocated to low- and high-stimulus paradigms using a standard cycle of trains of stimuli lasting 30 seconds at 30 Hz with an interstimulus interval of 5 minutes. After a 12-week baseline, the stimulus was applied for 14 weeks, including an initial period during which the stimulus was ramped up to the appropriate value. The reduction in seizure frequency was 24.5% for the high-stimulation group and 6.1% for the low-stimulation group ($P = 0.01$). A second trial (E05) was reported in 1998 involving 196 patients, and here there was a 28% reduction for the high-stimulation group and a 15% reduction for the low-stimulation group ($P = 0.04$) when the groups were compared. When the groups were compared with their baseline performance, both high- and low-stimulation groups achieved a significant result ($P = 0.0001$) (Handforth *et al* 1998). Salinsky *et al* reported results from an open-extension trial of 100 patients from the E03 study and noted that those patients who had a good response in the first 3 months maintained that response to 12 months, whereas those patients who did not respond at first remained unresponsive at 12 months (Salinsky *et al* 1996). In an abstract summarizing the outcome from 454 patients in all five trials, data were available for 440 patients and 96.7% had continued treatment to 1 year, 84.7% to 2 years, and 71.2% to 3 years. The median percentage seizure relief was 35% at 1 year, 43.3% at 2 years, and 44.1% at 3 years (Morris and Pallagi 1998). Although rapid cycling is used by many groups, especially in children, and benefits some patients, there is no clear indication at present as to which patients do better with this variation of the treatment.

The treatment has also been applied to children, and Hornig *et al* reported the results from 19 children in 1997 (Hornig *et al* 1997) and have recently updated this to the results from 60 children in an abstract in 1998 (Hornig and Murphy 1998). Follow-up to 18 months was available for at least 49 of these patients. The continuation rate was 95%. The predominant seizure type was complex partial seizures in 57% and generalized tonic–clonic seizures in 27%. A mean reduction in seizure frequency of 23% was noted at 3 months and the equivalent figures at 6, 12, and 18 months were 31%, 34%, and 42%, respectively. Although benefits have been reported in both children and adults with Lennox–Gastaut syndrome the original speculation by Hornig *et al* that they did better than other groups with vagus nerve stimulation is probably unfounded. In our own small series of children with epileptic encephalopathy followed up for 2 years, there was an improvement in seizure control in only 4 patients at 12 months after implantation. However at 2 years after implantation the results have been encouraging; the overall median percentage reduction in seizure frequency was 43% ($P = 0.02$) (Parker *et al* 1999). A group of 16 children was also reported by Lundgren *et al* from Lund in Sweden. Eight of the children had partial complex seizures and the remaining 8 had generalized seizures; 4 of these patients had Lennox–Gastaut syndrome. Six of these 16 children had a greater than 50% reduction in their seizure frequency and one was seizure-free. The seizure severity score also decreased and 6 children had a 50% or more improvement in their quality of life. Improvements in each of these three areas did not necessarily coincide (Lundgren *et al* 1998a).

Other benefits have been reported from vagus nerve stimulation. In the second randomized controlled trial reported by Handforth there were improvements in global evaluation scores that were statistically significant (Handforth *et al* 1998). In the 12 children reported by Hornig *et al* there were improvements in global rating scores in 11 of the children, although it has to be admitted that these scores were compiled by the families (Murphy *et al* 1995). Changes in cognitive performance have not been documented. Most papers report no change in the anticonvulsant regime of most patients.

CONCLUSION

Vagus nerve stimulation has a place in the treatment of drug-resistant epilepsy even though the precise indications for its use, and the mechanism of its action, still require considerable elucidation.

KEY POINTS

1. Direct or indirect stimulation of the nervous system is a potential method for the treatment of chronic drug-resistant epilepsy.

2. Stimulation is better than lesioning because it is adjustable and reversible. Stimulation is worse than lesioning in that it requires more supervision, expensive hardware, and is therefore more expensive.

3. Cerebellar stimulation is of unproven value.

4. Thalamic stimulation is probably of value, but at present requires more evaluation and in particular a properly organized, controlled trial.

5. Vagus nerve stimulation has proved to be effective in a variety of epileptic syndromes. More information is needed about its underlying mechanism and its effectiveness in various epileptic syndromes.

REFERENCES

Agnew WF, McCreery DB (1990) Considerations for safety with chronically implanted nerve electrodes. *Epilepsia* **31**:S27–S32.

Anonymous (1995) A randomized controlled trial of chronic vagus nerve stimulation for treatment of medically intractable seizures. The Vagus Nerve Stimulation Study Group. *Neurology* **45**:224–230.

Asconape JJ, Moore DD, Zipes DD, Hartman LM (1998) Early experience with vagus nerve stimulation for the treatment of epilepsy: cardiac complications. *Epilepsia* **39**(Suppl 6):193.

Ben-Menachem E (1996) Modern management of epilepsy: Vagus nerve stimulation. *Baillière's Clinical Neurology* **5**(4):841–848.

Ben-Menachem E, Manon-Espaillat R, Ristanovic R *et al* (1994) Vagus nerve stimulation for treatment of partial seizures: 1. A controlled study of effect on seizures. First International Vagus Nerve Stimulation Study Group. *Epilepsia* **35**:616–626.

Ben-Menachem E, Hamberger A, Hedner T *et al* (1995) Effects of vagus nerve stimulation on amino acids and other metabolities in the CSF of patients with partial seizures. *Epilepsy Research* **20**:221–227.

Chase MH, Sterman MB, Clemente CD (1966) Cortical and subcortical patterns of response to afferent vagal stimulation. *Experimental Neurology* **16**:36–49.

Chase MH, Nakamura Y, Clemente CD (1967) Afferent vagal nerve stimulation: neurographic correlates of induced EEG synchronisation and desynchronisation. *Brain Research* **5**:236–249.

Chase MH, Nakamura Y (1968) Cortical and subcortical EEG patterns of response to afferent abdominal vagal stimulation; neurographic correlates. *Physiology and Behaviour* **3**:605–610.

Chen R, Gerloff C, Classen J, Wassermann EM, Hallett M, Cohen LG (1997) Safety of different inter-train intervals for repetitive transcranial magnetic stimulation and recommendations for safe ranges of stimulation parameters. *Electroencephalography and Clinical Neurophysiology: Electromyography and Motor Control* **105**:415–421.

Chkhenkeli SA (1978) Inhibitory influences of caudate stimulation on the epileptic activity of human amygdala and hippocampus during temporal lobe epilepsy. *Physiology Human and Animal* **4**:406–411.

Chkhenkeli SA, Sramka M (1989) Therapeutic stimulation of the non-specific thalamic system for the treatment of some forms of epilepsy [Abstract]. *IXth Congress of Neurological Surgery, Delhi*.

Cooke PM, Snider RS (1995) Some cerebellar influences on electrically-induced seizures cerebral seizures. *Epilepsia* **4**:19–28.

Cooper IS, Upton AR (1985) Therapeutic implications of modulation of metabolism and functional activity of cerebral cortex by chronic stimulation of the cerebellum and thalamus. *Biological Psychiatry* **20**:811–813.

Cooper IS, Upton AR, Amin I (1980) Reversibility of chronic neurologic deficits. Some effects of electrical stimulation of the thalamus and internal capsule in man. *Applied Neurophysiology* **43**:244–258.

Davis R, Gray EF (1980) Technical problems and advances in the cerebellar-stimulating systems used for reduction of spasticity and seizures. *Applied Neurophysiology* **43**:230–243.

Davis R, Kudzman J, Ratzan K (1982) Management of infected cerebellar stimulation systems. *Neurosurgery* **10**:340–343.

Dempsey EW, Morison RS (1942) The production of rhythmically recurrent cortical potentials after localised thalamic stimulation. *American Journal of Physiology* **135**:293–300.

Easton A, Walker B, Gale K (1996) Influence of activity in nucleus tractus solitarus (NTS) on seizure manifestations [Abstract]. *Epilepsia* **37** (Suppl 5):68.

Espinosa JA, Aiello M, Naritoku DK (1998) Revision and removal of stimulating electrodes after long-term therapy with vagus nerve stimulation. *Epilepsia* **39** (Suppl 6):192.

Fisher RS, Uematsu S, Krauss GL *et al* (1992) Placebo-controlled pilot study of centromedian thalamic stimulation in treatment of intractable seizures. *Epilepsia* **33**:841–851.

Fisher RS, Uthman BM, Ramsay RE *et al* (1993) Alternative surgical techniques for epilepsy. In: Engel J (ed) *Surgical Treatment of the Epilepsies*, 2nd edn, pp 549–564. New York: Raven Press.

Fisher RS, Mirski M, Krauss GL (1997) Brain stimulation In: Engel JJ, Pedley TA (eds) *Epilepsy: A Comprehensive Textbook*, pp 1867–1875. Philadelphia: Lippincott-Raven.

Galvez-Jimenez N, Lozano A, Tasker R, Duff J, Hutchison W, Lang AE (1998) Pallidal stimulation in Parkinson's disease patients with a prior unilateral pallidotomy. *Canadian Journal of Neurological Sciences* **25**:300–305.

Goddard GV, McIntyre DC, Leech CK (1969) A permanent change in brain function resulting from daily electrical stimulation. *Experimental Neurology* **25**:295–330.

Hablitz JJ, Wray DV (1977) Modulation of cerebellar electrical and unit activity by low-frequency stimulation of the caudate nucleus in chronic cats. *Experimental Neurology* **55**:289–294.

Handforth A, DeGiorgio CM, Schachter SC *et al* (1998) Vagus nerve stimulation therapy for partial-onset seizures: a randomized active-control trial. *Neurology* **51**:48–55.

Henry TR, Bakay RA, Votaw JR *et al* (1998) Brain blood flow alterations induced by therapeutic vagus nerve stimulation in partial epilepsy: I. Acute effects at high and low levels of stimulation. *Epilepsia* **39**:983–990.

Hornig G, Murphy JV (1998) Vagal nerve stimulation: Updated experience in 60 pediatric patients [Abstract]. *Epilepsia* **39**(Suppl 6):169.

Hornig GW, Murphy JV, Schallert G, Tilton C (1997) Left vagus nerve stimulation in children with refractory epilepsy: an update. *Southern Medical Journal* **90**:484–488.

Ko D, Heck C, Grafton S *et al* (1996) Vagus nerve stimulation activates central nervous system structures in epileptic patients during PET H2(15)O blood flow imaging [see comments]. *Neurosurgery* **39**:426–430; discussion 430–431.

Krahl SE, Clark KB, Smith DC, Browning RA (1998) Locus coeruleus lesions suppress the seizure-attenuating effects of vagus nerve stimulation. *Epilepsia* **39**:709–714.

Leijten FS, van Rijen PC (1998) Stimulation of the phrenic nerve as a complication of vagus nerve pacing in a patient with epilepsy. *Neurology* **51**:1224–1225.

Liu M, Schellenberg AG, Patterson T, Bigelow DC, Stecker MM (1998) Intraoperative bronchospasm induced by stimulation of the vagus nerve. *Anesthesiology* **88**:1675–1677.

Lockard JS, Congdon WC, DuCharme LL (1990) Feasibility and safety of vagal nerve stimulation in monkey model. *Epilepsia* **31**:S20–S26.

Lundgren J, Amark P, Blennow G, Stromblad LG, Wallstedt L (1998a) Vagus nerve stimulation in 16 children with refractory epilepsy. *Epilepsia* **39**:809–813.

Lundgren J, Ekberg O, Olsson R (1998b) Aspiration: a potential complication to vagus nerve stimulation. *Epilepsia* **39**:998–1000.

Magnes J, Morruzzi G, Pompeiano O (1961) Synchronisation of the EEG produced by low frequency electrical stimulation in the region of the solitary tract. *Archives Italiennes de Biologie* **99**:33–67.

Mirski M, Fisher RS (1994) Electrical stimulation of the mamillary nuclei increases seizure threshold to pentylenetetrazol. *Epilepsia* **35**:1309–1316.

Monnier M, Kalberer M, Krupp P (1960) Functional antagonism between diffuse reticular and intralaminary recruiting projections in the medial thalamus. *Experimental Neurology* **2**:271–289.

Morris G, Pallagi J (1998) Long-term follow-up of 454 patients with epilepsy receiving vagus nerve stimulation [Abstract]. *Epilepsia* **39** (Suppl 6):93.

Murphy JV, Hornig G, Schallert G (1995) Left vagal nerve stimulation in children with refractory epilepsy. Preliminary observations. *Archives of Neurology* **52**:886–889.

Mutani R (1969) Experimental evidence for the existence of an extrarhinencephalic control of the activity of the cobalt rhinencephalic epiletogenic focus. Part 1. The role played by the caudate nucleus. *Epilepsia* **10**:337–350.

Naritoku DK, Terry WJ, Helfert RH (1995) Regional induction of fos immunoreactivity in the brain by anticonvulsant stimulation of the vagus nerve. *Epilepsy Research* **22**:53–62.

Oakley JC, Ojemann GA (1982) Effects of chronic stimulation of the caudate nucleus on a prexisting alumina seizure focus. *Experimental Neurology* **75**:360–367.

Parker APJ, Polkey CE, Binnie CDB, Madigon C, Ferrie CD, Robinson RO (1999) Vagal nerve stimulation in epileptic encephalopathies. *Pediatrics* (in press).

Penfield W, Jasper H (1954) *Epilepsy and the Functional Anatomy of the Human Brain*. Boston: Little Brown.

Penry JK, Dean C (1990) Prevention of intractable partial seizures by intermittent vagal stimulation in humans: Preliminary results. *Epilepsia* **31**:40–43.

Puizillout JJ (1986) Noyeau du fasiceau solitaire, serotonine et regulation de vigilance. *Revue Electroencephalogrie et de Neurophysiologie Clinique* **16**:95–106.

Puizillout JJ, Foutz AS (1976) Vago-aortic nerves stimulation and REM sleep: evidence for a REM triggering and REM maintenance factor. *Brain Research* **111**:181–184.

Ramsay RE, Uthman BM, Augustinsson LE *et al* (1994) Vagus nerve stimulation for treatment of partial seizures: 2. Safety, side effects, and tolerability. First International Vagus Nerve Stimulation Study Group. *Epilepsia* **35**:627–636.

Rutki P (1990) Anatomical, physiological and theoretical basis for the antiepileptic effect of vagus nerve stimulation. *Epilepsia* **31**:1–6.

Salinsky MC, Burchiel KJ (1993) Vagus nerve stimulation has no effect on awake EEG rhythms in humans. *Epilepsia* **34**:299–304.

Salinsky MC, Uthman BM, Ristanovic RK, Wernicke JF, Tarver WB (1996) Vagus nerve stimulation for the treatment of medically intractable seizures. Results of a 1-year open-extension trial. Vagus Nerve Stimulation Study Group. *Archives of Neurology* **53**:1176–1180.

Steinhoff BJ, Stodieck SR, Zivcec Z, *et al* (1993) Transcranial magnetic stimulation (TMS) of the brain in patients with mesiotemporal epileptic foci. *Clinical Electroencephalography* **24**:1–5.

Stoica I, Tudor I (1967) Effects of vagus afferents on strychnine focus of the coronal gyrus. *Rev Roum Neurol* **4**:287–295.

Stoica I, Tudor I (1968) Vagal trunk stimulation influences on epileptic spiking focus activity. *Rev Roum Neurol* **5**:203–210.

Takaya M, Terry WJ, Naritoku DK (1996) Vagus nerve stimulation induces a sustained anticonvulsant effect. *Epilepsia* **37**:1111–1116.

Talairach J, Bancaud J (1974) Approche nouvelle de la neurochirurgie de l'epilepsie. *Neurochirurgie* **20** (Suppl 1):19.

Terry WJ, Takaya M, Naritoku DK (1996) Regional changes in brain glucose metabolism in rats following anticonvulsant stimulation of the vagus nerve [Abstract]. *Epilepsia* **37**(Suppl 5):117.

Trenerry MR, Jack CR Jr, Sharbrough FW, *et al* (1993) Quantitative MRI hippocampal volumes: association with onset and duration of epilepsy, and febrile convulsions in temporal lobectomy patients. *Epilepsy Research* **15**:247–252.

Uthman BM, Wilder BJ, Penry JK *et al* (1993) Treatment of epilepsy by stimulation of the vagus nerve. *Neurology* **43**:1338–1345.

Van Buren JM, Wood JH, Oakley J, Hambrecht F (1978) Preliminary evaluation of cerebellar stimulation by double-blind stimulation and biological criteria in the treatment of epilepsy. *Journal of Neurosurgery* **48**:407–416.

Velesco M, Velasco F, Velasco AL, Lujan M, Vazques del Mercado J (1989) Epileptiform EEG activities of the centromedian thalamic nuclei in patients with intractable partial motor, complex partial, and generalized seizures. *Epilepsia* **30**:295–306.

Velasco AL, Boleaga B, Santos N, Velasco F, Velasco M (1993a) Electroencephalographic and magnetic resonance correlations in children with intractable seizures of Lennox–Gastaut syndrome and epilepsia partialis continua. *Epilepsia* **34**:262–270.

Velasco F, Velasco M, Velasco AL, Jimenez F, Genton P, Portera-Sanchez A (1993b) Effect of chronic electrical stimulation of the centromedian thalamic nuclei on various intractable seizure patterns: I. Clinical seizures and paroxysmal EEG activity. *Epilepsia* **34**:1052–1064.

Velasco M, Velasco F, Velasco AL, Velasco G, Jimenez F (1993c) Effect of chronic electrical stimulation of the centromedian thalamic nuclei on various intractable seizure patterns: II. Psychological performance and background EEG activity. *Epilepsia* **6**:1065–1074.

Velasco F, Velasco M, Velasco AL, Jimenez F, Marquez I, Rise M (1995) Electrical stimulation of the centromedian thalamic nucleus in control of seizures: long-term studies. *Epilepsia* **36**:63–71.

Wilder BJ, Schmidt RP (1965) Propagation of epileptic discharge from chronic neocortical foci in monkeys. *Epilepsia* **6**:296–309.

Woodbury JW, Woodbury DM (1990) Effects of vagal nerve stimulation on experimentally induced seizures in rats. *Epilepsia* **31**:S7–S19.

Wright GDS, McLellan DL, Brice JG (1985) A double-blind trial of chronic cerebellar stimulation in twelve patients with severe epilepsy *Journal of Neurology, Neurosurgery and Psychiatry* **47**:769–774.

Zanchetti A, Wang SC, Morruzzi G (1952) The effect of vagal afferent stimulation on the EEG pattern of the cat. *Electroencephalography and Clinical Neurophysiology* **4**:357–361.

Zuccarello M, Sawaya R, Lukin R, deCourten-Myers G (1986) Spontaneous cerebellar hematoma associated with chronic cerebellar stimulation. Case report. *Journal of Neurosurgery* **65**:860–862.

Anesthesia for epilepsy surgery

56

PB HEWITT

INTRODUCTION

When surgery for epilepsy was first developed, local anesthesia was used to permit identification of the area of cortex where the epileptic focus originated. This also made it possible to test whether the resection would impair speech or motor function and to ascertain the subjective effects of stimulation of the exposed cortex before its excision. The team from the Montreal Neurological Institute (Gilbert *et al* 1966) defined the following criteria for anesthetic management during temporal lobe surgery:

1. The patient must be conscious and as alert as possible to enable the surgeon to elicit responses on stimulation of the motor, sensory, and speech areas of the brain.
2. Drugs or agents that suppress or distort cortical electrical activity should not be used. This included the use of nitrous oxide, which Gilbert *et al* considered to depress the electrocorticogram.
3. The anesthetist must be sufficiently alert to interpret unusual sensations, such as those similar to the patient's aura, when certain areas of the brain are stimulated.
4. The patient must, however, be sedated and comfortable during a very prolonged procedure performed under a field block.

Preoperative investigation and intraoperative electrocorticography (ECoG) have now developed a level of sophistication that enables the area that can be resected to be defined safely, yet effectively, without requiring further tests on a conscious patient during surgery. Therefore, on most occasions resections can be carried out under general anesthesia. Although the effects of direct cortical stimulation in a conscious patient are interesting they seldom affect the decision on the extent of the resection which is required, so local anesthesia is now rarely indicated. Some of the investigations carried out prior to resective surgery require general anesthesia with special features.

MAIN CONSIDERATIONS FOR GENERAL ANESTHESIA

The anesthetic requirements for any intracranial procedure must be satisfied when epilepsy surgery, or any investigation entailing intracranial intervention, is carried out. An intravenous infusion must be set up using a cannula large enough for blood transfusion (14G or 16G in adults, 18G may be adequate in children less than 10 years old).

Standard monitoring must include arterial pressure, ECG, heart rate, end-tidal carbon dioxide, arterial oxygen saturation (using pulse oximetry) and neuromuscular block regulated by using a peripheral nerve stimulator. Induction of anesthesia is followed by tracheal intubation, then intermittent positive pressure ventilation of the lungs is instituted with a mechanical ventilator, muscle relaxation being maintained with a nondepolarizing neuromuscular blocking agent. Nitrous oxide, oxygen, and a low concentration of a volatile anesthetic agent are used to maintain anesthesia.

Avoidance of increases in intracranial pressure and provision of rapid recovery of consciousness after operation are important. Maintenance of heat balance requires special attention during long procedures.

SPECIAL CONSIDERATIONS IN PATIENTS WITH EPILEPSY

The special requirements for patients with epilepsy include consideration of the preoperative anticonvulsant drugs and their interactions with anesthetic drugs and other medications. Appropriate perioperative management of the medical treatment is also important because of the risk of convulsions during the period of recovery from the anesthetic. There is seldom the question of space-occupying lesions in patients from specialized programs for epilepsy surgery. Although such lesions may present with epilepsy they are usually treated on their own merits. Particular problems that may present difficulties during the induction of anesthesia include behavioral problems, causing difficulties in cooperation, and dental problems, which are associated especially with chronic phenytoin therapy. Many inhaled anesthetics and intravenous analgesics have both pro- and anticonvulsant actions in humans. Although these effects are poorly understood, and biologic variability may determine an individual patient's response, such actions do need to be taken into consideration (Modica *et al* 1990).

ANESTHESIA FOR PREOPERATIVE INVESTIGATIONS

BRAIN IMAGING

Computerized tomography (CT) is normally performed without anesthesia. Cerebral angiography, which is seldom required now, is carried out under local anesthesia, plus sedation if necessary, or with a standard technique of general anesthesia (Cruickshank 1994).

Magnetic resonance imaging (MRI) may require sedation or full general anesthesia in young children or those with behavior disorders. Midazolam (0.5–0.75 mg kg^{-1}, given orally) has been recommended in the USA for sedation or premedication, but is not currently marketed for administration by this route in the UK.

General anesthesia presents significant problems because of the necessity to avoid the use of ferromagnetic materials within the vicinity of the scanner (Nixon *et al* 1986; Patteson and Chesney 1992; Peden *et al* 1992). Special anesthetic and monitoring equipment are therefore required

and a second anesthesiologist may be necessary so that one anesthesiologist remains in the scanning room with the patient, while the other stays outside to monitor and control equipment which cannot be operated within the magnetic field. All the staff entering the area must leave items made of ferromagnetic material (e.g. pagers and watches) and items that would be damaged by the magnetic field (e.g. credit cards) outside the area. Anesthetic equipment taken into the magnetic field needs to be made of appropriate materials (e.g. aluminum gas cylinders, plastic trolleys). Plastic laryngoscopes, however, still present problems because their batteries contain ferromagnetic materials.

Special monitoring equipment is available, such as pulse oximeters with long fiberoptic probes for application to an extremity. Leads are passed through radiofrequency (RF) screens to monitors outside the field. Electrocardiographic traces are susceptible to distortion and local burns may occur at electrode sites. All monitoring leads, for example to connect noninvasive blood pressure measurement cuffs, or end-tidal carbon dioxide monitoring sampling tubes, must be extra long to reach through the RF windows to the monitoring area.

Anesthetized patients will usually require tracheal intubation to maintain a clear airway while in the MRI tube. Preformed Ring, Adair, Elwyn (RAE, Mallinckrodt) tubes or nasotracheal tubes may be easier to fix securely than standard orotracheal tubes. Laryngeal mask airways (LMAs) may be used for patients where spontaneous ventilation is to be maintained during the imaging procedure (Rafferty *et al* 1990). However, LMAs do not protect the air passages against the risk of inhalation of regurgitated gastric contents or permit the safe use of intermittent positive pressure ventilation (IPPV) during imaging. Inhalational or intravenous techniques with spontaneous or controlled ventilation may be used depending upon clinical circumstances and individual preferences but, whatever the choice, the same standards of care and monitoring as employed in the operating room must be provided.

NEUROPHYSIOLOGY

Standard electroencephalography (EEG) using scalp electrodes can be achieved in most patients without anesthesia; a sleep EEG is often helpful in defining focal abnormalities, but if sedation is necessary, it may be prescribed by the neurophysiologist if sufficiently experienced in this field.

Investigations with an invasive component such as the insertion of foramen ovale or sphenoidal electrodes require a brief period of anesthesia with a smooth recovery. Occasionally, more often with sphenoidal electrodes, a period of pharmacologic activation may be required during the recordings. In the past this was carried out using intermittent intravenous thiopental or methohexital while the anesthesiologist endeavored to maintain a clear airway without hindering the positioning of the electrodes. A standard anesthetic facemask cannot be used because it would intrude into the area where the electrodes are to be inserted. A tracheal tube is undesirable for a brief procedure and is not generally indicated. On occasions, difficulty may be encountered with positioning an LMA, or with maintenance of satisfactory spontaneous ventilation in the presence of an LMA. In this case, or if there is thought to be a risk of regurgitation of gastric contents (e.g. with an obese patient), it is safer to proceed to orotracheal intubation to secure the airway. Occasionally an electrode will penetrate the pharyngeal or buccal mucosa producing hemorrhage, and a pharyngeal pack may be needed to provide extra airway protection.

A total intravenous anesthetic (TIVA) technique can prove very stressful for both patient and anesthetist because adequate oxygenation and airway maintenance are difficult to guarantee without tracheal intubation. Anesthesia for this investigation has, however, been facilitated in recent years by the use of the LMA (Brain 1983; Ammar and Towey 1990). Maintenance of anesthesia with intermittent boluses or infusion of propofol (2,6-diisopropylphenol, Diprivan®) (Roberts *et al* 1988) helps to provide a light level of anesthesia with tolerance of the LMA yet not interfering with EEG recording or rapid awakening.

Major invasive procedures such as placing of 'mat' electrodes over the surface of the cortex and of 'depth' electrodes inserted via a craniotomy necessitate general anesthesia. Conventional general anesthesia as employed for any craniotomy is used for these procedures. Muscular relaxation produced with an infusion of atracurium provides a useful background for controlled ventilation because of the flexibility of the duration of action (Eagar *et al* 1984) and rapid recovery from the neuromuscular block (Pearce *et al* 1984).

CAROTID AMYTAL TEST

In cooperative adults and older children, the entire procedure of arterial catheterization and intracarotid amobarbital (Amytal, amylobarbitone sodium) injection is usually carried out under local anesthesia alone. In young or apprehensive patients, general anesthesia may be produced with a total intravenous technique using propofol, *either* with incremental doses being administered as required *or* using the infusion regimen described by Roberts *et al* (1988). Alternatively, a neuroleptic technique with fentanyl and droperidol, or midazolam, alfentanil with midazolam, or full inhalational anesthesia with tracheal intubation or an LMA can be used. However, all of these alternatives will

lead to slower recovery and delay in achieving a sufficiently 'clear headed' state for cooperation with the test. Sometimes the carotid Amytal (amobarbital) test is used to look for the neurophysiologic state of bilateral secondary synchrony, in which circumstances light general anesthesia should be used. The patients will usually have been deliberately kept unsedated in order to be able to monitor their EEG. In young, uncooperative patients, this can make induction of anesthesia very challenging and inhalational induction with sevoflurane in oxygen may be the only practical option. Maintaining a very light level of anesthesia to facilitate useful EEG recordings requires skill and experience.

PENTOTHAL SUPPRESSION TEST

A Pentothal (thiopental) suppression test may be performed with EEG monitoring in order to detect secondary synchrony. During this test, incremental doses of sodium thiopental (Pentothal, Abbott; Intraval Sodium, Rhone-Poulenc Rorer) are administered via an indwelling intravenous cannula to produce sufficient electrical silence and thereby reveal persistent epileptiform activity, which is thought to represent the primary focus. An anesthesiologist must be present during this procedure to monitor cardiorespiratory function, maintain a clear airway, provide respiratory support when spontaneous breathing is depressed and, if necessary, carry out endotracheal intubation and IPPV. Thiopental administration will need to be halted if cardiorespiratory depression, as indicated by an excessive fall in blood pressure, occurs and appropriate treatment with intravenous fluids and vasopressor drugs given. Therefore the thiopental suppression test must be carried out in an area with full anesthetic, monitoring, and resuscitation facilities.

REPEAT ANESTHESIA

Patients may require multiple anesthetics over a period of weeks or months for a succession of tests followed by their definitive operation, so the problems of repeat anesthesia arise. Halothane should not be used for a second anesthetic within a short period of time; a minimum interval of 28 days (Adams *et al* 1986) or of three months (Committee of Safety of Medicines 1986) is recommended. Isoflurane is currently the preferred volatile agent for neurosurgical use owing to the lesser effect on cerebral blood flow, the more rapid postoperative recovery compared with halothane, and the absence of problems with repeat anesthesia. Enflurane was used prior to the introduction of isoflurane and, despite work implicating it as an

recording during corticography and avoidance of cumulative effects is helpful. After flushing the cannula with 0.9% saline, either the ultra-short-acting muscle relaxant succinylcholine or a short-to-medium-duration neuromuscular blocker such as atracurium or vecuronium in a $2 \times ED_{95}$ dose (Adams and Hewitt 1985) is used to produce satisfactory intubating conditions. (ED_{95} is that dose which produces 95% twitch depression and achieves sufficient muscle relaxation to permit surgery.)

Tracheal intubation

Intubation of the trachea, as for other neurosurgical procedures, is most satisfactorily secured with a cuffed, reinforced, polyvinylchloride orotracheal tube that is well secured to avoid any risk of movement during the procedure. Of course, any form of fixation which could compress the neck veins and produce venous engorgement must be avoided. Correct positioning must be confirmed in the normal way using end-tidal carbon dioxide monitoring, bilateral auscultation of the lungs, and observation of respiratory pressure when connected to the automatic lung ventilator.

Maintenance of anesthesia

Use of IPPV maintains end-tidal carbon dioxide concentrations at, or slightly below, physiologic levels. Marked hyperventilation and reduction of arterial carbon dioxide levels are not normally required for this type of neurosurgery, as the surgeons are not dealing with large space-occupying tumors, or very inaccessible lesions necessitating a marked reduction in cerebral blood volume. Indeed it is probably preferable to avoid hypocarbia because this may increase the likelihood of precipitating convulsive activity. Nitrous oxide and oxygen mixture, plus full neuromuscular blockade, is normally used as the background combination for the maintenance of anesthesia. To guarantee unconsciousness this mixture should be supplemented with a low concentration of a volatile agent. For many years halothane was used without major problems in anesthesia for epilepsy surgery, but the postoperative recovery of consciousness tended to be undesirably slow after long procedures, especially if repeated doses of thiopental had been used during corticography. There was also, of course, the worry that repeat anesthesia might be necessary following a halothane-based anesthetic for preoperative radiologic investigations.

When enflurane became available in the UK in the late 1970s it was clear that it held potential advantages over halothane for neurosurgery. There was more rapid recovery

of consciousness and less increase in cerebral blood flow at low concentrations (McDowall 1976; Prys-Roberts 1977) as well as the avoidance of the risk of halothane hepatitis. Halothane hepatitis is a rare phenomenon occurring once in every 10 000–30 000 anesthetic exposures (Rogers 1986). It occurs most often in women with obesity, and with short intervals between the administration of the agent (Dundee 1981). Jaundice appears between the sixth and tenth days postoperatively, and in 70% of patients massive hepatic necrosis ensues, leading to rapidly worsening hepatic encephalopathy and death. Most patients who develop halothane hepatitis have a history of pyrexia, leukocytosis, and raised serum transaminase levels after a previous exposure.

There was considerable interest in the effects of enflurane on the electroencephalogram as the agent had been shown to provoke cortical seizure activity which might be associated with clonic–tonic muscle activity in humans (Clark et al 1971; Stockard et al 1975). It had been demonstrated that hypocapnia enhanced these effects (Clark et al 1971). The consensus view was that these effects were not harmful although there had been reports of EEG abnormalities persisting for between 6 and 30 days in normal subjects (Burchiel et al 1977). There have been several individual reports of seizures occurring after enflurane anesthesia in patients with no previous history of epilepsy (Linde et al 1970; Neigh et al 1971; Ohm et al 1975; Kruczek et al 1980; Ng 1980; Rosenberg et al 1981; Allan 1984; Jenkins and Milne 1984; Yazji and Seed 1984; Grant 1986; Nicoll 1986; Modica et al 1990). In the absence of electroencephalographic evidence, and with the difficulty of excluding all other possible precipitating factors, it is very difficult to ascertain a causal relationship. Etiology of such seizures therefore remains in doubt.

In a randomized, blind, prospective study of such patients undergoing epilepsy surgery, no systematic differences were found between the intraoperative ECoG recordings of patients being given enflurane and those given halothane. Neither were there on comparison with their own conventional preoperative scalp EEGs reviewed by an electrophysiologist with very extensive experience in this field. A retrospective study revealed no significant difference between the incidence of postoperative seizures in patients whose anesthesia was maintained with enflurane compared with those given halothane. There was a tendency to an increased frequency of postoperative fits in patients who had neuroleptanesthesia and a reduction in patients whose resections had been carried out with local anesthesia supplemented by incremental doses of intravenous thiopental (Hewitt and Cripps 1984).

Isoflurane must now be regarded as the preferred volatile supplement. It has the least effect on cerebral blood flow when compared with other currently available agents, allows rapid postoperative awakening even after prolonged anesthesia, and has the lowest risk of problems with repeat anesthesia. Adequate depth of anesthesia is usually produced by concentrations between 0.5% and 2% isoflurane in nitrous oxide 66% with oxygen.

Muscle relaxation

Muscle relaxation can be obtained with atracurium (0.5–0.6 mg), then maintained with an infusion of around 0.5 mg kg^{-1} using 250 mg of atracurium diluted up to 50 ml with isotonic saline and administered using a syringe pump. Monitoring the neuromuscular block with a simple handheld peripheral nerve stimulator enables the anesthesiologist to establish the appropriate infusion rate. After 1 hour, if the twitch response is absent, the infusion should be slowed down by 0.1 mg kg^{-1} (to 0.4 mg kg^{-1}), or if the twitch response is increasing to more than 25% of the control height, the infusion rate should be increased by 0.1 mg kg^{-1} (to 0.6 mg kg^{-1}). Toward the end of the operation when the dura is being closed, or about 45 min before the conclusion of surgery, the infusion should be stopped and the neuromuscular block allowed to wear off. If the train-of-four response has returned to normal and response to tetanic stimulation is fully maintained, no reversal will be required. If any tetanic fade is apparent, neostigmine (2.5 mg) with glycopyrrolate (0.5 mg), should be given intravenously to restore full, normal muscle power.

Patients on anticonvulsant drugs may show resistance to the effects of nondepolarizing neuromuscular blocking drugs and therefore require increased dosage (Desai *et al* 1989).

Heat balance

Epilepsy surgery normally takes a minimum of 4 hours and can therefore involve significant heat loss in an operating theater which is normally maintained at 22°C. An overblanket, which can blow hot air maintained between 32 and 38°C (e.g. Bair–Hugger) over the patient, is therefore of great help. Any blood transfused should pass through a blood warmer to avoid further cooling of the patient.

Electrocorticography

Once the osteoplastic flap has been turned and the dura mater opened, electrocorticography will be performed to confirm the preoperative EEG findings and to delineate the affected region. During these recordings it is essential to avoid any action such as touching or moving of the patient or the electrodes and their connections which could cause artifacts on the ECoG. Liaison between the surgeon, anesthesiologist, and neurophysiologist is essential to provide consistent and stable background conditions on all occasions. Adequate neuromuscular block (as described above) and stable, light general anesthesia should be maintained throughout.

During the period of recording the neurophysiologist may ask the anesthesiologist to inject thiopental, or methohexital, to activate the ECoG. Administration of these drugs should be carried out at a slow and consistent rate (e.g. thiopental 25 mg every 30 s) until the required effects are obtained. This may mean taking the ECoG recording down to the stage of 'burst suppression'. The total dose of thiopental employed is usually around 4–6 mg kg^{-1} body weight, which may produce some hypotension and tachycardia. If this is a problem, it may be necessary to increase the rate of administration of intravenous fluid and reduce the inspired concentration of volatile anesthetic for a short period. After a period of recording from the cortical surface further electrodes may be placed at a greater depth (e.g. in the hippocampal region) and further recordings made before proceeding with the resection.

In all centers with a substantial volume of work, the most frequent resection is a resection of the anterior part of the temporal lobe. This produces minimal surgical stimulation during most of the procedure but dissection on the floor of the temporal fossa increases the level of stimulation and often requires an increase in the concentration of volatile anesthetic (e.g. isoflurane 1.5–2.0%) for a short time, or small incremental doses of an intravenous opioid (e.g. alfentanil 0.5 mg).

Blood loss is usually negligible and transfusion seldom required during these procedures, although it may be necessary if loss from the scalp and bone flaps is high during opening and closure. Patients who have had a previous procedure recently, such as mat electrode placement, may be anemic and require peroperative transfusion. Frontal and other cortical resections are managed similarly. Amygdalohippocampectomy is sometimes carried out instead of temporal lobectomy. This involves removal of a smaller mass of tissue from a less easily accessible site. If brain retraction produces changes in monitored parameters the surgeon should be told so that appropriate adjustments can be made.

Anatomic hemispherectomy, being a more radical and more extensive procedure, not only takes longer but is also associated with greater blood loss and always necessitates blood transfusion. Some of the alternatives, such as functional hemispherectomy (Villemure *et al* 1993) or hemispherotomy (Delalande *et al* 1993) are less extensive. The patients are often children and may be underweight for their years, in some cases severely cachectic (Brian *et al* 1990). It is therefore helpful to estimate circulating blood volume on the basis of 80–85 ml kg^{-1} body weight in the newborn, reducing to around 70 ml kg^{-1} body weight at puberty. A patient with a normal preoperative hemoglobin concentration should have losses greater than 15% of circulating volume replaced by blood transfusion (Smith 1998). A fluid administration set with calibrated burette (100–150 ml) should be used for patients weighing less than 25 kg to allow more accurate replacement of the losses while avoiding circulatory overload.

Transfusion fluids should be warmed to avoid further reduction in body heat of patients undergoing prolonged surgery. Whole blood is not often available nowadays; therefore, appropriate replacement of blood components to maintain the osmotic effect of the plasma proteins, to avoid fluid losses from the circulation into the tissues, as well as to replace lost clotting factors, must be carefully supervised (Smith 1998). If plasma substitutes, such as the gelatin preparations (e.g. Gelofusine, Haemaccel), are used it is important to remember that their effects are dissipated in 3–4 hours (Eller and Abrams 1998) and continued infusion in the postoperative period will be required to maintain their effect.

The patients invariably have a hemiparesis preoperatively and may be very debilitated from frequent fits. Careful positioning on the operating table is particularly important to avoid excess pressure on the bony prominences, which could lead to pressure sores.

POSTOPERATIVE CARE

At the conclusion of surgery and application of bandaging, neuromuscular block should have worn off adequately or have been antagonized (see above) and the depth of anesthesia lightened sufficiently for spontaneous respiration to be resumed. The adequacy of respiration should be checked by observing the pattern of breathing for absence of tracheal tug, or other signs of problems, and the continued monitoring of end-tidal carbon dioxide. If these are satisfactory the pharynx should be cleared by suction. Suction down the trachea should be avoided if the breath sounds are clear because any coughing produced by this stimulation will have an adverse effect by raising the intracranial pressure. Nitrous oxide administration is discontinued and 100% oxygen supplemented with sufficient isoflurane to prevent 'bucking' on the endotracheal tube. The tube is then taken out while applying positive pressure to the reservoir bag, in order to ensure that any secretions lodged around it in the larynx are expelled rather than inhaled when the tube is removed. The tip of the pharyngeal sucker should be kept positioned at the

back of the pharynx at this time in order to catch the plug of mucus, lodged between the cuff of the tube and the vocal cords, when it is expelled during this maneuver. Oxygen 100% is then given via an anesthetic facemask while the breathing and physiologic variables are checked. While the patient is still asleep the nonsteroidal anti-inflammatory drug (NSAID) diclofenac sodium (Voltarol) may be administered as a suppository (100 mg for an adult, 1 mg kg^{-1} for a child) to initiate postoperative pain relief. Such NSAIDs provide useful alternatives or adjuncts to opioids as they do not depress respiration, or impair gastrointestinal motility, and do not cause dependence.

The patient is transferred to the bed in the lateral recovery position. Following anatomic hemispherectomy it is preferable to position the patient with the operated side uppermost in order to avoid herniation of the remaining hemisphere through the falx. Oxygen should be administered via a disposable mask during transfer to the recovery room and arterial oxygen saturation monitored with a pulse oximeter.

Postoperative analgesia is often provided by codeine phosphate, initially given intramuscularly, in dosage of up to 60 mg 4-hourly in an adult patient. Intravenous use should be avoided because of histamine release. Prolonged use leads to constipation, therefore it is recommended to change to oral acetaminophern (paracetamol) analgesia as soon as possible. In children, the dosage of codeine phosphate is around 0.75 mg kg^{-1} body weight and may be administered orally or intramuscularly. Acetaminophen (paracetamol) may be used as supplementary postoperative analgesia in a dosage of 10–15 mg kg^{-1} body weight and has the advantage that it can be administered as an elixir (e.g. Panadol), oral suspension (e.g. Calpol), or as rectal suppositories, thus reducing the need for intramuscular injections.

Fluid balance is maintained using 4% dextrose in 0.18% saline solution at a rate of 2 ml kg^{-1} hour^{-1} intravenously until oral intake has been resumed. Blood transfusion will be required if intraoperative losses have not been replaced adequately in order to prevent development of hypovolemia with hypotension and tachycardia. The hemoglobin concentration or hematocrit should be checked on the first postoperative day. If the hemoglobin level is below 10 g dl^{-1} or hematocrit less than 0.35, further blood transfusion should be given before removing the intravenous cannula.

These patients are liable to have convulsions in the postoperative period because of the immediate effects of surgery. The patients therefore need to be nursed in a high-dependency area where nursing staff are always available to provide airway care, administer oxygen, prevent injury, and administer anticonvulsant therapy. The patient's regular preoperative anticonvulsants are recommended as soon as possible after the operation.

REFERENCES

Adams AP, Hewitt PB (1985) The new muscle relaxants: atracurium and vecuronium. In: Atkinson RS, Adams AP (eds) *Recent Advances in Anaesthesia and Analgesia*, Vol 15, pp 13–25. Edinburgh: Churchill Livingstone.

Adams AP, Campbell D, Clarke RSJ *et al* (1986) Halothane and the liver. *British Medical Journal* **293**:1023.

Allan NS (1984) Convulsions after enflurane. *Anaesthesia* **39**:605–606.

Ammar T, Towey R (1990) The laryngeal mask airway. *Anaesthesia* **45**:75.

Association of Anaesthetists of Great Britain and Ireland (1988) *Recommendations for Standards of Monitoring during Anaesthesia and Recovery*. London: Association of Anaesthetists.

Brain AIJ (1983) The laryngeal mask – a new concept in airway management. *British Journal of Anaesthesia* **55**:801–805.

Brian JE Jr, Deshpande JK, McPherson RW (1990) Management of hemispherectomy in children. *Journal of Clinical Anesthesia* **2**:91–95.

British National Formulary (1998) No. 34 (March); p 533. London: British Medical Association, Royal Pharmaceutical Society.

Burchiel KJ, Stockard JJ, Rowe MJ, Calverley RK, Smith NT (1977) Relationship of pre- and postanesthetic EEG abnormalities to enflurane-induced seizure activity. *Anesthesia and Analgesia* **56**:509–514.

Campkin TV, Turner JM (1980) *Neurosurgical Anaesthesia and Intensive Care*, p 144. London: Butterworths.

Clark DL, Hosnick EC, Rosner BD (1971) Neurophysiological effects of different anaesthetics in unconscious man. *Journal of Applied Physiology* **31**:884–891.

Committee on Safety of Medicines (1986) Halothane hepatotoxicity. *Current Problems* **18**:1–2.

Cruickshank S (1994) Anaesthesia for neuroradiology. In: Walters FJM, Ingram GS, Jenkinson J (eds) *Anaesthesia and Intensive Care for the Neurosurgical Patient*, pp 144–166. Oxford: Blackwell Science.

Delalande O, Pinard JM, Basdevant C, Plouin P, Dulac O (1993) Hemispherotomy: a new procedure for hemispheric disconnection [abstract]. *Epilepsia* **34**(Suppl 12): 140–141.

Desai P, Hewitt PB, Jones RM (1989) Influence of anticonvulsant therapy on doxacurium and pancuronium-induced paralysis. *Anesthesiology* **71** (Suppl): abstract 784.

Dundee JW (1981) Prospective study of liver function following repeat halothane and enflurane. *Journal of the Royal Society of Medicine* **74**:286–290.

Eagar BM, Flynn PJ, Hughes R (1984) Infusion of atracurium for long surgical procedures. *British Journal of Anaesthesia* **56**:447–452.

Eller EB, Abrams KJ (1998) Intravenous fluids. In: Adams AP, Hewitt PB, Grande CM (eds) *Emergency Anaesthesia*, 2nd edn, pp 62–72. London: Edward Arnold.

Gilbert RGB, Brindle GF, Galindo A (1966) Anesthetic management for surgery of temporal lobe epilepsy. In: *Anesthesia for Neurosurgery*, pp 132–137. Boston: Little Brown.

Grant IS (1986) Delayed convulsions following enflurane anesthesia. *Anaesthesia* **41**:1024–1025.

Hewitt PB, Cripps TP (1984) Anesthesia for epilepsy surgery. *British Journal of Anaesthesia* **56**:1308.

Hewitt PB, Chu DLK, Polkey CE, Binnie CD (1999) Effect of propofol on the electrocorticogram in epileptic patients undergoing cortical resection. *British Journal of Anaesthesia* **82**:199–202.

Jenkins J, Milne AC (1984) Convulsive reaction following enflurane anesthesia. *Anaesthesia* **39**:44–45.

Kruczek M, Albin MS, Wolf S, Bertoni JM (1980) Postoperative seizure activity following enflurane anesthesia. *Anesthesiology* **53**:175–176.

Linde HW, Lamb VE, Quimby CW, Homi J, Eckenhoff JE (1970) The search for better anesthetic agents. *Anesthesiology* **32**:555–559.

Manninen P, Contreras J (1986) Anesthetic considerations for craniotomy in awake patients. *International Anesthesiology Clinics* **24**:157–174.

McDowall DG (1976) Neurosurgical anesthesia and intensive care. In: Hewer L, Atkinson RS (eds) *Recent Advances in Anaesthesia*, Vol 12, pp 16–43. London: Churchill Livingstone.

Modica PA, Tempelhoff R, White PF (1990) Pro- and anticonvulsant effects of anesthetics (parts 1, 2). *Anesthesia and Analgesia* **70**:303–315, 433–444.

Neigh JL, Garman JK, Harp JR (1971) The electroencephalographic pattern during anesthesia with Ethrane. *Anesthesiology* **35**:482–487.

Ng ATH (1980) Prolonged myoclonic contractions after enflurane anesthesia – a case report. *Canadian Anaesthetists' Society Journal* **27**:502–503.

Nicoll JMV (1986) Status epilepticus following enflurane anaesthesia. *Anaesthesia* **41**:927–930.

Nixon C, Hirsch NP, Ormerod IEC, Johnson G (1986) Nuclear magnetic resonance imaging. Its implications for the anaesthetist. *Anaesthesia* **41**:131–137.

Ohm WW, Cullen BF, Amory DW, Kennedy RD (1975) Delayed seizure activity following enflurane anesthesia. *Anesthesiology* **42**:367–368.

Parke IJ, Stevens JF, Rice ACE *et al* (1992) Metabolic acidosis and fatal myocardial failure after propofol infusion in children. *British Medical Journal* **305**:613–616.

Patteson SK, Chesney JT (1992) Anesthetic management for magnetic resonance imaging: problems and solutions. *Anesthesia and Analgesia* **74**:121–128.

Pearce AC, Hewitt PB, Adams AP (1984) Atracurium as the sole muscle relaxant for neurosurgical procedures. *British Journal of Anaesthesia* **56**:1310.

Peden CJ, Menon DK, Hall AS, Sargentoni J, Whitwam JG (1992) Magnetic resonance for the anesthetist. II: Anaesthesia and monitoring in MR units. *Anaesthesia* **47**:508–517.

Prys-Roberts C (1977) Editorial: Old wine in new bottles. *British Journal of Anaesthesia* **49**:845–846.

Rafferty C, Burke AM, Cossar DF, Farling PA (1990) Laryngeal mask and magnetic resonance imaging. *Anaesthesia* **45**:590–591.

Roberts F, Dixon J, Lewis GTR, Tackley RM, Prys-Roberts C (1988) Propofol anaesthesia, induction and maintenance; a manual infusion scheme. *Anaesthesia* **43S**:14–17.

Rogers EL (1986) Liver disease. In: Adams AP, Hewitt PB, Rogers MC (eds) *Emergency Anaesthesia*, pp 310–325. London: Edward Arnold.

Rosenberg H, Clofine R, Bialik O (1981) Neurological changes during awakening from anesthesia. *Anesthesiology* **54**:125–130.

Smith GN (1998) Blood groups and blood transfusion. In: Adams AP, Hewitt PB, Grande CM (eds) *Emergency Anaesthesia*, 2nd edn, pp 33–47. London: Edward Arnold.

Smith M (1994) Anaesthesia for epilepsy and stereotactic surgery. In: Walters FJM, Ingram GS, Jenkinson J (eds) *Anaesthesia and Intensive Care for the Neurosurgical Patient*, pp 318–344. Oxford: Blackwell Science.

Smith M (1996) Anaesthesia in epilepsy surgery. In: Shorvon S, Dreifuss F, Fish D, Thomas T (eds) *The Treatment of Epilepsy*, pp 794–804. Oxford: Blackwell Science.

Smith M, Smith SJ, Scott C, Harness WFJ (1996) Activation of the electrocorticogram by propofol during surgery for epilepsy. *British Journal of Anaesthesia* **76**:499–502.

Stockard JJ, Burchiel K, Smith NT, Calverley RK, Eger EI II (1975) The effects of nitrous oxide and carbon dioxide on epileptiform EEG activity produced by enflurane. *Anesthesiology* **45**(Suppl):A309.

Villemure JG, Adams CBT, Hoffman HJ, Peacock WJ (1993) Hemispherectomy. In: Engel J (ed.) *Surgical Treatment of the Epilepsies*, 2nd edn, pp 511–518. New York: Raven Press.

Yazji NS, Seed RF (1984) Convulsive reaction following enflurane anaesthesia. *Anaesthesia* **39**:1249.

Seizure reduction

JM OXBURY AND CE POLKEY

The ideal outcome from the surgical treatment of epilepsy is an improved quality of life resulting from a complete absence of seizures without drug side-effects and unaccompanied by any new physical or cognitive/memory disability or serious psychiatric disturbance arising from the surgery. Unfortunately, this ideal is not always achieved! It has been said that epilepsy surgery, although it reduces the seizure frequency in most patients and cures some, is 'expensive, dangerous, and either unavailable or not acceptable to most patients' (Dasheiff et al 1994). Some of the dangers arise during the preoperative investigations. It is most important, therefore, that every patient contemplating surgical treatment or undergoing preoperative evaluation should at all stages be informed realistically about the probability of the benefits on the one hand and about the possible risks of permanent new disability on the other.

To inform the patient correctly, the physician must have a clear understanding of the probability of good outcome (seizure, physical, cognitive, and psychiatric) and of the possibility of unwanted effects. Needless to say, these depend upon a number of factors including the pathology underlying the epilepsy (see Chapter 42) and the type of surgery that may be offered. The cognitive/memory and quality of life issues, and the physical disabilities and psychiatric disturbances that may arise, are described in other chapters (58 to 63). This chapter is concerned only with seizure outcome. Seizure outcome is, however, central to overall outcome. Patients who are rendered seizure-free by surgery report significantly better emotional and psychosocial outcome than do those who are not rendered seizure-free even to the extent of only having isolated auras (Chapter 49). Furthermore, they see themselves as having the least handicap (O'Donoghue et al 1998) even though a significant proportion of them do experience difficulties when first faced with the seizure-free lifestyle (Bladin 1992).

There are no data derived from controlled trials of surgery versus nonsurgical measures to provide a basis for ideas about the possible benefits of surgery for good seizure outcome (Dasheiff et al 1994; Berg and Vickrey 1998). Wyler et al (1995), however, have set a standard for assessing different types of surgery by demonstrating superior seizure relief, without additional cognitive/memory deficit, from total as compared to partial hippocampectomy in a prospective randomized, and blinded trial. The pathology underlying the epilepsy consisted of various degrees of hippocampal sclerosis. During the first postoperative year, 69.4% of the total hippocampectomy group did not experience any seizure, including isolated auras, compared to only 38.2% of the partial hippocampectomy group. The difference was statistically significant ($P = 0.02$). A trend ($P = 0.07$) toward younger patients having a better outcome was also noted. As discussed below, complete freedom from seizures during the first year after surgery is a matter of considerable prognostic importance.

There have been two major retrospective studies comparing the outcome of patients who underwent surgery with others who were considered to be comparable but did not have surgery (Guldvog *et al* 1991; Vickrey *et al* 1995). The Norwegian study (Guldvog *et al* 1991) compared 201 patients who underwent surgery, predominantly temporal or frontal, during the period 1949–1988 with 185 matched patients of whom it was felt in retrospect that 38 were possible surgical candidates. The median duration of the follow-up was 9 years for both groups with ranges 2–29 years for the surgical group and 2–31 years for the nonsurgical group. The median preoperative seizure frequency of the surgical group (20/month) did not differ significantly ($P = 0.86$) from that for the 38 possible surgical candidates (30/month) who did not undergo surgery. By the last year of follow-up the median frequency had fallen to 0/month for the surgical group compared to 10/month for the others ($P = 0.0002$). The seizure outcome was better in the surgical group irrespective of preoperative seizure frequency, age, or the etiology of the epilepsy. However, a significantly greater proportion of the surgical group had acquired new neurologic deficit.

The Los Angeles study (Vickrey *et al* 1995) compared the outcome of 202 patients who were evaluated at UCLA and went on to surgery (mostly anterior temporal resections) with that of 46 patients who were evaluated but could not proceed to operation. Essentially, the findings were the same as for the Norwegian study. The surgically treated group had a greater fall in average monthly seizure frequency and consumed less medication.

SEIZURE OUTCOME GRADING

As has been pointed out by Spencer (1996), there are many pitfalls to predicting postoperative seizure outcome, especially long-term, let alone the relationship between any change in seizure frequency and/or seizure severity, compared to preoperatively, and quality of life. The comparison of results achieved by different centers, or by different surgical techniques, can be particularly difficult in the absence of a widely agreed system of seizure outcome grading. The difficulty is accentuated because the criteria for surgical selection can be far from uniform and are often not stated precisely beyond listing the investigations that have been carried out during the preoperative evaluation. Furthermore, duration of follow-up varies, but is usually short, and

groups are often heterogeneous for pathology and/or type of surgery.

OUTCOME CLASSIFICATION

Currently the most widely used system for classifying seizure outcome is that described by Engel *et al* (1993), shown in Table 57.1, which is a modification of the system described by Engel (1987). It is a 'combined' system and not strictly quantitative. Thus, it attempts both to classify postoperative seizure frequency and to specify whether or not a patient has derived benefit from the surgical intervention. The authors recognized that the attempt to cover both aspects introduces the disadvantages of subjective judgments. There are a number of particular problems.

● The distinction between a disabling seizure and a nondisabling seizure is a matter of opinion and to some extent a matter of national driving license regulations. In this classification, auras without impairment of consciousness and simple partial motor seizures that 'have no functional consequence' are considered to be nondisabling and there is specific mention that people prone to such seizures can legally drive. That is not, however, the case in the UK and various other countries, where a

Table 57.1 Classification of postoperative seizure outcome as described by Engel *et al* (1993).

Class 1   Free from disabling seizures. This excludes early postoperative seizures (first few weeks).
  A. Completely seizure-free since surgery
  B. Nondisabling simple partial seizures only since surgery
  C. Some disabling seizures after surgery, but free of disabling seizures for at least 2 years
  D. Generalized convulsion with antiepileptic drug withdrawal only

Class 2   Rare disabling seizures ('almost seizure-free').
  A. Initially free of disabling seizures but has rare seizures now
  B. Rare disabling seizures since surgery
  C. More than rare disabling seizures after surgery, but rare seizures for at least 2 years
  D. Nocturnal seizures only

Class 3   Worthwhile improvement. (Determination of 'worthwhile improvement' requires quantitative analyses of additional data such as percentage seizure reduction, cognitive function, and quality of life.)
  A. Worthwhile seizure reduction
  B. Prolonged seizure-free intervals amounting to more than half the follow-up period but not less than 2 years

Class 4   No worthwhile improvement. (Determination of 'worthwhile improvement' requires quantitative analyses of additional data such as percentage seizure reduction, cognitive function, and quality of life.)
  A. Significant seizure reduction
  B. No appreciable change
  C. Seizures worse

person who has suffered an epileptic attack, however mild, while awake, must refrain from driving until a completely seizure-free period of at least one year from the date of the attack has elapsed. On the other hand, nocturnal seizures are classed as disabling (class 2) in this classification. In the UK they need not be so. There, in the long-term, such seizures are often less disabling than occasional simple partial seizures because nocturnal seizures do not revoke the entitlement to drive provided there is at least a 3-year history of them unpunctuated by any awake seizures.

- Apart from nocturnal seizures, entry to class 2 outcome is dependent upon the disabling seizures being 'rare.' Clearly it is a subjective decision whether or not the seizures are rare and it would be difficult to be sure that the decision would be uniform across different epilepsy surgery centers.

- A similar problem arises with the decision whether or not any improvement has been 'worthwhile,' since that decision is not dependent upon seizure frequency alone but rather upon quality of life factors or perhaps even factors primarily effecting carers.

QUANTITATIVE MEASUREMENT OF SEIZURE FREQUENCY

Cessation of the seizures is the major goal. If it is achieved, then the length of the period for which it is maintained can be a measure. Otherwise, quantification of the frequency of the ongoing seizures is dependent upon the patient keeping accurate diary records with a separation at least between isolated auras or simple partial seizures, complex partial seizures, and those with secondary generalization. At its simplest, the precise number of seizures that have been experienced since the last attendance is recorded at each visit to the clinic or at each telephone communication. The advantage of a purely quantitative system is that it enables seizure frequency to be specified at regular intervals, such as annually, without any judgment whether the seizures are disabling or whether surgery has been beneficial. Those very important aspects can be addressed by other purpose-designed measuring systems such as quality of life scales. Furthermore, a purely quantitative system can be more easily used to plot change over time.

The percentage of patients achieving an at least 50% reduction in seizure frequency is a widely used measure in add-on drug trials (Marson et al 1996). It would, however, be too crude as a surgical outcome measure. Categorization of those experiencing postoperative seizures into, for instance, <5% of preoperative, 5% to <10%, 10% to <25%,

and 25% or more might be reasonable and would allow changes to be plotted over time.

Engel et al (1993) recognized that a purely quantitative measure of postoperative seizures accompanied by independent measures of quality of life and of cognitive and/or physical dysfunction could be preferable to the seizure outcome classification summarized in Table 57.1. As an alternative to the latter, they suggested a 'focused postoperative seizure scoring system' (see Table 57.2). This system has been validated by the Mayo Clinic/Medical School group (So et al 1997) and used by Ficker et al (1999) to plot changes in postoperative seizure control over time (see below).

SEIZURE SEVERITY

Seizure severity is particularly difficult to measure. Various scales have been developed in an attempt to quantify this factor, but the International League Against Epilepsy Commission on Outcome Measurement (ILAE 1998) was unable to recommend the use of any one as a standard outcome measure.

FACTORS INFLUENCING POSTOPERATIVE SEIZURE FREQUENCY

A number of factors have the potential to affect the prognosis for the relief of seizures following excisional surgery.

Table 57.2 Scoring system for postoperative seizure frequency as proposed by Engel et al (1993) with minor modifications[a]

Score	
0	Seizure-free off AED[c]
1	Seizure-free, need for AED unknown
2	Seizure-free, needs AED to remain so
3	(Nondisabling)[b] simple partial seizures
4	(Nondisabling)[b] nocturnal seizures only
5	1–3/year
6	4–11/year
7	1–3/month
8	1–6/week
9	1–3/day
10	4–10/day
11	>10/day but not status epilepticus
12	Status epilepticus without barbiturate coma

[a] The authors point out that within categories 5–11 separate seizure types (simple partial, complex partial, secondarily generalized) can be scored independently.
[b] Parentheses not in the original proposal of Engel et al (1993).
[c] AED, antiepileptic drugs.

Those that will be considered here are the locus and type of the resection, the nature of the pathology that is removed, and the age at surgery.

LOCUS OF SURGERY

Prior to the advent of MRI and to the widespread appreciation that the excision of pathology was central to successful epilepsy surgery, operative strategy largely depended upon the resection of an epileptogenic zone defined by using complex EEG techniques. During this era, outcome with respect to seizures was mostly assessed in relation to the locus of the excision (Engel 1987).

Data collected by Professor Engel based on 6009 patients who underwent epilepsy surgery at around 100 centers across the world during the period 1986–1990 revealed the percentage who became seizure-free, depending on the locus of the surgery, as follows (Engel *et al* 1993):

Anterior temporal lobectomy	67.9%
Amygdalohippocampectomy	68.8%
Extratemporal nonlesional resection	45.1%
Extratemporal lesional resection	66.6%
Hemispherectomy	67.4%
Multilobar resection	45.2%
Corpus callosotomy	7.6%

The difference in outcome from extratemporal resections according to whether they were 'lesional' (that is they removed pathology) or nonlesional is a clear testament to the need to remove pathology to achieve complete seizure relief. The lower success rate from multilobar excisions compared with hemispherectomy is probably due to the former being restricted and consequently giving only an incomplete resection of the pathology. It is likely that the majority of the temporal resections would have included pathologic tissue, making them equivalent to extratemporal lesional resections. Provided that pathology is resected, therefore, the site of resection appears to have little influence on seizure outcome.

PATHOLOGY COMPLETELY REMOVABLE BY RESTRICTED RESECTIONS

The complete removal of definite pathology, usually from within a single lobe of the brain, is the most powerful factor underlying the complete abolition of seizures without adding neurologic deficit.

The need to remove pathology to achieve the greatest success from temporal lobe resections has been recognized, although not necessarily by all, at least since Falconer (1971) and need not be reiterated here. For extratemporal

excisions, the Engel *et al* (1993) data (see above) showed a 66.6% success rate for lesional cases, where pathology was removed, compared to only 45.1% for nonlesional cases. In line with this view, Polkey and his colleagues have reported that a focal abnormality on neuroimaging is the only favorable prognostic factor for a good outcome from frontal resections (Ferrier *et al* 1999). Furthermore, Scott *et al* (1999) have suggested that if high-quality MRI does not reveal pathology, the patient should be carefully counseled before proceeding to further investigation because in that circumstance there is only a low probability that successful surgery will be feasible.

There is some variation in outcome according to the nature of the pathology (Cascino *et al* 1993; Berkovic *et al* 1995) and whether it is completely excised (Fried and Cascino 1993). The latter authors concluded that complete removal of the pathology is the most important factor determining successful postoperative seizure control and that excision of the presumed epileptogenic zone without resection of the pathology gives dismal results.

Hippocampal sclerosis/mesial temporal sclerosis

Resection of the sclerotic medial temporal lobe structures from patients with predominantly unilateral hippocampal sclerosis renders around 80% seizure-free or virtually so (see Chapter 11). Factors associated with a particularly high probability of achieving complete freedom from seizures include:

- A history of a prolonged convulsion or multiple convulsions when aged 6 months to 4 years (Abou-Khalil *et al* 1993). Such a history is associated with a high probability that the hippocampus will be severely sclerotic (Sagar and Oxbury 1987).
- Strictly unilateral hippocampal smallness (sclerosis) as determined by measurement of the volumes of the hippocampi in relation to brain volume (see Chapter 44). In the study of Arruda *et al* (1996) the numbers in Engel class 1 at least 1 year after surgery were 85.1% for those with unilateral atrophy, 47.1% for bilateral atrophy even though asymmetric, and 50% for those with normal volumes on both sides.
- Concordance between the laterality of the major hippocampal atrophy as seen on MRI, strictly unilateral anterior/medial temporal lobe epileptiform discharges on noninvasive interictal EEG, and the neuropsychologic carotid amytal data, making ictal EEG monitoring unnecessary (Holmes *et al* 1996).
- Surgery in childhood, when aged <16 years (Oxbury *et al* 1996).

- Total resection of the sclerotic hippocampus (Wyler *et al* 1995).

Both Berkovic *et al* (1995) and Spencer (1996) have commented that late seizure recurrence after several years of freedom from seizures is more common after surgical treatment for hippocampal sclerosis than with foreign-tissue pathology such as benign or low-grade tumor.

Dual pathology

Around 15% of surgical candidates have MRI evidence of a reduced hippocampal volume, indicative of sclerosis, in association with other pathology, most often a neuronal migration defect or a porencephalic cyst (Cendes *et al* 1995; Raymond *et al* 1995). The second pathology may be temporal or extratemporal. Both the hippocampal and the extrahippocampal pathology need to be removed to give the best probability of freedom from seizures (Li *et al* 1999). Unsuccessful surgical treatment of hippocampal sclerosis has been attributed in some cases to the presence of cortical dysgenesis subsequently detected by quantitative MRI block analysis but not detected preoperatively by standard high-resolution MRI (Sisodiya *et al* 1997).

Malformations of cortical development

Sisodiya, Squier, and Anslow review the surgical treatment of intractable epilepsy due to malformations of cortical development (MCD) in Chapter 10. Under the heading of MCD they include focal cortical dysplasia, microdysgenesis, polymicrogyria, lissencephaly, heterotopia, schizencephaly, hemimegalencephaly, and tumors/hamartomas. In this chapter, tumors/hamartomas are considered separately from the other forms of MCD.

The data cited by Sisodiya and colleagues in their Table 10.1 show that, excluding tumors/hamartomas, most of those for whom surgery achieves prolonged complete freedom from seizures have focal cortical dysplasia. Nevertheless, they constitute a small number. English-language references yielded only 31 such cases reported with adequate detail. Depending upon the extent of the pathology, and on the neurologic status of the patient preoperatively, the surgery may be a more or less extensive focal resection, or hemispherectomy may be necessary. There are also reports of occasional patients with polymicrogyria (Bruton 1988), schizencephaly (Silbergeld and Miller 1994), lissencephaly (Hirabayashi *et al* 1993), and heterotopia (Verity *et al* 1982; Lindsay *et al* 1987) who have had a successful outcome from surgery. Hemispherectomy was

the surgery for heterotopia. Complete freedom from seizures has also been reported after hemispherectomy for hemimegalencephaly (DiRocco 1996; Guerrini *et al* 1996). Overall, the success rate with focal resections for MCD is <50% (Hirabayashi *et al* 1993), although Kuzniecky *et al* (1991) did report a greater success in purely temporal lobe patients.

As with other pathology, the probability of good outcome is maximized if a complete resection can be achieved. Unfortunately, with MCD it is not always possible to assess the extent of the pathology by neuroimaging techniques. Consequently, MRI is less reliable for surgical planning and the extent of the resection must rely heavily on neurophysiologic data obtained intraoperatively or derived from preoperative EEG monitoring with intracranial electrodes. Thus, Duchowny and colleagues have reported (Whiting *et al* 1998) that, although the overall rate of freedom from seizures is only around 33%, complete removal of the epileptogenic zone as defined by subdural EEG recordings gives a success rate >60%.

Dysembryoplastic neuroepithelioma (DNT)/hamartoma

DNT are essentially benign tumors that contain glial and neuronal elements without tumor matrix and are primarily nonneoplastic malformations of tissue development (Wolf *et al* 1995). Daumas-Duport *et al* (1988) in their original description of DNT reported that around 75% became seizure-free postoperatively. A similarly good outcome has been recorded in subsequently reported series (Kirkpatrick *et al* 1993; Raymond *et al* 1994). Some cases present in early childhood and surgery at age <10 years can achieve abolition of the epilepsy in up to 90% without impairment of intellectual development (Knight *et al* 1988).

Ganglioglioma

Gangliogliomas are composed of neoplastic neural and glial cells. Morris *et al* (1998) reviewed 38 cases with a ganglioglioma (26 temporal lobe) who underwent surgical treatment for intractable epilepsy at the Cleveland Clinic. Twenty of 32 (63%) were in Engel class 1 at 2 years after surgery. Preoperative factors that were statistically significantly indicative of good seizure outcome were a young age and a short duration of seizure history at the time of operation. The authors recommended early surgical intervention for children with intractable epilepsy due to suspected ganglioglioma.

Oligodendroglioma and low-grade astrocytoma

Spencer (1996) has reviewed long-term outcome in 67 cases of low-grade glioma treated surgically for intractable epilepsy at the Yale University School of Medicine: 75% achieved 2–10 years of continuous freedom from seizures. The period of remission usually commenced during the first postoperative year.

Cavernous angioma

The literature review of Moran *et al* (1999) suggests that surgical treatment renders around 85% patients seizure-free irrespective of the cerebral locus of the cavernoma. The duration of the seizure history was statistically significantly shorter in those who became seizure-free than in those who did not. The authors' own series of 16 patients treated by lesionectomy (2 occipital, 1 parietal, 10 temporal, 2 frontal) or temporal lobectomy (1) followed for a mean of 3.2 years gave 7 temporals in Engel class 1 or 2; none of those situated extratemporally achieved class 1.

PATHOLOGY USUALLY NECESSITATING HEMISPHERECTOMY

Wilson (1970) reported that hemispherectomy completely or substantially relieved the epilepsy in 82% people (average age 13 years) who had presented with intractable epilepsy associated with a spastic hemiplegia of early childhood onset. Around half of them had their epilepsy on the basis of a porencephalic cyst secondary to middle cerebral artery territory infarction prenatally or perinatally. Most of the others had cerebral hemiatrophy following a febrile illness with severe convulsions during early childhood (the HHE syndrome). Unfortunately the operation had to be abandoned owing to the high incidence of late complications due to obstructive hydrocephalus often associated with CNS hemosiderosis. Fortunately, it has subsequently been possible to develop surgical techniques that permit hemispherectomy without these complications (see Chapter 53).

Holthausen *et al* (1997) reviewed the outcome from hemispherectomy in 333 patients treated at 11 different European and North American epilepsy surgery centers using surgical techniques introduced since the late 1970s. Overall, around 69% became seizure-free. There was some variation according to the nature of the underlying pathology and possibly also to the surgical technique used. Dysplasia was the pathology in the largest number (99), followed by Rasmussen encephalitis (83), vascular (46), 'hemiatrophy' (44), and Sturge–Weber syndrome (28). The median age at surgery was <11 years in all pathology groups. Unfortunately, the length of the postoperative follow-up was rather short in that patients could enter the study with a minimum of only 6 months postsurgery. Nevertheless, this is a study of major importance because most epilepsy surgery centers, even those with special expertise in hemispherectomy, cannot approach comparable numbers and often have a predilection for treating a particular pathology (see also, Chapter 53).

Dysplasia

Freedom from seizures was judged to have resulted in 56.6% of those with this pathology in the multicenter study. It should, however, be stressed that follow-up may have been short. The age at operation was particularly young (median 1.7 years, range 0.2–11.8). Three out of four with polymicrogyria and heterotopia were still completely seizure-free more than 3 years after hemispherectomy in the Oxford series mentioned by Sisodiya and colleagues in Table 10.2 (Chapter 10) – as was one with lissencephaly and heterotopia but not the one with focal cortical dyplasia. This gives an overall success rate of around 65% in this small series. In the multicenter study there was no suggestion of a statistically significant relationship between outcome and the presence of epileptiform discharges over the 'good' hemisphere preoperatively.

Hemimegalencephaly

With this condition, hemispherectomy may give a higher success rate, up to 64% achieving Engel class 1 or 2 (Holthausen *et al* 1999). Nevertheless, the patients mostly remain severely disabled in other ways.

Sturge–Weber syndrome (SWS)

In the multicenter study around 86% of those with SWS were considered to have become seizure-free or virtually so after hemispherectomy. Surgery was often undertaken at a very young age (median 0.9 years, range 0.1–9.8). Early surgery has been advocated especially if seizures cannot be controlled during the first year of life, since good cognitive development can be achieved if the epilepsy is abolished and medication can be withdrawn (Engel *et al* 1998; Graveline *et al* 1999). Hemispherectomy may not be necessary if the leptomeningeal angiomatosis is restricted to the posterior part of the hemisphere.

Prenatal and perinatal cerebral infarction/hemorrhage and the hemiconvulsions, hemiplegia, and epilepsy (HHE) syndrome

Both these conditions (vascular and hematrophy) achieved remission rates of around 75% in the multicenter study. Surgery was at mean age 8.2 years for the vascular group and 10.6 years for the HHE syndrome group. This approximates to the success rate for seizure relief reported by Wilson (1970).

Rasmussen encephalitis

Of those with Rasmussen syndrome who underwent hemispherectomy at median age 8.5 years (range 3.3–17.8) in the multicenter study, 75% were considered to be seizure-free or essentially so postoperatively. This is similar to the success rate at Johns Hopkins as reported by Vining (1999). Partial hemisphere resections are usually unsuccessful but may be useful for obtaining a tissue diagnosis before moving on to hemispherectomy provided that it is initially appreciated that this latter will very probably be necessary.

COMPLETENESS OF REMOVAL OF PATHOLOGY

The mechanisms whereby pathology leads to seizures are not understood, but there are various examples of how complete removal of pathology results in a greater likelihood of a more complete relief from the epilepsy.

Thus, Wyler *et al* (1995) have shown in a prospective randomized and blinded trial that total hippocampectomy renders seizure-free a statistically significantly higher proportion of patients with hippocampal sclerosis than does only partial hippocampectomy. Arruda *et al* (1996) have shown that seizure relief after the removal of sclerotic hippocampus is most likely to be followed by complete cessation of the epilepsy if the contralateral hippocampus is normal. Presumably the presence of even mildly sclerotic hippocampus on the nonoperated side is an example of unavoidably remaining pathology. As has been mentioned above, the relatively poor results of surgery for cortical dysplasia are probably because some dysplastic tissue remains *in situ* postoperatively. Likewise, surgery for Rasmussen encephalitis rarely relieves the epilepsy unless the whole affected hemisphere is removed.

It is not entirely clear whether just the pathology or in addition possibly epileptogenic tissue peripheral to the pathology must be removed to achieve the best outcome. Fried and Cascino (1998) conclude that when it is functionally feasible the resection should include some margin around the pathology ('extended lesionectomy'). They do not, however, make specific recommendations concerning how the extent of this margin should be determined.

AGE AT SURGERY

Children

Hemispherectomy is mostly carried out on children or young adolescents. This policy is at least partly determined by the conditions for which it is the indicated treatment. Thus, in Rasmussen encephalitis it is used not only to achieve control of very severe epilepsy but also to try to halt, and to some extent reverse, progressive cognitive decline in a disease that has a predilection for children. In children with vascular or HHE pathology, hemispherectomy is often carried out because the severe epilepsy is accompanied not only by hemiplegia but also by seriously disruptive behavior and antiepileptic drug intoxication. The usual outcome is not only a marked reduction in the frequency of the seizures, if not a complete cessation of the epilepsy, but also a marked improvement in behavior, cognitive gains, and alleviation of the drug intoxication. My personal experience of the Oxford hemispherectomy patients is that the few operated at ages above 16 years make slow, and possibly incomplete, recoveries compared to those operated when younger. So, for hemispherectomy there is little choice but that it should be mostly carried out in childhood or early adolescence.

Falconer (1972) clearly stated his belief that the results of surgery for mesial temporal sclerosis were better when carried out on those aged <16 years than in patients 2–4 decades older. Nevertheless, 25 years later many surgical series report patients operated for this pathology at a mean age 25–35 years after what for many of them has been 20–30 years of intractable epilepsy putting them at social disadvantage. As Spencer (1996) states the contention that earlier epilepsy surgery may produce more beneficial results 'is often stated, but never proved.'

Most children who enter into remission after apparently intractable epilepsy do so within 3 years of its onset, and few who have been referred as candidates for possible epilepsy surgery gain significantly improved seizure control through the correction of apparent omissions of medication (Duchowny 1995). Lindsay *et al* (1984) reviewed people they had ascertained when their complex partial seizure disorder had commenced at age <11 years and who had not remitted by age 16 years. The review was carried out 19–29 years after ascertainment. Only 15% had either remitted spontaneously or achieved adequate control on medication and 16% were dead. In contrast, 85% of 19 children, many of them referred by Janet Lindsay, who underwent temporal lobe epilepsy surgery for mesial temporal sclerosis when aged <16 years were in Engel class 1 at 5 years after surgery (Oxbury *et al* 1996). Statistically significantly more of them were seizure-free off medication than were equivalent patients operated as adults. Some of these children were included in the mixed pathology group operated during 1973–1988 and reported by Adams *et al* (1990), of whom overall 66% became seizure-free. As with the cases reported by Blume *et al* (1997), and in contrast to those reported by Gilliam *et al* (1997), none of the Oxford children underwent intracranial EEG monitoring. The overall outcome was much as in the other series listed by Spencer (1996). As with most other aspects of epilepsy surgery, there are no proper controlled trial data, but it does seem that the child with intractable epilepsy due to mesial temporal sclerosis has a better chance with surgery than without provided that the criteria for surgery are fulfilled.

When MRI of a child with intractable focal epilepsy shows a tumor, albeit a probably indolent or benign dysembryoplastic neuroepithelioma, most would agree that early surgery is advisable if the lesion is situated in a location where removal is unlikely to cause neurologic deficit. Not only is there a high probability that the epilepsy will be alleviated but also apparent indolence cannot be guaranteed.

The more elderly

Data presented by McLachlan *et al* (1992) suggest that the outcome from epilepsy surgery in those aged >45 years may not be so good as in younger adults but that surgery can nevertheless be worthwhile in carefully selected cases.

POSTOPERATIVE PREDICTION OF SUBSEQUENT OUTCOME

SEIZURES DURING THE FIRST TWO POSTOPERATIVE YEARS

Complete freedom from seizures during the early years after surgery is a matter of considerable importance. Elwes *et al* (1991), using actuarial statistics, found that 90% of those who were to achieve a one-year remission after en bloc anterior temporal lobectomy did so within 2 years of the surgery. Ninety percent of those who had not experienced any seizure during the first 2 postoperative years remained seizure-free after a median follow up of 41.5 months.

Seizures within the first postoperative week were excluded. Also, subsequent seizures consisting of auras, defined as short-lived premonitory symptoms with no disturbance of cognitive or motor function, were discounted. The pathology underlying the epilepsy in these patients was various, including mesial temporal sclerosis and 'lesions.' Similarly, Wingkun *et al* (1991) reported that 40–50% of those who have a seizure, again excluding isolated auras, during the first year (including the first postoperative week) after temporal or extratemporal resections continue to have an average of one or more seizures per month during postoperative years 2 to 5. Furthermore, most of the other 50–60% continue to have seizures during these years, albeit less frequently.

Some patients do manifest the running-down phenomenon whereby seizures during the early postoperative years ultimately remit to be followed by prolonged periods of freedom (Salanova *et al* 1996). Ficker *et al* (1999), using the seizure frequency score summarized in Table 57.2, surveyed 214 patients who had undergone temporal lobe excisions at the Mayo Clinic to assess change during the postoperative period by comparing seizure frequency scores between consecutive postoperative years. Improvement was seen in 4.7% patients who had undergone temporal excisions compared to 15% of 59 patients who had undergone frontal resections, the difference being significant ($P = 0.009$). Improvement among the temporal group tended to be maintained, in that 90% of those who had shown improvement obtained scores <5 at their most recent follow-up (mean 3–4 years postsurgery). Deterioration was seen in 11% of the temporals compared to 5.1% of the frontals. Most changes (80% for the temporals and 50% for the frontals) occurred between the first and the second postoperative years. A tendency for control to deteriorate was associated with an older age at surgery among the temporals. The findings are concordant with those of Elwes *et al* (1991).

LONGER-TERM OUTCOME

Rougier *et al* (1992) used a nonhomogenous Markov chain model to take account of both the intravariability of postsurgical outcome and the differences in duration of follow-up in a group of 100 consecutive cortical resections (76 temporal, 23 frontal, 1 parietal). The outcome was estimated to be of major benefit when freedom from seizures was combined with the absence of any new handicap consequent upon the surgery. They estimated that there is a 56% chance of those treated surgically achieving this good state at 5 years postsurgery.

KEY POINTS

1. The ideal outcome from surgery is improved quality of life, resulting from a complete absence of seizures without drug side-effects unaccompanied by any new disability arising from the surgery. Seizure outcome is central to overall outcome, in that patients who are rendered seizure-free report significantly better emotional and psychosocial outcome than do those who are not even to the extent of only having isolated auras. The complete removal of definite pathology is the most powerful factor underlying the complete abolition of seizures without adding neurologic deficit.

2. The most widely used system for classifying seizure outcome is that described by Engel *et al* (1993). It is a combined system, and not strictly quantitative, that attempts both to classify postoperative seizure frequency and to specify whether benefit has been derived. The advantage of a purely quantitive system is that seizure frequency may be specified at regular intervals, such as annually, without any judgment as to whether the seizures are disabling or whether surgery has been beneficial.

3. In general, around 65–70% of appropriately selected patients who have various forms of pathology fully removed become seizure-free, irrespective of whether the removal is from a temporal lobe or is extratemporal. Such a success rate, or better, should be achieved by focal excisions of hippocampal sclerosis, benign tumors (oligodendroglioma, dysembryoplastic neuroepithelioma, and ganglioglioma), and cavernous angioma. Similar success rates may be achieved by hemispherectomy for pre- or perinatal stroke, HHE syndrome, Sturge–Weber syndrome, Rasmussen encephalitis, and hemimegalencephy.

4. A number of factors are associated with a particularly high probability of achieving complete freedom from seizures following surgery for hippocampal sclerosis. They include a history of a prolonged childhood febrile convulsion; strictly unilateral hippocampal smallness as determined by volume measurement; concordance between the imaging, EEG, and neuropsychologic data; surgery at a young age; and total hippocampal removal.

5. Surgery in childhood or early adolescence is particularly efficacious when the pathologic basis of the epilepsy is hippocampal sclerosis, dysembryoplastic neuroepithelioma, or ganglioglioma. Success rates with malformations of cortical development may be considerably lower. Overall, surgery at ages over 45 years may be less successful.

6. Complete freedom from seizures during the first 2 years after epilepsy surgery (excluding the first postoperative week) gives a very good prognosis for continuing freedom from seizures. In contrast, around 50% of those who experience a complex or secondarily generalized seizure during the first postoperative year beyond the first week, will continue to experience at least occasional seizures.

REFERENCES

Abou-Khalil B, Andermann E, Andermann F, Olivier A, Quesney LF (1993). Temporal lobe epilepsy after prolonged febrile convulsions: excellent outcome after surgical treatment. *Epilesia* 34:878–883.

Adams CBT, Beardsworth ED, Oxbury SM, Oxbury JM, Fenwick PBC (1990) Temporal lobectomy in 44 children: outcome and neuropsychological follow-up. *Journal of Epilepsy* 3 (Suppl 1):157–168.

Arruda F, Cendes F, Andermann F (1996) Mesial atrophy and outcome after amygdalohippocampectomy or temporal lobe removal. *Annals of Neurology* 40:446–450.

Berg AT, Vickrey BG (1998) Outcome measures. In: Engel J Jr, Pedley TA (eds) *Epilepsy: A Comprehensive Textbook*, Vol 2, pp 1891–1899. Philadelphia: Lippincott-Raven.

Berkovic SF, McIntosh AM, Kalnins RM, *et al* (1995) Preoperative MRI predicts outcome of temporal lobectomy: an actuarial analysis. *Neurology* 45:1358–1363.

Bladin PF (1992) Psychosocial difficulties and outcome after temporal lobectomy. *Epilepsia* 33:898–907.

Blume WT, Girvin JP, McLachlan RS, Gilmore BE (1997) Effective temporal lobectomy in childhood without invasive EEG. *Epilepsia* 38:164–167.

Bruton CJ (1988) *The Neuropathology of Temporal Lobe Epilepsy* (Institute of Psychiatry Maudsley Monographs 31). Oxford: Oxford University Press.

Burgerman RS, Sperling MR, French JA, Saykin AJ, O'Connor MJ (1995) Comparison of mesial versus neocortical onset temporal lobe seizures: neurodiagnostic findings and surgical outcome. *Epilepsia* 36:662–670.

Cascino GD, Boon PAJM, Fish DR (1993). Surgically remediable lesional syndromes. In: Engel J Jr (ed) *Surgical Treatment of the Epilepsies*, 2nd edn, pp 77–86. New York: Raven Press.

Cendes F, Cook MJ, Watson C, *et al* (1995) Frequency and characteristics of dual pathology in patients with lesional pathology. *Neurology* 45:2058–2064.

Dasheiff RM, Ryan CW, Lave JR (1994). Epilepsy brain surgery: a Pittsburgh experience. *Seizure* 3:197–207.

Daumas-Duport C, Scheithauser BW, Chodkiewicz JP, Laws ER, Vedrenne C (1988) Dysembryoplastic neuroepithelial tumour: a surgically curable tumor of young patients with intractable partial seizures. *Neurosurgery* 23:545–556.

DiRocco C (1996) Surgical treatment of hemimegalencephaly. In: Guerrini R, Andermann F, Canapicchi R, Roger J, Zifkin BG, Pfanner P (eds) *Dysplasias of Cerebral Cortex and Epilepsy*, pp 295–304. New York: Lippincott-Raven.

Duchowny M (1995) Epilepsy surgery in children. *Current Opinion in Neurology* 8:112–116.

Elwes RDC, Dunn G, Binnie CD, Polkey CE (1991). Outcome following resective surgery for temporal lobe epilepsy: a prospective follow up study of 102 consecutive cases. *Journal of Neurology, Neurosurgery and Psychiatry*, 54:949–952.

Engel J Jr (1987) Outcome with respect to epileptic seizures. In: Engel J Jr (ed) *Surgical Treatment of the Epilepsies*, pp 553–571. New York: Raven Press.

Engel J Jr, Van Ness PC, Rasmussen TB, Ojemann LM (1993) Outcome with respect to epileptic seizures. In: Engel J Jr (ed) *Surgical Treatment of the Epilepsies*, 2nd edn. pp 609–621. New York: Raven Press.

Engel J Jr, Cascino GD, Shields WD (1998). Surgically remediable syndromes. In: Engel J Jr, Pedley TA (eds) *Epilepsy: A Comprehensive Textbook*, Vol 2, pp 1687–1696. Philadelphia: Lippincott-Raven.

Falconer MA (1971) Genetic and related aetiological factors in temporal lobe epilepsy: a review. *Epilepsia* 12:13–31.

Falconer MA (1972). Place of surgery of temporal lobe epilepsy during childhood. *British Medical Journal* 2:631–635.

Ferrier CH, Engelsman J, Alarcon G, Binnie CD, Polkey CE (1999). Prognostic factors in presurgical assessment of frontal lobe epilepsy. *Journal of Neurology, Neurosurgery and Psychiatry* 66:350–356.

Ficker DM, So EL, Mosewich RK, Radhakrishnan K, Cascino GD, Sharbrough FW (1999) Improvement and deterioration of seizure control during the postsurgical course of epilepsy surgery patients. *Epilepsia* 40:62–67.

Fried I, Cascino GD (1993) Lesional surgery. In: Engel J Jr (ed) *Surgical Treatment of the Epilepsies*, 2nd edn, pp 501–509. New York: Raven Press.

Fried I, Cascino GD (1998) Lesionectomy. In: Engel J Jr, Pedley TA (eds) *Epilepsy: A Comprehensive Textbook*, pp 1841–1850. Philadelphia: Lippincott-Raven.

Gilliam F, Wyllie E, Kashden J et al (1997) Epilepsy surgery outcome: comprehensive assessment in children. *Neurology* 48:1368–1374.

Graveline C, Hwang PA, Fitzpatrick T, Jay V, Hoffman HJ (1999) Sturge–Weber syndrome: implications of functional studies on neural plasticity, brain maturation, and timing of surgical treatment. In: Kotagal P, Luders HO (eds) *The Epilepsies. Etiologies and Prevention*, pp 61–70. San Diego: Academic Press.

Guerrini R, Dravet C, Bureau M, *et al* (1996) Diffuse and localised dysplasias of the cerebral cortex: clinical presentation, outcome, and proposal for a morphologic MRI classification based on a study of 90 patients. In: Guerrini R, Andermann F, Canapicchi R, Roger J, Zifkin BG, Pfanner P (eds) *Dysplasias of Cerebral Cortex and Epilepsy*, pp 255–270. New York: Lippincott-Raven.

Guldvog B, Loyning Y, Hauglie-Hanssen E, Flood S, Bjornaes H (1991). Surgical versus medical treatment for epilepsy. I. Outcome related to survival, seizures, and neurologic deficit. *Epilepsia* 32:375–388.

Hirabayashi S, Binnie CD, Janota I, Polkey CE (1993) Surgical treatment of epilepsy due to cortical dysplasia: clinical and EEG findings. *Journal of Neurology, Neurosurgery and Psychiatry* 56:765–770.

Holmes MD, Dodrill CB, Ojemann LM, Ojemann GA (1996) Five-year outcome after epilepsy surgery in non-monitored and monitored surgical candidates. *Epilepsia* 37:748–752.

Holthausen H, May TW, Adams CBT et al (1997) In: Tuxhorn I, Holthausern H, Boenigk HE (eds) *Pediatric Epilepsy Syndromes and Their Surgical Treatment*, pp 749–773. London: John Libbey.

Holthausen H, Tuxhorn I, Pieper T, Pannek H, Lahl R, Oppel F (1999) Hemispherectomy in the treatment of neuronal migrational disorders. In: Kotagal P, Luders HO (eds) *The Epilepsies. Etiologies and Prevention*, pp 93–102. San Diego: Academic Press.

ILAE (1998) ILAE Commission on Outcome Measurement in Epilepsy, 1994–1997. Final Report. *Epilepsia* 39:213–231.

Kirkpatrick PJ, Honavar M, Janota I, Polkey CE (1993) Control of temporal lobe epilepsy following en bloc resection of low-grade tumors. *Journal of Neurosurgery* 78:19–25.

Knight ES, Oxbury JM, Oxbury SM, Middleton JA (1998). Cognitive development in children under 12 years of age after temporal lobe epilepsy surgery (TLES) for dysembryoplastic neuroepithelial tumour (DNET). *Epilepsia* 39 (Suppl 6):172.

Kuznieckky R, Garcia JH, Faught E, Morawetz RP (1991) Cortical dysplasia in temporal lobe epilepsy: magnetic resonance imaging correlations. *Annals of Neurology* 29:293–298.

Li LM, Cendes F, Andermann F et al (1999) Surgical outcome in patients with epilepsy and dual pathology. *Brain* 122:799–805.

Lindsay J, Ounsted C, Richards P (1984) Long-term outcome in children with temporal lobe seizures. V. Indications and contra-indications for neurosurgery. *Developmental Medicine and Child Neurology* 26:25–32.

Lindsay J, Ounsted C, Richards P (1987) Hemispherectomy for childhood epilepsy: a 36-year study. *Developmental Medicine and Child Neurology* 29: 592–600.

McLachlan RS, Chovaz CJ, Blume W, Girvin JP (1992) Temporal lobectomy for intractable epilepsy in patients over age 45 years. *Neurology* 42:662–665.

Marson AG, Kadir ZA, Chadwick DW (1996) New antiepileptic drugs: a systematic review of their efficacy and tolerability. *British Medical Journal* 313:1169–1174.

Moran NF, Fish DR, Kitchen N, Shorvon S, Kendall BE, Stevens JM (1999) Supratentorial cavernous angiomas and epilepsy: a review of the literature and case series. *Journal of Neurology, Neurosurgery and Psychiatry* 66:561–568.

Morris HH, Matkovic Z, Estes ML et al (1998) Ganglioglioma and intractable epilepsy: clinical and neurophysiologic features and predictors of outcome after surgery. *Epilepsia* 39:307–313.

O'Brien TJO, Kilpatrick C, Murrie V, Vogrin S, Morris K, Cook MJ (1996) Temporal lobe epilepsy caused by mesial temporal sclerosis and temporal neocortical lesions. A clinical and electroencephalographic study of 46 pathologically proven cases. *Brain* 119:2133–2141.

O'Donoghue MF, Duncan JS, Sander JWAS (1998) The subjective handicap of epilepsy. A new approach to measuring treatment outcome. *Brain* 121: 317–343.

Oxbury JM, Adams CBT, Fenwick PBC, Oxbury SM (1996) Surgery in childhood gives best chance to 'cure' drug-resistant temporal lobe epilepsy due to severe hippocampal sclerosis. *Epilepsia* 37 (Suppl 5):209.

Raymond AA, Halpin SFS, Alsanjari N et al (1994) Dysembryoplastic neuroepithelial tumour. Features in 16 patients. *Brain* 117:461–475.

Raymond AA, Fish DR, Sisodiya SM, Alsanjari N, Stevens JM, Shorvon SD (1995) Abnormalities of gyration, heterotopias, tuberous sclerosis, focal cortical dysplasia, microdysgenesis, dysembryoplastic neuroepithelial tumour and dysgenesis of the archicortex in epilepsy. Clinical, EEG, and neuroimaging features in 100 adult patients. *Brain* 118:629–660.

Rougier A, Dartigues J-F, Commenges D, Claverie B, Loiseau P, Cohadon F (1992) A longitudinal assessment of seizure outcome and overall benefit from 100 corticectomies for epilepsy. *Journal of Neurology, Neurosurgery and Psychiatry* 55:762–767.

Sagar HJ, Oxbury JM (1987) Hippocampal neuron loss in temporal lobe epilepsy: correlation with early childhood convulsions. *Annals of Neurology* 22:334–340.

Salanova V, Andermann F, Rasmussen T, Olivier A, Quesney L (1996) The running down phenomenon in temporal lobe epilepsy. *Brain* **119**:989–996.

Scott CA, Fish DR, Smith SJM (1999) Presurgical evaluation of patients with epilepsy and normal MRI; role of scalp video-EEG telemetry. *Journal of Neurology, Neurosurgery and Psychiatry* **66**:69–71.

Silbergeld DL, Miller JW (1994) Resective surgery for medically intractable epilepsy associated with schizencephaly. *Journal of Neurosurgery* **80**:820–825.

Sisodiya SM, Moran N, Free SL *et al* (1997) Correlation of widespread preoperative magnetic resonance imaging changes with unsuccessful surgery for hippocampal sclerosis. *Annals of Neurology* **41**:490–496.

So EL, Radhakrishnan K, Silbert PL, Cascino GD, Sharbrough FW, O'Brien PC (1997) Assessing changes over time in temporal lobectomy: outcome by scoring seizure frequency *Epilepsy Research* **27**:119–125.

Spencer SS (1996) Long-term outcome after epilepsy surgery. *Epilepsia* **37**: 807–813.

Verity CM, Strauss EH, Moyes PD, Wada JA, Dunn HG, Lapointe JS (1982) Long term follow-up after cerebral hemispherectomy: neurophysiologic, radiologic, and psychologic findings. *Neurology* **32**:629–629.

Vickrey BG, Hays RD, Rausch R *et al* (1995) Outcomes in 248 patients who had diagnostic evaluations for epilepsy surgery. *Lancet* **346**:1445–1449.

Vining EPG (1999) Rasmussen's syndrome. In: Kotagal P, Luders HO (eds) *The Epilepsies. Etiologies and Prevention*, pp 283–288. San Diego: Academic Press.

Whiting SE, Jayakar P, Duchowny M *et al* (1998) The utility of subdural EEG patterns to define the epileptogenic zone in children with cortical dysplasia. *Epilepsia* **39** (Suppl 6):65.

Wilson PJE (1970) Cerebral hemispherectomy for infantile hemiplegia. Report of 50 cases. *Brain* **93**:147–180.

Wingkun EC, Awad IA, Luders H, Awad CA (1991) Natural history of recurrent seizures after resective surgery for epilepsy. *Epilepsia* **32**:851–856.

Wolf HK, Wellmer J, Muller MB, Wiestler OD, Hufnagel A, Pietsch T (1995) Glioneuronal malformative lesions and dysembryoplastic neuroepithelial tumours in patients with chronic pharmacoresistant epilepsies. *Journal of Neuropathology and Experimental Neurology* **54**:245–254.

Wyler AR, Hermann BP, Somes G (1995) Extent of medial temporal resection on outcome from anterior temporal lobectomy: a randomised prospective study. *Neurosurgery* **37**:982–990.

Physical complications of epilepsy surgery 58

CE POLKEY

Any interventional procedure, either for investigation or for treatment, must be accompanied by risk of complications, although there is considerable debate about the precise meaning of that term, which may be interpreted differently by the physician and by the patients and their relatives. The complications from any intervention, and their practical consequences, will also vary with the patient's physical and intellectual state prior to intervention.

Complications can be discussed in relation to several areas. First, there are the general complications of surgery that relate to all procedures. Many of the complications and contraindications to surgery do not apply to the group of patients undergoing these interventions for intractable epilepsy, who usually do not suffer from any other disease and on the whole are aged less than 60 years, the majority less than 40 years. In general, minor respiratory problems, diabetes, etc, can be safely managed by modern anesthesia, but these matters are dealt with in detail in Chapter 56.

Special mention must be made of the potential problems from blood loss, fluid and electrolyte balance, and heat loss in infants and small children, which are dealt with in relation to the specific procedures. However, it is unlikely that patients being considered for epilepsy surgery will have gross contraindications to the procedure or to anesthesia.

It also has to be recalled that at present a high profile is given to audit of surgical procedures, both within professional groups and by patient groups. It is therefore necessary, when discussing a particular procedure with patients and their relatives, to ensure that complications are discussed openly and at a senior level. Both the level of complications encountered in general experience, and those encountered by the particular group concerned should be mentioned.

The general complications of intracranial surgery include hemorrhage, infection, and ischemia and, in addition, a number of small complaints that may be related to the fashioning of the craniotomy and so on.

Although not strictly a physical complication, changes in epileptic status as a result of intervention may be important in the short term.

Finally, there is the question of the possibility of a neurologic defect and the important distinction between those effects that are predicted and were expected and those whose occurrence is rare or completely unexpected. In general in neurosurgery and other branches of surgery there has been debate about the level of complications that should be accepted as expected and therefore about which the patient and their relatives are entitled to be warned, and those complications that are totally unexpected and therefore about which the patient cannot be advised. Because most epilepsy surgery or invasive diagnostic procedures are a matter of choice rather than involving decisions made under pressure of clinical circumstances, the concept and application of informed consent is especially important. A person taking such consent must be sufficiently senior and experienced as to be competent for that task, and the person giving it must have understood the explanation and implications. It may be impossible to achieve this in one session. It is especially important that any such discussion should include the particular experience or facilities of the group undertaking the procedure, since these will influence the possible frequency and severity of complications. It is not clear what legal validity the present operation consent form used in the UK has. It is common sense to make sure that it is countersigned by the operating surgeon or equivalent. A written record that a discussion has taken place regarding the purpose of the procedure and possible complications should exist and if appropriate the actual complications should be listed. In the Sidaway case it was hoped that an objective frequency of any complications would be suggested above which the patient must be warned. However, after appeal to the House of Lords it was stated that the surgeon must only warn of those complications that a reasonable body of professional practitioners would warn the patient of, and that – in the UK at any rate – is where the matter stands (Anonymous 1985). This is in keeping with the Bolam test, which uses the proposition that practitioners cannot be accused of negligence if they act in accordance with practice accepted at the time by a responsible body of medical opinion (Anonymous 1957). It is therefore clear that the level of warning is a matter for discretion by a responsible practitioner who has to draw the line between giving sufficient information to allow the patient to make an informed decision and warning patients in such a way as to deter them from accepting interventional treatment. This is especially true of complex investigations, which should not be pursued if the patient is unwilling to accept the outcome, including complications, of the proposed ultimate therapeutic procedure.

COMPLICATIONS OF PREOPERATIVE TESTS

There are two groups of tests that have the potential for serious unwanted physical effects. These are the intracarotid sodium amytal test, which involves angiography, and the insertion of various numbers and types of intracranial electrodes.

INTRACAROTID SODIUM AMYTAL TEST

Whatever the eventual target vessel, the approach is transfemoral and, because modern neuroradiologists are extremely skillful, and because most patients in the preoperative

assessment program are young and fit, complications at the puncture site and in threading the catheter up the aorta are almost unrecorded. The general level for spasm or consequent embolism in the femoral artery or its branches is that of the procedures overall and is very low, as is the occurrence of neurologic complications. A survey of recent literature describing cerebral angiography indicates an incidence of around 1–5% for some kind of transient problem, with transient neurologic problems having an incidence of 0.5–1% and permanent neurologic problems an incidence of 0.1–0.3% (Grzyska et al 1990; Kachel et al 1991; Waugh and Sacharias 1992). Among at least 150 amytal tests over 20 years, we have had no permanent complications; one patient aged 42 developed a mild and transient paraparesis thought to be due to the dislodging of an intimal plaque blocking a lumbar branch of the aorta. In the same group there were five patients (>3%) with evidence of transient neurologic deficit (all a mild hemiparesis) resolving over periods between 2 hours and 36 hours. They were all commenced on steroids but were not given anticoagulants.

There are a number of valid criticisms of the standard Wada test in which the injection is made into the internal carotid artery and a number of modifications of the test, called selective amytal tests, have been described. Although their theoretical justification is not simple, they have in common selective catheterization of small arteries or sometimes balloon occlusion by combination of these to restrict the circulation of the amytal to the medial temporal structures. Borchgrevink et al in Oslo describes selective injection into the middle cerebral artery trunk as being more satisfactory than internal carotid artery catheterization (Borchgrevink et al 1993). Jack et al were the first to describe selective catheterization of the posterior circulation. This has given rise to some complications (Jack et al 1988; Rausch et al 1993). Wieser describes a balloon occlusion method applied with no problems (Wieser et al 1989). A patient undergoing the standard ICSA test should therefore be advised that the complication rate is low and that no permanent effects have been seen. Advice to patients undergoing a selective test needs to be given more carefully and, where appropriate, should include local data for the procedure.

As far as tests for bilateral secondary synchrony are concerned, there is no advantage to a selective test. In these patients, however, there may be dangers in the total dose of amytal or other intravenous anesthetic agents used, especially if an isoelectric EEG recording is necessary, and there should be careful consultation with the anesthetist about the care and monitoring of these patients during the test and during recovery.

MINOR INVASIVE RECORDING

This includes sphenoid electrodes, which are free of permanent effects, although there may be transient discomfort.

Epidural peg electrodes

These are not commonly used. In a personal report by Wyllie, quoted by Pilcher (Pilcher *et al* 1993), bacterial colonization was seen in 22%, a hematoma on CT in one patient, and two patients were sufficiently anaemic to require transfusion.

Foramen ovale electrodes

These are placed through the foramen ovale, and therefore through the trigeminal nerve fibers, to lie in the ambient cistern between the medial temporal structures and the brain stem. The method was originally conceived and described by Wieser (Siegfried *et al* 1985; Wieser *et al* 1985) and has come into use in a number of centers (Kuzniecky *et al* 1990; Awad *et al* 1991). Clearly, the correct technique is important and most centers treating substantial numbers of patients now use smooth multicontact (four to six contacts) electrodes introduced through a suitable cannula (Wieser and Moser 1988). There are unpublished anecdotal reports of death from hemorrhage and complete avulsion of the trigeminal nerve when unsuitable electrodes or cannulas have been used. The chief complications are damage to the nerve usually during insertion, hemorrhage within the subarachnoid or subdural space, usually of no consequence, misplacement of the electrode within the cerebral substance with or without significant hemorrhage, and finally infection. We have investigated over 200 patients with these electrodes, the majority having bilateral placements over the last 6 or 7 years. Temporary swelling of the face and some transient numbness in the nerve distribution occurs in some of these patients and is related to the skill of the operator. However, in recent times we have found it prudent to limit the number of attempts at placement. In a small proportion of patients (not more than 5%) it is impossible to insert the electrodes on one or the other side and then another attempt may be made some weeks later. We now feel that no more than two attempts are appropriate and if they are not successful we proceed to subdural strips. Among these patients are a small number (less than 2%) with permanent numbness in one or more divisions in the fifth nerve and only one with persistent facial pain. Wieser reports transient perioral dysesthesiae in 9% of a series of 101 patients (Wieser *et al* 1993). Misplacement of the electrode is difficult to diagnose with certainty; in some patients the electrode clearly curves across the floor of the middle fossa, indicating proper placement, but in others it takes a straighter course that could indicate penetration of the brain substance. Known penetration of the brain with clinical consequences has been seen by us on only four occasions and there were serious consequences in only two of these patients. In one there was a disorder of eye movement that resolved completely, and in the other a capsular hemorrhage resulted in a permanent hemiparesis. Wieser reported one transient pontine syndrome and one subarachnoid hemorrhage in his group of 101 patients (Wieser *et al* 1993). Stefan has reported serious problems in a group of patients who had previously undergone temporal lobe surgery (Schuler *et al* 1993). Our patients are covered with antibiotics and we ensure that the electrode is not penetrating the buccal mucosa. We have had about five cases of frank meningitis (2%), including one unsuccessful placement, all of which responded to appropriate treatment. Wyllie reports 2 cases in 32 patients (Schuler *et al* 1993).

INVASIVE RECORDING

The use of both subdural and intracerebral electrodes, either separately or in combination, has potentially serious risks in terms of infection and intracranial hemorrhage, extradural, subdural, and intracerebral. These are well documented elsewhere in the book.

Infection and CSF leakage during invasive monitoring

Although these problems are seen during minor invasive recording with foramen ovale electrodes and subtemporal strips, they are much commoner with large arrays and numbers of electrodes. In all cases prophylactic antibiotics are used from just before insertion until after removal. Meningitis has occurred, even with unsuccessful insertion, in less than 1% of foramen ovale insertions and responds well to antibiotics.

With the subdural electrode arrays and intracerebral placement of depth electrodes, infection is much more of a risk. The electrode leads should be brought out through an incision remote from that used for access, and the electrodes should be left in place for as short a time as possible. Leakage of CSF, especially along the nonreactive leads from subdural electrodes, is almost impossible to prevent. However, it will often diminish considerably, or cease, after the first 24 hours, especially if the head is kept elevated. When such leakage is great, the frequent changing of bandages will help to prevent colonization by secondary organisms and also prevent the offence that poor hygiene can give to others.

Because patients with intracerebral or subdural electrodes may have their craniotomies opened several times, there tends to be an accumulation of organized and granulation tissue that is more prone to infection. The occurrence of swelling of the wound, or discharge, should never be attributed solely to superficial wound infection.

Invasive recording comprises the placement of electrodes in the subdural space, within the brain substance, commonly referred to as depth electrodes, and combinations of the two. Such electrodes are used chiefly for recording but occasionally for stimulation. Provided the parameters of current and voltage are controlled, there are no known adverse effects of this kind of stimulation. To avoid entering the subdural space, Goldring pioneered the use of extradural plastic grids in children (Goldring and Gregorie 1984).

SUBDURAL ELECTRODES

The use of these varies in number, location, and size. The majority consist of plastic strips or mats, but in groups who use combined subdural and depth electrodes the subdural electrodes may be thin reeds or wire bundles. The complications are increased with increasing size and number of electrodes and the duration of implantation. Subdural or subarachnoid hemorrhage is rare; care must be taken when the electrodes have to be passed into inaccessible areas, such as the medial surface of the hemisphere, to advance them with caution. Blood collecting in the subdural space or even extradurally is uncommon because of careful technique and also because the bulk of the electrodes tends to discourage this. We have seen a substantial collection in 3 of 66 grid implantations (4.5%). Wyler *et al* report no such complications in 350 patients (Wyler *et al* 1991).

Infection is clearly a risk in any situation where cables have to come to the outside and can be minimized by three maneuvers: the use of antibiotic cover; bringing the cables out of the site remote from the main incision; and minimizing the duration of the implantation. We have also made it our custom, whenever possible, to carry out the definitive procedure when the electrodes are removed. Dural closure after placement of the electrodes is rarely a problem but there is always bound to be a point of potential CSF leakage when the cables come out and CSF will track along them. Elevation of the head and changing of soiled dressings is all that can be done to control this. On one occasion out of 35 major grid implantations we have seen an adverse reaction consisting of brain swelling in a young woman with a severe frontal injury previously operated elsewhere. Other centers report an incidence of frank meningitis or other intracranial infection following subdural implantation

of 1% or less. Wyler reported that they had an overall infection rate of 0.85% and that the particular antibiotic (cefazolin) that was given to half of the patients had no influence on this infection rate. The average implantation time in their series was 4.5 days; we try to keep it to less than 4 days (Wyler *et al* 1991). In 66 implantations, immediate infection was seen in 6 patients (9%) and at a late stage after further therapeutic surgery in 3 patients (4.5%).

INTRACRANIAL (DEPTH) ELECTRODES

Centers using depth electrodes report an incidence of infection of about 2%. The variation is not great, Van Buren reporting the cumulative data from 879 patients pooled from 14 centers as a rate of 1.3% (Van Buren 1987); later figures culled by Pilcher *et al* give an average of 1.75% (Pilcher *et al* 1993).

Other complications of depth electrode insertion will be discussed in relation to the approach used by the surgeon. There are three common approaches: the orthogonal approach, in which the electrodes are inserted from a lateral direction usually through individual drill holes in the skull; the axial approach, in which they are inserted parallel to the midline, usually through bifrontal entry points; and the posterior approach, in which they are inserted along the length of the hippocampus from an occipital entry point. This latter has produced visual field defects that are not seen with other approaches (Spencer 1987). Neurologic deficit can occur as a consequence of depth electrode insertion and is usually assumed to be due to hemorrhage, either occult or overt. Whether it is necessary to have a detailed angiographic map while placing depth electrodes is not clear and may depend upon the approach. Clearly, in the orthogonal approach, where major vessels are certain to lie in the trajectory of the electrode, it is essential, especially if the entry points are through twist-drill holes. Even in this situation, demonstrable hemorrhage has been reported in 1%. In the other approaches, the electrodes traverse areas free of major vessels, except at their insertion point where the cortical vessels are visible. The overall occurrence of cerebral hemorrhage in the pooled data collected by Van Buren in 1987 indicates an incidence of 1.9% for transient hemorrhage, with permanent effects in 0.8% (Van Buren 1987). Inspection of the detailed reports from various centers at the First Palm Desert Symposium indicates a variation between 3% and 1%. Centers using the orthogonal approach tended also to carry out angiography to guide the insertion. The suggestion made by Pilcher *et al* that the incidence of cerebral hemorrhage as a result of depth electrode implantation is less when the orthogonal approach is used (1–2%) than when other approaches are used (2–3%) appears to be true, although whether this is due to the approach alone or to other factors is not clear (Pilcher *et al* 1993).

It would be logical to suppose that the complication rate for the use of depth electrodes will be related to the number of penetrations, and therefore some workers have sought to reduce this risk by using combined subdural and depth electrodes, thereby reducing the average number of electrodes inserted in each patient. Van Veelen *et al* (1990), using no more than two electrodes per side in 28 patients, report no hemorrhage. In our series of 56 patients using combined subdural and depth electrodes, with 4–6 depth electrodes on each side, we have suffered three significant episodes of deep hemorrhage, which we attribute to details of the electrode insertion technique.

Death attributable to invasive procedures is very rare. Figures in the literature suggest none for the Wada test and minor invasive procedures and very low levels (Van Buren 1987) for major invasive procedures.

Drug withdrawal

There are dangers in the drug withdrawal necessary to provoke seizures because of the increased seizure activity that results and the possible consequences of this. A delicate balance is necessary because, if the patient experiences frequent seizures or status epilepticus, not only may the seizures be unrepresentative of their habitual seizures but the electrographic recordings may deteriorate so as to be uninterpretable for the purpose for which they are being obtained. Patients who have had their medication reduced and who have been sleep-deprived can become moody and difficult. In addition, very occasionally, there may be significant periods of confusion and very rarely frankly psychotic behavior.

THERAPEUTIC PROCEDURES: INTRODUCTION

Mortality in modern series of epilepsy surgery is low. At the first Palm Desert Symposium figures of around 0.5% were given for temporal lobectomy and similar figures were quoted by Pilcher for the Second Symposium (Van Buren 1987; Pilcher *et al* 1993). The ILAE global report gives no mortality from 35/40 centers and a mean direct operative mortality of 1% from the remaining five centers (Anonymous 1997). It might be thought that there would be more mortality in series of children's operations, but Ventureyra and Higgins report no mortality in 47 chil-

Table 58.1 Perioperative mortality in Maudsley Hospital epilepsy surgery series 1976–1998.

Procedure		Deaths	
	No.	No.	%
Temporal lobe resections	386	2	0.52
Other resections	120	1	0.83
Hemispherectomies	47	1	2.1
Total	553	4	0.72

Note: There were no deaths from intracranial electrode insertion (n = 126) or from functional surgery (n = 89).

dren, mean age 6 years (Ventureyra and Higgins 1993); Adelson and colleagues report one death in a neonate among 33 children, mean age 7 years (Adelson *et al* 1992); and Morrison *et al* report one death in 79 children, mean age 9 years (Rougier *et al* 1992). In our own series there were no deaths from operations to place intracranial electrodes or from functional surgery. In our 553 resective operations there were 4 perioperative deaths (0.72%) and 13 late deaths (2.9%); the details are given in Table 58.1. There were two unexplained deaths among the perioperative deaths, in both cases cerebral edema supervened in the first few hours after surgery and at postmortem examination no cause of death was established. One patient underwent a totally uneventful right 'en bloc' temporal lobectomy. The other patient underwent a hemispherectomy and at autopsy the remaining hemisphere of that patient was grossly abnormal in addition to the edema. Without going into detail, some care is necessary in children, where blood loss is of some importance especially in relation to the major sinuses.

GENERAL NEUROSURGICAL COMPLICATIONS

The complications of craniotomy are equally likely with an investigatory or a therapeutic procedure. Indeed, with an investigatory procedure, such as the insertion of subdural mats, the possibility of hemorrhage may be increased because of the short interval between opening and closing the head, reducing the efficacy of natural hemostasis. In general, in therapeutic craniotomies, the risk of extradural hematoma is low, in our series 0.5–1%. It presents in the classical way, is treated by rapid evacuation, and usually has no permanent sequelae. Subdural hematomas are even rarer in therapeutic operations, although they are somewhat commoner after mat insertion. The acute and chronic consequences of hemispherectomy, and their prevention, are dealt with in detail in Chapter 53.

The incidence of infection is relatively low, being put at between 1.3% and 3.4% by Van Buren and in the later assessment by Pilcher at around 0.5% (Van Buren 1987; Pilcher *et al* 1993). As already noted, in our series it is commoner when intracranial monitoring has been used. Occasionally the patient appears to have meningitis or a meningitic reaction, but more commonly it appears in the extradural space, often involving the bone flap. Although there may be evidence of it in the immediate postoperative period, it can take months or years to declare itself. The routine use of prophylactic antibiotics has reduced it to a level that is still greater than for routine craniotomies for other purposes. In our institution we would attribute this to two reasons. The first is the relative length of epilepsy operations, usually extending to greater than 5 hours. The second is the use of ECoG, which introduces a potential pathway for infection and also increases the number of people and movements in the operating theater. Treatment of established infection employs well-established principles of isolating the responsible organism, using vigorous appropriate antibiotic treatment and the surgical removal of dead and infected tissue where necessary. In temporal lobe surgery we have reduced the infection rates by covering any mastoid air cells with a pericranial graft as soon as they are exposed. No patient in our series has died or come to permanent harm from infection. It does not appear to affect the seizure outcome of the operation, but the misery it can cause to all parties should not be underestimated.

INTRACRANIAL RESECTIVE SURGERY

Accepting the levels of general neurosurgical complications described, it is necessary to look in some detail at the particular problems associated with specific resections, which generally speaking produce physical neurologic deficit, changes in intellectual ability, or psychiatric morbidity. This chapter is concerned chiefly with physical defects, that is, neurologic complications. For this purpose we will divide these into frontal, temporal, parietal and central, occipital, and major resections and hemispherectomy. Where appropriate, reference will be made to additional complications from operating in the dominant hemisphere. It hardly needs to be said that the avoidance of complications by careful subpial dissection of the cortex (possibly using the CUSA) and proper respect for the arterial and venous blood supply with skeletalization where appropriate will help to reduce postoperative scarring and unexpected or apparently unexplained ischemic damage.

Frontal lobe resection

These are, of course, unilateral frontal lobe resections; bifrontal resections for epilepsy are not done. Proper technique would ensure no damage to the medial surface of the remaining hemisphere or its blood supply. Even with formal resection it is theoretically possible to avoid damage to the olfactory tract. Unless the resection encroaches upon the gyrus anterior to the precentral gyrus in a nondominant hemisphere, it is unlikely to produce any hemiparesis. Of course, in the dominant hemisphere the region of Broca's area must be respected and it is recommended by Crandall that such resections should be carried out under local anesthesia (Crandall 1987). However Olivier and Awad suggest that this is not always reliable and that anatomically the posterior 2.5 cm of the third frontal convolution should be spared (Olivier and Awad 1993). Resection from the supplementary motor area (SSMA) can sometimes result in a reversible syndrome of contralateral neglect or hemiparesis, mutism, and diminished spontaneous movements. Recovery occurs over some weeks.

Temporal lobe resections

Mortality and nonneurological morbidity

Peroperative mortality is low, around 0.39% in the pooled material described at the First Palm Desert Symposium (Van Buren 1987). In the latest review it is put at less than 1%, with some centers such as the Montreal Neurological Institute (MNI) reporting no deaths in 526 cases (Pilcher *et al* 1993). In our own series there have been only two postoperative deaths (0.52%); one patient developed a deep vein thrombosis and then hemorrhaged as a result of anticoagulant therapy, and another patient had unexplained cerebral edema at the end of uneventful surgery with no apparent cause at autopsy. Other nonneurological complications are acceptably low and perhaps the commonest is postoperative infection, which is given at 0.5% in the Second Palm Desert Symposium (Pilcher *et al* 1993).

Late mortality following temporal lobe surgery is a different matter. Jensen notes that there is an excess mortality among chronic epileptics, around 59.4 deaths per 1000 patients, and that suicide was a common cause of death in this group (Jensen 1975a). However, although the early postoperative deaths in the operated patients were low, there were 50 late deaths in 2282 patients, 21.9 per 1000 or around 2%. Of these, 31 were either suicide or epilepsy and these patients tended to be those who had not benefited from surgery. Taylor and Marsh, reporting on the deaths in Falconer's series, noted that there had been 37 deaths in 193 patients (19%) and that 23 of these deaths were either in circumstances that related to epilepsy or by suicide, half the suicides occurring in patients who were seizure-free (Taylor and Marsh 1977). In our 305 consecutive temporal lobe resections there were 17 other deaths (5.6%), 13 of which were epilepsy related, and 6 of these were sudden and unexpected with no cause found at autopsy (SUDEP). It is clear that surgery reduces the excess mortality among drug-resistant epileptics but does not remove it completely.

Neurologic sequelae

The neurologic sequelae of temporal lobe resections are now acceptably low. Lesionectomy and neocortical removal are least likely to produce such problems so long as the superior temporal gyrus is respected. The sequelae of combined neocortical and deep removal and of selective mesial resections are similar and, on the whole, since the inception of temporal lobe surgery the complication rate has fallen. There is no point in a detailed history of this except to note that resection of the insular cortex was found at an early stage, by the MNI, to run a high risk of hemiparesis – called manipulation hemiplegia because it probably resulted from manipulation of branches of the middle cerebral artery – without any increased improvement in seizure relief (Penfield *et al* 1961). The commonest neurologic sequelae of temporal lobe resection are a contralateral hemiparesis or hemiplegia, a contralateral visual field defect, and a homolateral third-nerve palsy or paresis. Jensen provides a good summary of the experience up to 1975 (Jensen 1975b) and subsequent results are to be found in the two Palm Desert Symposia (Van Buren 1987; Pilcher *et al* 1993). The avoidance of hemiplegia or hemiparesis must be related mainly to vascular causes, especially in selective mesial resections. In combined resections the risk varies between zero and 1–2%, being lower in larger series; in selective amygdalohippocampectomy it varies between less than 0.5% in the Zurich series to 4.2% in our series, and two transient hemiparesis (3.2%) in Renella's series (Renella 1989).

Falconer and Wilson showed that the relationship between the length of a temporal lobe resection and the subsequent visual field cut was due to the course of the visual fibers around the temporal horn (Falconer and Wilson 1958). Such visual field defects relate to the disruption of the fibers in the roof of the temporal horn (Babb *et al* 1982). Awad and his colleagues in their analysis of postoperative MRI scans showed that the more lateral the resection the more likely it was to produce a deficit, although there was no close correlation between the size

of the resection and the severity of the visual field defect (Katz *et al* 1989). The size of the defect cannot be predicted with resections of less than 7.5 cm (Pilcher *et al* 1993). Spencer's extended lobectomy does not produce more visual field defects than the standard operation (Spencer *et al* 1984). Rarely, visual field defects may result from vascular causes, although neither Yasargil nor Renella report any hemianopia following selective amygdalohippocampectomy.

Central and parietal resections

Any question of resection from the central area, that is, the primary motor or sensory area, must carry some risk of loss of function and this risk will be related to the pathology of the underlying disease process, which may have already produced a disability or displaced the cortex away. But it will also be related to the ability to identify these areas, which can now be done noninvasively with MRI and AC-PC coordinates (Olivier and Awad 1993) or possibly with functional MRI. Alternatively, mapping by stimulation during chronic intracranial recording (Wyler 1992), or directly at the surgery, will achieve the same effect. In spite of these precautions, unexpected deficits may occur. Although these could be due to wrong identification of the primary areas, it may also occur if secondary vascular damage takes place because an artery or vein passing through a resected area is damaged, a mechanism postulated by Olivier (Olivier and Awad 1993). In the same review, Olivier notes that, when there is no voluntary hand movement, position sense is absent, and there is paresis of the lower limb, then the whole central area can be resected. It has to be recalled that it is equally important to identify the postcentral gyrus in order to avoid profound proprioceptive loss in the hand or arm, which can be more disabling than pure motor loss.

It is possible to carry out resections in some areas of motor function with acceptance of some deficit. However, resection of the hand area always produces deficit of fine motor movements and should be avoided. Opinions vary about resection of the nondominant face area, but any resection should be limited superiorly to 2–3 mm below the thumb area. It is also possible to resect some of the nondominant parietal lobe without apparent effect except for some transient sensorimotor dysfunction (Pilcher and Rusyniak 1993).

In the dominant hemisphere, resections from the posterior temporal or parietal region run the risk of receptive aphasia, dyslexia, dysgraphia, and dyscalculia. For this reason, resections from these areas are usually avoided.

Occipital resections

Occipital resections are rare; there are three series in the literature and the largest number of patients described is 42. Attempting to avoid a visual field defect by carrying out a temporal resection where the discharges spread into that area rather than an occipital resection was found to be of limited benefit by Palmini *et al* (1993). In two of the series it is noted that there were already preoperative visual field defects, 56% in one series (Williamson *et al* 1992) and 59% in the other (Salanova *et al* 1992). In the second series the visual field defect was completed in all patients and five others acquired a defect, also complete, making an overall incidence after operation of 76%. Bidzinski also noted that a complete occipital resection always produced some visual field defect (Bidzinski *et al* 1992). However, two of the patients undergoing lesionectomy described by Cascino *et al* had no defect (Cascino *et al* 1990). Williamson *et al* (1992) note that most patients adapted to their visual field defect within one year of surgery.

Major resections

These are defined as resections that involve more than one anatomic lobe. The creation of such a space within the cranial cavity does not itself create any special problems, although the patients tend to be more constitutionally ill and cerebrally irritable postoperatively than those undergoing lesser resections. The creation or persistence of neurologic deficits, especially limb dysfunction such as hemiparesis or hemisensory loss, visual field defects, or deterioration of speech function, is often related to the original pathology, which may already have produced such defects. By and large they can only be judged for each individual patient, but with one exception they are unlikely to be substantially increased by the resection. The exception is any form of cortical dysplasia or hemimegalencephaly-type syndrome where function may be preserved in the presence of severe epileptic disorder.

Hemispherectomy

Although hemispherectomy is a serious operation, it is likely that the mortality rate of 4% quoted at the First Palm Desert Symposium (Ribaric 1991) probably includes series of patients operated upon over a long period of time and more recent series do not have such mortality (Rodhan *et al* 1992). Nevertheless, in small children it can present a complex and serious anesthetic problem (Brian 1990).

It is impossible to discuss this topic without some reference to the various techniques available that are aimed at reducing serious side-effects, and to the underlying pathology, which determines the extent of the additional damage inflicted by the surgery. In our practice, and most others, patients coming to hemispherectomy or equivalent operation fall into three groups. The first is those with a major hemispheric insult at a very early age that is not progressive. Examples of this are *in utero* vascular occlusion, the consequences of a major venous thrombosis, etc., and Sturge–Weber disease. These patients usually have a complete infantile hemiplegia and average to low cognitive function. Their neurologic status is usually unchanged by surgery and their cognitive function can be unchanged or improved (Beardsworth and Adams 1988). The second group are those with Rasmussen disease (Rasmussen *et al* 1958) where the hemiplegia may not be complete and there may be no visual field defect.

Complications with regard to technique relate to the difficulties of such a major operation in infants and young children and to the fate of the large space created. In infants and young children problems may arise with regard to blood loss, which, even if the operation is conducted carefully, may be sufficient to require transfusion. The worst problem is venous bleeding, which may be torrential and difficult to control in the short term. The position of the head has to be a compromise between too much elevation, which would risk air embolism, and too little, which would increase venous pressure, making hemostasis more difficult to secure. Two simple maneuvers may help. The first is to ensure that all veins draining into major venous sinuses are divided close to the brain surface, leaving a suitable stump to coagulate if the initial coagulation is not secure and minimizing the risk of tearing the sinus. The second is to take particular care in the posterior dissection around the tent, where tributaries may lead into the great vein of Galen or straight sinus. There is also a theoretic possibility that maneuvers to control severe bleeding from the superior sagittal sinus may lead to thrombosis of this sinus, although I have not seen it personally.

As is well known, and dealt with elsewhere in this book, there are a number of variants of hemispherectomy that were devised to overcome the well-documented consequences of classical hemispherectomy as described by Krynauw (1950). These complications of hemosiderosis and associated conditions occur even with modern techniques (Oppenheimer and Griffith 1966; Rasmussen 1973). The remedies include subtotal hemispherectomy (Rasmussen 1975), functional hemispherectomy (Sass *et al* 1992), and exclusion of the space from the CSF pathways as suggested by Adams (1983). They all seem to be effective in this regard. Functional hemispherectomy also has less risk of major venous hemorrhage. Some patients, 4 out of 35 in our series, may require shunting of the remaining ventricle after modified hemispherectomy. Another solution, more recently proposed, is that of hemispherectomy where fiber tracts are divided to isolate the hemisphere without major tissue resection (Delalande *et al* 1993). The results with regard to seizure control are said to be good and no large space is created, nor is there any risk of substantial blood loss, which may be important in small children. Holthausen has reviewed the results of hemispherectomy and notes that changes in limb function are related to the original pathology and the stage of myelination. Patients with acquired lesions lose more function after hemi spherectomy than patients with developmental problems (Holthausen *et al* 1997).

FUNCTIONAL SURGERY

These procedures can be divided into three groups: interruption of fiber tracts as in callosotomy and multiple subpial transection; stereotactic creation of lesions within the brain; and stimulation of deep brain and other nervous system structures.

CALLOSAL SECTION

Complications from callosal section depend upon the extent of the section and the nature of the underlying disease process. When carried out as an alternative to hemispherectomy in unilateral hemisphere disease, it is clearly sensible to approach the midline from the damaged side. Also, in those patients there is more likely to be mixed cerebral speech dominance, which may have important consequences as we shall see later. Finally, planning of the approach may be important and this will depend upon whether a total or partial section is intended. In any event, the approach should be made so as to avoid interruption of major tributaries to the superior sagittal sinus. From here the complications may be divided into acute and chronic and in both cases they are related to the extent of the resection, being minimal with a truncal section and greatest with an anterior two-thirds or total section. Venous ischemia or even thrombosis, when unilateral, would manifest itself as a hemiparesis with the possible addition of focal seizures. There may be transient paresis, usually affecting one leg, due to retraction on the medial surface of the hemisphere. More serious, however, is the risk of akinetic mutism, probably the result of bilateral anterior cerebral artery spasm. In the first report by Van Wagenen and Bogen in 1940 there were two patients out

of ten who acquired an hemiparesis, thought to be due to cerebral venous thrombosis (Van Wagenen and Herren 1940). However, the Dartmouth group reported a series of eight patients in 1977 with a very high complication rate that they attributed to the attempts to carry out an extensive one-stage operation (Wilson *et al* 1977). They therefore modified their procedure by staging it, performing a less extensive callosotomy, and using the operating microscope. In this second series the complication rate was much lower (Wilson *et al* 1982). However, even in series published in the late 1980s and 1990s there is still a significant incidence of both general complications and neurologic complications, although they tend to be transient. Thus, Kimball *et al* report three deaths in 52 operations including one air embolism and one extradural hematoma (Kimball *et al* 1989). The MNI, reporting 43 operations, had no deaths but some complications in 16 patients, including 3 patients with transient weakness of the right leg and 4 with decreased speech output, also transient (Oguni *et al* 1991). In a series from Memphis of 80 patients undergoing 90 procedures, there were 2 deaths, one from air embolism, and 5 significant complications. In a French series of 26 children, transient complications were recorded in 30%, all of which resolved within 3 months (Pinard *et al* 1991). In our own series of 27 patients undergoing anterior callosotomy, there have been two instances of acute anterior cerebral ischemia, both of which recovered completely. We have had transient limb weakness in a few patients and an extradural hematoma in one. In summary, the risk of death at callosotomy seems to be between zero and 6%, that of permanent neurologic deficit less than 5%, but that of transient deficit up to 5%.

The possible and complex cognitive complications of callosal section are seen in two areas. The first comprises changes in speech function in patients of mixed cerebral dominance for speech, where interhemispheric communication is essential for the proper comprehension and production of speech and related functions. This was first reported by Sass *et al* (1990). It has been suggested, but is by no means the universal opinion, that a carotid amytal test to establish speech dominance should precede the surgery in every case and the operation, especially total section, refused to those of mixed dominance.

Finally, callosal section may produce an alteration in the patient's fit pattern so that certain kinds of seizures such as myoclonic jerks or absent seizures may be more frequent.

MULTIPLE SUBPIAL TRANSECTION

This is a relatively new procedure that has proved effective in the hands of the originator and is used by a number of groups but has resulted in few publications. It is used in eloquent areas. There have been occasional hematomas in a published series but no lasting changes. Both Morrell (Morrell *et al* 1989) and Rougier (Rougier *et al* 1996) reported transient sensory changes in their patients.

STEREOTACTIC LESIONS

The creation of lesions in apparently normal brain to control epilepsy by modification of brain activity has been proposed and has been performed for many years by a number of methods. Generally speaking, they are directed at temporal and extratemporal targets. The clear sources of complications specific to this group must be poor placement of the target and hemorrhage at the target site or along the track of the probe (Young 1990).

Recently there have been reports of stereotactically directed radiosurgery for epilepsy, but these are too few and too recent to allow assessment of possible complications (Barcia-Solorio *et al* 1992; Heikkinen *et al* 1992).

STIMULATION

Clearly the use of chronic indwelling stimulating electrodes will run the risk of complications commonly associated with such apparatus. These must include implant failure and infection, which are relatively rare and occur with the same frequency as with any other implanted device. When the stimulating electrodes are intracranial, there is also the possibility of CSF leakage. Deep brain stimulation for epilepsy has been directed at two targets, the cerebellum and the thalamic nuclei.

Cerebellar stimulation was introduced by Cooper (1973) but subsequently shown to be ineffectual (Wright *et al* 1985). Complications were rare; there were anecdotal reports of sudden death but these occur in epilepsy anyway. Deep brain stimulation has also been applied to the thalamic nuclei, more recently by Velasco *et al* (1995). The same potential complications must exist as with stereotactic lesioning, mainly malposition of the electrodes and hemorrhage.

Vagus nerve stimulation was first introduced in 1990 (Uthman *et al* 1990) and by 1998 over 2500 implantations had been made worldwide. The complication rate has been very low. There have been instances of infection, transient vocal cord paralysis, and of SUDEP, although the incidence of the latter is not thought to be greater than it would be in the group of severe epileptics who are being treated with this device (Handforth *et al* 1998).

KEY POINTS

1. The physical complications of epilepsy surgery are well documented.
2. The complications related to investigations are infrequent and occur only in major invasive procedures such as carotid amytal tests or intracranial electrode insertion. Mortaility is zero and morbidity is 5–10% and only severe in half of these patients.
3. Complications of therapeutic procedures are general and local. General complications are infection and hemorrage which affect 1–2% of the patients and usually resolve without permanent sequelae.
4. Mortality in the perioperative period is low, <0.5% for temporal lobe resections rising to 2% for hemispherectomy. Late mortality is significant, up to 5% in temporal lobe resections.
5. The neurological sequelae of focal resections, including temporal lobe resections, vary with the site of the resection, but unexpected deficits occur in 1–2% of cases.
6. The mortality and morbidity from functional surgery is equally low.

REFERENCES

Adams CBT (1983) Hemispherectomy – a modification. *Journal of Neurology, Neurosurgery and Psychiatry* **46**:617–619.

Adelson PD, Peacock WJ, Chugani HT *et al* (1992) Temporal and extended temporal resections for the treatment of intractable seizures in early childhood. *Pediatric Neurosurgery* **18**(4):169–178.

Anonymous (1957) *Bolam vs Friern Hospital Management Committee* 1 WLR 582.

Anonymous (1985) *Sidaway vs Governors Bethlem Royal Hospital* 1 AC 871.

Anonymous (1997) A global survey on epilepsy surgery, 1980–1990: a report by the Commission on Neurosurgery of Epilepsy, The International League Against Epilepsy. *Epilepsia* **38**(2):249–255.

Awad IA, Assirati JAJ, Burgess R, Barnett GH, Luders H (1991) A new class of electrodes of 'intermediate invasiveness': preliminary experience with epidural pegs and foramen ovale electrodes in the mapping of seizure foci. *Neurological Research* **13**:177–183.

Babb TL, Wilson CL, Crandall PH (1982) Asymmetry and ventral course of the human geniculo-striate pathway as determined by hippocampal visual evoked potentials and subsequent visual field defects after temporal lobectomy. *Experimental Brain Research* **47**:317–328.

Barcia-Salorio JL, Barcia JA, Hernandez G, Lopez-Gomez L, Roldan P (1992) Radiosurgery of epilepsy. *Acta Neurochirugica* **117**:109(Abstract).

Beardsworth ED, Adams CBT (1988) Modified hemispherectomy for epilepsy. Early results in 10 cases. *British Journal of Neurosurgery* **2**:73–84.

Bidzinski J, Bacia T, Ruzikowski E (1992) The results of the surgical treatment of occipital lobe epilepsy. *Acta Neurochirurgica Wien* **114**:128–130.

Borchgrevink HM, Nakstad PH, Bjorneas H, Bakke SJ (1993) Superselective amytal anaesthesia by the medial and posterior cerebral arteries improved localisation of function in epileptic patients prior to neurosurgical intervention [Abstract]. *Epilepsia* **34**:S2:34.

Brian JE Jr, Deshpande JK, McPherson RW (1990) Management of cerebral hemispherectomy in children. *Journal of Clinical Anesthesia* **2**:91–95.

Cascino GD, Kelly PJ, Hirschorn KA, Marsh WR, Sharbrough FW (1990) Stereotactic resection of intra-axial cerebral lesions in partial epilepsy. *Mayo Clinic Proceedings* **65**:1053–1060.

Cooper I (1973) Chronic stimulation of the paleo-cerebellum in humans. *Lancet* **i**:206.

Crandall PH (1987) Cortical resections. In: Engel J (ed) *Surgical Treatment of the Epilepsies*, pp 377–404. New York: Raven Press.

Delalande O, Pinard JM, Basdevant C, Plouin P, Dulac O (1993) Hemispherotomy: a new procedure for hemispheric disconnection [Abstract]. *Epilepsia* **34**(Suppl 2):140.

Falconer MA, Wilson JL (1958) Visual field changes following anterior temporal lobectomy: their significance in relation to 'Meyer's loop' of the optic radiation. *Brain* **81**:1–14.

Goldring S, Gregorie EM (1984) Surgical management of epilepsy using epidural mats to localise the seizure focus. *Journal of Neurosurgery* **60**:457–466.

Grzyska U, Freitag J, Zeumer H (1990) Selective cerebral intraarterial DSA. Complication rate and control of risk factors. *Neuroradiology* **4**:296–299.

Handforth A, DeGiorgio CM, Schachter SC, *et al* (1998) Vagus nerve stimulation therapy for partial-onset seizures: a randomized active-control trial. *Neurology* **51**(1):48–55.

Heikkinen ER, Heikkinen MI, Sotaniemi K (1992) Stereotactic radiotherapy instead of conventional epilepsy surgery. A case report. *Acta Neurochir Wien* **119**:159–160.

Holthausen H, Strobl K, Pieper T, Teixeira VA, Oppel F (1997) Prediction of motor functions post hemispherectomy. In: Tuxhorn I, Holthausen H, Boenigk H (eds) *Paediatric Epilepsy Syndromes and Their Surgical Treatment*, pp 785–798. London: John Libbey.

Jack CR, Nichols DA, Sharbrough FW, Marsh WR, Petersen RC (1988) Selective posterior cerebral amytal test for evaluating memory function before surgery for temporal lobe seizure. *Radiology* **168**:787–793.

Jensen I (1975a) Temporal lobe epilepsy. Late mortality in patients treated with unilateral temporal lobe resections. *Acta Neurologica Scandinavica* **52**:374–380.

Jensen I (1975b) Temporal lobe surgery around the world. Results, complications, mortality. *Acta Neurologica Scandinavica* **52**:354–373.

Kachel R, Jahn U, Schiffmann R, Basche S (1991) Complications in cerebral angiography. A study of 6698 cerebral angiographies [in

German]. *Revista Medico-Chirurgicala a Societatii de Medici Si Naturalisti Dinlasi* **1–2**:97–105.

Katz A, Awad IA, Kong AK et al (1989) Extent of resection in temporal lobectomy for epilepsy. II. Memory changes and neurologic complications. *Epilepsia* **30**:763–771.

Kimball S, Walker GG, Wyler AR (1989) Corpus callosotomy: Anterior versus staged anterior and posterior callosal sectioning. *Epilepsia* **30**:729.

Krynauw RA (1950) Infantile hemiplegia treated by removing one cerebral hemisphere. *Journal of Neurology, Neurosurgery and Psychiatry* **13**:243–267.

Kuzniecky R, Faught E, Morawetz R (1990) Surgical treatment of epilepsy: initial results based upon epidural electroencephalographic recordings. *Southern Medical Journal* **6**:637–639.

Morrell F, Whisler WW, Bleck TP (1989) Multiple subpial transection. A new approach to the surgical treatment of focal epilepsy. *Journal of Neurosurgery* **70**:231–239.

Oguni H, Olivier A, Andermann F, Comair J (1991) Anterior callosotomy in the treatment of medically intractable epilepsies: a study of 43 patients with a mean follow-up of 39 months. *Annals of Neurology* **30**:357–364.

Olivier A, Awad IA (1993) Extratemporal resections. In: Engel J (ed) *Surgical Treatment of the Epilepsies*, 2nd edn, pp 489–500. New York: Raven Press.

Oppenheimer DR, Griffith HB (1966) Persistent intracranial bleeding as a complication of hemispherectomy. *Journal of Neurology, Neurosurgery and Psychiatry* **29**:229–240.

Palmini A, Andermann F, Dubeau F et al (1993) Occipitotemporal epilepsies: evaluation of selected patients requiring depth electrodes studies and rationale for surgical approaches. *Epilepsia* **34**:84–96.

Penfield W, Lende RA, Rasmussen T (1961) Manipulation hemiplegia, an untoward complication in the surgery of focal epilepsy. *Journal of Neurosurgery* **18**:769–776.

Pilcher WH, Rusyniak G (1993) Complications of epilepsy surgery. In: Silberg DI, Ojemann GA (eds) *Epilepsy Surgery*, pp 311–325. Philadelphia: W.B. Saunders.

Pilcher WH, Roberts DW, Flanigin HF *et al* (1993) Complications of epilepsy surgery. In: Engel J (ed) *Surgical Treatment of the Epilepsies*, 2nd edn, pp 565–581. New York: Raven Press.

Pinard JM, Delande, Jambaque I, Chiron C, Plouin P, Dulac O (1991) Anterior and total callosotomy in epileptic children: Prospective one-year follow-up study. *Epilepsia* **32**(Suppl 1):54.

Rasmussen T (1973) Post-operative superficial hemosiderosis of the brain, its diagnosis, treatment and prevention. *American Neurological Association* **98**:133–137.

Rasmussen T (1975) Surgery for epilepsy arising in regions other than the frontal or temporal lobes. In: Purpura DP, Penry JK, Walter RD (eds) *Advances in Neurology*, Vol 8 *Neurosurgical Treatment of the Epilepsies*, pp 207–226. New York: Raven Press.

Rasmussen T, Obozewski J, Lloyd-Smith D (1958) Focal seizures due to chronic localised encephalitis. *Neurology* **8**:435–445.

Rausch R, Silfvenius H, Wieser HG, Dodrill CB, Meador KJ, Jones-Gotman M (1993) Intraarterial amobarbital procedures. In: Engel J (ed) *Surgical Treatment of the Epilepsies*, 2nd edn, pp 341–358. New York: Raven Press.

Renella RR (1989) Outcome of surgery. Anonymous *Microsurgery of the Temporal Region*, pp 158–164. Wien: Springer-Verlag.

Ribaric II (1991) Reappraisal of the results of 'restricted temperofrontal resections' in selected epileptic patients. *Epilepsia* **32**(Suppl 1).

Rodhan NR, Kelly PJ, Cascino GD, Sharbrough FW (1992) Surgical outcome in computer-assisted stereotactic resection of intra-axial cerebral lesions for partial epilepsy. *Stereotactic and Functional Neurosurgery* **58**:172–177.

Rougier A, Sundstrom L, Claverie B *et al* (1996) Multiple subpial transection: report of 7 cases. *Epilepsy Research* **24**(1):57–63.

Rougier A, Saint-Hilaire JM, Bouvier G *et al* (1992) Research and surgical treatment of epilepsy [in French]. *Neuro-Chirurgie* **38**(Suppl 1):1–112.

Salanova V, Andermann F, Olivier A, Rasmussen T, Quesney LF (1992) Occipital lobe epilepsy: electroclinical manifestations, electrocorticography, cortical stimulation and outcome in 42 patients treated between 1930 and 1991. Surgery of occipital lobe epilepsy. *Brain* **115**:1655–1680.

Sass KJ, Novelly RA, Spencer DD, Spencer SS (1990) Postcallosotomy language impairments in patients with crossed cerebral dominance. *Journal of Neurosurgery* **72**:85–90.

Sass KJ, Sass A, Westerveld M *et al* (1992) Specificity in the correlation of verbal memory and hippocampal neuron loss: dissociation of memory, language, and verbal intellectual ability. *Journal of Clinical and Experimental Neuropsychology* **14**:662–672.

Schuler P, Neubauer U, Schulemann H, Stefan H (1993) Brain-stem lesions in the course of a presurgical re-evaluation by foramen-ovale electrodes in temporal lobe epilepsy. *Electroencephalography and Clinical Neurophysiology* **86**:301–302.

Siegfried J, Wieser HG, Stodieck SRG (1985) Foramen ovale electrodes: A new technique enabling presurgical evaluation of patients with mesiobasal temporal lobe seizures. *Applied Neurophysiology* **48**:408–417.

Spencer DD (1987) Depth electrode implantation at Yale University. In: Engel J (ed) *Surgical Treatment of the Epilepsies,* pp 603–607. New York: Raven Press.

Spencer DD, Spencer SS, Mattson RH, Williamson PD, Novelly RA (1984) Access to the posterior medial temporal structures in the surgical treatment of temporal lobe epilepsy. *Neurosurgery* **15**:667–671.

Taylor DC, Marsh SM (1977) Implications of long-term follow-up studies in epilepsy: With a note on the cause of death. In: Penry JK (ed) *Epilepsy. The Eighth International Symposium,* pp 27–34. New York: Raven Press.

Uthman BM, Wilder BJ, Hammond EJ, Reid SA (1990) Efficacy and safety of vagus nerve stimulation in patients with complex partial seizures. *Epilepsia* **31**:S44–S50.

Van Buren JM (1987) Complications of surgical procedures in the treatment and diagnosis of epilepsy. In: Engel J (ed) *Surgical Treatment of the Epilepsies,* pp 465–475. New York: Raven Press.

Van Veelen CMW, Debets C, Van Huffelen AC *et al* (1990) Combined use of subdural and intracerebral electrodes in preoperative evaluation of epilepsy. *Neurosurgery* **26**:93–101.

Van Wagenen WP, Herren RY (1940) Surgical division of commissural pathways in the corpus callosum. *Archives of Neurology and Psychiatry* **44**:740–759.

Velasco F, Velasco M, Velasco AL, Jimenez F, Marquez I, Rise M (1995) Electrical stimulation of the centromedian thalamic nucleus in control of seizures: long-term studies. *Epilepsia* **36**:63–71.

Ventureyra EC, Higgins MJ (1993) Complications of epilepsy surgery in children and adolescents [Review]. *Pediatric Neurosurgery* **1**:40–56.

Waugh JR, Sacharias N (1992) Arteriographic complications in the DSA era. *Radiology* **1**:243–246.

Wieser HG, Moser S (1988) Improved multipolar foramen ovale electrode monitoring. *Journal of Epilepsy* **1**:13–22.

Wieser HG, Elger C, Stodieck SRG (1985) The 'foramen ovale electrode': a new recording method for the preoperative evaluation of patients suffering from mesio-basal temporal lobe epilepsy. *Electroencephalography and Clinical Neurophysiology* **61**:314–322.

Wieser HG, Valvanis A, Roos A, Isler P, Renella RR (1989) "Selective" and "superselective" temporal lobe Amytal tests: I Neuroradiological, neuroanatomical and electrical data. In: Manelis J (ed) *Advances in Epileptology*, Vol. 17, pp 20–27. New York: Raven Press.

Wieser HG, Quesney LF, Morris HH (1993) Foramen ovale and peg electrodes. In: Engel J (ed) *Surgical Treatment of the Epilepsies,* 2nd edn, pp 331–339. New York: Raven Press.

Williamson PD, Thadani VM, Darcey TM, Spencer DD, Spencer SS, Mattson RH (1992) Occipital lobe epilepsy: clinical characteristics, seizure spread patterns, and results of surgery. *Annals of Neurology* **31**:3–13.

Wilson DH, Reeves A, Gazzaniga M, Culver C (1977) Cerebral commissurotomy for control of intractable seizures. *Neurology* **27**:708–715.

Wilson DH, Reeves AG, Gazzaniga M (1982) 'Central' commissurotomy for intractabler generalised: Series two. *Neurology* **32**:687–697.

Wright GDS, McLellan DL, Brice JG (1985) A double-blind trial of chronic cerebellar stimulation in twelve patients with severe epilepsy. *Journal of Neurology, Neurosurgery and Psychiatary* **47**:769–774.

Wyler AR (1992) Subdural strip electrodes in the surgery of epilepsy. In: Luders H (ed) *Epilepsy Surgery,* pp 395–398. New York: Raven Press.

Wyler AR, Walker G, Somes G (1991) The morbidity of long term seizure monitoring using subdural strip recording. *Journal of Neurosurgery* **74**:734–737.

Young RF (1990) Brain stimulation. In: Friedman WA (ed) *Stereotactic Neurosurgery*, pp 865–879. Philadelphia: W.B. Saunders.

Neuropsychologic function following frontal excisions

RG MORRIS AND EC MIOTTO

Since the nineteenth century the profound behavioral disturbances following damage to the frontal lobes have been well known, perhaps the classic historical example being Phineas Gage, the patient studied by Harlow (1848, 1868). It was only in the twentieth century that the new psychometric procedures could be used to investigate the cognitive basis for these disturbances; for example, Weigl's (1941) early finding of mental flexibility impairment on a simple color-form sorting task in a patient with bilateral frontal lobe damage (see also Rylander 1939; Halstead 1940).

Our knowledge in this area has been advanced considerably with the advent of the frontal lobe excision as treatment for epilepsy, starting with the famous case studies of Penfield and Evans (1935) and then those reported by Hebb (Hebb 1939, 1941; Hebb and Penfield 1940). These early studies were instrumental in establishing that selective lesions of the prefrontal cortex have only a slight effect on intellectual functioning as measured using standardized tests, a view that has been confirmed by a number of studies since then (e.g. Milner 1964, 1975), including the finding that mnemonic deficits readily shown with temporal lobe lesions do appear to be present.

However, it was only in the modern era of psychology that cognitive function following frontal lobe excisions were investigated in much more depth, revealing important areas of deficit. Perhaps a key landmark for this was in 1962, with Milner's follow-up of the patient K.M., originally operated

on in 1938 by Penfield (Milner et al 1968). This patient showed a strikingly impaired performance on the Wisconsin card sorting test (see Chapter 31), with an unusual degree of perseverative behavior, sorting almost all of the 128 cards to form. Additional data were obtained for unilateral cases (Milner 1963, 1964), showing a pattern of exacerbated perseverative behavior on this task. There followed numerous studies in which various neuropsychologic deficits were 'discovered' including, for example, impaired attention, initiation of cognitive activity, problems with sequencing and temporal ordering, and difficulties with response inhibition, mental flexibility, and problem solving (Milner 1995).

PREFRONTAL CORTICAL EXCISIONS AND COGNITION

The frontal lobe excision for the treatment of frontal lobe epilepsy involves seeking to preserve the region of the motor cortex and sparing the speech area of Broca in the language-dominant hemisphere. Beyond this there is considerable heterogeneity. The excisions do not necessarily follow the functional boundaries within the prefrontal cortex, for obvious reasons, although some studies have been able to group patients according to whether they invade particular regions, for example, dorsolateral, orbitofrontal, or mesial cortices. Indeed, a combination of clinical and functional neuroimaging studies and work with nonhuman primates has suggested an approximate functional differentiation of different regions. It is thought that the ventromedial prefrontal cortex is involved in decision-making processes, with the lateral prefrontal cortex having a major role in the coordination and sequencing of behavior, including planning and working memory. Competing theoretic frameworks may suggest different cognitive mechanisms relating to the prefrontal cortex (Roberts *et al* 1996), but there is considerable agreement concerning what types of cognitive deficits exist in postsurgery patients. The aim of this review is to consider these, with additional reference to the authors' own work in this area; the main areas considered include working memory and self-ordered action, the temporal organization of memory, problem solving and simulation of everyday planning or organization, all areas of function that have been linked with the prefrontal cortex.

WORKING MEMORY AND SELF-ORDERED ACTION

Investigations of both patients' and nonhuman primates' lesions has implicated the prefrontal cortex in working memory function (Goldman-Rakic 1996). This is the ability to hold 'on line' information for temporal use or for the purposes of computation. Such a function is thought to be a key component of cognition, since it enables a person to direct and control cognitive activity in a coherent manner. In nonhuman primates, dorsolateral lesions result in working memory impairment, for example, on the delayed-response test, designed to measure temporary storage of spatial location (Goldman-Rakic and Rosvold 1970; Goldman-Rakic 1987). In both humans and animals, the presence of a deficit depends in part on the precise location of the lesion and also the extent to which the material held in memory requires active monitoring or manipulation (Petrides 1996).

This latter phenomenon is seen in humans with prefrontal excisions. Simple spatial memory tasks such as the *Corsi block span*, in which the patient observes the examiner tap out a sequence of moves on an array of blocks and has to repeat this sequence immediately (see Chapter 31), do not consistently show deficits in frontal excision patients (e.g. Owen *et al* 1990). Those that require self-order 'searching' or strategy formation can produce substantial deficits.

For example, Petrides and Milner (1982) presented subjects with stacks of cards on which a set of 6, 8, 10, or 12

stimuli were displayed in a matrix array. For each stack the stimuli used remained constant, but their position in the matrix varied from card to card. The object was to go through the stack selecting an item at random, but taking care on subsequent cards not to select the same one twice. Verbal and nonverbal versions of this task were constructed, using words, high or low imagery (e.g. *lemon* or *attitude*), representational drawings (e.g. of a *pair of shoes* or a *suitcase*), or abstract designs. For the two 'word' conditions left frontal (LF) excision patients were significantly impaired relative to normal controls, but not right frontal (RF) patients. Generally, patients with temporal lobe lesions were not impaired on these conditions, the exception being patients with extensive right hippocampal (RTH) lesions with low imagery material. For the representational drawings, despite being an easier task, both LF and RF groups were impaired, the severity of impairment increasing markedly with the number of stimuli used on the cards.

A spatial task containing the main feature of self-ordered pointing was developed by Morris when working with Professor Trevor Robbins in Cambridge (Morris *et al* 1988) and has been subsequently modified in the form of a computer game, the *Executive-Golf Task* (Feigenbaum *et al* 1996; Miotto *et al* 1996). The task (see Fig. 59.1) simulates a 'game of golf' with the patient searching for holes in which a 'golfer' is predicted to 'putt' a ball, avoiding returning to this place in subsequent searches. Patients make their responses using a touch-sensitive screen, initially trying each hole in turn until successful. At this point, the golfer is seen to putt the ball into this particular hole. The patient then searches for another hole, the main rule being remembering not to return to a hole that has already been used by the golfer. A series of searches follows until all the holes have had balls 'putted' into them. The main similarity with the Petrides and Milner (1982) task is that the patient chooses which holes to explore and must apply the same 'don't go back to' rule to avoid error.

In a preliminary study, Owen *et al* (1990; see also Owen *et al* 1996) found a deficit in frontal lobe excision patients studied at the Maudsley Hospital London, under the care of Professor Charles Polkey. More recently, Miotto *et al* (1996) tested 20 frontal lobe excision patients (9 RF; 11 LF) on the executive-golf test, and their data can be compared to those in patients with the left and right *en bloc* temporal lobectomy (20 LTL; 20 RTL) investigated by Feigenbaum *et al* (1996). Both frontal groups were clearly impaired in comparison to their respective normal controls, the RF patients being significantly more impaired than the LF patients (see Fig. 59.2). The latter difference is not easily accounted for by the possibility of larger lesions in the

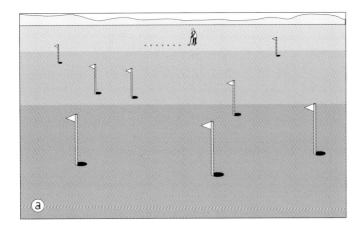

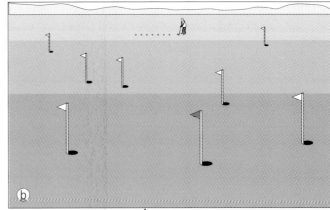

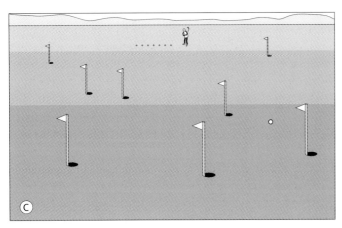

Fig. 59.1 The executive-golf task. The photographs show the layout of the task. (a) The computer is waiting for the subject to select a spatial location. (b) An incorrect location has been chosen and the flag turns a different color. (c) The correct hole has been selected (bottom right-hand corner) and feedback is provided by the golfer 'putting' the ball into this hole (*published with permission*).

RF group, since size of lesion did not appear to correlate with impairment. The LTL patients were not impaired, but there was a significant impairment in the RTL patients, attributed to their known deficit in spatial memory.

A feature of both the self-ordered pointing and executive-golf tasks is the use of systematic strategies to aid performance. An identifiable strategy in the executive-golf task is to follow a predetermined search path in which the patient begins each search with the same location (golf-hole), skipping holes that have been 'putted' into in previous trials. Most normal controls adopt this strategy. Miotto *et al* (1996) measured the strategy in their study and found that only the RF patients showed a significant impairment. Furthermore, when this measure is covaried in the original analysis of between-search errors, the difference between the LF and RF groups disappears, but both groups still show impairment. In contrast, the RTL and LTL patients tested by Feigenbaum *et al* (1996) show no impairment in strategy formation. An example of impaired strategy is given in Fig. 59.3, with an example of an orderly series of searches by a control subject (G.F., top panels), contrasting with the lack of strategy shown by the RF patient B.K. (bottom panels). For G.F. the starting position remains the same for each search until this partic-

ular 'hole' has been successful and then the subject switches to another, while for B.K. the starting position and search pattern varies in an unsystematic fashion. Miotto *et al* (1997) explored what would happen in these patients if the search path was constrained by the task, thus preventing the development of a systematic search strategy.

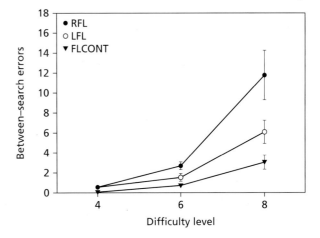

Fig. 59.2 Between-search errors on the executive-golf task comparing right frontal lobe (RFL), left frontal lobe (LFL) and controls (FLCONT). Level of difficulty refers to the number of locations used (*published with permission*).

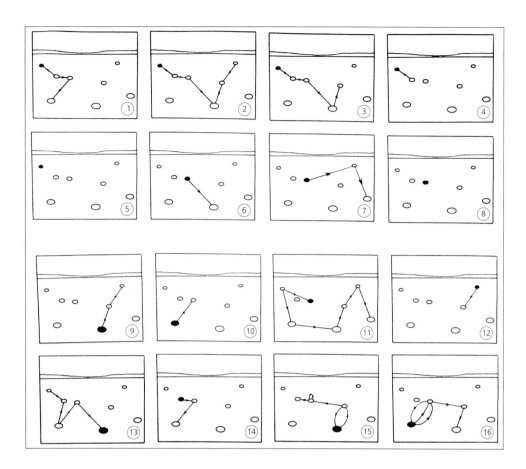

Fig. 59.3 Strategy formation on the executive-golf task. The top panels show an example of orderly searches by a control subject (G.F.). The starting position is indicated by the 'black' hole and the direction of search by arrows. The subject starts initially using one position for each search until this position is successful, and then switches to another starting position. The bottom search paths (panels 9–16) illustrate the more random nature of searches in a frontal lobe excision patient (B.K.). Note the random starting position and the presence of between-search errors (*published with permission*).

A further spatial working memory task was developed, now called the *Owl Spatial Working Memory Task*. In the form of a computer game, the aim is to search around an imaginary 'wood' to find 'owls'. In this case, the computer presents only two locations at a time, providing a limited choice in terms of attempting to discover where the owl might be. The patient is required to find each owl but avoid selecting previous successful locations when they appear. This task revealed an impairment in both the RF and LF patients, but no statistical difference between the two patient groups overall, suggesting again that when strategy is taken into account, the deficit exists with lesions in either hemisphere.

The tasks reviewed in this section show a common deficit, which perhaps relates to the 'monitoring' or 'editing' of previous response, rather than holding on-line mnemonic information *per se*. A deficit is seen with lesions in both hemispheres in all of the nonverbal tasks, but only in the left group with the word self-ordered task. The core deficit in this task, however, may transcend the modality of presentation or type of material and relate to the executive component within working memory. Superimposed on this are the presence of strategy, that may invoke superordinate cognitive processes, depending on how the task is designed.

THE TEMPORAL ORGANIZATION OF MEMORY

In daily life, many activities require planning of complex sequences of action over a broader time frame, perhaps minutes, hours, or days. To do so, they must retain the temporal order of events, either when reconstructing past experiences or planning for the future.

This ability was first tested in patients with frontal lobe excisions by Corsi (cited in Milner and Petrides 1984), using tests of recency discrimination. Here, the patient is presented with a series of items (for example words, pictures of objects, or abstract paintings). Following a certain number of presentations, sets of two out of the previous list may be presented and the patient has to indicate which was most recent. Corsi found that LF patients were significantly impaired when the stimuli were verbal, whereas RF patients were impaired most with pictorial and abstract painting tests. In contrast, when the patients were presented with repeated stimuli, paired with novel ones, and asked to indicate whether an item had been seen before (two-choice recognition), there were no impairments. However, patients with temporal lobe lesions showed impairment with the latter procedure. An additional finding was that LF patients whose lesions encroached on the dorsolateral region were the ones who tended to show the verbal recency discrimination deficit.

Swain *et al* (1988) have pointed out that, in these and other such tasks (Ladavas *et al* 1979; Shimamura *et al* 1990), the relationship between the items in the recency discrimination task is arbitrary, the material arranged in a pseudo-random order by the examiner. In everyday life, the order in which events occur may not be random, but governed by known principles of organization. Knowledge about the approximate sequencing of frequently experienced events is thought to be stored within semantic memory in the form of scripts (Schank and Abelson 1977; Schank 1979). For example, when visiting a restaurant, there are a certain number of routine or ritual activities that are well known and can be used to guide the behavior of a person. Patients with frontal lobe excisions have been shown to have difficulty generating the components of scripts (Godbout and Doyon 1995) and determining the correct order of script items when asked to arrange events in a 'typical order' (Sirigu *et al* 1996).

The extent to which memory for the order of events is impaired in frontal lobe excision patients when they form part of a well-known script was investigated by Swain *et al* (1988). They presented patients with a story conforming to a high-frequency script (in this case about a shopping trip). They were not found to be impaired when asked to order a series of target words relating to key elements of the story or reorder a series of sentences representing the events. In contrast, when presented with a story that did not conform to a well-known script (in this case a space adventure story), they did show an impairment in ordering. When the patients were split into those with left versus right excisions, the right group was found to be more severely impaired on ordering for the novel stories. This difference was less pronounced when asked to order the sentences. Additionally, Swain *et al* (1988) found that recognition memory for the material was unimpaired, in line with previous studies that show a lack of deficit for this type of memory. The pattern of deficit on ordering cannot be attributed to the ordered story being easier, given that the controls tended to be worse on this condition.

This deficit may suggest a role for the prefrontal cortex in the retrieval of certain types of information about order, possibly when there are arbitrary temporal relations between events. This could either be in situations where the temporal relations are weak, and thus more susceptible to brain damage, or the prefrontal cortex could have the specific role (among others) of representing arbitrary sequences. In either case, the results predict difficulties in remembering the order of events, when they deviate from a familiar scenario.

PROBLEM SOLVING

The inability to organize and plan behavior in a coherent fashion is a frequent feature of patients with frontal lobe damage. Attempts have been made to capture this difficulty in the laboratory, including, for example, use of variations on the *Tower of Hanoi* (ToH) task to measure problem-solving ability.

This test, derived from an ancient puzzle, requires the patient to rearrange 'beads' or 'discs' threaded onto a series of rods to achieve a goal state (Fig. 59.4). The test involves planning, because the optimal approach is to think ahead in order to solve each problem in the minimum number of moves. Several versions of this test have been developed, including the Tower of London (ToL), which involves rearranging colored beads. This test has been shown to be sensitive to anterior lobe brain damage initially by Shallice and McCarthy (Shallice 1982), who found that patients with left anterior hemisphere lesions of mixed etiology were specifically impaired. A subsequent study by Owen *et al* (1990) using a computerized test found a deficit in patients with frontal excisions (left and right), but no increase in the time taken to plan moves (the opposite pattern was found for Parkinson's disease in a study by Morris *et al* 1988).

THE GOAL–SUBGOAL CONFLICT

The ToH test and the ToL variant invoke a range of cognitive processes, including basic perceptual and motor functions. Additionally, the problem-solving aspect involves processes associated with specific strategies and a working memory component, as the patient stores the solution to a particular problem during execution. Typically, in generating solutions to problems a normal person will split the solution up into 'subgoals' and combine these into a sequence in what is called a 'hill climbing' strategy (Simon 1975). When confronted with the ToH *de novo* it is thought that new algorithms have to be constructed to provide the approach or solutions to deal with it or the construction of a new schema or procedure. The prefrontal cortex is proposed to be intimately involved in this process (Shallice and Burgess 1996).

In order to explore these aspects, the authors (Morris *et al* 1997a, b) developed a computerized version of a three-disc ToH using 3-D graphics to represent the discs, rods, and plinths (Fig. 59.4). In the first study, a series of problems was devised comprising practice and then four or five move levels (where the number of moves represents the topographic distance between the starting state and goal arrangement). The test explored the following features:

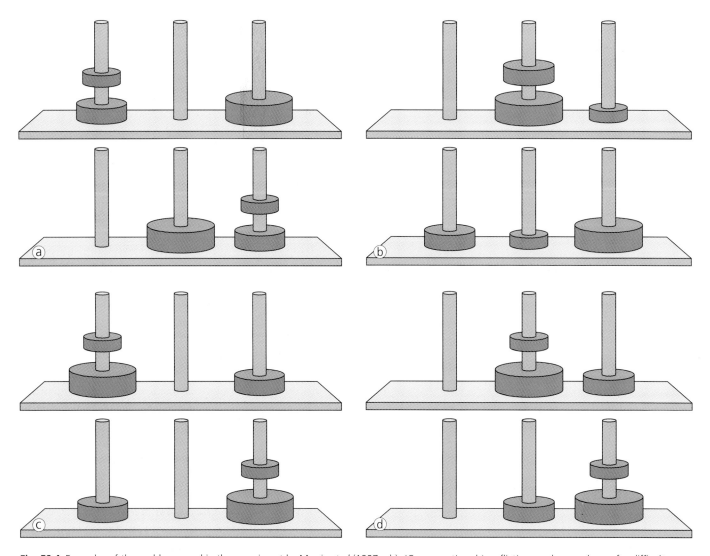

Fig. 59.4 Examples of the problems used in the experiment by Morris *et al* (1997a, b). 'Congruent' and 'conflict' examples are shown for difficulty levels 4 and 5. The aim is to shift the bottom 'discs' in each array so as to match the top arrangement using the touch-sensitive screen.

1. *The type of problem.* In certain instances, a problem will create a scenario where the initial move or sequence of moves is apparently in the opposite direction from the overall goal. This is termed a 'goal–subgoal conflict' and has been posited as a reason for failure on the ToH associated with frontal lobe damage, the explanation being that the patient is unable to inhibit (incorrectly) going in the direction of the goal (Goel and Grafman 1995). Alternately, the goal–subgoal conflict requires novel schemata, not so readily derived if the prefrontal cortex is damaged. Performance on problems where the first move was apparently in the same direction (*congruent*) or away (*conflict*) from the goal was tested.

2. *Motor function.* A motor control task was implemented in which the patient was 'led' by the computer through the exact moves needed to solve each problem. The movement times generated could then be used to subtract from the problem-solving times to see whether the patient was slower in 'thinking' over and above and perceptual or motor deficit (based on Morris *et al* 1988).

3. *Spatial memory.* The patient was shown a sequence of moves and then had to repeat them from memory. The sequence was increased until systematic failure followed, determining the span of the patient.

The performance of 21 frontal lobe excision (10 RF, 11 LF) patients was examined and compared to 40 temporal lobe patients (20 RTL, 20 LTL) and 35 normal controls. They were tested on firstly four, and then five move problems (level 4 and 5), with four problems at each level, two involving congruent and two conflict problems. The results are shown in Fig. 59.5. This shows that on the initial level 4, there is a clear deficit with the conflict problems

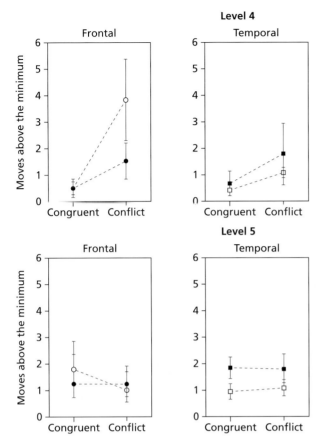

Fig. 59.5 Mean moves above the minimum on the computerized Tower of Hanoi test for five groups (LF, RF, LT, RT, and controls) on the 'congruent' and 'conflict' conditions, split according to four- and five-move problems.

but that this is seen only in the LF group. The other three patient groups are unimpaired in relation to the controls. However, when the patients reach level 5 the LF deficit disappears and is replaced by one in the RTL patients, but on both congruent and conflict problems. The thinking times, adjusted to take out the perceptual and motor components, as indicated above, suggested that with the level 4 moves, the conflict problems resulted in longer planning times and subsequent execution, but this was not seen for five-move problems.

It seems that when the LF patients first confront the conflict problems at level 4 they are slower to generate ways to deal with them, revealing an impairment. With the subsequent level 5 problems, the conflict is no longer 'novel' and the problems are perhaps dealt with using now-established procedures or strategies. In the RTL patients, the deficit on level 5 is due to the additional memory load caused by a longer start to goal-solution paths, corresponding to the known spatial memory deficit in this group. This overall pattern is less likely to be explained by problems with response inhibition, as mooted by Goel and Grafman

(1995). Specifically, this would suggest that the slower planning time on the conflict condition would be lost, but this was not the case.

The cause of impairment appears to be different in the RTL group, as indicated by the results of the memory span measure. While this revealed a deficit in the LF and RTL groups, when performance on this measure was covaried in the original ToH analysis, the deficit in the LF group remained, suggesting that it was independent of memory difficulty, while it disappeared in the RTL group, suggesting that it was related.

The goal–subgoal deficit in the LF group 'echoes' the left anterior impairment on the ToL found by Shallice and McCarthy in 1982; it is also congruent with SPECT neuroimaging data obtained by Morris et al (1993) which showed left dorsolateral lobe activation associated with a critical 2-min period during which normal subjects had started on level 4 move problems. In the ToL set of problems, goal–subgoal conflicts exist in the level 4 problems, but have never been systematically explored.

PATH LENGTH AND SELECTION EQUIVOCATION

The tasks cited above have relatively small distances between the start and finish. Longer solution paths, however, might be expected to place a greater demand on working memory and are perhaps more akin to planning in everyday life. For example, the three-disc ToH described above has a problem space that can be increased up to seven moves (Fig. 59.6). Problems of this size generate more uncertainty in terms of the correct intermediate subgoal. Indeed, in many problems there are more than one plausible route, and the need to determine the most efficient one can be termed *selection equivocation*. Figure 59.6 shows how long sequences of moves must involve movement between three domains, determined by the position of the largest disc (left, middle, or right). The two main routes always diverge, one going clockwise, the other anticlockwise round the ring made up by joining the domains. The two routes can either be *similar* in length (Fig. 59.6a) or *dissimilar* (Fig. 59.6b). If the two routes differ more substantially in length, the failure to choose the right one would predict a larger deficit.

Morris et al (1998) investigated whether ToH problems with larger solution paths resulted in a different pattern of deficit in temporal lobe patients, and whether selection equivocation was a significant factor. Exactly the same frontal and temporal lobe patients that were investigated by Morris et al (1997a, b) were included in this study, which compared six- and seven-move problems either with

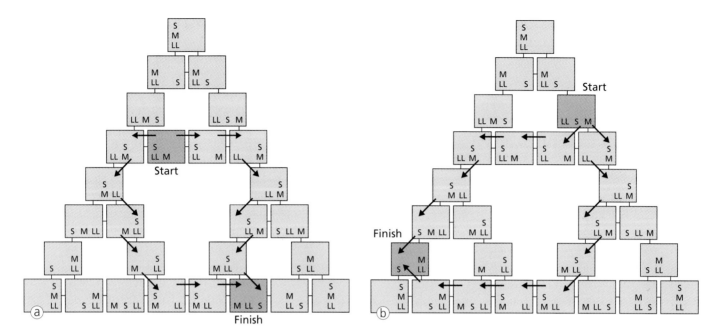

Fig. 59.6 The problem spaces for the three-disc Tower of Hanoi. Each box represents a particular arrangement of the discs, with the lines between boxes representing links between arrangements created by moving a single disc. The disc sizes are represented by letters (S = small; M = medium; LL = large) and their relative positions are represented spatially. (a) Figure shows two alternative routes between starting and goal position for a 'similar length' problem; (b) figure represents the routes of a 'different length' problem (*published with permission*).

similar or dissimilar lengths. Practice on the task was provided with three, four, and five more problems before reaching this length.

This revealed a distinct pattern of result common to the six- and seven-move problems, which showed that the RF group were impaired, but to the same extent on the similar and dissimilar length conditions at both difficulty levels 6 and 7. The LF patients, previously impaired on the level 4 goal–subgoal conflict conditions, showed no impairment. The RTL group were impaired, but only in the dissimilar condition.

One way of interpreting this finding is that the frontal lobe patients are inefficient in their choice of solution path irrespective of problem equivocation. The RTL group might have a selective deficit, precisely because their spatial memory impairment makes it difficult for them to 'track down' the solution path and remember an outcome in order to select the most efficient route.

Why, then, should the RF patients show an impairment, rather than the LF patients? One possibility is that the left prefrontal cortex is involved in more immediate system that deals with novelty, as outlined above. With repeated exposure, this factor dissipates. However, with longer solution paths, the problems become more complex and necessitate the need to develop specific spatial strategies, which may be reliant on the right prefrontal cortex, just as strategy formation was related to the RF group studied by Miotto *et al*

1996) (some of these strategies have been identified originally in detail by Simon (1975), but include for example, moving the largest disc into position first). It is possible that frontal lobe patients are deficient in developing these strategies in the same way as a similar cohort of patients failed to do so on the executive-golf task (Miotto *et al* 1996).

DISCUSSION

The above studies illustrate the complexity of investigating problem-solving abilities in patients with frontal lobe damage, even those with clear frontal lobe excisions. Like all planning tasks, the ToH or ToL involve a complex mixture of cognitive components that may rely on different regions of the brain for support. Nevertheless, the current study illustrates the interaction between prefrontal (problem solving) and temporal lobe (mnemonic) processes, dissociated by studying these patient groups together.

EVERYDAY PLANNING

The use of laboratory tests of planning has been encouraged by the clear impairment in the planning and organization of behavior in everyday life. There are many case reports of this; for example, Penfield and Evans (1935) describe the behavior of a 44-year-old lady who had undergone a right frontal lobectomy as follows:

> 'She had planned to get a simple supper for one guest (Dr Penfield) and four members of her own family. She looked forward to it with pleasure and had a whole day for preparation. This was a thing that she could have done with ease ten years before. When the appointed hour arrived, she was in the kitchen, the food was all there, one or two things were on the stove, but the salad was not ready, the meat had not been started and she was distressed and confused by her long continued effort alone … with help the task of preparation was quickly completed and the occasion went off successfully' (p 131).

While clinicians will relate anecdotes of a similar nature in many other patients, it is only recently that tests aimed at 'simulating' this type of difficulty in the laboratory have been used in clinical practice. For example, Shallice and Burgess (1991) developed the *multiple errands task* in which the patient is taken out into a shopping precinct and undertakes a series of errands, ranging in complexity from buying a packet of throat pastilles to obtaining the necessary material/information to send a postcard. This highlighted grossly inefficient strategies in brain-injured patients even when they were of high intellectual function.

Recently, the authors (Miotto and Morris 1998) developed a 'board game' task aimed at simulating planning activity, but in the laboratory, in the same vein as Shallice and Burgess (1991). This is the *Virtual Planning Test* (VIP) . The patient has to plan 4 days' worth of activities, in advance of a notional journey abroad. Some of the activities relate specifically to the current context of the week; for example, paying the electricity bill. Others relate to the journey; for example, going to the bank to buy traveler's checks. Some also have to be done by a specific time in the week or in preparation for completing other activities. For part of a day (morning or afternoon) the patient can select two activities only. In order to emphasize the planning component of the task, and to make it a more realistic simulation of everyday planning, once the activities for a single day have been chosen, the patient cannot go back on them. They therefore have to think in advance to ensure all the required activities are done in time. There are also distracter activities, defined as plausible activities, but not those specified as having to be done by the examiner. Some of these activities relate to the 4 days (e.g. 'stay indoors and take it easy for a while') or to the journey (e.g. 'buy a film for your camera').

Twenty-five patients with frontal lobe excisions were investigated on this task (ten RF; nine LF; six bifrontal), compared to intelligence quotient (IQ) matched controls. The results showed a clear impairment in the frontal lobe group, with the specificity of the deficit higher than that found in comparable tests of executive functioning, for example, the Wisconsin card sorting test. Additionally, an analysis of the errors made showed that when the patients did make errors they were differentially more prone to select distracter items that related to the 4 days. This tendency to go for more 'proximal' types of activity is consistent with the general characteristics of distractibility associated with the frontal lobe syndrome. This phenomenon, termed *contextual proximity*, may suggest a lower level of threshold of activation for schemata directing behavior, consistent with a breakdown of a supplementary central control mechanism, the supervisory attentional system (SAS), as suggested originally by Shallice (1982). In contrast with previous studies using similar patient groups, there were no differences in terms of the extent of deficit when comparing lesions in different hemispheres or prefrontal locations. This may be due to the complexity of the planning task, which could call into play the coordination of a variety of cognitive activities all supported by separate systems or regions within the prefrontal cortex.

COMMENT

The complexity of the prefrontal cortex is illustrated by the range of deficits found in patients with frontal lobe excisions, where the term 'executive' function has been used as a catch-all phase as a way of grouping them together. The foundations for understanding in these deficits have been layed through detailed studies of patients with surgical lesions as treatment for epilepsy, stemming principally from the Montreal Neurological Institute. As the studies reviewed above show, there are many aspects that are as yet still not fully understood. The symbiotic relationship between basic neuroscience and monitoring the outcome of treatment for epilepsy will continue in the future, with the frontal excision patient perhaps still providing an important opportunity to understand the neuroanatomic significance of the frontal cortex.

KEY POINTS

1. The effects of prefrontal surgical lesions for epilepsy have been investigated in some depth. An experimental approach to this field was heralded by the follow up of patient K.M. by Milner in 1962. The higher order function of the prefrontal cortex has been delineated by studying such patients.

2. Deficits in self-ordered 'searching' are associated with prefrontal lobe lesions and these have recently been demonstrated in relation to spatial search, involving spatial working memory.

3. Prefrontal cortical lesions can cause impairment in remembering the temporal order of events, but recent studies suggest that it is not the case when there is a semantic structure (for example, a familiar story line) linking the events.

4. Problem solving impairments are observed in patients with prefrontal lesions, specifically on the Tower of Hanoi or Tower of London tests. Recent studies suggest that left prefrontal damage may be associated with processing the 'novelty' aspect of planning, whilst that on the right is associated with the monitoring aspects.

5. Recent research has attempted to measure in the laboratory 'everyday' problems in problem solving or planning through the game 'simulation.' Tests such as the Virtual Planning Test indicate deficits in this area, but no specific association with the side or site of surgical lesion.

REFERENCES

Feigenbaum JD, Polkey CE, Morris RG (1996) Deficits in spatial working memory after unilateral temporal lobectomy in man. *Neuropsychologia* **34**:163–176.

Godbout L, Doyon J (1995) Mental representations of knowledge following frontal-lobe or posterolandic lesions. *Neuropsychologia* **33**:1671–1696.

Goel V, Grafman J (1995) Are the frontal lobes implicated in 'planning' functions? Interpreting data from the Tower of Hanoi. *Neuropsychologia* **33**:623–643.

Goldman-Rakic PS (1987) Circuitry of primate prefrontal cortex and regulation of behavior by representational memory. In: Plum F (ed.) *Handbook of Physiology: the Nervous System*, Vol 5, pp 373–417. Bethesda, MD: American Physiology Society.

Goldman-Rakic PS (1996) The prefrontal landscape: implications of functional architecture for understanding human mentation and the central executive. *Philosophical Transactions of the Royal Society of London B*, **351**:1445–1453.

Goldman-Rakic PS, Rosvold HE (1970) Localisation of function within the dorsolateral prefrontal cortex of the rhesus monkey. *Experimental Neurology* **27**:291–304.

Halstead WC (1940) Preliminary analysis of grouping behavior in patients with cerebral injury by the method of equivalent and nonequivalent stimuli. *American Journal of Physiology* **96**:1263–1294.

Harlow JM (1848) Recovery from the passage of an iron bar through the head. *Boston Medicine and Surgery Journal* **39**:289–293.

Harlow JM (1868) Recovery from the passage of an iron bar through the head. *Massachusetts Medical Society Publications* **2**:327–346.

Hebb DO (1939) Intelligence in man after large removal of cerebral tissue: report of four left frontal cases. *Journal of General Psychology* **21**:73–87.

Hebb DO (1941) Human intelligence after removal of cerebral tissue from the right frontal lobe. *Journal of General Psychology* **25**:257–264.

Hebb DO, Penfield W (1940) Human behavior after extensive bilateral removals from the frontal lobes. *Archives of Neurology and Psychiatry* **44**:421–436.

Ladavas E, Umilta C, Provinciali L (1979) Hemisphere-dependent cognitive performance in epileptic patients. *Epilepsia* **20**:493–502.

Milner B (1963) Effects of different brain lesions on card sorting. *Archives of Neurology* **9**:90–100.

Milner B (1964) Some effects of frontal lobectomy in man. In: Warren JM, Akert K (eds) *The Frontal Granular Cortex and Behavior*, pp 313–334. New York: McGraw-Hill.

Milner B (1995) Aspects of frontal lobe functioning. In: Jasper HH, Riggio S, Goldman-Rakic PS (eds) *Epilepsy and the Functional Anatomy of the Frontal Lobe*, pp 67–84. New York: Raven Press.

Milner B, Petrides M (1984) Behavioural effects of frontal-lobe lesions in man. *Trends in Neurosciences*, **7**:403–407.

Milner C (1975) Psychological aspects of focal epilepsy and its neurosurgical management. In: Purpura DP, Penry JK, Walter RD (eds) *Advances in Neurology*, Vol 8, pp 229–221. New York: Raven Press.

Milner B, Corkin S, Teuber HL (1968) Further analysis of the hippocampal amnesic syndrome: 14-year follow-up study of H.M. *Neuropsychologia* **6**:215–234.

Miotto EC, Morris RG (1998) Virtual planning in patients with frontal lobe lesions. *Cortex*, **34**: 639–657.

Miotto EC, Bullock P, Polkey CE, Morris RG (1996) Spatial working memory and strategy formation in patients with frontal lobe excisions. *Cortex* **32**:613–630.

Morris RG, Downes, JJ, Sahakian BJ, Evenden JL, Heald A, Robbins TW (1988). Planning and spatial working memory in Parkinson's disease. *Journal of Neurology, Neurosurgery and Psychiatry*. **51**:757–766.

Morris RG, Ahmed S, Syed GM, Toone BK (1993) Neural correlates of planning ability: frontal activation during the Tower of London test. *Neuropsychologia* **31**:1367–1378.

Morris RG, Miotto EC, Feigenbaum JD, Bullock P, Polkey CE (1997) The effect of goal–subgoal conflict on planning ability after frontal and temporal lesions in humans. *Neuropsychologia* **35**:1147–1157.

Morris RG, Miotto EC, Feigenbaum JD, Bullock P, Polkey CE (1998) Planning ability after frontal and temporal lobe lesions in humans: the effect of selection equivocation and working memory load. *Cognitive Neuropsychology* **14** (7):1007–1027.

Owen AM, Downes JJ, Sahakian BJ, Polkey CE, Robbins TW (1990)

Planning and spatial working memory following frontal lesions in man. *Neuropsychologia* **20**:249–262.

Owen AM, Morris RG, Sahakian BJ, Polkey CE, Robbins TW (1996) Double dissociations of memory and executive functions in a self-ordered working memory tasks following frontal lobe excision, temporal lobe excisions and amygdalohippocampectomy in man. *Brain* **119**:1597–1615.

Penfield W, Evans J (1935) The frontal lobe in man: a clinical study of maximum removals. *Brain* **58**:115–133.

Petrides M (1996) Specialized systems for the processing of mnemonic information within the primate frontal cortex. *Philosophical Transactions of the Royal Society of London* B **351**:1455–1462.

Petrides M, Milner B (1982) Deficits on subject-ordered tasks after frontal- and temporal-lobe lesions in man. *Neuropsychologia* **20**:249–262.

Roberts AC, Robbins TW, Weiskrantz L (1996) Executive and cognitive functions of the prefrontal cortex: introduction. *Philosophical Transactions of the Royal Society of London* B **351**:1389–1395.

Rylander G (1939) *Personality Changes after Operations of the Frontal Lobes.* London: Oxford University Press.

Schank RC (1979) *Reminding and memory organization: an introduction to MOPS.* Research Report No. 170. New Haven: Yale University, Department of Computer Science.

Schank RC, Abelson RP (1977) *Scripts, Plans and Understanding.* Hillsdale, NJ: Erlbaum.

Shallice T (1982) Specific impairments of planning. *Philosophical Transactions of the Royal Society of London* B **298**:199–209.

Shallice T, Burgess PW (1991) Deficits in strategy application following frontal lobe damage in man. *Brain* **114**:727–741.

Shallice T, Burgess PW (1996) The domain of supervisory processes and temporal organisation of behaviour. *Philosophical Transactions of the Royal Society of London* B **351**:1405–1412.

Shimamura AP, Janowksy JS, Squire LR (1990) Memory for the temporal order of events in patients with frontal lobe excisions and amnesic patients. *Neuropsychologia* **28**:803–813.

Simon HA (1975) The functional equivalence of problem-solving skills. *Cognitive Psychology* **7**:268–288.

Sirigu A, Zalla T, Pillon B, Grafman J, Dubois B, Agid Y (1996) Encoding of sequence and boundaries of scripts following prefrontal lesions. *Cortex* **32**:297–310.

Swain SA, Polkey CE, Bullock P, Morris RG (1988) Recognition memory and memory for order in script-based stories following frontal lobe excisions. *Cortex* **34**: 25–45.

Weigl E (1941) On the psychology of so-called processes of abstraction. *Journal of Abnormal Social Psychology* **36**:3–33.

Cognitive and memory changes after temporal lobe excisions

SM OXBURY

This chapter describes the changes in cognition and memory resulting from temporal lobe excisions for the relief of epilepsy. Thus it focuses on work in which neuropsychologic assessment was carried out both pre- and postoperatively. Studies that analyze function in postsurgical patients only provide important insights into localization of function. They help to guide further research and provide clues as to those functions that may be usefully evaluated in future pre- and postoperative work, but they cannot throw light on the important questions concerning the effects of the surgery. Thus they cannot contribute specifically to the analysis of factors that are associated with, and hence may be used to predict, change.

Over the last 10–15 years there have been huge advances in the endeavor to measure the neuropsychologic outcome of temporal lobe operations and to identify factors that may help to predict change in individual patients, particularly memory decline. Early pre/postoperative studies tended to group patients according to side of excision and to concentrate almost exclusively on laterality differences. Postoperative seizure relief was taken into account in some studies, and the Montreal group under Professor Brenda Milner's guidance have focused on differences related to the extent of the hippocampal removal, although this distinction has been used more often in postoperative studies than in evaluation of pre/postoperative change. The importance of the nature and extent of the underlying pathology, of the preoperative neuropsychologic status of the patient, and of

whether functional tissue was to be included in the excision began to be addressed in the mid-1980s. Much is now known about the influence of these and other related parameters on neuropsychologic outcome. The possibility of relating change to the extent and the location of excisions has also developed with the introduction of more restricted removals and the greater opportunity to image the brain postoperatively. Other factors, such as the functional intactness of the contralateral temporal lobe structures and gender differences in cognition have also come into play.

The main emphasis has been on memory. It has long been established firstly that the anterior temporal lobes, and particularly the medial structures, play a very important role in memory, especially in the acquisition of new information. Secondly, there is a hemispheric asymmetry with the left language-dominant anterior temporal lobe having a specific role in the registration and recall of verbal material and the right nondominant side being specialized to some degree for visuospatial and nonverbal material. Other cognitive functions have been evaluated, frequently in terms of an overall intelligence quotient (IQ) score, and there has been a good deal of work on language that may be vulnerable in dominant hemisphere operations. Examination of executive function is a fairly new area and this interest has arisen out of the observation that many temporal lobe epilepsy patients are impaired on executive function tasks preoperatively.

Methodological issues in pre/postoperative comparisons

include test–retest reliability, including practice effect which is particularly salient for tests of memory and learning as discussed in Chapter 46, and regression to the mean (Chelune *et al* 1991; Hermann *et al* 1991a). Group results are important in showing general trends and in providing evidence of change despite individual variance. However, there is also the question of what is a clinically significant change in terms of the quality of life of the individual patient. In neuropsychologic test measures, this is often defined operationally as one standard deviation of difference between the pre- and the postoperative scores. The length of follow-up interval is important. Early follow-up studies within about 1 month of the surgery may show impairments that are not apparent later, and this has to be remembered when interpreting results in such circumstances.

INTELLIGENCE AND GENERAL MEASURES OF COGNITIVE FUNCTION

Modest increases in full-scale IQ have been reported after anterior temporal lobectomy particularly where seizure outcome is good (Rausch and Crandall 1982) and possibly more often after right nondominant than after left dominant operations (Novelly *et al* 1984). It has been suggested that such changes reflect improved function of the non-operated hemisphere (Powell *et al* 1985). Indeed, Rausch and Crandall (1982) found improved scores on performance measures after left anterior temporal lobectomy (ATL) but not after right, and improved verbal IQ after right ATL but not after left. Verbal IQ also improved after right ATL in Ivnik *et al*'s (1987) study. Performance IQ and the perceptual organization factor derived from the Wechsler Adult Intelligence Scale-Revised (WAIS-R) improved after both right and left ATL, but the latter measures may be particularly susceptible to practice effects. Hermann and Wyler (1988a) emphasized that the majority of cognitive measures remain stable across surgery. They examined individual changes, operationally defined as a gain or loss of one or more standard deviation in an individual's score, in 64 cognitive measures. On this criterion, intelligence scores remained stable in 85% of patients, and two-thirds of the 15% changes were gains. The only significant laterality effect was on a visual-spatial measure where there were more losses after nondominant ATL than after dominant. This result has not been replicated and the authors suggested that it reflected the larger excisions in the nondominant temporal lobe. Memory scores showed more losses than gains as was to be expected in a temporal lobe surgery series (see below for detailed discussion). More

recently Phillips and McGlone (1995) have reported a similar study designed to identify clinically significant change (a gain or loss of one or more standard deviation as above) in individuals. They too found that most indices (68%) remained stable. There were very few changes in intelligence test scores and the number of gains and losses were approximately equal.

Hermann and Wyler (1988a) found age at operation to be associated with change in these general cognitive measures, with younger patients showing more improvement than older ones. Other factors, including gender, side of operation, and seizure outcome were not related.

The influence of specific pathologies on these intelligence measures has also been considered. McMillan *et al* (1987) found no significant IQ changes after ATL in patients with hippocampal sclerosis nor in the 'other pathology' group taken as a whole. Similarly, Kirkpatrick *et al* (1993) found no significant change in Verbal IQ or Performance IQ in 31 patients having ATL for tumor-related epilepsy, mostly attributable to dysembryoplastic neuroepithelial tumor. More recently, however, Seidenberg *et al* (1998) examined a range of cognitive measures in patients having standard ATL. They were grouped according to whether they had the syndrome of medial temporal lobe epilepsy (MTLE) characterized by classical hippocampal sclerosis, early childhood febrile convulsions, and a subsequent relatively early onset of the habitual epilepsy (see Chapter 11) or non-MTLE without evidence of other structural pathology. There was also a control group of patients with epilepsy who did not have surgery but who were tested on two occasions. This allowed a statistical computation of regression-based z scores for change, controlling for the effects of practice, measurement error, and regression to the mean. The results showed that the majority of changes occurred in the left non-MTLE patients. These included a drop in the verbal-comprehension factor derived from the Verbal IQ scale of the WAIS-R. This change was not related to seizure outcome. The authors discuss the possibility that these left non-MTLE patients, who have had essentially normal dominant anterior and medial temporal lobe structures removed, have suffered a reduced ability to retrieve information from long-term semantic memory in addition to the anterograde verbal memory decline detailed below.

Intuitively one would expect that the extent of anterior temporal lobe excision would affect neuropsychologic outcome and in particular that the greater the cortical excision the greater the chance of disturbing cognitive functions other than memory. This has been suggested for naming in dominant temporal lobe removals but was not found to affect other cognitive measures (Katz *et al* 1989; Wolf *et al*

1993). Oxbury *et al* (1995), however, compared cognitive outcome in patients with left hippocampal sclerosis grouped according to type of operation, selective amygdalohippocampectomy, or *en bloc* temporal lobectomy. The patients having selective surgery did better in terms of Verbal IQ at 2-years follow-up. This latter result, together with Seidenberg *et al*'s (1998) finding, suggests that the dominant anterior temporal lobe is involved in the processing and retrieval of verbal semantic information, and that there are indeed verbal disadvantages to the removals despite the small differences found in these studies. More restricted excisions would seem to be desirable whenever possible for the relief of the epilepsy.

LANGUAGE FUNCTION

As a general rule temporal lobe surgery does not seriously impair language function, but some risks are recognized after dominant hemisphere operations. There may be transient dysphasia in the acute phase. In a small number of patients this persists and is clinically significant. There may be a less significant but persisting increase in word-finding difficulty in a larger proportion of patients.

The evidence for mild but persisting effects has been conflicting. Hermann and colleagues (Hermann and Wyler 1988b; Hermann *et al* 1991b) reported pre/postoperative change in performance on the multilingual aphasia examination (MAE) at 6 months after ATL. The groups having dominant hemisphere surgery did not decline in language test scores in either study and, indeed, receptive language scores improved significantly, albeit by a small amount in absolute terms. Verbal fluency increased in the first study but not in the second, where variability in scores was considered to be attributable to the statistical phenomenon of regression to the mean. Similarly, Davies *et al* (1994, 1995) using the Boston naming test (BNT), verbal fluency tests, and subtests from the WAIS-R, reported no decline in naming or fluency at 1 year post-operation. In their first study, the extent of the lateral cortical resection was guided by stimulation mapping to spare the language areas and varied between 3 and 9 cm. There was a marginal drop in the ability to define words in the WAIS-R vocabulary test. In the second study, where a more standard ATL was performed without stimulation mapping of language areas, those having left dominant surgery gained significantly in verbal fluency and marginally in object naming.

On the other hand, Langfitt and Rausch (1996), using the more sensitive extended version of the BNT, found significant exacerbation of word-finding difficulty at 1 year post-operation in 30% of those who had undergone dominant left ATL. The group having right ATL improved their naming performance by a small but significant amount. Decline was associated with older age at surgery and with the postoperative interval, those tested earlier tending to show greater decline. Nevertheless, six of the seven identified as having significant decline were tested approximately 1 year after surgery. The deficit was of the 'tip of the tongue' type, with circumlocutions being fairly common, and phonemic cues often effective. This was similar to the preoperative pattern. The left ATL group included five right language-dominant patients, none of whom showed a decline in naming. Seidenberg *et al* (1998), in their comparison of patients with and without the syndrome of MTLE, reported significant postoperative language decline at 6 months after ATL in the left operated group without MTLE but not in those with MTLE nor in the right operated patients. The impairment was seen in the MAE naming subtest but not in aural comprehension. Language outcome was not related to seizure outcome.

Clinically apparent dysphasia in the acute postoperative period is not uncommon after dominant ATL and is usually transient. It is often attributed to local brain swelling around the site of the excision (Davies *et al* 1994) and usually resolves within weeks. Katz *et al* (1989) reported that after left dominant ATL, 5 of 29 patients developed mild dysphasia which was not completely resolved at discharge from hospital. This disturbance was not associated with the extent of the resection. Whether any had persisting problems at 1-year follow-up is not stated. Stafiniak *et al* (1990) studied acute change in language function following ATL and related it to the presence or absence of early risk factors. Early risk was defined as a CNS insult, such as a febrile convulsion, encephalitis or head trauma, suffered at or before the age of 5 years. At 2–3 weeks post-operation, left ATL patients without early risk showed a decline in naming scores relative to all other groups. Six of the ten such patients demonstrated a >25% decline, while no patients with early risk showed decline to that extent if at all. The deficit was typically of the 'word selection' type. Patients could often describe the objects but not provide the name, and some were aided by phonemic cueing. Atypical language representation determined by intracarotid sodium amobarbital tests was identified in 27% of the ATL patients. All but one of these had early risk, and none suffered naming decline. Saykin *et al* (1995) subsequently studied a larger sample and employed a wider range of language tests, six measures including the BNT. Again, they found a significant decline in language function only in the left group without early risk. The change occurred selectively in naming as compared to other linguistic functions. Inspection of these data suggest that average BNT scores in this group were down by more than three standard deviations at 3 weeks post-operation.

The incidence of persistent and clinically significant language change after left dominant ATL has been estimated as 6–10% (Pilcher *et al* 1993). It has usually been attributed to some individuals having language zones extending more anteriorly than others. Hermann *et al* (1994) reviewed 84 cases of left dominant ATL performed without functional mapping of language zones. As a group they were significantly but only slightly worse on the MAE naming test 6 months postoperatively as compared to preoperatively. Within the group, however, 7% had larger negative changes than the worst decline after any right temporal lobectomy. This figure is consistent with the Pilcher *et al* (1993) estimate. Furthermore it demonstrates that the analysis of group change can obscure the detection of a subset of patients who clearly have negative outcomes.

MEMORY

The importance of temporal lobe structures for anterograde memory function is well known, as already described in Chapter 30, and memory impairment in patients who have had unilateral temporal lobe surgery is well recognized. Such deficits have been characterized as showing laterality and material specificity. Thus, verbal memory deficits are seen after left operations and nonverbal deficits after right operations, although in the present state of our knowledge the former association appears to be more robust than the latter. It has also long been established that memory disorders may exist preoperatively and may be exacerbated by surgery. The important question in terms of neuropsychologic outcome is in what circumstances do aspects of memory deteriorate as a result of surgery and can this be avoided? The ability to predict change is fundamental to informed preoperative counseling of patients. In this context verbal memory and left temporal lobe surgery have been studied to a much greater extent than nonverbal memory and right temporal lobe surgery. The association between verbal memory impairment and left temporal lobe damage is a more consistent finding and hence a more promising area for analysis, and verbal memory decline after left temporal lobe surgery may sometimes be quite marked and troublesome. Right temporal lobe surgery patients seldom complain of nonverbal or spatial memory impairment. Indeed, at the Second International Palm Desert Conference on Epilepsy

Surgery, patients undergoing dominant ATL were considered to be those most at risk of neuropsychologic morbidity (Dodrill *et al* 1993).

VERBAL MEMORY

Most studies reporting pre/postoperative change in verbal memory have used standard tests of anterograde memory. These are usually:

1. Story recall tasks such as the logical memory from the Wechsler memory scale (WMS).
2. Verbal learning tasks including: word pairs (paired associate learning from WMS); word lists (auditory verbal learning test, California verbal learning test; Bushke–Fulds selective reminding test).

Various scores derived from these tests have been used to evaluate changes and their relationship to other factors. The majority of studies have restricted their patient groups to those with left hemisphere language dominance as demonstrated by carotid amobarbital testing.

VERBAL MEMORY CHANGE AFTER LEFT TEMPORAL LOBE SURGERY

Factors associated with verbal memory change include the following.

Hippocampal pathology

Verbal memory change is related to the pathologic status of the excised hippocampus. Thus Rausch (1987) reported that those with little or no hippocampal sclerosis showed greater verbal memory decline after left ATL than those with more marked pathology. Similarly, Oxbury and Oxbury (1989), using combined verbal memory scores from story recall and paired associate learning, showed very significant postoperative decline on all measures in patients whose excision specimens had contained virtually normal hippocampus. Those patients with classical severe hippocampal sclerosis did not decline in the immediate memory score although they did show some decline in the delayed memory score. Others have reported comparable findings in story recall (Hermann *et al* 1992) and word list learning (Helmstaedter and Elger 1996). Employing volumetric magnetic resonance imaging (MRI) parameters as a measure of hippocampal atrophy, Trenerry *et al* (1993) even reported some improvement in story recall scores after excision of particularly atrophic left hippocampal formation. Resection of relatively nonatrophic left hippocampal formation was followed by poor verbal memory outcome. This pattern was again confirmed by Sass *et al* (1994) using a different verbal memory measure, the selective reminding test (a form of word-list learning), where those with severe hippocampal neuron loss did not change significantly but those with only mild to moderate hippocampal neuron loss showed significant deterioration.

Most recently Seidenberg *et al* (1998), in a well-controlled study, used a wide range of measures to compare neuropsychologic outcome following ATL in patients with and without the syndrome of MTLE. They found that the most significant declines occurred in the left non-MTLE group with verbal memory being the most substantial area of decline, again confirming the relationship between verbal memory decline and removal of nonsclerotic hippocampus.

Preoperative neuropsychologic status

It has often been observed that patients who have the most intact verbal memory preoperatively show the greatest postoperative decline (Powell *et al* 1985; Rausch 1987; Ivnik *et al* 1988). More specifically Chelune *et al* (1991), using several verbal memory measures derived from the WMS together with word-list learning, showed that higher preoperative performances were associated with larger decrements in postsurgical scores. Similar findings have been reported by Hermann *et al* (1991a, 1995), Helmstaedter and Elger (1996), and Davies *et al* (1998) using word-list learning tasks, and also by Jokeit *et al* (1997) using story recall.

This now well-established finding is a reflection of the effect of removing functional tissue and is substantially related to the pathologic status of the hippocampus as described above. Those without hippocampal pathology have higher preoperative verbal memory function (see Chapter 30) and are at a greater risk of memory decline when nonsclerotic functional tissue is removed.

Age at seizure onset

An association between age at seizure onset and verbal memory outcome after left temporal lobe surgery has been shown in some studies. Saykin *et al* (1989) reported that patients with early onset (mean = 1.9 years) did not decline in story recall after left ATL, whereas those with later onset (mean = 16.0 years) did. Similarly, Wolf *et al* (1993) and Hermann *et al* (1995) found a greater postoperative decline in story recall and word-list learning to be associated with later age of onset. On the other hand, Jokeit *et al* (1997) found early epilepsy onset to be associated with an increased risk to memory function, although in contrast early probable age at temporal lobe

damage was associated with better memory prognosis after left-sided surgery. Davies *et al* (1998) found no association between age at onset and verbal memory decline following left ATL.

Inconsistencies in these findings are probably due to differences in patient populations, particularly the pathologic make-up of the groups, and possibly to test selection or to the parameters chosen for analysis from those tests and the treatment of the results. Where it is found, the age of onset effect, whereby those with early seizure onset show less verbal memory decline postoperatively than those with later onset, is at least partly related to the factors discussed above. Early onset of recurrent seizures is a typical feature of the syndrome of MTLE, which is characterized by hippocampal sclerosis, and we have already seen that after left ATL such patients have better verbal memory outcome than those without hippocampal sclerosis. This is very clearly illustrated in Seidenberg *et al*'s (1998) report where left MTLE patients were shown to be at much less risk of verbal decline than the left non-MTLE patients. The average age of onset in the groups was 6.7 years and 20.5 years, respectively.

Age at operation

Older age at surgery has been considered to be associated with poorer memory outcome (Blakemore and Falconer 1967), and this corresponds to impressions in clinical practice, at least in the Oxford experience. Age at surgery, however, and age at onset are correlated and so it is possible that younger age at surgery is more associated with the presence of hippocampal sclerosis, which we know gives a more favorable memory outcome. Saykin *et al* (1989) found no age at surgery effect, despite their clear age at onset effect. Their follow-up, however, was carried out 1 month after surgery when changes are far from stabilized and this might have influenced the findings. More recently Hermann *et al* (1995) have examined some of these factors in order to determine their unique predictive relation to pre/postoperative verbal memory decline. Using both story recall and word-list learning they found that age at surgery significantly predicted decline. This was seen specifically in word-list learning. Helmstaedter and Elger (1996, 1998) also found significant age at surgery effects in a word-list learning test. Patients aged >30 years, but not those aged <15 years, were particularly at risk in the acquisition phase. On the other hand the consolidation/retrieval score deteriorated in all age groups. Thus we may conclude that older age at surgery is indeed a factor in poor verbal memory outcome after left ATL.

Gender

A number of studies in recent years have addressed the question of gender differences in outcome from temporal lobectomy. A female advantage in verbal memory outcome after left ATL has been reported by Geckler *et al* (1993). Trenerry *et al* (1995), using story recall, and Davies *et al* (1996), using word-list learning, also found that verbal memory was less likely to decline after left ATL in females than in males. Berenbaum *et al* (1997), however, found that women were superior to men on the word-list learning both pre- and postoperatively but did not differ in the extent of their pre/postoperative change. It seems too early to draw any firm conclusions in this area.

Seizure outcome

Continuing seizures have been considered to contribute to reduced verbal memory after left ATL. Recent work, however, does not indicate that it is a major factor. Both Sass *et al* (1994) and Seidenberg *et al* (1998) found verbal memory decline to be independent of seizure outcome. In both studies, outcome was related to the presence or absence of hippocampal sclerosis and Seidenberg *et al*'s (1998) data comparing left operated patients with and without the syndrome of MTLE demonstrate this very clearly. Both groups showed equal decline. Similarly, Jokeit *et al* (1997) found patients who became seizure-free did not differ in memory change from patients who continued to have seizures, but good preoperative memory was a strong predictor of postoperative loss. Helmstaedter and Elger (1996), however, report a relationship between continuing seizures and one measure of verbal memory, the recognition score in their list-learning task. There was no association for the other verbal memory measures which declined in left ATL patients.

Thus, although continuing seizures may have some effect on verbal memory functioning after surgery, their importance is minor compared to that of the functional and structural integrity of the excised tissue.

Extent of excision

One would expect that the extent of both the medial and the lateral temporal excision would influence the degree of verbal memory decline. This has not, however, been found consistently for ATL. Katz *et al* (1989) found no correlation between story recall and size of total resection, nor size of resection in basal, inferolateral, or superolateral quadrants, but the extent of medial resection approached significance. In contrast, Helmstaedter and Elger (1996) found decline in both acquisition and recognition in word-list learning to be associated with the extent of the lateral neocortical excision. Wolf *et al* (1993) did not find any association between verbal memory decline and the extent of either medial or lateral cortical resection.

On the other hand, comparisons between amygdalo-hippocampectomy and ATL have produced some results. Goldstein and Polkey (1993) compared outcome after amygdalohippocampectomy and temporal lobectomy. After left operations, story recall scores declined with no difference between the surgical groups. Decline in paired-associate learning, however, was greater after temporal lobectomy than after amygdalohippocampectomy. The authors point out the difference was marginal. They also raised the possibility that these cognitive differences may have been explained by differences in pathology since their groups were not matched in this respect. Oxbury *et al* (1995) compared *en bloc* temporal lobectomy and selective amygdalo-hippocampectomy in groups matched for hippocampal pathology, and found less verbal memory decline after amygdalohippocampectomy than after temporal lobectomy at 2-year follow-up.

Hill (1998) found impaired performance on the word-list learning selective reminding test with no difference between the groups, but ATL were more impaired than selective amygdalohippocampectomy on an experimental version of story recall (Frisk and Milner 1990). She then devised a task in which story context was used to facilitate selective reminding word-list learning. Those who had undergone selective amygdalohippocampectomy were able to benefit but the performance of the ATL patients did not improve at all. This work was done on postoperative patients only, so it is possible that the differences would have been present preoperatively, but it nevertheless suggests that the combination of deficits in different aspects of verbal memory seen after standard temporal lobectomy, as opposed to restricted medial excisions, may be particularly handicapping.

Helmstaedter *et al* (1996) also found differences in verbal memory outcome after left ATL, selective amygdalohippocampectomy, and temporocorticolesionectomy. Both the ATL and the selective amygdalohippocampectomy groups declined in delayed recall and recognition scores on word-list learning, but there was an additional decline in immediate recall in the ATL group. In contrast there was no change in verbal memory after temporocorticolesionectomy in which only pathologic tissue was removed. The authors conclude that the medial and lateral temporal structures subserve different aspects of verbal memory, and also that the declines seen are related to the removal of still-functioning brain tissue.

This last comment emphasizes yet again the importance of the pathologic and functional status of tissue to be excised. The point is made very forcefully by Chelune (1995) in relation to medial resections when he says: 'A large resection may produce no more effect on memory than a small resection if the hippocampus is highly dysfunctional'. In addition, the above findings suggest that although selective amygdalohippocampectomy as opposed to ATL does not protect against verbal memory decline, it may have a somewhat lesser effect than ATL where there is a risk of added deficit consequent upon removal of lateral neocortex. The extent to which differential functions of medial and lateral structures in aspects of verbal memory and learning can be teased apart on the basis of present evidence is discussed by Helmstaedter et al (1997).

The structural and functional integrity of the contralateral temporal lobe

There is some evidence that verbal memory decline after dominant left temporal operations is partly related to the intactness of the right temporal lobe. This stems from studies using various markers of right temporal lobe integrity. Using MRI volumetrics, Trenerry et al (1993) reported that not only the size of the left hippocampus but also that of the right was associated with postoperative verbal memory and learning capacity. In a second study, Trenerry et al (1996a) examined outcome in patients with symmetrical hippocampal volumes. Both those with bilaterally nonatrophic hippocampi and those with bilaterally atrophic hippocampi declined in verbal memory after left ATL. Those with bilateral hippocampal atrophy tended to show the greater decline although the difference did not reach significance. This differs from the usual finding that those with left hippocampal sclerosis decline less than those without hippocampal sclerosis and suggests that the additional atrophy in the right hippocampus has affected verbal memory outcome. Parallel conclusions may be drawn from data from carotid amobarbital studies. Jokeit et al (1997) found impaired right hemisphere memory function to be a significant predictor of verbal memory decline after left temporal lobectomy, and Loring et al (1995) found that symmetrical carotid amobarbital memory scores were associated with verbal memory decline. Preoperative neuropsychologic performance suggestive of right temporal lobe dysfunction was related to poor outcome in verbal memory measures in a study by Helmstaedter and Elger (1996).

VERBAL MEMORY CHANGE AFTER RIGHT TEMPORAL LOBE SURGERY

In general, right temporal lobe surgery is not deleterious to verbal memory. Indeed, there have been several reports of improvements in verbal memory postoperatively (Rausch and Crandall 1982; Novelly et al 1984; Hermann et al 1995; Helmstaedter and Elger 1996; Trenerry et al 1996a). In several other studies verbal memory does not change.

There are some reports, however, indicating that verbal memory decline may occur after right temporal lobectomy in some circumstances. For example, in the Novelly et al (1984) study improvement did not occur in those with poor seizure outcome and this group tended to decline in verbal memory at later follow-up. Incisa della Rocchetta et al (1995) related poor verbal memory after right temporal lobectomy to abnormality in the left temporal lobe as demonstrated by MRI spectroscopy. This was a postoperative study only and it is not known whether the poor verbal memory in these right temporal lobe patients predated the surgery. Davies et al (1998) report the risk of verbal memory decline after right temporal lobectomy to be greater in older patients with low IQ. All these findings suggest that factors beyond the right temporal lobe are involved. There are also hints that removal of a nonsclerotic right nondominant hippocampus could have a mild effect on verbal memory. There is a tendency for those without hippocampal sclerosis to decline in verbal memory (Oxbury and Oxbury 1989; Hermann et al 1992; Seidenberg et al 1996). This, however, is insubstantial compared to the losses after removal of nonsclerotic left dominant hippocampus.

NONVERBAL MEMORY CHANGES AFTER TEMPORAL LOBE SURGERY

Right temporal lobe operations

Impaired memory for nonverbal stimuli in patients who have had right temporal lobe surgery has been demonstrated for many types of material that cannot easily be coded in words. These include nonsense figures, stylus maze learning (both visual and tactual), faces, spatial location (Kimura 1963; Corkin 1965; Milner 1965, 1968; Smith and Milner 1981; Pigott and Milner 1993; Jones-Gotman et al 1997; Nunn et al 1998). These findings certainly point to a range of nonverbal memory function associated with the right anterior temporal lobe, both cortical and medial structures. Few of the studies, however, have addressed the question relevant to epilepsy surgery practice – whether and in what circumstances the deficits are actually caused by the surgery or whether they are present preoperatively.

Taylor (1969) reported pre/postoperative decline in right temporal lobectomy patients in recall of the complex Rey figure. Until quite recently much of the work in the pre- and postoperative assessment of temporal lobe surgery patients has focused on figural recall tasks, mainly the Rey figure, the visual reproduction of figures from the WMS, and occasionally the Benton visual retention test. All these figures are considered to be largely verbally encodable but have been used because of the paucity of more appropriate standard clinical tests.

These figural memory tests have not yielded reliable or consistent findings. Reports have included mild decline after right temporal lobectomy (Novelly *et al* 1984), no change (Rausch and Crandall 1982; Naugle *et al* 1993) and improvement (Saykin *et al* 1989). No significant association between figural memory change and the pathologic status of excised hippocampus has been shown (Rausch and Babb 1993; Trenerry *et al* 1993; Wyler *et al* 1995). There was, however, a slight trend in this direction in two studies (Hermann *et al* 1992, Seidenberg *et al* 1998). Trenerry *et al* (1996b) found an association between removal of nonatrophic right hippocampus and visual memory decline in females but not in males. Preoperative level of performance has not been associated with postoperative change (Chelune *et al* 1991). There was no significant association between the extent of the medial or the cortical excision and figural memory in the study of Katz *et al* (1989). Likewise, Wyler *et al* (1995) did not find any association between the extent of the right hippocampal excision and figural memory change in a blinded, randomized ATL trial comparing large and small hippocampal excisions.

A face memory task has shown a significant but modest postoperative decline after right but not left ATL, but performance on this task was not associated with the extent of the hippocampal removal nor the presence or absence of hippocampal sclerosis (Wyler *et al* 1995).

Figural *learning* tasks, utilizing a series of abstract designs presented over several trials, may be more useful. Trenerry *et al* (1993) found pre-/postoperative decline in visual learning in those whose operations included the excision of a nonatrophic right hippocampus. Gleissner *et al* (1998) found that the group with right hippocampal sclerosis, who were impaired on this task preoperatively, did not decline further after selective amygdalohippocampectomy, nor was there any decline in patients without hippocampal sclerosis, none of whom had hippocampal

removals. These latter were mostly tumor cases undergoing lesionectomy. These authors were not able to test further their claim that this type of learning is a hippocampal function by examining some patients from whom nonatrophic hippocampus was removed and who would have been expected to decline. Using postoperative patients only, Majdan *et al* (1996) have found right temporal lobectomy patients to be impaired on a similar figural learning task. The results of these studies suggest that the deficit, when it is seen, affects initial learning more than delayed recall or recognition.

It is possible that greater understanding of the role of the medial and cortical structures of the right temporal lobe and the effects of surgical removal will come to light as more work is focused on figural learning and spatial learning and memory tasks. Nevertheless, at a purely clinical level it is fair to say that patients who have had right temporal lobe epilepsy surgery including medial removals do not often complain of memory disturbance postoperatively, particularly those with a typical history of medial temporal lobe epilepsy and hippocampal pathology.

Left temporal lobe operations

In general, left temporal lobe operation is not considered to have an adverse effect on nonverbal memory tasks. Thus Rausch and Crandall (1982) found no change in visual reproduction scores after left ATL, and Novelly *et al* (1984) found that after a mild early postoperative decline nonverbal memory improved significantly in relation to the preoperative level in those with good seizure outcome. Some reports, however, describe a less favorable outcome in specific groups. In Novelly *et al*'s (1984) study those with poor seizure outcome suffered a loss in visual reproduction scores. Saykin *et al* (1989) found an unexpected decline in figural memory in left temporal lobectomy patients with early onset epilepsy and attributed it to 'a crowding effect'. On the other hand, other studies have shown that the risk is greater in those who have nonsclerotic left hippocampus removed (Hermann *et al* 1992; Trenerry *et al* 1993; Seidenberg *et al* 1998). These findings have been dismissed as merely reflecting *verbal* memory deficit since the test material is considered to be easily verbalizable. An alternative explanation is that these mild losses after removal of intact hippocampus reflect some sort of general memory decline additional to any material-specific factor. This could be analogous to the mild verbal memory loss after removal of nonsclerotic right hippocampus described in a previous section.

SEVERE AMNESIA

There is a small risk that unilateral temporal lobectomy will cause a severe and lasting generalized memory impairment (Penfield and Milner 1958; Loring *et al* 1994). This severe amnesic syndrome is a disabling condition unlike the relatively mild, material-specific disorders described above. It consists of a global anterograde amnesia, such that the patient is unable to learn new material or to remember ongoing daily events, while general intelligence is preserved. It is associated with a preexisting abnormality in the medial structures, especially the hippocampus, of the non-operated temporal lobe (Penfield and Mathieson 1974; Warrington and Duchen 1992). An excision that includes the medial structures then deprives the patient of adequate function bilaterally. When there are doubts about the structural and functional integrity of the temporal lobe contralateral to the proposed surgery, then it is necessary to demonstrate by carotid amobarbital tests that this hemisphere can support memory function (see Chapter 47). As far as the author is aware, in all the reported cases of the development of severe amnesia following temporal lobe surgery since the introduction of carotid amobarbital memory tests, the test criterion has been failed.

A case of a patient who developed the severe amnesic syndrome as a late complication of successful left temporal lobectomy has been described (Oxbury *et al* 1997). This young man had been seizure-free and neuropsychologically intact for 8 years postoperatively until a mild head injury provoked a return of seizures. These became uncontrolled leading to a bout of status epilepticus, which caused severe cell loss in the right hippocampus thus depriving him of hippocampal function bilaterally.

EXECUTIVE FUNCTION

Preoperative studies have shown deficits in temporal lobe epilepsy patients on the Wisconsin card sorting test and on verbal fluency, both traditionally regarded as executive function tasks reflecting frontal lobe function (see Chapters 30 and 31). This has prompted interest in whether the performance of such patients is modified by temporal lobe surgery.

WISCONSIN CARD SORTING TEST

Several studies have reported pre- and postoperative results on the Wisconsin card sorting test (Hermann and Wyler 1988a; Trenerry and Jack 1994; Hermann and Seidenberg 1995; Tuunainen *et al* 1995; Seidenberg *et al* 1998). None have reported postoperative decline. Improvements were reported in all studies but did not always reach statistical significance. These findings do not support a specific role for the anterior temporal lobe or the hippocampus in this executive function task, since excision did not exacerbate the preoperative deficits even when apparently normal tissue was excised. Rather, Hermann and Seidenberg (1995) found that in those who were impaired preoperatively change was significantly related to seizure outcome, there being a greater number of improvements among those who had become seizure-free. This finding supports the hypothesis that the original deficits are attributable to distal effects of the temporal lobe focus.

CHILDREN

DEVELOPMENTAL LEVEL AND INTELLIGENCE

Temporal lobectomy in children does not affect developmental level or IQ in the short term (Adams *et al* 1990; Szabó *et al* 1998). Meyer *et al* (1986) evaluated 50 children over intervals ranging from 6 months to 10 years. They too found no overall IQ change but a shorter interval between seizure onset and surgery was associated with IQ increase postoperatively. In Oxford, Oxbury *et al* (1996) have followed 28 children over 5 years after temporal lobe surgery carried out when they were aged <16 years. Seventeen had right operations and eleven left. Pathology was hippocampal sclerosis in 14 and dysembryoplastic neuroepithelial tumor (DNT) in 10. IQ was average preoperatively and maintained this level over the 5-year period. Recently the same group have reported the cognitive outcome in a specific group of children, those who had temporal lobe surgery for DNT, and were aged <12 years at operation (Knight *et al* 1998). Five of these children were aged <6 years at surgery and in most of these, preoperative developmental quotient (DQ) was compared with postoperative IQ. Defining a significant change as one standard deviation in score (i.e. 15 points of DQ or IQ), no child changed significantly over the 5-year period, showing that they continued to make cognitive progress at the rate predicted by their preoperative levels. The one possible exception was the only preschool child who underwent left-sided surgery. She dropped 14 IQ points over 5 years, so conclusions about very young children with a left-sided tumor should be guarded. Individual discrepancies between Verbal IQ and Performance IQ ranged widely and were unrelated to laterality of pathology.

MEMORY

The WMS memory quotient did not change overall in the Meyer *et al* (1986) series, but girls improved while boys worsened slightly. Verbal and nonverbal subtests, however, were not analyzed separately in relation to laterality. Adams *et al* (1990) found decreased verbal memory 6 months after left-sided operations but not right, and no change in either group on delayed reproduction of the Rey figure. Szabó *et al* (1998) examined 14 children who had undergone temporal lobe resections aged <13 years at a similar postoperative stage. They found a decrease in immediate verbal memory scores in those who had higher preoperative memory function and who underwent a left temporal lobe resection. Postoperative decreases in delayed memory were independent of preoperative ability or side of operation. Helmstaedter and Elger (1998) examining changes in verbal memory after left ATL included 12 children aged <15 years. In these they reported improved acquisition/learning in a word-list learning task, in contrast to older patients, but the consolidation/retrieval score deteriorated in all age groups. At 5-year follow-up, Oxbury *et al* (1996) found a decline in paired-associate learning compared to preoperatively in the left temporal group but not in the right. Nonverbal memory improved in both groups. Thus memory in children is vulnerable to deterioration after temporal lobe epilepsy surgery, particularly verbal memory after left-sided operations and this is not a transient effect.

LANGUAGE

Language was assessed in the Adams *et al* (1990) study. Six weeks after left-sided surgery children had slightly, but significantly, lower scores than preoperatively on a naming test. This had recovered at 6 months. No changes were evident in two verbal comprehension tasks, the test for the reception of grammar (TROG) and the token test. In the right, but not the left, operated group significant improvement was seen on the TROG at 6 months. At 5-year follow-up the token test scores were normal in both groups (Oxbury *et al* 1996). Object naming had improved in the right operated group but not in the left.

KEY POINTS

1. There is little if any effect on measures of intelligence and general cognitive function.
2. Language function is not usually affected although there have been reports of around 7% of patients developing a persistent and clinically significant dysnomic disorder after left dominant anterior temporal lobectomy. There may be a mild persisting increase in word-finding difficulty in up to 30% of patients.
3. Verbal memory is particularly likely to decline following left temporal lobe surgery if preoperative verbal memory and learning is good, if normal hippocampus is excised. It is less likely to do so when seizure onset has been at a young age, when surgery is undertaken at a young age, and when the contralateral hippocampus is intact. Seizure outcome is not a major factor in this respect.
4. Removal of severely sclerotic left hippocampus from patients whose verbal memory is already poor does not usually precipitate any marked change.
5. Selective amygdalohippocampectomy does not protect against verbal memory decline but can be less deleterious than a combined removal of medial and lateral structures.
6. Any nonverbal memory decline after right nondominant surgery is usually relatively asymptomatic.
7. Severe disabling amnesia is a rare complication and occurs when the contralateral temporal lobe structures cannot support memory.
8. Executive function does not decline.
9. Temporal lobe surgery in children does not appear to interrupt the normal development of intelligence and general cognitive ability, at least in those aged >6 years at operation and preschool children having right-sided operations. The risks to memory are similar to those in adults.

REFERENCES

Adams CBT, Beardsworth ED, Oxbury SM, Oxbury JM, Fenwick PBC (1990) Temporal lobectomy in 44 children: outcome and neuropsychological follow-up. *Journal of Epilepsy* **3** (Suppl 1):157–168.

Berenbaum SA, Baxter L, Seidenberg M, Hermann B (1997) Role of the hippocampus in sex differences in verbal memory: memory outcome following left anterior temporal lobectomy. *Neuropsychology* **11**(4):585–591.

Blakemore CB, Falconer MA (1967) Long-term effects of anterior temporal lobectomy on certain cognitive functions. *Journal of Neurology, Neurosurgery and Psychiatry* **30**:364–367.

Chelune GJ (1995) Hippocampal adequacy versus functional reserve: predicting memory functions following temporal lobectomy. *Archives of Clinical Neuropsychology* **10**:413–432.

Chelune GJ, Naugle RI, Lüders H, Awad IA (1991) Prediction of cognitive change as a function of preoperative ability status among temporal lobectomy patients seen at 6-month follow-up. *Neurology* **41**:399–404.

Corkin S (1965) Tactually guided maze learning in man. Effects of unilateral cortical excisions and bilateral hippocampal lesions. *Neuropsychologia* **3**:339–351.

Davies KG, Maxwell RE, Jennum P et al (1994) Language function following subdural grid-directed temporal lobectomy. *Acta Neurologica Scandinavica* **90**:201–206.

Davies KG, Maxwell RE, Beniak TE, Destafney E, Fiol ME (1995) Language function after temporal lobectomy without stimulation mapping of cortical function. *Epilepsia* **36**(2):130–136.

Davies K, Hermann B, Bush A, Wyler A (1996) Prediction of episodic memory loss in individuals following anterior temporal lobectomy using a regression model. *Epilepsia* **37** (Suppl 5):130.

Davies KG, Bell BD, Bush AJ, Wyler AR (1998) Prediction of verbal memory loss in individuals after anterior temporal lobectomy. *Epilepsia* **39**(8):820–828.

Dodrill CB, Jones-Gotman M, Loring D, Sass KJ (1993) Postscript: contributions of neuropsychology. In: Engel J Jnr (ed.) *Surgical Treatment of the Epilepsies*, 2nd edn, pp 309–312. New York: Raven Press.

Frisk V, Milner B (1990) The relationship of working memory to the immediate recall of stories following unilateral temporal or frontal lobectomy. *Neuropsychologia* **28**:121–135.

Geckler C, Chelune G, Trenerry M, Ivnik R (1993) Gender-related differences in cognitive status following temporal lobectomy. *Archives of Clinical Neuropsychology* **8**:226–227.

Gleissner U, Helmstaedter C, Elger CE (1998) Right hippocampal contribution to visual memory: a presurgical and postsurgical study in patients with temporal lobe epilepsy. *Journal of Neurology, Neurosurgery and Psychiatry* **65**:665–669.

Goldstein LH, Polkey CE (1993) Short-term cognitive changes after unilateral temporal lobectomy or unilateral amygdalohippocampectomy for the relief of temporal lobe epilepsy. *Journal of Neurology, Neurosurgery and Psychiatry* **56**:135–140.

Helmstaedter C, Elger CE (1996) Cognitive consequences of two-thirds anterior temporal lobectomy on verbal memory in 144 patients: a 3-month follow-up study. *Epilepsia* **37**(2):171–180.

Helmstaedter C, Elger CE (1998) Functional plasticity after left anterior temporal lobectomy: reconstitution and compensation of verbal memory functions. *Epilepsia* **39**(4):399–406.

Helmstaedter C, Elger CE, Hufnagel A, Zentner J, Schramm J (1996) Different effects of left anterior temporal lobectomy, selective amygdalohippocampectomy, and temporal cortical lesionectomy on verbal learning, memory and recognition. *Journal of Epilepsy* **9**:39–45.

Helmstaedter C, Grunwald TH, Lehnertz K, Gleißner U (1997) Differential involvement of left temporolateral and temporomesial structures in verbal declarative learning and memory: evidence from temporal lobe epilepsy. *Brain and Cognition* **35**:110–131.

Hermann B, Seidenberg M (1995) Executive system dysfunction in temporal lobe epilepsy: effects of nociferous cortex versus hippocampal pathology. *Journal of Clinical and Experimental Neuropsychology* **17**(6):809–819.

Hermann BP, Wyler AR (1988a) Neuropsychological outcome of anterior temporal lobectomy. *Journal of Epilepsy* **1**:35–45.

Hermann BP, Wyler AR (1988b) Effects of anterior temporal lobectomy on language function: a controlled study. *Annals of Neurology* **23**:585–588.

Hermann HP, Wyler AR, Vanderzwagg R et al (1991a) Predictors of neuropsychological change following anterior temporal lobectomy. role of regression toward the mean. *Journal of Epilepsy* **4**:139–148.

Hermann BP, Wyler AR, Somes G (1991b) Language function following anterior temporal lobectomy. *Journal of Neurosurgery* **74**:560–566.

Hermann BP, Wyler AR, Somes G, Berry AD III, Dohan FC (1992) Pathological status of the mesial temporal lobe predicts memory outcome from left anterior temporal lobectomy. *Neurosurgery* **31**(4):652–657.

Hermann BP, Wyler AR, Somes G, Clement L (1994) Dysnomia after left anterior temporal lobectomy without functional mapping: frequency and correlates. *Neurosurgery* **35**(1):52–57.

Hermann BP, Seidenberg M, Haltiner A, Wyler AR (1995) Relationship of age at onset, chronologic age, and adequacy of preoperative performance to verbal memory change after anterior temporal lobectomy. *Epilepsia* **36**(2):137–145.

Hill V (1998) *Memory function and the temporal lobes.* Unpublished DPhil thesis. University of Oxford.

Incisa della Rocchetta A, Gadian DG, Connelly A et al (1995) Verbal memory impairment after right temporal lobe surgery: role of contralateral damage as revealed by ^{1}H magnetic resonance spectroscopy and T2 relaxometry. *Neurology* **45**:797–802.

Ivnik RJ, Sharbrough FW, Laws ER (1987) Effects of anterior temporal lobectomy on cognitive function. *Journal of Clinical Psychology* **43**(1):128–137.

Ivnik RJ, Sharbrough FW, Laws ER (1988) Anterior temporal lobectomy for the control of partial complex seizures: information for counselling patients. *Mayo Clinic Proceedings* **63**:783–793.

Jokeit H, Ebner A, Holthausen H et al (1997) Individual prediction of change in delayed recall of prose passages after left-sided anterior temporal lobectomy. *Neurology* **49**:481–487.

Jones-Gotman M, Zatorre RJ, Olivier A et al (1997) Learning and retention of words and designs following excision from medial or lateral temporal lobe structures. *Neuropsychologia* **35**(7):963–973.

Katz A, Awad IA, Kong AK et al (1989) Extent of resection in temporal lobectomy for epilepsy. II. Memory changes and neurologic complications. *Epilepsia* **30**(6):763–771.

Kimura D (1963) Right temporal lobe damage. *Archives of Neurology* **8**:264–271.

Kirkpatrick PJ, Honavar M, Janota I, Polkey CE (1993) Control of temporal lobe epilepsy following *en bloc* resection of low-grade tumors. *Journal of Neurosurgery* **87**:19–25.

Knight ES, Oxbury JM, Oxbury SM, Middleton JA (1998) Cognitive development in children under 12 years of age after temporal lobe epilepsy surgery (TLES) for dysembryoplastic neuroepithelial tumor (DNET). *Epilepsia* **39** (Suppl 6):172.

Langfitt JT, Rausch R (1996) Word-finding deficits persist after left anterotemporal lobectomy. *Archives of Neurology* **53**:72–76.

Loring DW, Hermann BP, Meadow KJ et al (1994) Amnesia after unilateral temporal lobectomy: a case report. *Epilepsia* **35**(4):757–763.

Loring DW, Meador KJ, Lee GP et al (1995) Wada memory

asymmetries predict verbal memory decline after anterior temporal lobectomy. *Neurology* **45**:1329–1333.

McMillan TM, Powell GE, Janota I, Polkey CE (1987) Relationships between neuropathology and cognitive functioning in temporal lobectomy patients. *Journal of Neurology, Neurosurgery and Psychiatry* **50**(2):167–176.

Majdan A, Sziklas V, Jones-Gotman M (1996) Performance of healthy subjects and patients with resection from the anterior temporal lobe on matched tests of verbal and visuoperceptual learning. *Journal of Clinical and Experimental Neuropsychology* **18**:416–430.

Meyer FB, Marsh WR, Laws ER, Sharbrough FW (1986) Temporal lobectomy in children with epilepsy. *Journal of Neurosurgery* **64**:371–376.

Milner B (1965) Visually guided maze learning in man: effects of bilateral hippocampal, bilateral frontal and unilateral cerebral lesions. *Neuropsychologia* **3**:317–338.

Milner B (1968) Visual recognition and recall after right temporal lobe excision in man. *Neuropsychologia* **6**:191–209.

Naugle RI, Chelune GJ, Cheek R, Lüders H, Awad IA (1993) Detection of changes in material-specific memory following temporal lobectomy using the Wechsler Memory Scale-revised. *Archives of Clinical Neuropsychology* **8**:381–395.

Novelly RA, Augustine EA, Mattson RH *et al* (1984) Selective memory improvement and impairment in temporal lobectomy for epilepsy. *Annals of Neurology* **15**:64–67.

Nunn JA, Polkey CE, Morris RG (1998) Selective spatial memory impairment after right unilateral temporal lobectomy. *Neuropsychologia* **36**:837–848.

Oxbury JM, Oxbury SM (1989) Neuropsychology, memory and hippocampal pathology. In: Reynolds EH, Trimble MR (eds) *The Bridge Between Neurology and Psychiatry*. London: Churchill Livingstone.

Oxbury JM, Adams CBT, Oxbury SM, Carpenter KN, Renowden SA (1995) *En bloc* temporal lobectomy v selective amygdalohippocampectomy as treatments for intractable epilepsy due to hippocampal sclerosis. *Journal of Neurology, Neurosurgery and Psychiatry* **59**:200.

Oxbury SM, Creswell CS, Oxbury JM, Adams CBT (1996) Neuropsychological outcome after temporal lobe epilepsy surgery in children under 16 years of age: 5-year follow-up. *Epilepsia* **37** (Suppl 5):183.

Oxbury S, Oxbury J, Renowden S, Quier W, Carpenter K (1997) Severe amnesia: an unusual late complication after temporal lobectomy. *Neuropsychologia* **35**(7):975–988.

Penfield W, Mathieson G (1974) Memory: autopsy findings and comments on the role of the hippocampus in experiential recall. *Archives of Neurology* **31**:145–154.

Penfield W, Milner B (1958) Memory deficit produced by bilateral lesions in the hippocampal zone. *Archives of Neurology and Psychiatry* **79**:475–497.

Phillips NA, McGlone J (1995) Grouped data do not tell the whole story: individual analysis of cognitive change after temporal lobectomy. *Journal of Clinical and Experimental Neuropsychology* **17**(5):713–724.

Pigott S, Milner B (1993) Memory for different aspects of complex visual scenes after unilateral-temporal or frontal lobe resection. *Neuropsychologia* **13**:1–15.

Pilcher WH, Roberts DW, Flanigan HF *et al* (1993) Complications of epilepsy surgery. In: Engel J Jnr (ed.) *Surgical Treatment of the Epilepsies*, 2nd edn, pp 565–581. New York: Raven Press.

Powell GE, Polkey CE, McMillan TM (1985) The new Maudsley series of temporal lobectomy. I: Short-term cognitive effects. *British Journal of Clinical Psychology* **24**:109–124.

Rausch R (1987) Anatomical substrates of interictal memory deficits in temporal lobe epileptics. *International Journal of Neurology* **21–22**:17–32.

Rausch R, Babb TL (1993) Hippocampal neuron loss and memory scores before and after temporal lobe surgery for epilepsy. *Archives of Neurology* **50**:812–817.

Rausch R, Crandall PH (1982) Psychological status related to surgical control of temporal lobe seizures. *Epilepsia* **23**:191–202.

Sass KJ, Westerveld M, Buchanan CP, Spencer SS, Kim JH, Spencer DD (1994) Degree of hippocampal neuron loss determines severity of verbal memory decrease after left anteromesiotemporal lobectomy. *Epilepsia* **35**(6):1179–1186.

Saykin AJ, Gur RC, Sussman NM, O'Connor MJ, Gur RE (1989) Memory deficits before and after temporal lobectomy: effects of laterality and age of onset. *Brain and Cognition* **9**:191–200.

Saykin AJ, Stafiniak P, Robinson LJ *et al* (1995) Language before and after temporal lobectomy: specificity of acute changes and relation to early risk factors. *Epilepsia* **36**(11):1071–1077.

Seidenberg M, Hermann B, Dohan FC, Wyler A, Perrine A, Schoenfeld J (1996) Hippocampal sclerosis and verbal encoding ability following anterior temporal lobectomy. *Neuropsychologia* **34**:699–708.

Seidenberg M, Hermann B, Wyler AR, Davies K, Cohan FC, Leveroni C (1998) Neuropsychological outcome following anterior temporal lobectomy in patients with and without the syndrome of mesial temporal lobe epilepsy. *Neuropsychology* **12**(2):303–316.

Smith ML, Milner B (1981) The role of the right hippocampus in the recall of spatial location. *Neuropsychologia* **19**:781–793.

Stafiniak P, Saykin AJ, Sperling MR *et al* (1990) Acute naming deficits following dominant temporal lobectomy: prediction by age at first risk for seizures. *Neurology* **40**:1509–1512.

Szabó CA, Wyllie E, Stanford LD *et al* (1998) Neuropsychological effect of temporal lobe resection in preadolescent children with epilepsy. *Epilepsia* **39**(8):814–819.

Taylor LB (1969) Psychological assessment of neurosurgical patients. In: Rasmussen T, Marino R (eds) *Functional Neurosurgery*, pp 165–180. New York: Raven Press.

Trenerry MR, Jack CR (1994) Wisconsin card sorting testing performance before and after temporal lobectomy. *Journal of Epilepsy* **7**:313–317.

Trenerry MR, Jack CR, Ivnik RJ *et al* (1993) MRI hippocampal volumes and memory function before and after temporal lobectomy. *Neurology* **43**:1800–1805.

Trenerry MR, Jack CR, Cascino GD, Sharbrough FW, Ivnik RJ (1995) Gender differences in post-temporal lobectomy verbal memory and relationships between MRI hippocampal volumes and preoperative verbal memory. *Epilepsy Research* **20**:69–76.

Trenerry MR, Jack CR, Cascino GD, Sharbrough FW, So EL (1996a) Bilateral magnetic resonance imaging-determined hippocampal atrophy and verbal memory before and after temporal lobectomy. *Epilepsia* **37**(6):526–533.

Trenerry MR, Jack CR, Cascino GD, Sharbrough FW, Ivnik RJ (1996b) Sex differences in the relationship between visual memory and MRI hippocampal volumes. *Neuropsychology* **10**(3):343–351.

Tuunainen A, Nousiainen U, Hurskainen H (1995) Preoperative EEG predicts memory and selective cognitive functions after temporal lobe surgery. *Journal of Neurology, Neurosurgery and Psychiatry* **58**:674–680.

Warrington EK, Duchen LW (1992) A reappraisal of a case of persistent global amnesia following right temporal lobectomy: a clinicopathological study. *Neuropsychologia* **30**:437–450.

Wolf RL, Ivnik RJ, Hirschorn KA, Sharbrough FW, Cascino GD, Marsh WR (1993) Neurocognitive efficiency following left temporal lobectomy: standard versus limited resection. *Journal of Neurosurgery* **79**:76–83.

Wyler A, Hermann B, Somes G (1995) Extent of medial temporal resection on outcome from anterior temporal lobectomy: a randomized prospective study. *Neurosurgery* **37**:982–991.

Cognitive and memory changes after hemispherectomy

61

ES KNIGHT AND SM OXBURY

Hemispherectomy is mostly used to treat patients whose drug-resistant epilepsy is associated with predominantly unilateral hemisphere pathology giving rise to a hemiplegia. The aim is to achieve freedom from seizures by removing the damaged hemisphere without exacerbating the preexisting neurologic deficits. Medication can then be withdrawn and any cognitive decline that has begun may be arrested or reversed. This chapter reviews the postoperative neuropsychologic changes seen in these circumstances.

Reports of early series of anatomic hemispherectomy (Krynauw 1950; McFie 1961; Griffith and Davidson 1966; Wilson 1970; Lindsay *et al* 1984) clearly indicated that the surgical outcome was mostly successful. The seizures usually ceased, disruptive behavior was abolished or substantially improved, and there were some worthwhile cognitive gains especially amongst those whose preoperative level was not too severely impaired. The quality of life of both the patients and their families usually improved. The original surgical procedure was used less when it became clear that it had late complications, including death, due to recurrent intracranial bleeding leading to hemosiderosis and obstructive hydrocephalus (Oppenheimer and Griffith 1966). The operation has been reintroduced in various modified forms, each designed to avoid the late complications, including hemidecortication (Ignelzi and Bucy 1968), modified anatomic hemispherectomy (Adams 1983), functional hemispherectomy

(Rasmussen 1983), and hemispherotomy (Delalande *et al* 1993).

NEUROPSYCHOLOGIC OUTCOME FOLLOWING CURRENT SURGICAL TECHNIQUES

MIXED-PATHOLOGY STUDIES

Patients born with structural abnormalities of the brain, including early or *in utero* stroke, Sturge–Weber syndrome, and cortical dysplasia, or those who acquire major unilateral hemisphere damage in their early years, are major groups who undergo hemispherectomy. Their seizure onset can be as early as the first month of life (Vining *et al* 1990) but may be delayed for a few years. As in the earlier series, follow-up data are often presented in series comprised of patients with various pathologies, including those mentioned together with acute encephalitis leading to hemiplegia and intractable seizures, and the progressive encephalitis of Rasmussen's syndrome.

Villemure and Rasmussen (1990) have stated that the physiologic result of functional hemispherectomy is equivalent to anatomic hemispherectomy for control of seizures, so it is reasonable to expect that the behavioral and neuropsychologic outcome will be similar at least for groups of otherwise comparable patients. Thus Tinuper *et al* (1988) described outcome after intervals of 4–13 years in 14 cases. Preoperative intelligence quotient (IQ) in nine testable patients ranged from 36 to 84. In those without preoperative independent ictal discharge from the opposite hemisphere, behavior and social skills substantially improved and a mean increase of 10 IQ points occurred.

Beardsworth and Adams (1988) published early results after modified anatomic hemispherectomy and noted that seizure outcome was good, motor function was unaffected, and family life improved with the cessation of seizures. Some children also showed considerable cognitive gains postoperatively. Lindsay (1990), describing a series of 18 patients half of whom overlapped with the Beardsworth and Adams series, noted that surgery halted any preoperative cognitive regression and that there was a steady and sustained IQ rise in some. In a more recent review of 25 patients operated on by Adams who had reached their fifth postoperative year, Oxbury *et al* (1995) found significant and continuing IQ gains in those patients, about half of the group, who could be assessed preoperatively on the children's Weschler scales (WPPSI or WISC). Their preoperative full-scale IQ range was 40–81; the greatest gain appeared to take place between 6 months and 2 years after surgery with an average change of 10 points compared to their preoperative scores. At 5 years this had risen to 15 points (Fig. 61.1). The ceiling was about IQ 80. Those with early or *in utero* stroke and relatively late seizure onset tended to fare best, but numbers were too small to show significance. Those with more severe disabilities who could only be assessed on developmental scales continued to develop over the follow-up period but did not show the accelerated gains seen in those who were less handicapped. Exceptions were two children with Sturge–Weber syndrome: in one the disease began to affect the unoperated hemisphere and the child deteriorated, while the other, a boy with virtually no expressive speech, made remarkable speech progress after left hemispherectomy at the age of 9 years (described by Vargha-Khadem *et al* 1997). Considering the whole group, preoperative IQ or developmental quotient was significantly related to age at seizure onset, those with greater impairment having an earlier age of onset of seizures than those less impaired.

Vining *et al* (1997) have reported the outcome from hemispherectomy in 58 children, 27 with Rasmussen's syndrome, 24 with various developmental abnormalities – cortical dysplasias/hemimegalencephalies – and 7 with Sturge–Weber syndrome or other congenital vascular problems. Seizure outcome was related to etiology: the

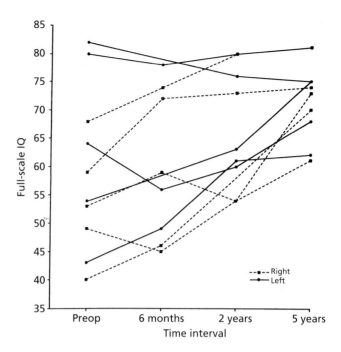

Fig. 61.1 Full-scale IQ preoperatively and at various postoperative intervals of children testable preoperatively on Weschler scales. (Preop vs. 6 months, *P* < 0.05; preop vs. 5 years, *P* < 0.05; 2 years vs. 5 years, *P* < 0.05.)

Rasmussen's group were 89% seizure-free compared to 67% in each of the other groups. They also reported outcome in terms of a 'burden of illness' score composed of seizure frequency, motor disability, and intellectual handicap. In these terms, outcome was very successful in 44, successful in 7, and only minimally successful in 3. Vining *et al* favor early surgery.

The psychologic findings in mixed-pathology series are very similar to those of the earlier series of unmodified hemispherectomies, discounting of course the unfortunate patients who developed late complications in those series. It is unclear why IQ may continue to rise well after the immediate postoperative period. Various explanations have been put forward. The improvement may arise because the function of the intact hemisphere is no longer disrupted by abnormal electrical discharges from the pathologic hemisphere, allowing learning to take place. Indeed, Tinuper *et al* (1988) related good outcome and postoperative IQ rise to normal EEG in the opposite hemisphere. They also suggest that drug dose reduction may be important. Preoperatively, behavior problems may have interfered with psychologic testing, and improved behavior and cooperation postoperatively may enhance performance (Beardsworth and Adams 1988). Although this may be a contributory factor it is unlikely to provide the whole explanation, since the behavioral improvement usually takes place long before the major cognitive gains are seen. Various factors may influence the cognitive outcome for an individual. Thus, preoperative IQ level influences the final postoperative cognitive level (Wilson 1970); not surprisingly, those who start better end up better, and postoperative gains occur less often in the most severely handicapped (Oxbury *et al* 1995). The health of the unoperated hemisphere is likely to be paramount and is probably related to several of the above points. In general, the side of hemispheric damage is not found to influence either the preoperative or the postoperative IQ level.

SPECIFIC-PATHOLOGY STUDIES

Sturge–Weber syndrome

The congenital vascular malformation of the leptomeninges in this syndrome can affect both hemispheres but is unilateral in the majority of cases and is usually limited to the parietooccipital region. The cortical damage may be progressive leading to irreversible mental and physical disability.

The outcome from surgical intervention is often favorable. The prognosis, however, is variable, being better when the pathology involves only one hemisphere (Zupanc 1996). Erba and Cavazzuti (1990) reported on twelve new patients with Sturge–Weber syndrome, three of whom were treated surgically, two by hemidecorticectomy in early infancy (9 and 12 months, respectively) and one by parietooccipital resection at 7 years. The two infants became seizure-free and compensated well for the motor deficit. Their scores on the Bayley scale of infant development prior to surgery had reflected no progress in cognitive or motor function. Following surgery, development was well documented and shown to parallel that of normal infants. They functioned within the normal IQ range, and at age 6 and 7 respectively were at normal schools. A similar result had been reported by Hoffman *et al* (1979) in an earlier series of six hemispherectomies performed in infants under 1 year of age. At follow-up ranging from 1 to 13 years, one had died after a deteriorating postoperative course, four were seizure-free, and one had only occasional seizures. The surviving children had normal IQ (range 82–99). In contrast a seventh child who also had onset of seizures in infancy did not have surgery until the age of 8 years. He became seizure-free but remained mentally handicapped (IQ 52 at 8 years follow-up). Hoffman *et al* concluded that IQ seems dependent on the promptness of surgery after the onset of seizures. They also suggest that the younger the patient at surgery the higher the eventual IQ. The results were less good in those treated by a more limited selective cortical excision (Hoffman *et al* 1979).

Rasmussen's syndrome

Hemispherectomy is also effective in this progressive condition. It affects previously normal children and usually begins in the first decade of life. The pathology involves progressively larger areas of the cerebral cortex but remains unilateral. The child experiences the onset of focal seizures, which become uncontrolled, and a progressive loss of hemispheric function leading to hemiplegia and intellectual deterioration. Smaller surgical removals are seldom effective and to date only hemispherectomy has been reported to eliminate seizures. Perhaps, in the future, the treatment will be medical rather than by such a radical surgical procedure (Hart *et al* 1994; Rogers *et al* 1994; Adcock *et al* 1997).

The cognitive effects of the condition depend partly on which cerebral hemisphere is involved. Taylor (1991) describes preoperative neuropsychologic decline and gives data on 32 cases treated in Montreal by various cortical excisions, 7 eventually having complete hemispherectomy. The mean preoperative IQ in those with left hemisphere disease (66.8) was slightly lower than in the right hemisphere group (72.2). Age at onset was about 6 years for both left and right groups, but whereas surgery was first performed an average of 3.5 years after onset in the right group, this interval was 9 years in the left group. The known association between language function and the dominant hemisphere and between visuospatial skills and the nondominant hemisphere was apparent, but not as marked as might have been expected. Taylor's study makes it clear how difficult it is to get a true preoperative evaluation, because by the time the decision to operate is made the child is often too ill with frequent seizures or epilepsia partialis continua for assessment to be possible. Earlier assessments may reflect a lesser degree of damage than has actually occurred by this stage.

A recent abstract (Pulsifer *et al* 1997) described neuropsychologic and psychosocial outcome following hemispherectomy in more than 60 patients with Rasmussen's syndrome, 24 of whom (8 left and 16 right) were evaluated both pre- and postoperatively. Left hemisphere cases had lower IQ than right hemisphere cases, but there was no significant relation between the side of operation and IQ change. In contrast to some of the findings in patients with developmental abnormalities, the greatest IQ gain occurred in those with the lowest preoperative IQ, suggesting, perhaps, that these children had their potential suppressed the most. The best cognitive outcome was associated with later onset of the disorder and shorter seizure history.

The so-called 'transfer' of language to the right hemisphere is an issue of much importance in children with Rasmussen's syndrome affecting the left hemisphere. Cases of speech developing in the right when it was previously located in the left, and the left hemisphere is then removed, have been described. This transfer may result in a general depressing effect on cognition due to the 'crowding' of the right hemisphere. Taylor (1991) reported that postoperative neuropsychologic function remained near the preoperative levels, suggesting that surgery has little effect on intellectual function. However, the timing of the operation is likely to be influenced by the extent of the condition and is usually undertaken in patients with Rasmussen's syndrome when the disease is well progressed and the hemisphere is no longer functionally viable.

Right hemisphere surgery and significant neuropsychologic deficit is seldom discussed. In the Oxford series of hemispherectomy for this condition, left visuospatial neglect postoperatively was observed in two cases who had surgery relatively early in the course of their disease. This was not a transient phenomenon as a copy of the Rey complex figure 2 years after surgery demonstrates (Fig. 61.2). This boy was 7 years old at operation and too ill for assessment close to that time, but neglect had not been observed at assessment 6 months earlier. Ten years later, despite a full-scale IQ of 80 which places him in good-outcome groups, he still has considerable visuospatial problems.

The timing of operation in patients with this disease has yet to be resolved and is made more difficult by the fact that there is individual variation in its rate of progression. Vining *et al* (1990) advocate that hemispherectomy should be offered when the nature and course of the illness become clear and before irreparable harm is done by intractable seizures and medication. Waiting too long can cause problems. Three cases were reported demonstrating that by waiting many years, and therefore experiencing many years of seizures and medication, the outcome was less favorable. Vining *et al* argue that hemiplegia will eventually occur, therefore posing the question of whether it is really worse for a child to have the hemiplegia earlier, but have a shorter period of seizures and medication, rather than continue to use the hand for a little longer but continue having seizures and deteriorating cognitively. They later reported on 12 children who underwent hemispherectomy and were followed up at an average of 9 years (Vining *et al* 1993). Early rather than late operation had allowed children to resume a more normal life. Early operation may also prevent some of the intellectual decline that accompanies uncontrolled seizures and their treatment.

The decision of when to operate is also made more difficult in children with left-sided disease because of the issue of language representation. Taylor (1991) reported that in those with left-hemisphere disease, and in whom language

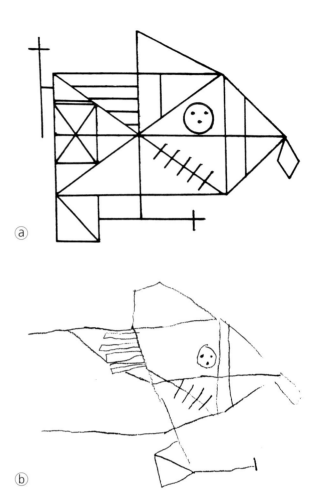

Fig. 61.2 (a) The Rey–Osterrieth complex figure and (b) the copy made by a 9-year-old boy 2 years after right hemispherectomy for Rasmussen's syndrome, demonstrating marked left visuospatial neglect.

lateralization had been determined by sodium amobarbital tests, half had speech represented on the right at the time of surgery. Seven out of eight of these children had started the disease when younger than 6 years. In contrast, those who had damage to the left language-dominant hemisphere starting after their sixth birthday continued to have language on that side. Little is known about the ability of speech to switch to the right hemisphere as continuing deterioration occurs in the left hemisphere. Therefore it remains unclear whether it is better to delay operation, in order to allow such speech transition from left to right as is possible, or whether nothing is lost in the long term by the sudden destruction of the speech area by surgical intervention in a young child. A case is described of a 10-year-old girl who still had some language on the left at the time of undergoing left hemispherectomy but whose speech continued to improve steadily, even though it was limited immediately after the surgery.

Monitoring the course of the illness with repeated assessments may help, not only in deciding when surgery ought to be considered but also how extensive it should be, although in general any intervention short of hemispherectomy is likely to be unsuccessful. Neuropsychologic evaluation is critical, especially in ascertaining speech lateralization.

FACTORS AFFECTING NEUROPSYCHOLOGIC OUTCOME

It appears that hemispherectomy in these cases rarely results in neuropsychologic decline. It is sometimes followed by worthwhile gains. At least as important as pre- to postoperative change, however, is the level of cognitive function ultimately reached. Possible relevant determinant factors are type of pathology, age at seizure onset, age at operation, duration of seizure history, and seizure outcome. Holthausen *et al* (1997) have shown that seizure outcome is related to pathology but not to age at onset or duration of seizure history, while acknowledging that the last two factors may influence cognitive outcome.

There are hints that those with early vascular pathology may do particularly well, especially when seizure onset is relatively late allowing a period of seizure-free development in the case of early stroke (McFie 1961; Wilson 1970; Oxbury *et al* 1995), and in Sturge–Weber syndrome when early onset is followed by early surgery. Those with hemimegalencephaly, a severe form of cortical neuronal migration disorder, do not appear to do well, possibly because of a high probability of pathology in the unoperated hemisphere, thus limiting successful outcome on all measures. Neuropsychologic outcome in Rasmussen's syndrome is complicated by variable age of onset and rate of progression, and the fact that subtotal resections are rarely undertaken early in the disease when it would exacerbate both neurologic and neuropsychologic deficits, at least in the short term. However, there are suggestions that a shorter seizure history is associated with higher cognitive level eventually.

The most appropriate view at present may be that of Vargha-Khadem and Mishkin (1997), who concluded from their study of language development in a mixed-pathology group that 'the sooner drug-resistant seizures are abolished by surgery the more favorable the cognitive developmental outcome, including the outcome for speech and language'.

EXCEPTIONAL CASES

Unusually high IQ

The majority of studies suggest that functioning with one hemisphere results in a general lowering of intellect due to 'crowding', and that the upper limit of ability in these circumstances is seldom above average and most often in the IQ 80–90 range. Smith and Sugar (1975) described a person who had been treated by left hemispherectomy when $5\frac{1}{2}$ and who at 26 years old had verbal IQ of 126 and performance IQ of 103. Furthermore, his performance on a large battery of other tests was in the average range. He illustrates how excellent verbal abilities, superior language and verbal reasoning skills, and considerable visuospatial skills, can be acquired after left hemispherectomy at an early age. Griffiths and Davidson (1966) described a case of right hemispherectomy at age 19 whose Wechsler scores were verbal IQ 101 and performance IQ 63 preoperatively, and verbal IQ 121 and performance IQ 91 15 years later. Both these cases are remarkable in the ability of one hemisphere alone to sustain these levels of ability and in the very considerable gains made in those cognitive domains usually mediated by the absent hemisphere.

Late right-hemisphere language development

Work on children with Rasmussen's syndrome suggests that language has lateralized by the age of 6 years (see above). The case of a boy described by Vargha-Khadem *et al* (1997), however, suggests that language can develop in the right hemisphere as late as the age of 9 years following left hemispherectomy for Sturge–Weber syndrome.

This child had failed to develop speech throughout his early life, and comprehension of single words remained at the level of 3–4 years. After the left hemispherectomy at age $8\frac{1}{2}$ years he began to acquire speech and language. When he was aged nearly 15 years some components of his receptive and expressive language scores placed him at an age equivalent of 8–10 years, while his IQ was 52 (VIQ = 59, PIQ = 53). Although the results indicate definite limits to the cognitive and linguistic capacity of the right hemisphere alone, his achievements provide valuable information that early childhood is not as critical for the acquisition of speech and language as had been thought.

SUMMARY

Hemispherectomy is a drastic measure with the possibility of postoperative complications, yet because of the devastating effects of seizures and medication and associated cognitive decline, at present it remains the treatment of choice for children with uncontrolled hemiplegic epilepsy. The cognitive outcome following hemispherectomy is determined to a great extent by the underlying pathologic substrate and its clinical course and characteristics. However, it is clear that the outcome is very often favorable both in terms of seizure relief and improved cognitive function.

KEY POINTS

1. Hemispherectomy for uncontrolled hemiplegic epilepsy based on unilateral multilobar pathology achieves favorable seizure outcome. Candidates are mostly children of below average cognitive ability extending down to the severely handicapped range and may demonstrate intellectual decline preoperatively.

2. With early static pathology IQ may rise over an extended postoperative period. This improvement is more likely to occur in those with less preoperative cognitive impairment, postoperative cessation of seizures and normal EEG in the unoperated hemisphere.

3. Hemispherectomy for the progressive condition of Rasmussen's syndrome is not followed by further cognitive decline. The neuropsychologic status depends only partly on laterality of disease. Issues relating to the optimum time for surgery in terms of achieving the best neuropsychologic outcome are not resolved.

4. The final cognitive level achieved after hemispherectomy appears to have an upper limit of IQ 80–90, apart from rare exceptional cases. Factors partially associated with higher eventual cognitive outcome are higher preoperative intellectual ability, later age at seizure onset, shorter duration of seizure history, type of pathology, and good postoperative seizure outcome.

REFERENCES

Adams CBT (1983) Hemispherectomy – a modification. *Journal of Neurology, Neurosurgery and Psychiatry* **46**:617–619.

Adcock J, Oxbury J, Beeson D *et al* (1997) Comparison of treatment of Rasmussen's encephalitis with plasmapheresis versus hemispherectomy. *Epilepsia* **38**(Suppl 8):189 (Abstract S.073).

Beardsworth E, Adams C (1988) Modified hemispherectomy for epilepsy: early results in 10 cases. *British Journal of Neurosurgery* **2**:73–84.

Delalande O, Pinard JM, Basdevant C, Plouin P, Dulac O (1993) Hemispherotomy: a new procedure for hemispheric disconnection. *Epilepsia* **34**:140.

Erba G, Cavazzuti V (1990) Sturge–Weber syndrome: natural history and indications for surgery. *Journal of Epilepsy* **3**(Suppl):287–291.

Griffith H, Davidson M (1966) Long-term changes in intellect and behavior after hemispherectomy. *Journal of Neurology, Neurosurgery and Psychiatry* **29**:571–576.

Hart Y, Cortez M, Andermann F *et al* (1994) Medical treatment of Rasmussen's syndrome (chronic encephalitis and epilepsy): effect of high-dose steroids or immunoglobulins in 19 patients. *Neurology* **44**:1030–1036.

Hoffman HJ, Hendrick EB, Dennis M, Armstrong D (1979) Hemispherectomy for Sturge–Weber syndrome. *Child's Brain* **5**:233–248.

Holthausen H, May TW, Adams CBT *et al* (1997) Seizures post-hemispherectomy. In: Tuxhorn I, Holthausen H, Boenigk H (eds) *Paediatric Epilepsy Syndromes and Their Surgical Treatment*, pp 749–773. London: John Libbey.

Ignelzi RJ, Bucy PC (1968) Cerebral hemidecorticectomy in the treatment of infantile cerebral hemiatrophy. *Journal of Nervous Mental Disease* **147**:14–30.

Krynauw R (1950) Infantile hemiplegia treated by removing one cerebral hemisphere. *Journal of Neurology, Neurosurgery and Psychiatry* **13**:243–267.

Lindsay J (1990) Hemispherectomy outcome. *Journal of Epilepsy* **3**(Suppl):253–256.

Lindsay J, Glaser G, Richards P, Ounsted C (1984) Developmental aspects of focal epilepsies of childhood treated by neurosurgery. *Developmental Medicine and Child Neurology* **26**:574–587.

McFie J (1961) The effects of hemispherectomy on intellectual functioning in cases of infantile hemiplegia. *Journal of Neurology, Neurosurgery and Psychiatry* **24**:240–249.

Oppenheimer D, Griffith H (1966) Persistent intracranial bleeding as a complication of hemispherectomy. *Journal of Neurology, Neurosurgery and Psychiatry* **29**:229–240.

Oxbury S, Zaiwalla Z, Adams C, Middleton J, Oxbury J (1995) Hemispherectomy in childhood: serial neuropsychological follow-up and prolonged improvement. *Epilepsia* **36**(Suppl 3):S24.

Pulsifer M, Brandt J, Vining E, Picarello K, Freeman J (1997) Intellectual functioning after cerebral hemispherectomy for Rasmussen's syndrome. *Epilepsia* **38**(Suppl 8):215–216.

Rasmussen T (1983) Hemispherectomy for seizures revisited. *Canadian Journal of Neurological Sciences* **10**:71–78.

Rogers S, Andrews P, Gahving L *et al* (1994) Antibodies to glutamate receptor GluR3 in Rasmussen's encephalitis. *Science* **265**:648–651.

Smith A, Sugar O (1975) Development of above-normal language and intelligence 21 years after left hemispherectomy. *Neurology* **25**:813–818.

Taylor LB (1991) Neuropsychological assessment of patients with chronic encephalitis. In: Andermann F (ed.) *Chronic Encephalitis and Epilepsy: Rasmussen's Syndrome*, pp 111–121. Boston: Butterworth-Heinemann.

Tinuper P, Andermann F, Villemure J, Rasmussen T, Quesney L (1988) Functional hemispherectomy for treatment of epilepsy associated with hemiplegia: rationale, indications, results and comparison with callosotomy. *Annals of Neurology* **24**:27–34.

Vargha-Khadem F, Mishkin M (1997) Speech and language outcome after hemispherectomy in childhood. In: Tuxhorn I, Holthausen H, Boenigk H (eds) *Paediatric Epilepsy Syndromes and Their Surgical Treatment*, pp 774–784. London: John Libbey.

Vargha-Khadem F, Carr L, Isaacs E, Brett E, Adams C, Mishkin M (1997) Onset of speech after left hemispherectomy in a 9-year-old boy. *Brain* **120**:159–182.

Villemure J, Rasmussen T (1990) Functional hemispherectomy: methodology. *Journal of Epilepsy* **3**(Suppl):177–182.

Vining E, Freeman J, Carson B, Brandt J (1990) Hemispherectomy in children: the Hopkins experience, 1968–1988, a preliminary report. *Journal of Epilepsy* **3**(Suppl):169–176.

Vining E, Freeman J, Brandt J, Carson B, Uematsu S (1993) Progressive unilateral encephalopathy of childhood (Rasmussen's syndrome): a reappraisal. *Epilepsia* **34**(4):639–650.

Vining E, Freeman J, Pillas D *et al* (1997) Why would you remove half the brain? The outcome of 58 children after hemispherectomy – the Johns Hopkins experience: 1968–1996. *Pediatrics* **100**:163–171.

Wilson P (1970) Cerebral hemispherectomy for infantile hemiplegia: a report of 50 cases. *Brain* **93**:147–180.

Zupanc M (1996) Update on epilepsy in pediatric patients. *Mayo Clinic Proceedings* **71**:899–916.

Cognitive and memory changes after posterior hemisphere excisions

S HENLEY AND SM OXBURY

Excisions from the posterior part of a hemisphere have the potential to interfere with the important cognitive functions subserved by the cortex of the posterior parietal and occipital and parietooccipitotemporal junction areas. On the left language-dominant side these include semantic aspects of language, comprehension, reading, writing, calculation, constructional and other praxis, probably some aspects of spatial function as suggested by recent functional imaging, and the combination of a disturbance in identifying objects visually (optic aphasia), dyslexia, and color anomia accompanying right homonymous hemianopia from left occipital damage. On the right nondominant side they include visuospatial disorders, including left neglect, and problems in visual perception and facial recognition.

Posterior hemisphere excisions constitute a relatively small proportion of the surgical operations carried out to treat epilepsy. Thus, in Olivier's (1988) series of 526 operations, less than 2% were in the parietal and occipital areas. It is not surprising, therefore, that published pre- and postoperative neuropsychologic studies of patients having posterior excisions are sparse. Furthermore, the small number, together with the factors of side, site, and extent of excision which could lead to a wide range of impairments, almost certainly result in there being too few patients in any one center who are sufficiently similar to be grouped together very meaningfully.

As in all epilepsy surgery, the nature of the pathology and the functional status of the tissue to be excised are important factors underlying neuropsychologic outcome.

Some pathologies, such as a cavernous angioma, may allow more circumscribed removal than others, such as cortical dysplasia, and do not contain functional tissue. Neurosurgical procedures frequently include functional mapping in these eloquent areas and, indeed, it is considered essential in several circumstances, particularly in proposed dominant hemisphere excisions (Olivier 1988). The few available published series including posterior excisions are not very detailed in terms of specific neuropsychologic functions tested and have tended to report overall measures. It has not always been clear that the neuropsychologic test battery has included tests designed to demonstrated the specific functions of the particular area under consideration.

SERIES REPORTED IN THE LITERATURE

Three studies have reported the neuropsychologic outcome of posterior excisions (Table 62.1). Wannamaker and Matthews (1976) reported two patients who had surgery on a parietal lobe out of a total of 14 patients undergoing surgery for their epilepsy. The patients were tested on the battery developed by Halstead (1947) and some tests of motor ability and sensory discrimination (Matthews et al 1970). The summary statement of the postsurgery neuropsychologic profile of each patient was classified as indicating that the patient was improved (I), not changed

Table 62.1 Neuropsychologic outcome in 11 individuals following posterior hemisphere excisions.

Author	Age at epilepsy onset (years)	Age at surgery (years)	Resection[a]	Pathology	Follow-up	Seizure frequency[b] (per month)		Neuropsychology		Impairment index[e] (Pre/Post)	Tests[f]
						Preoperative	Postoperative	Preoperative (VIQ/PIQ)[c]	Postoperative[d] (VIQ/PIQ)[c]		
Wannamaker and Matthews (1976)	17	22	RP	Tuberous sclerosis	1 month	60	0		NC	2/4	
	7	28	LP	Edema	48 months	12	17		W	8/10	
Adler et al (1991)	median 0.25	median 12.6	P	Cortical malformation	median 8 years		0		NC		
			P	Cortical malformation			0		–		
			P	Vascular malformation			0		–		
	median 9	median 16.6	O	Tumor	median 8.1 years		≥75%		M		
			O	Atrophy			≥75%		–		
			O	Cortical malformation			≥75%		–		
			O	Vascular malformation			0		NC		
			O	Nonspecific			Slight improvement		NC		
Gilliam et al (1997)	3 months	11	O	Dysplasia	6 months	60	60	55/46	46/49		WISC/WPPSI

[a] L = left, R = right, P = parietal, O = occipital.
[b] ≥ 75% = at least a 75% reduction in seizure frequency.
[c] VIQ = verbal IQ, PIQ = performance IQ.
[d] I = improved, NC = no change, M = improved but with new deficits, W = worse.
[e] Impairment index used by Wannamaker and Matthews (1976).
[f] WPPSI = Wechster Preschool and Preliminary Scale of Intelligence.

(NC), or worse (W) overall on the battery used. They also measured the frequency with which the patient passed a cut-off point for 10 tests in the battery which had been shown to discriminate between brain-damaged and non-brain-damaged subjects. This 'impairment index' ranged from 0–10, with 10 indicating the highest level of neuropsychologic impairment. Both patients appear to have deteriorated.

Adler *et al* (1991) reported the results of 35 patients who underwent surgery for extratemporal partial epilepsy, three of whom had surgery on a parietal lobe, and five of whom had surgery on an occipital lobe. Patients were given a postoperative 'performance' rating usually based on neuropsychologic test results (actual tests are not stated) but in some cases incorporating an index of social functioning as measured by reports from school, employers, or parents. Compared to preoperative performance patients were classified as improved (I), not changed (NC), worse (W), or improved but with new unexpected neurologic deficits (M). On the whole, neuropsychologic status did not deteriorate after posterior excisions.

Finally, Gilliam *et al* (1997) assessed the outcome of 33 children who underwent surgery for epilepsy, one of whom had occipital surgery and both pre- and postoperative neuropsychologic testing consisting of Weschler Intelligence Scale for Children (WISC) verbal and performance intelligence quotient (IQ). The child did not deteriorate significantly after surgery.

It can be seen from Table 62.1 that the seizure outcome for parietal patients was good, with four out of the five becoming seizure-free after surgery with only one unchanged. Of those who became seizure-free, two showed improvement neuropsychologically while one was unchanged. Only one patient became worse neuropsychologically. The left parietal patient of Wannamaker and Matthews (1976) gained no seizure relief and became worse neuropsychologically.

Of the occipital patients, only one patient became free of seizures although three had an improvement of more than 75%, and one had a slight improvement (approximately 25%) while one was unchanged. Three of the six had no change in neuropsychologic measures, including the patient who became seizure-free. The other three patients improved although one (Adler *et al* 1991) is classified as 'improved but with new and unexplained neurological deficits'. What these new deficits are is not stated.

Overall out of the eleven patients for whom neuropsychologic data are available, five (45%) showed improvement after surgery and two (18%) were worse. Also interesting is the finding that improvement was not necessarily accompanied by complete relief of the seizures.

The data are difficult to interpret because it is hard to control for factors such as age of onset and the side of the excision which are known to affect surgical outcome. Furthermore, neuropsychologic data have been compared across studies but each study used different criteria to classify patients and therefore what is reported as improved by one may not have been considered so by another. Each study also used a range of tests but only reported a general outcome; it would be interesting to see how individual test performances were affected by surgery.

PREVIOUSLY UNREPORTED OXFORD SERIES

In the authors' Oxford epilepsy surgery series, there are nine patients who have had posterior hemisphere excisions. Their details and pre- and postoperative neuropsychologic data are shown in Tables 62.2 and 62.3 Table 62.2 shows an overall cognitive measure and Table 62.3 goes into more detail of the specific tests. All the patients were tested on the Weschler Adult Intelligence Scale (WAIS) or WISC as well as on measures of language function (naming, comprehension, reading, and spelling) and on various tests of verbal and nonverbal memory (including the Rey copy and recall and Benton visual retention test). All preoperative assessments were made in the 9 months prior to surgery with the exception of patient 7, where the assessment was made 15 months before operation. Table 62.3 shows neuropsychologic changes defined as a fall or rise in postoperative as compared to preoperative scores equal to or greater than one standard deviation, where standard scores were based on age-appropriate norms for the patients at the time of the relevant assessment. Thus, in the younger patients, no change means that they have actually continued to make considerable gains in cognitive development in order to keep up with their peers.

Using the overall full-scale IQ measure there were no significant changes (Table 62.2). Table 62.3 shows relatively few significant changes considering the large number of measures employed. Thus performance was generally consistent with the preoperative level, and there were more gains than losses.

In some cases performance declined initially and then recovered. The greatest fluctuations were seen in the two youngest patients (cases 4 and 7). At 6 months follow-up, patient 7 showed significant drops in WISC-revised (WISC-R) subtests: digit span, vocabulary, arithmetic, comprehension, picture arrangement, and block design. At 2 years digit span, arithmetic, and comprehension were

Table 62.2 Neuropsychologic outcome following posterior hemisphere excisions: Oxford series.

No.	Sex[a]	Age at epilepsy onset (years)	Age at surgery (years)	Handedness[b]	CD[c]	Resection[d]	Pathology[e]	Latest follow-up (years postop)	Seizure outcome (Engel grade)	Visual field defect[f] Preoperative	Postoperative	FSIQ[g] (Pre/Post)	Tests
1	M	20 months	14	L	L	LO	Cortical dysplasia	2	2	Partial RHH	Complete RHH	97/96	WISC-R/WAIS-R
2	F	>=10	15	L	L	RO	Porencephalic cyst	6	1	Partial LLQ	Partial LHH	84/87	WISC/WAIS
3	M	7	10	R		RO	DNT	6 months	1	None	Partial LLQ	107/104	WISC-R
4	M	<=6	7	R		LP	Grade II astrocytoma	5	1	None	None	112/112	WISC-R
5	F	8	19	R	L	LP	Porencephalic cyst	5	2	None	None	81/90	WAIS-R
6	F	8	16	L	Bi L>R	LP	Benign cystic astrocytoma	5	2	None	Partial RLQ	85/81	WISC-R/WAIS-R
7	F	<=7	9	R		LP	Calcified angiomatosis	2	3	None	Partial LLQ	113/111	WISC-R
8	M	3.6	19	L	Bi	RP	Cortical dysplasia	5	4	None	Partial LLQ	74/72	WAIS-R
9	M	18	35	R	L	RP	DNT	6 months	1	None	None	109/101	WAIS-R

a M = male, F = female.
b L = left, R = right.
c CD = cerebral dominance, where tested, Bi = bilateral.
d O = occipital, P = parietal.
e DNT = dysembryoplastic neuroepithelioma.
f HH = homonymous hemianopia, LQ = lower quadrantic.
g FSIQ = full-scale IQ.

Table 62.3   Neuropsychologic changes following posterior hemisphere excisions: Oxford series.

No.	Resection[a]	VIQ/PIQ[b]			Verbal and language tests	Calculation[c]	Visuospatial and perceptual tests	Memory
		Preoperative	6 months	Latest				
1	LO	105/91	107/87	107/87	WAIS-R comprehension and spelling improved. Reading rate, but not accuracy or comprehension, declined, related to enlarged visual field defect		Rey copy and picture arrangement improved	
2	RO	80/90	75/86	87/89	Reading improved		Picture completion declined	Visual recall improved
3	RO	101/115	98/112		Spelling improved		Object assembly and Rey copy declined	Verbal memory improved. Visual recall declined
4	LP	100/124	100/95	102/121	WISC-R information improved although similarites declined. Reading and spelling improved, with reading now exceeding chronological age level	WISC-R arithmetic improved	Block design and object assembly declined initially but improved from 6 months. Rey copy improved	Digit span declined. Rey recall improved
5	LP	82/84	83/87	85/100	Object naming improved		Block design and object assembly improved. Rey copy declined mildly. PIQ improved overall	Verbal memory improved
6	LP	79/83	80/94	78/89	Reading improved	BAS test scores rose from 8.5 years to 13.6 years. WISC-R age scores fell	Block design dropped at 6 months but was back to preop level at 2 years. Picture arrangement dropped at 6 months but was above preop level at 2 years. Rey copy improved	Visual recall improved Digit span declined
7	LP	116/107	98/94	103/119	WISC-R comprehension declined although performance on shortened token test was unchanged. Reading and spelling progressed and were at average levels			
8	RP	76/75	76/79	71/74	12-point drop in VIQ mainly attributable to decline in arithmetic and digit span	WAIS-R arithmetic declined		Visual recall improved
9	RP	107/111	95/113					Benton improved. Immediate story recall and digit span dropped

[a] L = left, R = right, O = occipital, P = parietal.
[b] VIQ = verbal IQ, PIQ = performance IQ.
[c] BAS = British Ability Scales.

measures, but also of using all the data, which the categorical approach of psychiatric diagnosis cannot. All widely used quality of life measures include a number of items covering mental health. For example, the first epilepsy surgery-specific quality of life instrument, the 55-item epilepsy surgery inventory (ESI-55), contains five items which concern emotional well-being and another five which define role limitation due to emotional problems (Vickrey 1993). This measure was developed by taking a validated general health-related quality of life measure, the Rand 36-item health survey, and making it epilepsy surgery-specific with the inclusion of relevant additional items. The same rationale led to the development of the quality of life in epilepsy (QOLIE) inventory where the target population was patients with low to moderate seizure frequency. In other words, quality of life studies contain useful information about both mental health and psychosocial outcomes of surgery.

Earlier studies of psychiatric and psychosocial outcomes of epilepsy surgery were retrospective (Horowitz and Cohen 1968; Taylor and Falconer 1968; Jensen and Larsen 1979). There have also been some more recent prospective studies (Rausch and Crandall 1982; Hermann *et al* 1992; Seidman-Ripley *et al* 1993; McLachlan *et al* 1997), and one carried out by Vickrey *et al* (1995) using a combination of prospective and retrospective measures. Improvement in psychosocial function follows relief of seizures in a proportion of patients. Several studies have shown that complete relief of seizures leads to improved psychosocial function (Rausch and Crandall 1982; Dodrill *et al* 1992; Hermann *et al* 1992; Seidman-Ripley *et al* 1993; Vickrey *et al* 1995; Kellett *et al* 1997; McLachlan *et al* 1997). Rausch and Crandall (1982) followed 40 patients for a year, comparing a group who achieved complete remission of seizures with those who did not. They also had a smaller comparison group of patients who were referred for surgery but in whom investigations failed to localize a focus. They found that only patients with a seizure-free outcome improved psychosocially compared to those with a satisfactory (>75% seizure reduction) result. Seidman-Ripley *et al* (1993) used the Washington psychosocial seizure inventory (WPSI) in a prospective 1-year study of 30 patients, half of whom became seizure-free postoperatively. Only those who did so improved psychosocially.

Hermann *et al* (1992), in their prospective study of the psychosocial status of 97 patients after anterior temporal lobectomy, found that the most powerful predictors of overall postoperative psychosocial outcome were the adequacy of a patient's preoperative psychosocial adjustment, and a seizure-free outcome. Earlier work from the same group had found that complete cessation of seizures was most closely associated with major improvements in emotional and behavioral function. In this 1992 study, the rank sum of scores on the Minnesota multiphasic personality inventory (MMPI), the (WPSI), and the general health questionnaire (GHQ) was held to represent a composite 'total psychosocial adjustment' score. These instruments were administered preoperatively and 6–8 months after the operation. Postoperatively, this score correlated with the preoperative score. The postoperative score was also found to correlate with a completely seizure-free outcome. The seizure-free patients were compared with those who achieved a merely satisfactory outcome, that is greater than 75% seizure reduction; they did significantly better, corroborating the finding of Rausch and Crandall (1982). One major demerit of this study was the brief interval to postoperative assessment.

Vickrey *et al* (1995) performed an interesting study of outcomes from epilepsy surgery in 248 patients who entered the evaluation protocol of the University of California Los Angeles epilepsy surgery program. A total of 175 patients had undergone temporal lobe resection, while a comparison group of 46 could not go on to surgery because a focus could not be identified. Mean follow-up was 4.8 years and there was quality of life assessment both in prospective form and retrospectively with the ESI-55. There was no significant improvement in the prospective quality of life ratings, but an improvement in 5 of 11 domains of the retrospective quality of life instrument (the ESI-55), not including overall quality of life. The same group found that patients with a curative result scored significantly better than those with continuing seizures on the subscores of the ESI-55, and that patients with seizures of lesser severity scored in between (Vickrey *et al* 1992).

PSYCHIATRIC STUDIES

There have been fewer studies looking at psychiatric sequelae of surgery (Taylor and Falconer 1968; Jensen and Larsen 1979; Bladin 1992) and they come to a variety of conclusions. The older studies diagnosed patients according to the clinical judgment of the investigator or the consensus of opinion reflected in the clinical notes. More modern studies have, for the most part, used the operationalized criteria developed over the past 25 years. In the multiaxial classification of the Diagnostic and Statistical Manual of Mental Disorders of the American Psychiatric Association (DSM) versions III, IIIR, and IV, only the first two limbs are relevant in considering these studies. Axis I contains clinical disorders or mental illnesses such as anxiety, depression, and schizophrenia. Axis II describes enduring abnormalities which are nevertheless not mental illnesses; that is, personality disorders and mental retardation. Taylor and Falconer (1968) followed up 100 temporal lobectomy patients retrospectively. They reported that in this series of patients, a significant number of whom were referred by psychiatrists, 87 were psychiatrically abnormal preoperatively, with 30 being 'neurotic', 48 'psychopathic', 16 psychotic, and 5 having an 'epileptic' personality (two diagnoses were made in 12 of the cases). The proportion of normal patients postoperatively went from 17 to 32, but there was little or no improvement in the psychoses, a finding common to the studies; 37 patients went on to psychiatric admission at some point after their operation.

In their prospective study, Jensen and Larsen (1979) assessed 74 patients between 1 and 11 years postoperatively and looked at previous notes relating to their mental state preoperatively. No systematic diagnostic classification appears to have been used but 85% of the patients had been psychiatrically abnormal preoperatively, although most of this abnormality was made up of the rather nonspecific category of 'behavioral disturbance'.

Jensen and Larsen found that 69% of patients manifested a disorder in the follow-up period and that this reduction in psychiatric morbidity from preoperative levels was mainly due to a drop in the number of behaviorally disturbed patients. The number of schizophrenia-like psychoses, on the other hand, rose from 15 to 27% of the sample. For the patients as a whole, psychiatric disorder postoperatively was associated with a poor surgical result in terms of seizure control.

Bladin (1992) used DSM-III criteria for psychiatric diagnoses in 107 patients at a mean follow-up of 4 years. Significant postoperative anxiety is reported to have been suffered by 54% of patients, although it is not stated at what point after the operation these anxiety symptoms were experienced, how long they lasted, whether they amounted to an anxiety disorder as such and, if so, what types of anxiety disorder were present. Bladin also found such postoperative anxiety to be more common in patients who had undergone left temporal lobectomy. In addition, there were five patients who had suffered a depressive episode, and three who had been treated for paranoid psychosis. This is not an entirely satisfactory study as there is no obvious distinction drawn between symptoms and disorders. Assuming that some disorders were diagnosed, their exact nature is not revealed. The very great preponderance of anxiety over depressive symptoms is hard to explain, but the author draws attention to the problems experienced by patients in adjusting to successful surgical outcome. The results of this study are individual and also interesting, in that they demonstrate the importance of mood symptoms after surgery, with psychosis being much less common.

McLachlan *et al* (1997) conducted a 2-year prospective study of 51 patients undergoing temporal lobectomy using a comparison of medically treated patients. Assessment was by means of the ESI-55, and significant improvements were found in patients with at least a 90% reduction in seizure frequency. Such improvements, however, often only became evident in the second postoperative year. Kellett *et al* (1997) carried out a retrospective postal survey of 94 patients who had undergone epilepsy using a health-related quality of life measure, which included domains concerned with anxiety, depression, self-esteem, and balance of affect. They also found that complete cessation of seizures was associated with a substantially better psychosocial outcome.

In the authors' own study, the general practitioners (GPs) of 179 patients who had undergone temporal lobe surgery at the Maudsley Hospital, London, between 1976 and 1989 were contacted to establish details of mental health problems and diagnoses over the postoperative period (McEvedy *et al* 1993). The GPs of 132 of the 179 patients responded and the mean postoperative interval was 8 years. Of those 132 patients, 51% were seizure-free, but 74% continued on anticonvulsant medication (Table 63.1); 45% had received a psychiatric diagnosis in the follow-up period (diagnoses shown in Table 63.2), with two-thirds of these having suffered with a mood disorder, and approximately the same proportion having been under the care of a psychiatrist, lending weight to the GP psychiatric diagnoses.

Associations were found between continuing seizures and the presence of a mental health problem, specifically a mood disorder. There were also positive associations between right-sided operation on the one hand and the presence of a mental health problem, and a mood disorder on the other. Mental health problems in 44% of patients postoperatively is a high proportion, although not out of the realm of figures from previous similar

Table 63.1 Characteristics of 132 patients whose GPs responded.

Characteristic	Number	%
Sex		
M	64	48.5
F	68	51.5
Side of operation		
Right	60	45.5
Left	72	54.5
Type of operation		
Anterior resection	109	82.6
Amygdalohippocampectomy	23	17.4
Seizure-free	69	52.3
Taking anticonvulsants	98	74.2
Psychiatric diagnosis	58	44.6

Table 63.2 Principal psychiatric diagnosis in the 58 patients with mental health problems.

Diagnosis	Number of cases	%
Affective disorders		
Depression	17	29.4
Anxiety disorder	5	8.6
Mixed anxiety and depressive disorder	15	25.9
Nonaffective disorders		
Postictal psychosis	5	8.6
Personality disorder	8	13.8
Deliberate self-harm	2	3.4
Learning disability	2	3.4
Other	4	6.9
Total	58	100.0

studies. Perhaps more importantly, it is placed in context by studies of the previous psychiatric histories and current psychiatric status of epilepsy surgery candidates (Victoroff 1994; Manchanda et al 1996). In his study of 60 epilepsy surgery candidates, Victoroff (1994) found that 70% had a history of a DSM-IIIR axis I diagnosis, 58% a history of a depressive disorder, and 32% a history of an anxiety disorder (Victoroff 1994). Manchanda et al (1996) assessed 300 treatment-refractory patients who are potential epilepsy surgery candidates, and who had been admitted for investigation. Some 47% of the patients were psychiatric 'cases', with axis I diagnoses, i.e. a mental illness, in 29%, and a personality disorder in 18%. Anxiety disorders were present in 11% and were the most common mental illness found. Further information on the five patients who had experienced psychotic episodes was obtained from the psychiatrists who had treated them. With one exception, these appeared to be postictal psychoses. This finding of psychotic episodes in only 4% of cases postoperatively is in keeping with other more recent studies.

The finding of an association between right-sided operation and mood disorder is intriguing. The bulk of the literature favors the right hemisphere's role in the recognition of emotions, in dealing with negative emotions and in control of emotional expression (Silberman and Weingartner 1986). There appears to be a difference in the form of emotional information that each hemisphere is able to interpret. It may be that an intact left hemisphere is needed for the verbal expression of mood states and that, without this, a form of 'emotional agnosia' results. It may therefore be that the link between right-sided operated patients and subsequent affective disorder represents not so much a vulnerability of these patients as a peculiar invulnerability of the left-sided patients to affective disorder.

The study of McEvedy et al (1993) was not able to shed light on the psychologic outcome of those with a satisfactory, but not seizure-free, outcome, since they only compared the seizure-free with the rest.

PSYCHIATRIC CONTRAINDICATIONS TO EPILEPSY SURGERY

Fenwick (1987) surveyed 50 units worldwide, and of the 20 which replied, one-third recognized at least one absolute psychiatric contraindication. In the main, this constituted either psychosis or a severe disturbance of personality. Although the course of preexisting psychosis is not affected by surgery, such patients appear to achieve no worse a seizure outcome than others. Therefore, in as much as their quality of life is adversely affected by their seizure disorder present in addition to their psychosis, it does not seem reasonable to observe an inflexible bar on their consideration for surgery. Severe personality disorder, on the other hand, is likely to be bound up with the poor preoperative psychosocial adjustment which predicts poor psychosocial outcome, and reluctance to operate on such patients seems more reasonable.

EPILEPSY SURGERY IN CHILDHOOD

Some of the principal issues in this area concern whether or not there is an optimal age of the patient or stage in the development of a child's seizure disorder for operation. This matter is properly dealt with elsewhere in this book, but there are some considerations to be put from a psychosocial perspective. The first is that adults with intractable epilepsy presenting for surgical evaluation will usually have a long history of a severe seizure disorder, and that this will have inevitably led to a variety of coping strategies, and will often have resulted in psychologic and social disability. This latter may well have become part of the patient's psychologic constitution and persists regardless of seizure outcome after surgery. The second point is that if one takes this first conjecture to be intuitively correct, namely that children will have accrued less in the way of irremediable functional disability than adults with seizure disorders of comparable severity, then it follows not that the seizure outcome of operated children need be better in order to justify surgery in childhood, but that it must simply be no worse.

CONCLUSION

Previous studies of psychologic outcome from epilepsy surgery have mostly been concerned to evaluate the role of relief of seizures on psychosocial rehabilitation. There have been attempts, mentioned above, to chart specifically psychiatric outcomes of surgery (Taylor and Falconer 1968; Jensen and Larsen 1979; Bladin 1992). Perhaps the principal difficulties have been (a) the great differences in psychiatric outcome reported in older and more modern studies, (b) the lack of adequate control groups, (c) the absence of standardized diagnostic categories in earlier studies, and (d) the lack of long-term prospective studies. The latter points do not explain the marked difference in, for example, the rates of postoperative psychosis between earlier studies, e.g. the first Maudsley series reported by Taylor and Falconer (1968) or the Danish series of Jensen and Larsen (1979) on the one hand (both reporting around 20%) and the consensus of modern studies which find it to be comparatively uncommon (5% or less). The most obvious explanation for the conflicting results lies in the differing patient populations operated on over time. Interest in epileptic psychosis (arising from its perceived heuristic value for schizophrenia research) has perhaps been the focus of psychiatric attention for too long, and this needs to be placed in the context of the much more prevalent mood disorders, and difficulties in personal and social adjustment.

Bladin's (1992) study, like the authors' own, finds affective disorders to be the most common problem postoperatively in modern epilepsy surgery practice. Most likely these differences between older and more recent studies are principally due to differences in patient selection. Of the previous studies of psychiatric outcome, both Taylor and Falconer (1968) and Jensen and Larsen (1979) are agreed that continuing seizures are associated with a poor psychiatric outcome.

One finding common to several of the studies is that good preoperative psychosocial adjustment predicts good postoperative function. One of the clearest conclusions, and not the less important for being intuitively correct, is that a curative result from surgery is associated with, and presumably leads to, good postoperative psychosocial function. The findings in patients with improvements in seizure frequency (but not a curative result) are less clear-cut. As might be expected, they tend to lie between those with curative results and those with less than a 75% reduction in seizure frequency (Vickrey et al 1992; Malmgren et al 1997). Lesser seizure severity postoperatively also improves seizure outcome. An important lesson seems to be that postoperative adjustment takes time and that follow-up studies need to allow for this (Lindsay et al 1984; McLachlan et al 1997; Blumer et al 1998). Any follow-up study which limits itself to a period of a year or less is probably going to give misleading results for this reason.

To end on a note which looks ahead, questions in this area of the psychologic outcomes of epilepsy surgery which, in the authors opinion, demand further research are: (a) Why does satisfactory but not seizure-free outcome not lead to significant psychosocial improvement? This in turn is related to: (b) How is improvement in psychosocial function realized, and how can a program of postoperative rehabilitation assist patients to achieve it?

KEY POINTS

1. Potential epilepsy surgery candidates are a psychiatrically morbid population: 30% have a current mental illness and 70% a history of mental illness.

2. There are problems in synthesizing a view of psychiatric and psychosocial outcome research because of the differences in patient selection and assessment between older and newer studies. There is also a lack of data on long-term outcome assessed prospectively.

3. In current epilepsy surgery practice, postoperative mood disorders are common, at 30–50%. postoperative psychosis is significantly less frequent than previously, at 5% or less.

4. Good preoperative psychosocial function prefigures good outcome postoperatively. A curative result from surgery is associated both with good psychosocial function and good psychiatric outcome. There is also some effect found for reduction in seizure severity.

REFERENCES

Bladin PF (1992) Psychosocial difficulties and outcome after temporal lobectomy. *Epilepsia* **33**:898–907.

Blumer D, Wakhlu S, Davies K, Hermann B (1998) Psychiatric outcome of temporal lobectomy for epilepsy: incidence and treatment of psychiatric complications. *Epilepsia* **39**:478–486.

Dasheiff RM (1989) Epilepsy surgery: is it an effective treatment? *Annals of Neurology* **25**:506–509

Dodrill CB, Batzel LW, Griffith NC *et al* (1992) Surgical outcome: psychosocial changes after surgery for epilepsy. In: Luders H (ed.) *Surgery of Epilepsy*, pp 661–667. New York: Raven Press.

Elwes RDC, Dunn G, Binnie CD, Polkey CE (1991) Outcome following respective surgery for temporal lobe epilepsy: a prospective follow-up study of 102 consecutive cases. *Journal of Neurology, Neurosurgery and Psychiatry* **54**:949–952.

Engel J (ed.) (1993) *Surgical Treatment of the Epilepsies*, 2nd edn. New York: Raven Press.

Fenwick PBC (1987) Postscript: what should be included in a standard psychiatric assessment. In: Engel J (ed.) *Surgical Treatment of the Epilepsies*, pp 505–510. New York: Raven Press.

Fenwick PBC (1988) Psychiatric assessment and temporal lobectomy. *Acta Neurologica Scandinavica* **87**:96–101.

Fenwick PBC (1994) Psychiatric assessment and temporal lobectomy. In: Hermann B, Wyler AR (eds) *The Surgical Management of Epilepsy*. Stoneham, MA: Butterworth Heinemann.

Hermann BP, Wyler AR, Somes G (1992) Preoperative psychological adjustment and surgical outcome are determinants of psychosocial status after anterior temporal lobectomy. *Journal of Neurology, Neurosurgery and Psychiatry* **55**:491–496.

Horowitz MJ, Cohen FM (1968) Temporal lobe epilepsy, effect of lobectomy on psychosocial functioning. *Epilepsia* **9**:23–41.

Jensen I, Larsen JK (1979) Mental aspects of temporal lobe epilepsy, follow-up of 74 patients after resection of a temporal lobe. *Journal of Neurology, Neurosurgery and Psychiatry* **42**:256–265.

Kellett MW, Smith DF, Baker GA, Chadwick DW (1997) Quality of life after epilepsy surgery. *Journal of Neurology, Neurosurgery and Psychiatry* **63**:52–58.

Lindsay J, Ounsted C, Richards P (1984) Long-term outcome in children with temporal lobe seizures. V: Indications and contraindications for neurosurgery. *Developmental Medicine and Child Neurology* **26**:25–32.

Malmgren K, Sullivan M, Ekstedt G, Kullberg G, Kumlien E (1997) Health-related quality of life after epilepsy surgery: a Swedish multicenter study. *Epilepsia* **38**:830–838.

Manchanda R, Schaefer B, McLachlan RS (1996) Psychiatric disorders in candidates for surgery for epilepsy. *Journal of Neurology, Neurosurgery and Psychiatry* **61**:82–89.

McEvedy CJB, Polkey CE, Fenwick PBC (1993) Psychiatric outcome following temporal lobectomy for intractable epilepsy. *Epilepsia* **34**(Suppl 2):67.

McLachlan RS, Rose KJ, Derry PA *et al* (1997) Health-related quality of life and seizure control in temporal lobe epilepsy. *Annals of Neurology* **41**:482–489.

National Institutes of Health (1990) Consensus Conference. Surgery for epilepsy. *Journal of the American Medical Association* **264**:729–733.

Rausch R, Crandall PH (1982) Psychological status related to surgical control of temporal lobe seizures. *Epilepsia* **23**:191–202.

Seidman-Ripley JG, Bound VK, Andermann F *et al* (1993) Psychosocial consequences of postoperative seizure relief. *Epilepsia* **34**: 248–254.

Silberman EK, Weingartner H (1986) Hemispheric lateralization of functions related to emotion. *Brain and Cognition* **5**:322–353.

Taylor DC, Falconer MA (1968) Clinical, socioeconomic and psychological changes after temporal lobectomy for epilepsy. *British Journal of Psychiatry* **114**:1247–1261.

Vickrey BG (1993) A procedure for developing a quality of life measure for epilepsy surgery patients. *Epilepsia* **34**(Suppl 4):S22–S27.

Vickrey BG, Hays RD, Graber J, Rausch R, Engel JJ, Brook RH (1992) A health-related quality of life instrument for patients evaluated for epilepsy surgery. *Medical Care* **30**:299–319.

Vickrey BG, Hays RD, Rausch R *et al* (1995) Outcomes in 248 patients who had diagnostic evaluations for epilepsy surgery. *Lancet* **346**:1445–1449.

Victoroff J (1994) DSM-III-R psychiatric diagnoses in candidates for epilepsy surgery: lifetime prevalence. *Neuropsychiatry, Neuropsychology, and Behavioral Neurology* **7**:87–97.

Economics

independent of those related to the epilepsy. For example, the incremental cost for treating epilepsy that develops after a stroke depends as much on the severity of the stroke as the severity of the epilepsy. An individual with a severe permanent neurologic deficit after a stroke requires considerable expenditures independent of the costs of treating the seizures; indeed, epilepsy treatment might be a minor and insubstantial portion of the total costs. Another individual might sustain no permanent deficit after a stroke other than epilepsy, so the epilepsy-related costs might be the only ongoing expenses after acute treatment has finished. When determining costs, should an economist view the latter patient as having only stroke-related costs since the seizures are a consequence of the stroke, or divide the cost into separate epilepsy and stroke components? How one apportions costs among illnesses will impact total expense for any one illness. There are no easy ways to fairly apportion costs in this circumstance.

COST ESTIMATES

In addition to defining the affected population, a number of economic issues must be considered when calculating costs. There are different ways of assessing expense of illness, and one must consider more than the straightforward medical expenses incurred in the course of treating an illness. Also, costs can be assessed using an 'incidence-based' approach, a longitudinal analysis over the course of the disease, or using a 'prevalence-based' approach, which looks at costs cross-sectionally at a single time.

There are three major components of cost of an illness: direct costs, indirect costs, and psychologic or intangible costs (Shorvon 1996; Jacoby et al 1998). Direct costs are those medical and nonmedical expenses directly incurred on account of the illness. Direct medical costs include physician fees, hospital fees, medications, diagnostic tests, and surgical treatment. Direct nonmedical costs include rehabilitation and vocational training, special education, residential and community care, transportation for care, home modifications, and social services. The indirect costs are those due to reduced productivity, such as unemployment or underemployment, sick leave, excess mortality, social transfer payments, and care for relatives with epilepsy. They are very difficult to measure. Intangible costs include such detriments as social and psychologic effects and impairment in quality of life. Measurement of these costs is impossible.

In developing estimates of cost, one can either calculate costs of an average patient, or subdivide patients into various categories to allow for different severities of illness. Begley et al (1994) proposed a model that accounts for varying degrees of severity of illness in people with epilepsy. They defined six levels of illness, ranging from mild to severe. For example, some individuals promptly enter remission, and after a period of treatment no longer have health care expenses for the illness. At the other end of the spectrum, some have frequent uncontrolled seizures requiring recurrent hospitalization or even institutionalization. These individuals have substantial direct and indirect lifelong costs. With good epidemiological data, patients can be assigned to an appropriate category and costs calculated for each type of patient. This approach permits a more accurate assessment of costs for specific cohorts of patients with epilepsy, and aids in cost–benefit analyses. One can determine where money is being spent, and thence how to maximize return on investment.

ECONOMIC APPRAISAL STUDIES

The study of the relative value of various treatments with respect to their costs are known as economic appraisal studies. By placing a value on different interventions, a comparison can be made among the treatments. There are several ways of appraising economic costs: cost minimization, cost-effectiveness, cost–utility, and cost–benefit (Robinson 1993a, 1993b, 1993c, 1993d). These analyses can be applied to epilepsy and the reader is referred to the articles by Robinson (1993a, 1993b, 1993c, 1993d) for greater detail. Cost minimization analysis compares treatments of presumed equal efficacy, while the others incorporate not only monetary input but outcome or output, allowing for different efficacy or outcome among treatments.

In cost minimization analysis (Robinson 1993a), costs for various treatments are directly compared. It is assumed that the therapeutic outcome of the different interventions is identical. In epilepsy, this sort of analysis might be most easily applied to drug therapy if one assumes that efficacy is similar. However, efficacy may not be identical, and differing side-effects might influence outcome. Despite these limitations, this type of analysis can be useful when comparing different therapies which are used clinically in identical situations because it is believed that they are of equal value.

In cost-effectiveness analysis (Robinson 1993b) outcomes are measured in natural units (e.g. seizure frequency, mortality rates) and different interventions are not assumed to produce the same outcome. As long as differences in outcome can be measured, this type of analysis can be used. If one measures seizure frequency, then cost for a specific amount of seizure reduction could be calculated for different therapies. However, this model is limited by what can be studied, and does not account well for more intangible aspects of outcome or multiple types of outcome.

Cost–utility analysis (Robinson 1993c) combines different types of outcome into a single measure, a utility measure, of patient well-being. Then, comparisons are made between different treatments. The most popular scales used in cost–utility analyses are quality-adjusted life years and health-related quality of life measures, which incorporate costs of treatment and calculate economic benefit for various aspects of outcome. This analysis has been applied to epilepsy surgery (Silfvenius *et al* 1995; King *et al* 1997), and has the advantage of providing a measure that can be used to compare cost-effectiveness for treating different conditions. For example, one can compare the cost per quality-adjusted life year for treating diabetes or aneurysms with that of epilepsy surgery. However, cost–utility methods have many inherent biases, particularly when deriving the composite outcome measures, and they may inappropriately generalize about quality of life across patient groups (Shorvon 1996).

Cost–benefit analysis (Robinson 1993d) uses monetary values both for cost and in measuring outcome, and thereby provides an estimate as to the economic cost or loss to society for a particular intervention. The other analysis methods (cost–utility and cost-effectiveness) do not express outcome and input in similar units, and so cannot give this information. With cost–benefit analysis, for example, outcome is measured in dollars gained from increased income from higher productivity or reduced mortality (yielding prolonged productivity). However, economic productivity is a poor measure of the worth of human life. This method gives especially short shrift to the elderly, who may not be economically productive. Similarly, an intervention in a young child may yield relatively little economic benefit because of discounting (a method that gives little value to gains realized far in the future), yet the benefit is real. Nonetheless, cost–benefit analysis can be adjusted for these factors (though with inherent bias) and offers useful information when comparing therapies.

Cost appraisal studies have only been completed thus far mainly for epilepsy surgery, which is outside the scope of this chapter. Medical therapy, however, requires similar attention. The antiepileptic drugs that have come into use in the 1990s are far more expensive than older drugs. It is important to assess the efficacy and appraise the cost-effectiveness of new and older drugs for rational utilization of economic resources.

COST OF EPILEPSY

This section reviews the direct and indirect components of the cost of epilepsy. Examples will be shown of costs calculated for national populations. It must be emphasized that most of the figures cited below are estimates, because of the aforementioned limitations. Though reasonably precise accounting might be made for medical expenditures in some circumstances, imprecise diagnoses, inappropriate apportionment of costs, and inability to accurately measure indirect and intangible costs limit expense calculations.

DIRECT COSTS

Direct costs are those medical and nonmedical expenses attributable to epilepsy (Table 65.1). They account for perhaps one-third of the total economic cost of epilepsy, a similar proportion to that for neurologic illness as a whole in the United States noted by the National Foundation for Brain Research (Begley *et al* 1994). Some aspects of direct costs are relatively easy to obtain, for they are accessible through physician or patient records, patient questionnaires, insurance records, or national databases in countries with centralized health systems. This approach has been used in the United Kingdom and other European countries (Cockerell *et al* 1995; Gessner *et al* 1995; Jacoby *et al* 1998). Another approach to determining direct costs is to model care parameters using expert determinations regarding what constitutes appropriate care for the illness. These per capita cost estimates are then extrapolated based upon

Table 65.1 Direct costs for epilepsy.

Medical evaluation and treatment	Nonmedical treatment
Emergency services	Special education
Ambulance	Vocational training
Accident ward staff	Transportation for special needs
Inpatient hospital evaluation	Residential and community care
At time of diagnosis	Social services
After initial diagnosis	Home modification
General practitioner evaluation	
Specialist physician consultation	
Diagnostic services	
CT or MRI scan	
EEG	
Blood tests, miscellaneous testing	
Drug treatment	
Evaluation of drug reaction	
Serum levels, etc.	
Surgical evaluation	
Surgical treatment	
Physical rehabilitation	
Ancillary physician consultations	

known prevalence or incidence rates in the population being studied (Begley *et al* 1994; Banks *et al* 1995).

The initial evaluation when epilepsy is first diagnosed varies in expense, depending upon economic resources of the country, the individual, and vagaries of national practice. In a poor Third World country, the cost may be minimal, whereas in the United States, an expensive and litigious country, costs can be quite high (Begley *et al* 1994). A first seizure might lead to summoning an ambulance, evaluation in an accident ward, and inpatient hospitalization. In addition to the accident ward physician, a generalist might admit a patient to the hospital, a specialist (neurologist or neurosurgeon) may see the patient, and an expensive diagnostic evaluation then may be completed. This would include blood studies, magnetic resonance imaging (MRI) or CT scan or both, and an EEG.

After the initial evaluation is complete and epilepsy is diagnosed, regular treatment is required. The duration of this treatment depends upon the severity of the epilepsy and its natural history. Regular physician visits, periodic laboratory testing, and antiepileptic drugs are regular expenses during this time. However, seizure exacerbations and drug reactions can lead to additional hospitalizations, ambulance journeys, diagnostic evaluations, and additional specialist referrals. The refractory patient might consider epilepsy surgery, which entails added expense. In contrast, the well-controlled patient might have medication successfully withdrawn without further seizure recurrence, and have no expenses beyond those of the first few years. Other patients might remain controlled provided they continue to take medication, but still have a relatively low ongoing expense over the years.

Antiepileptic drugs are a major cost factor through the years, because of direct drug expense and the cost of monitoring the medication. The recent development of new drugs, while beneficial to some patients, may further add cost, since newer agents are considerably more expensive than older drugs. Variation in physician practice in different countries influences costs, as some agents are more popular than others depending upon country. Moreover, there is a wide variation in the cost of antiepileptic drugs from one country to the next depending upon resources and government policy. Table 65.2 lists some commonly prescribed drugs and their costs in different countries. As is obvious from the table, phenobarbital is two orders of magnitude cheaper than some other drugs, under which circumstances, whether the added incremental cost of some drugs is worthwhile remains to be determined. A cost–benefit analysis comparing different drugs would be worthwhile, and might aid in more effectively allocating resources. Presuming equal benefit, then the more expensive drugs should be reserved for only those who do not respond to cheaper drugs or who cannot tolerate them. However, if efficacy is not equal, then a more efficacious agent could be a better choice even if it is more expensive for both monetary and nonmonetary reasons.

For example, O'Neill *et al* (1995) published a study comparing the cost-effectiveness of vigabatrin, lamotrigine, and clobazam. They calculated the cost per successfully treated patient and compared efficacy of the drugs based upon controlled trials in the literature, which were generally part of preclinical testing protocols. Efficacy was defined as the proportion of patients with at least a 50% reduction in seizure frequency. They suggested that lamotrigine and vigabatrin cost 40% more than clobazam. However, caution should be used in interpreting this study, for there are several assumptions to which all might not agree. First, a 50% seizure reduction is not necessarily a therapeutic response and might be considered a treatment failure. Second, no trials compared one drug to another, but rather to placebo, so it is not possible to fairly compare the drugs.

Shakespeare and Simeon (1998) performed an economic analysis using data from a trial in the UK that directly compared carbamazepine and lamotrigine for partial and secondarily generalized seizures. They found that carbamazepine cost one-third as much as lamotrigine (£179 vs. £522) after allowing for costs associated with adverse effects. Therefore, while studies comparing drugs (Hughes and Cockerell

Table 65.2 Monthly antiepileptic drug expense in US dollars.[a]

Medication	USA	UK	Europe	Chile	Uruguay
Phenobarbital	0.99	0.70	3	5	9.3
Phenytoin	5.40[b]/16	4.10	4	16	17.40
Carbamazepine	28[b]/32	8.39	20.40	43	121.50
Valproate	40[b]/67	16.01	24.30	25	45.90
Lamotrigine	49.80	97.89	145	50	254.80
Gabapentin	—	136.90	—	—	—
Oxcarbazepine	—	—	160	50	189.60

[a]Data adapted from Jallon (1997) and Shorvon (1996).
[b]Generic costs.

1996; Heaney *et al* 1998) are important steps in developing a rational economic approach to drug prescription, more work is needed in this direction.

Estimates of direct expense have been made in several countries. Using a model that estimates health resource usage, Begley *et al* (1994) have calculated that lifetime direct medical costs for a cohort diagnosed with epilepsy in the United States in 1990 will be approximately $1.14 billion. Average cost per patient was $20 352, ranging from $4272 for the least affected to $138 602 for those non-institutionalized people with frequent seizures. Patients whose seizures were not in complete remission, while comprising only 15% of the population, accounted for 50% of the cost. Drug treatment was the expensive item on the bill, followed by physician visits and inpatient hospital costs (Table 65.3). Direct nonmedical expenses were not calculated in this study.

A prevalence-based approach was used in the UK, and contrasts with the incidence-based study described in the previous paragraph (Jacoby *et al* 1998). A group of 789 children and adults with epilepsy were evaluated, and both direct medical and nonmedical costs were ascertained (Table 65.4). The total annual direct cost was £1.23 billion (UK), with a per annum cost of £1568 per person. The

greatest expense to the health service was inpatient care (58%), and drug costs were second-most expensive, accounting for 23% of health service costs. Nonhealth direct costs were substantial and represented 56% of total direct costs, the bulk of these costs deriving from day care and, to a much lesser extent, remedial schooling. As shown in Table 65.4, costs correlate best with underlying seizure frequency. Costs for patients with seizures occurring monthly or more often were approximately eight times those of patients who had not experienced seizures in the preceding year. Hence, people with frequent seizures, though accounting for only one quarter of all patients, accounted for over half of direct cost.

Another report estimated annual direct expenditures in Australia at $238 million (Australian) total for 1992, which averages to $2340 (Australian) (Banks *et al* 1995). Sixty-one percent of these expenditures were for direct medical care, and 39% were for direct nonhealth care. Inpatient hospital expenditures were highest ($71.3 million Australian), and drug expenses were second highest, at $25.8 million (Australian). A Swiss study (Gessner *et al* 1995) estimated total direct costs at 229 million Swiss francs, a rate of approximately 6200 francs per patient. As in the US and UK, refractory individuals, though only 15–20% of the patients, consumed half of expenditures. Gessner *et al* (1995) also compared costs of epilepsy with those of ischemic heart disease and rheumatic diseases. They found that ischemic heart disease costs 2.7 times as much as epilepsy though the prevalence is six times higher. In contrast, rheumatic diseases cost 10 times as much as epilepsy, yet afflict less than half the number of people as epilepsy.

INDIRECT COSTS

Indirect costs, summarized in Table 65.5, embody the loss of society due to productivity losses, in contrast to direct costs which represent expenditures made by society for

Table 65.3 Lifetime direct medical costs of epilepsy in the US.[a]

Item	Percent of total cost
Medication	37.7
Outpatient physician visits	19.2
Inpatient hospital	14.1
EEG	6.7
CT/MRI	4.2
Emergency services	4.0
Drug reaction (including hospitalization)	3.6
Serum level tests	1.0

[a]These incidence-based lifetime cost estimates are for a US cohort diagnosed in 1990 (Begley *et al* 1994). These figures only account for the medical portion of direct expenses and do not include nonmedical direct expenses.

Table 65.4 Direct medical and nonmedical costs by seizure severity.[a]

Parameter	Number of seizures in past year			
	0 (n = 377)	<1/month (n = 204)	>1/month (n = 204)	All patients (n = 785)
Total health care costs	£61 235	£168 319	£311 118	£540 672
Cost per patient, total health care costs	£162	£825	£1525	£689
Total health and nonhealth care direct costs	£167 198	£347 890	£715 719	£1 231 050
Cost per patient, total health and nonhealth care direct costs	£443	£1705	£3508	£1568

[a]All costs are expressed in pounds sterling. Adapted from Jacoby *et al* (1998).

Table 65.5 Indirect costs for epilepsy.

Unemployment
Reduced productivity
    Underemployment
    Reduced activity days
    Time cost of treatment
    Sick leave
Excess mortality
Transfer payments
Loss by relatives to care for people with epilepsy

people with an illness (Shorvon 1996; Jacoby *et al* 1998). Indirect costs account for as much as two-thirds of the total economic cost of epilepsy in industrialized nations. Epilepsy imposes indirect costs on three levels: that of the patient, of his or her family, and of society. For example, patients may suffer from reduced earning capacity, family members may lose income because of time spent caring for an ill relative, and society might incur the expense of transfer payments and the loss of the potential of a citizen to contribute fully, both in economic and noneconomic ways.

People with epilepsy are underemployed and unemployed more often than the general population. On average, they suffer unemployment rates double those of their fellow citizens (Hauser and Hesdorffer 1990; Silfvenius *et al* 1995; Jacoby *et al* 1998). This is particularly true for those with incompletely controlled seizures, who may have even higher unemployment rates (Jacoby *et al* 1998). Epilepsy surgery series report unemployment in over 25% of patients with uncontrolled epilepsy (Silfvenius *et al* 1995; Sperling *et al* 1995). Productivity losses due to underemployment or unemployment may be estimated using an average earnings estimates, employing age- and gender-based work force participation rates. Also, people with uncontrolled seizures starting in childhood have lower levels of educational attainment, which can lead to reduced earning capacity in adult life.

If seizures are in remission or relatively infrequent, there may be no obvious loss in productivity (Jacoby *et al* 1998). However, the existence of epilepsy may lead someone to restrict their choice of careers because of perceived limitations in their capabilities, leading to reduced income in spite of full-time gainful employment. Even when fully employed, there is a time cost for epilepsy. Work time may be lost when someone has a seizure. Time must be taken to visit the doctor and have occasional diagnostic tests, and this may contribute to loss of pay or loss of productivity. Productivity due to lost time can be estimated from patient surveys and patterns of physician and diagnostic test utilization. It is difficult to accurately estimate this figure, because not all people take time off work for this purpose, but may engage in health care activities during vacation time, in the evening, or make up lost work time on another day. The impact of lost work time is potentially more significant in undeveloped countries than in developed countries. If the patient cannot work or loses time from their job, family income may suffer to the point of affecting nutrition, whereas social benefits will often secure the good health of the patient and their family in a developed country.

Mortality is another major indirect cost factor. The mortality rate in epilepsy is approximately double that of the general population (Hauser and Hesdorffer 1990). Premature deaths reduce the available work force and therefore represent a loss of output and productivity. Transfer payments are sometimes also included as an indirect cost. These are payments made to people as social security, welfare, food allowances, and medical care. They represent a shift of financial resources from one segment of the population to another, and as such diminish available funds for investment and increase tax rates. Since nearly all funds in transfer payments are spent by recipients, they still contribute to economic output though less so than if the money was not recycled by the government.

Begley *et al* (1994) have shown that indirect costs in their US cohort comprised 63% of the total cost of epilepsy. Of a total lifetime cost of nearly $3 billion for their cohort, indirect costs accounted for $1.86 billion. Seventy-six percent of the $1.86 billion was attributed to morbidity (unemployment, etc.), and the remainder to mortality costs. Of interest, only 15% of patients had recurrent seizures, but they accounted for 91% of indirect costs. Eighty-five percent of their patients were in remission, and they accounted for only 9% of the indirect costs.

A total of 1628 patients were enrolled in the National Epilepsy Survey in the United Kingdom (Cockerell *et al* 1995). In that study, indirect costs totaled £5.1 million annually out of a total cost of £7.1 million. Excess mortality accounted for nearly 8% of the indirect costs, with unemployment accounting for the rest. In Australia, it has been estimated that over $216 million (Australian) are spent per annum on indirect costs, of a total of $455 million (Australian) (Beran and Banks 1995). A Swiss estimate (Gessner *et al* 1995) of indirect costs caused by underemployment was 125 million Swiss francs, 35% of total expenses. However, this estimate did not include losses due to mortality or transfer payments, and so is a low estimate.

Indirect costs will vary from country to country depending upon general health of the population, medical resources available to treat epilepsy, per capita income, and the level of societal support for disabled or ill individuals. Estimates are not available for less developed countries.

INTANGIBLE COSTS

These costs include the social and psychologic costs of epilepsy. People with epilepsy have reduced marriage rates and reproduce less often (Hauser and Hesdorffer 1990). They have lower scores on quality of life scales (Vickrey *et al* 1995; Van Hout *et al* 1997), suffer a greater degree of social isolation, and have lower satisfaction levels. In many societies, people with epilepsy are stigmatized and cannot fully partake of life's large and small pleasures.

CONCLUSION

The economic costs of epilepsy are substantial, and it would be desirable to minimize this high cost. Since the bulk of the costs are indirect (Swingler *et al* 1994) and are mostly incurred as a result of uncontrolled seizures, prompt and effective medical intervention may have the potential to reduce overall costs. That is, it may be cost-effective to spend more money on direct medical costs to stop seizures in a target population with high indirect expenses. Conversely, rationing of direct health care monies in industrialized nations may have the effect of raising net societal costs, by denying or delaying effective

care (e.g. expensive drugs or surgery) and so causing high indirect costs. The challenge in Third World countries with limited resources is similar. In those countries, cost-effective treatment is even more important to maximize access to health care. It is critical to establish which treatments are effective to lessen indirect costs; it is clear this is best accomplished by stopping seizures, which is the factor that weighs most heavily with regard to cost (Van Hout *et al* 1997).

Since unemployment costs comprise the majority of indirect costs, the best strategy for reducing these costs would be to improve employment prospects in people with epilepsy. This would produce significant fiscal benefits for both the individual and the state.

Whether new epilepsy research will reduce the overall costs of epilepsy is doubtful. New technology and treatments have irresistibly increased expenses over the years, and costs are likely to rise in the foreseeable future. Economic analysis offers a good chance of rationally spending health care dollars to maximize return for investment. However, economic factors are only one part of the equation for deciding health expenditures. The intangible costs and benefits have an equally powerful claim on our consideration too. Human health cannot and must not be reduced to simple matters of dollars and cents, and humanistic concerns and values must take precedence.

KEY POINTS

1. Many illnesses compete for limited health care dollars. Since financial resources directly impact a people's health, social function, and life expectancy, it is important to understand the economics of these illnesses to better allocate health care funds.
2. Accurate knowledge of the epidemiology of epilepsy is necessary to arrive at meaningful cost estimates. Epilepsy is among the most common of neurologic diseases and care must be taken to fairly attribute costs when individuals suffer more than one neurologic impairment.
3. Refactory patients, though only 15–20% of the patients, consume half of the expenditures. The US estimates on average more than $20 000 lifetime cost per patient, ranging from $4272 for well controlled individuals to $138 602 for non-institutionalized people with frequent seizures.
4. Direct costs, which include both medical costs, such as special education and transportation, account for approximately one-third of the total economic cost of epilepsy.
5. Indirect costs account for perhaps two-thirds of the toal cost of epilepsy. This is due to productivity losses from unemployment, decreased educational attainment, and increased mortality among other factors. Unemployment represents the largest proportion of these costs.

REFERENCES

Banks GK, Regan KJ, Beran RG (1995) The prevalence and direct costs of epilepsy in Australia. In: Beran RG, Pachlatko C (eds) *Cost of Epilepsy*, pp 39–48. Baden: Ciba-Geigy Verlag.

Begley CE, Annegers JF, Lairson DR, Reynolds TF, Hauser WA (1994) Cost of epilepsy in the United States: a model based on incidence and prognosis. *Epilepsia* **35**:1230–1243.

Beran RG, Banks GK (1995) Indirect costs of epilepsy in Australia. In: Beran RG, Pachlatko C (eds) *Cost of Epilepsy*, pp 49–54. Baden: Ciba-Geigy Verlag.

Cockerell OC, Hart YM, Sander JWAS, Shorvon SD (1995) The cost of epilepsy in the United Kingdom. In: Beran RG, Pachlatko C (eds) *Cost of Epilepsy*, pp 27–38. Baden: Ciba-Geigy Verlag.

Gessner U, Sagmeister M, Horisberger B (1995) The economic impact of epilepsy in Switzerland. In: Beran RG, Pachlatko C (eds) *Cost of Epilepsy*, pp 67–74. Baden: Ciba-Geigy Verlag.

Hauser WA, Hesdorffer DC (1990) *Epilepsy: Frequency, Causes and Consequences*. Landover, MD: Epilepsy Foundation of America.

Heaney DC, Shorvon SD, Sander JW (1998) An economic appraisal of carbamazepine, lamotrigine, phenytoin, and valproate as initial treatment in adults with newly diagnosed epilepsy. *Epilepsia* **39** (Suppl 3):S19–S25.

Hughes D, Cockerell OC (1996) A cost-minimization study comparing vigabatrin, lamotrigine and gabapentin for the treatment of intractable partial epilepsy. *Seizure* **5**:89–95.

Jacoby A, Buck D, Baker G, McNamee P (1998) Uptake and costs of care for epilepsy: findings from a UK regional study. *Epilepsia* **39**:776–786.

Jallon P (1997) Epilepsy in developing countries. *Epilepsia* **38**:1143–1151.

King JT, Sperling MR, Justice AC, O'Connor MJ (1997) A cost-effectiveness analysis of anterior temporal lobectomy for intractable temporal lobe epilepsy. *Journal of Neurosurgery* **87**:20–28.

O'Neill BA, Trimble MR, Bloom DS (1995) Adjunctive therapy in epilepsy: a cost-effectiveness comparison of alternative treatment options. *Seizure* **4**:37–44.

Robinson R (1993a) Economic evaluation and health care: costs and cost-minimization analysis. *British Medical Journal* **307**:726–729.

Robinson R (1993b) Economic evaluation and health care: cost-effectiveness analysis. *British Medical Journal* **307**:793–795.

Robinson R (1993c) Economic evaluation and health care: cost-utility analysis. *British Medical Journal* **307**:859–862.

Robinson R (1993d) Economic evaluation and health care: cost-benefit analysis. *British Medical Journal* **307**:924–926.

Shakespeare A, Simeon G (1998) Economic analysis of epilepsy treatment: a cost minimization analysis comparing carbamazepine and lamotrigine in the UK. *Seizure* **7**:119–125.

Shorvon S (1996) Models of economic appraisals in epilepsy. In: Pachlatko C, Beran RG (eds) *Economic Evaluation of Epilepsy Management*, pp 19–26. London: John Libbey.

Silfvenius H, Lindholm L, Saisa J, Olivecrona M, Uvebrant P, Christianson S-A (1995) Cost of and savings from pediatric epilepsy surgery: a Swedish study. In: Beran RG, Pachlatko C (eds) *Cost of Epilepsy*, pp 83–106. Baden: Ciba-Geigy Verlag.

Sperling MR, Saykin AJ, Roberts DF, French JA, O'Connor MJ (1995) Occupational outcome after temporal lobectomy for refractory epilepsy. *Neurology* **45**:970–977.

Swingler RJ, Davidson DLW, Roberts RC, Moulding F (1994) The cost of epilepsy in patients attending a specialist epilepsy service. *Seizure* **3**:115–120.

Van Hout B, Gagnon D, Souetre E *et al* (1997) Relationship between seizure frequency and costs and quality of life of outpatients with partial epilepsy in France, Germany, and the United Kingdom. *Epilepsia* **38**:1221–1226.

Vickrey BG, Hays RD, Rausch R *et al* (1995) Outcomes in 248 patients who had diagnostic evaluations for epilepsy surgery. *Lancet* **346**:1445–1449.

The health economics of epilepsy surgery

H SILFVENIUS

Traditionally, the outcomes of therapeutic and palliative epilepsy surgery are judged by their effects in reducing seizure frequency (Engel *et al* 1993). However, even some early reports of epilepsy surgery included attempts to evaluate the outcome in socioeconomic, personality, and rehabilitation-related terms (Falconer *et al* 1955; Guillaume and Mazars 1956; Green *et al* 1958; Savard and Walker 1965; Taylor and Falconer 1968). More recently, health-related quality of life (HRQoL) and health economics have provided new methodologies to evaluate the outcome of epilepsy surgery. At a first glance, epilepsy surgery seems more costly than antiepileptic drug (AED) treatment alone. But the crucial question is whether AED treatment, in suitable patients, is as effective as epilepsy surgery in improving long-range HRQoL and reducing cost, or whether epilepsy surgery is an extra expenditure on top of the cost of pharmacotherapy. This survey will discuss the health economics of epilepsy surgery in light of the developments in the field. Although epilepsy surgery is a fairly expensive, high-technology exercise in developed countries, it can be shown that not utilizing it is even more costly. In developing countries, epilepsy surgery has been accomplished at low cost.

DEFINITIONS

Care programs consume resources through which society expects health improvement. No society expects health care without investment. The resources consumed by health care include capital investment among the direct costs, although this, and the cost of administration, is rarely dealt with in the epilepsy surgery literature. The economic loss due to loss of production, referred to below as production-loss, from unemployment or underemployment, or from premature mortality is an indirect cost, of which the expenditure for disability pensions or allowances, i.e. the transfer cost, is a part. Such loss of production caused by disease is calculated from the productive period of a society's population, accepted as between 16 and 65–70 years of age. Production-loss may also be defined as a net production-loss, which, combined with consumption-loss, would be termed gross production-loss. Private and public consumption consumes a considerable portion of the gross national product (GNP); for example, currently 80% in Sweden. The valued consumption-loss from mortality is therefore estimated as the net production-loss/0.20 (SNRA 1997). Intangible costs include disease burdens that are difficult to define economically, such as pain, social stigmatization, health-related restrictions in life, etc. (Pachlatko 1993). The expected improvement in health can be measured 'in natura', i.e. as seizure outcome, in utilities 'quality adjustment,' and in 'currency' (Drummond *et al* 1987).

Four methods of evaluating the health economic consequences of care are defined: cost-minimization, cost-effectiveness, cost–benefit, and cost–utility; the last three of these measures are commonly used.

Cost-effectiveness analysis would measure seizure reduction or reduced number of disability days (in a long perspective, disability-adjusted life-years (DALYs) or years lived with disability (YLDs)). Prolonged life or reduced mortality can be assessed with years of life lost (YLLs). The marginal cost ratio of cost per health output defined by DALY, YLD, or YLL would evaluate the cost-effectiveness of care (Murray 1994). It does not, however, address complications in similar terms. Murray (1994) specified the health economic use of DALYs as 'to aid in: setting health service priorities, setting health research priorities, identifying disadvantaged groups and targeting on health interventions, to provide a comparable measure of output for intervention, programme and sector evaluation and planning.' This description fits well with the long clinical tradition of promoting epilepsy care.

A cost–benefit study would evaluate the consequences in monetary terms of the 'human capital' by examining whether society gained anything by reducing production-loss through care resource allocation. The concept of 'human capital-investment in man-human wealth' is, according to Mooney's (1977) citation of Schultz (1971), 'the leading exponent of the concept,' that 'people enhance their capabilities as producers and as consumers by investing in themselves.' Becker (1964), cited by Mooney, suggests that 'activities that influence future monetary and psychic income by increasing the resources in people ... are called investment in human capital.' Schultz responded to the opposition against the concept of human capital that it 'stems from a feeling that there is something morally and/or ethically wrong in treating man as some sort of capital – a concept previously ascribed only to machines, buildings and other "things".' The 'human capital concept' is utilized most frequently in education, health, and training (Mooney 1977). Cost–benefit analyses of pediatric care are of particular interest as they project the expected benefit (reduced direct/indirect costs) to society, i.e. the taxpayers of the future. The elderly do not fit into the care consumption–benefit reasoning, in spite of which they are taken care of on ethical grounds. Generally speaking,

cost–benefit views guide decisions on the allocation of resources (Pachlatko and Beran 1996).

A cost–utility analysis addresses the outcome using QALYs, i.e. accumulated healthy days in relation to a care program (Kriedel 1980). QALYs are one way of expressing a positive care outcome; reduced DALYs/YLDs/YLLs would similarly evaluate the change (Murray 1994). Discounting in health economics, commonly 5%, is used for future cost effects of a care program as related to resources consumed today. Purchasing-power parity (PPP) ratios can be used for comparison of costs and savings from health care in developed and in developing countries (Murray and Lopez 1994; Murray *et al* 1994).

Direct cost is readily accepted by the medical profession, especially by those familiar with the administration of health care. Costs of capital investment, health care technology, drugs, care, and transportation are part of direct cost. Furthermore, there is little problem in accepting care costs for children and the elderly who are not contributing to the current production in society. However, when health economics refers to the indirect cost from unemployment and underemployment, and to mortality, a mental barrier rises against the presentation of production as a provider of resources and as the balance on which the direct and indirect cost is weighed. Fluctuations in employment rate would themselves cause the value of the human capital resource to fluctuate, depending on whether care was given in a financially strong period or at time of recession. The reduction in indirect cost from care would accordingly wax and wane and be difficult to maintain as a reference. A basic point is that society's wealth pays the cost, and wealth can be composed of national resources, external loans, production of work and services, etc. The human capital, as defined in health economics (Becker 1964; Schultz 1971), is capable of contributing its share to the society's wealth (GNP) that can be expressed as currency. Over a long period, the GNP may remain unchanged, rise, or decrease (Lecomber 1978). Short-range fluctuations, comparable to stock market volatility, would accordingly also have a bearing on the direct cost (see discounting). At a time of recession, with increased unemployment, society usually acts by reducing direct and transferral costs in order to drive the financial situation toward higher employment rates.

COST OF EPILEPSY

Epidemiology is the basis for health economic estimations of the cost of epilepsy and epilepsy care (DHEW 1978; Silfvenius *et al* 1991; Cockerell *et al* 1994; Begley *et al*

1995, 1997; Langfitt 1997; van Hout *et al* 1997). According to current views, remission is obtainable in 70–80% of newly diagnosed epilepsy patients (Cockerell *et al* 1994; Alving 1995). Despite the reduction in adverse effects and improved HRQoL that antiepileptic drugs administered by experts have brought about, unemployment and unchanged excess mortality from severe epilepsy seem not to have changed substantially (Elwes *et al* 1991; Jalava *et al* 1997; Nilsson *et al* 1997).

The median prevalence of active epilepsy from adult populations treated medically is reported to be 5–8/1000. A study population for assessing health economics of epilepsy includes institutionalized, incident population 50–122/100 000/year, prevalence of active epilepsy 5/1000, and lifetime prevalence 3–5% of general population (Cockerell *et al* 1994). In a specialized epilepsy center, 2–5% of the patients are said to be candidates for epilepsy surgery, and 7–18% of epilepsy patients followed by neurologists are estimated to be surgical candidates (Genton *et al* 1993; Constantino and Armon 1994). Even today, adult patients have commonly suffered from seizures for a decade or more prior to epilepsy surgery and have been burdened economically, to a greater degree than the general population, by unemployment. Excess mortality in epilepsy constitutes, through loss of production, an extra financial loss to society. Partial seizures have been reported to have a standardized mortality rate (SMR) of 1.5 (Olafsson *et al* 1998). Severe epilepsy in children has an urgent need for surgical evaluation using advanced diagnostics and epilepsy surgery, to remove or reduce the negative influences of epilepsy on education or training and future productive life. Jalava *et al* (1997) found significant problems in social adjustment and competence in adults whose epilepsy started in childhood. The unemployment rate among adults with epilepsy was reported to be increased 2–3.5 times compared to the control population, being higher in the presence of associated handicap (Elwes *et al* 1991). Pediatric epilepsy surgery has been proved to accomplish health economic savings Silfvenius 1995a; (Silfvenius *et al* 1995; Wyllie 1995). Following a good outcome from pediatric epilepsy surgery, there is an opportunity to correct deficient childhood education and vocational training and thus achieve long-range health economic savings for the child, the family, and society.

An economic evaluation is pertinent for the 'patient–care provider–society' grouping, expressing the relationship between 'demand–supply–financing.' The earliest health economic survey of epilepsy was that published in 1975 in the United States (DHEW 1978). Begley *et al* (1995) updated this and other data to 1990 prices. They summarized the cost for AEDs, residential care, vocational rehabilitation, special education, and research to US$13.4

billion, the cost for 6 days of hospitalization to US$532 million, and that for visits by physicians to US$76.7 million. Begley *et al* (1994) also estimated the cost of epilepsy in the United States. The average initial direct cost per patient was US$4272, and the long-range cost for intractable epilepsy per patient was US$138 602. These authors' most recent prognostic estimation of indirect cost suggests a cost of US$3000–9000 per patient per annum, and a lifetime cost (until remission or death) of US$20 000. They further expect a wide range in percentage between direct and indirect cost, the latter one often considered to be the larger one (Begley *et al* 1997). Silfvenius *et al* (1991) estimated the annual cost to society of epilepsy in Sweden, at 1990 prices: the direct cost was US$49 million, and the indirect cost US$150 million. Cockerell *et al* (1994) calculated the consumption of medical care for the United Kingdom, basing their calculations on two national epilepsy populations, and specifying direct and indirect costs. The annual direct cost was £0.65 million; the cost for schooling and residential care was £1.57 million. The total annual indirect cost was £5.1 million, of which the transfer payments amounted to £2.0 million. The authors arrived at an annual direct cost per patient of £535 (during the first year £611), and for the United Kingdom £147 million (patients in their first year £18 million). The total indirect cost, excluding transferrals, was £4167 per patient, and £1144 million for the United Kingdom as a whole.

Recently, a 3-month joint study from France, Germany, and the United Kingdom addressed the cost issue in 300 patients with partial epilepsy. Using a scale that placed patients in five groups according to their seizure frequency, the authors showed that mean total direct cost for those who were seizure-free was US$437, and for those with more than one seizure/day US$1026. The mean total indirect cost for the patients who were seizure-free was US$326, but for those patients with more than one seizure/day it was US$1055. Extrapolating the authors' data suggests that the mean total annual cost for the patients who were seizure-free could be less than US$3120, and for those with more than one seizure/day around US$8684 (van Hout *et al* 1997). Pfäfflin and May (1997) studied the impact of epilepsy on employment and restriction in daily life on persons with epilepsy in Germany, through a questionnaire to general practitioners engaged in epilepsy care. Severe epilepsy was noted in 22%, and 66% of these patients reported restrictions in daily life. The employment rate (54%) among persons with epilepsy was much lower than in the general population (81%) (cf. Elwes *et al* 1991). When patients with moderately severe epilepsy in another study were asked to list their concerns about living – on a blank sheet of paper and thus uninfluenced by investigators' views – the four most frequent concerns listed were driving (64%), independence (54%), employment (51%), and social embarrassment (33%). Listing only the most important concern gave three choices: driving (28%), employment (21%), and independence (9%) (Gilliam *et al* 1997a).

Under optimal circumstances, epilepsy surgery leads to discontinuation of AEDs, which produces a reduction in direct cost. Partial reduction in seizure frequency can accomplish a partial health economic gain, while permanent surgical morbidity and mortality leads to a health economic loss. A comparative assessment of clinical and health economic aspects of failure of surgical and medical care necessitates methodological evaluation to establish comparable success–failure ratings for medical and surgical treatments. Both treatments reveal inherent shortcomings in the attempt to suppress epilepsy completely, a challenge for future care. Morris *et al* (1997) analyzed the cost involved in urgent or emergency admission to hospital by studying the total charges and lengths of stay. They observed that the mean length of stay for an admission to internal medicine was 3.61 days as compared to 2.25 days for admission to a neurology facility. The mean total charges for the care by physicians in internal medicine was US$7856; for the neurologists it was US$4606. This study convincingly underlines the improved efficacy of expert care. In a comparison of the outcome of surgical and medical treatments of epilepsy, the clinical and health economic aspects of improved treatment of status epilepticus, by which direct cost and excess mortality (indirect cost) could be reduced, should be considered (Town *et al* 1997; van Hout *et al* 1997). In addition, emergency care of status epilepticus includes transportation costs, which should be included in the valuation.

The Commission on Neuroimaging of the International League Against Epilepsy (ILAE) recently made recommendations for the neuroimaging of patients with epilepsy (ILAE 1997a). Compared with other literature in the field, because it has to have a global perspective, the report understandably has a low 'cost profile.' The providers of facilities for epilepsy surgery may base their initial estimates of investment and direct cost on that recommendation.

The burden of epilepsy has also been addressed in a global perspective using QALY/DALY methodologies. Studies by the World Health Organization (WHO) underscore the differences in health and care between developed and developing societies (Murray 1994; Murray and Lopez 1994). Differences in epilepsy mortality and disease burden, as expressed by DALY, have been compared between established market economies and developing countries,

the latter having higher values (Murray 1994). Such a measure, equalling an assessment of reduced QALY, can quantify the difference accomplished by care. Epilepsy institutions are today operating in many countries, and most of those countries operate market economies. Their annual budgets, as well as those of residential care facilities, would give examples of the cost of care and rehabilitation of people with severe epilepsy (Thompson and Oxley 1988; Cockerell *et al* 1994).

ECONOMIC VALUATION OF EPILEPSY SURGERY DIAGNOSTICS

Since the 1980s, epilepsy surgery has spread within developed countries with access to advanced, expensive technologies. Organization, technology, level of expertise, selection of candidates, and annual production are crucial factors in determining the clinical and health economic profile of an epilepsy surgical center/comprehensive epilepsy center (ESC). A comprehensive epilepsy center with low productivity would have a limited capacity to take care of surgical candidates with a severe seizure situation as compared to a comprehensive epilepsy center with an annual turnover above the 'critical number of patients' necessary to evaluate and treat complicated cases properly (Wieser and Siegel 1992). The ILAE Commission on European Affairs has published 'Appropriate Standards of Epilepsy Care Across Europe.' Following its recommendation, an epilepsy surgery center should perform a minimum of 25 surgical procedures a year to qualify for recognition (Brodie *et al* 1997). This recommendation lays a good basis for an economic appraisal of an established diagnostic/care organization itself and of its output. An American consensus report on the organization of epilepsy surgery centers was issued in 1990 (Anonymous 1990).

The seemingly high direct cost of epilepsy surgery has been addressed in various ways, for example, by suggesting simplified diagnostics, preference for certain surgical investigations, and weighing of the direct cost against the postoperative savings in direct and indirect cost. The direct cost of epilepsy surgery is related to the diagnostic and surgical facilities, level of expertise, care organization, and results. Advanced facilities are generally available at ESCs in developed countries and cost utilities of this technology can be studied. A comparison of annual reports of ESCs would give insight into capital investment, administrative cost, care cost, and the possibility of health economic valuation of care results. Such data would be useful in comparing care and cost profiles with epilepsy institutions with medical, rehabilitatory, and residential care. The 'natural history of epilepsy' could thereby be assessed at an early stage from both medical and surgical points of view.

Concentration of resources into a new care facility or organization can improve epilepsy surgery, reduce diagnostic and surgical costs, enhance cost-effectiveness, and increase cost–benefit, especially if generally accepted for use. The predictive value of diagnostic technology has been studied in an attempt to evaluate investment and improvement of outcome (Mayes *et al* 1994). Electrophysiology, one of the cornerstones of epileptology, contributes two of three significant outcome predictors that could be seen as indicators of expert diagnostics and contributing to secondary cost gains. These predictors were quantified interictal epileptiform activity, ictal EEG abnormality, and neuroimaging data. It has further been found that noninvasive low-cost presurgical investigations suffice for successful anterior temporal lobectomy (Kilpatrick *et al* 1995). Tissue pathology, abnormality on imaging, and EEG are useful predictors of the outcome of anterior temporal lobectomy (Elwes *et al* 1995). Interictal EEG and convergent interictal sleep EEG and MRI findings can also predict successful epilepsy surgery (DellaBadia *et al* 1995; Roubina *et al* 1995). Prolonged EEGs in children and outpatient video-EEG monitoring can provide high-quality, cost-gain recordings (Rose 1995). Digitalized video-EEG may accomplish cost reduction as compared to analog recording (Hope *et al* 1996). Video-EEG reduces medical care resources and costs in patients with nonepileptic psychogenic seizures (Rose *et al* 1996).

Unilateral mesial temporal lobe atrophy seen on appropriate MRI investigation, and EEG abnormality, strongly predict ipsilateral seizure onset (Cendes *et al* 1995). Fast FLAIR MRI is diagnostically more sensitive than conventional MRI (Jack *et al* 1995; Ruggieri *et al* 1995). The diagnostic capacities of volumetric MRI (vMRI) and PET match each other (Radtke *et al* 1995). MRI spectroscopy and vMRI converge in predictive value in nonlesional temporal lobe epilepsy (Xue *et al* 1995). Volumetric MRI reliably detects mesial temporal atrophy and predicts surgical success (Cook *et al* 1995). Functional MRI (fMRI) detects metabolic changes during seizures, and can be used in accurately delimiting vital areas of the sensorimotor, visual, auditory, Broca, and Wernicke cortices using various functional testing techniques (Ives *et al* 1995; Lee *et al* 1995; Sirven *et al* 1995). Good predictability of ictal SPECT with surgical outcome has likewise been reported (Berkovic *et al* 1995). Magnetoencephalography (MEG), an expensive new technique under refinement, combined with EEG may locate seizure generators in hidden cortical banks, or in deep-seated structures (Paetau *et al* 1994; Stefan *et al* 1994). The cost-effectiveness of the presurgical use of MEG has been evaluated (Aung *et al* 1995; Roberts *et al* 1995). Cost reduction could occur because of a reduction in the scope and number of preoperative tests in lesional epilepsy surgery, in the case of diagnostic convergence in temporal lobe epilepsy, in early epilepsy surgery, and in large hemisphere lesions. Neuropsychology is another integral part of epilepsy surgery diagnostics and outcome evaluation. Sawrie *et al* (1998) studied the predictive role of discriminative presurgical neuropsychologic testing within five cognitive domains in adults. The predictive rate for patients to become seizure-free after a left anterior temporal lobectomy was 80%, with a positive predictive power of 92.11% above the base rate. The comparable figures for right anterior temporal lobectomy were 83.33% for seizure freedom, with a predictive power of 89.66%. Chelune *et al* (1998) queried whether low IQ would predict outcome after anterior temporal lobectomy. Analyzing 1034 cases of a joint study, they found a statistically significant lower IQ score, of only a few points (2.3). Noteworthy was that patients with IQ ≤ 75 proved to have a nearly fourfold increase in risk for continued seizures. However, the authors did not consider this finding as a basis for not performing epilepsy surgery.

Stewart *et al* (1997) determined the diagnostic and surgical cost in relation to the extent of diagnostic procedures both in anterior temporal lobectomy and in extratemporal epilepsy surgery. The minimum cost of an inpatient EEG study without epilepsy surgery was US$1576, while in those admitted twice for EEG and epilepsy surgery the comparative mean cost was US$21 454. Invasive EEG increased the cost to the range of US$50 739–89 688. The direct cost of the extratemporal epilepsy cases investigated and operated, with *longer* hospitalization than for the anterior temporal lobectomy cases, was US$74 151 and US$89 688, respectively.

HEALTH ECONOMIC EVALUATION OF EPILEPSY SURGICAL PROCEDURES

An early health economic estimate of epilepsy and epilepsy surgery was included in the 1975 DHEW-NIH study of cost (DHEW 1978). The direct cost for an epilepsy surgery procedure was then estimated at US$50 000. Silfvenius *et al* (1991) reported the direct cost of epilepsy surgery, from a national Swedish survey of four university hospitals in 1988–1990, and at 1990 prices it ranged between US$36 000 and US$46 000. International reports from 1993–1994 suggested that the direct cost for epilepsy surgery varied between US$21 800 and US$86 500 (Rainwater *et al* 1993; Ecker and Snead 1994). Intraoperative identification of eloquent cortices with electrical stimulation can avoid other costly diagnostic tests (Silbergeld and Ojemann 1993). The cost of epilepsy surgery has been compared with care for other conditions using DRG-classifications and ranges between US$16 000 and US$65 000 (Kasunic *et al* 1995).

New MRI technology has radically simplified presurgical assessment. Currently, the surgical procedure is more accurately targeted in relation to etiology, especially in lesional epilepsy surgery. The cost of epilepsy surgery interventions will vary with the length of the procedure and the technological demands. Epilepsy surgery in 'silent' brain areas would be faster and cheaper than lengthy procedures in vital cortices demanding elaborate preoperative and intraoperative diagnostic and surgical measures. Modifying a traditional surgical technique, like anatomic hemispherectomy, into a shorter procedure, hemispherotomy, will reduce not only theatre cost but also hospitalization length as the latter procedure provides a speedier recovery (Delalande *et al* 1995). As has already been suggested, a reduced need for presurgical evaluation and concomitant cost reduction could therefore apply to lesional epilepsy surgery, in case of diagnostic convergence in temporal lobe epilepsy, in early epilepsy surgery, and in large hemisphere lesions. A reduced diagnostic need also applies to palliative epilepsy surgery such as corpus callosum section and implantation of vagus nerve stimulation (VNS). By contrast, multiple subpial transection (MST), although a fairly short surgical procedure, demands advanced presurgical work-up, which puts it in the same cost category as other comprehensive resective epilepsy surgery (Langfitt 1997).

EPILEPSY SURGERY OUTCOME

A COST PERSPECTIVE

Considering all resective epilepsy surgery procedures and MST, freedom from seizures is achieved in 45–90% of patients; 20–35% of cases improve; while 10–20% of the operated attain no improvement, or even experience worsening of their seizure situation and are burdened by new permanent morbidity (0–10%), or may progress to mortality (0–10%) (Andermann *et al* 1991; Primrose and Ojemann 1991; Van Ness, 1991; Talairach *et al* 1992). Success from radical pediatric epilepsy surgery is obtained in 50–75% of children operated (Villemure *et al* 1993; Delalande *et al* 1995; Schramm *et al* 1995; Tuxhorn *et al*

1997). A global ILAE survey of epilepsy surgery (1980–1990) revealed similar outcome scores (ILAE 1997b). Reoperation, an extra direct cost, yields freedom from seizures in 45–50% and is justified both clinically and on economic grounds (Germano *et al* 1993; Polkey *et al* 1993). For the surgically oriented mind, reoperation is basically comparable to a change of AED in the medical treatment of intractable epilepsy. The results of resective epilepsy surgery in children and adults are comparable (Lüders 1992; Engel *et al* 1993; Tuxhorn *et al* 1997). Palliative epilepsy surgery, corpus callosum section, and VNS, in patients unsuited for resective epilepsy surgery or in whom resective epilepsy surgery has failed, can also be evaluated with QALY/DALY methodologies (Dodrill *et al* 1992). The diagnostic mortality approximates 0.5%, the surgical mortality 0–10%, and they are related to the procedures (Engel *et al* 1993; Pilcher *et al* 1993). The permanent diagnostic and surgical morbidity is 0–10%. If epilepsy surgery stops seizures at the expense of impaired cognition and/or emotional stability, then it is of limited help in restoring HRQoL, especially in persons highly dependent on such capacities. Neuropsychology has detected improved, unchanged, or impaired cognition after anterior temporal lobectomy. Impaired verbal memory after left anterior temporal lobectomy (ATL) is seen in cases where there is minimal mesial temporal lobe sclerosis, or none at all (Seidenberg *et al* 1995). Nonverbal memory can be reduced after right anterior temporal lobectomy (Morris *et al* 1995). A verbal deficit may be present prior to left temporal lobectomy and may progress after surgery (Helmstaedter *et al* 1995; Saykin *et al* 1995). Word finding and memory deficits have been found in 25% of patients after ATL (Langfitt and Rausch 1995). Others have found no postoperative memory decline in two-thirds of cases (Phillips and McGlone 1995). Unchanged or improved memory after ATL has been reported, as well as preoperative language and memory impairment in left temporal lobe epilepsy (Davies *et al* 1994, 1995). About one-third of patients undergoing surgery for temporal lobe seizures experience significant memory impairment (Baxendale *et al* 1996). Long-range neuropsychologic and psychosocial risks of epilepsy surgery have been emphasized (Rausch 1995). Fortunately, disabling memory deficit is rare, but a significant head trauma after surgery may render the patient globally amnestic (Oxbury *et al* 1997). The surgical risks of a psychiatric complication are minor and the condition is medically treatable. Such complications do prolong the recovery period and do increase both direct and indirect cost (Hermann *et al* 1993; Blumer *et al* 1996). Improved emotional and overall life adjustment has also been noted after ATL (Rayport and Ferguson 1995). It has been found that in 65% of seizure-free patients the behavioral disturbances were resolved promptly by epilepsy surgery (Snars *et al* 1995).

In adults, epilepsy surgery is often performed late after seizure onset (10–20 years). During such a long period of time the social status declines and the disabilities of a patient with intractable epilepsy may increase and they may incur stigmatization. Children with epilepsy, and their families, experience social restrictions that tend to be difficult to normalize after successful surgery (Silfvenius *et al* 1995a; Thorbecke 1997). The preoperative delay will also *increase* the cost of illness, and demand more elaborate and expensive diagnostics. A significant difference in seizure outcome has been noted after extratemporal lesional surgery in younger compared with older age groups with epilepsy (Smith *et al* 1995). Successful epilepsy surgery reduces direct and indirect costs, but reduction in expenditures can also be gained from partial seizure relief measured by DALY/QALY. An incremental cost-effectiveness ratio of US$25 700/QALY was found for a typical 30-year-old epilepsy patient as compared to US$16 500 for a 72-year-old person with knee arthroplasty or US$32 400 for antihypertensive therapy for a 50-year-old patient (King *et al* 1994). The cost-effectiveness of epilepsy surgery for temporal lobe seizures is said to compare favorably with other health technologies (Langfitt 1997). The ATL study of King *et al* (1997) indicated that evaluation for ATL provided an average of 1.1 additional QALYs compared with AED treatment, at an additional cost of US$29 800 and a cost-effectiveness ratio of US$27 200/QALY, a value comparable to that of other accepted medical and surgical treatments.

QUALITY OF LIFE, EDUCATION/TRAINING, AND EMPLOYMENT

New measures of epilepsy surgery outcome have been proposed that emphasize the need for a closer 'patient-family to caregiver' relation with better preoperative definition of expectation, outcome, and rehabilitation (Taylor *et al* 1997). The authors argued that 'Until recently, no record has been made, before surgical treatment of epilepsy, of what *exactly* the patient or the patients' caregiver was hoping to achieve beyond seizure relief or of what the surgical team wished to achieve by the operation.' Wilson *et al* (1998) published a report on this topic related to ATL. Analyses of HRQoL and of health economics underscore a holistic view of epilepsy surgery, an obvious view that had been taken by some surgeons in the field many years ago. The need for a deep understanding of the patient's and their family's expectation of a pending operation is easy to

grasp because of the expected rapid change that is about to take place. Differences will easily be detected and compared. A similar holistic attitude is also needed in medical treatment of epilepsy, especially if AEDs are inefficient in improving the patient's seizure situation within an acceptable period. Expectations of AED treatment that later proves to be failing will turn into disappointment over the years and end as burnt-out expectations of life qualities. Both underselling and overselling of medical or surgical treatments should be guarded against. Satisfaction or dissatisfaction by the individual or family is evaluated in relation to the expectation of a surgical procedure. The often unquantified practical expressions of the traditional seizure outcome of the patient or their family may agree or disagree with the preoperative expectation. An unchanged postoperative seizure situation and a new neurologic complication will certainly topple the preoperative optimistic expectation. Likewise, there may be disappointment if, in spite of a successful outcome in regard to seizures, there is no improvement in HRQoL or employment.

The HRQoL, a measure of change in life from epilepsy care, has attracted methodological interest, particularly as regards anterior temporal lobectomy (Vickrey *et al* 1992, 1995; Vickrey 1993; Langfitt 1995; Schulz *et al* 1995; Schwartz *et al* 1995; Cramer *et al* 1996; Wiebe *et al* 1997). A cross-cultural translation of a QoL-protocol is now available (Perrine *et al* 1998). The ILAE Commission on Outcome Measurement In Epilepsy, 1994–1997, Final Report addresses two sectors relevant to surgical treatment: epilepsy surgery itself and HRQoL (Baker *et al* 1998). HRQoL may be expressed in QALY/DALY terms as already described. Recent studies have reported the following experiences in relation to epilepsy surgery. A patient's satisfaction with epilepsy surgery is dependent upon its effect on seizures, absence of neurologic deficits, change in working ability, and other postoperative factors (Guldvog 1994). An overall improvement has been reported after epilepsy surgery in social functioning and patient satisfaction and other concordant experiences (McEvedy *et al* 1993; Michaelis *et al* 1995; Paglioli-Netu *et al* 1995; Ribaric *et al* 1995). Seidman-Ripley *et al* (1993) found that even a partial improvement in seizure relief carries psychosocial improvement. This can be assessed with QALY/DALY methodologies and converted into health economic terms.

Problems in getting employment may impede other beneficial effects of epilepsy surgery. Epilepsy surgery influences HRQoL more favorably than does medical management (McLachlan *et al* 1994; Baca *et al* 1995). A higher HRQoL rating after epilepsy surgery in seizure-free patients has been reported (Malmgren and Sullivan 1995). Epilepsy surgery is more efficient than AEDs alone in improving HRQoL (Kellet *et al* 1996; Loring *et al* 1996; McLachlan *et al* 1996; McMackin *et al* 1996; Palas *et al* 1996; Stoddard *et al* 1996; Thorbecke 1996). Wilson *et al* (1998) found that among patients who had undergone ATL, seizure freedom was their foremost expectation (72%), followed by driving (45%), new activities (38%), and employment (35%). When studying the expectation distribution postoperatively among the successes, the percentages of 'driving' and 'new activities' increased slightly. The surgical failures, on the other hand, had an increased percentage in 'new activities' and in other expectations of a psychosocial nature. Using a statistical regression analysis, Gilliam *et al* (1997b) evaluated clinical variables with HRQoL after epilepsy surgery. The authors found both better role function and better mental health, which were significantly associated with employment and driving. Lassouw *et al* (1997) studied HRQoL after epilepsy surgery. The highest impact on HRQoL was the hope of being employed, and for occupational opportunities (18.1%). In 25% of the cases the working situation improved. Kellett *et al* (1997) statistically analyzed 94 patients who had had epilepsy surgery, in regard to employment *inter alia*. They noted that the seizure-free patients had an odds ratio of becoming employed of 8.38 relative to those who had undergone evaluation but no epilepsy surgery. Improvements in these regards would reduce the indirect cost. Recent reports on employment have described short-range results that may be extrapolated (Engel *et al* 1993). Epilepsy surgery patients employed preoperatively continue to be so postoperatively, or maintain their employment status (Augustine *et al* 1984; Vermeulen *et al* 1993). Presurgical self-reports have shown preference for passivity, dependency, and poor patient compliance in participation in postoperative evaluation of occupational rehabilitation (Callanan *et al* 1994). One investigation showed that employment postoperatively was increased by 21% (Buelow and Kaiser 1993). A study of reoperation for temporal lobe seizures showed all patients to be unemployed prior to the reoperation, whereas afterwards 85% were working (Germano *et al* 1993). However, limited functional gain in employment after epilepsy surgery has also been seen (Batzel *et al* 1993). Early epilepsy surgery has a positive effect on vocational or educational outcome, and often improves the occupational status (Sperling *et al* 1994; Walker *et al* 1994). Preoperative employment and good seizure outcome were correlated with improved employment after extratemporal lobectomy but not after ATL (Van Ness *et al* 1994). A favorable psychosocial outcome after epilepsy surgery was seen in almost 80% of these patients, who were living independently and gainfully employed

(Dewar *et al* 1994). One study found that 84% of the seizure-free patients were employed or attending school (Fielstein *et al* 1994). On the other hand, Vickrey *et al* (1995), found no significant differences in preoperative and postoperative employment status. It has been noted that the formerly unemployed improved their situation and that early epilepsy surgery favored postoperative employment (Helmstaedter *et al* 1995). An increase in the probability of working full-time postoperatively is enhanced by working or studying during the year prior to epilepsy surgery, or having further education after surgery (Reeves *et al* 1995). Sperling *et al* (1995b) evaluated employment after ATL in 73 patients and noted that unemployment declined postoperatively by 14%, all seizure-free patients being employed; patients with remaining but reduced seizures, also had increased employment after ATL. Of 13 students at time of ATL, 11 had graduated and 9 were employed. Crawford and Gage (1997) conducted a study on QoL issues related to epilepsy surgery. They found little difference between preoperative (58.1%) and postoperative work status (61.3%). Doherty *et al* (1997) studied 32 patients who had undergone anterior temporal lobectomy. In regard to employment, 56% held jobs preoperatively, 63% postoperatively at 2 years, and 77% at 5 years. Furthermore, they noted a decreasing trend in clinic postoperative visits. Lendt *et al* (1997) reported the effects of epilepsy surgery on preoperative and postoperative socioeconomic status in 151 patients, some of whom were children. They noted that 49% of the pupils or students became trainees and employees after surgery, that 82% of the formerly employed continued their working, that 34% of those formerly unemployed found a job, and that the preoperative unemployment decreased by 16%. The effect of epilepsy surgery on employment supplemented with health economic evaluation has been reported by some authors (Silfvenius *et al* 1995b; Reeves *et al* 1997; Silfvenius 1999). The latter compared the preoperative and postoperative income after ATL in 86 adults, finding a significant increase only in those with an annual income in the range of US$20000–39999. An increased income has been quantified after successful epilepsy surgery in adults, and to some extent also in those scored as surgical failures (Silfvenius *et al* 1995a). Similarly, successful pediatric epilepsy surgery is cost-effective for both the child and the parents (Silfvenius *et al* 1995a, 1997b).

Disabling postoperative neurologic and psychiatric complications should be taken into account when evaluating the cost-effectiveness of epilepsy surgery. The neurologic complications of epilepsy surgery, apart from the cognitive effects, should be evaluated against the complications of epilepsy itself, especially poorly controlled epilepsy. Epilepsy surgery leading to abolition of seizures reduces the excess mortality (Sperling *et al* 1995a).

The outcome from corpus callosum section (CCS) in regard to seizures is inferior to that of resective epilepsy surgery (Engel *et al* 1993). Nevertheless, partial behavioral and psychosocial improvement may follow CCS, the care giver's load is lessened, and resources can partly be reallocated. VNS is now accepted as a choice after failed resective epilepsy surgery, and after CCS, or under other circumstances. The cost of the VNS implant plus the other care costs can be summed and compared with the postoperative fractional change in direct or indirect cost evaluated by QALY/DALY (Damiano and Dodrill 1997). Cost studies on epilepsy surgery indicate that, in addition to being medically and ethically highly motivated, epilepsy surgery is a good health economic investment.

EPILEPSY SURGERY AND HUMAN CAPITAL: UNEMPLOYMENT A DISEASE BURDEN, CARE A COST SAVING

Improved education or vocational training and reduced part-time or full-time unemployment or underemployment are the cost–benefits to society from a radically or partially improved seizure situation. Such cost–benefits are apparent within the direct and indirect cost sectors.

Use of seizure-free rate as an effectiveness measure showed that epilepsy surgery is cheaper than AED treatment alone. Epilepsy surgery resulted in 57% seizure-free patients versus 12% for AEDs alone, equivalent to a net saving of US$58 300 per epilepsy surgery patient (Wiebe *et al* 1994). A European study found the cost of medical care to be three times higher in patients with intractable epilepsy, compared with those who were well-controlled (Popovic

and Ribaric 1995). The direct cost of medical treatment over a period of 50 years is 30 times higher than the cost of epilepsy surgery. The seemingly high initial cost for advanced diagnostics should be seen in a longer perspective during which costs may be reduced (Rentz *et al* 1996). In Sweden the reduction in life-long indirect cost after successful pediatric epilepsy surgery has been put at US$250 000 per treated child (Silfvenius *et al* 1995a). Evidence for an increased income has similarly been established for operated adults (Silfvenius *et al* 1995b, 1997a,b; Silfvenius and Olivecrona 1998) (Table 66.1 and Fig. 66.1).

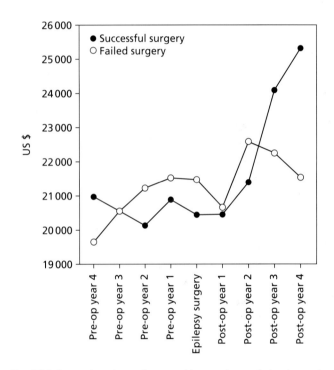

Fig. 66.1 Pre- and postoperative annual income by surgical outcome in 70 adult Swedish epilepsy patients. The mean year of epilepsy surgery was 1988. Data are expressed in 1994 prices.

Table 66.1 Estimated future lifetime production of 228 successfully operated non-handicapped epileptic children (discounting 5%).

Grown-up boys, *n* = 114	
Full-time working, 92%	
105 men, annual income 150 000 SEK × 50 productive years	288 million SEK (US$ 36 million)
Part-time working, 8%	
9 men, annual income 90 000 SEK × 50 productive years	15 million SEK (US$ 1.87 million)
Grown-up girls, *n* = 114	
Full-time working, 60%	
68 women, annual income 100 000 SEK × 50 productive years	124 million SEK (US$ 15.5 million)
Part-time working, 40%	
46 women × annual income 60 000 SEK × 50 productive years	50 million SEK (US$ 6.25 million)
Costs for epilepsy surgery, 74 000 SEK × 228 children	−17 million SEK (−US$ 2.12 million)
Lifetime production, grown-up nonepileptic children	460 million SEK (US$ 57.5 million)

65% surgical success rate of 350 children = 228.

Changes in employment status (indirect cost) after epilepsy surgery were referred to in the text above. Langfitt (1997) estimated the cost-effectiveness of anterior temporal lobectomy. He arrived at the following lifetime discounted (5%) cost of treatment care per patient: presurgical evaluation, morbidity, and anterior temporal lobectomy cost US$47 002; total follow-up cost US$62 361; the grand total amounting to US$109 362. Begley *et al* (1994, 1995, 1997) have described the methodology of their incident prognostic direct cost model for the cost of epilepsy in the United States, derived from data collected during 1995–1998. The authors characterize 620 patients with complex partial seizures divided into three subgroups having early remission, and another three subgroups with intractable seizures, and related each patient category to care and disease evolution. A comprehensive cost evaluation is structured to cost: hospital inpatient care, medical and surgical (ATL), inpatient and outpatient physician visits, drug treatment, hospital emergency care, ambulance transport, and diagnostic procedures. It helps to evaluate the outcome of palliative resective epilepsy surgery (clinical outcome classes 3–4), and of CCS and VNS procedures, and could bring new insights into reallocation of resources within epilepsy care relevant to the demand for personnel for residential care and to changes in underemployment in families with a severely ill member with epilepsy.

EPILEPSY SURGERY IN DEVELOPING COUNTRIES

Restricted availability of equipment, due to high capital cost, at epilepsy surgery centers in developing countries and their present utilities provide examples of low-cost epilepsy surgery. A recent report from Colombia reported the annual budget of comprehensive medical (outpatient and inpatient care), surgical, and rehabilitational and schooling programs at an epilepsy surgery center to range between US$1270 and US$ 2080 (Fandino-Franky *et al* 1995). The mean direct cost, including diagnostics, per epilepsy surgical procedure was US$1700 (Fandino-Franky *et al* 1995; Fandino-Franky 1997; Fandino-Franky and Silfvenius 1998). The direct cost of therapeutic pediatric epilepsy surgery in Colombia was similarly reported to be US$2808 by Fandino-Franky (1997). In South Africa the cost was about one-fifth of that in the United States (Kies 1995). Rao *et al* (1997) reported the results of newly commenced anterior temporal lobectomy activity in India, probably also at low cost. Epilepsy surgery is increasingly being performed in developing countries, and accomplishes outcomes comparable to those in developed countries.

Most of the publications on epilepsy surgery related to health economics focus on direct cost, a few on indirect cost, but hardly any on capital investment, administration, or consumption-loss. For developing countries, the cost of capital investment is a considerable obstacle and should, together with depreciation of the value of equipment, be incorporated in the assessment of direct costs. It will soon be possible to compare in health economic terms the epilepsy surgery outcomes of developed and developing countries using the PPP method (Murray *et al* 1994).

SUMMARY

Health-related quality of life (HRQoL) and health economics express in broad perspectives the burden of epilepsy and the effects of care. Both methods have recently been used in evaluating the outcome of epilepsy surgery. In addition, health economics can evaluate whether care resources are being used adequately, and also identify inefficient services. In the suitable candidate, refraining from epilepsy surgery perpetuates the socioeconomic burden for the patient and their family and is also a waste of the health resources of the community. The cost of epilepsy surgery is related to the costs of the applied technology and level of expertise, the costs of maintaining an organization to bring the candidates for surgery to the assessment programs, and the economic consequences, both good and bad, of the outcome of the surgery. Advances in epilepsy surgery may reduce cost and enhance the cost-effectiveness or benefit of these interventions. Both in adults and children who are suitable candidates for epilepsy surgery, the outcome may have a more favorable influence on HRQoL and health costs than continuing medical treatment alone. Successful epilepsy surgery achieves an overall improvement in social functioning and patient satisfaction. The cost-effectiveness of epilepsy surgery for temporal lobe seizures compares favorably with results from other health technologies. The indirect cost of epilepsy, due to unemployment and untimely death, are much reduced by successful epilepsy surgery, and to a lesser degree by partially successful surgery. Operated adults often gain an increase in income. Epilepsy surgery in children has long-range positive socioeconomic effects and is a health economic saving for the community. There are encouraging reports of low-cost epilepsy surgery in developing countries.

KEY POINTS

1. The outcome of epilepsy surgery is commonly scored by seizure reduction, and at times expressed socioeconomically. Health economics is a recent outcome evaluation.

2. Care consumes resources: a direct cost. Unemployment and mortality is an indirect cost, and includes the expenditure for disability pensions.

3. Two methods here mentioned to evaluate health economics consequences of care are cost-effectiveness and cost–benefit. A cost-effectiveness analysis would measure seizure reduction as disability-adjusted-life-years (DALY). Reduced mortality can be assessed with years of life lost (YLLs). A cost–benefit study would evaluate if society did gain anything from reduced production loss through care resource allocation.

4. Epidemiology sets the basis for health economics estimations of cost. Remission is said to be high in newly diagnosed patients, but umemployment and mortality from severe epilepsy seem unchanged. Recent reports have dealt with health economics on individual and societal levels.

5. Epilepsy surgery utilizes advanced technology. Organization, expertise, selected candidates, and annual production are crucial factors in determining the health economics profile of epilepsy surgery.

6. Recent direct costs of excisional epilepsy surgery have ranged between US$16 000 and 86 500. A simple, low-cost presurgical evaluation could apply to lesional epilepsy surgery, in some cases of temporal lobe epilepsy, early epilepsy surgery and large hemisphere lesions.

7. Resective epilepsy surgery achieves freedom from seizures in 45–90%. If seizures are stopped at the price of impaired cognition, it is of limited help. Improved, unchanged, or impaired cognition after epilepsy surgery has been reported. For adults in whom epilepsy surgery is performed late after seizure onset the social status declines, the disabilities increase and stigmata incur. Children with epilepsy and their families experience social restrictions difficult later to normalize.

8. Some patients continue to work after epilepsy surgery; in others employment increases, schooling/ training may improve, while still others experience no change. Increased income has also been qualified. Successful pediatric epilepsy surgery is found cost-effective for the child and family.

9. Improved education/vocational training, reduced part- or full-time unemployment are societal cost–benefits from an improved seizure situation, effects apparent in the direct/indirect cost sectors. The high initial costs for advanced epilepsy surgery diagnostics should be seen in a long perspective of cost reduction. The estimated cost-effectiveness of epilepsy surgery as a lifetime cost of care per patient, including evaluation and morbidity equalled US$17 002, the total follow-up amounted to US$62 361.

10. High capital cost in developing countries and available utilities give examples of low-cost epilepsy surgery, a fraction of that in the rich world.

REFERENCES

Alving J (1995) What is intractable epilepsy. In: Johannessen *et al* (eds) *Intractable Epilepsy*, pp 1–12. Petersfield, UK and Bristol, PA: Wrightson Biomedical Publishing.

Andermann F, Rasmussen TB, Villemure J-G (1991) Hemispherectomy: results for control of seizures in patients with hemiparesis. In: Luders H (ed) *Epilepsy Surgery*, pp 625–632. New York: Raven Press.

Anonymous (1990) National Institutes of Health Consensus Conference. Surgery for Epilepsy. *Journal of the American Medical Association* **264**:729–733.

Augustine EA, Novelly RA, Mattson RH *et al* (1984) Occupational adjustment following surgical treatment of epilepsy. *Annals of Neurology* **15**:68–72.

Aung M, Sobel DF, Gallen CC *et al* (1995) Potential contribution of bilateral magnetic source imaging to the evaluation of epilepsy surgery candidates. *Neurosurgery* **37**:1113–1120; discussion 1120–1121.

Baca S, Babu S, Spencer SS (1995) Health related quality of life in epilepsy surgery patients. *Epilepsia* **36**(Suppl 4):96 (Abstract).

Baker GA, Camfield C, Camfield P *et al* (1998) Commission on outcome measurement in epilepsy, 1994–1997: Final report. *Epilepsia* **39**:213–231.

Batzel L, Ojemann G, Ojemann L *et al* (1993) Vocational outcome in epilepsy surgery. *Epilepsia* **34**(Suppl 6):25 (Abstract).

Baxendale SA, Van Paeschen W, Thompson PJ *et al* (1996) Prediction of postoperative memory decline in temporal lobectomy: a multivariate analysis. *Epilepsia* **37**(Suppl 5):181.

Becker GS (1964) *Human Capital, A Theoretical and Empirical Analysis with Special Reference to Education*, pp 121–122. New York: National Bureau of Economic Research.

Begley CE, Annegers JF, Lairson DR *et al* (1994) Cost of epilepsy in the United States: a model based on incidence and prognosis. *Epilepsia* **35**:12340–12343.

Begley CE, Annegers JF, Lairson DR *et al* (1995) The lifetime cost of epilepsy in the United States: a model based on incidence and prognosis. In: Beran RG, Pachlatko Ch (eds) *Cost of Epilepsy. Proceedings of the 20th International Epilepsy Congress*, pp 17–26. Wehr/Baden: Ciba-Geigy Verlag.

Begley CE, Anneggers JF, Lairson DR *et al* (1997) Estimating the cost of epilepsy in the United States. *Epilepsia* **38**(Suppl 8):242.

Berkovic SF, McIntosh AM, Kalnins RM *et al* (1995) Preoperative MRI predicts outcome of temporal lobectomy: an actuarial analysis [see comments]. *Neurology* **45**:1358–1363.

Blumer D, Wakhlu S, Davies K (1996) Psychiatric complications and their treatment in a series of 50 patients with unilateral temporal or frontal lobectomy for epilepsy. *Epilepsia* **37** (Suppl 5):17.

Brodie MJ, Shorvon SD, Canger R *et al* (1997) Commission on European Affairs: appropriate standards of epilepsy care across Europe. *Epilepsia* **38**:1245–1250.

Buelow JM, Kaiser L (1993) Correlation study of postsurgical patients' ability to work, perceived surgical benefits and seizure tendency. *Epilepsia* **34**(Suppl 6):24 (Abstract).

Callanan MA, Morrell MJ, Barry J (1994) Willingness to participate in occupational and educational rehabilitation after epilepsy surgery. *Epilepsia* **35**(Suppl 8):56 (Abstract).

Cendes F, Arruda F, Dubeau F *et al* (1995) Relationship between mesial temporal atrophy and ictal and interictal EEG findings in a series of 250 patients. *Epilepsia* **36**(Suppl 4):23 (Abstract).

Chelune GJ, Naugle RI, Hermann BP *et al* (1998) Does presurgical IQ predict seizure outcome after temporal lobectomy? Evidence from the Bozeman Epilepsy Consortium. *Epilepsia* **39**:314–318.

Cockerell OC, Hart YM, Sander WAS *et al* (1994) The cost of epilepsy in the United Kingdom: an estimation based on the results of two population-based studies. *Epilepsy Research* **18**:249–260.

Constantino TME, Armon C (1994) What percentage of patients with epilepsy followed by neurologists might be epilepsy surgery candidates? *Epilepsia* **35**(Suppl 8):47 (Abstract).

Cook MJ, O'Brien TJ, Kilpatrick C *et al* (1995) Volumetric MRI hippocampal asymmetry reliably detects hippocampal sclerosis and predicts a good post-operative outcome. *Epilepsia* **36**(Suppl 4):167 (Abstract).

Cramer JA, Perrine K, Devinsky O *et al* (1996) A brief questionnaire to screen for quality of life in epilepsy: The QOLIE-10. *Epilepsia* **37**:577–582.

Crawford PA, Gage MJ (1997) Epilepsy surgery: Does it make a difference? *Epilepsia* **38**(Suppl 8):234.

Damiano AM, Dodrill CB (1997) Quality of life with vagus nerve stimulation. *Epilepsia* **38**(Suppl 8):236.

Davies KG, Maxwell RE, Jennum P *et al* (1994) Language function following subdural grid-directed temporal lobectomy. *Acta Neurologica Scandinavica* **90**:201–206.

Davies KG, Maxwell RE, Beniak TE (1995) Language function after temporal lobectomy without stimulation mapping of cortical function. *Epilepsia* **36**:130–136.

Delalande O, Pinard JM, Jalin CL *et al* (1995) Surgical results of hemispherotomy. *Epilepsia* **36**(Suppl 3):241 (Abstract).

DellaBadia JR, Bell WL, Mathews VP *et al* (1995) Assessment of interictal EEG and MRI as screening tools for surgical candidacy. *Epilepsia* **36**(Suppl 4):14 (Abstract).

Dewar SR, Eliashiv SD, Engel J Jr *et al* (1994) Seizure control and psychosocial outcome following surgical treatment of temporal lobe epilepsy associated with lesions. *Epilepsia* **35**(Suppl 8):100 (Abstract).

DHEW (1978) *Plan of Nationwide Action on Epilepsy*. Department of Health, Education and Welfare, National Institutes of Health, DHEW publication no. (NIH) 79–1115, Washington, DC.

Dodrill CB, Batzel LW, Fraser RT (1992) Psychosocial changes after surgery for epilepsy. In: Lüders H (ed) *Epilepsy Surgery*, pp 661–668. New York: Raven Press.

Doherty K, Gates JR, Penovich E *et al* (1997) Temporal lobectomy and postoperative outcome rationale. *Epilepsia* **38**:235.

Drummond MF, Stoddardt GL, Torrance GW (1987) *Methods for the Economic Evaluation of Health Care Programmes*. Oxford: Oxford University Press.

Ecker M, Snead OC III (1994) Cost-effectiveness of epilepsy surgery in children: preliminary data. *Epilepsia* **35**(Suppl 8): 49 (Abstract).

Elwes RDC, Marshall J, Battie A *et al* (1991) Epilepsy and employment: a community based survey in an area of high unemployment. *Journal of Neurology, Neurosurgery and Psychiatry*, **54**:200–203.

Elwes RDC, Dunn G, Binnie CD *et al* (1995) Noninvasive predictors of outcome after temporal lobectomy. *Epilepsia* **36**(Suppl 3):253 (Abstract).

Engel J JR, Van Ness PC, Rasmussen TR *et al* (1993) Outcome with respect to epileptic seizures. In: Engel J Jr (ed) *Surgical Treatment of the Epilepsies*, 2nd edn, pp 609–621. New York: Raven Press.

Falconer MA, Hill D, Meyer A *et al* (1955) Treatment of temporal-lobe epilepsy by temporal lobectomy (A survey of findings and results). *Lancet* **268**:827–835.

Fandino-Franky J (1997) The cost of epilepsy surgery in children in developing countries. *Epilepsia* **38**(Suppl 7):22.

Fandino-Franky J, Silfvenius H (1998) World-wide disparities in epilepsy care: a Latin American outlook. *Epilepsia* (in press).

Frandino-Franky J, Torres M, Vergara J *et al* (1995) Low-cost epilepsy surgery in Colombia. *Epilepsia* **36**(Suppl 3):243.

Fielstein EM, Roth DL, Williams KL *et al* (1994) Long-term vocational outcome in seizure-free patients. *Epilepsia* **35**(Suppl 8):44 (Abstract).

Genton P, Thomas P, Guerrini R (1993) How many candidates for epilepsy surgery? *Epilepsia* **34**(Suppl 6):33 (Abstract).

Germano IM, Olivier A, Jones-Gotman M *et al* (1993) Psychosocial outcome after reoperation for temporal lobe epilepsy. *Epilepsia* **34**(Suppl 6):25 (Abstract).

Gilliam F, Kuzniecky R, Faught E *et al* (1997a) Patient-validated content of epilepsy-specific quality-of-life measurement. *Epilepsia* **38**:233–236.

Gilliam F, Kuzniecky R, Faught E *et al* (1997b) Association of clinical variables with quality of life after epilepsy surgery. *Epilepsia* **38**(Suppl 3):162.

Green JR, Steelman HF, Duisberg REH *et al* (1958) Behavior changes following radical temporal lobe excision in the treatment of focal epilepsy. *Research Publication of the Association for Research in Nervous and Mental Disease* **36**:295–315.

Guillaume J, Mazars G (1956) Indications and results of surgical treatment of temporal epilepsy. *Sem hôp* **32**:2013–2018.

Guldvog B (1994) Patient satisfaction and epilepsy surgery. *Epilepsia* **35**:579–584.

Helmstaedter C, Lendt M, Elger CE (1995) Epilepsy surgery and socioeconomic status: A three-year follow up study in 168 patients. *Epilepsia* **36**(Suppl 3):179 (Abstract).

Hermann B, Somes G, Walker G *et al* (1993) Psychosis after temporal lobe surgery. *Epilepsia* **34**(Suppl 6):71 (Abstract).

Hope VT, Husian AM, Mebustr KA (1996) Cost analysis of analog versus digital electroencephalography. *Epilepsia* **37**(Suppl 5):61.

ILAE (1997a) Commission on Neuroimaging of the International League Against Epilepsy. (1997 Recommendation for neuroimaging of patients with epilepsy.) *Epilepsy Research* **38**:1255–1256.

ILAE (1997b) A Global Survey On Epilepsy Surgery, 1980–1990: A report by the Commission on Neurosurgery of Epilepsy, The International League Against Epilepsy. *Epilepsia* **38**:249–255.

Ives J, Warach S, Schlaug G *et al* (1995) EEG triggered functional MRI shows potential to reveal focal abnormality in generalized epilepsy. *Epilepsia* **36**(Suppl 4):172 (Abstract).

Jack CR, Hammond C, Rydberg J *et al* (1995) Comparison of Flair to spin echo MRI in detection of mesial temporal sclerosis. *Epilepsia* **36**(Suppl 4):25 (Abstract).

Jalava M, Sillanpää M, Camfeld C *et al* (1997) Social adjustment and competence 35 years after onset of childhood epilepsy: a prospective controlled study. *Epilepsia* **38**:708–722.

Kasunic K, Smith B, Elisevich K *et al* (1995) Comparison of costs between epilepsy surgery patients and other patients within DRGs 001, 024 and 025. *Epilepsia* **36**(Suppl 4):95 (Abstract).

Kellett MW, Smith DF, Baker GA *et al* (1996) Quality of life and employment following epilepsy surgery. *Epilepsia* **37**(Suppl 5):8.

Kellett MW, Smith DF, Baker GA *et al* (1997) Outcome and psychosocial status following epilepsy surgery. *Epilepsia* **38**(Suppl 3):246.

Kies BM (1995) Economic aspects of epilepsy in South Africa. *Epilepsia* **36**(Suppl 3):178 (Abstract).

Kilpatrick C, Cook M, Kaye A *et al* (1995) Noninvasive investigations successfully select patients for temporal lobectomy. *Epilepsia* **36**(Suppl 3):97 (Abstract).

King JT, Sperling MR, O'Connor MJ (1994) Is anterior temporal lobectomy for medically intractable temporal lobe epilepsy 'cost-effective'? *Epilepsia* **35**(Suppl 8):46 (Abstract).

King JT, Sperling MR, Justice AC, O'Connor MJ (1997) A cost-effectiveness analysis of anterior temporal lobectomy for intractable temporal lobe epilepsy. *Journal of Neurosurgery* **87**:20–28.

Kriedel T (1980) Cost benefit analysis of epilepsy clinics. *Social Sciences and Medicine* **14**:35–39.

Langfitt JT (1995) Comparison of the psychometric characteristics of three quality of life measures in intractable epilepsy. *Quality of Life Research* **4**:101–114.

Langfitt JT (1997) Cost-effectiveness of anterotemporal lobectomy in medically intractable complex partial epilepsy. *Epilepsia* **38**:154–163.

Langfitt JT, Rausch R (1995) Word-finding deficits persist after left anterotemporal lobectomy. *Archives of Neurology* **53**:72–76.

Lassouw G, Doelman J, Janssen G *et al* (1997) Quality of life as outcome measure for epilepsy surgery. *Epilepsia* **38**(Suppl 3):162.

Lecomber R (1978) Social costs and the national accounts. In: Pearce DW (ed) *The Valuation of Social Cost*, pp 164–197. London: George Allen and Unwin.

Lee CC, Jack CR, Riederer SJ (1995) Functional magnetic resonance imaging with standard hardware: results in 18 epilepsy patients. *Epilepsia* **36**(Suppl 4):172(Abstract).

Lendt M, Helmstaedter C, Elger CE *et al* (1997) Pre- and postoperative socioeconomic development of 151 patients with focal epilepsies. *Epilepsia* **38**:1330–1337.

Loring DW, Meador KJ, Lee GP *et al* (1996) Quality of life before and after epilepsy surgery in patients with complex partial seizures. *Epilepsia* **37**(Suppl 5):7.

Lüders H (ed) (1992) *Epilepsy Surgery*, pp **625–632**. New York: Raven Press.

Malmgren K, Sullivan M (1995) Quality of life after epilepsy surgery: a Swedish multicenter follow-up study. *Epilepsia* **36**(Suppl 3):171(Abstract).

Mayes BN, Vanlandingham K, Lewis DV *et al* (1994) Predictors of temporal lobectomy outcome: a multivariate analysis. *Epilepsia* **35**(Suppl 8):153(Abstract).

McEvedy J, Ffytche D, Elwes R, *et al* (1993) Psychosocial outcome of temporal lobectomy for epilepsy. *Epilepsia* **34**(Suppl 6):116(Abstract).

McLachlan S, Derry PA, Girvin JP *et al* (1994) Prospective controlled assessment of quality of life following temporal lobectomy. *Epilepsia* **35**(Suppl 8):46(Abstract).

McLachlan RS, Derry PA, Rose KJ *et al* (1996) Prospective controlled study of surgical versus medical management of temporal lobe epilepsy. *Epilepsia* **37**(Suppl 4):121.

McMackin D, Burke T, Philips J *et al* (1996) The relationship between age at surgery and identity functioning following temporal lobectomy for intractable epilepsy. *Epilepsia* **37**(Suppl 5):7.

Michaelis K, Klamus J, Ellis M *et al* (1995) Patients' perception of outcome after surgery. *Epilepsia* **36**(Suppl 3):187(Abstract).

Mooney GH (1977) *The Valuation of Human Life*. London: Macmillan.

Morris G, Hartz A, Guse C *et al* (1997) Cost-effective care of seizures. *Epilepsia* **38**(Suppl 8):243.

Morris RG, Abrahams S, Polkey CE (1995) Recognition for words and faces following unilateral temporal lobectomy. *British Journal of Clinical Psychology* **34**:571–576.

Murray CJL (1994) Quantifying the burden of disease: the technical basis for disability-adjusted life years. In: Murray CJL, Lopez AD (eds) *Global Comparative Assessments in the Health Sector. Disease Burden Expenditures and Intervention Packages* (Collected articles from the Bulletin of the World Health Organization), pp. 3–19. Geneva: WHO.

Murray CJL, Lopez AD (1994) Quantifying disability: data, methods and results. In: Murray CJL, Lopez AD (eds) *Global Comparative Assessments in the Health Sector. Disease Burden, Expenditures and Intervention Packages* (Collected articles from the Bulletin of the World Health Organization), pp. 55–96. Geneva: WHO.

Murray CJL, Govindaraj R, Musgrove P (1994) National health expenditures: a global analysis. In: Murray CJL, Lopez AD (eds) *Global Comparative Assessments in the Health Sector. Disease Burden, Expenditures and Intervention Packages* (Collected articles from the Bulletin of the World Health Organization), pp. 141–156. Geneva: WHO.

Nilsson L, Tomson T, Farahman BY *et al* (1997) Cause-specific mortality in epilepsy: a cohort study of more than 9000 patients once hospitalized for epilepsy. *Epilepsia* **38**:1062–1068.

Olafsson E, Hauser WA, Gudmunsson G (1998) Long-term survival of people with unprovoked seizures: a population-based study. *Epilepsia* **39**:89–92.

Oxbury S, Oxbury J, Renowden S *et al* (1997) Severe amnesia: an unusual late complication after temporal lobectomy. *Neuropsychologia* **35**(7):975–988.

Pachlatko Ch (1993) Economic aspects of epilepsy – an introduction. In: Beran RG, Pachlatko Ch (eds) *Cost of Epilepsy, ILAE Commission on Economic Aspects of Epilepsy. Proceedings of the 20th International Epilepsy Congress*, Oslo, pp 11–16. Baden: Ciba-Geigy Wehr/Verlag.

Pachlatko CH, Beran RG (eds) (1996) *Economic Evaluation of Epilepsy Management*. London: John Libbey.

Paetau R, Hämäläinen M, Hari R *et al* (1994) Comparison of magnetoencephalography, functional MRI, and motor evoked potentials in the localization of the sensory-motor cortex. *Epilepsia* **35**:275–284.

Paglioli-Netu E, Da Costa J, Palmini A *et al* (1995) Psychosocial profiles of epileptic patients rendered seizure free after anterior temporal lobectomy are similar to those of patients well controlled on medication. *Epilepsia* **36**(Suppl 4):104(Abstract).

Palas J, Gates JR, Doherty K (1996) A longitudinal study of social outcomes in epilepsy patients after focal resection. *Epilepsia* **37**(Suppl 5):8.

Perrine K, Devinsky O, Bryant-Comstock L *et al* (1998) Development and cross-cultural translations of a 31-item quality of life in epilepsy inventory. *Epilepsia* **39**:81–88.

Pfäfflin M, May TW (1997) Impact of epilepsy on employment and restriction in daily life. *Epilepsia* **38**(Suppl 3):103.

Phillips NA, McGlone J (1995) Grouped data do not tell the whole story: individual analysis of cognitive change after temporal lobectomy. *Journal of Clinical and Experimental Neuropsychology* **17**:713–724.

Pilcher WH, Roberts DW, Flanigin HF *et al* (1993) Complications of epilepsy surgery. In: Engel J Jr (ed) *Surgical Treatment of the Epilepsies*, 2nd edn, pp 565–581. New York: Raven Press.

Polkey CE, Awad IA, Tanaka T *et al* (1993) The place of reoperation. In: Engel J Jr (ed) *Surgical Treatment of the Epilepsies*, 2nd edn, pp 663–668. New York: Raven Press .

Popovic M, Ribaric II (1995) Direct costs of epilepsy. *Epilepsia* **36**(Suppl 3):178(Abstract).

Primrose DC, Ojemann GA (1991) Outcome of resective surgery for temporal lobe epilepsy. In: Luders H (ed) *Epilepsy Surgery*, pp 601–612. New York: Raven Press.

Radtke RA, Lee N, Hanson MW *et al* (1995) Comparison of volumetric hippocampal MRI and FDG-PET: correlation with surgical outcome. *Epilepsia* **36**(Suppl 4):75(Abstract).

Rainwater MR, Ricker BR, Temkin NR *et al* (1993) Direct medical costs and cost savings with epilepsy surgery. *Epilepsia* **34**(Suppl 2):116(Abstract).

Rao B, Rhadhakrishnan K, Thomas S *et al* (1997) Epilepsy surgery in a developing country. *Abstract, 11th International Congress of Neurological Surgery, Amsterdam*, p. 136.

Rausch R (1995) Neuropsychological and psychosocial follow-up of patients with temporal lobectomy surgery for intractable epilepsy. *Epilepsia* **36**(Suppl 4):138(Abstract).

Rayport M Ferguson SM (1995) Psychiatric findings after temporal lobe surgery: A prospective study. *Epilepsia* **36**(Suppl 3):100(Abstract).

Reeves AL, So EL, Evans RW *et al* (1995) Factors predictive of work status after anterior temporal lobectomy (ATL) for intractable epilepsy. *Epilepsia* **36**(Suppl 4):85(Abstract).

Reeves AL, So EL, Evans RW *et al* (1997) Factors associated with work outcome after anterior temporal lobectomy for intractable epilepsy. *Epilepsia* **38**:689–695.

Rentz AM, Halpern MT, Murray M *et al* (1996) Cost of illness of epilepsy by disease severity. *Epilepsia* **37**(Suppl 5):87.

Ribaric II, Popovic M, Vukojevic S (1995) Psychosocial status in patients operated on for intractable complex partial seizures. *Epilepsia* **36**(Suppl 3):187(Abstract).

Roberts T, Rowley H, Kucharczyk J (1995) Applications of magnetic source imaging to presurgical brain mapping. *Neuroimaging Clinics of North America* **5**:251–266.

Rose DF (1995) Eight and 24 hour video/EEG in children: economic cost vs diagnostic gain. *Epilepsia* **36**(Suppl 4):111(Abstract).

Rose ML, Martin RC, Gilliam FG *et al* (1996) Improved healthcare resource utilization and costs following video/EEG telemetry confirmed nonepileptic psychogenic seizure diagnosis. *Epilepsia* **37**(Suppl 5):10.

Roubina S, Ellis M, Klamus J *et al* (1995) Can interictal EEG predict successful temporal lobectomy for epilepsy? *Epilepsia* **36**(Suppl 3):254(Abstract).

Ruggieri P, Comair Y, Ross J *et al* (1995) The utility of fast flair imaging in epilepsy. *Epilepsia* **36**(Suppl 4):25(Abstract).

Savard RJ, Walker E (1965) Changes in social functioning after surgical treatment for temporal lobe epilepsy. *Social Work* **10**:87–95.

Sawrie SM, Martin RC, Gilliam FG *et al* (1998) Contribution of neuropsychological data to the prediction of temporal lobe epilepsy surgery outcome. *Epilepsia* **39**:319–325.

Saykin AJ, Stafiniak P, Robinson LJ *et al* (1995) Language before and after temporal lobectomy: specificity of acute changes and relation to early risk factors. *Epilepsia* **36**:1071–1077.

Schramm J, Behrens E, Entzian W (1995) Hemispherical deafferentation: an alternative to functional hemispherectomy. *Neurosurgery* **36**:509–515; discussion 515–516.

Schultz TW (1971) Investment in human capital. *American Economic Review* **1**.

Schulz R, Ebner A, Schuller M *et al* (1995) Analysis of postoperative seizure recurrence after 65 temporal lobe partial resections [in German]. *Nervenarzt* **66**:901–906.

Schwartz CE, Cole B, Vickrey BG, *et al* (1995) The Q-TWiST approach to assessing health-related quality of life in epilepsy. *Quality of Life Research* **4**:135–141.

Seidenberg M, Hermann B, Schoenfeld J *et al* (1995) Identification of subjects who undergo significant cognitive change following anterior temporal lobectomy. *Epilepsia* **36**(Suppl 4):135(Abstract).

Seidman-Ripley JG, Bound VK, Andermann F *et al* (1993) Psychosocial consequences of postoperative seizure relief. *Epilepsia* **34**:248–254.

Silbergeld DL, Ojemann GA (1993) The tailored temporal lobectomy. *Neurosurgery Clinics of North America* **4**:273–281.

Silfvenius H (1995) Current state of affairs; epilepsy surgery in children and adolescents. In: Aldenkamp AP, Dreifuss FE, Renier W *et al* (eds) *Epilepsy in Children and Adolescents*, pp 183–203. Boca Raton, FL: CRC Press.

Silfvenius H (1999) In: Pachlatko Ch, Bevan RG (eds) *Economic Aspects of Epilepsy: An Overview. Epilepsia* (Suppl).

Silfvenius H, Olivecrona M (1998) Health economical gain of epilepsy surgery. In: Avezaat *et al* (eds) *Stereotactic and Functional Neurosurgery* Bologna: Monduzzi Editore, pp 93–105.

Silfvenius H, Dahlgren H, Jonsson E *et al* (1991) Epilepsy surgery [in Swedish]. The Swedish Council on Technology Assessment in Health Care.

Silfvenius H, Lindholm L, Säisä J *et al* (1995a) Costs of and savings from pediatric epilepsy surgery; a Swedish study. In: Beran RG, Pachlatko Ch (eds) *Cost of Epilepsy. Proceedings of the 20th International Epilepsy Congress*, pp 83–106. Wehr/Baden: Ciba-Geigy Verlag.

Silfvenius H, Säisä J, Olivecrona M *et al* (1995b) Socioeconomic aspects of adults operated on for epilepsy. *Epilepsia* **36**(Suppl 3):178(Abstract).

Silfvenius H, Säisä J, Olivecrona M *et al* (1997a) Income, employment and epilepsy surgery: a Swedish study. In: Beran RG, Pachlatko CH (eds) *Economic Evaluation of Epilepsy Management*, pp. 73–89. Sydney. John Libbey.

Silfvenius H, Säisä J, Olivecrona M *et al* (1997b) Health economical aspects of paediatric epilepsy surgery In: Tuxhorn I, Holthausen H, Boenigk H (eds) *Paediatric Epilepsy Syndromes and Their Surgical Treatment*, pp 26–32. London: John Libbey.

Sirven JI, Detre J, French JA *et al* (1995) Functional magnetic resonance imaging of simple partial and subclinical seizures in the evaluation of epilepsy surgery patients. *Epilepsia* **36**(Suppl 4):172(Abstract).

Smith JR, Lee MR, King DW *et al* (1995) Relationship of age at surgery to outcome of ablative epilepsy surgery. *Epilepsia* **36**(Suppl 4):140(Abstract).

Snars J, Somerville E, Batchelor J *et al* (1995) Psychological morbidity after anterior temporal lobectomy for intractable temporal lobe epilepsy. *Epilepsia* **36**(Suppl 3):218(Abstract).

SNRA (1997) Vägverkets samhällsekonomiska kalkylmodell. Ekonomisk teori och värderingar. Swedish National Road Administration. Economical Calculation Model, Economical Theory and Valuation, Publication No. **130** [in Swedish]. Sweden: Section on planning of road transportation system.

Sperling MR, Roberts D, Saykin AJ, *et al* (1994) Occupational outcome after anterior temporal lobectomy correlates with seizure control. *Epilepsia* **35**(Suppl 8):47(Abstract).

Sperling MR, Liporace JD, French JA *et al* (1995a) Epilepsy surgery and mortality from epilepsy. *Epilepsia* **36**(Suppl 4):140(Abstract).

Sperling MR, Saykin AJ, Roberts FR *et al* (1995b) Occupational outcome after temporal lobectomy for refractory epilepsy. *Neurology* **45**:970–977.

Stefan H, Schuler P. Abraham-Fuchs K *et al* (1994) Magnetoencephalographic evaluation of children and adolescents with intractable epilepsy. *Acta Neurologica Scandinavica Supplementum* **152**:83–88.

Stewart R, Kasunic K, Elisevich K *et al* (1997) Clinical care pathways and associated costs in a surgical epilepsy program. *Epilepsia* **38**(Suppl 3):89–90.

Stoddard KR, Westerveld M, Sass KJ *et al* (1996) Effects of surgery on quality of life in epilepsy. *Epilepsia* **37**(Suppl 5):7.

Talairach J, Bancaud J, Bonis A *et al* (1992) Surgical therapy for frontal epilepsies. In: Chauvel P, Delgado-Escueta AV, Halgren E, *et al* (eds) *Frontal Lobe Seizures and Epilepsies (Advances in Neurology)* **57**: 707–732. New York: Raven Press.

Taylor DC, Falconer MA (1968) Clinical, socio-economic, and psychosocial changes after temporal lobectomy for epilepsy. *British Journal of Psychiatry* **114**:1247–1261.

Taylor DC, Neville BGR, Cross JH (1997) New measures of outcome needed for the surgical treatment of epilepsy. *Epilepsia* **38**:625–630.

Thompson PJ, Oxley J (1988) Socioeconomic accompaniments of severe epilepsy. *Epilepsia* **29**:9–18.

Thorbecke R (1996) Quality of life in the social domain and outcome after temporal lobe resection: a prospective study. *Epilepsia* **37**(Suppl 4):9.

Thorbecke R (1997) Social outcome after temporal lobe surgery in adolescents compared to adults. In: Tuxhorn I, Holthausen H, Boenigk H (eds) *Paediatric Epilepsy Syndromes and Their Surgical Treatment*, pp 326–333. London: John Libbey.

Town AR, Boggs JG, Waterhouse EJ *et al* (1997) Natural history of untreated status epilepticus. *Epilepsia* **38**(Suppl 8):210

Tuxhorn I, Holthausen H, Boenigk H (eds) (1997) *Paediatric Epilepsy Syndromes and Their Surgical Treatment*. London: John Libbey.

Van Ness PC (1991) Surgical outcome for neocortical (extrahippocampal) focal epilepsy. In: Luders H (ed) *Epilepsy Surgery*, pp 613–624. New York: Raven Press.

Van Ness PC, Seleman S, Stagno S (1994) Employment after epilepsy surgery for neocortical localization related seizures. *Epilepsia* **35**(Suppl 8):48(Abstract).

van Hout B, Gagnon D, Souetre E *et al* (1997) Relationship between seizure frequency and costs and quality of life of outpatients with partial epilepsy in France, Germany and the United Kingdom. *Epilepsia* **38**:1221–1226.

Vermeulen J, Alpherts WC, Aldenkamp AP (1993) Results of the neurosurgical treatment of patients with drug-resistant epilepsy: psychosocial aspects [in Dutch]. *Nederlands Tijdschrift voor Geneeskunde* **137**:2251–2254.

Vickrey BG (1993) A procedure for developing a quality-of-life measure for epilepsy surgery patients. *Epilepsia* **34**(Suppl 4):S22–27.

Vickrey BG, Hays, RD, Graber J *et al* (1992) A health-related quality of life instrument for patients evaluated for epilepsy surgery. *Medical Care* **30**:299–319.

Vickrey BG, Hays RD, Engel J Jr *et al* (1995) Outcome assessment for epilepsy surgery: the impact of measuring health-related quality of life. *Annals of Neurology* **37**:158–166.

Villemure J-G, Adams CBT, Hoffman HJ *et al* (1993) Hemispherectomy. In: Engel J Jr (ed) *Surgical Treatment of the Epilepsies*, 2nd edn, pp 511–518. New York: Raven Press.

Walker JA, Bruce AV, Laxer KD *et al* (1994) Early age surgery is associated with improved vocational and educational outcome. *Epilepsia* **35**(Suppl 8):46(Abstract).

Wiebe S, Blume W, Girvin J *et al* (1994) Economic evaluation of temporal lobe epilepsy. *Epilepsia* **35**(Suppl 8):46(Abstract).

Wiebe S, Rose K, Derry P *et al* (1997) Outcome assessment in epilepsy: comparative responsiveness of quality of life and psychosocial instruments. *Epilepsia* **38**:430–438.

Wieser HG, Siegel AM (1992) Guidelines for comprehensive epilepsy centers. *Proceedings of the Round Table held during the 2nd International Zurich Epilepsy Symposium*, p. 91.

Wilson SJ, Saling MM, Kincade P *et al* (1998) Patient expectations of temporal lobe surgery. *Epilepsia* **39**:167–174.

Wyllie E (1995) Surgery for catastrophic localization-related epilepsy in infants. In: Wyllie E (ed) *Epilepsy in Children and Young Adults: Controversies and Recent Advances Epilepsia* **37**(Suppl 1):22–25.

Xue M, Najm I, Comair Y *et al* (1995) Proton magnetic resonance spectroscopy and volumetry are predictive of seizure outcome in patients with TLE. *Epilepsia* **36**(Suppl 4):83(Abstract).